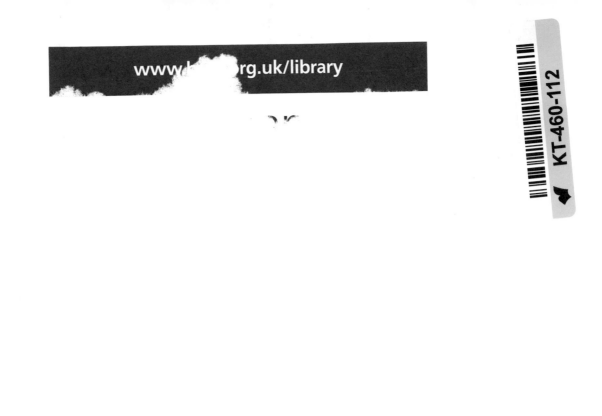

General Surgery

Second Edition

Kirby I. Bland · Michael G. Sarr ·
Markus W. Büchler · Attila Csendes ·
O. James Garden · John Wong
Editors

General Surgery

Volume 1

Principles and International Practice

Second Edition

With 190 Figures and 193 Tables

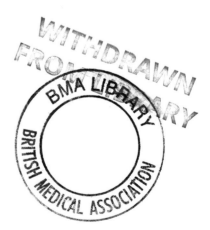
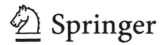

Editors

Kirby I. Bland, MD
Fay Fletcher Kerner Professor and Chairman
Department of Surgery
Deputy Director, Comprehensive Cancer Center
University of Alabama School of Medicine
Birmingham, AL
USA

Markus W. Büchler, MD
Professor of Surgery and Chairman
Department of General and Visceral Surgery
University of Heidelberg
Heidelberg
Germany

Attila Csendes, MD, FACS (Hon)
Professor of Surgery and Chairman
Department of Surgery
University Hospital
Santiago
Chile

Michael G. Sarr, MD
James C. Mason Professor of Surgery
Department of Surgery
Mayo Clinic College of Medicine
Rochester, MN
USA

O. James Garden, MBChB, MD, FRCS (Ed), FRCP (Ed), FRACS (Hon)
Regius Professor of Clinical Surgery
Department of Clinical and Surgical Sciences
The University of Edinburgh
Royal Infirmary of Edinburgh
Edinburgh
UK

John Wong, BSc (Med (Syd)), MBBS (Syd), PhD (Syd), MD (Hon (Syd)), FRACS, FRCS (Edin), FRCS (Glasg), FACS (Hon)
Chair Professor
Department of Surgery
The University of Hong Kong
Queen Mary Hospital
Hong Kong
China

ISBN: 978-1-84628-832-6   e-ISBN: 978-1-84628-833-3
Print and e-bundle ISBN: 978-1-84800-139-8

British Library Cataloguing in Publication data
A catalogue record for this book is available from the British Library

Library of Congress Control Number: 2008937563

Springer Science+Business Media
springer.com

Printed on acid-free paper

9 8 7 6 5 4 3 2 1 0

To the surgical residents and practicing general surgeons with whom we have had the privilege of teaching the art, science, and practice of surgery.

Preface

The editors of *General Surgery: Principles and International Practice* acknowledge the essential contribution for the general surgeon and resident-in-training of an accessible, concise, and state-of-the-art volume that explores and documents evolutionary principles for the practice of surgery. The editors further acknowledge the physical, psychologic, and socioeconomic importance of surgical diseases and their impact on society. These facts are evident in that the scientific community continues to witness extraordinary advances in the therapy of both benign and malignant surgical diseases of various organ sites. Much of this progress has been especially evident over the past decade. Implicit in these advances are new concepts and techniques of management that allow the surgeon to integrate this discipline with medicine, pharmacology, immunology, biostatistics, pathology, genetics, medical and radiation oncology, and diagnostic radiology and imaging. Further, each of these major disciplines contributes a small component for the diagnostic and therapeutic approaches to clinical care; hence, the comprehensive planning, integration, and provision of patient care throughout preoperative, intraoperative, and postoperative phases of care remains essential in the successful practice of our specialty.

The editors, therefore, acknowledge that the aim of this work is to provide an illustrative, instructive, and comprehensive textbook that depicts the rationale of basic operative principles essential to surgical therapy. Many treatises are available currently that integrate scientific rationale, clinical trials, multidisciplinary approaches, and outcomes with anatomic and technical maneuvers for the management of surgical diseases. In organizing this textbook, the editors chose authors renowned in the disciplines for illustrating, informing, and depicting in a comprehensive fashion the surgical therapy expectant for metabolic, infectious, endocrine, and neoplastic derangements in adult and pediatric patients *from a truly international and multi-continental perspective*. The editors and authors were chosen carefully from across geographies as also from multi-cultural and diverse locations. While the authors consider this text to be inclusive regarding the technical and operative considerations for preoperative, intraoperative, and postoperative care, its purpose should not be intended to replace standard textbooks of surgery, nor should it be considered complete in its coverage of pathophysiologic disorders. In contrast, this text is organized to familiarize practicing surgeons, residents, and fellows with state-of-the-art surgical principles and techniques that are essential to contemporary practice. Therefore, the tenor of the book has been developed to co-exist with other major surgical reference texts that are dedicated – some in a more comprehensive fashion – to the therapy of individual organs and systemic diseases. Our book is much more a "working text" for the practicing surgeon with emphasis on diagnosis and treatment.

All chapters in *General Surgery: Principles and International Practice* include a condensed bibliography of highly selective journal articles, reviews, and texts. In this manner of attempting to be concise, we hope to provide precise focus for the education of the reader relative to accepted surgical principles involved in patient management. Moreover, the editors have sought to provide a counterviewpoint for the selection of therapy by presenting at the opening of each chapter, a list of "Pearls and Pitfalls" that highlight particular concerns.

The organization of the text is designed for easy access. The editors have developed 13 sections, each representing an important branch of surgical science: General Principles, Trauma and Burns,

Critical Care, Head and Neck, Gastrointestinal, Pediatric, Oncology, Endocrine, Gynecology, Vascular, Endovascular Therapy, Geriatric, and Management of Surgical Specialties Requiring Care of the General Surgeon. The majority of chapters provide pertinent, though not exhaustive, summaries of anatomy and physiology, a history of the surgical illness, and stages of operative approaches with relevant technical considerations outlined in a manner that is easily understandable. Complications are reviewed typically when appropriate for the organ system, disease, or problem. The text is supported amply by line drawings and photographs that depict relevant anatomic or technical principles. Although some overlap exists among related chapters, the editors have made every attempt to minimize duplicative or repetitious discussions, except when controversial or state-of-the-art issues are presented. Moreover, the editors have also attempted to ensure that accurate presentations and illustrations depict properly the most complex problems confronted by the general surgeon.

Finally, in an attempt to address advanced and contemporary concepts, this text has been organized to address in detail expeditious, safe, and anatomically accurate operations that incorporate standard as well as evolving surgical principles and techniques. These principles have been tested in the clinics of valid scientific knowledge and are well-supported by time-tested approaches that have been provided by practicing surgeons. The editors are grateful for having the opportunity to respond to the challenge of developing this truly *international* text and are indeed hopeful that our readers will find this book to be a repository of insightful, useful, and timely information.

Kirby I. Bland
Michael G. Sarr
Markus W. Büchler
Attila Csendes
O. James Garden
John Wong

Acknowledgements

The editors are grateful to have been entrusted with the responsibility of developing this textbook for the international world of surgery. The organization and publication of this text required the knowledge and assistance of many persons. To all our residents in surgery, research fellows, and international physicians in the five universities in which they were trained and practice, the editors acknowledge an intellectual debt. We appreciate their reviews, critiques, and criticism that allowed the formulation of *General Surgery: Principles and International Practice.* We are grateful for their constant encouragement and assistance in the preparation of this tome.

We thank our Co-Editors – Professors Büchler, Csendes, Garden, and Wong, who provided invaluable critiques, overviews, and advised the assimilation and management of separate chapters into the sections to which they were assigned. Their services have been invaluable to the successful organization of this text, truly reflecting its international scope. Further, we acknowledge the assistance of our Associate Editors: Dr. Loring W. Rue III (University of Alabama at Birmingham); Dr. Michael L. Kendrick (Mayo Clinic College of Medicine); Professor Chung-Mau Lo (The University of Hong Kong); and Dr. Jens Werner (University of Heidelberg), who provided incalculable time and effort overseeing the accuracy and timeliness of this publication.

The editors also acknowledge the significant support offered by our individual editorial assistants, who provided the day-to-day contacts, oversight, and management of manuscripts that were submitted in each international office. We specifically acknowledge Irmgard Alffermann in the office of Professor Büchler (Heidelberg, Germany), Leslie M. Benson and Kan Moore in the office of Dr. Bland (Birmingham, Alabama), Penny Earle in the office of Professor Garden (Edinburgh, United Kingdom), Deborah I. Frank in the office of Dr. Sarr (Rochester, Minnesota), and Isabel Zamorano in the office of Professor Csendes (Santiago, Chile). Each of these editorial assistants provided invaluable service that is appreciated highly by the editors and allowed Springer to publish this tome in a timely and organized fashion.

Finally, the editors acknowledge the foresight and support provided by Melissa Morton of Springer Science + Business Media who in conjunction with us, also saw the need of such an international approach to a textbook on surgery and to suggest and allow us to begin the organization of this volume. The assistance and organizational skills of Stephanie Sakson are also to be specifically acknowledged due to her extraordinary attention and diligence to the task at hand. Ms. Sakson's oversight allowed the assimilation of the book from its inception and ensured its completion.

Kirby I. Bland, MD
Michael G. Sarr, MD

Table of Contents

Volume 1

Volume 2

Editors

Kirby I. Bland, MD
Fay Fletcher Kerner Professor and
Chairman
Department of Surgery
Deputy Director,
Comprehensive Cancer Center
University of Alabama School of Medicine
Birmingham, AL
USA

Markus W. Büchler, MD
Professor of Surgery and Chairman
Department of General and Visceral
Surgery
University of Heidelberg
Heidelberg
Germany

Attila Csendes, MD, FACS (Hon)
Professor of Surgery and Chairman
Department of Surgery
University Hospital
Santiago
Chile

Michael G. Sarr, MD
James C. Mason Professor of Surgery
Department of Surgery
Mayo Clinic College of Medicine
Rochester, MN
USA

**O. James Garden, MBChB, MD, FRCS (Ed),
FRCP (Ed), FRACS (Hon)**
Regius Professor of Clinical Surgery
Department of Clinical and Surgical Sciences
The University of Edinburgh
Royal Infirmary of Edinburgh
Edinburgh
UK

**John Wong, BSc (Med (Syd)), MBBS (Syd),
PhD (Syd), MD (Hon (Syd)), FRACS,
FRCS (Edin), FRCS (Glasg), FACS (Hon)**
Chair Professor
Department of Surgery
The University of Hong Kong
Queen Mary Hospital
Hong Kong
China

Associate Editors

Michael L. Kendrick, MD
Assistant Professor of Surgery
Department of Surgery
Mayo Clinic College of Medicine
Rochester, MN
USA

Chung-Mau Lo, MBBS (HK), MS, FRCS (Edin)
FACS, FHKAM (Surg)
Chin Lan-Hong Professor in Hepatobiliary and
Pancreatic Surgery
Department of Surgery
The University of Hong Kong
Hong Kong SAR
China

Loring W. Rue III, MD
Professor and Vice Chair
Chief, Section of Trauma, Burns & Surgical
Critical Care
University of Alabama School of Medicine
Birmingham, AL
USA

Jens Werner MD, MBA
Professor of Surgery
Department of General, Visceral, and
Transplant Surgery
University of Heidelberg
Heidelberg
Germany

Contributors

Cary B. Aarons, MD
General Surgery Resident
Department of Surgery
Boston University Medical Center
Boston, MA, USA

Hernando Abaunza O., MD, FACS
Professor
Department of Surgery
Universidad Nacional de Colombia / Hospital
Militar Central,
Bogota, Colombia

Herand Abcarian, MD, FACS
Turi Josefsen Professor and Head
Department of Surgery
University of Illinois at Chicago
Chicago, IL, USA

Mario A. Abedrapo Moreira, MD
Department of Surgery
Clinical Hospital
University of Chile
Santiago, Chile

Donald J. Adam, MD, FRCSEd (Gen Surg)
Senior Lecturer in Vascular Surgery
Department of Vascular Surgery
University of Birmingham
Birmingham, UK

Göran Åkerström, MD, PhD
Professor
Department of Surgical Sciences
University Hospital
Uppsala, Sweden

Christopher L. Amling, MD
Professor of Surgery and Director

Division of Urology
Department of Surgery
University of Alabama at Birmingham
Birmingham, AL, USA

John B. Ammori, MD
Senior Resident
Department of Surgery
University of Michigan
Ann Arbor, MI, USA

Patricio Andrades, MD
Research Associate
Department of Surgery
University of Alabama at Birmingham
Birmingham, AL, USA

Åke Andrén-Sandberg, MD, PhD
Professor of Surgery
Department of Surgery
Karolinska University Hospital at Huddinge
Stockholm, Sweden

Laurence Annet, MD, PhD
Department of Radiology
Saint-Luc University Hospital
Université Catholique de Louvain
Brussels, Belgium

Xabier A. de Aretxabala, MD, FACS
Professor
Department of Surgery
Clinic Hospital University of Chile
Santiago, Chile

Nimmi Arora, MD
Research Fellow, Division of General Surgery
Department of Surgery
New York Presbyterian Hospital
New York, NY, USA

Supreeta Arya, MD
Associate Professor and Consultant Radiologist
Department of Radiodiagnosis
Tata Memorial Hospital
Mumbai, India

Yutaka Atomi, MD, PhD, FACS
Professor of Surgery
Department of Surgery
School of Medicine
Kyorin University
Tokyo, Japan

Wing-Yan Au, MD, FRCPE
Professor
Department of Medicine
Queen Mary Hospital
Hong Kong, China

Simon P. Bach, MD, FRCS
Clinical Lecturer and Honorary Registrar
Division of Colorectal Surgery
Department of General Surgery and Trauma
John Radcliffe Hospital
Oxford, UK

Charles M. Balch, MD, FACS
Professor of Surgery
Oncology & Dermatology
Deputy Director for Clinical Trials & Outcomes
Johns Hopkins Institute for Clinical &
Translational Research
Johns Hopkins Medicine
Baltimore, MD, USA

Glen C. Balch, MD
Assistant Professor
Department of Surgery
Memorial Sloan Kettering Cancer Center
New York, NY, USA

Paul E. Bankey, MD, PhD
Director of the Trauma Institute and Associate
Professor of Surgery
Department of Surgery
University of Rochester Medical Center
Rochester, NY, USA

Philip S. Barie, MD, MBA, FCCM, FACS
Professor of Surgery and Public Health
Department of Surgery and Public Health
Weill Medical College of Cornell University
New York, NY, USA

Renald Barry, MB, ChB, MMed(Surgery)
Professor/Chief Specialist
Department of Surgery
University of the Free State
Bloemfontein, South Africa

David E. Beck, MD
Chairman, Department of Colon and Rectal
Surgery
Ochsner Clinic Foundation
New Orleans, LA, USA

James M. Becker, MD, FACS
James Utley Professor and Chairman
Department of Surgery
Boston University Medical Center
Boston, MA, USA

Jacques Belghiti, MD
Professor
Department of Digestive Surgery
Hospital Beaujon
Clichy, France

Orlin N. Belyaev, MD
Assistant Physician
Department of Surgery
St. Josef Hospital
Ruhr University Bochum
Bochum, Germany

David A. Berg, MD
Fellow, Colorectal Surgery
Department of Surgery
Temple University Hospital
Philadelphia, PA, USA

Walter L. Biffl, MD, FACS
Associate Professor
Department of Surgery
Denver Health Medical Center/University of
Colorado-Denver
Denver, CO, USA

Kirby I. Bland, MD
Fay Fletcher Kerner Professor and Chairman
Department of Surgery
Deputy Director, Comprehensive Cancer
Center
University of Alabama School of Medicine
Birmingham, AL, USA

**Kenneth D. Boffard, MB, Bch, FRCS, FRCS
(Edin), FRCPS(Glas), FCS(SA), FACS**
Professor and Clinical Head
Department of Surgery
Johannesburg Hospital, University of the
Witwatersrand
Johannesburg, South Africa

Anne Marie Boller, MD
Fellow, Division of Colon and Rectal Surgery
Department of Surgery
Mayo Clinic Foundation
Rochester, MN, USA

Luigi Bonavina, MD
Associate Professor
Department of Surgery
University of Milan
Milan, Italy

Raul Martin Bosio, MD
General Surgery Resident
Department of Surgery
University of Toledo
Toledo, OH, USA

**Rudolph G. Botha, MBChB, DA(SA), MMed
(Surgery)(UFS), CMSA**
Principal Specialist and Senior Lecturer
Department of Surgery
Universitas Hospital
University of the Free State
Bloemfontein, South Africa

Andrew J. M. Boulton, MD, DSc(Hon), FRCP
Professor of Medicine and Consultant
Physician in Diabetes
Department of Medicine
Manchester Royal Infirmary
Manchester, UK

Stephen A. Boyce, BA, MBBS, MRCS
Specialist Registrar
Department of Surgery
University of Edinburgh
Royal Infirmary of Edinburgh
Edinburgh, UK

Andrew W. Bradbury, MD, FRCSEd
Professor
Department of Vascular Surgery
Birmingham Heartlands Hospital
Birmingham, UK

Italo Braghetto, MD, FRCS
Professor
Department of Surgery
Clinical Hospital
University of Chile
Santiago, Chile

Graham Branagan, MS, FRCS
Specialist Registrar and Consultant
Department of Surgery
Salisbury District Hospital
Salisbury, UK

Stacy A. Brethauer, MD
Fellow, Advanced Laparoscopic and Bariatric
Surgery
Department of General Surgery
Cleveland Clinic
Cleveland, OH, USA

L. D. Britt, MD, MPH, FACS
Chairman, Brickhouse Professor of Surgery
Department of Surgery
Eastern Virginia Medical School
Norfolk, VA, USA

Rebecca C. Britt, MD
Assistant Professor
Department of Surgery
Eastern Virginia Medical School
Norfolk, VA, USA

Ayesha S. Bryant, MSPH, MD
Assistant Professor
Division of Cardiothoracic Surgery
Department of Surgery
University of Alabama at Birmingham
Birmingham, AL, USA

Markus W. Büchler, MD
Professor of Surgery and Chairman
Department of General and Visceral Surgery
University of Heidelberg
Heidelberg, Germany

Patricio Burdiles, MD, FACS
Chief, Digestive Surgical Unit
Department of Surgery
Clinical Hospital
University of Chile
Santiago, Chile

Jean M. Butte, MD
Faculty of Medicine
Department of Digestive Surgery

Pontificia Universidad Católica de Chile
Santiago, Chile

Juan Luis Calisto, MD
Department of Laparoscopic Surgery
Clinica Anglo Americana
Lima, Peru

Alejandro Campos Gutierrez, MD
Assistant Professor of Surgery
Department of Surgery
Clinical Hospital University of Chile
Santiago, Chile

Fábio Guilherme Campos, MD, PhD
Department of Gastroenterology
University of São Paulo Medical School
São Paulo, Brazil

Miguel Caracoche, MD
Department of Surgery
Hospital de Clínicas "José de San Martín"
Universidad de Buenos Aires
Buenos Aires, Argentina

Gordon L. Carlson, BSc, MBChB, MD, FRCS
Professor
Department of Surgery
University of Manchester
Hope Hospital
Manchester, UK

Susan W. Caro, MSN, RNC, APNG
Director, Family Cancer Risk Service
Vanderbilt-Ingram Cancer Center
Vanderbilt University Medical Center
Nashville, TN, USA

William R. Carroll, MD, FACS
Professor
Division of Otolaryngology, Head & Neck
Surgery
Department of Surgery

University of Alabama at Birmingham
Birmingham, AL, USA

Ross Carter, MBChB, MD, FRCS
Consultant General Surgeon
Department of Surgery
Glasgow Royal Infirmary
Glasgow, UK

Stephen D. Cassivi, MD, MSc, FRCSC, FACS
Associate Professor of Surgery
Department of Surgery
Mayo Clinic and Foundation
Rochester, MN, USA

Jerry R. Castro, MD
Fellow
Department of Head and Neck Service
Memorial Sloan-Kettering Cancer Center
New York, NY, USA

Ivan Cecconello, MD
Professor and Chairman
Department of Digestive Surgery
São Paulo University School of Medicine
São Paulo, Brazil

Robert J. Cerfolio, MD, FACS, FACCP
Professor and Chief
Section of Thoracic Surgery
Department of Surgery
University of Alabama at Birmingham
Birmingham, AL, USA

Herbert Chen, MD, FACS
Associate Professor
Department of Surgery
University of Wisconsin
Madison, WI, USA

Miin-Fu Chen, MD, FACS
Professor and Director
Department of General Surgery

Chang-Gung Memorial Hospital
Chang-Gung University
Taoyuan, Taiwan
Republic of China

Steven L. Chen, MD, MBA
Department of Surgical Oncology
John Wayne Cancer Institute
Santa Monica, CA, USA

Daniel Cherqui, MD
Professor and Chief
Department of Digestive Surgery
CHU Henri Mondor
Creteil, France

Silas M. Chikunguwo, MD, PhD, ASCP
Fellow, Advanced Laparoscopic and Bariatric
Surgery
Department of Surgery
Cleveland Clinic Foundation
Cleveland, OH, USA

Eugene A. Choi, MD
Instructor in General Surgery
Department of Surgical Oncology
University of Texas
Houston, TX, USA

Kathleen K. Christians, MD
Associate Professor of Surgery
Department of Surgery
Medical College of Wisconsin
Milwaukee, WI, USA

Kent-Man Chu, MBBS, MS, FRCS(Ed), FACS
Professor of Surgery
Department of Surgery
University of Hong Kong
Queen Mary Hospital
Hong Kong, China

Louise C. H. Chin, MBBS, MRCP
Department of Diabetes and Endocrinology
Manchester Royal Infirmary
Manchester, UK

William G. Cioffi, MD, FACS
Professor and Chair
Department of Surgery
Brown Medical School
Providence, RI, USA

Orlo H. Clark, MD, FACS
Professor
Department of Surgery
UCSF/Mt. Zion Medical Center
San Francisco, CA, USA

Sue Clark, MD, FRCS
The Polyposis Registry
St. Mark's Hospital
Harrow, UK

Douglass B. Clayton, MD
Resident, Division of Urology
Department of Surgery
University of Alabama at Birmingham
Birmingham, AL, USA

Richard Cohen, MBBChir, BSc, MD, FRCS
Consultant Colorectal Surgeon
Department of Colorectal Surgery
University College Hospital
London, UK

Lisa M. Colletti, MD
Professory of Surgery
Department of Surgery
University of Michigan Medical School
Ann Arbor, MI, USA

Joachim Conze, MD, PhD
Consultant in General Surgery
Department of Surgery

University Hospital of the RWTH
Aachen, Germany

Willy Coosemans, MD, PhD
Professor
Department of Thoracic Surgery
University Hospital Leuven
Leuven, Belgium

C. Clay Cothren, MD, FACS
Director, Surgical Critical Care Fellowship
Department of Surgery
Denver Health Medical Center
Denver, CO, USA

Henry M. Cryer, MD, PhD, FACS
Professor in Surgery
Chief of Trauma and Critical Care
Department of Surgery
David Geffen School of Medicine at UCLA
Los Angeles, CA, USA

Attila Csendes, MD, FACS (Hon)
Professor of Surgery and Chairman
Department of Surgery
University Hospital
Santiago, Chile

José Eduardo M. Cunha, MD
Department of Gastroenterology
São Paulo University School of Medicine
São Paulo, Brazil

Paul M. Dark, BSc, MBChB, PhD, FCEM, FRCS
Senior Lecturer
Intensive Care Department
Hope Hospital
University of Manchester
Manchester, UK

Kimberly A. Davis, MD, FACS
Associate Professor of Surgery
Department of Surgery

Yale University School of Medicine
New Haven, CT, USA

Malcolm M. DeCamp, MD
Chief, Division of Cardiothoracic Surgery
Department of Surgery
Beth Israel Deaconess Medical Center
Boston, MA, USA

Georges Decker, MD
Department of Thoracic Surgery
University Hospital Leuven
Leuven, Belgium

Paul De Leyn, MD, PhD
Professor and Thoracic Surgeon
Department of Thoracic Surgery
University Hospital Gasthuisberg Leuven
Leuven, Belgium

Ronald P. DeMatteo, MD
Vice Chair, Department of Surgery
Head, Division of General Surgical Oncology
Memorial Sloan-Kettering Cancer Center
New York, NY, USA

Michael J. Demeure, MD, MBA
Professor of Surgery
Department of Surgery
Arizona Health Sciences Center
University of Arizona
Tucson, AZ, USA

Daniel T. Dempsey, MD, FACS
George S. Peters, MD and Louise C. Peters Chair
in Surgery
Department of Surgery
Temple University School of Medicine
Philadelphia, PA, USA

Claude Deschamps, MD, FRCSC, FACS
Professor of Surgery and Chair
Department of Surgery

Mayo Clinic and Foundation
Rochester, MN, USA

Clifford S. Deutschman, MS, MD, FCCM
Professor of Surgery
Department of Anesthesiology & Critical Care
University of Pennsylvania School of Medicine
Philadelphia, PA, USA

Nicolás A. Devaud, MD
Department of Digestive Surgery
Pontificia Universidad Católica de Chile
Santiago, Chile

Costanzo A. DiPerna, MD
Department of Surgery
Vallejo Medical Center
Kaiser Permanente
Vallejo, CA, USA

J. Michael Dixon, BSc(Hon), MBChB, MD, FRCSEng, FRCSEd, FRCPEd(Hon)
Consultant Surgeon and Senior Lecturer
in Surgery
Edinburgh Breast Unit
Western General Hospital
Edinburgh, UK

Matthew R. Dixon, MD
Fellow
Department of Colon and Rectal Surgery
University of Minnesota
St. Paul, MN, USA

Matteo Donadon, MD
Clinical Research Fellow
Department of Surgical Oncology
The University of Texas MD Anderson
Cancer Center
Houston, TX, USA

Elvis S. Donaldson Jr., MD
Lexington Gyn-Oncology

Central Baptist Hospital
Lexington, KY, USA

John H. Donohue, MD
Professor of Surgery
Division of Gastroenterologic
and General Surgery
Mayo Clinic Foundation
Rochester, MN, USA

Leona B. Downey, MD
Assistant Professor of Medicine
Section of Medical Oncology
University of Arizona
Arizona Cancer Center
Tucson, AZ, USA

Henning Dralle, MD, FRCS
Professor of Surgery and Chairman
Department of General, Visceral and Vascular
Surgery
Martin Luther University Halle-Wittenberg
Halle, Germany

Quan-Yang Duh, MD
Professor of Surgery
University of California-San Francisco
Department of Surgical Service
Veterans Affairs Medical Center
San Francisco, CA, USA

Mark D. Duncan, MD, FACS
Associate Professor of Surgery
Department of Surgery
Johns Hopkins Bayview Medical Center
Baltimore, MD, USA

François Durand, MD
Staff Surgeon
Department of Hepatology
Hospital Beaujon
Clichy, France

Luis A. Durand, MD
Department of Internal Medicine
Hospital de Clínicas "José de San Martín"
Universidad de Buenos Aires
Buenos Aires, Argentina

Roelf S. Du Toit, MBChB, MMed (Surgery), FCS(SA)
Professor/Chief Specialist
Department of Surgery
University of the Free State
Bloemfontein, South Africa

Soumitra R. Eachempati, MD, FACS
Associate Professor of Surgery
and Public Health
Department of Surgery and Public Health
Weill Medical College of Cornell University
New York, NY, USA

Matthew J. Eagleton, MD
Assistant Professor of Surgery
Department of Vascular Surgery
Cleveland Clinic Lerner College of Medicine
Cleveland, OH, USA

Pedro F. Escobar, MD
Department of Gynecologic Oncology
Lee Cancer Care
Lee Memorial Hospital
Fort Myers, FL, USA

Douglas B. Evans, MD
Professor of Surgery
Department of Surgery
University of Texas MD Anderson Cancer Center
Houston, TX, USA

Sheung Tat Fan, MBBS, MS, MD, PhD, DSc, FRCS, FACS, FCSHK, FHKAM
Professor and Chairman of Hepatobiliary
Surgery
Head, Department of Surgery

University of Hong Kong
Queen Mary Hospital
Hong Kong, China

Mark B. Faries, MD
Director, Translational Tumor Immunology
Department of Surgical Oncology
John Wayne Cancer Institute
Santa Monica, CA, USA

David R. Farley, MD
Professor
Department of Surgery
Mayo Clinic Foundation
Rochester, MN, USA

Victor W. Fazio, MB, MS, FRACS, FACS, FRCS
Rupert B, Turnbull Jr. MD Professor
Chairman, Department of Colorectal Surgery
Cleveland Clinic Foundation
Cleveland, OH, USA

**Kenneth C.H. Fearon, MBChB, MD, FRCPS
(Glas), FRCPS(Ed), FRCPS(Eng)**
Professor of Surgical Oncology
University of Edinburgh
Royal Infirmary of Edinburgh
Edinburgh, UK

Robert J. Feezor, MD
Fellow, Division of Vascular Surgery and
Endovascular Therapy
Department of Surgery
University of Florida College of Medicine
Gainesville, FL, USA

Daniel L. Feingold, MD, FACS
Assistant Professor of Surgery
Section of Colon and Rectal Surgery
Columbia University
New York, NY, USA

Markus Feith, MD
University Lecturer
Department of Surgery
Technical University Munich
Munich, Germany

Volker Fendrich, MD
Assistant Physician
Department of Visceral, Thoracic,
and Vascular Surgery
University of Marburg
Marburg, Germany

Paula Ferrada, MD
General Surgery Resident
Department of General Surgery
Beth Israel Deaconess Medical Center
Harvard University
Boston, MA, USA

Ricardo Ferrada, MD, MPH, FACS
Professor
Department of Surgery
University of Valle
Cali, Colombia

Pedro Ferraina, MD, PhD, FACS
Professor and Chairman
Department of Surgery
Hospital de Clínicas "José de San Martín"
Universidad de Buenos Aires
Buenos Aires, Argentina

Ariel Ferraro, MD
Department of Surgery
Hospital de Clínicas "José de San Martín"
Universidad de Buenos Aires
Buenos Aires, Argentina

Ian G. Finlay, MB ChB, BSc FRCS
Consultant Colorectal Surgeon
Department of Coloproctology
Glasgow Royal Infirmary
Glasgow, UK

John L. R. Forsythe, MD, MBBS, FRCS(Eng), FRCS(Ed)
Consultant Transplant Surgeon
Transplant Unit
Royal Infirmary of Edinburgh
Edinburgh, UK

Robert R. Franklin, MD, FACOG
Fellow, American College of Obstetricians and Gynecologists
Obstetrical & Gynecologic Associates, P.A., Houston, TX, USA

Robert D. Fry, MD
Chairman
Department of Surgery
Hospital of the University of Pennsylvania
Philadelphia, PA, USA

Peter A. Gaines, MBChB, FRCP, FRCR
Consultant Radiologist
Sheffield Vascular Institute
Northern General Hospital
Sheffield, UK

Henning A. Gaissert, MD
Research Fellow, Division of Thoracic Surgery
Department of Surgery
Harvard Medical School
Boston, MA, USA

Susan Galandiuk, MD
Director
Section of Colon and Rectal Surgery and Price Institute of Surgical Research
University of Louisville School of Medicine
Louisville, KY, USA

Joaquim Gama-Rodrigues, MD, PhD
Associate Professor of Surgery
Department of Gastroenterology
University of São Paulo
São Paulo, Brazil

Richard L. Gamelli, MD, FACS
Robert J. Freeark Professor and Chairman
Department of Surgery
Loyola University Medical Center
Maywood, IL, USA

Sidhu P. Gangadharan, MD
Staff Surgeon
Department of Surgery
Beth Israel Deaconess Medical Center
Boston, MA, USA

O. James Garden, MBChB, MD, FRCS(Ed), FRCP(Ed), FRACS(Hon)
Regius Professor of Clinical Surgery
Department of Clinical and Surgical Sciences
The University of Edinburgh
Royal Infirmary of Edinburgh
Edinburgh, UK

Keith E. Georgeson, MD
Joseph M. Farley Professor of Surgery
Director, Division of Pediatric Surgery
Department of Surgery
University of Alabama at Birmingham
Birmingham, AL, USA

Silvio Ghirardo, MD
Fellow
Department of Head and Neck Service
Memorial Sloan-Kettering Cancer Center
New York, NY, USA

Jean-François Gigot, MD, PhD, FRCS
Professor
Surgical Hepatobiliary and Pancreatic Division
Saint-Luc University Hospital
Brussels, Belgium

M. Sean Grady, MD
Charles Harrison Frazier Professor
Department of Neurosurgery

University of Pennsylvania
Philadelphia, PA, USA

Theresa A. Graves, MD
Assistant Professor
Department of Surgfery
Brown University Medical School
Providence, RI, USA

Jhanelle Gray, MD
Assistant Professor
Department of Medical Oncology
H. Lee Moffitt Cancer Center
and Research Institute
Tampa, FL, USA

**S. Michael Griffin, MBBS, MD, FRCS(Eng),
FRCS(Ed)**
Professor of Gastrointestinal Surgery
Northern Oesophagogastric Unit
Royal Victoria Infirmary
Newcastle upon Tyne, UK

Robert Gryfe, MD, PhD, FRCSC
Colorectal Surgical Oncologist
Department of Surgery
Mount Sinai Hospital
University of Toronto
Toronto, Canada

Angelita Habr-Gama, MD, PhD
Professor of Surgery
Department of Gastroenterology
University of São Paulo
São Paulo, Brazil

Jason F. Hall, MD
Department of Surgery
Harvard Medical School
Massachusetts General Hospital
Boston, MA, UK

**John P. Harris, MS, FRACS, FRCS, FACS,
DDU(Vascular)**
Professor of Vascular Surgery
Department of Surgery
The University of Sydney
Sydney, Australia

Merwe Hartslief, MBChB, M.Med
Department of Surgery
University of the Free State
Bloemfontein, South Africa

Richard J. Heald, M.Chir, FRCS
Director of Surgery
Pelican Cancer Foundation
North Hampshire Hospital
Basingstoke, UK

Per Hellman, MD, PhD
Associate Professor
Department of Surgical Sciences
University Hospital
Uppsala, Sweden

Juan Hepp, MC
Department of Surgery
Clínica Alemana Santiago
Santiago, Chile

David N. Herndon, MD
Jesse H. Jones Distinguished Chair in Burn
Surgery
Department of Surgery
University of Texas Medical Branch
Galveston, TX, USA

**Yik-Hong Ho, MBBS Hons (Qld), MD (Qld),
FRCS Ed, FRCS (Glasg), FRACS, FAMS, FI CS**
Professor and Head of Surgery
Department of Surgery
School of Medicine
James Cook University
Townsville, Queensland Australia

Richard Hodin, MD
Professor
Department of Surgery
Harvard Medical School
Massachusetts General Hospital
Boston, MA, USA

Robert L. Holley, MD
Associate Professor
Department of Obstetrics and Gynecology
University of Alabama at Birmingham
Birmingham, AL, USA

Yves Horsmans, MD, PhD
Professor
Department of Gastro-Enterology
Saint-Luc University Hospital
Université Catholique de Louvain (UCL)
Brussels, Belgium

Scott G. Houghton, MD
Department of Surgery
Mayo Clinic and Foundation
Rochester, MN, USA

Catherine Hubert, MD
Surgical Hepatobiliary and Pancreatic Division
Saint-Luc University Hospital
Université Catholique de Louvain (UCL)
Brussels, Belgium

Jörg Hutter, MD
Senior Physician
Department of Surgery
Paracelsus Private Medical University
Salzburg, Austria

Luis A. Ibañez, MD
Professor of Surgery and Head
Department of Digestive Surgery
Pontificia Universidad Católica de Chile
Santiago, Chile

Kamal M. F. Itani, MD
Professor
Department of Surgery
Boston University
Chief of Surgery
Boston VA Healthcare System
West Roxbury, MA, USA

Carlos Eduardo Jacob, MD, PhD
Department of Gastroenterology
Digestive Surgery Unit
University of São Paulo Medical School
São Paulo, Brazil

Ajay Jain, MD
Assistant Professor
Department of Surgery
Johns Hopkins University
Baltimore, MD, USA

Hans Jeekel, MD, PhD
Professor
Department of Surgery
Erasmus Medical Center
Rotterdam, The Netherlands

W. Scott Jellish, MD, PhD
Professor
Department of Anesthesiology
Loyola University Medical Center
Maywood, IL, USA

James W. Jones, MD, PhD
Visiting Professor of Medical Ethics
Center for Medical Ethics and Health Policy
Baylor College of Medicine
Houston, TX, USA

William D. Jordan Jr., MD
Professor and Chief
Vascular Surgery & Endovascular Therapy
Department of Surgery
University of Alabama at Birmingham
Birmingham, AL, USA

José Jukemura, MD
Department of Biliary & Pancreatic Surgery
Faculty of Medicine
University of Sao Paulo
São Paulo, Brazil

Vikram S. Kashyap, MD, FACS
Associate Professor of Surgery
Department of Vascular Surgery
Cleveland Clinic Foundation
Cleveland, OH, USA

Debra L. Kennamer, MD
Professor
Department of Anesthesiology and Pain
Medicine
University of Texas MD Anderson Cancer Center
Houston, TX, USA

Dong Yoon Keum, MD, PhD
Department of Thoracic and Cardiovascular
Surgery
Dongsan Medical Center
Keimyung University
Daegu, South Korea

Jawaid A. Khan, MBBS, MS, FRCS(Edin)
Professor
Department of General Surgery
Mission of Mercy Hospital & Research Institute
(formerly AG Hospital)
Calcutta, India

Peter Kienle, MD
Consultant
Department of Surgery
University of Heidelberg
Heidelberg, Germany

Patrick K. Kim, MD
Assistant Professor
Department of Surgery
University of Pennsylvania School of Medicine
Trauma Center at Penn
Philadelphia, PA, USA

Andrew N. Kingsnorth, BSc, MS, FRCS, FACS
Professor of Surgery
Department of General Surgery/Upper
GI Surgery
Peninsula Medical School
Derriford Hospital
Plymouth, UK

James K. Kirklin, MD
Professor & Director
Division of Cardiothoracic Surgery
Department of Surgery
University of Alabama at Birmingham
Birmingham, AL, USA

Masaki Kitajima, MD, PhD, FACS, FRCS, ASA
Professor
Department of Surgery
School of Medicine
Keio University
Tokyo, Japan

V. Suzanne Klimberg, MD
Professor
Department of Surgery
Chief, Breast Surgical Oncology
University of Arkansas for Medical Sciences
Little Rock, AR, USA

Hanns-Peter Knaebel, MD, MBA
Executive Vice President, Marketing & Sales
Clinical Science
Aesculap AG
Tuttlingen, Germany

Niels A. P. Komen, MD
Department of Surgery
Erasmus Medical Center
Rotterdam, The Netherlands

Owen Korn, MD, FACS
Associate Professor
Department of Surgery
Clinical Hospital University of Chile
Santiago, Chile

Aleksandra Kuciejewska, MRCP
Breast Unit
Royal Marsden London
London, UK

Lorrie A. Langdale, MD
Associate Professor
Department of Surgery
University of Washington and VA-Puget Sound
Health Care
Seattle, WA, USA

Julie R. Lange, MD, ScM
Assistant Professor of Surgery and Oncology
Department of Surgery
Johns Hopkins Medicine
Baltimore, MD, USA

David W. Larson, MD
Assistant Professor of Surgery
Department of Surgery
Division of Colon and Rectal Surgery
Mayo Clinic Foundation
Rochester, MN, USA

Andrew Latchford, BSc, MRCP
Research Fellow
The Polyposis Registry
St. Mark's Hospital
Harrow, UK

Alexis Laurent, MD, PhD
Department of Digestive Surgery
CHU Henri Mondor
Créteil, France

Christopher J. LeCroy, MD
Vascular Fellow
Department of Surgery
University of Alabama at Birmingham
Birmingham, AL, USA

Cheong J. Lee, MD
Department of General Surgery
University of Michigan
Ann Arbor, MI, USA

James A. Lee, MD
Assistant Professor
Division of Endocrine Surgery
Department of Surgery
UCSF Mt. Zion Medical Center
San Francisco, CA, USA

Jason T. Lee, MD
Assistant Professor of Surgery
Division of Vascular Surgery
Stanford University Medical Center
Stanford, CA, USA

Wei-Chen Lee, MD
Department of Liver Surgery and
Transplantation
Chang-Gung Memorial Hospital
Chang-Gung University
Taoyuan, Taiwan
Republic of China

Stanley P. L. Leong, MD, FACS
Professor
Department of Surgery
University of California
San Francisco, CA, USA

Toni Lerut, MD, PhD
Professor
Department of Thoracic Surgery
University Hospital Gasthuisberg Leuven
Leuven, Belgium

Joshua M. Levine, MD
Assistant Professor
Co-Director, Neurocritical Care Program
Department of Neurology
University of Pennsylvania
Philadelphia, PA, USA

Raymond H. S. Liang, MD, FRCPE, FRCPG, FRCP, FRACP, FHKCP, FHKAM (medicine)
S. H. Ho Professor in Haematology and Oncology
Li Ka Shing Faculty of Medicine
University of Hong Kong
Hong Kong, China

Sherry J. Lim, MD
Fellow, Surgical Oncology
University of Texas MD Anderson
Cancer Center
Houston, TX, USA

Anne Y. Lin, MD
Assistant Professor of Surgery
Section of Colorectal Surgery
Washington University School of Medicine
Louis, MO, USA

Chi-Leung Liu, MBBS, MS, MD, FRCS, FACS
Associate Professor
Department of Surgery
University of Hong Kong
Queen Mary Hospital
Hong Kong, China

Chung-Yau Lo, MBBC(HK), MS(HK), FRCSC (Edin.), FACS
Chief of Endocrine Surgery
Department of Surgery
University of Hong Kong Medical Centre
Queen Mary Hospital
Hong Kong, China

Yaira Lopez, MD
Resident, Digestive Surgery
Department of Surgery
Clinical Hospital
University of Chile
Santiago, Chile

Reginald V. N. Lord, MD
Consultant Surgeon
Department of Surgery
St. Vincent's Hospital Sydney
University of New South Wales
Sydney, Australia

Alain Luciani, MD
Department of Imagerie Medicale
CHU Henri Mondor
Creteil, France

François I. Luks, MD, PhD
Professor of Pediatric Surgery
Department of Surgery
Brown Medical School
Providence, RI, USA

Marcel C. C. Machado, MD, FACS
Professor
Department of Surgery
University of Sao Paulo
Sao Paulo, Brazil

Andreas Machens, MD
Associate Professor of Surgery
Department of General, Visceral and Vascular Surgery
Martin Luther University Halle-Wittenberg
Halle, Germany

J. Scott Magnuson, MD, FACS
Assistant Professor
Division of Otolaryngology, Head & Neck Surgery
Department of Surgery
University of Alabama at Birmingham
Birmingham, AL, USA

Thomas H. Magnuson, MD
Professor
Department of Surgery
Johns Hopkins Bayview Medical Center
Baltimore, MD, USA

Eric J. Mahoney, MD
Instructor
Department of Surgery
Brown Medical School
Providence, RI, USA

Rakesh K. Mangal, MD, FACOG
Obstetrical & Gynecological Associates, P.A.
Department of OB/Gyn & Reproductive
Endocrinology & Infertility
Texas Woman's Hospital
Houston, TX, USA

James M. Markert, MD, MPH
Professor and Director
Division of Neurosurgery
Department of Surgery
University of Alabama at Birmingham
Birmingham, AL, USA

David J. Maron, MD
Assistant Professor of Clinical Surgery
Department of Surgery
Hospital of the University of Pennsylvania
Philadelphia, PA, USA

John C. Marshall, MD, FRCSC, FACS
Professor of Surgery
Departments of Surgery & Critical Care
Medicine
St. Michael's Hospital
Toronto, Canada

Lorna P. Marson, MD, FRCS
Senior Lecturer in Transplant Surgery
Transplant Unit
Royal Infirmary of Edinburgh
Edinburgh, UK

Mary C. McCarthy, MD
Professor
Division of Trauma, Critical Care, and
Emergency Surgery
Department of Surgery
Wright State University Boonshoft School of
Medicine
Dayton, OH, USA

Laurence B. McCullough, PhD
Professor of Medicine and Medical Ethics
Associate Director for Education
Center for Medical Ethics and Health Policy
Baylor College of Medicine
Houston, TX, USA

Lisa K. McIntyre, MD
Assistant Professor
Department of General Surgery
Harborview Medical Center
Seattle, WA, USA

Colin J. McKay, MBChB, MD, FRCS
Senior Lecturer
Department of Surgery
Glasgow Royal Infirmary
Glasgow, UK

Elisabeth C. McLemore, MD
General Surgery Resident
Department of Colorectal Surgery
Cleveland Clinic Florida
Weston, FL, USA

Robin S. McLeod, BSc, MD, FRCSC, FACS
Professor of Surgery
Department of Surgery & HPME
University of Toronto
Toronto, Canada

Kelly M. McMasters, MD, PhD
Sam and Lolita Weakley Professor and
Chairman
Department of Surgery
University of Louisville School of Medicine
Louisville, KY, USA

Donald E. Meier, MD
Associate Professor
Department of Pediatric Surgery
Texas Tech University Medical School at El Paso
El Paso, TX, USA

Genevieve B. Melton-Meaux, MD
Assistant Professor
Department of General Surgery
Johns Hopkins Bayview Medical Center
Baltimore, MD, USA

Miguel Angel Mercado, MD
Professor and Chief
Department of Surgery
Instituto Nacional de Ciencias Medicas y
Nutricion
Mexico City, Mexico

Agneta Montgomery, MD, PhD
Associate Professor
Department of Surgery
University of Lund
Malmö University Hospital
Malmö, Sweden

Frank G. Moody, MD
Professor
Department of Surgery
University of Texas Medical School
Houston, TX, USA

Ernest E. Moore, MD, FACS
Chief of Surgery and Trauma Services
Denver Health System
Vice Chair, Department of Surgery

University of Colorado Health Sciences Center
Denver, CO, USA

Frederick A. Moore, MD, FACS, FCCM
Division Head, Surgical Critical Care and Acute
Care Surgery
Department of Surgery
Methodist Hospital
Houston, TX, USA

Brendan John Moran, MCh, FRCSI, FRCS
Consultant Colorectal and General Surgeon
Department of General Surgery
North Hampshire NHS Trust
Basingstoke, UK

Toshiyuki Mori, MD, FACS
Associate Professor
Department of Surgery
School of Medicine
Kyorin University
Tokyo, Japan

Gareth J. Morris-Stiff, MBBCh, MD, MCh, FRCS
Specialist Registrar
Department of Laparoscopic Surgery
Princess of Wales Hospital
Bridgend, UK

Melinda M. Mortenson, MD
Surgical Oncology Fellow
Department of Surgical Oncology
University of Texas MD Anderson Cancer
Center
Houston, TX, USA

Neil J. Mortensen, MD, FRCS
Professor
Department of Colorectal Surgery
John Radcliffe Hospital
Oxford, UK

Donald L. Morton, MD
Chief, Melanoma Program
John Wayne Cancer Institute,
Santa Monica, CA, USA

Michael W. Mulholland, MD, PhD
Frederick A. Coller Distinguished Professor
Department of Surgery
University of Michigan
Ann Arbor, MI, USA

Christophe A. Müller, MD
Department of Surgery
St. Josef Hospital Bochum
Ruhr University Bochum
Bochum, Germany

Pamela N. Munster, MD
Medical Oncologist
Department of Interdisciplinary Oncology
H. Lee Moffitt Cancer Center and Research Institute
Tampa, FL, USA

Christopher S. Muratore, MD
Assistant Professor
Division of Pediatric Surgery
Brown University Medical School
Providence, RI, USA

Emma L. Murray, MBChB, BSc Hons
Edinburgh Breast Unit
Western General Hospital
Edinburgh, UK

Chrispen D. Mushaya, MBChB(UZ), FCS(ECSA)
Department of Surgery
The Townsville Hospital
Townsville, Australia

Philippe Nafteux, MD
Department of Thoracic Surgery
University Hospital Leuven
Leuven, Belgium

Mario S. Nahmod, MD
Department of Surgery
Hospital de Clínicas "José de San Martín"
Universidad de Buenos Aires
Buenos Aires, Argentina

Lena M. Napolitano, MD, FACS, FCCP, FCCM
Professor
Department of Surgery and Surgical Critical Care
University of Michigan Health System
Ann Arbor, MI, USA

Leslie Karl Nathanson, MBChB, FRACS
Department of Surgery
Royal Brisbane Hospital
Brisbane, Australia

A. Ross Naylor, MBChB, MD, FRCS
Professor in Vascular Surgery & Consultant Vascular Surgeon
Department of Surgery
Leicester Royal Infirmary
Leicester, UK

Heidi Nelson, MD
Professor of Surgery
Division of Colon and Rectal Surgery
Mayo Clinic College of Medicine
Rochester, MN, USA

Edmund A. M. Neugebauer, PhD
Director and Chairman for Surgical Research
Faculty of Medicine
Institute for Research in Operative Medicine
University Witten/Herdecke
Cologne, Germany

Fritz U. Niethard, MD
Professor
Orthopädische Universitätsklinik
Klinikum der Rheinisch-Westfälisch-
Technischen Hochschule
Aachen, Germany

Yuji Nimura, MD
President
Aichi Cancer Center Hospital and
Research Institute
Nagoya, Japan

Hideki Nishio, MD
Lecturer
Department of Surgery
Nagoya University Graduate School of
Medicine
Nagoya, Japan

Santhat Nivatvongs, MD
Professor of Surgery
Division of Colon and Rectal Surgery
Mayo Clinic College of Medicine
Rochester, MN, USA

Nora F. Nugent, MBBCh, BAO, MRCSI
Department of Plastic Surgery
Cork University Hospital
Wilton, Cork, Ireland

Gustavo S. Oderich, MD
Assistant Professor of Surgery
Division of Vascular Surgery
Mayo Clinic College of Medicine
Rochester, MN, USA

Mamerhi O. Okor, MD
Assistant Professor
Division of Neurosurgery
Department of Surgery
University of Alabama at Birmingham
Birmingham, AL, USA

Hector Orozco, MD, FACS
Professor and Chairman
Surgical Division
Instituto Nacional de Ciencias Medicas y
Nutricion
Mexico City, Mexico

James W. Orr Jr., MD, FACOG, FACS
Medical Director
Department of Obstetrics and Gynecology
University of South Florida
Fort Myers, FL, USA

Sandra Osorio Veliz, MD
Instructor
Department of Surgery
Clinical Hospital University of Chile
Santiago, Chile

Mary F. Otterson, MD, MS, FACS
Professor of Surgery
Division of General Surgery
Medical College of Wisconsin
Milwaukee, WI, USA

Kenneth Ouriel, MD, FACS, FACC
Professor of Surgery
Cleveland Clinic Foundation,
Cleveland, OH USA
CEO, Sheikh Khalifa Medical City
Abu Dhabi, UAE

C. Keith Ozaki, MD, FACS
Associate Professor
Department of Surgery
University of Florida College of Medicine
Gainesville, FL, USA

Robert T. A. Padbury, MBBS, FRACS, PhD
Director
Division of Surgical and Specialty Services
Flinders Medical Centre
Bedford Park, Australia

David L. Page, MD
Professor of Pathology and Preventive Medicine
Department of Pathology
Vanderbuilt University Medical Center
Nashville, TN, USA

Martín Palavecino, MD
Fellow, HPB Surgery and Liver Transplantation
General Surgery Service
Hospital Italiano de Buenos Aires
Buenos Aires, Argentina

Edward E. Partridge, MD
Professor
Department of Obstetrics and Gynecology,
Director, Comprehensive Cancer Center
University of Alabama at Birmingham
Birmingham, AL, USA

Kepal N. Patel, MD
Assistant Professor
Division of Endocrine Surgery
Department of Surgery
NYU School of Medicine
New York, NY, USA

Juan Pekolj, MD, PhD, FACS
Chief of HPB Surgery Section
General Surgery Service
Hospital Italiano de Buenos Aires
Buenos Aires, Argentina

Glenn E. Peters, MD
Professor and Director
Division of Otolaryngology, Head & Neck
Surgery
Department of Surgery
University of Alabama at Birmingham
Birmingham, AL, USA

Robin K. S. Phillips, MS, FRCS
Professor and Director
The Polyposis Registry
St. Mark's Hospital
Harrow, UK

Henrique Walter Pinotti, MD
Professor
Department of Surgery
Faculty of Medicine
University of Sao Paulo
São Paulo, Brazil

Peter W. T. Pisters, MD
Professor of Surgery
Department of Surgical Oncology
University of Texas MD Anderson
Cancer Center
Houston, TX, USA

Henry A. Pitt, MD
Professor
Department of Surgery
Indiana University
Indianapolis, IN, USA

Luis Poggi, MD, FACS
Department of Laparoscopic Surgery
Clinica Anglo Americana
Lima, Peru

Raphael E. Pollock, MD, PhD
Division Head, Surgery
Department of Surgical Oncology
University of Texas M.D. Anderson Center
Houston, TX, USA

John R. Porterfield Jr., MD, MSPH
General Surgery Resident
Department of Surgery
Mayo Clinic College of Medicine
Rochester, MN, USA

John J. Poterucha, MD
Associate Professor of Medicine
Division of Gastroenterology and Hepatology
Mayo Clinic College of Medicine
Rochester, MN, USA

Francesco P. Prete, MD
Department of Surgical Sciences
University of Foggia
Foggia, Italy

Richard A. Prinz, MD, FACS
Professor and Chairman
Department of General Surgery
Rush Medical College
Chicago, IL, USA

Igor Proscurshim, BS
Department of Gastroenterology
University of São Paulo Medical School
São Paulo, Brazil

Robert V. Rege, MD
Professor and Chairman
Department of Surgery
The University of Texas Southwestern Medical
Center at Dallas
Dallas, TX, USA

Donald A. Reiff, MD, FACS
Assistant Professor
Section of Trauma, Burns & Surgical Critical
Care
Department of Surgery
University of Alabama at Birmingham
Birmingham, AL, USA

Feza H. Remzi, MD, FACS, FASCRS
Department of Colorectal Surgery
Cleveland Clinic
Cleveland, OH, USA

Götz M. Richter, MD
Professor
Department of Radiology
University of Heidelberg
Heidelberg, Germany

Diego Rivera, MD
Attending Surgeon
Hospital Universitario del Valle
Cali, Colombia

Ivan S. Roa, MD
Chief
Department of Pathology
Clinica Alemana Santiago
Universidad de la Frontera
Santiago, Chile

Bradley M. Rodgers, MD
Chief, Division of Pediatric Surgery
Department of Surgery and Pediatrics,
University of Virginia Children's Hospital
Charlottesville, VA, USA

Phillip Y. Roland, MD, FACOG, FACS
Assistant Professor
Department of Gynecologic Oncology
Florida Gynecologic Oncology
Ft. Myers, FL, USA

Laurence Z. Rosenberg, MD, BS
Southeastern Plastic Surgery and
Department of Surgery
Florida State University School of Medicine
Tallahassee, FL, USA

Matthias Rothmund, MD, FACS
Chief and Professor
Department of Visceral, Thoracic,
and Vascular Surgery
University of Marburg
Marburg, Germany

Theresa W. Ruddy, MD
Department of General Surgery
Rush University Medical Center
Chicago, IL, USA

Loring W. Rue III, MD, FACS
Professor and Vice Chair
Chief, Section of Trauma, Burns & Surgical
Critical Care
University of Alabama at Birmingham
Birmingham, AL, USA

Theodore J. Saclarides, MD
Professor of Surgery
Department of General Surgery
Rush University Medical Center
Chicago, IL, USA

Yoshiro Saikawa, MD, PhD
Department of Surgery
School of Medicine
Keio University
Tokyo, Japan

George H. Sakorafas, MD, PhD
Surgeon and Lecturer
4th Department of Surgery
Athens University Medical School
Athens, Greece

Priya Sampathkumar, MD
Consultant, Division of Infectious Diseases
Mayo Clinic College of Medicine
Rochester, MN, USA

William Sanchez M., MD, FACS
Associate Professor of Surgery
Universidad Militar Nueva Granada
Hospital Militar Central
Bogota, Colombia

Michael G. Sarr, MD
James C. Mason Professor of Surgery
Department of Surgery
Mayo Clinic College of Medicine
Rochester, MN, USA

Anja Schaible, MSc
Department of Surgery
University Hospital
Heidelberg, Germany

Philip R. Schauer, MD
Professor
Department of General Surgery
Cleveland Clinic
Cleveland, OH, USA

Deborah Schrag, MD, MPH
Elizabeth and Felix Rohatyn Chair for
Junior Faculty
Department of Medicine
Memorial Sloan-Kettering Cancer Center
New York, NY, USA

Volker Schumpelick, MD
Professor
Department of Surgery
University Clinic Aachen
Aachen, Germany

James M. Seeger, MD
Professor and Chief
Division of Vascular Surgery and Endovascular
Therapy
Vice Chairman, Department of Vascular
Surgery
University of Florida
Gainesville, FL, USA

Anthony J. Senagore, MD, MS, MBA
Professor
Department of Surgery
College of Human Medicine
Michigan State University
Lansing, MI, USA

Francis Seow-Choen, MBBS, FRCSEd, FAMS, FRCS
Senior Consultant Colorectal Surgeon
Seow-Choen Colorectal Center
Mt. Elizabeth Medical Centre
Singapore

Jatin P. Shah, MD, PhD, FACS
Chief, Head and Neck Service
Elliot W. Strong Chair in Head and Neck
Oncology
Memorial Sloan Kettering Cancer Center
New York, NY, USA

Jonathan Shenfine, MBBS, FRCS
Northern Oesophagogastric Unit
Royal Victoria Infirmary
Newcastle upon Tyne, UK

Shailesh V. Shrikhande, MD, MBBS, MS
Associate Professor and Consultant Surgeon
Department of Gastrointestinal Surgical
Oncology
Tata Memorial Hospital
Maharashtra, India

J. Rüdiger Siewert, MD
Chairman of the Board of Directors
University Hospital Heidelberg
Heidelberg, Germany

Lelan F. Sillin III, MD, MS (Ed), FACS
Professor of Surgery and Vice Chair of
Educational Affairs
Department of Surgery
School of Medicine and Dentistry
University of Rochester
Rochester, NY, USA

Diane M. Simeone, MD
Professor
Department of Surgery
University of Michigan
Ann Arbor, MI, USA

Rache M. Simmons, MD, FACS
Associate Professor
Department of Surgery
New York Presbyterian Hospital Weill Medical
College
New York, NY, USA

Bhuvanesh Singh, MD, PhD
Director, Laboratory of Epithelial Cancer
Biology
Department of Surgery
Memorial Sloan-Kettering Cancer Center
New York, NY, USA

Richard J. E. Skipworth, BSc(Hons), MBChB, MRCS(Ed)
Clinical Research Fellow
University of Edinburgh
Royal Infirmary of Edinburgh
Edinburgh, UK

Samuel J. A. Smit, MBChB, MMed(Surgery)
Principal Specialist/Sr Lecturer
Department of Surgery (G72)
University of the Free State
Bloemfontein, South Africa

Ian E. Smith, MD, FRCP, FRCPE
Professor of Cancer Medicine
Royal Marsden Hospital London
London, UK

Martin D. Smith, MBBCh(Wits), FCS(SA)
Adjunct Professor
Department of Surgery
Chris Hani Baragwanath Hospital
University of the Witwatersrand
Johannesburg, South Africa

Wade R. Smith, MD
Director, Orthopaedic Trauma
University of Colorado School of Medicine
Denver Health Medical Center
Denver, CO, USA

Carmen C. Solórzano, MD, FACS
Associate Professor of Surgery
Department of Surgery
Rush Medical College
Chicago, IL, USA

Gonzalo Soto Debeuf, MD
Department of Surgery
Clinical Hospital
University of Chile
Santiago, Chile

Jenny Speranza, MD
Assistant Professor
Division of Colorectal Surgery
Department of Surgery
Cleveland Clinic Florida
Weston, FL, USA

Lewis Spitz, MBChB, PhD, MD(Hon), FRCS, FRCPCH, FAAP(Hon), FCS(SA)(Hon)
Emeritus Nuffield Professor of Paediatric Surgery
Department of Paediatric Surgery
Institute of Child Health (University College London)
London, UK

Philip F. Stahel, MD
Associate Professor
Department of Orthopedic Surgery
Denver Health Medical Center
University of Colorado School of Medicine
Denver, CO, USA

Michael J. Stamos, MD, FACS, FASCRS
Professor of Surgery

Chief, Division of Colon and Rectal Surgery
Department of Surgery
UC Irvine Medical Center
Orange, CA, USA

Hubert J. Stein, MD, FACS
Chairman
Department of Surgery
University Hospital Salzburg
Salzburg, Austria

J. Michael Straughn Jr., MD
Assistant Professor
Department of Obstetrics and Gynecology
University of Alabama at Birmingham
Birmingham, AL, USA

Arthur F. Stucchi, PhD
Associate Research Professor
Department of Surgery, Pathology and Laboratory Medicine
Boston University School of Medicine
Boston, MA, USA

Michael Stumpf, MD
Department of Surgery
University Hospital
Rhenish-Westphalian Technical University-Aachen
Aachen, Germany

Paul H. Sugarbaker, MD, FACS, FRCS
Director of Surgical Oncology
Peritoneal Surface Oncology Program
Washington Cancer Institute
Washington Hospital Center
Washington, DC, USA

Masanori Sugiyama, MD, PhD
Professor
Department of Surgery
School of Medicine
Kyorin University
Tokyo, Japan

Timothy M. Sullivan, MD, FACS, FACC
Professor of Surgery
Department of Vascular / Endovascular Surgery
North Central Heart Institute
Sioux Falls, SD, USA

Yutaka Suzuki, MD, PhD
Department of Surgery
School of Medicine
Kyorin University
Tokyo, Japan

Flavio Roberto Takeda, MD
Research Fellow
Digestive Surgery Department
São Paulo University School of Medicine
São Paulo, Brazil

Eric P. Tamm, MD
Associate Professor
Department of Diagnostic Radiology
University of Texas MD Anderson Cancer
Center
Houston, TX, USA

**Kok-Yang Tan, MBBS(Melb), MMed
(Surgery), FRCS(Edin), FAMS**
Associate Consultant, Colorectal Service
Department of Surgery
Alexandra Hospital
Singapore

John L. Tarpley, MD
Professor
Department of Surgery
Vanderbilt University School of Medicine
Nashville, TN, USA

**Kumaran Thiruppathy, MBBS (Lon),
MRCS, BSc (Hon)**
Department of General Surgery
University College London Hospital
London, UK

Jon S. Thompson, MD
Professor and Vice Chair
Department of Surgery
University of Nebraska Medical Center
Omaha, NE, USA

Margaret Thompson, MD
Breast Fellow and Instructor
Department of Surgery/Division of Breast
Surgical
University of Arkansas for Medical Sciences
Little Rock, AR, USA

**Joe J. Tjandra, MD, FRACS, FRCS, FRCPS,
FASCRS**
Late Associate Professor of Surgery
Department of Colorectal Surgery
Royal Melbourne Hospital
Victoria, Australia

S. Rob Todd, MD, FACS
Assistant Professor
Department of Surgery
Methodist Hospital
Houston, TX, USA

Thomas F. Tracy Jr., MD
Vice Chairman, Department of Surgery
Division of Pediatric Surgery
Brown Medical School
Hasbro Children's Hospital
Providence, RI, USA

Waldemar H. Uhl, MD, FRCS
Professor
Department of Surgery
St. Josef Hospital Bochum
Bochum, Germany

Marshall M. Urist, MD
Professor of Surgical Oncology
Department of Surgery
University of Alabama at Birmingham
Birmingham, AL, USA

Takashi Uruno, MD
Department of Surgery
UCSF Medical Center at Mt. Zion
San Francisco, CA, USA

Bernard E. Van Beers, MD, PhD
Professor of Radiology
Department of Medical Imaging
Saint-Luc University Hospital
Université Catholique de Louvain (UCL)
Brussels, Belgium

**C. Andrew van Hasselt, MBChB(Rand),
MMed(Otol), FRCS, FRCS(Edin), FCS(SA),
FHKAM(Otol)**
Professor
Department of Otorhinolaryngology, Head and
Neck Surgery
Prince of Wales Hospital
Shatin, N.T. Hong Kong

Dirk Van Raemdonck, MD, PhD, FETCS
Associate Professor of Surgery
Department of Thoracic Surgery
University Hospital Gasthuisberg Leuven
Leuven, Belgium

R. Edward Varner, MD
Director, Female Pelvic Medicine &
Reconstructive Surgery
Department of Obstetrics and Gynecology
University of Alabama School of Medicine
Birmingham, AL, USA

Luis O. Vasconez, MD
Professor and Director
Division of Plastic Surgery
Department of Surgery
University of Alabama at Birmingham
Birmingham, AL, USA

Jean-Nicholas Vauthey, MD, FACS
Professor of Surgery
Department of Surgical Oncology
University of Texas MD Anderson Cancer
Center
Houston, TX, USA

Gary A. Vercruysse, MD
Assistant Professor of Surgery
Division of Trauma, Surgical Critical Care &
Burns
Grady Memorial Hospital
Atlanta, GA, USA

Jacobus S. Vermaak, MBBCh(Wits)
Department of Surgery
Chris Hani Baragwanath Hospital
University of the Witwatersrand
Johannesburg, South Africa

Alexander C. Vlantis, FCS(SA), FCS(HK)
Department of Surgery
The Chinese University of Hong Kong
Prince of Wales Hospital
Hong Kong, China

Huamin Wang, MD, PhD
Assistant Professor
Department of Pathology
University of Texas MD Anderson
Cancer Center
Houston, TX, USA

Andrew L. Warshaw, MD
W. Gerald Austen Professor and Chair
Department of Surgery
Massachusetts General Hospital
Boston, MA, USA

Randal S. Weber, MD, FACS
Professor and Chairman
Department of Head and Neck Surgery
University of Texas MD Anderson
Cancer Center
Houston, TX, USA

William I. Wei, MS, FRCS, FRCSE, FACS, FRACS, (Hon) FHKAM, (ORL, Surg)
Li Shu Pui Professor of Surgery
Chair in Otorhinolaryngology
The University of Hong Kong
Hong Kong, China

Markus Weißkopf, MD
Head of Spine Center
Hospital of Orthopaedic Surgery Schwarzach
Schwarzach, Germany

Richard O. Wein, MD, FACS
Assistant Professor
Department of Otolaryngology–Head and Neck Surgery
Tufts- New England Medical Center
Boston, MA, USA

Jens Werner, MD
Professor of Surgery
Department of General and Visceral Surgery
University of Heidelberg
Heidelberg, Germany

Steven D. Wexner, MD, FACS, FRCS, FRCS(Ed)
Chairman
Department of Colorectal Surgery
Cleveland Clinic Florida,
Weston, FL, USA

Malcolm H. Wheeler, MD, FRCS
Retired Professor of Endocrine Surgery
University Hospital of Wales
Cardiff, UK

Richard L. Whelan, MD
Associate Director
Section of Colorectal Surgery
Columbia University
New York, NY, USA

Alastair Windsor, MBBS, MD, FRCS, FRCS(Ed)
Colorectal Surgery Consultant
Department of Surgery
University College Hospital
London, UK

Bruce G. Wolff, MD
Professor of Surgery
Chair, Division of Colon and Rectal Surgery
Mayo Clinic College of Medicine
Rochester, MN, USA

W. Douglas Wong, MD, FRCS(C), FACS
Chief, Colorectal Service
Department of Surgery
Memorial Sloan-Kettering Cancer Center
New York, NY, USA

John Wong, MBBS(Syd), PhD(Syd), Hon MD(Syd)FRACS, FRCS(Edin), FRCS(Glasg), Hon FACS
Chair Professor
Department of Surgery
The University of Hong Kong
Queen Mary Hospital
Hong Kong, China

Douglas E. Wood, MD
Professor and Chief
General Thoracic Surgery
Department of Surgery
University of Washington
Seattle, WA, USA

Randy J. Woods, MD
Assistant Professor
Division of Trauma, Critical Care, and
Emergency Surgery
Department of Surgery
Wright State University School of Medicine
Miami Valley Hospital
Dayton, OH, USA

Henry Yeh, MD
Department of Colorectal Surgery
Epworth and Royal Melbourne Hospitals
Melbourne, Australia

Tonia M. Young-Fadok, MD, MS, FACS, FASCRS
Professor of Surgery
Chair, Division of Colon and Rectal Surgery
Mayo Clinic
Phoenix, AZ, USA

S. Mahmood Zare, MD
Assistant Professor
Department of Surgery
Boston VA Healthcare System
West Roxbury, MA, USA

Christopher K. Zarins, MD
Chidester Professor of Surgery
Division of Vascular Surgery
Stanford University Medical Center
Stanford, CA, USA

Nicholas J. Zyromski, MD
Assistant Professor of Surgery
Department of Surgery
Indiana University
Indianapolis, IN, USA

General Principles

1 Anesthesia and Risk Management

W. Scott Jellish

Pearls and Pitfalls

- An adequate review of systems is key to determining physical health and providing an assessment of perioperative risk. A few extra minutes spent obtaining an adequate history will reduce the ordering and expense of unnecessary tests.
- The value of exercise tolerance and the ability to accomplish 4 metabolic equivalents (METS) of activity can be used to predict complication rates for many surgeries.
- The ability to intubate and ventilate a patient is of primary importance and weighs heavily on the assessment of risk.
- Electrocardiograms (ECGs) are useful, not as a screening tool, but as a modality for obtaining a more accurate medical assessment of patients in high-risk groups.
- Avoid the technology trap. Nonselective batteries of tests will often
  - Fail to uncover pathologic conditions
  - Detect abnormalities that do not necessarily improve outcome
  - Increase medicolegal liability because of poor follow-up
- Low serum albumin is a marker of increased pulmonary complications and should be measured in all patients suspected of poor diet or hypoalbuminemia.
- A patient's emotional and psychiatric needs are as important as physical status in assessing perioperative risk and postoperative outcome. These variables should be thoroughly evaluated.

Risk assessment by the anesthesiologist is a complex task incorporating numerous physical and laboratory findings. Physical status and the ability of the patient to withstand the stress of the surgical procedure must be determined. The assessment of risk is based on the knowledge of prevalence rates of unwanted consequences in population groups sharing the same characteristics or risk factors. The preoperative interview should educate the patients about anesthesia perioperative care and pain treatment to reduce anxiety and facilitate recovery. The complex interaction between perceived risk, benefit, and the acceptance of that risk is influenced by characteristics such as familiarity, control, catastrophe potential, and level of knowledge. Medical counseling during the presurgical assessment is used to obtain pertinent information about the patient's medical history, as well as physical and mental condition. The care plan is determined and guided by patient choices, which helps relieve anxiety and establish mutual trust.

Important Goals For Preoperative Preparation Prior to Surgery

Risk management involves identification of risk and either avoiding conditions which predispose the patient to that risk, or developing a means to alter the consequences of an action or event which usually leads to an adverse outcome. Factors that affect risk include: the nature and duration of the illness requiring the operation, other comorbidities, age, nutritional status, as well as the type of operation considered. The American Society of Anesthesiologists Task Force on Preanesthesia Evaluation issued a Practice Advisory which focuses on the timing of the evaluation, choice of tests, and the recommendation that no tests beyond a physician evaluation be ordered for patients undergoing minimally invasive surgical procedures. It is the task of the anesthesiologist to assess risk and formulate an acceptable plan which will anticipate potential problems, increase patient safety, produce an acceptable operating field, and provide a stable and pain-controlled postoperative environment.

The preoperative assessment is based on a thorough and efficient fact-finding process. The ultimate goals are to reduce the morbidity associated with surgery, increase the quality, decrease the costs of perioperative care, and restore the patient quickly to their preoperative level of functionality. This assessment includes decisions for noninvasive testing to better estimate risk and determine patients who might benefit from specific preoperative procedures. Indirect studies of perioperative morbidity over four decades have shown that perioperative patient conditions are significant predictors of postoperative morbidity. The fact finding methods used by anesthesiologists to assess surgical risk include: an adequate history, physical exam, and finally, confirmatory laboratory tests as directed by the history and physical exam. This not only improves outcomes but also reduces costs. It is the medical history that will give the most information concerning the patient and their ability to undergo the surgical procedure. The history has been demonstrated to give primary information concerning a patient's physical state in approximately 60% of cases. It should include both acute and chronic aspects of the patients health and should be focused on the upcoming surgical procedure. The first key aspect of the acute history is exercise tolerance. Patients are usually asked if they can climb two flights of stairs, which is 4 METS of activity. An inability to perform 4 METS of activity should arouse suspicion of congestive heart failure or coronary disease. The METS criteria are primarily based on studies that found that the complication rate for noncardiac surgery in elderly patients doubled if they were unable to complete 4 METS of activity. Other studies have demonstrated that the 4 METS rule can be used to predict complication rates in vascular and bariatric surgery, among others. Information concerning medications is the second key consideration and includes questions about supplements and why they are taken. Questions determining vitality, mobility, and fitness are also asked, along with a review of systems focusing on chronic disease, history of hospitalization and surgeries, family history, and social history.

A major factor that is always considered in a patient undergoing surgery is age. Although much of the increased morbidity related to age is appropriately attributable to comorbidity and the extent of the existing disease, a patient >80 years of age will have a reduced physiologic reserve. Numerous studies have found a significant increase in mortality after surgery beginning at the age of 70. The highest rate of anesthetic complications occurs in an age group >75 and among those with the greatest number of comorbidities. Thirty six percent of patients over 70 had nonfatal complications after surgery. In patients undergoing vascular procedures, the single best predictor of death, pulmonary edema, cardiac arrest, or myocardial infarction was age >70.

To assess operative risk, the anesthesiologist must also include a physical examination of the patient. In most instances, pertinent physical findings have already been established by the primary care or general medicine physician. However, there are some instances where the anesthesiologist discovers a previously undiagnosed finding (murmur, bruit, etc.) that may require further investigation. There are a few physical features that are important to the anesthesiologist which directly affect intraoperative risk, namely the anatomy of the airway and the body habitus of the patient, as it pertains to the anatomical features which could increase the difficulty of a regional anesthetic.

The ability to intubate and ventilate a patient for a surgical procedure is of primary importance to the anesthesiologist and weighs heavily in the assessment of risk criteria. Closed claims analysis reveals that 85% of airway-related incidents involve brain damage or death, and as many as one-third of deaths attributable solely to anesthesia have been related to the inability to maintain a patent airway. Numerous complications and morbidities are associated with endotracheal intubation (❥ *Table 1-1*). Malformations of the face, acromegaly, cervical spondylosis, occipito-atlanto-axial disease, tumors of the airway, and long-term diabetes producing stiff joint syndrome carry added risk. Head movement and the ability to hyperextend the neck producing a thyromental distance of >6.5 cm would be consistent with a normal airway and easy mask ventilation. The ability of the patient to prognath the jaw and an inter-incisor gap of >5 cm would provide evidence of a large mouth opening which is suggestive of an easy laryngoscopy. Tooth morphology, especially "buck" teeth, may make the intubation extremely difficult. Loose teeth should also be identified as they could become easily dislodged and aspirated during intubation, adding considerable morbidity to the surgical procedure.

◻ Table 1-1

Complications of endotracheal intubation (Reprinted from Mallampati, 1997. With permission)

During intubation	Evident after extubation
Laryngospasm	Laryngospasm
Laceration, bruising of lips, tongue and pharynx	Aspiration of secretions, gastric contents, blood or foreign bodies
Fracture, chipping, dislodgement of teeth or dental appliances	Glottic, subglottic or uvular edema
Perforation of trachea or esophagus	Dysphonia, aphonia
Retropharyngeal dissection	Paralysis of vocal cords or hypoglossal, lingual nerves
Fracture or dislocation of cervical spine	Sore throat
Trauma to eyes	Noncardiogenic pulmonary edema
Hemorrhage	Laryngeal incompetence
Bacteremia	Soreness, dislocation of jaw
Aspiration of gastric contents or foreign bodies	Tracheomalacia
Endobronchial or esophageal intubation	Glottic, subglottic or tracheal stenosis
Dislocation of arytenoid cartilages or mandible	Vocal cord granulomata or synechiae
Hypoxemia, hypercarbia	
Bradycardia, tachycardia	
Hypertension	
Increased intracranial or intraocular pressure	

With tube in situ
Accidental extubation
Endobronchial intubation
Obstruction or kinking
Bronchospasm
Ignition of tube by laser device or cautery
Aspiration
Sinusitis
Excoriation of nose or mouth

The visibility of the oropharyngeal structures is assessed in the sitting position without phonation. Mallampati constructed a staging system to predict difficult tracheal intubation. This system was modified by El Ganzouri et al. to further estimate the success rate of intubation. A Class I designation is made when faucial pillars, soft palate, and uvula are visualized and would be consistent with a normal-appearing airway. Visualization of the faucial pillars and soft palate with an obstructed view of the uvula by the base of the tongue is consistent with a Class II airway. This designation is also considered low-risk for laryngoscopy and intubation. The Class III airway is characterized by visualization of the soft palate only and carries a higher risk for difficult intubation. The Class IV airway with visualization of the hard palate only is considered the most difficult to intubate and carries the highest risk of perioperative morbidity. Any patient diagnosed as having obstructive sleep apnea or in whom it is suspected on the basis of clinical signs (obesity, limited mouth opening, or a large tongue) should be treated as having a difficult airway until proven otherwise.

The next major anesthetic assessment of perioperative risk involves the cardiovascular system and the patient's fitness to undergo the procedure without major morbidity and mortality. The type and duration of surgery, particularly the risk of large blood loss, volume shifts, violation of visceral cavities, or vascular procedures, account for major surgical procedures with the greatest potential for complications (❯ *Table 1-2*). In addition, certain timing factors may influence the risk of the surgical procedure. Cardiac complications are 2–5 times more likely to occur with surgeries in the emergency setting than when done electively (Mozaffarian, 2005). Patients presenting for cardiac procedures (bypass, valve replacement, etc.) assume a higher risk of cardiac-related morbidity and mortality by the nature of their surgery.

The patient that presents for noncardiac surgery poses the biggest problem for the assessment of fitness to undergo a surgical procedure. History-taking alone often provides enough information to

◻ Table 1-2

Cardiac risk stratification for noncardiac surgical procedures[a] (Reproduced from ACC/AHA Guideline Update for Perioperative Cardiovascular Evaluation for Non-Cardiac Surgery – Executive Summary, 2002, American Heart Association. With permission)

Stratification
High (reported cardiac risk often >5%)
Emergent major operations, particularly in the elderly
Aortic and other major vascular procedures
Peripheral vascular procedures
Anticipated prolonged surgical procedures associated with large fluid shifts and/or blood loss
Intermediate (reported cardiac risk generally <5%)
Carotid endarterectomy
Head and neck procedures
Intraperitoneal and intrathoracic procedures
Orthopedic procedures
Prostate surgery
Low[b] (reported cardiac risk generally <1%)
Endoscopic procedures
Superficial procedure
Cataract removal
Breast procedures

[a] Cardiac risk signifies combined incidence of cardiac death and nonfatal myocardial infarction.
[b] Does not generally require further preoperative testing.

determine a patient's risk of complications for the proposed surgery. Questions directed toward the occurrence of any previous myocardial infarction and the presence and frequency of any precipitating or potentiating factors involving any chest discomfort, may be an indication of ischemia. Questions should also be directed towards symptoms of heart failure (orthopnea, paroxysmal nocturnal dyspnea, and dyspnea on exertion) and the results of previous cardiac tests. The physical exam should include the measurement of vital signs and evidence of peripheral vascular disease (carotid or femoral bruits or diminished pulses). The lung fields should be examined for decreased breath sounds, rales, or rhonchi. The patient with a suspicious history who has symptoms or physical evidence of unstable angina, congestive heart failure, or rhythm disturbances is at high risk for a myocardial event. High-cardiac-risk patients need further investigation to determine functional status or if the degree of myocardial ischemia will be altered by subsequent therapy. The additional diagnostic procedures performed in high- or intermediate-risk patients help the anesthesiologist determine the extent of intraoperative monitoring, the anesthetic plan, and even if the procedure should be avoided altogether.

An ECG sometimes uncovers occult disease in older adults, but it rarely shows clinically important abnormalities in younger asymptomatic patients without cardiac risk factors. The usefulness of the preoperative ECG depends on the information it provides physicians to identify cardiac risk, quantify abnormalities in known risk, and make decisions about perioperative therapy. Routine ECGs in asymptomatic women under 50 and men under 40 are usually not indicated.

Patients who benefit from a preoperative ECG manifest one or more of the following conditions: chest pain not ascribed to any etiology, angina or anginal equivalents, history of congestive heart failure, high blood pressure, diabetes or symptoms of dysrhythmias, shortness of breath, history of smoking, inability to exercise, or need for vascular surgery. Abnormalities on ECG that have the potential to alter management of perioperative care are: atrial flutter or fibrillation; first , second , or third-degree AV block; ST segment changes suggestive of myocardial ischemia; premature ventricular and atrial contractions; LV or RV hypertrophy; short P–R interval; Wolf Parkinson-White syndrome; prolonged QT; peaked t waves; and small voltage indicative of cardiomyopathy. The consensus exists that ECGs are useful, not as a screening tool, but as a tool for obtaining a more accurate medical assessment of patients in otherwise high-risk groups.

Further cardiac studies to stratify risk may be most beneficial for patients who are considered to be at intermediate risk of cardiac complications. These tests may also be indicated for patients with known or suspected coronary artery disease who are undergoing high-risk procedures and in whom functional status and stability of ischemia is difficult to assess. Testing the low-risk patient undergoing low-risk surgery is an exercise in futility. There are some generally accepted principles regarding what exactly is an effective screening test. It must be accurate and able to detect the target condition earlier than without screening and with efficient accuracy to avoid producing large amounts of false-positive or false-negatives. The test should improve the likelihood of favorable health outcomes compared to treating patients once they present with signs or symptoms of the disease. The threshold for ordering these tests should reflect the cardiac risk of the planned procedure.

The ECG exercise treadmill test is useful in patients who can exercise but is rarely applicable to patients with ischemic lower extremities. Studies have demonstrated that standard exercise stress tests were falsely positive for significant coronary artery disease in 40% of patients and falsely negative in 15%. Many times, the patient cannot achieve the maximum predicted heart rate because of dyspnea or claudication. Thus in a population with a high prevalence of coronary artery disease, a positive exercise stress test only slightly increases the likelihood of coronary artery disease and a negative test correlates poorly with the absence of heart disease. Therefore interest has increased in other noninvasive tests for cardiac risk stratification.

Holter monitoring or ambulatory ECG for detecting *asymptomatic ischemia* is not widely used, but its findings may correlate well with those of exercise testing and dipyridamole-thallium scans (DTS) in predicting adverse cardiac events. The ST changes indicative of ischemia (1 mm ST depression for at least 1 min) often can be seen at heart rates below those obtained by conventional stress testing. Several studies have concluded that ischemia detected during Holter monitoring was a reliable predictor of postoperative cardiac events even after all other risk factors were controlled. Comparisons of exercise tolerance tests, Holter monitoring, and cardiac catheterization in patients with stable angina revealed that patients with positive Holter results had a greater likelihood of having multi-vessel coronary artery disease. The advantages of Holter monitoring to identify high-risk patients for cardiac complications include its availability, ease of interpretation, and low cost. However, it is used the least in clinical practice to assess perioperative risk. It is of no value in patients with pre-existing ECG abnormalities that obfuscate determinations of ST segment depression.

Pharmacological stress testing should be considered for patients with an abnormal ECG (including left and possibly right bundle branch block and a history of myocardial infarction). It should also be considered for those taking digoxin and in those who cannot exercise to acceptable levels. As with all tests, their predictive value to determine adverse cardiac outcome is important. Relative risk is the probability of an adverse event where the test is negative. A high score determines a high risk of a cardiac event, whereas a score of 1 implies that risk is similar whether the test is positive or negative. Relative risk scores have been developed for noninvasive cardiac tests and help determine the effectiveness of these tests for prediction of poor outcome. Studies of cardiac risk using DTS suggest that patients with normal studies have a low risk for cardiac complications (good negative predictive value); however, the prognostic implications of an abnormal scan are less well established. Prospective studies to determine the efficacy of DTS on predicting intraoperative myocardial ischemia or infarct suggest a close relationship between reversible defects and adverse cardiac outcome. The sensitivity of the exam, however, appears to be in the presence or absence of coronary artery disease, but not ischemia. The combined median relative risk score for this test was 4.6. However, recent reports demonstrate no correlation between redistribution defects and adverse cardiac outcome or risk of perioperative ischemia. Thus routine DTS screening is not recommended for determination of adverse cardiac outcome.

Radionucleide ventriculography (RNVG) and assessment of left ventricle function and ejection fraction (EF) can predict perioperative cardiac morbidity in patients undergoing vascular procedures. In addition to determining EF, the scan can show ventricular wall motion abnormalities and systolic and diastolic dysfunction. Pasternak et al. demonstrated that a calculated EF of less than 35% was associated with a perioperative myocardial infarction rate of 20%. The combined relative risk with this stipulated EF was 3.7, delineating a positive result. Although not all studies have substantiated the accuracy of RNVG for predicting postoperative cardiac mortality, measurement of EF using this technique is one of the strongest predictors of overall and late survival after vascular surgery.

Dobutamine stress echo (DSE) was developed as a tool for assessing the presence of coronary artery disease. The exam is composed of the administration of a pharmacologic inotropic agent (dobutamine) which increases heart rate and myocardial contractility, thereby increasing myocardial oxygen (O_2) consumption. If O_2 demand outstrips supply, myocardial dysfunction will be evident by echocardiographic evidence of hypokinesis, akinesis, or dyskinesis. The development of new wall motion abnormalities following dobutamine is considered indicative of significant heart disease.

This test is recommended in patients with intermediate clinical predictors (prior MI, compensated CHF, diabetes, and mild angina) with poor functional capacity (<4 METS) or intermediate clinical predictors with moderate or excellent functional capacity (>4 METS) and high surgical risk. DSE and DTS appear to have comparable specificity and sensitivity; however, relative risk scores generated from numerous outcome studies were demonstrated to average 6.2 for DSE, which suggests the test may be more effective for predicting an adverse cardiac event.

Coronary artery plaque burden and coronary calcium evaluation using electron beam computed tomography (EBCT) has recently been touted to be diagnostic for coronary artery disease risk. The test examines coronary plaque burden and found that those with coronary calcium scores >1,000 all had elevation of cardiac troponin-T perioperatively. However, EBCT's ability to reduce morbidity and mortality has not been demonstrated, and more importantly, the cost-effectiveness and consequences of negative tests and false-positives are unknown. Thus it is not recommended as a screening tool for perioperative cardiac morbidity.

Coronary angiography is not recommended for risk assessment in patients going for noncardiac surgery unless they have clinical evidence of coronary artery disease and are undergoing moderate- to high-risk surgical procedures. If coronary artery disease or cardiac dysfunction is severe enough to request coronary angiography, the anesthesiologist presumes the risk to be high and the patient in question will undergo a cardiac event during surgery. The anesthesiologist also presumes a coronary artery bypass graft (CABG) or percutaneous transluminal coronary angioplasty (PTCA) will be performed if appropriate lesions are found. The presence of significant coronary stenosis does not always indicate that an MI is unavoidable or that invasive monitoring is required because the involved artery may supply a scar or its stenosis may be compensated by collaterals. The use of coronary angiography to assess risk for perioperative morbidity and mortality is not supported at present and studies to evaluate its use are ongoing.

The evaluation of pulmonary function is also important in assessing patient risk for surgery. In fact, recent recommendations from the American College of Physicians stress that patients be evaluated for the presence of the following risk factors for postoperative pulmonary complications: chronic obstructive pulmonary disease, age >60 years, ASA physical status II or greater, functional dependence, and congestive heart failure (Roizen, 1993). Obesity and mild or moderate asthma were not significant risk factors. Pulmonary complications are the most common form of postoperative morbidity expressed by patients who undergo abdominal and thoracic procedures. In addition to pneumonia, postoperative pulmonary complications include massive lobar collapse due to mucous plugging, pneumonitis, atelectasis, and a combination of one or more of these problems. The high incidence of these complications and their associated costs make it imperative that patients at increased risk be identified and pulmonary function optimized prior to the surgical procedure. The anesthesiologist may request pulmonary function tests to assess risk prior to intrathoracic procedures to determine if the patient will tolerate loss of functional lung units. The calculation of percent predicted volume has increased the accuracy of spirometry as a preoperative tool for evaluating pulmonary risk. The risk assessment by the anesthesiologist will also include methods to reduce pain and techniques to preserve viable lung function postoperatively.

Abdominal procedures produce a 30% incidence of pulmonary complications. In addition to dysfunction of the abdominal musculature, abdominal surgery impairs diaphragmatic function, which further reduces FRC. The preoperative evaluation of pulmonary risk in the patient undergoing abdominal surgery should include age, general health performance, weight, coexisting pulmonary morbidity and the type and approach for the surgery. Spirometry is indicated in patients in whom severe pulmonary dysfunction is evident as a means to assess whether they may need pulmonary rehabilitation prior to surgery. Other procedures that have a high risk of pulmonary complications include prolonged surgeries (>3 h), neurosurgery, head and neck surgery, vascular surgery, emergency surgery, and aortic aneurysm repair.

A low serum albumin (<3.5 g/dl) is also a marker of increased risk for postoperative pulmonary complications and should be measured in all patients who are clinically suspected of hypoalbuminemia. Other tests have also been suggested to estimate pulmonary risk. Spirometry diagnoses obstructive lung disease but does not translate into an effective risk predictor for patients. Comparisons of spirometric studies with clinical data have not consistently demonstrated it to be superior to history and physical exams in predicting postoperative pulmonary complications. Chest radiographs are frequently used as part of a routine preoperative evaluation of risk. The evidence suggests, however, that clinicians may predict most abnormal preoperative chest radiographs by history and physical exams and that this test only rarely provides unexpected information. Chest radiographs are helpful for patients with known cardiopulmonary disease and those older than 50 who are undergoing upper abdominal, thoracic, or abdominal aortic aneurysm surgery.

The numerous factors considered in the perioperative assessment of risk make exchange of information sometimes difficult and hard to convey. A generalized scoring system of risk allows groups of patients to be stratified according to the severity of their illness before treatment is begun and enables better analysis of morbidity and mortality for these groups. A risk scoring system should have several prerequisites: (1) simple to use; (2) applicable to most general surgery cases; (3) used for both elective and emergency procedures; and (4) universally accepted to assess both morbidity and mortality. The scoring system most often used by anesthesiologists to assess risk is the American Society of Anesthesiologists Physical Status classification. Patients are allocated to one of five categories based on their medical history and physical examination without the use of any specific tests. A physical status I (PS I) designates a normal healthy patient while a PS IV individual has incapacitating disease that limits lifestyle and is a threat to life. PS V patients are moribund and not expected to survive more than 24 h. An "E" designation is added to denote an emergency procedure with an associated increase in risk. Postoperative morbidity and mortality rise with increased ASA grade, and if age is added as a covariable, the scoring system has an even better predictive effect (❯ Table 1-3).

◘ Table 1-3

American Society of Anesthesiologists Classification (Qaseem et al., 2006)

ASA class		Rates of PPCs class definition by class (%)
I	A normally healthy patient	1.2
II	A patient with mild systemic disease	5.4
III	A patient with systemic disease that is not incapacitating	11.4
IV	A patient with an incapacitating systemic disease that is a constant threat to life	10.9
V	A moribund patient who is not expected to survive For 24 h with or without operation	N/A

ASA = American Society of Anesthesiologists; NA = not applicable; PPC = postoperative pulmonary complication.

◘ Table 1-4

Goldman's nine independent variables associated with perioperative cardiac events (Data from Goldman et al., 1977)

- Age over 70 years
- Myocardial infarction in the preceding 6 months
- Perioperative third heart sound or jugular venous distention
- Significant valvular aortic stenosis
- Emergency surgery
- Intraperitoneal, intrathoracic, or aortic operation
- More than five premature ventricular beats per minute documented at any time before operation
- Rhythm other than sinus or the presence of atrial premature contractions on preoperative electrocardiogram
- One or more markers of poor general medical condition

The Goldman Cardiac Risk Index was designed to predict the risk of cardiac complications following noncardiac surgery. Nine factors are considered to give a total score of 0–53 (❯ *Table 1-4*). Scores are then grouped into four risk classes. Originally, Goldman was critical of the ASA classification system as being poorly defined and subjective, but it has proved to be as good as the more cumbersome Goldman classification which is not routinely used today by anesthesiologists. Other classification systems, such as the Pulmonary Complication Risk and the Prognostic Nutritional Risk scoring systems are used to determine operative risk based on prolonged preoperative hospitalizations of debilitated patients. These scoring systems are too wide-ranging and not specific enough to be used as the basis for individual decision-making concerning the patient about to undergo surgery and are rarely used by anesthesiologists.

Once the assessment of operative risk has been determined the anesthesiologist should also make specific recommendations concerning the discontinuation of oral intake and the reduction of aspiration risk. Metoclopramide, ranitidine, and sodium citrate may be given prior to the scheduled surgery to reduce the risk of aspiration, especially if the patient has a condition which predisposes them to passive reflux of stomach contents (e.g. hiatal hernia, gastroesophageal reflux disease). If the airway is judged acceptable to proceed with direct laryngoscopy, cricoid pressure is used and a rapid sequence induction performed to obtain a patent airway. These procedures done correctly will reduce the risk of aspiration and the accompanying increase in morbidity and mortality associated with such an occurrence.

The physical and mental state of the anesthesiologist is another variable, though not assessed at the time of the preoperative visit that affects the overall risk of the surgical procedure. Human errors affect patient safety in two ways: (1) they increase the probability of accident initiators; and (2) they increase the probability of a failure to properly respond to a problem. Anesthesiologists can experience a number of potential problems that could affect patient outcome. Fatigue and sleep deprivation affect vigilance and the recognition of problems as they occur during the operation. Suitability factors may also be present in which the person lacks the appropriate personality, temperament, or ability to perform anesthesia. Cognitive problems occur in which individuals cannot process all of the information presented to them at a particular time. In addition, the individual may try to cut corners or be careless. Detractors in the operating room could also increase risk to the patient. Social conversations, noise, and considerations of upcoming cases may distract the anesthesiologist from events that occur during the surgical procedure, which may lead to increased morbidity. Aging also affects the operating team, in which case the abilities of both the surgeon and anesthesiologist decline. Lack of continuing education and unfamiliarity with new techniques put the older anesthesiologist at a distinct disadvantage when dangerous situations arise. These human factors could ultimately increase the risk of a particular surgical procedure to a much greater extent than predicted by risk assessments obtained from medical history and laboratory testing.

The final portion of the preoperative risk assessment involves the explanation of risk to the patient and their acceptance of the perceived risk. This explanation also includes discussion of the anesthetic plan and agreement of that plan with the patient and surgeon. The assessment of surgical risk is the best guess of what might happen from a combination of past clinical experiences, cohort data from groups of patients with similar problems, and the patient's own comorbidities. Medical counseling and decision-making is largely about handling these risks. However simple the awaited surgical procedure, it is a very important event in the patient's life. Though small, there is a certain level of risk associated with the simplest surgical interventions, and the patient has a legal right to secure information including risk factors that are specific to their particular case. The patient's agreement to undergo the surgical procedure utilizing the anesthetic technique discussed, is perceived as a contract between physician and patient that is governed by mutual trust established during the preoperative visit. At a time when the patient's right to decide his or her own medical management is becoming more prevalent, the preoperative assessment and the estimate of operative risk play a vital role in the informed consent process and is the cornerstone to a successful surgical outcome.

Selected Readings

Archer C, Levy AR, McGreor M (1993) Value of routine perioperative chest x-rays: a meta-analysis. Can J Anaesth 40:1022–1027

Eagle KA, Berger PB, Calkins H, et al. (2002) ACC/AHA guideline update for perioperative cardiovascular evaluation for noncardiac surgery – executive summary: a report of the American College of Cardiology/American Heart Association Task Force on Practice Guidelines (Committee to Update the 1996 Guidelines on Perioperative Cardiovascular Evaluation for Noncardiac Surgery). Circulation 105:1257–1267

El-Ganzouri AR, McCarthy RJ, Tuman KJ, et al. (1996) Preoperative airway assessment: predictive value of a multivariate risk index: Anesth Analg 82:1197–1204

Goldman L, Caldera DL, Nussbaum SR, et al. (1977) Multifactorial index of cardiac risk in noncardiac surgical procedures. N Engl J Med 297:845–850

Kertai MD, Boersma E, Bax JJ, et al. (2003) A meta-analysis comparing the prognostic accuracy of six diagnostic tests for predicting perioperative cardiac risk in patients undergoing major vascular surgery. Heart 89:1327–1334

Mallampati SR (1997) Airway management. In: Barash PG, Cullen BF, Stoelting RF (eds) Clinical anesthesia, 3rd edn. J.B. Lippincott, Philadelphia, PA, p 587

Mozaffarian D (2005) Electron-beam computed tomography for coronary calcium – a useful test to screen fro coronary artery disease? JAMA 294(22):2897–2900

Pasternak LR, Arens JF, Caplan RA, et al. (2002) Task force on preanesthesia evaluation. Practice advisory for preanesthesia evaluation: a report by the American Society of Anesthesiologists Task Force on Preanesthesia Evaluation. Anesthesiology 96:485–496

Pasternak PF, Imparato AM, Riles TS, et al. (1985) The value of the radionuclide angiogram in the prediction of perioperative myocardial infarction in patients undergoing lower extremity revascularization procedures. Circulation 72(Suppl II):13–17

Pate-Cornell ME, Lakats LM, Murphy DM, et al. (1997) Anesthesia patient risk: a quantitative approach to organizational factors and risk management options. Risk Analysis 17:511–523

Qaseem A, Snow V, Fitterman N, et al. (2006) Risk assessment for and strategies to reduce perioperative pulmonary complications for patients undergoing noncardiothoracic surgery: a guideline from the American College of Physicians. Ann Intern Med 144:575–580

Reilly DF, McNeely MJ, Doerner D, et al. (1999) Self-reported exercise tolerance and the risk of serious perioperative complications. Arch Intern Med 159:2185–2192

Roizen MF (1993) The usefulness of the perioperative electrocardiogram. J Clin Monit 9:101–103

Sgura FA, Kopecky SL, Grill JP, et al. (2000) Supine exercise capacity identifies patients at low risk for perioperative cardiovascular events and predicts long-term survival. Am J Med 108:334–336

Srinivas M, Roizen MF, Barnard J, et al. (1994) Relative effectiveness of four preoperative tests for predicting adverse cardiac outcomes after vascular surgery: a meta-analysis. Anesth Analg 79:422–433

2 Fluids and Electrolytes

Kimberly A. Davis · Richard L. Gamelli

Pearls and Pitfalls

- Total body water accounts for 60% of body weight – 40% as the intracellular compartment and 20% as the extracellular compartment.
- 5% of body weight is the intravascular compartment.
- In adults, daily maintenance volume is 25–30 ml/kg containing about 1 mEq/kg sodium and 1/2 mEq/kg potassium.
- Volume deficit is the most common fluid disorder in the surgical patient.
- All fluid losses are isotonic except for urine and sweat/evaporation, thus most replacement fluids should be isotonic.
- Isotonic fluid losses are due most commonly to vomiting, diarrhea, nasogastric suctioning, gastrointestinal fistulae, and sequestration of fluids in soft tissue injuries and infections.
- Hyponatremia may result from SIADH (or the syndrome of inappropriate secretion of anti-diuretic hormone) related to head trauma; correction involves free water restriction.
- Hypernatremia from loss of free water from diabetes insipidus or high output renal failure requires a slow correction of serum sodium.
- Hyperkalemia from renal failure can be treated by intravenous calcium gluconate, insulin/glucose infusion, potassium exchange resins, and hemodialysis.
- After hemorrhage, fluid and protein move from the interstitium to the plasma, so-called transcapillary plasma refill, resulting in restoration of plasma volume and protein concentration, but with reduced oxygen carrying capacity due to decrease in total red cell mass, i.e., a normovolemic anemia.
- The primary goal of resuscitation is restoration of normal tissue perfusion through volume expansion.
- Ringers lactate is the best fluid for acute resuscitation; hypotonic fluids and those containing glucose should be avoided.
- Inadequate restoration of circulating volume can cause persistent acidosis, systemic inflammatory response syndrome, multiple organ dysfunction system, multi-system organ failure, and even death.

Introduction

The great French physiologist, Claude Bernard, was the first to recognize that human beings lived in two very different environments: the external environment, and the "milieu intérieur," in which the tissues lived. Another 50 years passed before it was known that this internal environment was closely protected by several intrinsic mechanisms. The outcome of these protective mechanisms was termed "homeostasis" by Walter Cannon, a professor of physiology at Harvard. At the crux of this "milieu intérieur" is the maintenance of normal fluid and electrolyte balance.

Administration and replacement of the body's fluid and electrolytes represents a fundamental component of a surgeon's practice. An understanding of the complex mechanisms of homeostasis is necessary, as most diseases and many injuries, including operative trauma, alter the physiology of fluids and electrolytes within the body. Redistribution of body fluids from one compartment to another, as is seen in response to inflammation, infection, and traumatic injury, usually results in a decrease in the volume of circulating extracellular fluid, and subsequent hypoperfusion or "shock". During resuscitation of patients from shock, a strong working knowledge of normal fluid and electrolyte balance is paramount to assure rapid restoration of circulating volume, and the prevention of the untoward sequelae of the systemic inflammatory response syndrome (SIRS) and multisystem organ failure (MSOF).

Distribution of Body Fluids

Roughly 60% of body mass is made up of water, although this percentage varies with age and sex. The total percentage of body water decreases with increasing age, and women tend to have a lower percentage of body water than men. Body water is divided classically into two fluid compartments: the intracellular compartment (two thirds or 40% total body water) and the extracellular compartment (one third or 20% total body water) (❍ *Fig. 2-1*). The intracellular space is represented predominantly by muscle mass, in which the major cations are magnesium and potassium, buffered by bicarbonate and negatively charged proteins. The extracellular space has sodium and chloride as its main ions and is further subdivided into the plasma (one quarter or 5% of total body water) and the interstitium (three-quarters or 15% of total body water). Water is freely diffusable across semi-permeable membranes, keeping osmotic forces in balance. The forces that drive fluid movement between compartments are the relative Starling forces between the intracellular and extracellular fluid compartments.

◨ Figure 2-1
Body water distribution

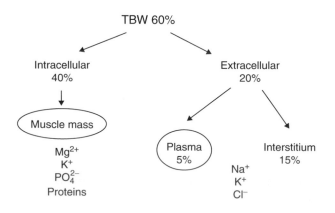

Regulation of Normal Homeostasis

Fluid and Electrolyte Balance

The delicate balance of fluid and electrolytes is normally controlled by the kidneys and the neuroendocrine system. Usually, fluid input and output are equal or in balance. When input exceeds output, the term "positive balance" is employed. Conversely, in those patients in whom output exceeds input, the term "negative balance" is applied.

Most intake of water is liquid, with only a third derived from solids, while output is usually classified as either *sensible* or *insensible*. Sensible losses are measurable and include urine (800–1,500 ml per day), feces (150 ml per day), and sweat (200–1,000 ml per day). Insensible losses are non-measurable and involve evaporation of water from the lungs (exhaled air) and diffusion of water through the skin. Up to 8–12 ml/kg/day is lost through the skin and respiratory tract as insensible loss in the normal human being. Although fairly fixed, insensible loss varies with body temperature, ambient temperature, activity, and daily fluid intake.

The Kidney

Although the type and quantity of input is important, the composition of the "milieu intérieur" is maintained predominantly by the nature of the output; thus the kidneys serve as the primary organ for maintaining constancy of the internal environment. By varying the glomerular filtration rate, the kidneys are able to respond rapidly to changes in volume, solute content and composition of body fluids.

Normal kidney function involves filtration of approximately 180 l of plasma per day. Sodium is resorbed preferentially in the proximal tubule in conjunction with bicarbonate and other divalent cations. The loop of Henle is responsible predominantly for the resorption of water and sodium in conjunction with chloride. In the distal tubule, however, active sodium resorption is coupled with excretion of potassium and hydrogen ion under the control of aldosterone, thus representing a sodium/potassium or sodium/hydrogen exchange. The collecting duct, under the control of ADH (antidiuretic hormone, or arginine vasopressin) results in the resorption of water, and subsequent concentration of the urine. Thus, the maintenance of normal fluid and electrolyte balance is dependent on the formation of a large quantity of glomerular filtrate that is almost completely resorbed from the renal tubules prior to excretion.

Neuroendocrine Control of Renal Function

Changes in fluid and electrolyte balance and renal function normally occur daily as a result of variations in intake and output, or abnormally after injury or illness. Both the volume and composition of body fluids are monitored continuously by receptors and transduced via the neuroendocrine system into changes in renal handling of water and electrolytes. Effective circulating volume is monitored continuously by arterial and renal baroreceptors and by atrial stretch receptors. When effective circulating volume decreases, activity from these receptors decreases, releasing a tonic inhibition from the neuroendocrine system, mediated by increased secretion of adrenocorticotropic hormone (ACTH), resulting in increased aldosterone secretion, and increased secretion of renin, resulting in increased formation of angiotensin. Aldosterone, synthesized, stored, and secreted by the adrenal gland, increases sodium and chloride resorption and potassium excretion in the kidney. Angiotensin, in addition to being a potent vasoconstrictor and myocardial stimulant, stimulates release of ADH, resulting in resorption of free water and augmenting the release of aldosterone. The net effect of these neuroendocrine pathways is to restore circulating volume and maintain normal body fluid and electrolyte balance.

Maintenance of Normal Fluid Balance

Baseline requirements for healthy human beings must account for both insensible losses (approximately 750 ml of pure water per day) and sensible losses of hypotonic fluids of (approximately 350 ml per day). Additionally, a normal person must excrete approximately 600 mOsm per day via the urine to maintain normal body composition secondary to metabolism. The minimal volume of urine necessary to accomplish this varies widely based on the ability of the kidney to concentrate urine, but approximates 500–800 ml per day. Therefore, under normal conditions, the average 70 kg male requires between 1,500 and 2,500 ml of fluid per day, or about 25–30 ml/kg body weight per day (❷ *Table 2-1*).

The healthy human being also requires a minimal amount of sodium chloride to maintain a normal balance. When human beings are stressed to conserve sodium, they do so at the expense of potassium via the sodium/potassium exchange in the kidney related to aldosterone secretion. Thus, an intake of approximately 60–100 mEq of sodium are necessary per day to prevent excess potassium loss, or approximately 1 mEq/kg body weight. With adequate maintenance doses of sodium, urinary potassium loss will be about 30–60 mEq per day, or approximately 0.5 mEq/kg body weight per day.

Conditions of Abnormal Fluid Loss

Any abnormal fluid losses (replacement) must be added to the daily fluid and electrolyte requirements described above. Most replacement represents losses of transcellular fluids, with varied electrolyte compositions. Normal concentrations found in several body fluids are listed in ❷ *Table 2-2*. Abnormally high secretion of any of these fluids, particularly those from the gastrointestinal tract, is a major cause of fluid and electrolyte disturbances in surgical patients. Knowledge of the electrolyte composition and volume of the body fluid lost is vital in determining replacement therapy. The electrolyte compositions of commonly available replacement fluids are listed in ❷ *Table 2-3*. Common metabolic disturbances from fluid loss and suggested volume replacement are listed in ❷ *Table 2-4*.

◻ Table 2-1

Maintenance fluid requirements for the surgical patient

Body weight	Fluid requirement
For 0–10 kg	100 ml/kg/day
For 10–20 kg	50 ml/kg/day
For > 20 kg	20 ml/kg/day
For 70 kg adult	2,500 ml/day

◘ Table 2-2

Electrolyte compositions of body fluids (mEq/l)

	Na^+	K^+	Cl^-	HCO_3^-	Volume (ml)	Osmolality (mOsm/l)
Saliva	10	26	10	30	1,000	Variable
Stomach	60[a]	10	130	0	1,500	280
Duodenum	140	5	80	0	1,500	280
Ileum	140	5	104	30	3,000	280
Colon	60	35	40	0	750	280
Pancreas	145	5	75	115	1,000	280
Bile	145	5	100	35	1,000	280
Sweat	50	5	55	0	500	Variable
Blood	140	5	100	24	5,000	280

[a]Varies with acid secretion; in patients with achlorhydria or after acid-secreting inhibition, sodium approaches 130 mEq/l.

◘ Table 2-3

Electrolyte composition of replacement fluids (mEq/l)

Solution	pH	Na^+	Cl^-	K^+	Ca^{2+}	Other components	Osmolality (mOsm/l)
Lactate Ringers (LR)	5	130	109	4	3	Lactate 28 mEq/l	280
NS	4	154	154	0	0		308
D5LR	5	130	109	4	3	Dextrose 50 g/l, lactate 28 mEq/l	560
D5NS	4	154	154	0	0	Dextrose 50 g/l	588
D5.45NS	4	77	77	0	0	Dextrose 50 g/l	434
D5.25NS	4	34	34	0	0	Dextrose 50 g/l	357

◘ Table 2-4

Replacement fluids for the management of common metabolic disturbances

Source of fluid	Metabolic disturbance	Suggested replacement
Gastric	Hypochloremic, hypokalemic metabolic alkalosis	D5NS with 20 mEq/l KCl
Pancreatic	Acidemia, hypoproteinemia	LR (bicarbonate may be supplemented in D5 water)
Small bowel	Hypovolemia	LR
Colon (diarrhea)	Hypokalemic metabolic acidosis	D5NS with 20 mEq/l KCl

One practical approach to addressing abnormal fluid and electrolyte losses divides the types of loss into alterations in volume, concentration, composition and/or distribution.

Alterations in Volume

If isotonic fluid is added to or lost from body fluids, the volume of extracellular fluid is changed. Sudden loss of an isotonic fluid, such as an intestinal fluid, results in an acute decrease in extracellular fluid volume without changing intracellular fluid volume. As long as the osmolarity between the two compartments remains identical, no net movement of fluid from the intracellular to the extracellular space will occur.

In contrast, the sudden loss of circulating blood volume is different than the loss of an isotonic salt solution. Hemorrhage results in decreased cardiac output with the resultant total body ischemia, which cannot be corrected until blood volume is restored. In the absence of transfusion therapy, this correction requires movement of fluid and protein from the interstitium to the plasma, or "transcapillary plasma refill". Transcapillary refill is triggered initially by a fall in capillary hydrostatic pressure, resulting in the movement of protein-free fluid from the interstitium to the plasma space. A second phase involves the movement of protein into the plasma space in support of plasma oncotic pressure. This change restores plasma volume and protein concentration, but with a reduced oxygen carrying capacity due to the decrease in total red cell mass, i.e., a normovolemic anemia. Transcapillary refill can sustain a relatively fixed level of plasma volume, equal to about two-thirds of the initial plasma volume, irrespective of the rate of bleeding. Plasma refill reaches 33% by 30 min after hemorrhage and 50% by 3 h, allowing a fairly rapid restoration of circulating blood volume.

The diagnosis of an abnormal volume status is clinical. Hypovolemia, or volume deficit, is the most common fluid disorder in the surgical patient. Disorders resulting in a loss of isotonic fluid include vomiting, diarrhea, nasogastric suctioning, and gastrointestinal fistulae. Other causes include sequestration of fluids (third spacing) secondary to soft tissue injuries (e.g., trauma, postoperative) and infections, intra-abdominal and retroperitoneal inflammation, intestinal obstruction, and burns. Signs and symptoms of volume deficit include, but are not limited to, altered mental status, hypotension, tachycardia, decreased skin turgor, and hypothermia. Oliguria secondary to renal hypoperfusion is a common barometer of hypovolemia.

Hypervolemia, or volume *excess,* may be iatrogenic or secondary to cirrhosis, renal failure, or congestive heart failure. Both plasma and interstitial volumes are increased. Symptoms include ascites, pulmonary edema, and peripheral edema.

Alterations in Concentration

If water is added or lost from the extracellular space, the concentration of osmotically active particles will change. In contrast to the intracellular space, in the extracellular space, sodium represents 90% of the osmotically active particles. Therefore, selective changes in total body water are reflected by sodium concentration. A change in the concentration of osmotically active particles will necessitate the movement of water from one compartment to another to restore osmotic balance across membranes.

Hyponatremia (sodium < 130 mEq/l) is associated with free water excess. Symptoms of hyponatremia include central nervous system signs of increased intracranial pressure and tissue edema. It is important to recognize that severe hyponatremia may be associated with oliguric renal failure, which may not be reversible if therapy is delayed. In the surgical patient, acute hyponatremia usually reflects one of two iatrogenic errors. The first is infusion or ingestion of a large volume of free water at a time when high levels of ADH inhibit compensatory diuresis. This setting is most common early in the postoperative period when there may be a high level of ADH in response to pain and anxiety. The second setting occurs with the use of hypotonic fluids to replace isotonic fluid losses. In the trauma patient with a head injury, hyponatremia may herald the development of SIADH, or the "syndrome of inappropriate ADH" secretion. The need for therapy depends on the severity of associated symptoms. Free water restriction can return sodium concentrations toward normal; however, in selected patients, free water restriction is not adequate, and supplementation with salt-containing solutions (and on occasion with hypertonic (3%) sodium chloride) is necessary to return serum sodium levels to normal.

Hypernatremia (sodium > 145 mEq/l) results from excessive free water loss and can be extra-renal or renal in nature. Extra-renal free water loss results from an increase in metabolism from any cause, particularly fever. Evaporative water loss, either through open wounds or through the administration of un-humidified oxygen to hyperventilating patients (particularly those with a tracheostomy), can also result in dehydration and resultant hypernatremia. Hypernatremia can also result from increased renal water loss. High output renal failure due to ischemia/reperfusion damage to the distal tubules and collecting ducts impairs water resorption. Additionally, loss of the ability to release ADH from the central nervous system, such as occurs after some severe head injuries, can impair water resorption (diabetes insipidus). Finally high osmotic loads, due to the iatrogenic administration of mannitol, glycosuria from poorly controlled diabetes, or excess urea from high nitrogen diets, can result in an osmotically driven diuresis with subsequent free water loss.

Treatment of hypernatremia is directed toward restoring normal osmolality of body fluids, carefully and relatively slowly, because the central nervous system tolerates over-vigorous adjustments in sodium concentration poorly. The volume of free water needed to replace a patient's deficit should be calculated from the following formula and replaced over 2–3 days.

$$\text{Free water deficit} = (\text{total body water}) \times ([Na^+_{patient}]/[Na^+_{normal}]) - (\text{total body water})$$

Alterations in Composition

The concentration of most other ions in the extracellular space can change without affecting osmolarity. These changes represent alterations only in composition and do not cause fluid shifts. Of particular importance are concentration changes in potassium or in acid-base balance, via changes in hydrogen ions.

The normal intake of potassium per day is 50–100 mEq, and in the absence of hypokalemia, the majority of this intake is secreted in the urine. About 98% of the potassium in the body is located in the intracellular compartment, at concentrations of 150 mEq/l. Although the amount of extracellular potassium is relatively small, normal potassium concentrations are critical for myocardial and neuro-muscular function.

Hypokalemia (<3.5 mEq/l) is the most common electrolyte abnormalities in post-surgical patients, resulting from excessive renal secretion, movement of potassium intracellularly, prolonged administration of potassium-free intravenous solutions or nutrition with ongoing obligatory renal losses, and loss via increased gastrointestinal secretions, particularly colonic (i.e. diarrhea). Renal excretion of potassium is increased when large volumes of sodium ion are resorbed via the normal cation exchange mechanisms of the kidney. Potassium requirements after large isotonic volume replacement are increased, probably through the above mechanism. Additionally, potassium becomes very important in acid-base balance, as movement of potassium in or out of the cell occurs in response to changes in hydrogen ion concentration in the blood. Because alkalosis causes net movement of potassium out of cells, severe metabolic alkalosis may exacerbate hypokalemia, as the kidney will compensate for the alkalosis by increasing hydrogen ion resorption at the expense of potassium. Finally, excessive loss of gastrointestinal fluid can result in profound hypokalemia (see ❥ *Table 2-1*).

Symptoms of hypokalemia include muscle weakness, paralytic ileus, and, if severe, cardiac dysrhythmias. Treatment involves potassium replacement, although no more than 40 mEq/l of potassium may be added to intravenous fluids in the absence of electrocardiographic monitoring. Potassium replacement must be undertaken cautiously in patients with acute or chronic renal insufficiency.

Hyperkalemia (>5 mEq/l) is encountered rarely in patients with normal renal function. Most factors in surgical patients that affect potassium metabolism result in excess secretion of potassium and the tendency toward hypokalemia, except in the patient with abnormal renal function, where hyperkalemia can be a serious concern. Symptoms of hyperkalemia include nausea, vomiting, intestinal colic, and diarrhea. Electrocardiographic abnormalities of mild to moderate hyperkalemia include peaked T-waves. Cardiac dysrhythmias occur at concentrations >7 mEq/l and include atrial asystole, with subsequent ventricular tachycardia and/or fibrillation. Temporary suppression of myocardial irritation related to hyperkalemia can be accomplished with the administration of 1 g of 10% calcium gluconate intravenously, and/or by the concomitant administration of glucose and insulin (50 g glucose with 10 units insulin intravenously), which drives potassium intracellularly. Definitive treatment involves cation exchange resins (Kayexalate) or hemodialysis to remove potassium from the patient.

Acid-base balance: The pH of normal body fluids is maintained within a narrow range of 7.37–7.42, which is necessary to maintain normal body functions. This regulation of pH occurs despite a large daily production of both organic and inorganic acids by normal metabolism. Three mechanisms regulate acid-base metabolism: rapid buffering of acids by salts of weak acids (the bicarbonate buffer system), rapid elimination of acids via the lungs (expired CO_2), and slow elimination of acids by the kidneys (renal compensation).

The pH of the extracellular space is a function of the ratio of bicarbonate salt (HCO_3^-) to carbonic acid (H_2CO_3, which in turn is related to the pCO_2). In simple terms, a ratio of 20:1 between bicarbonate and H_2CO_3 will result in a normal pH via an efficient system of buffering. In metabolic acidosis, the concentration of bicarbonate decreases, resulting in a relative excess of carbonic acid. Respiration then rapidly increases, eliminating larger amounts of carbonic acid as water and CO_2, attempting to return the ratio to 20:1. The reverse occurs in a metabolic alkalosis. In contrast, respiratory acidosis and alkalosis are produced by disturbances in ventilation, resulting in a change in pH from normal values of 0.08 for each 10 mmHg change in pCO_2. Compensation is primary renal, but this compensation is relatively slow. In respiratory acidosis (pCO_2 >45 mmHg), chronic renal compensation results in a 3.5 mEq increase in HCO_3^- for each 10 mmHg increase in pCO_2, but can take up to 72 h to occur fully. Similarly, in respiratory alkalosis (pCO_2 < 35 mmHg), renal compensation yields a 5 mEq decrease in HCO_3^- for each 10 mmHg decrease in pCO_2. Common abnormalities of acid-base metabolism in the surgical patient and their causes are shown in ❥ *Table 2-5*.

Alterations in Distribution

In the surgical patient, the decrease in circulating volume due to "third space" losses is of particular importance. Third space loss refers to fluid that extravasates into a compartment other than the

■ Table 2-5
Common abnormalities of acid-base metabolism

Acid-base disorder	Defect	Common cause	Serum bicarbonate concentration	Physiologic compensatory mechanism
Metabolic acidosis	Acid gain or base loss	Lactate, diabetes, diarrhea, fistulae, azotemia	Decreased	Pulmonary (rapid)
Metabolic alkalosis	Base gain or acid loss	Vomiting, NG suction, diuretics	Increased	Pulmonary (rapid)
Respiratory acidosis	CO_2 retention (hypoventilation)	Sedation, COPD	Decreased	Renal (slow)
Respiratory alkalosis	Excessive CO_2 loss (hyperventilation)	Pain, agitation, mechanical ventilation	Increased	Renal (slow)

intracellular or extracellular compartments. Classically, third spacing occurs only with massive ascites, burns, bowel obstruction, peritonitis, and crush injuries. Inflammatory conditions of the abdomen and retroperitoneum, including pancreatitis, also result in significant intraperitoneal fluid and bowel wall edema. The magnitude of fluid loss from these conditions can be difficult to appreciate without the realization that the peritoneum alone has a 1 m^2 surface area, such that a slight increase in thickness due to edema and peritonitis will result in a functional loss of several liters of fluid. Similar large volume losses can occur with severe infections of the soft tissue, such as necrotizing fasciitis, with burn wounds, and with severe crush injuries. Finally, sepsis or SIRS can cause a diffuse capillary leak, with a resultant loss of large volumes of intravascular fluids into the interstitium. In all cases, volume resuscitation is the therapy of choice to restore intravascular volume.

Fluid Replacement Therapy

In surgical patients, fluids are used for either maintenance or resuscitation. Because each has a different goal, the composition of and approach to administration of fluids for maintenance or resuscitation are different fundamentally. Maintenance fluids supply the ongoing fluid and electrolyte requirements of the patient. Resuscitative fluids administered to patients in hypovolemic shock should replace existing fluid deficits, as well as ongoing abnormal fluid losses. Initial resuscitative fluids should be isotonic crystalloid solutions, such as normal saline and/or lactated Ringers, administered in bolus form, starting with approximately 30 ml/kg or 2,000 ml in an average-sized adult or 20 ml/kg in a child.

Hypovolemia, or the loss of intravascular volume, results in inadequate perfusion to the tissues of the body, with the resultant inability to supply metabolic demands and remove metabolic wastes. The primary goal of resuscitation, therefore, is to restore normal tissue perfusion rapidly through volume expansion. During resuscitation, administration of fluids containing glucose will result in hyperglycemia, with a resultant osmotic diuresis; because urine output is a measure of adequacy of visceral perfusion, such an osmotic diuresis might be viewed incorrectly as adequate resuscitation, thereby prolonging the shock period. Therefore, glucose-containing fluids should be avoided in the acute resuscitation of the hypovolemic patient.

Lactated Ringers (LR) solution is isotonic, readily available, inexpensive, and does not aggravate pre-existing electrolyte abnormalities. LR administration does not worsen the lactic acidosis normally present in shock. As volume is restored, lactate is mobilized to the liver and metabolized to bicarbonate, leading to a mild metabolic alkalosis 1–2 days after massive resuscitation with LR. In addition, mild to moderate hyponatremia may also occur, because LR has only 130 mEq/l of sodium. Normal saline (NS) is also an effective resuscitation fluid, particularly in patients with head trauma in whom hyponatremia must be avoided. Hypernatremic, hyperchloremic metabolic acidosis is possible after massive resuscitation with NS, particularly in children and in patients with large burns or severe trauma. Resuscitation with hypotonic fluids should be avoided because these fluids dilute the intravascular space and result in an osmotic pressure gradient with a higher osmotic pressure in the interstitial space, drawing water into the interstitium, and the goal of intravascular volume restoration will not be accomplished.

Inadequate restoration of circulating volume can lead to a cascade of related complications, including persistent acidosis, SIRS, MODS, multi-system organ failure, and eventual death. Traditionally, endpoints of resuscitation have been normalization of hemodynamic parameters, restoration of adequate urine output (0.5 ml/kg/h), and return of normal mental status; however, with the understanding that hypoperfusion can exist with normotension, better markers of tissue perfusion have been sought. Monitoring and optimizing oxygen delivery and mixed venous oxygen saturation via use of pulmonary artery catheters will improve outcome after major surgical procedures. Rapid correction of metabolic acidosis with normalization of base deficits after resuscitation from trauma has also improved survival. The adequacy of resuscitation can also be assessed and survival improved by the correction of abnormalities in gastric intramucosal pH (pHi) measured by gastric tonometry. Finally, a renewed interest has developed in the use of non-invasive near infrared absorption spectroscopy in the trauma patient to assess tissue oxygenation (a marker of oxygen transport) at the end-organ level. Although the ideal marker of adequate resuscitation remains elusive, better techniques to monitor specific end-organ perfusion in the future will allow better optimization of resuscitative efforts.

Selected Readings

Drucker WR, Chadwick CDJ, Gann DS (1981) Transcapillary refill in hemorrhage and shock. Arch Surg 116:1344–1353

Elliot DC (1998) An evaluation of endpoints of resuscitation. J Am Coll Surg 187:536–547

Henry S, Scalea TM (1999) Resuscitation in the new millennium. Surg Clin North Am 79(6):1259–1267

Maynard N, Bihari D, Beale R, et al. (1993) Assessment of splanchnic oxygenation by gastric tonometry in patients with acute circulatory failure. JAMA 270:1203–1210

Porter JM, Ivatury RR (1998) In search of the optimal end points of resuscitation in trauma patients: a review. J Trauma 44:908–914

Shoemaker WC, Kram HB, Appel PL (1990) Therapy of shock based on pathophysiology, monitoring and outcome prediction. Crit Care Med 18:S19–S25

3 Nutritional Support in the Surgical Patient

Richard J. E. Skipworth · Kenneth C. H. Fearon

Pearls and Pitfalls

- Manage well-nourished elective patients according to "stress-free" Enhanced Recovery After Surgery (ERAS) principles with optimal pain relief, pro-active management of gut function and early mobilization.
- Allow oral fluids until 2 h prior to operation to decrease dehydration, and consider routine pre-operative oral carbohydrate and fluid loading to promote post-operative anabolism.
- Employ thoracic epidural anesthesia to reduce sympathetic activation, prevent paralytic ileus, control pain on movement, and promote mobilization.
- Recommence feeding early in the post-operative period. If voluntary nutritional intake is inadequate, supplement with artificial nutritional support.
- Use enteral nutrition in preference to parenteral nutrition in patients with functioning gastrointestinal (GI) tracts.
- Commence early oral/enteral nutritional support in all malnourished surgical patients to reduce the effects of the stress response and prevent post-operative complications.
- Modern perioperative care means that even if the patient is *moderately* malnourished, pre-operative nutritional support is likely to be of limited benefit. Instead, proceed with surgery and plan for adequate *post-operative* and *post-discharge* nutritional support.
- In patients who are *severely* malnourished, it is often prudent to review the appropriateness of surgical intervention.
- Consider carefully the likely clinical course of a post-operative patient who develops complications. If likely total downtime of gut function from time of surgery is > 5–7 days, always institute artificial nutritional support (especially if the patient has pre-existing malnutrition).

Introduction

Patients undergoing major surgery are at high risk of malnutrition due to the combination of perioperative starvation and activation of both the immune system and the neuroendocrine stress response. Starvation reduces the anabolic substrate available to the patient, whereas the immune/stress response induces whole-body catabolism. In particular, the stress response to surgery and trauma is associated with a significant increase in metabolic rate, glucose and fatty acid utilization, gluconeogenesis, and skeletal muscle protein degradation. These factors all contribute to the depletion of protein, lipid and carbohydrate stores and deterioration in nutritional status. In turn, poor nutritional status is linked with adverse outcome via the effects of tissue wasting and impaired organ function. Loss of power and the increased fatigability of wasted skeletal muscle delays mobilization and affects respiratory and cardiac function, whereas impaired immune function confers increased susceptibility to infection. Thus, malnourished surgical patients are at increased risk of cardiorespiratory embarrassment, chest and wound infections, prolonged hospitalization and death.

Maintenance/optimization of nutritional status is an integral component of standard surgical and trauma care. Nutritional supplementation for surgical patients, if administered appropriately, can be shown to enhance outcome and improve patient quality of life in a cost-effective manner. However, nutritional care should not simply be viewed as the provision of perioperative or post-injury feeding. Rather, it should be seen as a global strategy of metabolic control, nutritional support and early mobilization, the aim of which is to maximize the rate of recovery and the final nutritional/functional status of the patient.

This chapter will review the basic physiology underlying the metabolic stress response to injury, and detail the clinical administration of artificial nutritional support. In particular, this chapter will describe the guidelines by which surgeons should manage patients of varying pathology and nutritional status. In this way, the reader can develop a strategic understanding of what aspects of clinical care are important, and acquire the appropriate knowledge to manage them.

The Metabolic Stress Response to Surgery and Trauma: The "Ebb and Flow" Model

Any bodily injury, be it operative or accidental, is not only associated with local effects, but is also accompanied by a systemic metabolic response. The main features of this metabolic response are initiated by the immune system, cardiovascular system, sympathetic nervous system, ascending reticular formation and limbic system. However, the metabolic stress response may be further exacerbated by anesthesia, dehydration, starvation (including pre-operative fasting), sepsis, acute medical illness, or even severe psychological stress, and thus any attempt to limit or control these other factors is beneficial to the patient.

In 1930, Sir David Cuthbertson divided the metabolic response to injury into "*ebb*" and "*flow*" phases (❷ *Fig. 3-1*). The ebb phase begins at the time of injury, and lasts for approximately 24–48 h. It may be attenuated by proper resuscitation, but not completely abolished. The ebb phase is

◘ Figure 3-1
Phases of the metabolic stress response to injury (After Cuthbertson)

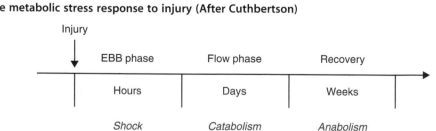

characterized by hypovolemia, decreased basal metabolic rate, reduced cardiac output, hypothermia, and lactic acidosis. The predominant hormones regulating the ebb phase are catecholamines, cortisol and aldosterone (following activation of the renin-angiotensin system). The magnitude of this neuro endocrine response depends on the degree of blood loss and the stimulation of somatic afferent nerves at the site of injury. The main physiological role of the ebb phase is to conserve both circulating volume and energy stores for recovery and repair.

Following resuscitation, the ebb phase evolves into a hypermetabolic flow phase. This phase involves the mobilization of body energy stores for recovery and repair, and the subsequent replacement of lost or damaged tissue. It is characterized by increased basal metabolic rate (hypermetabolism), increased cardiac output, raised body temperature, increased oxygen consumption, and increased gluconeogenesis. The flow phase may be subdivided into an initial catabolic phase, lasting approximately 3–10 days, followed by an anabolic phase, which may last for weeks if extensive recovery and repair are required following serious injury. During the catabolic phase, the increased production of counter-regulatory hormones (including catecholamines, cortisol, insulin and glucagon) and inflammatory cytokines (e.g. interleukin [IL]-1, IL-6 and tumor necrosis factor [TNF]-α) result in significant fat and protein mobilization, leading to significant weight loss and increased urinary nitrogen excretion (❷ *Fig. 3-2*). The increased production of insulin at this time is associated with

❏ Figure 3-2
Key initiators and mechanisms resulting in patient catabolism during the flow phase of the metabolic stress response

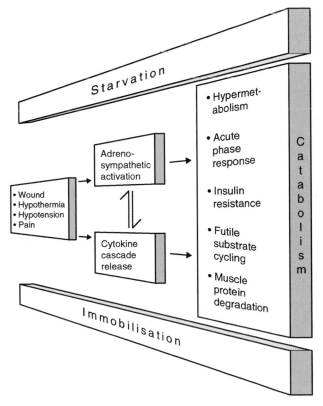

significant *insulin resistance* and therefore injured patients often exhibit poor glycemic control. The combination of pronounced or prolonged catabolism, in association with insulin resistance, places patients within this phase at increased risk of complications, particularly infectious and cardiovascular. Obviously the development of complications will further aggravate the neuroendocrine and inflammatory stress responses, thus creating a vicious catabolic cycle.

Key Catabolic Elements of the Flow Phase of the Metabolic Stress Response

There are several key elements of the flow phase which determine largely the extent of catabolism and thus govern the nutritional requirements of the surgical patient (❯ *Fig. 3-2*).

Hypermetabolism

The majority of trauma patients (except possibly those with extensive burns) demonstrate energy expenditures approximately 15–25% above predicted healthy resting values (i.e. 1,500–2,500 kcal/day). The predominant cause appears to be a complex interaction between the central control of metabolic rate and peripheral energy utilization. In particular, central thermodysregulation (caused by the pro-inflammatory cytokine cascade); increased sympathetic activity; abnormalities in wound circulation (ischemic areas produce lactate which must be metabolized by the ATP-consuming hepatic Cori cycle; hyperemic areas cause an increase in cardiac output); increased protein turnover; and nutritional support may all increase patient energy expenditure. Theoretically, patient energy expenditure could rise even higher than observed levels following surgery or trauma, but several features of standard intensive care (including bed rest, paralysis, ventilation and external temperature regulation) counteract the hypermetabolic driving forces of the stress response. Furthermore, the skeletal muscle wasting experienced by patients with prolonged catabolism actually limits the volume of metabolically active tissue.

Alterations in Skeletal Muscle Protein Metabolism

Muscle protein is continually synthesized and broken down each day, with an average turnover rate in humans of 1–2%, and with a greater amplitude of changes in protein synthesis (±twofold) than breakdown (±0.25-fold) during the diurnal cycle. Under normal circumstances, synthesis equals breakdown and muscle bulk remains constant. Physiological stimuli that promote net muscle protein accretion include feeding (especially extracellular amino acid concentration) and exercise. Paradoxically, during exercise, skeletal muscle protein synthesis is depressed, but increases again during rest and feeding.

During the catabolic phase of the stress response, muscle wasting occurs due to an increase in muscle protein degradation (via enzymatic pathways), coupled with a decrease in muscle protein synthesis. The major site of protein loss is peripheral skeletal muscle, although nitrogen losses do also occur in the respiratory muscles (predisposing the patient to hypoventilation and chest infections) and in the gut (reducing gut motility). Cardiac muscle appears to be mostly spared. Under extreme conditions of catabolism (e.g. major sepsis), urinary nitrogen losses can reach 20 g per day; this is equivalent to *600–700 g loss of skeletal muscle per day*.

The predominant mechanism involved in the wasting of skeletal muscle is the ATP-dependent ubiquitin proteasome pathway, although the lysosomal cathepsins and the calcium-calpain pathway play facilitatory and accessory roles.

Clinically, a patient with skeletal muscle wasting will experience asthenia, increased fatigue, reduced functional ability, decreased quality of life, and an increased risk of morbidity and mortality. In critically ill patients, muscle weakness may be further worsened by the development of critical illness myopathy, a multi-factorial condition that is associated with impaired excitation-contraction-coupling at the level of the sarcolemma and the sarcoplasmic reticulum membrane.

Alterations in Hepatic Protein Metabolism: The Acute Phase Protein Response (APPR)

In response to inflammatory conditions, including surgery, trauma, sepsis, cancer or autoimmune conditions, circulating peripheral blood mononuclear cells secrete a range of pro-inflammatory cytokines, including IL-1, IL-6, and tumor necrosis factor (TNF)-α. These cytokines, in particular IL-6, promote the hepatic synthesis of positive acute phase proteins, e.g. fibrinogen and C-reactive protein (CRP). The APPR represents a "double edged sword" for surgical patients as it provides proteins important for recovery and repair, but only at the expense of valuable lean tissue and energy reserves.

In contrast to the positive acute phase reactants, the plasma concentrations of other liver export proteins such as albumin (the negative acute phase reactants) fall acutely following injury. However, rather than represent a reduced hepatic synthesis rate, the fall in plasma concentration of negative acute phase reactants is thought, principally, to reflect increased transcapillary escape, secondary to an increase in micro-vascular permeability. Thus, increased hepatic synthesis of positive acute phase reactants is not compensated for by reduced synthesis of negative reactants.

Insulin Resistance

Following surgery or trauma, post-operative hyperglycemia develops as a result of increased glucose production combined with decreased glucose uptake in peripheral tissues. Decreased glucose uptake is a result of insulin resistance that is transiently induced within the stressed patient. Suggested mechanisms for this phenomenon include the action of pro-inflammatory cytokines, and the decreased responsiveness of insulin-regulated glucose transporter proteins. The degree of insulin resistance is proportional to the magnitude of the injurious process. Following routine upper abdominal surgery, insulin resistance may persist for approximately 2 weeks.

Post-operative patients with insulin resistance behave in a similar manner to individuals with Type II diabetes mellitus, and are at increased risk of sepsis, deteriorating renal function, polyneuropathy, and death.

The mainstay management of insulin resistance is intravenous insulin infusion. Insulin infusions may be used in either an *intensive* approach (i.e. sliding scales are manipulated to *normalize* the blood glucose level) or a *conservative* approach (i.e. insulin is administered when the blood glucose level exceeds a defined limit and discontinued when the level falls). Studies of post-operatively ventilated patients in the intensive care unit (ICU) have suggested that maintenance of normal glucose levels using intensive insulin therapy can significantly reduce both morbidity and mortality (Fearon and Luff, 2003). Furthermore, intensive insulin therapy is superior to conservative insulin approaches in reducing morbidity rates. However, the mortality benefit of intensive insulin therapy over a more conservative approach has not been proven conclusively. The observed benefits of insulin therapy are probably simply as a result of maintenance of normoglycemia, but the glycemia-independent actions of insulin may also exert minor, organ-specific effects (e.g. promotion of myocardial systolic function).

The Identification of Patients at Increased Risk of Nutritional Depletion

Ideally, all surgical patients should receive pre-operative nutritional screening. However, formal screening is not performed commonly in clinical practice. A recent study has suggested that only 33% of UK centers performing upper GI cancer resections perform routine pre-operative nutritional screening by dietetic staff (Murphy et al., 2006). However, in the same study, 75% of centers stated that they would commence routinely pre-operative nutritional support if a patient was found to be malnourished on admission. It therefore seems vital that medical staff encourage and are capable of performing basic nutritional assessment, and are also able to identify risk factors that predispose the surgical patient to an increased risk (❷ *Table 3-1*).

Simple and inexpensive measures of nutritional status that indicate patients are at increased risk include body weight loss >10%, body mass index (BMI) <18 kg/m², and the well-recognized, but non-specific risk index of significant hypoalbuminemia (<30 g/l).

An alternative method of assessment is to measure functional status and thus make an indirect judgment regarding nutritional status. Subjective assessment of functional status is usually performed using a score of performance status (PS), e.g. Karnofsky performance score (KPS) or the World Health Organisation (WHO) score. These are the most robust treatment risk indices in medical oncology and are easily applied in the pre-operative surgical setting. Objective techniques of functional status assessment involve direct measurements of mobility or muscle power (e.g. hand-grip dynamometry, which is a highly accurate prognostic indicator in surgical patients).

Malnutrition scoring systems are available (e.g. prognostic inflammatory nutritional index [PINI], mini-nutritional assessment [MNA]), but they are not readily used in clinical practice. Furthermore, a variety of strategies have been suggested for screening patients for malnutrition in the community, but it is not clear whether their implementation reduces morbidity or mortality.

◻ **Table 3-1**

Risk factors associated with nutritional depletion

- Old age
- Physical inactivity
- Cancer
- Upper gastrointestinal surgery
- Ongoing sepsis
- Impaired oral intake

The Aim of Nutritional Support in the Surgical Patient

For well-nourished patients, the primary objective of post-operative care is the restoration of normal GI function to allow adequate food intake and rapid recovery. This objective should be carried out within the context of an "enhanced recovery after surgery (ERAS)" protocol or "fast track" surgery program. Within these multimodal codes of surgical practice, strategies are taken to minimize the surgical stress response and to avoid traditional principles of surgical care which have been shown to have no benefit, or are actually detrimental, to the rapid recovery of the patient (❍ *Fig. 3-3*). In particular, strict attention is paid to pain control, early mobilization and the promotion of GI function (❍ *Table 3-2*). Furthermore, the patient is well-counseled and encouraged to take an active role in their own post-operative recovery. To date, most ERAS programs have targeted patients undergoing GI (primarily colon) surgery, and have shown that the implementation of modern "stress-fee" surgical practice can minimize deterioration in physiological function and reduce time to hospital discharge. Indeed, use of an epidural (which allows for dynamic pain control, early mobilization, reduction of post-operative ileus, and blockade of the neuroendocrine stress response) combined with early enteral feeding can result in elective abdominal surgery where the patient remains in positive nitrogen balance with no net losses.

In at-risk malnourished patients, the aim of perioperative nutritional support is to avoid the post-operative complications and increased mortality which are associated with malnutrition (❍ *Fig. 3-4*). In these individuals, evidence suggests that artificial nutritional support can reduce the length of stay, decrease morbidity, improve quality of life, and consequently limit the cost of health care resources. However, to achieve these goals, one must know when (and how) to administer the relevant nutritional support. In contrast with surgical practice in the 1970s and 1980s, modern "stress-free"

◨ Figure 3-3
Key elements of the Enhanced Recovery After Surgery (ERAS) protocol. CHO = carbohydrate; NSAIDs = non-steroidal anti-inflammatory drugs

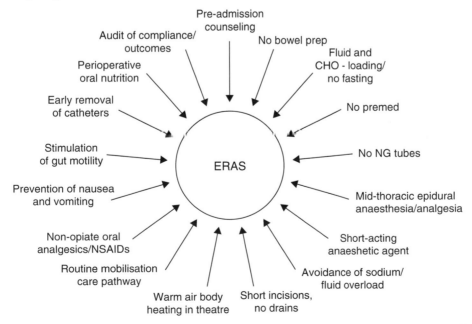

■ Table 3-2

Main objectives of the Enhanced Recovery After Surgery (ERAS) protocol

- Optimize pain relief
- Optimize gut function
- Early mobilization

■ Figure 3-4

Effects of weight loss on patient outcome

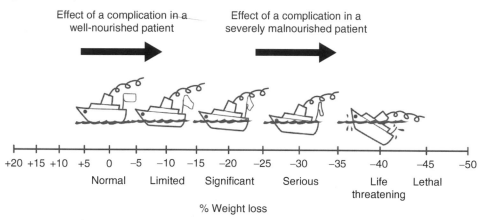

% Weight loss

anesthesia/perioperative care means that from a strategic viewpoint, even if the patient is *moderately* malnourished, *pre-operative* nutritional support is of limited benefit. Instead, the best management is to proceed with surgery, and once the primary pathology has been dealt with, provide the patient with aggressive *post-operative* nutritional support.

In patients who are *severely* malnourished, it is often prudent to review operative strategy and consider in benign disease whether there are any medical options that could be followed. In severely malnourished patients with malignant disease, consideration should be given to whether the patient has been understaged and if resectional surgery is really the appropriate path to follow (e.g. consider downstaging or stenting).

Nutritional Management of Well-Nourished and Malnourished Surgical Patients

The Well-Nourished Surgical Patient

Patients should be managed within the context of an ERAS protocol, with an emphasis on dynamic pain relief, early mobilization and the restoration of normal GI function. As well as adhering to the principles of "stress-free" surgery, it is important for the surgeon to have a global strategy to maintain patients' food intake. Key issues are shown in (❷ *Fig. 3-3*) and include:

- *Avoid routine placement of nasogastric decompression tubes.* Nasogastric tubes are of no proven benefit and prevent restoration of normal food intake.

- *Avoid routine use of bowel preparation except in special circumstances* (e.g. low anterior resection with covering loop ileostomy). If bowel preparation is used, provide the patient with simultaneous low residue oral nutritional supplements.
- *Provide oral fluids up to 2 h prior to operation and consider routine use of oral carbohydrate and fluid loading.* The latter has been proven to reduce post-operative insulin resistance and thus allows the patient to respond to nutritional support more effectively.
- *Use strategies to reduce post-operative ileus.* Routine use of a thoracic epidural blocks reflex sympathetic inhibition of small bowel mobility and is proven to improve gut function post-operatively.
- *Avoid excessive administration of intravenous saline in the intra-operative and post-operative period.* Intravenous saline is proven to cause gut edema, delayed gastric emptying, and worsened patient outcome. Start the patient on oral fluids on the first post-operative day and discontinue the intravenous infusion.
- *Feed the patient early in the post-operative period.* Many surgeons believe that oral feeding cannot be commenced until bowel movements have begun. Furthermore, many others believe that early feeding is associated with increased risks of anastomotic leakage. Neither of these perceptions has been proven on clinical studies. A meta-analysis of controlled trials of early enteral feeding versus nil by mouth after GI surgery concluded that there is no clear advantage to keeping patients nil by mouth after elective GI resection. Early feeding reduced both the risk of any type of infection and the mean length of stay in hospital. However, the risk of vomiting did increase in patients fed early. Therefore, post-operative feeding should be commenced early with prescription of adequate anti-emetics if required.

The provision of appetizing hospital food and access to sufficient nursing staff to help patients who have difficulty in eating is a key issue in helping patients return to a normal food intake. For patients with an anastomosis in the upper GI tract, ingestion of solid food may have to be delayed for several days (e.g. until contrast studies confirm an intact esophageal anastomosis). In the intervening period, patients can be given post-operative enteral feeding either via a jejunostomy or fine-bore nasoenteral feeding tube. This allows maintenance of nutritional status should the patient develop a post-operative complication that retards normal progression towards oral nutrition (e.g. an anastomotic leak). Upper GI cancer patients are often managed in this way. Following colorectal operations where the GI tract remains functional, solid food can be commenced without adverse effect on the first post-operative day. However, patients may find liquid supplements easier to take in the first instance. Generally, if oral nutrition is not re-established within 5–7 days post-operatively, enteral or parenteral feeding should be considered.

Post-operative energy and protein requirements depend on body composition, clinical status and mobility. However, an estimation of requirements is 30 kcal/kg/day and 1 g protein/kg/day for the average patient. Few patients require more than 2,200 kcal/day. Additional calories are unlikely to be used effectively and may constitute a metabolic stress.

The Moderately/Severely Malnourished Surgical Patient

Studies suggest that approximately 20–40% of surgical patients may already be malnourished on admission to hospital. Following surgery, these patients have a higher risk of complications, prolonged hospital stay, delayed recovery, and ultimately, increased mortality. The key issue in managing severely malnourished patients is that plans must always be in place to progress their nutritional status back up towards normality. If severely malnourished patients develop complications which inhibit nutritional support (e.g. abdominal sepsis from an anastomotic leak), their nutritional/metabolic problems can suddenly become major determinants of outcome (see ❯ *Fig. 3-4*).

Moderate or severely malnourished patients (e.g. weight loss >15%, BMI <18 kg/m², albumin <30g/l) should be identified by pre-operative nutritional screening and should then be referred to the unit dietician or dedicated nutrition team for consideration of not only perioperative, but also post-discharge, artificial nutritional support. This is because patients who are malnourished at the time of GI surgery can demonstrate evidence of deteriorating nutritional status for up to 2 months or more following hospital discharge. In these patients, the provision of nutritional advice and routine oral nutritional supplements (ONS) in the immediate post-operative period and ensuing 2 months has been shown to promote a more rapid recovery of nutritional status, physical function and quality of life. In contrast, the evidence supporting the short term routine use of ONS in patients who have a normal nutritional status is not clear.

Some patients may not tolerate an adequate intake of ONS in the post-operative period. Therefore, placement of a feeding jejunostomy at the time of surgery in malnourished patients at risk of complications is always a good pre-emptive maneuver. A non-functioning GI tract is an early indication to use total parenteral nutrition (TPN), in order to provide bedrock for progress and the gradual introduction of enteral feeding. Once enteral feeding is well tolerated, TPN can be withdrawn.

Despite the evident benefits of *post-operative* nutritional support, there is no clear proof that malnourished patients requiring surgery (e.g. Crohn's disease) benefit from prolonged *pre-operative* artificial nutritional support. Such patients are best treated by surgical correction of their pathology followed by intensive nutritional support in the post-operative period. In patients who are *severely* malnourished, it is often wise to reassess the necessity and appropriateness of surgery and consider any non-operative medical or palliative options.

Strategies for the nutritional management of well-nourished, moderately malnourished and severely malnourished patients in the post-operative period are summarized in ❯ *Fig. 3-5*.

The Surgical Patient with Post-Operative Complications

Surgery will induce a catabolic state within the patient, placing that individual at increased risk of complications. The development of post-operative complications will prolong or re-initiate the neuroendocrine and inflammatory stress responses, thus creating a vicious catabolic cycle, and elevating significantly protein and energy requirements. It is therefore vital that these patients receive adequate nutritional support.

The Practicalities of Artificial Nutritional Support

Although artificial nutritional support can be of undoubted benefit, it can also be associated with major complications. Therefore, nutritional support should be monitored closely and regularly (❯ *Table 3-3*). The measurements and frequency of monitoring depend on the individual patient, the

◘ Figure 3-5
Strategies for the nutritional management of well-nourished, moderately malnourished and severely malnourished patients in the post-operative period. ERAS = Enhanced Recovery After Surgery; EN = enteral nutrition; TPN = total parenteral nutrition

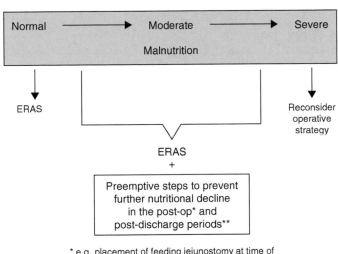

◘ Table 3-3
Methods to monitor surgical patients who are receiving artificial nutritional support

Status	Test	Frequency
Biochemistry	Electrolytes	Twice weekly
	Urea	
	Blood glucose	
	Liver function tests	
	Urinalysis	
Fluid balance	Fluid charts	Daily
	Weight	Once weekly
Nutritional status	Weight	Once weekly
	Nitrogen balance	
Nutritional intake	Nursing records	Daily
	Food and fluid charts	

route and the stage of feeding. Daily monitoring should be carried out in unstable patients or patients who have recently started nutritional support. A co-ordinated multidisciplinary team approach can reduce the incidence of complications and improve patients' overall quality of life. The choice of which form of support is appropriate to the individual patient will depend on patient disease status and the perceived risk of associated complications.

Oral Nutritional Supplements (ONS)

Provision of post-operative ONS containing 1.5 kcal/ml and 0.06 g/ml of protein have been shown to improve nutritional status, quality of life, and morbidity rate in malnourished patients undergoing GI surgery.

Enteral Nutrition (EN)

EN uses the physiological route of nutrient intake, is cheaper and generally safer, and should be the preferred method of nutritional support in the presence of a functioning GI tract. Most surgical patients can tolerate a standard whole protein feed (1 kcal/ml). A peptide or elemental formula can be considered in patients with significant malabsorption. Patients are generally commenced on 30–50 ml/h, increasing within 24–48 h as gastric aspirates fall and tolerance improves, until prescribed targets are reached.

If supplementation of an inadequate oral intake is required, then overnight feeding for 8–12 h may be sufficient and allows the patient to be mobile during the day. A pump should be used to control the rate of feed delivery, avoiding the abdominal cramps and bloating associated with bolus feeding.

EN can be administered via several different routes:

Nasogastric Feeding: The most appropriate route of enteral tube feeding for patients who require short-term support (e.g. less than 4 weeks) is via a fine-bore nasogastric (NG) tube.

Gastrostomy: Gastrostomy (endoscopic, radiological or surgical) should be reserved for mid- to long-term feeding. It is more comfortable than NG feeding and has a lower risk of tube misplacement or blockage. Major indications include neurological disorders and head and neck cancer. Contra-indications include sepsis, ascites and clotting disorders.

Jejunostomy: Tubes may be placed surgically or endoscopically. The most common indication is following major upper GI surgery. The jejunostomy is sited at the time of surgery and can be used for feeding within 12 h of surgery.

Parenteral Nutrition

Peripheral intravenous feeding (e.g. via a cannula) should only be used in the short-term. Central venous feeding, via either a peripherally-inserted central catheter (PICC line) or a catheter in a central vein, is the preferred route. A dedicated central venous feeding line minimizes infective complications. However, in suitable circumstances a triple lumen central line inserted under aseptic conditions and with a dedicated port for TPN can be used. Following insertion of a central venous line into the internal jugular or subclavian veins, a chest x-ray must be taken to exclude a pneumothorax and confirm the position of the catheter tip at or near the junction of the superior vena cava with the right atrium. Furthermore, care should be taken during line insertion to exclude arterial puncture and the risk of bleeding.

Mixtures of nutrients are usually combined in a single bag. Many pharmacies now use three or four standard regimens. The solutions contain fixed amounts of energy and nitrogen, and typically provide 1,800–2,400 kcals (50% glucose, 50% lipid) and 10–14 g nitrogen. The amount of electrolytes, vitamins and trace elements can be varied. In general, standard regimens are simpler, safer and cheaper than those prepared individually. However, nutritional requirements should always be determined in consultation with a dietician.

Historically, TPN has been associated with an increased risk of patient infection. These infections may have been the result of infected intravenous access, or a result of carbohydrate overloading and subsequent hyperglycemia. However, in many of these studies, the TPN solutions in question lacked glutamine. The subsequent addition of glutamine or glutamine dipeptides to standard TPN in order to enhance immune function has the potential to improve outcome.

TPN is of benefit in the treatment of severely malnourished patients and post-operative patients with GI complications. However, the routine use of post operative TPN is not beneficial in patients capable of eating within 5–7 days of an operation.

Daily biochemical monitoring must be undertaken when initially re-feeding the chronically severely malnourished patient because of the dangers of hypocalcemia and hypophosphatemia.

Immunonutrition

Feeds which contain immune-enhancing agents (e.g. arginine, branched chain amino acids, omega-3 fatty acids, dietary nucleotides) may be given pre-operatively and/or post-operatively. It has been suggested that these compound feeds may be particularly advantageous in the management of patients with cancer and multiple injuries, but evidence for both efficacy and cost-effectiveness is currently unclear. A meta-analysis has demonstrated that EN supplemented with immunomodulatory nutrients results in significant reduction in the risk of developing infectious complications but has no effect on mortality. Furthermore, other studies have suggested that some immunomodulatory formations are associated with an increased risk of mortality in critically ill patients.

Conclusion

Nutritional support should be considered as a global strategy of reducing nutritional depletion and maximizing patient recovery. The correct use of nutritional support can inhibit the deleterious effects of the metabolic stress response on patient nutrition; can accelerate recovery in elective surgical patients; and can be life-saving in malnourished patients, especially those who develop post-operative major complications. Further studies are required to optimize both the composition of current feeds and their application.

Selected Readings

Beattie AH, Prach AT, Baxter JP, Pennington CR (2000) A randomised controlled trial evaluating the use of enteral nutritional supplements postoperatively in malnourished surgical patients. Gut 46:813–818

Fearon KC, Luff R (2003) The nutritional management of surgical patients: enhanced recovery after surgery. Proc Nutr Soc 62:807–811

Fearon KC, Ljungqvist Von O, Meyenfeldt M, et al. (2005) Enhanced recovery after surgery: a consensus review of clinical care for patients undergoing colonic resection. Clin Nutr 24:466–477

Ljungqvist O, Fearon KC, Little RA (2005) Nutrition in surgery and trauma. In: Gibney MJ, Marinos E, Ljungqvist O, Dowsett J (eds) Clinical nutrition. Blackwell Science, Oxford, pp. 312–324

Murphy PM, Modi P, Rahamim J, et al. (2006) An investigation into the current perioperative nutritional management of oesophageal carcinoma patients in major carcinoma centers in England. Ann R Coll Surg Engl 88:358–362

Nygren J, Hausel J, Kehlet H, et al. (2005) A comparison in five European Centres of case mix, clinical management and outcomes following either conventional or fast-track perioperative care in colorectal surgery. Clin Nutr 24:455–461

O'Riordain MG, Falconer JS, Maingay J, et al. (1999) Peripheral blood cells from weight-losing cancer patients control the hepatic acute phase response by a primarily interleukin-6 dependent mechanism. Int J Oncol 15:823–827

O'Riordain MG, Fearon KC, Ross JA, et al. (1994) Glutamine-supplemented total parenteral nutrition enhances T-lymphocyte response in surgical patients undergoing colorectal resection. Ann Surg 220:212–221

Tambyraja AL, Sengupta F, MacGregor AB, et al. (2004) Patterns and clinical outcomes associated with routine intravenous sodium and fluid administration after colorectal resection. World J Surg 28:1046–1051

Van den Berghe G, Wouters P, Weekers F, et al. (2001) Intensive insulin therapy in the critically ill patients. N Engl J Med 345:1359–1367

Van den Berghe G, Wilmer A, Hermans G, et al. (2006) Intensive insulin therapy in the medical ICU. N Engl J Med 354:449–461

4 Abnormal Bleeding and Coagulopathies

Randy J. Woods · Mary C. McCarthy

Pearls and Pitfalls

- Resuscitation of the bleeding patient with isotonic saline solutions will rapidly dilute and deplete the clotting system.
- In patients who respond to fluids but appear to have continued moderate blood loss, angiography and embolization may be of value in stopping continued bleeding if deemed not to be surgically controllable.
- Prevention and correction of acidosis and hypothermia is essential for the optimal function of platelets and clotting factors.
- In the stable patient, using coagulation studies to guide component replacement is effective. However, in the face of massive hemorrhage, awaiting coagulation studies will prolong the duration of shock and coagulopathy.
- It is vital to anticipate the need for blood products. Patients arriving with a significant base deficit or ongoing hemorrhage will require FFP, platelets, and/or cryoprecipitate.
- Blood products and the best ICU care will not take the place of adequate surgical control of hemorrhage.
- Damage control procedures in the injured patient should be performed prior to the onset of coagulopathy. High-risk patients have an injury severity score >25, pH < 7.3, T $< 35°C$, systolic blood pressure <90 mmHg, base deficit >6, and lactate >4 mmol/l.

Recent advances in the care of the bleeding surgical patient have resulted in a significant decrease in the morbidity and mortality of major injuries. Concepts such as "damage control surgery," improved blood banking techniques, a better understanding of component therapy, and increased awareness of the impact of the "lethal triad" (hypothermia, acidosis, and coagulopathy) have enabled surgeons to successfully control severe hemorrhage. Understanding the physiology of the coagulation system, the clinical presentation of inherited and acquired coagulopathies, and appropriate treatment options enable the surgeon to provide optimal care for the bleeding patient.

Physiology of the Coagulation System

The traditional intrinsic and extrinsic model of the coagulation cascade has been replaced by the cell-based model, in which platelets, endothelium, and inflammatory cells interact in the production of thrombus and mature clot. Hemostasis is a three-stage process which includes: (1) primary hemostasis (initiation) occurs when activated platelets stimulated by the presence of tissue factor (TF) form a plug within minutes; (2) secondary hemostasis (amplification) occurs when the immature platelet plug is reinforced with fibrin strands; and (3) fibrinolysis, dissolves the clot after the vascular endothelium has been repaired, which occurs over a period of days.

In the current understanding of hemostasis, cells such as those of the vascular endothelium have acquired a larger role. Breakdown of the endothelial layer exposes collagen and TF to circulating platelets and leukocytes, causing the platelets to adhere and plug the disrupted vessel. Once activated, the platelets act as a catalyst for secondary hemostasis. Amplification occurs when the tissue factor stimulated cell membranes bind Factor VII and act as a catalyst for the large-scale production of thrombin. The activated platelets express adhesion molecules that interact with leukocytes causing activation and amplification of processes involving cytokines and cofactors. This crossover into the inflammatory system helps to explain the activation of both inflammation and coagulation in septic and bleeding patients. In systemic immune response syndrome (SIRS), circulating cytokines stimulate coagulation, causing the development of microemboli and progressing to multiple system organ failure (MSOF). This observation helps to explain how manipulating the coagulation system can result in improvement in organ failure due to SIRS or sepsis.

Clinical Presentation of Coagulopathies

Inherited Coagulopathies

In preparing for elective surgery or evaluating a trauma patient, a thorough history and physical exam should be performed. Questions about prior mucosal bleeding tendencies, easy bruising, or previous episodes of hemarthrosis have taken the place of routine coagulation testing. Further evaluation for bleeding dyscrasias should be prompted by positive responses to the pertinent review of systems or family history. In general, mucosal bleeding and subcutaneous bleeding are indicative of platelet dysfunction. Deep muscle bleeding or hemarthrosis is typical of factor deficiencies. The initial evaluation should consist of a complete blood count (CBC) assessing for anemia and a quantitative platelet count, protime (PT), activated partial thromboplastin time (aPTT), and a platelet function study.

Inherited platelet membrane receptor defects are not uncommon, with von Willebrand disease (vWD) being the most common deficiency. Occasionally the aPTT will be slightly elevated. It is important to identify the correct subtype of vWD so that proper treatment can be initiated.

Inherited factor deficiencies are also common, with the hemophilias being the most prevalent. Patients with hemophilia will have histories of hemarthrosis, spontaneous muscle hematomas, and gastrointestinal bleeding. Inherited deficiencies of factor VIII (hemophilia A) and factor IX (hemophilia B) require factor replacement and monitoring of treatment factor levels in the cases of trauma or surgery. In general, with the proper evaluation and perioperative factor replacement, elective and even acute surgical emergencies can be safely managed in patients with hemophilia.

Acquired Coagulopathies

Patients are now living longer and receiving chronic treatment for atrial fibrillation, carotid artery atherosclerosis, and valvular disease. Treatment may include drugs that interfere with the normal clotting cascade. Therefore, acquired coagulopathies are increasingly common. Active and otherwise healthy patients are receiving medications such as aspirin, warfarin, ibuprofen and other nonsteroidal anti-inflammatory drugs (NSAIDs), clopidogrel, and ticlopidine. Generally these medications have a good risk:benefit ratio. However, when a patient simply falls from the standing position, the risk of intracranial hemorrhage and death increases if rapid reversal of these agents is not initiated promptly.

Acquired platelet abnormalities are common and can be either qualitative (aspirin or clopidogrel therapy) or quantitative (myelodysplastic disorder). Platelet function studies can be helpful when a patient's medication history is unknown, for example, when they arrive in the emergency department with an intracranial hemorrhage after a fall at home. However, recent personal experience has demonstrated that a normal platelet function test does not guarantee that coagulation will proceed normally.

Hemodilutional Coagulopathy

Hemodilutional coagulopathy develops in patients with ongoing hemorrhage. If the coagulopathy is not treated promptly, the patient will deteriorate to irreversible shock. This may be related to a cellular change such as apoptosis or exhaustion of physiologic reserves. The factors of the lethal triad – hypothermia, acidosis and coagulopathy – may contribute to this resistant shock state. Resuscitation of the bleeding patient with isotonic saline solutions will rapidly dilute the components of the clotting system. Hemorrhage up to one blood volume and replacement with packed red blood cells (PRBC) alone will result in a 70% decrease in the coagulation factors. The remaining coagulation factors are usually sufficient to prevent a bleeding diathesis (Ingerslev and Hvid, 2006). However, acidosis and hypothermia are frequently seen in patients with traumatic shock and compound the problem. Ischemia-reperfusion injury to the endothelium after delayed or inadequate volume resuscitation or a soft tissue crush injury from blunt trauma can also result in significant consumption of factors. Early transfusion of packed red blood cells alone will result in depletion of coagulation factors and other components of successful clotting. One must keep in mind that the patient is bleeding more than just red blood cells. Component therapy using banked RBCs has replaced the use of fresh whole blood. Therefore the other coagulation elements must also be replaced.

In trauma patients, exsanguination is one of the leading causes of death (Lavoie et al., 2004). Ongoing hemorrhage and increased utilization of factors and other elements of the clotting cascade compound this problem. Early initiation of packed red blood cells and transfusion of fresh frozen plasma (FFP) or thawed plasma, cryoprecipitate, and platelets are needed to reverse the coagulopathy in actively bleeding patients. FFP contains all the essential clotting factors, including fibrinogen, although the fibrinogen level in FFP is less than that in cryoprecipitate. It is important to anticipate the use of FFP because it requires 30 min to thaw. The clotting factors in FFP are crucial for the conversion of fibrinogen to fibrin for clot formation. In the massively bleeding patient, fibrinogen will be one of the first factors to be depleted, and administration of cryoprecipitate may also be required. Cryoprecipitate is also stored frozen, but due to its smaller volume, can be available in 10–20 min.

Recombinant factor VIIa (rFVIIa) is a recent addition to the armamentarium to correct coagulopathy. Recombinant FVIIa is approved in the management of patients with hemophilia A who have demonstrated antibodies to factor VIII. Recombinant FVIIa does not have an approved indication for use in trauma surgical patients, although there have been studies showing benefit. There is also evidence that the use of rFVIIa improves coagulation studies and reduces the amount of blood loss.

Exogenous factor VII binds to circulating tissue factor (TF) at the site of the endothelial injury. Factor VII then activates factors IX and X, which ultimately results in a burst of thrombin generation.

Disseminated Intravascular Coagulation

Disseminated intravascular coagulation (DIC) is a consequence of an underlying disease and not a process itself (see ❷ *Table 4-1*). DIC should be thought of as systemic endothelial dysfunction in which the usually anticoagulant endothelium becomes a stimulus for a hypercoagulable state. Optimal results in the treatment of DIC are achieved following an aggressive search for its etiology and treatment. DIC stems from tissue factor (TF) expression on a multitude of cell surfaces. One possible source of TF is endothelial injury due to sepsis. As stated previously, the TF causes activation of factors VII and IX, which ultimately leads to thrombin generation. Unlike normal clotting events, the TF in DIC is not localized to the injured site, thereby causing a local process to become systemic. This uncontrolled activation of factors VII and IX causes activation of the clotting process at all levels. If the consumption of coagulation factors outpaces production, then uncompensated DIC occurs. The patient then becomes hypocoagulable and bleeding occurs. If the underlying cause of DIC is untreated, clotting factors will be consumed and fibrin split products (degradation products from the fibinolytic process) will increase. Platelet count and fibrinogen levels decrease, while PT/INR, aPTT, and D-dimer levels increase. Mortality in septic patients with DIC is double that of patients without DIC. As DIC progresses, fibrin microemboli occlude the microvasculature of end organs, resulting in local hypoperfusion and eventually MSOF.

The diagnosis of DIC depends on whether the patient is in a hypercoagulable state (consumption of clotting products matched by production) or hypocoagulable state (consumption outpaces the production). Signs of thrombosis include mental status changes, tissue ischemia (seen in the fingertips of the hand with a radial arterial line), renal insufficiency, respiratory failure, and gastrointestinal ulceration. Classic signs in the hypocoagulable state include intracranial bleeding, skin petechia and ecchymosis, mucosal bleeding, hematuria, and gastrointestinal bleeding. Retroperitoneal bleeding may be manifest by a falling hematocrit.

The treatment of DIC begins with resuscitation and rapid transfusion of PRBC, if indicated. Persistent shock will result in refractory DIC with increased mortality; prompt resuscitation is vital. In patients experiencing major thrombotic events (limb-threatening ischemia) heparin, or low molecular weight heparin may be beneficial. However, correcting the underlying etiology of the DIC is

◻ Table 4-1
Etiologies of DIC

Sepsis (gram-negative infection)
Traumatic shock
Delayed resuscitation in shock
Ischemic or necrotic tissue
Abscess
Cancers (acute leukemia and metastatic prostatic carcinomas)
Severe traumatic brain injury
Severe thermal injury
Fat embolism
Complicated birth
Transfusion reaction

paramount to successful recovery of the patient. Abnormal PT/INR should be corrected with FFP, severe thrombocytopenia (platelet count $<50,000/mm^3$) with platelet transfusions, and fibrinogen levels replenished to above 100 mg/dl with cryoprecipitate.

In the setting of sepsis-associated DIC with organ system dysfunction, activated protein C may be of benefit. In patients with Acute Physiology and Chronic Health Evaluation (APACHE) II Scores greater than 25, activated protein C shows promise in reversing organ dysfunction with an acceptable risk of bleeding.

Treatment

The initial treatment of the bleeding patient will depend upon the etiology of hemorrhage. Patients with inherited coagulopathies will need initial factor replacement and maintenance of therapeutic levels. A hematology consult may be helpful in management. However, patients who are bleeding due to prolonged or inadequate resuscitation from shock, massive transfusion, or an acquired coagulopathy need to be addressed differently.

First, the surgeon should ensure that blood loss is not the result of inadequate surgical control. When a patient's blood pressure is low and a damage control procedure is performed, bleeding may be controlled temporarily. With continued resuscitation, rewarming, and normalization of the blood pressure, bleeding that was initially controlled may resume. A return to the operating room may be needed to re-explore the operative field. Blood products and rigorous intensive care will not take the place of adequate surgical control of significant bleeding. In patients who respond to fluids but appear to have continued moderate blood loss, angiography and embolization may be valuable. This is especially true if the initial exploration did not reveal the bleeding source, or if bleeding is deep within the liver parenchyma, in the retroperitoneum, or along the pelvic sidewall from a complex pelvic fracture.

Laboratory studies such as PT/INR, aPTT, qualitative and quantitative platelet studies can be used to direct component replacement. Diffuse oozing in the operative site is an indicator of hypothermia and/or a platelet defect. Bloody return from operative drains can be caused by many factors. In a stable patient, using coagulation studies to guide component replacement is effective. However, in the face of massive hemorrhage, awaiting coagulation studies will prolong the duration of the coagulation abnormality. This results in continued blood loss, hypoperfusion, and further endothelial injury, with consequent DIC. In complex situations, thromboelastography (TEG) allows more rapid point-of-care testing for platelet function, enzyme activity, and fibrinolysis. Evaluating fibrinolysis may help in determining mild cases of DIC and prompt an earlier evaluation for an etiology.

Intraoperatively, packing the site of injury to control bleeding and truncating the procedure to concentrate on control of hypothermia and coagulopathy is necessary. Return to the operating room in 24–72 h for completion of the surgical procedure should be planned. In the majority of patients, aggressive rewarming and resuscitation is needed. Initially factor repletion is empiric, and later coagulation studies are used as a guide. Formulas for component replacement based on number of PRBC transfused can be wasteful (Ingerslev and Hvid, 2006). However, transfusion formulas are useful triggers to remind providers that PRBC are devoid of platelets or clotting factors. Ongoing clinical evidence of bleeding or laboratory assessment should guide further transfusion of blood products.

After control of hemorrhage and enteric spill in a damage control procedure, what remains in the short-term is aggressive correction of an acquired coagulopathy. In many institutions, the short

◘ Table 4-2

Protocol for use of activated recombinant factor Vii (rFVIIa)

Before using rFVIIa in the coagulopathic patient address
• Serum pH > 7.2
• Temperature $> 35°C$
• Platelet count $> 50,000$ mm^3
• Fibrinogen > 100 mg/dl
Initial dose of 100 mcg/kg body weight (may need to be repeated)

trip from the OR to the ICU is enough to result in a further delay in resuscitation. It may be helpful to delay transfer to the ICU and continue resuscitation in the OR. Rapid infusion devices that deliver 1–2 l/min of warmed blood and blood products can quickly replace needed factors. Care must be taken not to overload the patient, but this time spent before transfer can be lifesaving in the appropriate patient. Although surgical blood salvage (cell saver) should be used whenever possible, the recycled red blood cells will be critically low in essential clotting factors and platelets. Therefore, salvaged blood used in resuscitation will require FFP, platelets, and at times, cryoprecipitate to be administered in conjunction with recycled washed red blood cells.

Mentioned earlier, rFVIIa has been shown to reduce hemorrhage in trauma patients. More work needs to be done refining the optimal patient population, appropriate timing of the product, and the accompanying risks and complications. There is no consensus on the dosage of rFVIIa in trauma patients or those with intracranial hemorrhage. A randomized trial in trauma has recently been completed in the United States. Hypothermia and acidosis should be corrected prior to the administration of rFVIIa (Meng et al., 2003). The drug is very expensive, and therefore, most trauma centers have developed protocols for its use (see ❷ *Table 4-2*).

Although often difficult, preventing hypothermia and acidosis is the best strategy to minimize coagulopathy. Prompt resuscitation of patients reduces endothelial injury and decreases MSOF, infectious complications, and death. There are many tools at the surgeon's disposal to facilitate these goals. The surgeon should become familiar with the concepts reviewed here and be ready to initiate treatment promptly.

Selected Readings

Dutton RP, McCunn M, Hyder M, et al. (2004) Factor VIIa for correction of traumatic coagulopathy. J Trauma 57:709–718; discussion 718.

Erber WN, Perry DJ (2006) Plasma and plasma products in the treatment of massive haemorrhage. Best Pract Res Clin Haematol 19:97–112

Ingerslev J, Hvid I (2006) Surgery in hemophilia. the general view: patient selection, timing, and preoperative assessment. Semin Hematol 43:S23–S26

Lavoie A, Ratte S, Clas D, et al. (2004) Preinjury warfarin use among elderly patients with closed head injuries in a trauma center. J Trauma 56:802–807

MacLeod JB, Lynn M, McKenney MG, et al. (2003) Early coagulopathy predicts mortality in trauma. J Trauma 55:39–44

5 Blood Transfusion and Alternative Therapies

Henry M. Cryer

Pearls and Pitfalls

- Blood transfusion is substantially overutilized and has significant associated risk, including: transfusion reactions, transmission of blood borne pathogens, and immune suppression.
- The accepted transfusion "trigger" in euvolemic patients is 7 gm/dl for healthy individuals and 8–9 gm/dl for patients with co-morbidities associated with decreased cardiopulmonary reserve.
- Blood transfusion is an independent predictor of MOF, SIRS, increased infection, and mortality in patients with severe injuries and undergoing complex surgical procedures.
- Transfusion of only the amount of blood that maximizes immediate survival and minimizes late inflammatory complications is the goal of resuscitation.
- Trauma patients and other patients in hemorrhagic shock should be transfused based upon blood pressure, pulse, and other measurements of decreased perfusion rather than relying upon laboratory values.
- "The triad of death" including bleeding, hypothermia, and acidosis, leads to the "bloody vicious cycle" of hemorrhage, resuscitation, hemodilution, coagulopathy, and continued bleeding.
- "Damage control" strategies that control immediately life-threatening injuries and hemorrhage and wait until normal physiology has been restored in the ICU prior to definitive repair of injuries have been adopted to avoid the "bloody vicious cycle".
- Massive blood loss requires rapid decisions.
- Massive transfusion must be anticipated and massive transfusion protocols instituted prior to the development of coagulopathy.
- One proposed massive transfusion protocol utilizes a 1:1:1 ratio of PRBC, FFP and platelets. Alternate each unit of blood with FFP and then give 1 6-pack of platelets after each 6 units of blood.

Introduction

Blood transfusion is integral to the success of advanced surgical procedures on the heart, transplantation, joint replacement, major cancer resections, and major injury. When patients lose blood either from injury or an operation, blood transfusion has the obvious benefit of restoring oxygen carrying capacity to maintain the metabolic demands of organs and tissues. On the other hand, there are definite risks and consequences of the infusion of blood products including transfusion reaction, transmission of blood born pathogens, and immune suppression. As with any therapy, it is important to establish a risk-benefit profile for the various clinical situations in which blood transfusion is considered during the care of surgical patients.

Potential Benefits of Blood Transfusion

It is obvious that blood loss leads to lack of oxygen carrying capacity, decreased tissue perfusion, and ultimately organ failure and death if allowed to proceed below a critical threshold. This threshold is different depending on the circumstances in which bleeding occurs. Sudden loss of blood as occurs after major vascular injury can result in profound hemorrhagic shock and sudden death if control of bleeding and volume restoration do not occur rapidly. On the other hand, with gradual loss of blood as usually occurs during elective surgical operations, continuous intravascular volume repletion leads to euvolemic anemia rather than profound hemorrhagic shock. Under conditions of euvolemic anemia, it has been established that the lower threshold for hemoglobin concentration, below which organ function cannot be maintained, is in the neighborhood of 5–6 g/dl. This threshold may be somewhat higher in patients that have underlying decreases in physiologic reserve such as patients with coronary artery disease, or patients with chronic obstructive pulmonary disease. Signs and symptoms of decreased perfusion are rather subtle at a hemoglobin level of 5 g/dl, where hemodynamics are maintained, but decreases in mentation occur. By the time the hemoglobin reaches approximately 3 g/dl patients become comatose and begin to have ST segment changes indicative of impending myocardial infarction. Given these findings, the currently accepted blood transfusion trigger is a hemoglobin level of 7 g/dl in an otherwise euvolemic patient with relatively normal health. Patients with decreased physiologic reserve usually have a transfusion trigger somewhat higher at the 8–9 g/dl range. Patients undergoing acute blood loss should be transfused if active hemorrhage is not controlled and there is evidence of hypovolemia, such as decreased blood pressure and tachycardia.

Consequences of Blood Transfusion

The obvious benefit of blood transfusion is to improve oxygen carrying capacity and restore tissue perfusion with oxygen and nutrients. Counterbalancing these potential benefits are a number of deleterious consequences of blood transfusion. Immediate risks include allergic, febrile, and hemolytic transfusion reactions, acute pulmonary edema, and anaphylaxis. Delayed risks include transmission of Human Immunodeficiency Virus (HIV), Hepatitis C Virus (HCV), Hepatitis B Virus (HBV) and other as yet poorly characterized or undiscovered pathogens. The blood supply is regulated differently in different countries, so there is some variability in the risks of these complications. Estimates for Western countries are listed in ❷ *Table 5-1*. Over 10,000,000 units of packed red blood cells are transfused annually in the United States with only 30–40 deaths nationwide thought to be caused by these transfusions. This equates to roughly 1 death per 300,000 transfusions. It is important to remember this figure when considering alternatives to blood transfusion. The most dangerous complication is a major hemolytic reaction caused by ABO incompatibility resulting in the lysis of donor

◘ Table 5-1

Estimated risk of transfusion (Modified from Madjidpour, et al. 2005)

HIV	1:1.5M–1:4.7M
HBV	1:31K–1:205K
HCV	1:2M–1:3M
Bacterial sepsis	1:30K–1:140K
Malaria	1:4M
Acute hemolysis	1:13K
Delayed hemolysis	1:9K
TRALI	1:4K–1:500K
Mistransfusion	1:14K–1:18K

RBCs. The clinical presentation of ABO incompatibility is immediate occurring within minutes of the initiation of the blood transfusion. The patient becomes tachypneic, hypotensive and extremely anxious. There may be high fever, evidence of diffuse microvascular bleeding, the development of renal failure, disseminated intravascular coagulation (DIC) and death. This reaction usually results from a clerical error and occurs very rarely at a rate approximately 1 per 700,000 units of blood transfused. Treatment is to stop the transfusion immediately and support the circulation with intravenous fluids, mechanical ventilation and supportive care. Non-hemolytic febrile and other allergic reactions also occur with varying severity ranging from mild urticaria to severe lymphangioedema and acute lung injury (TRALI).

In trauma patients, blood transfusion has been identified as an independent predictor of multiple organ failure (MOF), systemic inflammatory response syndrome (SIRS), increased infection, and increased mortality. Furthermore, the cumulative risk appears to be linearly correlated with the number of units transfused, the length of storage time, and the presence of donor leucocytes. Whether blood transfusion is simply a surrogate measure of severity of hemorrhagic shock or it is the blood transfusion itself which leads to these problems has been difficult to ascertain. However, the distinction is somewhat moot, since the problem requiring multiple blood transfusions is always present when blood transfusion occurs. It is clear that transfusion of six or more units of blood during the first 24 hours (h) after injury is associated with a profound pro-inflammatory response and increased risk for MOF, infection and immune suppression. While there is also evidence that transfusion of even one unit of blood can increase the risk of these complications, the magnitude of the effect is less clear.

Immunosuppression is also a consequence of allogenic blood transfusion and in some studies is associated with increased risk of cancer recurrence after potentially curative surgery, as well as increased frequency of postoperative bacterial infection. Furthermore, this infection risk is higher in patients requiring blood transfusion with traumatic injury compared to those receiving transfusion during or after elective surgery. While the mechanism is still unclear, increased storage time of blood has been associated with the generation of inflammatory mediators and neutrophil activation. Leukoreduction of banked blood has the theoretic benefit of avoiding the immune effects associated with white blood cells and is now uniformly practiced in many European countries. Additionally, free hemoglobin, which occurs as a result of hemolysis of old red blood cells, increases significantly as blood storage time increases. This free hemoglobin can bind to nitric oxide and interfere with regulation of microvascular tone, leading to a mismatch of supply and demand in the microcirculation.

Guidelines for Blood Transfusion

Given the significant risk of allogenic blood transfusion, a risk-benefit analysis must be undertaken prior to the transfusion of blood. The American Society of Anesthesia has published a consensus practice guideline for peri-operative blood transfusion and adjuvant therapies and similar guidelines have been published in Europe. These guidelines focus on the peri-operative management of patients undergoing surgery or other invasive procedures in which significant blood loss occurs or is expected.

Preoperative Decisions Regarding Blood Transfusion

Pre-operative evaluation should include a review of prior medical records, a physical examination, an interview of the patient or family to identify risk factors, and a laboratory evaluation to include at least a hemoglobin level, hematocrit and coagulation profile. If patients have increased potential for organ ischemia, such as cardiorespiratory disease, this may influence the ultimate transfusion trigger. Patients taking anticoagulation medications such as clopidogrel, coumadin or aspirin may require increased transfusion of blood and non-red blood cell components such as fresh frozen plasma and platelets. Additionally, a pre-operative evaluation should include checking for the presence of congenital or acquired blood disorders, the use of vitamins or herbal supplements that may effect coagulation, (❍ *Table 5-2*) and previous exposure to drugs such as aprotinin that may cause an allergic reaction upon repeated exposure.

Congenital and acquired abnormalities in clotting must be identified and contingency plans made. The normal clotting cascade involves primary and secondary hemostatic mechanisms, and there is a delicate balance between factors which promote bleeding versus those that promote coagulation in the

◼ Table 5-2

Vitamins and herbal supplements that may affect blood loss (Blajchman, 2006)

Herbal supplements that decrease platelet aggregation
Bilberry
Bromelain
Dong quoi
Feverfew
Fish oil
Flax seed oil
Garlic
Ginger
Gingko biloba
Grape seed extract
Saw palmetto
Herbs that inhibit clotting
Chamomile
Dandelion root
Dong quoi
Horse chestnut
Vitamins that affect coagulation
Vitamin K
Vitamin E

peri-operative period. When small- or medium-sized blood vessels are injured or lacerated by injury or operation, the initial transection is usually followed by intense spasm. In addition, platelets are activated secondary to exposure to subendothelial collagen located in the injured vessel wall causing adherence and elaboration of coagulation factors, resulting in the formation of thrombin and cross linking of fibrin to form a platelet plug with cessation of bleeding after a minute or two (primary hemostasis). Subsequently, a waterfall coagulation cascade results in the conversion of fibrin to fibrin culminating in the formation of stable fibrin clot (secondary hemostasis). Counteracting the procoagulant pathway, a number of proteolytic enzymes are produced to promote inactivation of coagulation factors by a process of fibrinolysis. The balance between these systems results in a highly regulated and controlled hemostatic process. The delicate balance of this system can be adversely affected by a number of congenital coagulation defects as well as co-morbid conditions such as hepatic insufficiency, renal insufficiency, and drug treatment with clopidogrel, coumadin, aspirin, and alcohol.

The most common congenital abnormalities are hemophilia A (Factor VIII deficiency) and hemophilia B (Factor IX deficiency). Patients with these congenital defects are able to make a platelet plug by primary hemostasis but lack the ability to make a firm fibrin clot because of the defect in secondary hemostasis. Therefore, these patients must be supported through the peri-operative or peri-injury period with the infusion of commercial Factor VIII preparation or prothrombin complex concentrate which contains Factor IX, to maintain factor levels above 50% of normal during the peri-operative period.

Patients with hepatic insufficiency have a decrease in synthetic function of the liver with a resultant deficiency of all coagulation factors except for III and VIII. Additionally they have decreased platelet counts as a result of hypersplenism associated with portal hypertension. Moreover, the cirrhotic liver fails to adequately clear plasma activators of the fibrinolytic system, which may result in an enhanced fibrinolysis. These patients often need aggressive administration of fresh frozen plasma and platelets during the peri-operative period.

Patients with renal insufficiency differ from patients with hepatic insufficiency in that the primary defect in coagulation associated with renal disease involves primary rather than secondary hemostasis. The defect is the result of platelet dysfunction and impaired platelet vessel wall interaction. Unfortunately, platelet transfusions are of limited to no benefit because the transfused platelets are inactivated by the same toxins as the native platelets. Transfusion of cryoprecipitate and packed red blood cells has been shown to decrease the platelet defect, although the mechanism is not clear. Similar results have been seen when the hematocrit is raised by the use of recombinant erythropoietin (EPO). Desmopressin (DDAVP) has also been used to shorten bleeding times in patients with uremia.

As the population ages, the number of elderly patients undergoing surgery, as well as those who are injured, are increasing at a rapid rate. Many of these patients take clopidogrel, aspirin, coumadin, or other blood thinning agents for a variety of reasons. Elective surgery patients should discontinue anti-coagulation therapy prior to surgery for the effects of these drugs to dissipate. If the operation cannot be delayed, then administration of reversal agents such as vitamin K, prothrombin complex concentrate, platelets, recombinant activated Factor VII or fresh frozen plasma should be considered. Obviously, the risks of thrombosis versus the risks of increased bleeding must be weighed when altering the anti-coagulation status of these patients.

Coumadin, which has a half-life of approximately 40 h, acts by blocking the synthesis of vitamin K-dependent coagulation factors. Patients undergoing elective surgery can simply stop taking their coumadin several days prior to operation. On the other hand, trauma patients or patients undergoing emergency operation require active reversal with fresh frozen plasma. While vitamin K administration can reverse the effects of coumadin, the rate of correction is variable and markedly decreases the ability to recoumadinize the patient in the post-operative period. For this reason rapid correction of anti-coagulation from coumadin therapy is usually done with infusion of fresh frozen plasma using one unit of FFP to correct the PT by approximately 2 seconds.

Aspirin therapy causes anti-coagulation by inhibiting platelet function. The defect lasts for the lifespan of the platelet, which is approximately 10 days. Since the half-life of aspirin is quite short (less than 1 h), platelet transfusions are effective in reversing the defect acutely when necessary.

Clopidogrel effects last for a week or more. Platelet transfusion may be used to reverse the pharmacologic effects of clopidogrel when quick reversal is required, but the half-life of the drug is 8 h and it is in a steady state in the circulation. Recombinant-activated Factor VII has been shown to reverse the platelet inhibition associated with both clopidogrel and ASA and should be considered intraoperatively if platelet transfusion is not effective.

After the pre-operative assessment, patients should be informed of the potential risks and benefits of blood transfusions and their preferences elicited. If blood loss can be anticipated, it is important to ensure that blood and blood components are available for the patients' operative procedure. If sufficient time exists, pre-admission blood collection to prevent or reduce allogeneic blood transfusion should be considered. However, it must be acknowledged that adverse outcomes such as transfusion reaction due to clerical error or bacterial contamination may still occur with the use of autologous blood transfusion. If a patient cannot tolerate pre-operative anemia or sufficient time is not available for pre-operative blood donation, then banked blood products must be used.

Intra-Operative Blood Transfusion

The decision to transfuse blood during an operation depends on the patients' underlying physiologic status as well as the amount and rate of blood loss, and physiologic derangements. The amount of blood loss is usually monitored by the anesthesiologist's observation of the amount of blood collected in suction canisters and by weighing laparotomy pads. In addition, the anesthesiologist measures hemoglobin and hematocrit levels at regular intervals during the operation. The presence of inadequate perfusion and oxygenation of vital organs is assessed by measuring blood pressure, heart rate, ECG, temperature, and blood oxygen saturation levels continuously during the procedure. When excessive blood loss is anticipated, intra-operative red blood cell recovery should be considered. While transfusion triggers have been developed for the euvolemic anemic state in the intensive care unit during the postoperative period, the data are insufficient to precisely define a trigger for blood transfusion during an operation. Certainly blood transfusion should occur if the hemoglobin level is less than 6 g/dl and usually is not necessary when the level is greater than 10 g/dl. A visual assessment of the surgical field should be conducted on a regular basis to assess for excessive microvascular bleeding (coagulopathy). If adequate intravascular volume is maintained by the infusion of crystalloids and colloids and blood loss is slow, organ perfusion can usually be maintained with hemoglobin levels as low as 6 g/dl in an otherwise healthy individual. On the other hand, if rapid blood loss results in hypotension, the decision to transfuse red cells is made by anticipating the blood loss or on evidence of hypotension rather than a laboratory result.

When massive blood transfusion is required (ten or more units of packed red blood cells), attention must be given to preventing and managing coagulopathy. Coagulopathy should be prevented by transfusing platelets and fresh frozen plasma prior to the development of microvascular bleeding, if at all possible. Platelets should be transfused if the platelet count is below 50,000 cells/ml but may also be indicated despite an apparently adequate platelet count if there is known or suspected platelet dysfunction. Additionally, when active bleeding is ongoing, fresh frozen plasma should be administered when the international normalized ratio (INR) or activated partial thromboplastin time (APTT) is elevated. Cryoprecipitate should be given when fibrinogen concentrations are less than 80 mg/dl. Recombinant-activated Factor VII may also be indicated should component therapy not result in resolution of the coagulopathy. Disturbing reports of occasional thrombotic complications leading to stroke, myocardial infarction, and intestinal ischemia after rVIIa are emerging. Therefore, this agent should be used with restraint and reserved for patients with recalcitrant coagulopathy unresponsive to component therapy.

When blood loss approaches one blood volume (approximately 70 ml/kg) a massive transfusion protocol should be initiated. This protocol does not require abnormal laboratory values as a transfusion trigger, and usually involves infusion of one unit of fresh frozen plasma and one unit of platelets for each unit of red blood cell transfused. From a practical perspective, for each unit of packed red blood cells, one unit of fresh frozen plasma should be infused along with a 6-pack of platelets for every 6 units of packed red blood cells transfused.

Special considerations must be accounted for when dealing with injured patients arriving in hemorrhagic shock as a result of blood loss prior to patient arrival. In this situation a large degree of hemorrhage has already occurred leading to impaired physiology, poor organ perfusion, and compensatory responses to preserve blood flow to the brain and heart, which are likely already at maximal capacity. As a result of marked peripheral vasoconstriction and decreased blood pressure, bleeding may have already markedly slowed or even ceased. To successfully treat these patients intravascular volume must be restored simultaneously with control of hemorrhage. Prior to definitive control of hemorrhage there is a fine line between too little fluids, resulting in hypoperfusion with organ ischemia, and too much fluid, leading to re-bleeding as a result of "popping the clot." From a practical perspective, this means transfusing packed red blood cells and crystalloid solution at a rate which is slow enough to gradually increase blood pressure towards normal, while rapidly identifying the source of hemorrhage and stopping it. The second major consideration in this group of patients is the development of coagulopathy. These patients are often cold, acidotic, and hypotensive, all of which lead to coagulopathy. Ongoing hemorrhage and massive transfusion perpetuate the acidosis and hypothermia leading to the "bloody vicious cycle" with eventual death from exsanguination. Unlike the patient undergoing elective surgery where blood loss can be easily monitored and quantified, as well as anticipated, these patients generally meet the criteria for a massive transfusion protocol at the initiation of their therapy. Laboratory values have little to do with the management of these patients. They should be transfused in a 1:1:1 ratio, receiving a unit of fresh frozen plasma for each unit of packed red blood cells and a six pack of platelets for every six units of packed red blood cells transfused.

In addition to early institution of a massive transfusion protocol, these patients require active rewarming and adherence to the principles of damage control operation. Damage control refers to limiting the operation to stopping the bleeding prior to the development of coagulopathy and terminating the procedure prior to definitive repair of all injuries. Major bleeding vessels are rapidly repaired or ligated and hollow viscus injuries are stapled closed to prevent further contamination. The abdomen is closed with a temporary closure to prevent abdominal compartment syndrome and the patient is taken to the ICU to correct abnormal physiology. The patient is returned to the operating room 24–48 h later for definitive reconstruction.

Post-Operative Blood Transfusion

Once the critical emergency or elective operation is over, and active bleeding has been controlled, the patient usually ends up in an intensive care or other monitored environment with support of their vital organs and close monitoring of their physiology. Ideally, by the end of the operation or shortly after arrival in the intensive care unit the patient has been restored to a normal euvolemic state. A variety of physiologic compensation mechanisms including regional and microcirculatory changes in blood flow and a shift of the oxyhemoglobin dissociation curve to the right to decrease hemoglobin affinity for oxygen are in place which allow adequate oxygenation of tissues at a relatively anemic but normovolemic state. Factors such as increased cardiac output and decreased blood viscosity allow oxygen delivery to remain relatively unchanged until hemoglobin concentration falls below 7 g/dl. This level is much lower than the previously recommended 10 g/dl as a transfusion trigger and is supported by the prospective randomized transfusion requirements in critical care (TRICC) trial. While there is some variability between patients it appears that the 7 g/dl trigger provides sufficient oxygen carrying capacity for all patients except those with severe coronary artery disease. Most agree that patients with known cardiovascular disease should be transfused to a higher threshold in the 8.5–10 g/dl range. Whether similar transfusion triggers should be used for patients who are elderly, have nervous system problems, COPD, or renal disease remains to be determined. Practically, transfusion guidelines should take into account the patients' individual ability to tolerate and to compensate for an acute decrease in hemoglobin concentration. As there is no "universal" hemoglobin threshold that can serve for all patients, useful transfusion triggers should consider signs of inadequate tissue oxygenation that may occur depending on the patient's underlying diseases. Physiologic signs of inadequate oxygenation such as hemodynamic instability, oxygen extraction ratio > 50%, and myocardial ischemia, detectable by new ST-segment depressions > 0.1 mV, new ST-segment elevations > 0.2 mV or new wall motion abnormalities by transesophageal echocardiography have been suggested as triggers for transfusion. Ideally, transfusion should occur prior to the development of overt signs of ischemia.

Alternatives to Blood Transfusion

Given the risks of adverse outcomes associated with blood transfusion and the finite blood supply, strategies to minimize the need for blood transfusion must be pursued. Pre-operative donation of autologous blood (ABD) and injection of recombinant human erythropoietin (EPO), along with the cessation of anticoagulant drugs are the main options. In procedures with relatively predictable blood loss such as total joint replacement surgery, ABD has been shown to decrease the percent of patients receiving an allogeneic blood transfusion. On the other hand, only 50% of the ABD blood was actually transfused in that study, calling into question its cost effectiveness. The use of pre-operative EPO has been shown to reduce the need for allogeneic blood transfusion in anemic patients, but requires one week to become effective.

The primary techniques to minimize allogeneic blood transfusion include cell salvage techniques, acceptance of minimal hemoglobin levels, aggressive hemostatic techniques, and potentially artificial oxygen carriers. Blood salvage techniques have become commonplace, appear to be safe, and reduce the volume of homologous blood transfusion, but have not decreased the number of patients receiving homologous blood transfusion. The most common adjuvant hemostatic techniques include the application of agents such as fibrin glue and thrombin in a variety of preparations. There is ongoing research in this area which holds promise for the future. The development of artificial oxygen carriers to replace red blood cell transfusion is also promising, but has been disappointing to date. There are two main groups of artificial O_2 carriers: hemoglobin-based and perfluorocarbon emulsions. The hemoglobin molecule in hemoglobin-based artificial O_2 carriers needs to be stabilized to prevent dissociation of the $alpha_2beta_2$-hemoglobin tetramer into alphabeta-dimers in order to prolong intravascular retention and to eliminate nephrotoxicity. Other modifications serve to decrease O_2 affinity in order to improve O_2 off-loading to tissues. In addition, polyethylene glycol may be surface conjugated to increase molecular size. Finally, certain products are polymerized to increase the hemoglobin concentration at physiologic colloid oncotic pressure. Perfluorocarbons are carbon-fluorine compounds characterized by a high gas-dissolving capacity for O_2 and CO_2 and chemical and biologic inertness. Perfluorocarbons are not miscible with water and therefore need to be brought into emulsion for intravenous application. The most advanced products are in clinical phase III trials, but no product has achieved market approval yet in the US, Europe, or Canada.

Post-operatively, cell salvage, EPO, and acceptance of minimal hemoglobin values represent the most common alternatives to RBC transfusion. ICU-associated anemia is largely the result of the cumulative effects of blood loss and decreased RBC production. Blood loss in critically ill patients may be overt, occult, or due to phlebotomy. Decreased RBC production is the other major factor influencing the development of anemia. Decreased RBC production is due to the combined effects of abnormal iron metabolism, inappropriately low erythropoietin production, diminished response to erythropoietin, and direct suppression of RBC production.

Clinical trials have shown that compared with non-treated subjects, rHuEPO-treated ICU patients will have increased serum erythropoietin concentrations, increased reticulocyte counts, increased hemoglobin and hematocrit values, and require fewer RBC transfusions. These clinical trials have not detected significant differences in outcomes in association with rHuEPO, however. Retransfusion of unwashed RBCs collected from drains and chest tubes has been used effectively in a variety of settings. The reported complication rate is low, but so are the total number of patients reported. When considering alternatives to red blood cell transfusion one must remember the incredibly low mortality associated with banked blood. Studies to show an equivalent safety profile with alternatives will be most challenging.

Selected Readings

Blajchman MA (2006) The clinical benefits of the leukoreduction of blood products. J Trauma 60:583–590

Hebert TC, Wells G, Blajchman MA, et al. (1999) A multi-centered randomized control clinical trial of transfusion requirements in critical care. New Engl J Med 340:409–417

Practice Guidelines for Perioperative Blood Transfusion and Adjuvant Therapies (2006) An Updated Report by the American Society of Anesthesiologists Task Force on Perioperative Blood Transfusion and Adjuvant Therapies. Anesthesiology 105:198–208

Madjdpour C, et al. (2005) Perioperative blood transfusions. Value, risks, and guidelines. Anaesthesist, 54:67–80

6 Circulatory Monitoring

Eric J. Mahoney · Walter L. Biffl · William G. Cioffi

Pearls and Pitfalls

- Normal vital signs do not equate to circulatory adequacy.
- Tachycardia indicates a loss of 15–30% of blood volume, but can be blunted in the elderly, the athlete, pregnant women, and patients medicated with beta-blockers.
- Automated blood pressure devices lack accuracy when the systolic blood pressure is below 110 mmHg; use of a manual device in these settings is recommended.
- Monitor the mean arterial pressure (MAP), **NOT** the systolic blood pressure.
- Measure central venous pressure (CVP) and pulmonary capillary wedge pressure (PCWP) at end expiration.
- Beware that base deficits and lactic acidosis do not always occur secondary to hypoxia.
- Use oxygen delivery (DO_2) as a guide, not as an endpoint.

Introduction

The fundamental goal of circulatory monitoring is to assess the adequacy of tissue perfusion. At first glance, this would appear to be relatively straightforward – heart rate and blood pressure are easy to assess and to interpret. However, neither accurately reflects perfusion, and the assessment of circulatory adequacy becomes much more difficult with increasing severity or complexity of illness. With several methods available to evaluate a patient's circulatory status, the clinician must learn to utilize and to interpret various monitoring modalities. In this chapter, we will discuss each of these methods (❷ *Table 6-1*).

Physical Examination

Circulatory monitoring begins with the physical examination. Frequently, important signs will be noticed within the first 10 seconds of the examination. Although many of the signs discovered may be non-specific, taken as a whole they provide valuable information regarding the status of the patient. During severe circulatory compromise, a patient may be very anxious, confused, or obtunded. Jugular venous distension is a common sign of cardiogenic shock or volume overload. Increased sympathetic tone leads to tachycardia as well as peripheral vasoconstriction with associated cool, clammy skin. Dry mucous membranes, sunken eyes, and decreased skin turgor are signs of chronic hypovolemia. Additionally, decreased urine output in a patient is a compensatory mechanism whereby water

◘ Table 6-1
Means of circulatory monitoring

	Advantages	Disadvantages
Physical examination	Simple	Non-specific insensitive
Pulse	Accessible reliable	Age variation
		Influenced by:
		Medications
		Physiological status
		Insensitive to occult hypoperfusion
Noninvasive blood pressure monitoring (sphygmomanometry)	Accessible	Unreliable
	Good indicator of vital organ perfusion	Insensitive to occult hypoperfusion
		Influenced by:
		Poor cuff fit
		Limitations to auscultation
		Atherosclerosis
Invasive blood pressure monitoring (arterial lines)	Accurate	Invasive
	Continuous blood pressure Monitoring	Infectious risk
	Access for blood tests	Thrombosis/ischemic risk
		System malfunction
		Transducer height
		Dampening
		Mismatching
		Catheter whip
Pulmonary artery catheters	Assess volume status	Invasive
	Assess left heart function	Infectious risk
	Assess oxygen delivery (DO2) and oxygen uptake (VO2)	Thrombosis/embolism risk
		Cardiac conduction risks:
		Arrhythmias
		Complete heart block
		Ventricular perforation
		Pulmonary artery rupture
		Misinterpretation
Central venous pressure monitoring	Assess volume status	Invasive
	Assess right heart function	Infectious risk
		System malfunction
		Pneumothorax
		Hemothorax
		Chylothorax
		Brachial plexus injury
		Mediastinitis
		Affect by premorbid cardiac and pulmonary conditions
Serum lactic acid	Assess global perfusion	Non-specific
Serum base deficit	Assess global perfusion	Non-specific

excretion is minimized in an attempt to maintain blood volume. These physical characteristics must be elucidated by the examiner and properly evaluated with the objective information presented in order to treat the patient properly.

Pulse

The pulse should be assessed for rate, rhythm, and strength. The normal heart rate varies with age (❷ *Table 6-2*). Tachycardia is a fairly reliable marker of circulatory compromise. It may be a response to hypovolemia or cardiac ischemia; or it may also be a cause of circulatory compromise when a brief diastolic interval precludes adequate cardiac filling. In most cases, tachycardia and cutaneous vasoconstriction are early and predictable physiologic responses to hypovolemia. The appearance of tachycardia indicates a loss of 15–30% of circulating blood volume. With increasing blood loss, there is a progressive increase in heart rate and respiratory rate (❷ *Table 6-3*). An abnormal rhythm may also signify cardiac ischemia or be associated with compromised cardiac output, such as is the case with rapid atrial fibrillation or flutter. Whereas a strong distal pulse is reassuring, a thready pulse signifies circulatory compromise. The minimal systolic blood pressure may be estimated by the anatomic location of a palpable pulse (❷ *Table 6-4*). Finally, asymmetry of pulses is typical of pathologic processes such as atherosclerotic stenosis, arterial dissection, or other pathology.

One should be mindful of special circumstances during which the expected physiological responses to inadequate circulation may not be apparent. For example the elderly may be unable to mount the expected increase in heart rate or inotropy in order to respond to shock due to a decrease in sympathetic tone and reserve. Additionally, the use of beta-adrenergic antagonist medication or a

■ Table 6-2

Normal pulse rate variations with age

Age (years)	Infant	2–6	7–13	Adult (>13)
Normal pulse range (bpm)	140–160	120–140	100–120	60–100

■ Table 6-3

Estimated fluid and blood losses based on patient's presentation (Adapted from American College of Surgeons' Committee on Trauma, 2004. With permission)

	CLASS 1	CLASS II	CLASS III	CLASS IV
Blood loss (ml)	Up to 750	750–1,500	1,500–2,000	>2,000
Blood loss (% blood volume)	Up to 15%	15–30%	30–40%	>40%
Pulse rate (bpm)	<100	>100	>120	>140
Blood pressure (mmHg)	Normal	Normal	Decreased	Decreased
Respiratory rate	14–20	20–30	30–40	>40
Urine output (ml/h)	>30	20–30	5–15	Negligible
CNS/Mental status	Slightly anxious	Mildly anxious	Anxious, confused	Confused, lethargic
Fluid replacement (3:1 rule)	Crystalloid	Crystalloid	Crystalloid and blood	Crystalloid and blood

◼ Table 6-4

Approximate minimal systolic blood pressures based on palpable pulse locations

Pulse location	Radial	Brachial	Femoral	Carotid
Approximate SBP (mmHg)	90	80	70	60

cardiac pacemaker in this cohort of patients may prevent the tachycardic response to hemorrhage. Also, in young healthy athletic adults and in pregnant women, physiological adaptations result in a markedly expanded blood volume. Thus, relatively large amounts of blood loss may result in only modest elevations in heart rate. This relative hypervolemia provides an additional compensatory mechanism for the individual and limits the elevation in heart rate until a profound volume of blood is lost.

Blood Pressure

Non-invasive (Sphygmomanometry)

The blood pressure cuff is applied to a limb, usually the upper arm, and is inflated to a pressure that eliminates flow in the underlying artery as determined by auscultation or palpation of loss of a pulse. When the cuff is deflated and cuff pressure falls below systolic pressure, blood begins to flow through the artery again, but in turbulent fashion. This first audible sound is designated the systolic blood pressure. As the cuff is deflated, the artery will no longer be compressed, and flow will become laminar again and no longer be audible. The pressure at which this occurs is designated the diastolic pressure

The clinician must be wary of relying too heavily on sphygmomanometry for patient care. The arterial blood pressure "is one of the most common and most unreliable measurements in modern medicine." Cuff pressures can be misleading because this mode relies on the assumption that pressures in the cuff are the same as those in the encompassed artery. While this assumption is usually correct, errors often occur as the result of inappropriately sized cuffs. Although seldom checked, the length of the bladder of the cuff should be at least 80% of the circumference of the upper arm, and the width at least 40% of the circumference of the upper arm in order for the measurement to be accurate. If the bladder is too small, blood pressure measurements will be erroneously high; if too big, erroneously low. Patients with atherosclerotic disease may have falsely elevated readings due to non-compressible, calcified arteries. In the morbidly obese, due to a conical rather than cylindrical shape of the arm or a poor fit of the blood pressure cuff pressure, the readings may be falsely elevated. Furthermore, due to limitation on human hearing, listening for sounds generated from the artery (Korotkoff sounds) as the cuff deflates can be very inaccurate, especially during hypotension. On the other hand, automated blood pressure cuffs are not consistently accurate when systolic blood pressures are below 110 mmHg (American College of Surgeons' Committee on Trauma, 2004). For these reasons, direct intravascular monitoring may be preferred in critically ill patients.

Invasive (Arterial Lines)

Arterial lines are an invasive means of monitoring blood pressure that require the cannulation of an artery, but provide real-time assessment of the blood pressure. Indications for arterial line insertion include the need for continuous arterial pressure monitoring, arterial blood gas monitoring, and access for frequent blood tests. Although an improvement over sphygmomanometry, arterial lines too, can be inaccurate. After the artery is cannulated and the pressure transducer is calibrated, the transducer must be zeroed at the level of the right atrium or else reading will be erroneous: falsely elevated if the transducer is too low, falsely depressed if the transducer is too high.

The measured systolic pressure may be inaccurate due to mismatching between the catheter and the artery, catheter whip, or reflected pressure waves. Mismatching refers to the compliance of the catheter relative to the arterial wall. If the catheter tubing is too stiff compared to the artery, the systolic pressure will be higher and the diastolic lower than the actual pressure in the artery. Conversely, if the tubing is more compliant than the vessel, dampening of the pressure will occur, and the measured systolic pressure will be lower and the diastolic pressure higher. Catheter whip is due to movement of the catheter within the lumen of the vessel. This usually occurs when the catheter is placed in a relatively large vessel, such as the femoral artery, and can cause the measurements of systolic pressure to vary by approximately 20 mmHg. The systolic pressure is normally amplified in the periphery due to pressure waves being reflected back centrally from vascular bifurcations and stenotic vessels. As pathophysiologic atherosclerotic changes occur in the vessels, this amplification will be more pronounced and systolic pressures will be falsely elevated. Also, severe peripheral vasoconstriction may lower pressure in the distal arteries compared to the proximal arteries. Given these potential inaccuracies, it is wise to follow – and titrate therapy – to the mean arterial pressure, as it is relatively consistent throughout the vasculature and should be considered accurate.

Cannulation of an artery is not a completely benign procedure and can lead to serious complications. These include catheter-related bloodstream infections, pseudoaneurysms, and thromboembolism. The latter may lead to distal ischemia or necrosis. Therefore arterial catheters should be inserted in arteries with considerable collateral circulation, such as the radial artery, rather than brachial artery. Because ischemia of the hand is functionally devastating, one should always assess collateral circulation of the radial artery before cannulation by performing an Allen's test. Continuous intraarterial fluid infusion may also be employed to prevent catheter thrombosis.

Central Venous Pressure Monitoring

Central venous pressure (CVP) monitoring involves the measurement of pressure in a central vein (e.g. vena cava, subclavian vein, jugular vein). Although pressure does not always equate to volume, CVP is used to assess preload as well as right heart function. The transducer must be placed at the zero reference point, known as the phlebostatic axis, for central venous pressures to be accurate. This phlebostatic axis is the artificial point on the thorax where the fourth intercostal space meets the midaxillary line, and corresponds to the position of the right and left atria in the supine position.

Since the intrathoracic pressure varies with the respiratory cycle, the most accurate CVP measurement is made at end-expiration when the vascular transmural pressures approach zero. The practitioner must account for positive end-expiratory pressure (PEEP) in patients who are being mechanically ventilated because this may elevate the measured CVP. Alternatively, if the patient can tolerate it, the CVP may be measured with the PEEP temporarily discontinued.

Although the "normal" CVP is quoted as between 4–8 mmHg, the optimal CVP for circulatory adequacy depends on the function of the heart. In general, a sick patient with a low CVP (0–4 mmHg)

◘ Table 6-5

Factors leading to elevated CVP

Acute left sided myocardial infarction
Diseases with ejection fraction < 50%
Mitral or tricuspid value regurgitation
Pulmonary embolism
Tension pneumothorax
Pericardial tamponade

usually benefits from volume resuscitation, and a patient with a "normal" CVP (4–8 mmHg) may or may not benefit from additional fluid. When the CVP is > 8 mmHg, the clinician may need to use additional means to assess the circulatory adequacy and then make a therapeutic decision. Of particular significance is the change in CVP over time, e.g. after fluid resuscitation, and what affect this has on cardiac function, vital signs, tissue perfusion, and overall clinical status. Only a change of CVP of greater than 4 mmHg is considered clinically significant.

In a patient with normal cardiac function, CVP approximates the pulmonary capillary wedge pressure, which in turn approximates the left atrial end-diastolic pressure. However, there are multiple acute and chronic cardiac and pulmonary diseases that interfere with this relationship. These are listed in ❱ *Table 6-5*. In these cases, simultaneous assessment of right and left heart function with a pulmonary artery catheter may be helpful (see below).

When deciding to monitor CVP one must consider the risks of inserting a CVP catheter into the internal jugular or subclavian vein. These include pneumothorax, hemothorax, chylothorax, brachial plexus injury, and mediastinitis. Several studies have shown that ultrasound guided placement of intravenous catheters is the safest method of placement.

Pulmonary Artery Catheters (Pac)

Pulmonary artery catheters are useful in assessing the filling pressures of the left and right sides of the heart and in providing objective data on cardiac performance. These long catheters (110 cm in length) are passed through a central venous introducer or cordis and then "floated" into the right heart and pulmonary artery with the assistance of an inflatable balloon located just proximal to the tip of the catheter. The balloon can then be "wedged" in a smaller pulmonary artery. From the pulmonary artery catheter, a large amount of information can be obtained (❱ *Table 6-6*). Since the measuring port of the catheter lies just distal to the balloon, and taking into account the valveless pulmonary venous system, the pulmonary capillary wedge pressure approximates the left atrial pressure (except in cases of pulmonary hypertension) which will equal left-ventricular end diastolic pressure in patients with competent mitral valves.

One value that can be extrapolated from the PAC is the Oxygen Delivery (DO_2). This is defined as the product of the oxygen content and the cardiac output (CO):

$$DO_2 = CO \times 13.4 \times Hemoglobin \times SaO_2$$

Table 6-6

Clinical data available from pulmonary artery catheters (Adapted from Marino, 1998)

Central venous pressure	Stroke volume index
Pulmonary artery pressure	Left ventricular stroke work index
Pulmonary capillary wedge pressure	Right ventricular stroke work index
Cardiac output	Right ventricular ejection fraction
Cardiac index	Systemic vascular resistance
Oxygen delivery	Pulmonary vascular resistance
Oxygen uptake	Mixed venous oxygen saturation
Oxygen extraction ratio	

Oxygen delivery is typically reported as an indexed value (normal range 520–570 ml $O_2/min/m^2$); thus the cardiac index is used in the calculation. Also, one can calculate Oxygen Consumption (VO_2), which is defined as the difference in oxygen content between the arterial and mixed venous blood:

$$VO_2 = CO \times 13.4 \times \text{Hemoglobin}(g/dl) \times (SaO_2 - SvO_2)$$

The normal range for indexed VO_2 is 110–160 ml $O_2/min/m^2$. The ratio of the Oxygen Consumption to Oxygen Delivery is called the Oxygen Extraction Ratio (O_2ER):

$$O_2ER = (VO_2/DO_2) \times 100$$

The normal range for O_2ER is 20–30%. However, this is highly variable. When metabolic demands are increased or when oxygen delivery falls, the VO_2 increases and the O_2ER can reach 50–60% in order to maintain aerobic metabolism.

Previously, Shoemaker and colleagues identified values for cardiac index (4.5 $l/min/m^2$), DO_2 (600 ml $O_2/min/m^2$) and VO_2 (170 ml $O_2/min/m^2$) above which survival could be predicted in critically ill patients. However, subsequent randomized controlled trials by other researchers using these as endpoints of resuscitation were mixed as to any survivor benefit. In support of the aforementioned research, Shoemaker and Kern published a meta-analysis of randomized controlled trials that had evaluated resuscitation to normal or supranormal values. They concluded that successful resuscitation to supranormal physiologic values resulted in a significant reduction in organ failure and mortality but only among the most severely injured (i.e. those with $>$ 20% predicted mortality) and when initiated prior to the onset of organ failure. These results are supported by Boyd whose meta-analysis of six randomized studies concluded that there was an improvement in outcome, but again only when PAC-directed therapy was initiated prior to organ failure or sepsis. Balogh and colleagues cautioned that supranormal resuscitation was associated with a higher 24 h lactated Ringer's infusion requirement, with an increased incidence of abdominal compartment syndrome, multiple organ failure and mortality. Moreover, supranormal DO_2 values do not ensure adequate oxygen utilization. Moore et al. reported on a cohort of severely injured patients in whom a supranormal VO_2 was unattainable despite a supranormal DO_2. This group had a higher incidence of multiple organ failure that was theorized to be due to defective aerobic metabolism.

The Mixed Venous Oxygen Saturation (SvO_2) is the concentration of oxygen within the pulmonary artery and represents a mixture of blood returning from all parts of the body. As such, it is used as an indicator of global perfusion. The normal SvO_2 is approximately 75%. As with any physiologic variable of tissue oxygenation, it is nonspecific and is a function of oxygenation by the lungs, oxygen delivery by the cardiovascular system, and oxygen uptake by the tissues. A drop in SvO_2 could be due to deterioration in cardiac or pulmonary function, or an increase in O_2 consumption. On the other hand, the SvO_2 may be elevated in situations such as septic shock due to impaired tissue extraction and utilization of oxygen. Not even a normal SvO_2 ensures adequate oxygenation, and some advocate for concomitant lactic acid levels.

Consequently, the SvO_2 value is most helpful when it is (a) initially corroborated with another measure of perfusion, such as lactic acid; and (b) followed continuously over time. Technology exists now that provides real-time SvO_2 measurements utilizing specialized PACs that have a continuous SvO_2 monitor at the tip of the catheter. Any sudden or significant change in SvO_2 provides an early warning of a worsening condition and should prompt an aggressive search for its cause.

Similar to any invasive catheter, PACs are associated with risks such as bacterial contamination, thrombosis, and embolism. However, there are additional complications that are unique to PACs. During the manipulation of the catheter, ventricular dysrhythmias can be triggered, as well as valvular injury induced. In a patient with a pre-existing left bundle branch block, the catheter can lead to complete heart block by interfering with the right bundle branch conduction. Also, case reports of intracardiac catheter knotting have been reported.

The severe bleeding risks associated with PACs deserve special mention. The first is right ventricular perforation, which occurs due to overly aggressive insertion and can lead to pericardial tamponade and possibly death. The other is rupture of the pulmonary artery itself. This occurs when the balloon is placed (or migrates) too distally into the pulmonary artery or when the balloon is over inflated. The rupture presents suddenly as hemoptysis either during or immediately after inflation of the catheter balloon, and often mandates emergent thoracotomy with lung resection. Risk factors include pulmonary artery hypertension, advanced age, lung cancer, and coagulopathies (Bishop et al., 1993).

In addition to the risks of technical complications, several recent trials have questioned the clinical benefit of PACs. On the other hand, it has been suggested that the fault lies not with the PAC but with the interpretation of the data that it provides. The PAC is a tool with value primarily in patients whose clinical response to CVP-directed therapy is unexpected or in whom specific objective measures of cardiac performance are desired in order to direct inotropic or vasopressor therapy.

Serum Lactate

With hypoperfusion, aerobic metabolism cannot occur and anaerobic metabolism ensues. Pyruvate is therefore converted into lactic acid rather than being shunted into the tricarboxylic acid cycle. This lactic acid is released into the bloodstream and can be measured as an indicator of global perfusion. Multiple studies have demonstrated that elevated blood lactate is a reliable marker of hypoperfusion. Furthermore, failure to clear the lactate level to normal levels with 24 h was associated with a mortality of $> 75\%$.

One disadvantage of relying on blood serum lactate is that factors other than hypoperfusion may cause lactic acidosis. Lactic acidosis is classified as either Type A, Type B, or D-lactic acidosis. Type A includes syndromes associated with inadequate oxygen delivery, whereas type B lactic acidosis typically represents conditions during which lactic acidosis exists in the absence of hypoperfusion. A complete list is shown in ❯ *Table 6-7.*

◘ Table 6-7

Lactic acidosis

Type A
Circulatory insufficiency (shock, heart failure)
Severe anemia
Cholera
Mitochondrial enzyme defects
Carbon monoxide poisoning
Cyanide poisoning
Type B
Hypoglycemia (glycogen storage diseases)
Seizures
Diabetes mellitus
Ethanol
Severe hepatic insufficiency
Malignancy
Salicylates
Severe exercise
D-lactic acidosis
Short gut syndrome
Jejuno-ileal bypass operation

Base Deficit

The Base deficit is a measure of the number of millimoles of base required to correct the pH of a liter of whole blood to 7.40. The normal range of base deficit is $+3$ to -3 mmol/l. One may calculate the base deficit from the arterial blood gas as follows:

If $PaCO_2 < 40$

$$\text{Ideal } PaCO_2 \text{ (i.e. 40)} - \text{measured } PaCO_2 = \Delta PaCO_2$$

$$\textit{Then } \Delta PaCO_2 \times 0.008 = \text{calculated } \Delta pH$$

$$\textit{Then } (7.40 + \text{calculated } \Delta pH) - \text{measured pH} = \text{actual } \Delta pH$$

$$\textit{Then } \text{actual } \Delta pH \times 2/3 \times 100 = \text{Base deficit}$$

If $PaCO_2 > 40$

$$\text{Measured } PaCO_2 - \text{Ideal } PaCO_2 \text{ (i.e. 40)} = \Delta paCO_2$$

$$\text{Then } \Delta PaCO_2 \times 0.008 = \text{calculated } \Delta pH$$

$$\text{Then } (7.40 - \text{calculated } \Delta pH) - \text{measured pH} = \text{actual } \Delta pH$$

$$\text{Then } \text{actual } \Delta pH \times 2/3 \times 100 = \text{Base deficit}$$

Early on during hypovolemia, base deficit can be used as an indirect measurement of lactic acidosis. In seminal work done by Davis and colleagues (Davis et al., 1991), base deficit was shown to correlate with volume requirement as well as being a sensitive indicator of severity of shock and efficacy of resuscitation. However, the base deficit lacks specificity, and any condition that leads to acidemia (e.g. renal tubular acidosis, diabetic ketoacidosis) will lead to elevations in the base deficit.

Summary

Assessment of circulatory adequacy is an integral component of surgical care. Physical examination and assessment of vital signs may detect more profound circulatory deficits. However, there is a role for more invasive monitoring in critically ill patients. In complex patients who may be susceptible to occult hypoperfusion, monitoring of global indicators of perfusion can help guide resuscitation.

Selected Readings

Abramson D, Scalea TM, Hitchcock R, et al. (1993) Lactate clearance and survival following injury. J Trauma 35:584–588

American College of Surgeons' Committee on Trauma (2004) Advanced Trauma Life Support for Doctors (ATLS) Student manual, 7th edn. American College of Surgeons, Chicago, IL

Balogh Z, McKinley MA, Cocanour CS, et al. (2003) Supranormal trauma resuscitation causes more cases of abdominal compartment syndrome. Arch Surg 138:637–642

Bishop MH, Shoemaker WC, Appel PL, et al. (1993) Relationship between supranormal circulatory values, time delays, and outcomes in severely traumatized patients. Crit Care Med 21:56–63

Boyd O (2000) The high risk surgical patient: where are we now? Clin Intensive Care Special Issue:3–10

Burchard KW, Gann DS, Wiles CE (2000) The circulation, ch. 2. In: Burchard KW, Gann DS, Wiles CE (eds) The clinical handbook for surgical critical care. Parthenon, New York

Davis JW, Davis IC, Bennink LD, et al. (2003) Are automated blood pressure measurements accurate in trauma patients? J Trauma 55:860–863

Davis JW, Shackford SR, Holbrook TL (1991) Base deficit as a sensitive indicator of compensated shock and tissue oxygen utilization. Surg Gynecol Obstet 173:473

Davis JW, Shackford SR, Mackersie RC, et al. (1988) Base deficit as a guide to volume resuscitation. J. Trauma 28:146

DuBose, Thomas Jr D (1998) Acidosis and alkalosis, ch. 50. In: Fauci AS, Braunwald E, Isselbacher KJ, et al. (eds)

Harrison's principles of internal medicine, 14th edn. McGraw Hill, New York, pp 279–280

Elliott DC (1998) An evaluation of the endpoints of resuscitation. J Am Coll Surg 187:536–547

Friedman G, et al. (1995) Combined measurements of blood lactate concentrations and gastric intramucosal pH in patients with severe sepsis. Crit Care Med 23:1184–1193

Marino PL (1998) Hemodynamic monitoring, sec. 3. In: Marino PL (ed) The ICU book, 2nd edn. Williams & Wilkins, Baltimore, MD

Holcroft JW, Anderson JT (2005) Cardiopulmonary monitoring, sec. 6, ch. 4. In: American College of Surgeons (eds) ACS surgery principles and practice. WebMD Publishing, New York

Iberti TJ, et al. (1990) A multicenter study of physicians' knowledge of the pulmonary artery catheter. JAMA 264:2928–2932

Keenan, SP (2002) Use of ultrasound to place central lines. J Crit Care 17:126–137

Kern JW, Shoemaker WC (2002) Meta-analysis of hemodynamic optimization in high-risk patients. Crit Care Med 30:1686–1692

Moore FA, Haenel JB, Moore EE, et al. (1992) Incommensurate oxygen consumption in response to maximal oxygen availability predicts post-injury multiple organ failure. J Trauma 33:58–66

Shah MR et al. (2005) Impact of the pulmonary artery catheter in critically ill patients: meta-analysis of randomized clinical trials. JAMA 294:1664–1670

7 Acute Pain Management

Edmund A. M. Neugebauer

Pearls and Pitfalls

- Sufficient pain management is a prerequisite for enhanced patient recovery and for a reduction in postoperative morbidity and mortality.
- Pain assessment and documentation ("fifth vital sign") are fundamental prerequisites for adequate pain management.
- Opioids remain the fundamental group of analgesic drugs for the treatment of moderate to severe pain.
- Co-analgesics support the action of analgesics but are not sufficient alone for postoperative pain relief.
- Peripheral nerve blocks have the advantage of not compromising patient alertness.
- Local analgesics are very effective in epidural analgesia.
- Epidural local anesthetics lead to a decreased incidence of pulmonary infection and complications overall compared with opioids.
- Treatment of acute pain should be procedure-specific and treatment should be adapted to the measured pain intensity reported by the patient.
- Pain management is an interdisciplinary task requiring close liaison with all personnel involved in the care of the patient.
- Use of evidence-based clinical practice guidelines are recommended and should be adapted locally.

"Acute pain management is a basic human right."
(Professor M. I. Cousins, President, Australian and New Zealand College of Anaesthetists)

Although major efforts have been conducted to improve acute pain management in recent years, we are still far away in meeting this basic human right. In the USA and Europe, the results of studies dedicated specifically to both medical and postoperative patients in academic hospitals have shown unequivocally that pain remains undertreated. Pain should *not* be an accompanying phenomenon of medical treatments; in principle, the possibilities for adequate pain management are available to all. Sufficient pain therapy is an important prerequisite for enhanced patient recovery and will reduce the postoperative risk of morbidity and mortality. Moreover, a significant reduction in long-term morbidity can be achieved since moderate to severe pain has been demonstrated as an independent predictor for chronic postoperative pain. Adequate pain therapy is cost-effective; it is associated with a decrease in both intensive care and overall hospital stay. Studies have shown that up to 70% of patients present to hospital because of acute pain.

Furthermore, they associate the success of medical treatment with the relief of pain and it is of significant value from the patients' perspective.

Definition

Pain as defined by the International Association for the Study of Pain is "an unpleasant sensory and emotional experience associated with actual or potential tissue damage, or described in terms of such damage." Pain is subjective and is an individual, multifactorial experience influenced by culture, previous pain events, mood, beliefs, and an ability to cope. *Acute pain* is defined as "pain of recent onset and probable limited duration." It usually has an identifiable temporal and causal relationship to injury (trauma, operation) or disease (colic, peritonitis, etc.). *Chronic pain* persists commonly beyond the time of healing of an injury (>3–6 months) and frequently has no clear identifiable cause. Acute and chronic pain may represent a continuum.

Pathophysiological and Pharmacological Basics

Pain development and transduction involves multiple interacting peripheral and central mechanisms. The understanding of principles is important for the choice of medical treatments and will therefore be summarized briefly. The basis of each central nervous system function is the excitation–response relationship.

Peripheral level: Acute pain starts by tissue injury caused by mechanical, thermal, or chemical excitation. The detection of noxious stimuli requires activation of peripheral sensory organs (nociceptors) and transduction of the energy into electrical signals for conduction to the central nervous system. Nociceptive afferents are distributed widely throughout the body (skin, muscle, joints, viscera, meninges).

Spinal cord level: Once transducted into electrical stimuli, conduction of neuronal action potentials into afferent input and dorsal horn output follows. This signal conduction is called transmission in the spinal cord. The processing of pain on its way from excitation to perception is subject to several transformations. Tissue damage such as that associated with infection, inflammation, or ischemia, produces an array of chemical mediators (algetic substances such as prostaglandins, and histamines) that can sensitize nociceptors to increase pain perception. This increase in sensitivity is termed peripheral sensitization, which can also lead to central sensitization. In addition to the excitatory processes, inhibitory modulation occurs within the dorsal horn.

Central projecting level: A peripheral pain signal, which reaches the central nervous system after transduction, transmission, and transformation needs to be translated into pain perception. The areas of the brain involved are the limbic system, cortex (e.g. cingulate cortex, insula, prefrontal cortex), and thalamus. The perception and experience of pain is multifactorial and is further influenced by psychological and environmental factors of each individual. ❯ *Figure 7-1* gives a schematic representation of the nociceptor pathway.

For adequate pain management, it is necessary to be familiar with the main mechanisms of pain relief by the different analgesic drugs (❯ *Table 7-1* and ❯ *Fig. 7-2*). Analgesic drugs can be subdivided into five major categories.

■ Figure 7-1
Overview of the nociceptor pathway

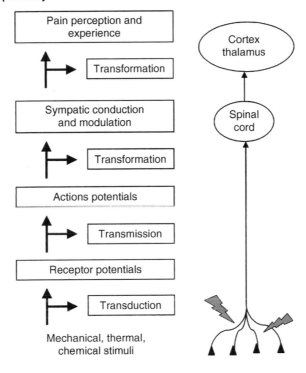

■ Table 7-1
Categories of analgesic drugs

- Non-opioids
- Opioids
- Local anesthetics
- Co-analgesics
- Adjuvant drugs

Non-opioid Analgesics

The basic action of most non-opioids (nonsteroidal anti-inflammatory drugs — NSAIDs) is the inhibition of the cyclooxygenase (COX) enzymes. Two subtypes of COX enzymes have been identified — the constitutive COX-1 and the "inducible" COX-2, and now a COX-3 is being investigated. Many of the effects of NSAIDs can be explained by inhibition of prostaglandin synthesis in peripheral tissues, nerves, and the central nervous system. Prostaglandins have many physiological functions including gastric mucosal protection, renal tubular function, intrarenal vasodilatation, bronchodilatation, and production of endothelial prostacyclin. Such physiological roles are mainly regulated by COX-1 and are a basis for many of the adverse effects associated with NSAID use. Tissue damage results in COX-2 production, leading to synthesis of prostaglandins that result in pain and inflammation. NSAIDs are

◘ Figure 7-2
Nociceptive pathway and therapeutic options of pain relief

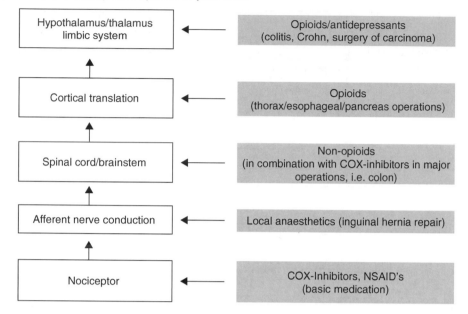

nonselective COX inhibitors that inhibit both COX-1 and COX-2 with a wide spectrum of analgesic, anti-inflammatory, antipyretic effects. Aspirin acetylates inhibit COX irreversibly but NSAIDs are reversible inhibitors of enzymes. The COX-2 inhibitors (e.g., parecoxib) have been developed to selectively inhibit the inducible form. Arylacid derivatives (diclofenac) and aryl propionic derivates (ibuprofen) are non-selective COX-inhibitors. Paracetamol (acetaminophen) and metamizol have additional central effects. A combination of paracetamol and NSAIDs has additive effects on postoperative analgesia.

Opioids

Opioids remain the central group of analgesic drugs for the treatment of moderate to severe acute pain and transmit their action via different types of receptors. Opioids can be differentiated into pure μ-agonists (morphine, oxycodone, fentanyl, tramadole), mixed agonists–antagonists (antagonistic at μ-receptors and agonistic at κ- and σ-receptors, e.g., pentazocin, tilidine), partial agonists with high affinity and small intrinsic activity at μ-receptors (buprenorphine), and pure antagonists (at μ-, κ-, and σ-receptors) such as naloxone.

The opioid receptors are located mostly at structures that are involved in transmission, transformation, and translation of afferent signals. A high density is found in the limbic system, the thalamus, the pons region, and the substancia gelatinosa in the dorsal horn. Clinically meaningful side effects are dose-related; once a threshold dose is reached, every 3–4 mg increase of morphine-equivalent dose per day is associated with one additional adverse event. The most significant adverse effects are sedation, pruritus, nausea, and vomiting. The risk can be reduced significantly by parallel application of NSAIDs and/or adjuvant drugs. In the management of acute pain one opioid is not superior to others but some opioids appear more effective in some patients than others.

Local Anesthetics

Local anesthetics exert their effects as analgesics by impeding neuronal excitation and/or conduction. Short-duration local anesthetics (lignocaine, plasma half-life 90 m) have to be differentiated from long-duration local anesthetics (bupivacaine, ropivacaine). The local anesthetic effect depends very much on the site of administration, the dose administered, and the presence or absence of vasoconstrictors. Local application of 20 ml 0.25% bupivacaine in the area of trocar incision sites in laparoscopic cholecystectomy or colectomy reduces postoperative pain intensity significantly.

Local anesthetics are very effective in epidural analgesia. The quality of pain relief from low-dose epidural infusion (bupivacaine 0.1%, ropivacaine 0.2%) is improved consistently from the addition of adjuvants such as opioids. The concept of fast-track recovery benefits most from the application of an epidural.

Co-Analgesics and Adjuvant Drugs

Co-analgesics support the action of analgesics but are not sufficient alone for postoperative pain management. However, they are extremely helpful in combination with opioids and NSAIDs, and can reduce postoperative analgesic requirements (❯ *Table 7-2*). Adjuvant drugs are mainly used to decrease side effects of analgesic drugs such as emesis, vomiting, and constipation.

Assessment and Documentation of Acute Pain

Pain assessment and documentation are fundamental prerequisites for adequate pain management. Regular assessment leads to improved pain management. Under routine clinical conditions measurement of pain intensity is sufficient and should be performed by visual analogue or numerical rating scales. Self-reporting of pain should be used whenever appropriate as pain is by definition, a subjective experience. In the pre- and postoperative setting scoring should include static (rest) and dynamic (pain on sitting, coughing) measurements at least two times a day and following treatment of pain to determine efficacy. The score should be documented in the patient's charts as the "fifth vital sign." Uncontrolled or unexpected pain requires reassessment of the diagnosis and consideration of alternative causes for pain.

◼ Table 7-2

Co-analgesics and their main functions

Antidepressant	Increase function of inhibitory transmitter (e.g., serotonin, noradrenalin) (i.e., aminotryptiline)
Anticonvulsive	Supportive in neuropathic pain syndromes (e.g., carbamacepine, gabapentine)
Muscle relaxant	Supportive in muscle pain and spasms (e.g., benzodiazepine)
Corticosteroid	Anti-inflammatory (e.g., dexamethasone)
Bisphosphonate	Supporative in bony pain syndromes after metastasis of tumors (e.g., clodronate, pamidronate)

General Pain Management Procedures

The surgeon has a special responsibility in the treatment of pain. Aside from pharmacological interventions, consideration should be given to the possibility of intervention before, during, and after surgery to optimize pain management.

Preoperatively, the surgeon has to provide procedural information to the patient that summarizes what will happen during treatment and it is necessary to obtain sensory experiences from the patient (patient expectations). Combined sensory and procedural information is effective in reducing negative effect and reports of procedure-related pain and anxiety. The placebo-effect plays an important role and should be used. Patient information and training regarding coping and relaxation strategies have been shown to reduce pain and distress. The patients should be convinced that their pain is of utmost importance to the treating team and that they can also contribute to the success of pain management (patient as partner/co-therapist).

Intraoperatively, all treatments to the patient should be performed under the philosophy of avoiding pain wherever possible (minimal invasive techniques, positioning, etc). Drains should be avoided and wound closure should be performed preferably with absorbable sutures.

Postoperatively, a whole array of preventive measures should be considered with respect to reducing pain and associated complications: early rehabilitation (fast-track), wound management, physiotherapy, cold/heat massage techniques, and removal of lines and drains as soon as possible.

Medical Pain Management Procedures

Peripheral Nerve Blockade

The main advantage of using peripheral nerve blockade techniques as compared to systemic drug therapy is that the use of local anesthetics does not compromise patient alertness and allows pain-free mobilization.

Peripheral nerve blocks may be used for diagnostic and therapeutic purposes. Important technical issues include the technique of nerve location, the type of catheter equipment, the amount of drug, and the duration of drug efficacy. Following diagnostic location of the nerve, a continuous blockade can be undertaken. Local anesthetics such as lidocaine, mepivocaine, or prilocaine have a 2 h duration of efficacy whereas bupivacaine and ropivacaine can produce pain relief for up to 12 h. Adjuvant techniques may prolong the duration of action. For example, wound infiltration with a long-acting local anesthetic agent provides effective analgesia following inguinal hernia repair but not for open cholecystectomy or hysterectomy. Continuous femoral nerve blockade provides postoperative analgesia and functional recovery superior to intravenous morphine with fewer side effects and is comparable to epidural analgesia following knee-joint replacement surgery.

Both single injection and continuous application carry the risk of neurological injury, intravascular injection, dislodgment, hematoma, and infection. The incidence of neurological injury following peripheral nerve blocks is 0.02–0.4%.

Epidural Analgesia

Epidural analgesia (i.e., the provision of pain relief by continuous administration of pharmacological agents into the epidural space via an indwelling catheter) has become a widely used technique for the management of acute pain after surgery and trauma. Regardless of the analgesic agent used, location of catheter, or the type of surgery, it provides better pain relief than parenteral opioid administration. Improved pain relief with epidural local anesthetics leads to a decreased incidence of pulmonary infection and other pulmonary complications overall when compared with systemic opioids. The combination of a low concentration of local anesthetic and opioid is superior to either of the drugs alone. The addition of small amounts of adrenaline (epinephrine) to such mixtures improves analgesia and reduces systemic opioid consumption. Administration of a local anesthetic into the thoracic epidural space results in improved bowel recovery, but this benefit is not consistent with lumbar administration. Adverse effects are uncommon but include permanent neurological damage, which is reported at 0.05–0.0005%, and epidural hematoma (0.0005%). Others include respiratory depression (1–15%) and hypotension (5–10%).

Systemic Analgesia

Necessary prerequisites for patient-orientated systemic pain therapy are good knowledge and understanding of the cause of pain (inflammation, spasm, type of operation or operative access, anxiety, or depression of the patient), the anatomy and pain transduction, and, based on this information, the necessary surgical, physical, psychological, or medical therapy. Whereas chronic pain treatment starts with non-pharmacological techniques (psychotherapy, TENS, etc.) followed by mild non-opioid analgesics, and, subsequently, strong opioids, the treatment of acute pain follows the reverse order (❯ *Fig. 7-3*).

Strong opioids combined with NSAIDs are used as first-line therapy to control pain when intensity is highest. Analgesic drugs given by the intravenous route have a more rapid onset of action compared

◻ Figure 7-3
WHO's pain ladder of acute and chronic pain therapy

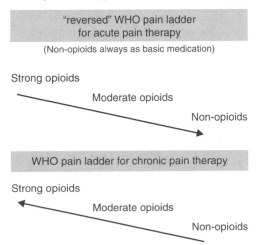

with most other routes of administration. Titration of opioid therapy for severe acute pain is best achieved using intermittent intravenous bolus doses (2–3 mg of morphine at 5 min intervals until relief of pain). Relative or absolute overdosing (also rapid injection) may lead to complications and side effects independent of the opioid used. However, the risk of overdosing with resultant respiratory depression is not an issue as long as the patient continues to experience pain. If it occurs, sufficient antagonists (naloxon 0.4 mg) should always be available and the sedation level should be assessed in parallel. Continuous infusion of opioids in the general ward setting is not recommended because of the increased risk of respiratory depression compared with other methods of parenteral opioid administration.

Non-opioid analgesics have an antipyretic and anti-inflammatory effect. They should be administered either solely (such as after minor operations) or in combination with opioids. Opioid and non-opioid drugs can be administered systemically by a number of different routes. The choice of route is determined by various factors including the overall condition of the patient but also by the ease of use, accessibility, speed of analgesic onset, duration of action, and patient acceptability. In general, the principle of individualization of dose and dosing intervals should apply to the administration of all analgesic drugs, whatever the route. Frequent assessment of the patient's pain and their response to treatment rather than strict adherence to a given dosing regimen is required if adequate analgesia is to be obtained.

Oral administration is straightforward, noninvasive, has good efficacy in most settings, and has a high patient acceptability. Other than in the treatment of severe acute pain, it is the route of choice for most analgesic drugs provided that there is no contraindication to its use. After major operations or trauma, the aim should be to change to the oral route as quickly as possible. The analgesic efficacy varies from one pain model to another and the administration of analgesics should be procedure-specific. Although still used commonly, intramuscular injection of analgesic agents is no longer recommended because of the significant risk of abscess formation, nerve lesions, and necrosis. Subcutaneous injection shares the same problem as intramuscular administration that absorption may be impaired in situations of poor perfusion. This leads to inadequate early analgesia and late absorption of the drug depot when perfusion is re-established. Rectal administration of drugs is useful when other routes are unavailable. Transdermal routes for opioid administration (fentanyl or buprenorphine patches) are not recommended for acute pain management due to safety concerns (respiratory depression) and the difficulties in short-term dose adjustments that may be required for titration.

The general rule is that the patient should determine their analgesic requirement within given limitations for all routes of administration. Patient-controlled analgesia (PCA) refers to methods of pain relief that allow the patient to self-administer small doses of an analgesic agent as required. This is not necessarily associated only to the use of programmable infusion pumps. Adequate analgesia needs to be obtained prior to commencement of PCA. Initial instructions for bolus doses should take into account individual patient factors such as history of prior opioid use and patient age. Individual prescriptions may need to be adjusted and drug concentrations should be standardized within each institution to reduce programming errors. A background infusion is not recommended in acute pain management.

Organization of Acute Pain Management

Pain management is an interdisciplinary undertaking. Successful management of acute pain requires close liaison with all personnel involved in the care of the patient and should include surgeons, anesthesiologists, and nurses. Effective acute pain management will only result from appropriate education and organizational structures for the delivery of pain relief. Clear-cut responsibilities between disciplines are mandatory and this may differ between countries or even hospitals. Effective organizational structures for the delivery of pain relief are often more important than the analgesic techniques themselves. In some institutions, acute pain services (APS) are responsible for managing more advanced methods of pain relief such as PCA and epidural analgesia. There is a wide diversity of APS structures (from low-cost nurse-based through to multidisciplinary services) with different responsibilities. A recent review of publications analyzing the effectiveness of APS concluded that its implementation is associated with a significant improvement of pain relief with a possible reduction of postoperative nausea and vomiting.

Marked improvements in conventional methods of pain relief can be expected by the introduction of evidence-based clinical practice guidelines. However, it is the implementation of guidelines and not their development, which remains the greatest obstacle to their use. Professional bodies in a number of countries have published guidelines for the management of acute pain. A procedure-specific approach is highly recommended such as the online PROSPECT group (www.postoppain.org). Resource availability, staff with pain management expertise, and the existence of formal quality assurance programs to monitor pain management are positive predictors of compliance with guidelines. Official guidelines need to be adapted for individual hospital requirements and the ward nurses play the most significant role in local adaptation. With their support, and that of clinical management and directors of surgical departments, national guidelines on acute pain management have been successfully translated into the initiative "Pain Free Clinic." The Cologne City Hospital, Merheim was the first in Germany to receive board certification by an external organization. This initiative can serve as a role model for other hospitals in improving the organization of acute pain management with benefit to the patients and the hospital.

Selected Readings

American Society of Anesthesiologists (2004) Practice guidelines for acute pain management in the perioperative setting. An updated report by the American Society of Anesthesiologists Task Force on Acute Pain Management. Anesthesiology 100:1573–1581

Australian and New Zealand College of Anaesthetists and Faculty of Pain Medicine (2005) Acute pain management: scientific evidence, 2nd edn. National Health and Medial Research Council. http://www.nhmrc.gov.au/publications/subjects/clinical.htm

Ballantyne IS, Carr DB, de Ferranti S, et al. (1998) The comparative effects of postoperative analgesic therapies on pulmonary outcome: cumulative meta-analyses of randomized, controlled trials. Anaesth Analg 86:598–612

Kehlet H (1997) Multimodal approaches to control postoperative pathophysiology and rehabilitation. Br J Anaesth 78:606–617

Kehlet H, Gray AW, Bonnett F, et al. (2005) A procedure-specific systematic review and consensus recommendations for postoperative analgesia following laparoscopic cholecystectomy. Surg Endosc 19:1396–1415

Neugebauer E (2005) Initiative Schmerzfreie Klinik – (k)eine vision. Der Schmerz 19:557

Neugebauer E, Hempl K, Sauuerland ST, et al. (1998) Situation der perioperativen Schmerztherapie in Deutschland – Ergebnisse einer repräsentativen, anonymen Umfrage von 1000 chirurgischen. Kliniken Chirurg 69:461–466

Veterans Health Administration D. o. D. Clinical practice guideline for management of postoperative pain (2002) http://www.oqp.med.va.gov/cqg/PAIN/PAIN_base.htm

Werner MU, Søholm L, Rotbøll-Nielssen, et al. (2002) Does an acute pain service improve postoperative outcome. Anaesth Analg 95:1361–1372

Zhao SZ, Chung F, Hanna P, et al. (2004) Dose-response relationship between opioids use and adverse effects after ambulatory surgery. Pain Symptom Manage 28:35–46

Trauma and Burns

8 Initial Evaluation of the Trauma Patient

Donald A. Reiff · Loring W. Rue III

Pearls and Pitfalls

- Based upon the mechanism of trauma, all possible injuries should be excluded through the pursuit of appropriate examinations and diagnostic studies to reduce the risk of unrecognized occult injury.
- Uncooperative and combative patients should be assumed hypoxic, under the influence of drugs and/or alcohol, or to have suffered significant head injury.
- When in doubt definitive control of the airway using an endotracheal tube is appropriate.
- Use an end-tidal carbon dioxide detection device, followed by auscultation, to determine adequate placement of the endotracheal tube.
- If the esophagus is inadvertently intubated while attempting airway control, leave the tube in place. This will protect the airway from gastric contents and eliminate the need for subsequent esophageal intubation.
- Large, persistent pleural air leaks may be caused by a disrupted mainstem bronchus. This injury will likely require a second tube thoracostomy, selective intubation of the uninjured bronchus by experienced personnel, and surgical repair.
- Proximal extremity injuries should have intravenous (IV) access obtained in the *contralateral* uninjured limb.
- A worsening base deficit is likely caused by unrecognized blood loss or inadequate volume resuscitation.
- Following blunt trauma, maintain spine precautions until the possibility of injury has been ruled out; apply cervical spine protection devices to patients who arrive without them.
- Failure to follow the ABCs of the primary survey for the multiply injured patient may seriously jeopardize survival; initial attention should *not* be directed toward the most dramatically obvious injury such as a mangled extremity.
- Failure to expose and examine the entire patient including the axillae, back, and perineum.
- Failure to perform a rectal examination and vaginal examination when appropriate.
- Failure to identify early signs of shock which include tachycardia, falling pulse pressure, and poor capillary refill. Compensatory mechanisms can maintain a normal systolic pressure until > 20–30% of the blood volume is lost.
- Placement of a subclavian central line on the *uninjured* side of a patient with thoracic trauma.
- Normal spine radiographs do not ensure the absence of osseous, ligamentous, or spinal injury. These diagnostic studies should be followed by a physical examination and comprehensive

neurologic assessment when the patient is not under the influence of intoxicating agents and allows a complete evaluation.

- Failure to obtain appropriate and adequate radiographs in a timely fashion.

Injury remains the leading cause of death for the first 4 decades of life and results in over 300,000 permanent disabilities each year. Federal data indicate that since 2003, expenses for trauma-related disorders exceed all other medical and surgical conditions in the USA. Often termed the "Golden Hour," outcomes for injured patients are enhanced by expeditious and appropriate surgical care rendered soon after injury. With the development of the Advanced Trauma Life Support (ATLS) protocols designed by the American College of Surgeons in 1978, a system for care of the acutely injured patient was developed, and using this template, physicians and surgeons have a guideline for rapidly evaluating and treating critically injured patients.

Initial Approach to the Injured Patient

Upon arrival of the injured patient to the resuscitation suite, a member of the trauma team should obtain the mechanism of injury and other pertinent clinical data in rapid and organized fashion. Simultaneously, the "primary survey," focusing on life-sustaining physiologic functions, is conducted while monitoring devices are placed on the patient. As the primary survey is underway, life-threatening injuries are treated when identified. Following completion of this initial survey, the "secondary survey," which consists of the traditional "head-to-toe" physical examination, is performed, radiographic studies are obtained, and a definitive management plan is formulated for the patient.

Primary Survey

Airway

The initial evaluation of the polytrauma patient begins with an assessment of airway adequacy. Signs of compromise should be sought in the primary survey and are usually evident by an injured patient's inability to communicate verbally. Alert and conversant patients who respond with a normal-sounding voice suggest no immediate problem with airway patency while those appearing agitated may be hypoxic or under the influence of alcohol and/or drugs, unable to protect their airways. Patients who are minimally responsive or obtunded may be hypercarbic, have suffered traumatic brain injury, or also may suffer from alcohol and/or drug intoxication.

A quick and effective technique to establish a patient's airway is the chin lift and jaw thrust maneuver, which is particularly helpful when the tongue is the obstructing agent. These actions displace the soft tissue anteriorly, opening the upper airway and allowing for air passage. Other techniques include the placement of an oropharyngeal or nasopharyngeal airway. Oropharyngeal airway should be restricted to obtunded patients as this device is not tolerated by awake patients. Nasopharyngeal airways are less likely to induce vomiting but should be avoided if facial or basilar skull fractures are suspected. While these maneuvers are temporarily effective in maintaining a patent airway, their use in the acutely injured patient is frequently suggestive of the need for definitive airway control.

All trauma patients are treated as "full stomachs" and a rapid-sequence method for intubation is recommended. This technique begins with pre-oxygenation of the patient while the induction and paralytic agents are being administered. Yankour suction should be available to clear the oropharynx and supraglottic region of all secretions. Instruments necessary for a surgical airway should be available in the event that intubation is unsuccessful. Properly applied cricoid pressure will minimize the risk of aspirating regurgitated gastric contents during mask ventilation. While maintaining inline cervical stabilization and under direct laryngoscopic or bronchoscopic visualization, the cuff of the endotracheal tube is positioned distal to the vocal cords. Correct placement of the endotracheal tube is confirmed using an end tidal carbon dioxide detection device, auscultation of the chest, and a chest radiograph.

If attempts at intubation fail or the oral and nasal routes are contraindicated due to maxillofacial injuries or anatomic distortion, a surgical airway is mandated. The surgical cricothyroidotomy remains the preferred technique in these emergency situations. The authors' preferred method for creating a cricothyroidotomy is using a modified Seldinger technique. A vertical skin incision is centered over the cricothyroid membrane, which is then sharply opened horizontally using the scalpel. A flexible bougie tube is passed through the cricothyroidotomy into the trachea acting as the guide over which a #6 shiley or 7–0 endotracheal tube is advanced and secured.

Breathing/Ventilation

Once the airway is adequately addressed, oxygenation and ventilation must be ensured. Oxygenation can be assessed with the noninvasive pulse oximeter and confirmed with an arterial blood gas measurement. Satisfactory ventilation can be evaluated by inspection, palpation, percussion, and auscultation of the chest. If inadequate ventilation is detected, the airway should be reassessed to ensure that the esophagus has not been intubated inadvertently. If ventilation remains inadequate, life-threatening chest injuries that impede ventilation must be considered. These conditions include a tension pneumothorax, massive hemothorax, open pneumothorax, and flail chest.

A *tension pneumothorax* can result from either blunt or penetrating trauma to the lung, bronchi, or trachea, allowing air to continually leak into the pleural space. This differs from a simple pneumothorax in that the lung parenchymal injury remains patent and no chest wall defect is produced to allow venting of the progressively accumulating pleural air. Consequently, with each breath, the patient generates negative intrathoracic pressure, progressively accumulating air into the pleural space, resulting in collapse of the ipsilateral lung. The resultant increased pleural pressure will ultimately shift the mediastinum to the contralateral side. This mediastinal shift results in vena caval distortion, thereby decreasing venous return to the heart, resulting in depressed cardiac output and hemodynamic instability. Patients appear anxious with tachycardia, hypotension, marked respiratory distress, absent ipsilateral breath sounds, tracheal deviation to the contralateral side, and neck vein distention. Consequently, *tension pneumothorax* is a clinical diagnosis. It is quickly treated by placing a large bore angiocath into the second intercostal space aligned with the mid-clavicular line so as to decompress the pleural space. Definitive treatment requires the placement of a tube thoracostomy attached to 20 cm of water suction.

A *massive hemothorax* can occur as the consequence of either blunt or penetrating trauma due to an injury to an intercostal or hilar vessel. Massive hemothorax is defined as 1,500 cc of blood loss into the hemithorax with subsequent compression of the lung. The diagnosis is established when shock is identified in concert with absent breath sounds and dullness to percussion on one side of the chest. The injury is treated by simultaneous restoration of the intravascular space with crystalloids and blood products and decompression of the pleural space with a large (#38 or #40 French) tube thoracostomy. A chest radiograph should be obtained following placement of the chest tube to ensure that the hemothorax has been completely evacuated. Decompression of the hemothorax allows for the apposition of the parietal and visceral pleura, which frequently results in cessation of ongoing blood loss from the majority of pulmonary and osseous sources. If more than 1,500 cc of blood is initially evacuated or if blood loss exceeds 200 cc/h for the next 2–3 h, a thoracotomy may be required to surgically address ongoing hemorrhage.

An *open pneumothorax* or "sucking chest wound" results from a defect in the chest wall that exceeds two thirds of the diameter of the trachea. Following the injury, which is typically penetrating trauma, the intrathoracic pressure will equate with the atmospheric pressure. With each subsequent inspiratory effort, air will preferentially follow the path of least resistance through the thoracic defect and into the pleural space. The injury can be initially controlled with placement of an occlusive dressing over the wound and securing it on three sides. This creates a flap valve where air is permitted to escape from the pleural space during expiration but no air is allowed to enter during inspiration. Tube thoracostomy should be performed at a site remote from the injury. Frequently, definitive surgical closure of the chest wall defect is required.

A *flail chest* is defined as a fracture of three or more consecutive ribs in two or more places, with or without sternal involvement, allowing for paradoxical respiratory motion. Frequently, a *flail chest* will have an associated hemo- or pneumothorax and will require the placement of a chest tube. Although there is a severe disruption of normal chest wall movement associated with the flail segment, the resulting physiologic derangement is the consequence of the underlying pulmonary contusion and poor respiratory mechanics related to chest wall pain. Treatment is directed at providing physiologic support of the gas exchange abnormalities and alleviating pain.

Parenteral analgesics, particularly with patient-controlled analgesia, is the mainstay of therapy and should be employed liberally. Some patients benefit from early placement of thoracic epidural catheters. Thoracic epidural analgesia for *flail chest* has been demonstrated to improve the patient's maximum inspiratory effort, tidal volumes, and vital capacity. In the event pulmonary toilet and ventilation are still suboptimal with epidural analgesia, mechanical ventilatory support is required. Ventilator support is best implemented early, as this has been demonstrated to reduce overall duration of ventilatory support as well as mortality (Gianna et al., 1993).

Circulation

With the airway secured and ventilation deemed adequate, the circulatory system is the next priority. Shock is best defined as inadequate delivery of oxygen to meet the metabolic demands of peripheral tissue. The most common etiology of shock for the trauma patient remains hemorrhagic shock, but other sources including cardiogenic, compressive (cardiac tamponade or tension pneumothorax), and neurogenic (spinal injury) must be considered. Following blunt trauma, hypovolemic shock is most often due to intraperitoneal blood loss, pelvic fractures, musculoskeletal injuries, and/or thoracic trauma. Hemorrhagic shock associated with penetrating trauma can result from a laceration of any major blood vessel causing external exsanguination through the wound or internal exsanguination into any of the major corporal compartments.

The treatment of shock begins first with its recognition. The hallmark clinical signs of shock include tachycardia, hypotension, narrowing of the pulse pressure, cutaneous vasoconstriction, oliguria, and mental status changes to include the spectrum from apprehension to obtundation. Following the recognition of shock, initial management includes gaining access to the vascular system and staunching obvious external hemorrhage. IV access is obtained by placing two large-bore short angiocaths in peripheral veins. Once IV access is obtained, phlebotomy can be performed for basic laboratory studies and type and cross match. Initial volume expansion is achieved with a 2 l bolus of warmed lactated Ringer's solution.

The volume required for the resuscitation of a patient is difficult to predict, but the "3 for 1 rule" can provide a rough approximation of a patient's initial fluid needs. This estimate assumes that a patient will need 3 cc of crystalloid for every cubic centimeter of blood loss. Patients in deep shock, or those who do not respond to their initial bolus of lactated Ringer should receive additional crystalloid boluses and early administration of blood products. The goal of any resuscitation strategy is reversal of the shock state and aggressive resuscitation should continue until adequate end organ perfusion and tissue oxygenation is achieved. Traditionally, the endpoints of shock resuscitation have been the restoration of normal blood pressure, heart rate, and adequate urinary output. Unfortunately, using these measures alone as a guide for adequate resuscitation may leave as many as 50–85% of trauma patients in "compensated" shock. In these situations, a patient's hemodynamic indices may be normal, but still have evidence of suboptimal tissue perfusion as demonstrated by the persistence of systemic acidemia, elevated lactate levels, and low mixed venous oxygen saturations. This situation can occur as blood flow and oxygen delivery is redistributed from the splanchnic bed to other critical organs such as the brain and heart. Recent resuscitation data suggest that in addition to restoring normal hemodynamic indices and urinary output, correction of the base deficit and restoring lactate levels to normal will result in significantly reduced mortality.

While fluid resuscitation is ongoing, the source of the circulatory collapse must be identified. Blood loss must first be excluded and may be as obvious as external hemorrhage or can occur occultly into any one or a combination of spaces to include the abdomen, thorax, retroperitoneum, or extremities. In the past, diagnostic peritoneal lavage (DPL) was the preferred technique used in the Emergency Department to exclude hemoperitoneum as a potential cause of hemodynamic instability. DPL remains a reliable study with reported sensitivities ranging from 90% to 96% and specificity from 99% to 100% (United States Medical Expenditures, 2003); however, this invasive and somewhat time-consuming procedure has been associated with nontherapeutic laparotomies. DPL will accurately identify hemoperitoneum but is unable to provide the source. Thus, a laparotomy is dictated for a solid organ injury that may have been better managed with nonoperative observation in an intensive care unit. In modern trauma centers, DPL's usefulness is limited because of readily available and rapid focused abdominal sonogram for trauma (FAST) and/or computerized tomography (CT) (Freedland et al., 1990).

FAST is a technique that surgeons can quickly master and is proving to be dependable, rapid, and noninvasive. The focused abdominal ultrasound is highly sensitive for detecting solid organ injury and is very reliable for identification of hemoperitoneum, with some studies demonstrating a sensitivity approaching 95% (Meyer et al., 1989). Its greatest value is realized in dealing with the hemodynamically unstable patient with multiple cavitary sources of potential blood loss. Ideally, efforts should be made to rapidly resuscitate and stabilize the patient in order to obtain a CT scan of the chest, abdomen, and pelvis, providing the clinician with definitive clinical information. Among patients in whom hemodynamic stability cannot be achieved and blood pressure liability precludes movement into an unsupervised setting such as the CT scanner, the FAST examination can quickly identify the presence or absence of a hemoperitoneum dictating the need for a laparotomy.

Pelvic fractures are an underappreciated source of blood loss in the polytrauma patient and blood loss can be of arterial, venous, and/or osseous origin. The patient can essentially exsanguinate from a pelvic fracture with the potential for several liters of blood to be sequestered in the retroperitoneum. Therapy begins with immobilization of the pelvis by applying a binder and/or providing surgical external fixation by an orthopedic specialist. This approach aligns the cancellous bone fragments and reduces the volume of the pelvis, thus allowing for a tamponade effect to arrest the venous and osseous hemorrhage. Failure to control hemorrhage in these circumstances is likely due to an arterial injury and may require angiography and therapeutic embolization. Femur fractures can be associated with 1,500 cc of blood loss and, similar to pelvic fractures, require immobilization as the initial treatment priority.

Neurologic Deficit/Exposure

The final aspect of the primary survey consists of identifying any gross neurologic deficit and exposing the patient completely. The Glasgow Coma Scale (GCS) is a detailed evaluation of function and an effective measure for evaluating the neurologic status of injured patients. The GCS is the sum of three components of assessment found in ❱ Table 8-1. Pupillary size, symmetry, and reaction to light are also assessed during the primary survey. These evaluations should occur early in the resuscitation process with frequent re-evaluations to document either patient improvement or deterioration. A worsening examination will prompt the need for additional therapy or diagnostic studies.

Among patients in whom brain injury is suspected with a concurrent depressed level of consciousness, steps should be taken urgently to definitively control the airway. Evidence supports that a single episode of hypoxemia is strongly associated with higher mortality and worse neurologic recovery. Similarly, a brief period of hypotension is correlated closely with poor long-term disability and worse mortality. Hyperventilation, previously employed for the head-injured patient, is currently contraindicated since it results in cerebral vasoconstriction and decreased cerebral perfusion, thus potentially worsening brain injury. Current recommendations regarding ventilation support promote avoidance of excessive hyperventilation maintaining a $PaCO_2$ of 30–35 mmHg. This level of carbon dioxide balances cerebral blood flow and intracranial pressure. Hyperventilation is withheld exclusively for those with evidence of elevated intracranial pressure and impending herniation.

Completion of the primary survey requires that the patient be completely disrobed so that any obvious external injury is not overlooked. After logrolling the patient, the back, perineum, and axillae are examined and a rectal examination is performed. Afterwards, warm blankets are placed over the patient to minimize the risk of hypothermia. Other measures to preserve body temperature include

☑ Table 8-1

Glasgow coma scale

Parameter	Score
Best motor response	
Normal	6
Localizes	5
Withdraws	4
Flexion	3
Extension	2
None	1
Best verbal response	
Oriented	5
Confused	4
Verbalizes	3
Vocalizes	2
None/Intubated	1
Eye opening	
Spontaneous	4
To command	3
To pain	2
None	1
Minor injury: 13–15	
Moderate injury: 9–12	
Severe injury: 8 or below	

heating the room, warming IV fluids and the inspired air in the ventilator circuit, and using environmental heaters such as the Bair Hugger. Hypothermia induces patient shivering to generate heat. This results in an increase in oxygen demand and worsening the shock state. Hypothermia can also impair both the primary and secondary hemostatic mechanisms.

Before beginning the secondary survey, the patient's clinical status should be reassessed by quickly reviewing all components of the primary survey with close attention to any alterations in vital signs and/or oxygen saturation. Additionally, basic radiographic and laboratory studies are performed. A minimum of three radiographic studies are performed for the trauma patient including an AP view of the chest and pelvis as well as a cross table lateral of the cervical spine. The information yielded from these studies is helpful in piecing together the clinical picture. Laboratory studies are frequently acquired when IV access is obtained. Additionally, an arterial blood gas should be drawn, usually from the femoral artery, to determine the extent of base deficit suggesting the degree of shock.

All severely injured patients should have a Foley catheter placed during their resuscitation. The only contraindication for Foley placement is a urethral injury which should be suspected with complex pelvic fractures, blood noted at the penile meatus, or a high-riding prostate detected during the rectal examination. If a urethral injury is suspected, a retrograde urethrogram is performed prior to the placement of the catheter.

A nasogastric (NG) tube is placed to decompress the stomach so as to reduce the risk of aspiration for intubated patients and those who are unable to protect their airways adequately due to CNS depression. Patients with midface instability or evidence of basilar skull fractures should have orogastric tubes placed instead of using the transnasal route to prevent potential iatrogenic injury.

Secondary Survey

The *secondary survey* consists of a review of the information regarding the injury mechanism, the patient's past medical history, and a complete "head to toe" physical examination. This portion of the evaluation should not begin until the primary survey has been completed, all life-saving interventions performed, and a satisfactory response to resuscitation observed. The physical examination needs to be performed in an organized and thorough manner beginning with the scalp and systematically moving caudally to the feet. Once completed, and based upon physical examination finding, the remainder of necessary diagnostic studies is obtained including radiographs of potential fractures, CT scans, and arteriograms.

CNS

As noted earlier, a brief neurologic examination is conducted during the primary survey. During the secondary survey, a more complete examination is performed evaluating the cranial nerves, motor strength of all extremities, spinal reflexes, and sensory losses to include pain, temperature, and proprioception from head to toe. Abnormalities identified in the physical examination should prompt further evaluation with a head CT or magnetic resonance imaging (MRI), as well as consultation with a neurosurgeon.

Blunt trauma patients should be assumed to have sustained a vertebral column injury until proven otherwise by an unequivocal physical examination and radiographic survey including CT imaging. Patients under the influence of alcohol and/or drugs and those with an abnormal GCS should remain in rigid cervical collars until their mental status has improved and a normal examination is demonstrated. The use of IV steroids in patients with spinal cord injury remains controversial. Current recommendations of a bolus followed by a continuous rate over a 23 h period are based upon a retrospective study demonstrating slight improvement in motor function of a single extremity in conjunction with steroid administration. Currently, prospective studies are underway in an effort to clearly define the usefulness and exact role of steroids following acute spinal cord injury.

Head

Because of the abundant blood supply, lacerations of the scalp and face can bleed briskly and are usually controlled during the primary survey with direct pressure or quick placement of temporary sutures. During the secondary survey, these injuries should be debrided, adequately cleansed with a surgical soap, and primarily closed. Extraocular motion should be assessed and the face should be closely examined for any asymmetry. Most facial fractures can be detected by palpation of the bony prominences while fractures of the midface can be detected by inserting a finger into the mouth examining for instability of the hard palate or incisors. Maxillary or mandibular fractures are suggested by malocclusion. The tympanic membranes and external auditory canals are inspected with an otoscope. The presence of a hemotympanum or cerebrospinal fluid otorrhea is diagnostic of a basilar skull fracture. Further evidence of a basilar skull fracture is suggested by bruising around the eyes and behind the ears, the so-called "Battle sign". If facial or basilar skull fractures are suspected, a CT scan of the face should be performed to confirm the diagnosis and better define the injury.

Neck

The neck is typically divided into three zones. Zone I extends from the clavicles to the base of the cricoid cartilage, zone II extends from the cricoid to the angle of the mandible, and zone III spans the region from the angle of the mandible to the base of the skull. These zones are of particular importance in managing the patient with penetrating trauma. Unstable patients require surgical exploration. Hemodynamically stable patients with penetrating injury to zone I or III, because of the inherent anatomic inaccessibility, are best approached with a diagnostic evaluation which may include arteriography, bronchoscopy, rigid esophagoscopy, and a barium swallow. A great deal of debate continues regarding management of zone II injuries, with some authors advocating diagnostic evaluation as with zone I and III injuries. Alternatively, because of the ease of accessibility and exposure, as well as the high incidence of serious injuries in this unprotected region, patients with wounds that penetrate the platysma often undergo surgical exploration.

Chest

The chest should be reevaluated in the secondary survey by inspection, palpation, percussion, and auscultation. The chest radiograph should be closely examined for rib fractures, soft tissue injury, pneumothorax, hemothorax, subcutaneous emphysema, deviation of the trachea or esophagus, and shifted or widened mediastinum. Following blunt trauma, the diagnosis of a diaphragmatic rupture is suggested by an elevated left hemidiaphragm, loculated hemopneumothorax, or visualization of the NG tube in the left hemithorax.

A transected thoracic aorta is commonly associated with deceleration injuries and is frequently fatal at the scene. Clinicians having a high index of suspicion based upon the mechanism of injury and appreciating the hallmark signs seen on chest radiographs can identify these injuries early in the resuscitation. Radiographic findings consistent with a transected aorta include a mediastinal width greater than 8 cm, fracture of the first or second rib, obliteration of the aortic knob, deviation of trachea and esophagus to the right, pleural cap, elevation and rightward shift of the right mainstem bronchus, and depression of the left mainstem bronchus. Suspicion of injury should lead to a helical CT of the chest with IV contrast. These new generation scanners are proving to be effective at identifying aortic injury accurately with few missed injuries (Porter and Ivatury, 1998). Timing of surgery is dependent upon the patient's overall condition. Patients with hemodynamic instability require immediate surgery while stable patients can be medically optimized in the intensive care unit prior to surgical repair.

Abdomen

The abdomen encompasses the pelvis, the retroperitoneum, and the peritoneal cavity. During the secondary survey, a thorough examination of the abdomen is conducted using the traditional approach of inspection, palpation, and percussion. Visual examination of the abdomen should reveal any penetrating injuries, lacerations, or contusions. The flank and back are examined during the *exposure* portion of the primary survey when the patient is carefully log rolled. The abdominal examination is completed by rocking the pelvis to assess for instability and pain. Among patients for whom an acute laparotomy is not indicated based upon physical examination alone, CT imaging of the chest, abdomen, and pelvis should be undertaken.

Penetrating injuries to the abdomen deserve special attention. It should be remembered that the diaphragm ascends to the level of the fourth intercostal space and thus any penetrating injury affecting the lower chest wall can potentially injure the intra-abdominal viscera. All gunshot wounds to the abdomen and lower chest should be explored. Stab wound to the anterior abdominal wall should be explored locally for the presence or absence of fascial penetration. If exploration reveals that the posterior fascia has been violated or if the exploration is indeterminate, patients should undergo exploratory celiotomy. Penetrating wounds to the flank have the potential to cause occult intra-abdominal injury and mandate, at a minimum, evaluation with a triple contrast CT study and serial examinations.

Extremities

The extremities should be examined for obvious fractures and lacerations. Suspected fractures should be radiographed and obvious fractures splinted as soon as possible. Assessment of the neurovascular status is of paramount importance. Hard signs of vascular trauma include active hemorrhage, distal pulse deficit, distal ischemia, and large or expanding hematomas. Among patients suffering fractures as a result of blunt force, persistent pulse discrepancies or hard signs following reduction of the fracture in the emergency department should prompt additional studies to eliminate the presence of a vascular injury. Patients with penetrating injury to an extremity should be carefully evaluated for the presence or absence of a hard sign of vascular injury and, if detected, surgical exploration is mandated (McKenney et al., 1996). Penetrating trauma in proximity to the major blood vessel without the "hard signs" is associated with a very low likelihood of significant vascular injury. Calculating an ankle/brachial index or performing color flow Doppler imaging and/or arteriography can be pursued. Prospective studies, however, have demonstrated that a thorough examination documenting the lack of "hard signs" of vascular injury is equally as sensitive as these diagnostic studies in determining the presence or absence of significant vascular injury. Motor or sensory deficits found on physical examination can result from either spinal cord injury, local peripheral nerve injury, or vascular injury with ischemia. Once vascular injury is excluded and the likely source of neurologic impairment is identified, appropriate consultation should be obtained.

Summary

A rapid and complete primary survey with early correction of life-threatening injuries has been shown to enhance patient survival and improve eventual outcomes. Delayed or inadequate resuscitation and unrecognized injuries ultimately will increase the patient's chance of developing multisystem organ dysfunction. Physicians who care for the acutely injured patient need to rehearse the steps of the primary and secondary survey until they become second nature to ensure that the "Golden Hour" is preserved and patient outcomes are enhanced.

Selected Readings

Boulanger BR, McLellan BA, et al. (1999) Prospective evidence of the superiority of a sonography-based algorithm in the assessment of blunt abdominal injury. J Trauma 47:632

Freedland M, Wilson RF, et al. (1990) The management of flail chest injury: factors affecting outcome. J Trauma 30:1460–1468

Frykberg ER, Dennis JW, et al. (1991) The reliability of physical examination in the evaluation of penetrating extremity trauma for vascular injury: results at one year. J Trauma 31:502–511

Gianna S, Waxman K, et al. (1993) Orotracheal intubation in trauma patients with cervical fractures. Arch Surg 128:903–906

McKenney MG, Martin L, et al. (1996) 1,000 consecutive ultrasounds for blunt abdominal trauma. J Trauma 40:607–612

Melton SM, Kerby JD, et al. (2004) The evolution of chest computed tomography for the definitive diagnosis of blunt aortic injury: a single-center experience. J Trauma 56:243–250

Meyer DM, Thal ER, et al. (1989) Evaluation of computed tomography and diagnostic peritoneal lavage in blunt abdominal trauma. J Trauma 29:1168–1170

Porter JM, Ivatury RR (1998) In search of the optimal end points of resuscitation in trauma patients: a review. J Trauma 44:908–914

United States Medical Expenditures (2003) United States Department of Health and Human Services – Agency for Healthcare Research and Quality. http://meps.ahrq.gov/CompendiumTables/TC_TOC.htm

9 Blunt Abdominal Trauma

Ricardo Ferrada · Diego Rivera · Paula Ferrada

Pearls and Pitfalls

- Patients suffering a high-energy trauma have solid viscera rupture in the abdomen and/or aortic rupture in the thorax until proven otherwise.
- Initial abdominal examination is inaccurate for detecting visceral injury, and especially so if the patient is in an altered mental state (alcohol, drugs, closed head trauma), pregnant, or paralyzed.
- Significant blunt abdominal trauma alone represents an indication for abdominal imaging.
- Fracture of the lower ribs ("abdominal ribs") should raise a very high suspicion of intra-abdominal injury.
- Do not forget the possibility of hollow organ injury, especially with deceleration forces or a potential seat belt injury.
- An "elevated" left hemidiaphragm or a left "hydro/hemothorax" must raise the possibility of diaphragmatic rupture.
- The ultrasonographic focused abdominal sonography for trauma (FAST) exam has replaced virtually the diagnostic peritoneal lavage because of its ease, speed, sensitivity, and ability to be repeated easily.
- Computed tomography (CT) is a reliable imaging modality for solid organ and pelvic injury but requires a patient with stable vital signs.
- Diagnostic peritoneal lavage (DPL) has essentially been replaced by the FAST, but DPL has some use when other tests are equivocal or when hollow organ injury is suspected.

General Considerations

Blunt abdominal trauma can be produced not only by direct contusion to the abdomen but also by deceleration injury or falls. Serious, devastating intra-abdominal injuries may be present despite the absence of external signs of trauma. This understanding underscores the importance of a complete evaluation in patients suffering high-energy trauma (❯ *Table 9-1*), including a thorough physical examination, the judicious use of diagnostic modalities, and careful follow-up. The physical examination is a crucial part of the initial evaluation; however, signs of clinically important blunt abdominal trauma are not reliable in severe trauma. Physical examination alone has a sensitivity of only ~35%, positive predictive value of 30–50%, and a negative predictive value of about 60%. If the Glasgow Coma Score is less than 7, the sensitivity of the physical examination is only 20%. Other circumstances

◘ Table 9-1

High-energy trauma

Fall from higher than 10 ft
Ejection from a vehicle
Motor vehicle crash at speeds exceeding 45 miles/h
Motorbike accident
Major fracture
First rib fracture
Lower costal rib fracture
Seat belt restraint mark

◘ Table 9-2

Unreliable physical examination

Alcohol or drug intoxication
Spinal cord injury
Pregnancy
Glasgow coma score <10
Multiple extra-abdominal injuries

in which the physical examination is unreliable include alcohol or drug intoxication, spinal cord injury, pregnancy, and multiple extra-abdominal injuries (❯ *Table 9-2*). Therefore, further investigation of the patient subjected to forces sufficient to have caused injury are necessary beyond just the physical examination, and the traumatologist must maintain a high index of suspicion of underlying intra-abdominal and intrathoracic injury.

In patients with lower rib fractures, called the "abdominal ribs," solid organ trauma should be suspected until proven otherwise. Splenic and/or hepatic injury is identified in 10–20%. As many as 40% of patients with hemoperitoneum show no findings on initial physical examination. For these reasons, the physical examination must be repeated serially by the same examiner, and consideration always given to diagnostic imaging (❯ *Figure 9-1*).

The most frequently injured organ as a result of blunt abdominal trauma is the spleen (40–55%), followed by the liver (35–40%). Although the hollow organs are injured less frequently (15%), delay in diagnosis results in high rates of morbidity and mortality with these injuries. The added difficulty in diagnosis of hollow organ injury on physical examination alone adds further complexity to management (❯ *Figure 9-2*).

Diagnostic Procedures

Defining the extent of injury after blunt abdominal trauma can be difficult even for an experienced surgeon without the aid of diagnostic procedures. In most cases, significant blunt abdominal trauma alone is an indication for a more thorough evaluation, including at least some imaging modality.

◙ Figure 9-1
Mesenteric rupture due to a blunt abdominal trauma with subtle signs. The bowel was ischemic and had to be resected

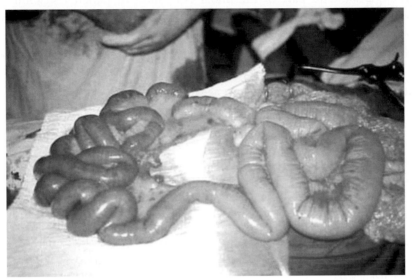

◙ Figure 9-2
Algorithm for Initial management

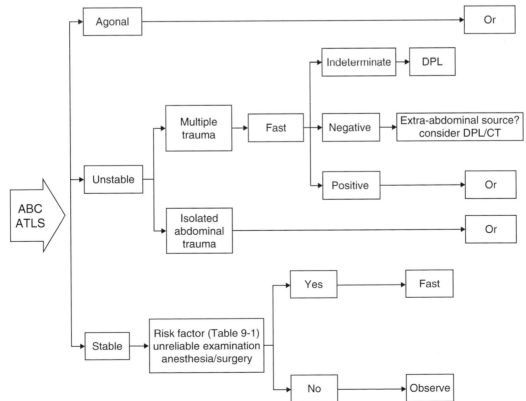

Radiography

Chest x-ray must be a standard part of the initial evaluation of patients sustaining potential blunt abdominal trauma. Concomitant thoracic visceral injuries may occur and must be considered as well. Signs of abdominal visceral or diaphragm rupture are rarely seen on x-ray, but an elevated hemidiaphragm, an air/fluid level in the chest, or other findings suggesting the presence of intra-abdominal viscera in the chest require investigation or celiotomy. Although a rare finding, pneumoperitoneum may indicate hollow viscus injury warranting laparotomy. Just as with the physical examination, the abdominal x-ray can be unreliable in underlying intra-abdominal injury. Nevertheless, review of the abdominal part of a pelvic x-ray screening for pelvic fracture is of potential use, especially in the patient who is unreliable.

Ultrasonography

In 1992, Tso and colleagues evaluated the use of ultrasonography (US) in 63 patients with blunt abdominal trauma. This preliminary study demonstrated a sensitivity of 69%, specificity of 99%, and accuracy rate of 96%, similar to CT and diagnostic peritoneal lavage (DPL) at the same institution. Rozycki and colleagues reported their outcomes subsequently and coined the term focused abdominal sonography for trauma (FAST) in 1,540 patients (1,227 with blunt injuries and 313 with penetrating injuries). With an overall sensitivity of 84% and a specificity of 99%, US was most sensitive and specific for the evaluation of hypotensive patients with blunt abdominal trauma (sensitivity 100%, specificity 100%).

US has become the surgeon's and traumatologist's "stethoscope" for patients with abdominal trauma. The advantages of this technique are that it is relatively easy to learn, cost-effective, noninvasive, takes only a few minutes, has no radiation, can be repeated as many times as needed, and can be performed simultaneously with the resuscitation effort.

The goal of the FAST exam is to detect fluid in easily accessible areas: precordial (intrapericardial), Morrison's pouch, left upper quadrant pouch of Douglas, and the pelvis. The estimated number of examinations that a non-radiologist must perform to acquire acceptable accuracy ranges from 100 to 400 US exams. FAST can detect a volume of fluid as low as 200 ml; however, injuries not resulting in hemoperitoneum or hollow visceral injury without extravasation of enough enteric content may be missed. There are notable limitations of the FAST exam which include: operator dependency, increased difficulty in the obese or distended patient, the patient with ascites or subcutaneous emphysema, and poor ability to recognize solid parenchymal or hollow visceral injuries without substantial extravasation of enteric content. One major advantage is that the FAST exam can be repeated serially and when clinical status changes. In the absence of clinical instability, a negative FAST can allow ongoing evaluation and treatment of extra-abdominal injuries (❯ *Figure 9-3*).

Computed Tomography

CT allows a complete and noninvasive assessment of the abdominal and pelvic cavities, retroperitoneal structures, soft tissues, and bones. CT is especially reliable for assessment of the liver and the spleen. In the kidney, CT allows assessment of not only the anatomy but the function as well. The accuracy in stable patients with blunt abdominal trauma is excellent, with a reported sensitivity and specificity approaching 98%. The negative predictive value is 99%, and thus a negative CT excludes very reliably

■ Figure 9-3
Algorithm for management according to the focused abdominal sonography for trauma (FAST) and computed tomography (CT) exam

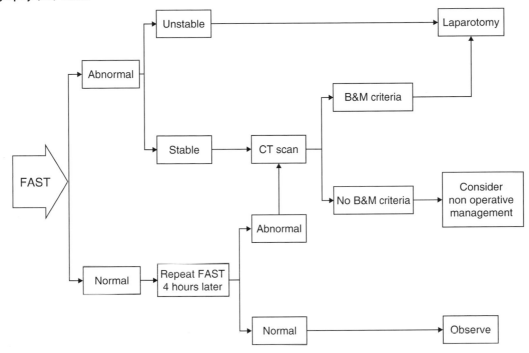

the need for an immediate laparotomy in the vast majority of patients. For these reasons, CT has become the favored diagnostic procedure in blunt trauma, and should be obtained in most patients, provided they are hemodynamically stable.

CT is particularly useful when the physical examination is unreliable or equivocal or when nonoperative management is considered in the setting of stable patients with a positive DPL or FAST exam. Several additional advantages of CT are that it is noninvasive, can define the location and extent of solid organ or retroperitoneal injuries, can detect ongoing bleeding when intravenous (IV) contrast is used, and does not require hemoperitoneum, as do DPL and FAST exams. Unless contraindicated, IV contrast agent should be used when CT is obtained for evaluation of blunt abdominal trauma to examine renal function as to get a better definition of solid parenchymal injury, blood flow, and extravasation. Detection of hollow visceral injuries is less accurate and less reliable, even with quality contrast-enhanced CT. Nevertheless, certain findings on CT may suggest strongly the presence of an underlying injury to hollow viscera or to the mesentery; these CT findings include pneumoperitoneum, leak of the contrast agent into the peritoneal cavity, thickening of bowel wall or the mesentery, and free fluid without solid visceral injury. If any of these signs are found or there is other suspicion of hollow viscus injury, either DPL or an emergent laparotomy should be performed.

Diagnostic Peritoneal Lavage

Prior to the advent of the FAST exam, DPL had become the gold standard for blunt abdominal trauma. Only 30 ml of blood can produce a microscopically positive test. DPL is very sensitive (sometimes possibly too sensitive) and thus not specific. When negative, clinically important intra-abdominal

☐ Table 9-3

DPL interpretation

Positive	RBC more than 100,000 mm^3
	WBC more than 500/mm^3
	Bile
	Bacteria
	Feces/intestinal content
Intermediate	RBC 50,000–100,000/mm^3
	WBC 100–500/mm^3

bleeding is highly unlikely. In contrast, DPL is oversensitive in that not all patients with a positive DPL have a serious enough injury to warrant operative intervention. Additional limitations of DPL include the inability to detect retroperitoneal injury or solid organ injury in the absence of hemoperitoneum, and it is contraindicated in advanced pregnancy or with a history of multiple previous laparotomies; a pelvic fracture can produce a false-positive exam in the absence of solid or hollow visceral injury. The indications for DPL are similar to those for CT. Currently, with the FAST exam, DPL is used only rarely unless FAST is either unavailable or equivocal or when CT is contraindicated.

Prior to performing a DPL, a nasogastric (NG) tube and urinary catheter must be inserted. The technique may be performed open or with a needle and wire passed into the intraperitoneal cavity using the Seldinger technique. Under local anesthesia, an incision midline below the umbilicus incision is performed. When a pelvic trauma is suspected or confirmed, the incision should be made above the umbilicus in order to avoid entering a potention pelvic hematoma. Once the skin and the fascia are incised, the wire and catheter are inserted, removing this wire as the peritoneum is penetrated, and the catheter is advanced toward the pelvis. If the technique is open, the peritoneum should be incised under direct visualization. After the catheter is inserted, aspiration with a 20 ml syringe is performed. If more than 10 ml of gross blood is obtained, the test is considered positive and terminated. Otherwise, 1,000 ml of 0.9% normal saline is instilled into the peritoneal cavity, the patient is turned gently from side to side if possible, and the fluid is drained by gravity. The DPL is considered positive when the return fluid is grossly bloody or evidence of enteric content is seen. If the fluid is pink or clear, a sample is sent to the laboratory for quantitative determination of red and white blood cells or signs; the criteria are outlined in ❷ *Table 9-3*.

Initial Management

For practical purposes, we classify trauma patients according to hemodynamic status as moribund (agonal), unstable, or stable.

Moribund or Agonal Patients

Moribund patients are those with no spontaneous ventilatory effort, no femoral pulse, and no response to painful stimuli. These patients require an emergent airway and strong consideration of immediate operative intervention for suspected hemorrhage. Accordingly, after assuring airway and breathing (the A and B of the ABCs of resuscitation), a laparotomy and/or a thoracotomy must be considered. Whether a resuscitative thoracotomy prior to laparotomy improves the survival rate of these patients is controversial. Some authors have recommended clamping of the thoracic aortic, even in the emergency room setting, prior to laparotomy (in the operating room) in patients with refractory hypotension and abdominal distension secondary to massive hemoperitoneum. The rationale for this approach is to increase upper torso and intracranial blood pressure immediately and to prevent cardiac arrest after release of abdominal wall tamponade during celiotomy. The mortality in this setting is exceedingly high, with very few survivors; many traumatologists do not believe in this approach. The patients are taken to an operating room immediately, placed supine, and the abdomen explored with other minimal maneuvers. During abdominal exploration, the finding of significant or ongoing intra-abdominal hemorrhage may require cross-clamping the aorta at the diaphragmatic hiatus if there had been no thoracotomy. The surgeon must pack and compress the bleeding area(s) and seek more stable conditions by infusing a large amount of IV fluid and blood. Most of these patients require a shortened procedure (so-called damage control) with transfer to a surgical critical care unit for stabilization and later definitive repair of the intraperitoneal injury if they survive.

Unstable Patients

Patients are considered unstable when any vital sign, such as pulse, ventilatory rate, or blood pressure, is significantly abnormal. The instability is produced by either respiratory compromise or hypovolemia, so the initial approach (the ABCs) must include the establishment of the airway, ventilation, and circulation with immediate control of any external bleeding and IV access. After the management of airway and breathing, the next step is fluid resuscitation with a warm, balanced salt solution. The authors start with a bolus of 1,500 ml in patients of 140 lb (70 kg) of weight. If a patient recovers skin color and the vital signs normalize, additional IV fluid is infused at a lower rate, according to the response in the pulse rate and amplitude and urine output. If stability is achieved, patients are managed according to the algorithm for stable patients. In contrast, if the vital signs do not recover or improve only temporarily with fluid resuscitation and blood transfusion, then ongoing hemorrhage should be suspected, and operative intervention may be indicated.

Stable Patients

Patients are judged to be stable when their vital signs are normal initially or when the vital signs return to normal after the initial IV bolus. A more detailed clinical history must then be obtained. Careful evaluation is necessary to define the extent of injury. The decision for continued observation or intervention is based on the mechanism of injury and findings on evaluation. The decision to treat by observation requires careful and repeated assessment. As the physical examination may not be reliable in a number of cases, serial examination will be crucial in decision making.

Subsequent Management after Initial Evaluation

The majority of patients with blunt abdominal trauma arrive with no clinical signs of abdominal trauma with the exception of pain and possibly abdominal wall ecchymosis. Management depends largely on the stability of the patient and findings of diagnostic procedures.

■ Table 9-4

Requirements for non-operative management

Hemodynamically stable
Absence of peritonitis
Contrast-enhanced CT without evidence of active bleeding
Monitoring in an intensive care unit
Staff available for repeated observation
Operation room available 24 h

In the group of stable patients, several situations require special mention. Patients who appear stable but have risk factors for potential serious injury mandate particularly careful observation, because delayed clinical deterioration may occur (❷ *Table 9-1*). Those who fell from more than 10 ft, were ejected from a vehicle, were involved in a motor vehicle crash of more than 45 miles/h, or were in a motorbike accident must be considered high-energy trauma. Subtle signs such as fracture of the first rib, abdominal wall ecchymosis from the seat belt ("seat belt sign"), or major fractures of long bones or pelvis also imply high-energy trauma and warrant close observation. Fractures of the lower "abdominal" ribs should suggest possible abdominal solid organ injury. In patients with a closed head injury, intoxication, drug abuse, or those who require neurosurgery or orthopedic surgery where the physical examination will be unreliable for several hours because of the anesthetic, some objective evaluation of the abdomen is necessary, such as a FAST exam, CT, or DPL. As noted previously, the FAST exam has become one of the most important tests in diagnosis of severe blunt abdominal trauma. When the first view is negative, if there are any doubts, the FAST can be repeated on multiple occasions.

A major advance in the last two decades has been the use of primary nonoperative management for solid viscera injury, as guided by initial imaging and clinical response. Good evidence suggests that nonoperative management in both children and adults is safe, and the results are better than with a laparotomy in selected cases. Appropriate candidates for nonoperative management are those without active bleeding from solid viscera injury without evidence of hollow viscus or mesenteric injury. Observation requires hemodynamically stable patients in whom ongoing evaluation and observation can be performed. Quality CT imaging, a monitored environment, and access to emergent intervention are required (❷ *Table 9-4*).

In selected patients with isolated solid viscera injury in whom contrast extravasation is seen either during the arterial or venous phase of the CT, a transcatheter arterial embolization may be considered. In contrast, nonoperative management should be abandoned in adults when hemodynamic status cannot be maintained after two units of packed red cells during the initial management or four units in the first 48 h, or if the embolization does not stop the extravasation at angiography.

The success rate of nonoperative management is high for isolated hepatic injury, but is less in splenic and especially renal injury, and is dependent on the extent of parenchymal injury (e.g., grade of liver and splenic injury). Risk factors for failure of nonoperative management includes the need for transfusion and free fluid over 300 ml in the abdominal cavity.

Selected Readings

ACEP Clinical Policies Committee, Clinical Policies Sub-committee on Acute Blunt Abdominal Trauma (2004)

Clinical policy: critical issues in the evaluation of adult patients presenting to the emergency department with acute blunt abdominal trauma. Ann Emerg Med 43:278–290

Blackbourne L, Soffer D, McKenney M, et al. (2004) Secondary ultrasound examination increases the sensitivity of the FAST exam in blunt trauma. J Trauma 57:934–938

Fang J, Wong Y, Lin B, et al. (2006) Usefulness of multidetector computed tomography for the initial assessment of blunt abdominal trauma patients. World J Surg 30:176–182

Ferrada R, Birolini D (1999) Penetrating abdominal trauma. Surg Clin N Am 79:1331–1356

Hoff WS, Holevar M, Nagy KK, et al. (2002) Practice management guidelines for the evaluation of blunt abdominal trauma: the EAST practice management guidelines group. J Trauma 53:602–615

Menegaux F, Tresallet C, Gosgnach M, et al. (2006) Diagnosis of bowel and mesenteric injuries in blunt abdominal trauma: a prospective study. Am J Emerg Med 24:19–24

Peitzman AB, Harbrecht BG, Rivera L, et al. (2005) Failure of observation of blunt splenic trauma in adults: variability in practice and adverse consequences. J Am Coll Surg 201:179–187

Rozycki G, Ballard R, Feliciano D, et al. (1998) Surgeon-performed ultrasound for the assessment of truncal injuries. Lessons learned from 1540 patients. Ann Surg 228:557–567

Velmahos G, Toutouzas K, Radin R, et al. (2003) Nonoperative treatment of blunt injury to solid abdominal organs. A prospective study. Arch Surg 138:844–851

10 Penetrating Trauma: Neck, Thorax, and Abdomen

Kenneth D. Boffard

Pearls and Pitfalls

Neck

- Never probe a wound in the neck if it is not bleeding—direct digital control may be preferable if it is.
- Always expect the worst.
- Always intubate early—the tube can be removed later if not needed.
- Paralyzing agents for airway control invite disaster.
- Always aim for proximal control of blood vessels.

Thorax

- All penetrating injuries of the abdomen may enter the chest (and vice versa). Assessment and investigation should therefore include both cavities, and include X-rays of the chest and abdomen.
- If the injury affects both the thorax and abdomen, unless *in extremis*, deal with the abdomen first.
- Fluid resuscitation must be mild to moderate.
- A double-lumen endotracheal tube will allow selective deflation of one lung, which may improve access and the ability to repair the injury.
- An emergency room thoracotomy will not revive a dead patient.

Abdomen

- Blood is not an irritant. Blood in the abdomen is not painful.
- Bowel sounds can still be present, even in the presence of significant visceral injury.
- If the injury penetrates the peritoneum or diaphragm, always assume that the penetration has caused damage on the "dark side."
- Be careful of underestimating the impending disaster of a distending abdomen in a shocked patient.
- All penetrating wounds come in pairs. If you find an entrance wound, there will be either an exit wound, or a missile left behind.
- Always use metal markers to mark penetrating wounds before X-ray. Marked wounds and missile fragments should correspond on the relevant X-rays and correlate with the suspected organ involved in the injury.

- With non-operative management, success is not predictable by grade of injury or computed tomography appearance, but only on physiological stability. In the presence of hemodynamic instability, prompt exploration of the abdomen becomes urgent.
- A negative laparotomy is better than a positive post-mortem.

Penetrating Injuries of the Neck

Introduction

The high density of critical vascular, aerodigestive, and neurologic structures within the neck makes the management of penetrating injuries difficult and contributes to the morbidity and mortality seen in these patients. However, there is a morbidity rate associated with exploration, and recently the policy of aggressive investigation and conservative surgery (including non-operative management) has become more common.

Management Principles

Current management of penetrating cervical injuries depends on several factors.

Primary Survey

Patients with signs of significant neck injury and hemodynamic instability will require prompt exploration. However, initial assessment and management of the patient should be carried out according to ATLS principles.

The major initial concern in any patient with a penetrating neck wound is early control of the airway. Appropriate protective measures for possible cervical spine injury must be implemented. A characteristic of neck injuries is rapid airway distortion with obstruction due to edema and hematoma, and often difficult intubation. The key to management is early intubation. The route of intubation must be considered carefully in these patients since it may be complicated by distortion of anatomy, hematoma, dislodging of clots, laryngeal trauma, and a significant number of cervical spinal injuries. These patients should be intubated as soon as possible, with appropriate neck protection. The use of paralyzing agents in these patients is contra-indicated, since the airway may be held open only by the patient's use of muscles. Abolishing the use of muscles in such patients usually results in the immediate and total obstruction of the airway, and no visibility due to the presence of blood, may be catastrophic. Ideally, local anesthetic spray should be used with sedation, and an immediate cricothyroidotomy below the injury should be considered when necessary. Tracheostomy should be reserved as a planned procedure in the operating theatre.

Control of hemorrhage should be undertaken by direct pressure where possible. If the neck wound is not bleeding, do not probe or finger the wound as a clot may be dislodged. If the wound is bleeding actively, then the hemorrhage can be controlled by direct digital pressure, or as a last resort, by a Foley catheter.

Secondary Survey

The injured area is often related to anatomical areas. The structures injured are those related to the particular anatomical areas (❯ *Fig. 10-1*). The neck is divided into:

- Posterior triangle
  - Behind the posterior border of sternomastoid muscle
- Anterior triangle, which is divided into
  - Zone I

◻ **Figure 10-1**
Investigation of penetrating injury to the anterior and posterior triangle of the neck

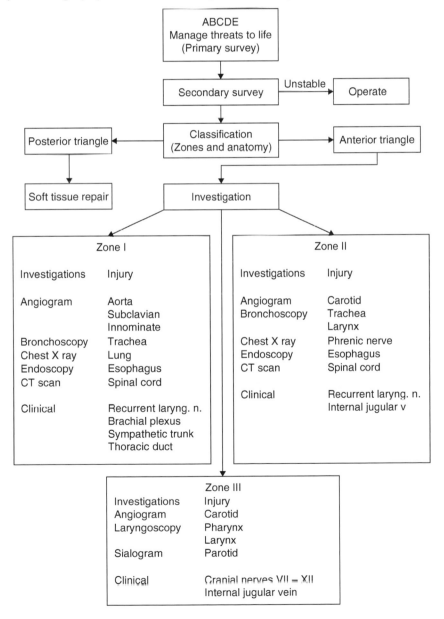

■ Figure 10-2
The anterior triangle of the neck showing the zones of the neck

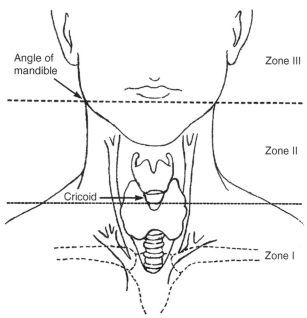

The area below the cricoid cartilage
- Zone II
  The area between the cricoid cartilage and the angle of the mandible
- Zone III
  The area above the angle of the mandible

Two immediate questions must be answered:

- Is the patient stable?
- Does the injury penetrate platysma?

If stable, the investigation can be based on index of suspicion, and anatomical probability of injury. Investigation will be based on the areas of the neck involved (❷ *Fig. 10-2*).

Management

In principle, all structures should be controlled and then repaired primarily. Arteries in Zones I and III will require proximal and distal control and probable repair. Subclavian artery injury carries specific risks. The key is proximal control with good exposure. Ideally this can be achieved with trans-femoral balloon control, but failing this, proximal control with thoracotomy or sternotomy and division of the clavicle (rarely excision) may be required. Veins can generally be tied off. All aerodigestive structures in Zone II should be repaired primarily with suitable (preferably suction) drainage.

Penetrating Injures of the Chest

It is best to artificially separate the "chest" and "abdomen" since there is a very high risk of injury to both cavities (❯ *Fig. 10-3*). Each penetrating injury should be marked with a metal marker taped to the skin prior to radiography. This will give helpful information of the risks of individual organ involvement (❯ *Fig. 10-4*).

Lethal injuries to the chest following penetrating injury include tension pneumothorax, massive bleeding (internally into the hemithorax, or externally), and cardiac tamponade.

Tension pneumothorax is diagnosed clinically with hypertympany on the side of the lesion, deviation of the trachea away from the lesion, and decreased breath sounds on the affected side. There is usually associated elevated jugular venous pressure in the neck veins. This is a clinical diagnosis, and once made an immediate needle thoracostomy or tube thoracostomy should be performed to relieve the tension pneumothorax.

The diagnosis of cardiac tamponade frequently is difficult to make clinically. It is usually associated with hypotension and elevated jugular venous pressure. There are usually muffled heart sounds, that are difficult to hear in a noisy resuscitation suite. Placing a central venous pressure (CVP) line with resultant high venous pressures can confirm the diagnosis, although a low CVP in a shocked patient does not exclude tamponade. If ultrasound is available, this is an extremely helpful diagnostic adjunct. Once the diagnosis is made, if the patient is hypotensive, the tamponade needs to be relieved as soon as possible, since ultimately decompensation is sudden. Needle pericardiocentesis may allow the aspiration of a few milliliters of blood, and this, along with rapid volume resuscitation to increase preload, can buy enough time to move to the operating room. However, in penetrating injury to the heart there is usually substantial clotting in the pericardium which may prevent aspiration. If there is no improvement, an urgent subxiphoid pericardial window, or thoracotomy is mandated.

◻ Figure 10-3
Patient with penetrating wound of the central torso

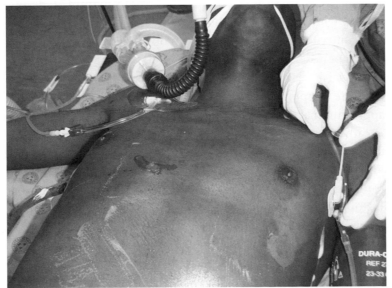

● Figure 10-4
X-ray of chest showing metal markers

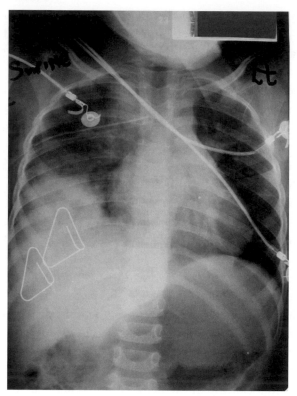

It is better to perform a thoracotomy in the operating room, either through an anterolateral approach or a median sternotomy, with good light and assistance and the potential for autotransfusion and potential bypass than it is to attempt heroic emergency surgery in the resuscitation suite. However, if the patient is in extremis with a systolic blood pressure below 40 mmHg, despite volume resuscitation, proceed immediately with a left anterior thoracotomy in an attempt to relieve the tamponade and control the penetrating injury to the heart. If there is an obvious penetrating injury, the pericardium is opened to relieve any tamponade, and if there is injury to either the left or right ventricle, the wound can be digitally controlled. As a last resort, a Foley catheter can be introduced into the hole and the balloon distended to create tamponade. The end of the Foley catheter should be clamped. Great care should be taken to apply minimal traction on the Foley catheter, just enough to allow sealing. Excessive traction will pull the catheter out, and extend the wound by tearing the muscle.

Once the bleeding is controlled, the wound can be easily sutured with pledgetted sutures, or temporarily, with skin staples.

Hemorrhage from intercostal vessels, secondary to penetrating wounds (or multiple fractured ribs), frequently will stop without operative intervention. This is also true for most bleeding from the pulmonary system. However, careful monitoring is essential using an intra-thoracic drainage with an underwater seal, and if the bleeding persists, then thoracotomy will be required to control the bleeding. It is helpful to attempt to collect shed blood from the hemothorax into an autotransfusion collecting device so that the massive hemothorax can be immediately autotransfused to the patient, and if time and expertise permit, a double lumen endotracheal tube, is very helpful.

Transmediastinal Gunshot Injuries

These injuries carry a high mortality. The management decisions will depend on the hemodynamic stability of the patient, determining the tract of the bullet, and the potential for structures along that tract to have been damaged.

- In the stable patient, the best examination is a CT scan with contrast. This will help to determine both the track of the bullet and assist in deciding whether other investigations are required.
- An angiogram and contrast study of the esophagus are the minimum investigations required in the stable patient. However, modern multi-slice CT scanning with contrast is a suitable alternative.
- Echocardiography (including a trans-esophageal echocardiogram) may be helpful if the tract is near the heart.

Penetrating Injuries of the Abdomen

The delayed diagnosis and treatment of abdominal injuries is one of the most common causes of preventable death from blunt or penetrating trauma. The deaths usually result from continuing, uncontrolled hemorrhage. Not all penetrating injuries of the abdomen will require surgical intervention if the patient is hemodynamically stable.

It is important to appreciate the difference between surgical resuscitation and definitive treatment for abdominal trauma. Surgical resuscitation includes the technique of "damage control," and implies completion of only that surgery necessary to save life by stopping bleeding and preventing further contamination or injury.

Resuscitation

Resuscitation of patients with suspected abdominal injuries should always take place within the ATLS context. Attention is paid to adequate resuscitative measures, including adequate pain control. Adequate analgesia (titrated intravenously) will never mask abdominal symptoms, and is much more likely to make abdominal pathology easier to assess, with clearer physical signs and a co-operative patient.

Diagnosis

Blood is not initially an irritant, and therefore it may be difficult to assess the presence or quantity of blood present in the abdomen. Bowel sounds may remain present for several hours after abdominal injury, or may disappear following trivial trauma. This sign is therefore particularly unreliable.

Investigation and assessment of the abdomen can be based on three groups:

1. The patient with a normal abdomen
2. An equivocal group requiring further investigation
3. The patient with an obvious injury to the abdomen

In the presence of hypotension, virtually all penetrating injuries to the abdomen should be explored promptly. Diagnostic modalities depend on the nature of the injury.

- Physical examination
- Diagnostic peritoneal lavage (DPL)
- Ultrasound—focused abdominal sonography for trauma (FAST)
- Contrast enhanced computed tomography scan (CECT)
- Diagnostic laparoscopy

The Hemodynamically "Normal" Patient

There is ample time for a full evaluation of the patient, and a decision can be made regarding surgery or non-operative management.

The Hemodynamically "Stable" Patient

The stable patient, who is not hemodynamically normal, will benefit from investigations aimed at establishing answers to the following:

- Has the patient bled into the abdomen?
- Has the bleeding stopped?

Thus, serial investigations of a quantitative nature will allow the best assessment of these patients. CECT scan is currently the modality of choice, although FAST also may be helpful, but is dependent on the operator.

The Hemodynamically "Unstable" Patient

Efforts must be made to define the cavity where bleeding is taking place, e.g. chest, pelvis or abdominal cavity. Diagnostic modalities are limited out of necessity, since it may not be practical to move an unstable patient to CT scan, even if readily available. DPL remains one of the most common, sensitive, cheapest, and readily available modalities to assess the presence of blood in the abdomen. Importantly, DPL can be performed without moving the patient from the resuscitation area. FAST is similarly useful, but is more operator dependent (be cautious if the operator is inexperienced in trauma patient handling). It must be emphasized that a negative DPL carries much greater importance than a positive one, since it gives a very clear indication whether the bleeding is intraperitoneal in nature in the unstable patient. This situation lends itself to FAST examination, as hemodynamic instability caused by intraperitoneal hemorrhage is likely to be found at FAST examination, which may be somewhat quicker than DPL.

Management—Surgical Strategies

Selective conservatism in the management of stab wounds of the abdomen is well established. The patient is reassessed for peritonism by the same surgeon at a specified interval—usually 4 hourly. Failure to improve implies the need for surgical exploration. However, a degree of surgical experience is required, and the more inexperienced the surgeon is in the management of penetrating trauma, the more the policy should lean toward operative intervention. For gunshot injury, the standard treatment is laparotomy.

Surgery for abdominal injury can conveniently be divided into

- Patients who are hemodynamically stable with easily repairable injuries; should undergo appropriate definitive surgery.
- Patients who are hemodynamically unstable, or who have difficult injury complexes; should have a damage control procedure as their default initial surgery.

Damage Control (Abbreviated Laparotomy)

"Damage control," (also known as "staged laparotomy") is a surgical strategy that sacrifices the completeness of the immediate repair to allow time to address the combined physiological impact of trauma and surgery. Once the physiology has been optimized, then the definitive surgery can proceed.

Following most major torso trauma, there is gross physiological instability, characterized by hypothermia, coagulopathy and acidosis. The priorities are therefore to control any ongoing hemorrhage, and limit contamination (e.g. by bile or bowel content). Thereafter, resuscitation takes place in the intensive care setting. Once stability has been achieved, the patient is returned to the operating room. Although the principles are sound, extreme care has to be exercised in over-utilization of the concept so that secondary insults to the viscera are minimized. Furthermore, enough appropriate surgery has to be carried out initially, in order to minimize activation of the inflammatory cascade and the consequences of SIRS and organ dysfunction.

The concept is not new, and livers were packed as long as 90 years ago, but with a failure to understand the underlying rationale, the results were disastrous. The concept was reviewed and the technique of initial abortion of laparotomy, establishment of intra-abdominal pack tamponade, and then completion of the procedure (once coagulation has returned to an acceptable level) proved to be life-saving. The concept of staging applies both to routine and emergency procedures, and can work equally well in the chest, pelvis and neck as in the abdomen.

Stage 1: Patient selection

Indications for damage control are shown in ❯ *Table 10-1*. Irrespective of the setting, a coagulopathy is the most common reason for abortion of a planned procedure, or the curtailment of definitive surgery. It is important to abort the surgery before the coagulopathy becomes obvious, and possibly irreversible.

◘ Table 10-1

Indications for damage control

Anatomical	Inability to achieve hemostasis
	Complex abdominal injury, e.g. of liver and pancreas
	Combined vascular, solid and hollow organ injury, e.g. aortic or caval injury
	Inaccessible major venous injury, e.g. retrohepatic vena cava
	Demand for non operative control of other injuries, e.g. fractured pelvis
	Anticipated need for a time consuming procedure
Physiological	Temperature < 34°C
Decline of physiological reserve	pH < 7.2
	Serum lactate > 5 mmol/l (N < 2.5 mmol/l)
	PT > 16 s
	PTT > 60 s
	> 10 units blood transfused
	Systolic BP < 90 mmHg for more than 60 min
Environmental	Operating time greater than 60 min
	Inability to approximate the abdominal incision
	Desire to reassess the intra-abdominal contents (directed relook)

Stage 2: Operative hemorrhage and contamination control
The primary objectives are:

- Hemorrhage control
- Control of contamination
- Temporary closure of the abdomen

Stage 3: Physiological resuscitation in the ICU
Priorities in the ICU are:

- Restoration of body temperature
- Correction of the clotting profile
- Repletion of blood and its components
- Optimization of oxygenation of tissues
- Avoidance of abdominal compartment syndrome

Stage 4: Operative definitive surgery
The patient is returned to the operating theater as soon as Stage 3 is achieved, which should take place within 48 h.
The timing is determined by:

- The indication for damage control in the first place
- The injury pattern
- The physiological response

Stage 5: Abdominal wall reconstruction
Once the patient has received definitive surgery, and no further operations are contemplated, then the abdominal wall can be closed.

Irrespective of the nature of both the initial and definitive surgeries which takes place, adjuncts such as adequate early nutrition (preferably enteral) optimized lung ventilation, tissue perfusion, and due attention to the immunosuppression associated with trauma patients will ensure the best possible outcome.

Selected Readings

Ellis BW, Paterson-Brown S (eds) (2000) Hamilton Bailey's emergency surgery, 13th edn. Arnold, London

Garden OJ, Paterson Brown S (ed) Abdominal Trauma (2005) Core Topics in General and Emergency Surgery: A companion to specialist surgical practice: 3rd edn. W.B. Saunders, London

Moore EE, Feliciano DV, Mattox LK (eds) (2004) Trauma, 5th edn. McGraw Hill, New York

Practice Management Guidelines. Eastern Association for the Surgery of Trauma www.east.org (accessed 2006)

Russell RCG, Williams NN, Bulstrode CJK (eds) (2004) Bailey and Love's short practice of surgery, 24th edn. Arnold, London

11 Vascular Trauma: Life-threatening Thoracoabdominal Injuries and Limb-threatening Extremity Injuries

C. Clay Cothren · Ernest E. Moore

Pearls and Pitfalls

- Prompt diagnosis based on injury mechanism and systematic evaluation in the emergency department for the 6 Ps:
  - Pallor
  - Paresthesia
  - Pulselessness
  - Paralysis
  - Pain
  - Poikilothermic
- Secure initial control of hemorrhage with digital compression
- Obtain early proximal and distal vascular control
- Arterial shunt quickly if delayed presentation
- Intraoperative angiography for diagnosis and evaluation of repair
- Presumptive fasciotomy
- Know regional nerve anatomy

Vascular injury can produce rapid exsanguination and threaten extremities or it may be a clinically silent time bomb with potentially disastrous consequences. Thus, a high index of suspicion, prompt diagnosis, and appropriate intervention are crucial to minimize associated morbidity and mortality. Although specific mechanisms of trauma should alert the practicing surgeon to unique injury patterns, identifying and managing the particular zone of injury is the most applicable information for the reader.

Thoracic Vascular Trauma

Almost a quarter of trauma-related deaths are due to thoracic injuries, and the vast majority of these injuries occur after penetrating mechanisms. Patients with penetrating wounds of the great vessels often present with massive hemorrhage or cardiac tamponade, while blunt injuries may be more subtle in their presentation. Hemodynamic instability and clinically significant chest tube output (>1,500 ml initial) represent indications for immediate thoracotomy. Mechanism of injury, patient symptoms, and clinical signs dictate ancillary imaging to evaluate for occult thoracic vascular injury.

Innominate Artery

Blunt innominate artery injury typically follows rapid deceleration mechanisms such as head-on motor vehicle collisions. The initial chest film may reveal a right-sided mediastinal hematoma (❯ *Fig. 11-1*) rather than the classic left-sided hematoma associated with descending thoracic aortic (DTA) injuries. The anatomy of the aortic arch and precise location and type of injury, either pseudoaneurysm or

◘ Figure 11-1

Post-injury imaging of the innominate artery reveals a right-sided mediastinal hematoma (a) and either a pseudoaneurysm or free extravasation at the innominate takeoff (b). Polytetrafluoroethylene (PTFE) "jump-graft" is placed between the proximal aorta and the distal, transected innominate artery, passing underneath the innominate vein (c)

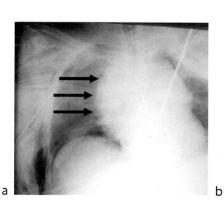
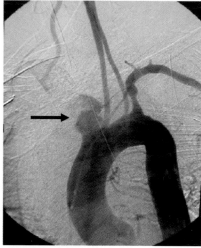
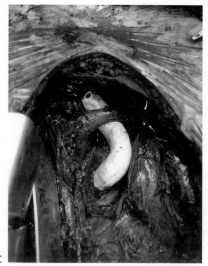

a   b

c

arterial avulsion, is clarified with angiography. The ideal operative approach is through a median sternotomy with or without a cervical extension. After thoracic entry and prior to exploration of the hematoma, an 8 mm polytetrafluoroethylene (PTFE) graft should be placed between the proximal aorta and the distal, transected innominate artery. Cardiac bypass and anticoagulation can be avoided with the use of a side-biting Satinsky clamp on the aortic arch during the proximal anastomosis. The innominate vein may be divided to acquire adequate visualization, or the tube graft can be passed underneath it. After graft interposition, the innominate injury is explored, controlled, and oversewn flush with the aortic arch. In patients sustaining penetrating injuries with hemodynamic instability or clinically significant chest-tube output, control of hemorrhage becomes the primary focus and may be obtained initially with digital control, followed by a side-biting Satinsky clamp beneath the area of injury, and then standard "jump-graft" off the proximal aorta.

Subclavian and Axillary Artery

Common patterns of injury to the subclavian artery are transection after a gunshot or stab wound to the upper chest, arterial thrombosis due to a blunt stretch injury, or direct injury due to a clavicular fracture. Only 21% of patients have an upper extremity pulse differential; therefore, patients considered high-risk due to mechanism or proximity should be evaluated with high-resolution computed tomography angiography (CTA) (❯ Fig. 11-2). As associated injuries of the brachial plexus are common, a thorough neurologic examination of the extremity is mandated prior to operative intervention. Adequate exposure of the proximal subclavian artery is best obtained via a median sternotomy on the right and a left anterior thoracotomy with upper sternal extension on the left. Repair of the distal subclavian artery is performed in two steps. To prevent exsanguination when approaching the injury, proximal arterial control is acquired with a 6 cm supraclavicular incision, encircling the subclavian artery with a vessel loop, while avoiding the phrenic nerve. Rapid exposure with a large hematoma may require proximal clavicular transection or resection. Adequate exposure of the injury is then obtained through an infraclavicular incision, extending out onto the upper arm as needed, with separation of the fibers of the pectoralis major muscle. Indiscriminate ligation or clamping for bleeding without

◘ Figure 11-2
Imaging of subclavian artery wounds show a suspicious hematoma in proximity to the vessels (a) or overt evidence of injury on angiography (b)

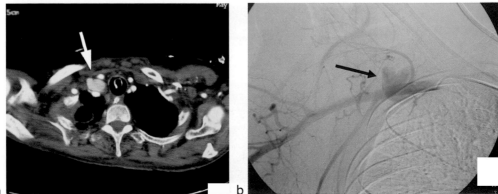

a   b

identification of the culprit vessel could result in inadvertent injury to the intertwined cords of the brachial plexus. Either a reversed saphenous vein graft or 6 mm PTFE graft is appropriate for repair.

Descending Thoracic Aorta

Approximately 10% of deaths after motor vehicle crashes (MVCs) are due to blunt tears in the DTA. The most common mechanisms are high-speed, head-on collisions or side impacts, although DTA injuries may be seen with autopedestrians' struck, fall, or crush injuries. Blunt injuries are located typically in the proximal descending aorta, just beyond the subclavian artery at the ligamentum arteriosum. Due to shear forces, there is typically partial transection of the aorta with containment by the pleural envelope preventing exsanguination. Occasionally complete transection or intimal dissection of the aorta with false lumen extension occurs. Suggestive findings on chest radiograph include loss of the aortic knob, mediastinal widening, apical capping, blurring of the aortopulmonary window, and deviation of trachea (❯ *Fig. 11-3*). Computed tomography (CT) and digital reconstructions are now the standard for definitive diagnosis. Patients with a concerning mechanism of injury should be started on intravenous beta-blockade in the emergency department prior to diagnostic

◘ Figure 11-3
Descending thoracic aortic (DTA) tears result in a widened mediastinum (a) on chest radiograph; computed tomography (CT) of the chest (b) documents partial aortic transection with intimal flap (solid arrow) and associated periaortic hematoma (dashed line)

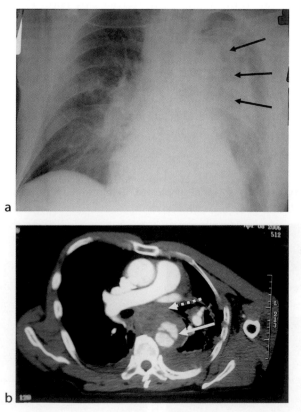

imaging to decrease shear stress on the aortic wall; a short-acting agent, e.g., esmolol, is the drug of choice, with the goal of decreasing systemic blood pressure to ≤ 100 mmHg and heart rate to < 100/min.

Current options for acute DTA tears include nonoperative management for minor injuries and endovascular stenting in patients with complex multisystem trauma, but operative repair remains the current standard. After double-lumen endotracheal intubation, operative access is acquired through a left posterolateral thoracotomy. The patient's hips are pivoted toward a supine 45° angle to provide access to the left femoral vessels for partial left heart bypass or femoral venoarterial bypass. Although primary repair with or without a graft patch is occasionally feasible, the majority of injuries require interposition grafting. Key pitfalls to be avoided during operation include the phrenic and vagus nerves during subclavian dissection and a left-sided recurrent laryngeal nerve (if present) during aortic repair. Centrifugal pumps for bypass do not require full systemic anticoagulation, but low-dose heparin (100u/kg) is usually administered unless there are substantive intracranial or spinal injuries or major solid organ injuries. Several clinical scenarios may modify the operative approach to the torn DTA. In the event of ongoing hemorrhage from concomitant abdominal trauma, emergent laparotomy is done prior to aortic repair, and unrelenting bleeding from pelvic fractures would similarly assume precedence. In patients with life-threatening intracranial bleeding or extensive right pulmonary contusion precluding left lung compression, the decision making becomes complicated. Nonoperative management with blood pressure control has proven safe and effective for some DTA tears, but head injury will not frequently permit hypotension. In these patients, endovascular stenting is probably the optimal management. In fact, endovascular repair may soon become the preferred treatment of DTA lesions.

Abdominal Vascular Trauma

A wide range of patient symptoms are encountered with intra-abdominal injuries, but most manifest some evidence of acute blood loss. With penetrating wounds to the abdomen, identification of the source of hemorrhage is usually accomplished at the time of emergent laparotomy. Initial vascular control should be accomplished with digital compression, with vascular clamps placed thereafter proximally and distally when feasible. Alternatively, if the vascular injury is contained, wide exposure and proximal/distal control should be gained before entering the hematoma. Associated open-bowel injuries, common with penetrating wounds, should be addressed by rapid stapling to minimize ongoing contamination. It is important to recognize that synthetic graft infections in the abdomen, despite associated gastrointestinal contamination, are rare.

Abdominal Aorta

Patients who survive to reach the operating room (OR) with a penetrating aortic wound frequently have a contained hematoma or free hemorrhage into the abdomen. For suprarenal aortic injuries, a left medial visceral rotation is essential for adequate exposure; if the injury is supraceliac, transecting the left crus of the diaphragm or performing left thoracotomy may be necessary. Due to lack of mobility of the abdominal aorta, few injuries are amenable to primary repair; small lateral perforations may be controlled with 4–0 prolene suture or a PTFE patch. But end-to-end interposition grafting with a PTFE tube graft is the most common repair. In contrast, blunt injuries are typically intimal tears of the infrarenal aorta and are exposed readily via a direct approach. To avoid future vascular-enteric fistulas, the vascular suture lines should be covered with mesentery or omentum.

Superior Mesenteric Artery and Vein

Penetrating wounds to the superior mesenteric artery (SMA) are encountered typically when exploring the abdomen for a gunshot wound, with "black bowel" and associated supramesocolic hematoma being pathognomonic (● *Fig. 11-4*). Blunt avulsion of the SMA is rare but should be queried in patients with a seatbelt-sign who have mid-epigastric pain or tenderness and associated hypotension. Operative approach, regardless of the etiology of injury, is based on the level of SMA injury. Fullen zone I injuries of the SMA, posterior to the pancreas, can be exposed by a left medial visceral rotation leaving the left kidney in situ. Fullen zone II SMA injuries, from the pancreatic edge to the middle colic branch, are approached via the lesser sac along the inferior edge of the pancreas at the base of the transverse mesocolon; the pancreatic body may be divided to gain proximal vascular access. More distal SMA injuries, Fullen zone III/IV, are approached directly and repaired within the mesentery.

For injuries of the SMA, temporary damage control with a Pruitt shunt can prevent bowel ischemia and edema; additionally, temporary shunting allows control of visceral contamination prior to placement of a PTFE graft. For definitive repair, end-to-end interposition with a reversed saphenous

☐ Figure 11-4

A supramesocolic hematoma (a) with associated "black bowel" (b) is pathognomonic for wounds to the superior mesenteric artery (SMA). Operative approach of Fullen zone I SMA injuries are exposed by a left medial visceral rotation, exposing the length of the aorta (c). Definitive repair is with a polytetrafluoroethylene (PTFE) graft from the aorta to the SMA past the point of injury (d)

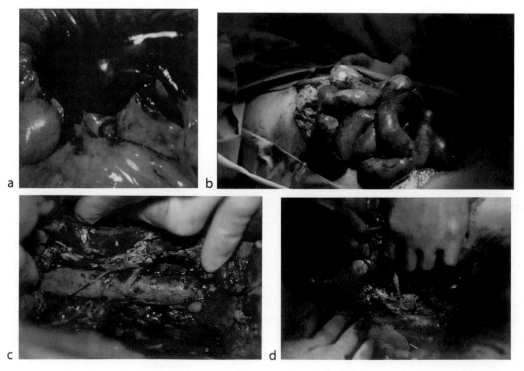

vein graft from the proximal SMA to the SMA past the point of injury can be done if there is no associated pancreatic injury. Alternatively, if the patient has an associated pancreatic injury, the graft should be tunneled from the distal aorta beneath the duodenum to the SMA. For proximal SMV injuries, digital compression for control of hemorrhage is followed by attempted venorrhaphy; ligation is an option in a life-threatening situation, but resultant bowel edema requires aggressive fluid resuscitation. Temporary abdominal closure and a second-look operation to evaluate bowel viability should be done.

Portal Triad

Penetrating wounds to the structures of the portal triad are the most common mechanism of injury, but blunt avulsions can occur. In general, the celiac axis to the level of common hepatic artery at the gastroduodenal arterial branch may be ligated due to extensive collaterals, but the proper hepatic artery should be repaired. The right or left hepatic artery, or in urgent situations the portal vein, may be ligated selectively, but associated ischemia of the liver parenchyma may necessitate delayed resection. If the right hepatic artery is ligated, cholecystectomy should also be performed. To gain access to the portal structures, control should first be gained with a Pringle maneuver prior to entering a hematoma; after defining the level of injury, vascular clamps facilitate exposure and should be used for proximal and distal control. Blindly suturing the porta is ill advised because of the proximity of the common bile duct. If the vascular injury is a stab wound with clean transection of the vessels, primary end-to-end repair is done. If the injury is destructive, temporary shunting should be performed followed by interposition-reversed saphenous vein graft. Blunt avulsions of the portal structures are particularly problematic if located at the hepatic plate, flush with the liver; control of hemorrhage at the liver can be attempted with directed packing or use of Fogarty catheters. If the avulsion is more proximal-flush with the pancreatic body border or if retropancreatic-the pancreas must be transected to gain access for control of the hemorrhage and repair.

Renovascular

Penetrating wounds to the renal pedicle are frequently destructive, and the initial priority is to control bleeding from the aorta and vena cava with Satinsky vascular clamps. In patients with multiple intra-abdominal injuries, nephrectomy is warranted. But the kidney should not be discarded until a normal functioning contralateral kidney is confirmed. The approach to blunt renal artery occlusion is controversial; renal salvage is rare if the warm ischemia time exceeds 5 h. Furthermore, most of these lesions are in the juxtaaortic renal artery and can be technically quite challenging.

Vascular Trauma of the Extremity

Often the extremities are placed at the bottom of the "to-do" list in patients with life-threatening multisystem trauma, only to find an ischemic limb hours later. Therefore, a high index of suspicion is warranted in patients with extremity fracture/dislocations; careful peripheral vascular examination, including Doppler pressure measurements comparing extremities, and associated neurologic examination is mandatory prior to transport to the OR or for ancillary imaging. Blunt trauma results in a stretch injury and subsequent occlusion of the artery at the level of the associated fracture or joint dislocation. Penetrating wounds can produce either vessel transection or a pseudoaneurysm. Motor/sensory defects may be the first sign of arterial injury due to ischemia, rather than an absent pulse. Additionally, imaging patients with soft signs or those with penetrating injuries in proximity to major vascular structures are important to avoid delays. Angiography, to discern between vessel spasm and overt injury, can be performed in the angiography suite or in the OR. "On-table" angiography in the OR facilitates rapid intervention, and is warranted in patients with evidence of ischemia on arrival in the emergency department. The notable exception is the patient with multiple fracture sites. Arterial access for "on-table" lower extremity angiography can be obtained percutaneously at the femoral vessels with a standard arterial catheter, via femoral vessel exposure and direct cannulation, or with exposure of the superficial femoral artery just above the medial knee. Once the vessel is repaired and restoration of arterial flow documented, completion angiography should be done in the OR if there is no palpable distal pulse. Vasoparalysis with verapamil, nitroglycerine, and papaverin may be employed. Fasciotomy, most often employed in the lower extremity, should be considered for all ischemic periods greater than 6 h or combined injury of named arteries and accompanying veins. Nonoperative management for small intimal flaps is appropriate, but repeated clinical follow-up is mandatory.

Brachial Artery

Brachial artery injuries are usually due to penetrating mechanisms (stab wounds, gunshot wounds, plate glass window laceration), and paramedics typically report substantial blood loss at the scene or pulsatile bleeding from the open wound. Blunt injuries with intimal dissections and secondary thrombosis may occur in patients with supracondylar fractures of the humerus. Although exploration is indicated in the majority of penetrating injuries, angiography may be helpful to diagnose blunt occlusions (❯ *Fig. 11-5*). Operative approach for a brachial artery injury is via a medial, upper extremity longitudinal incision; proximal control may be obtained at the axillary artery, and an S-shaped extension through the antecubital fossa provides access to the distal brachial artery. The segment of injured vessel is excised, and an end-to-end interposition using reverse saphenous vein is the procedure of choice. Upper extremity fasciotomy is required only rarely, unless the patient manifests preoperative neurologic changes, diminished pulse on revascularization, or extended time frame to operative intervention. Temporary shunting with a Pruitt-Inahara shunt may be useful for patient transport to an experienced facility.

External Iliac Artery

Transpelvic gunshot wounds or blunt injuries with associated pelvic fractures are the most common scenarios in patients with iliac artery injuries. Clinical examination and pulse measurements usually suggest the underlying injury, with confirmatory pelvic angiography employed occasionally (❯ *Fig. 11-6*). Operative exposure via a transabdominal approach affords access to the level of the inguinal ligament; a counterincision in the groin may be used to acquire more distal access. A Javid shunt can be used for damage control, with temporary shunting of the vessel. Definitive interposition

◘ Figure 11-5

Angiography confirms blunt brachial artery occlusion (a). On exploration via a medial upper extremity longitudinal incision, external bruising at the site of occlusion is evident (b). The injured vessel segment, with associated dissection and thrombosis, is excised (c) and an end-to-end interposition reversed saphenous vein graft is performed (d)

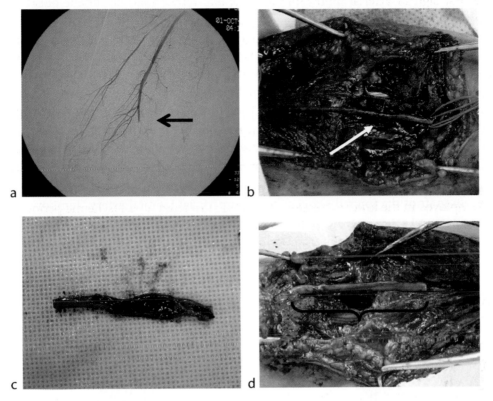

◘ Figure 11-6

Pelvic angiography reveals acute thrombosis of the left iliac artery (a) which is repaired with interposition tube grafting via a transabdominal approach (b)

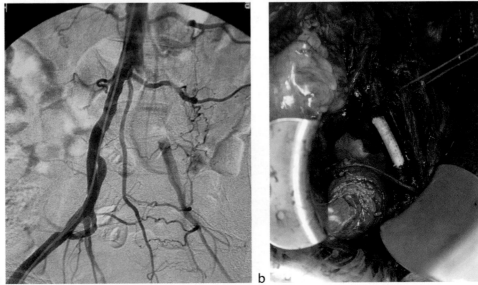

tube grafting with excision of the injured segment is appropriate. Careful monitoring for distal embolic events and reperfusion injury necessitating fasciotomy is imperative.

Superficial Femoral Artery

Although penetrating injury may result in transection with obvious signs of hemorrhage, a more insidious presentation of injury to the superficial femoral artery is seen in patients with a distal femur fracture after blunt trauma (❯ *Fig. 11-7*). The superficial femoral artery may either have intimal injury with thrombosis or complete blunt transection. Therefore, it is imperative to always ascertain ankle–ankle (A–A) indices after reduction of femur fractures in the trauma bay. If the A–A index is <0.9, angiography is indicated to evaluate for injury versus vessel spasm. Clearly, if the patient has a threatened foot, on-table angiography in the OR or operative exploration at fracture site should be performed. Typically, external fixation of the femur is performed followed by end-to-end reversed saphenous vein graft of the injured segment of the superficial femoral artery. Temporary shunting of the superficial femoral artery may be performed during orthopedic manipulation, particularly if there is a delay in recognition. Close monitoring for calf compartment syndrome is mandatory.

◻ Figure 11-7
Thrombosis of the superficial femoral artery occurs at the level of the distal femur fracture (a). After external fixation of the femur, a medial approach is used for exposure (b) and excision of the injured arterial segment (c)

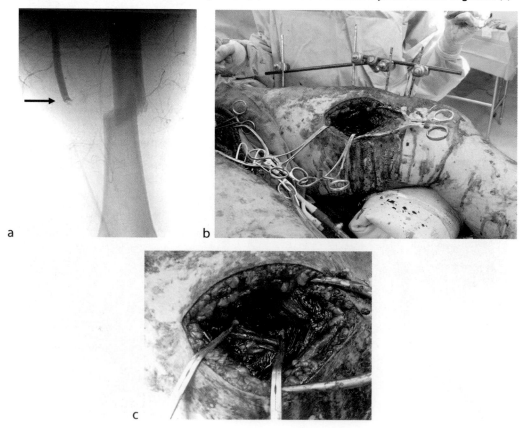

Popliteal Artery

Popliteal artery injuries are common after knee dislocations or supracondylar femur fractures in children (which clinically mimic knee dislocations). After relocation and maintaining alignment of the knee, clinical and pulse examination is performed. If the A–A index is <0.9, or if there are diminished pulses in the foot, angiography should be performed; however, clear ischemic compromise mandates immediate operative exploration. Preferred access to the popliteal space for an acute injury is the medial approach with one incision which allows detaching of the semitendinosus, semimembranosus, and gracilis tendons (❯ *Fig. 11-8*). Other options include a straight posterior approach with an S-shaped incision and a medial approach with two incisions. If the patient has an associated popliteal vein injury, this vein should be repaired first with a PTFE interposition graft while the artery is shunted. For an isolated popliteal artery injury, a reversed saphenous vein graft is performed either with an

❑ **Figure 11-8**
After reduction of a posterior knee dislocation, angiography should be performed to evaluate for a popliteal artery injury if the A–A index is <0.9 (a). Access to the popliteal vessel is either the medial approach (b) or the straight posterior approach with an S-shaped incision (c). Rapid temporary shunting in compromised extremities can be performed with a medial approach with two incisions (d)

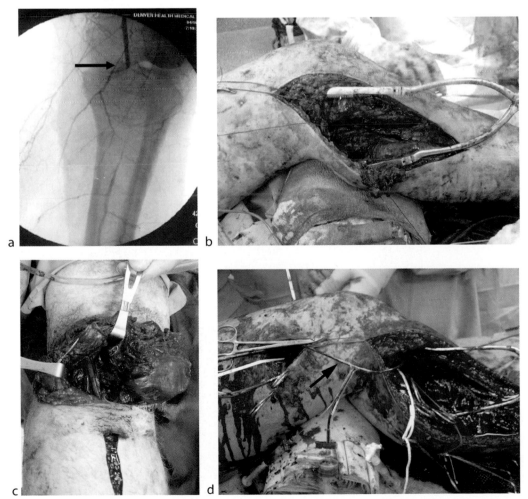

end-to-end or end-to-side proximal anastomosis and an end-to-end distal anastomosis. Compartment syndrome is common, and presumptive four-compartment fasciotomies are warranted in the majority of patients with combined arterial/venous injury.

Post-Injury Considerations

Although outcome is related to the technical success of the operation, in general the main cause of patient morbidity and mortality is associated soft tissue and nerve injury. Therefore, optimizing the patient's hemodynamic status, maintaining euthermia, and correcting coagulopathy are critical points of resuscitation. Prosthetic graft infections are rare complications, but preventing bacteremia is clearly imperative; administration of perioperative antibiotics and treatment of secondary infections are also indicated. Long-term arterial graft complications, such as stenosis or pseudoaneurysms, are uncommon, and routine graft surveillance is performed rarely. Consequently, long-term antiplatelet agents or antithrombotics are not routine.

Selected Readings

Carroll PR, McAninch JW, Klosterman P, Greenblatt M (1984) Renovascular trauma: risk assessment, surgical management, and outcome. J Trauma 30:547

Courcy PA, Brotman S, Oster-Grantie ML, et al. (1984) Superior mesenteric artery and vein injuries from blunt abdominal trauma. J Trauma 24:843

Dajee H, Richardson IW, Iype MO (1979) Seatbelt aorta: acute dissection and thrombosis of the abdominal aorta. Surgery 85:263

Feliciano DV (1998) Approach to major abdominal vascular injury. J Vasc Surg 7:730

Fullen WD, Hunt J, Altermeier WA (1972) The clinical spectrum of penetrating injury to the superior mesenteric arterial circulation. J Trauma 12:656

Johnston RH, Wall MJ, Mattox KL (1993) Innominate artery trauma: a thirty-year experience. J Vasc Surg 17:134

Kavic SM, Atweb N, Ivy ME, et al. (2001) Celiac axis ligation after gunshot wound to the abdomen: case report and review of the literature. J Trauma 50:738

Marin ML, Veith FJ, Panetta TF, et al. (1994) Transluminally placed endovascular stented graft repair for trauma. J Vasc Surg 20:466

Petersen SF, Sheldon GF, Lim RC (1979) Management of portal vein injuries. J Trauma 19:616

Reber PU, Patel AG, Sapio NLD, et al. (1999) Selective us of temporary intravascular shunts in coincident vascular and orthopedic upper and lower limb trauma. J Trauma 47:72

12 Thermal Injury

Nora F. Nugent · David N. Herndon

Pearls and Pitfalls

- Burn wounds can be categorized into superficial, partial-thickness, and full-thickness injuries to skin, depending on depth of injury to the epidermis and dermis.
- The severity of a burn is determined largely by the depth of injury and the extent or percentage of total body surface area involved.
- Areas such as the face, hands, feet, and perineum have special considerations in terms of functional and cosmetic outcomes.
- When assessing a large burn, a primary survey starting with airway, breathing, and circulation (ABC) must be done as in any trauma patient, with each problem encountered treated adequately.
- Early and adequate fluid resuscitation is vital and improves outcome in large burns.
- Burn patients may have sustained other injuries during their thermal injury. Do not forget to fully assess the patient.
- In circumferential, full thickness burns of the thorax and extremities, escharotomies may be necessary to allow adequate ventilation and circulation.
- In children and the elderly or incapacitated, consider non-accidental injury for suspicious injuries.
- Superficial and partial-thickness wounds may be treated with topical ointments and dressings.
- Deep dermal and full-thickness burns need surgical debridement and skin grafting. The wound may be covered temporarily with allo- or xenograft.

Basic Science

The pathophysiology of a thermal injury can be divided into that which occurs at a local level at the area of injury and the systemic response that occurs with a larger injury. Within the burn wound, three zones of injury have been described. An innermost zone of coagulation denotes an area of irreversible tissue loss, as a result of protein coagulation and denaturation. Surrounding this area is the zone of stasis, a region of potentially salvageable tissue. Damage has occurred, and there is decreased tissue perfusion. Resuscitation can prevent damage in this zone from becoming irreversible, however, conversely, inadequate resuscitation, infection, or excessive edema formation can convert possibly viable tissue to nonviable tissue. Prolonged decreased perfusion can lead to increased local tissue ischemia. Loss of tissue here can result in the burn wound deepening and widening. The outermost zone is the zone of hyperemia, in which as the name suggests, there is increased tissue perfusion, vasodilatation, and microvascular permeability. Inflammation and edema formation can take place here. This area of tissue recovers usually from injury.

After a burn reaches approximately 30% of the total body surface area, the effect of cytokine and inflammatory mediator release at the site of injury begins to have a systemic effect. Massive tissue edema can occur in burned tissue and also in unburned areas of soft tissue, intestine, lung, and muscle. The increased pressure in the tissue from the accumulated fluid can lead to decreased perfusion and subsequent ischemia, particularly in circumferential limb burns, especially full-thickness injuries, as deeper tissues (muscle, nerve) may become ischemic and require surgical release. This phenomenon occurs as a consequence of factors affecting control of transcapillary fluid shifts and fluid accumulation in the interstitium. Intravascular volume depletion transpires rapidly unless fluid resuscitation is adequate, although over-resuscitation can accentuate the edema formation. The rate of edema formation can be very rapid. Some of the factors involved include a marked increase in the rate of fluid and protein crossing into the interstitium, a marked increase in capillary permeability, inability to maintain a plasma-to-interstitial oncotic gradient, a decrease in interstitial pressure secondary to the release of osmotically active particles causing a vacuum effect pulling fluid in from plasma, and early disruption of the integrity of the interstitial space with disorder of collagen and hyaluronic acid structures and progressive increase in interstitial space compliance.

Myocardial contractility is decreased, possibly due to release of tumor necrosis factor α. The basal metabolic rate of the body increases to up to three times its original rate and leads to a catabolic state with loss of lean muscle mass. Downregulation of the body's immune response occurs, affecting both cell-mediated and humeral pathways. Bacterial translocation can arise from an impaired gastrointestinal mucosal barrier.

Carbon monoxide poisoning may also be present impairing oxygenation. Lung injury can occur as part of an inhalation injury or as a systemic reaction to the burn injury. Direct thermal injury from superheated gas and liquids can damage the upper airway. Airway obstruction and edema results from this topical epithelial injury and from the diffuse capillary leak associated with a cutaneous burn. Bronchospasm may be triggered by irritating chemicals inhaled, and small airway obstruction can result from sloughed epithelium, debris, and accumulated secretions, because the usual clearing ciliary mechanism is impaired. Alveolar collapse and atelectasis then occur as can pulmonary edema. This series of events leads to a high risk of tracheobronchitis and pneumonia, the end stage of which can be respiratory failure.

Clinical Presentation

The clinical presentation of thermal injury can vary depending on the causal agent and the depth and extent of the injury. An inhalation injury may accompany the cutaneous injury. The appearance of the burned area varies according to the depth of the burn (❯ *Table 12-1*).

First degree or superficial thermal injury involves only the epidermis. First degree burns present as pain and erythema of the skin, and generally heal within a week without scarring. Second degree or partial-thickness injury, which involves damage to both the epidermis and to a variable degree the underlying dermis, can be divided into superficial and deep categories. In superficial partial-thickness burns, the epidermis and no deeper than the upper third of the dermis is injured. Typically, there is blistering, and the wound is very painful, moist, and pink and blanches readily on pressure. Serous fluid usually oozes from the wound (❯ *Figs. 12-1* and ❯ *12-2*). Deep partial-thickness burns incur destruction of the epidermis and most of the dermis. These burns have a pink to white appearance and

◘ Table 12-1
Characteristics of different depths of thermal injury

Depth of burn	Skin appearance	Blisters	Capillary refill	Sensation
Superficial	Red	No	Rapid	Painful
Superficial partial thickness	Pink, moist	Yes	Present	Painful
Deep partial thickness	Pink, blotchy, dry	Sometimes	Slow	Reduced
Full thickness	White or black, dry	No	Absent	Absent

◘ Figure 12-1
Superficial burn to anterior chest from a scald injury

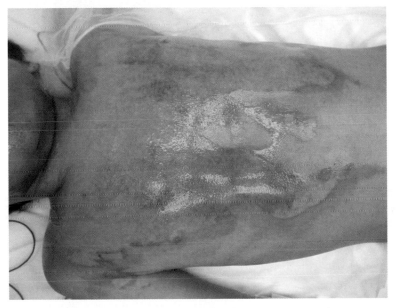

are not as painful as their more superficial counterparts because nerve endings have been injured. Capillary refill is reduced and may be very difficult to see.

Full-thickness or third degree injury is where the epidermis and the entire dermis are burned. The wound has a white, waxy appearance or a charred leathery eschar (❯ Fig. 12-3), is not painful because the nerve endings have been destroyed, and does not blanch on pressure. Coagulated vessels may be visible. Sometimes, it is very difficult to distinguish deep partial-thickness injury from third degree. Subdermal or fourth degree wounds occur when the injury has penetrated into the subcutaneous tissue and may involve muscle, tendon, or bone.

The mechanism of injury affects the clinical presentation and subsequent management. Flame injuries tend to produce full- or partial-thickness injuries. These burns may result from house fires or accidents with flammable substances such as gasoline. Scald injuries are common in children and tend to produce superficial and partial thickness injuries. Contact burns, which result from prolonged contact with a hot surface or contact with an extremely hot surface, tend to be deep dermal or full-thickness. These burns are seen usually in children or those who cannot remove themselves quickly from the source, such as the elderly, epileptics during a seizure, the disabled, or those under intoxication.

◘ Figure 12-2
Partial-thickness burn to forearm and hand

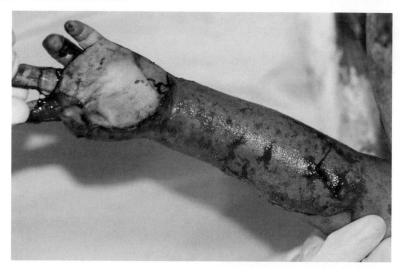

◘ Figure 12-3
Full-thickness burn to upper extremity. Escharotomies and fasciotomies have been performed

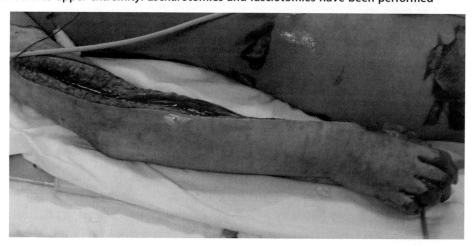

Electrical injuries vary in severity depending on the voltage of the power source. Low voltages, e.g. domestic electricity, usually cause small, deep contact entry and exit site burns. An alternating current crossing the myocardium has the potential to trigger cardiac arrhythmias. High voltages cause much more extensive tissue destruction. As well as entry and exit point burns, extensive muscle necrosis and nerve damage can occur along the path of the current. Limb loss may occur. Rhabdomyolysis from muscle damage and renal failure can also result from the injury. If the victim does not actually make contact with the power source, but is very close by, a flash injury can occur from an arc of current. The heat of the flash can cause superficial burns and can set clothing on fire resulting in deeper burns.

Chemical injuries occur as a result of contact with acids or alkalis, either in the workplace or the home. These burns tend to be deep and can penetrate tissue progressively if the chemical persists on the skin and continues to injure the tissue. Acid burns are painful and cause a coagulative necrosis and protein denaturation. Of note, hydrofluoric acid (used in glass etching) reacts with the body's calcium and can rapidly cause fatal hypocalcemia. Alkali burns induce a liquefactive necrosis and can penetrate deeper into tissues than acid. The onset of pain may be delayed, allowing the chemical longer contact with the skin before treatment is initiated.

Substantive inhalation injury usually presents with signs and symptoms of upper airway distress, such as stridor and dysphonia, from the resultant mucosal edema. Symptoms usually occur after some time has passed because it takes time for the edema to accumulate. Indications that an airway injury may have occurred include face and neck burns, singed nasal and facial hairs, and the presence of carbonaceous material in the mouth and upper airway. Symptoms of carbon monoxide poisoning may range from disorientation to obtundation and coma, depending on the extent of poisoning.

Diagnosis

Diagnosis of a thermal injury is based largely on history and physical examination. A thorough assessment and evaluation of the patient is essential. For a large burn, it may be necessary to begin emergency management while evaluating the patient concurrently.

In the history, the following information should be asked: the cause of the thermal injury, the time at which it occurred, whether the victim was in an enclosed space, and the duration of contact with the injuring agent. Any other injuries sustained at the time should be inquired about and sought after, because the patient may have other injuries sustained due to the nature of the injury, such as an explosion, or while trying to jump to escape from a burning house. Tetanus status should be established, and any first aid or other medical attention received at the scene enquired about. Allergies, medications, and pre-existing medical conditions also need to be known.

The severity of a burn injury is determined largely by the depth and extent of the burn injury. Notable exceptions to this include some chemical burns, such as hydrofluoric acid, and electrical injuries. The depth of injury is determined by the physical appearance of the cutaneous injury, and as discussed earlier can be classified into superficial, partial-thickness, and full-thickness injuries. This assessment is generally a clinical one, but techniques such as biopsies, laser Doppler studies, and ultrasonography, have been used in certain occasions to determine depth of injury.

The extent of burn injury is determined by calculating the percentage total body surface area (% TBSA) involved. Erythema or first-degree thermal injury is not included in this calculation. Several methods have been used to determine % TBSA involvement. The "rule of nines" can be used for a quick calculation, where each upper limb is 9%, each lower limb 18% etc. This general rule, however, does not take into account the different proportions of childrens' bodies. A Lund and Browder chart that has precalculated percentages for each body part for different age groups can also be used (❯ *Fig. 12-4*). For smaller burns, the patient's own hand can be used. The palmer surface has been estimated to be about 1% of the patient's body surface area, but this approach may overestimate burn size.

Assessment of airway involvement includes checking for singed nasal and facial hairs, dysphonia, and stridor, particularly if the burn took place in an enclosed space or if there are head and neck burns. Carbonaceous material may be present in the mouth and upper airway. Direct laryngoscopy and bronchoscopy may be indicated to supplement the diagnosis not only by allowing direct visualization of the upper airway and the tracheobronchial tree, but also by helping to assess edema and need for intubation. The chest radiograph will usually be remarkably normal. Carbon monoxide levels can be

◻ **Figure 12-4**
An example of a Lund and Browder chart used for assessment of % TBSA burn

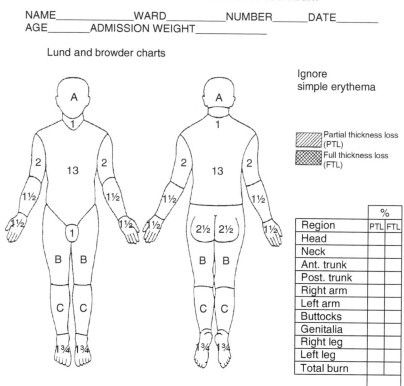

NAME_____WARD_____NUMBER_____DATE_____
AGE_____ADMISSION WEIGHT_____

Lund and browder charts

Ignore
simple erythema

Partial thickness loss (PTL)
Full thickness loss (FTL)

Region	%	
	PTL	FTL
Head		
Neck		
Ant. trunk		
Post. trunk		
Right arm		
Left arm		
Buttocks		
Genitalia		
Right leg		
Left leg		
Total burn		

Relative percentage of body surface area
affected by growth

Area	Age 0	1	5	10	15	Adult
A=½ of head	9½	8½	6½	5½	4½	3½
B=½ of one thigh	2¾	3¼	4	4½	4½	4¾
C=½ of one leg	2½	2½	2¾	3	3¼	3½

measured to assess for poisoning; however, time from exposure and use of supplemental oxygen will affect the interpretation of the value obtained.

Other important issues in the initial evaluation include assessment of the circulation and compartments of circumferentially burned limbs and limbs involved in the pathway of electrical injury. Pulses, capillary refill, temperature, swelling, movement, and sensation should be documented. A full neurologic exam should be undertaken. In electrical injuries, an electrocardiogram is imperative, the patient should be monitored for 24 h, and urine checked for myoglobin. Baseline blood gas, electrolyte, and hematologic values are obtained.

The possibility of non-accidental injury in pediatric thermal injuries must remain in the healthcare workers mind. Suspicious findings in the history include an evasive or changing story, a delay in seeking medical help, a story that does not fit with the age of the child or the pattern of injury, or lack of adequate supervision at the time of injury. There may be evidence of a "tide-line" and sparing of the flexion creases in an immersion type injury where the burn lines up when the child goes into the fetal position. Also, glove and stocking type injuries to hands and feet, deep contact burns, e.g. with an iron pattern, and no splash marks in a scald injury should arouse suspicion. Other injuries or evidence of past injuries and signs of neglect should be sought, and careful photography and documentation of the case undertaken. The child should be admitted to the hospital until the case can be assessed by the relevant authorities.

Treatment

First aid for a thermal injury consists of removing the victim from the source of injury in a manner that does not cause harm to the rescuer. Ignited clothing should be extinguished by getting the victim to drop to the ground and roll. Wet blankets can also be used. The clothing should then be removed. Electrical power sources should be sought and turned off before attempting to help the victim. Cooling measures should then be applied, such as running cool or lukewarm water. Very cold water or ice should be avoided because the blood flow to the burned area may be decreased, and the victim may become hypothermic.

The initial management of a major burn then follows that of a trauma patient with assessment of the ABCs, i.e., airway, breathing, circulation, as well as the cervical spine. Supplemental oxygen should be provided. If signs of inhalation injury are present or facial or neck burns are present, airway patency should be assessed. Stridor or other signs of acute respiratory distress indicate need for intubation. If a bronchoscopy is being done to evaluate the airway, an endotracheal tube can be passed over the scope and the patient intubated if necessary. Patients at risk for progressive edema, but without significant swelling, can be observed for 24–36 h; however, in established edema, intubation can be very difficult. Once a secure airway has been established, breathing needs to be re-assessed. In circumferential, full-thickness chest burns, ventilation may be impaired due to the reduced chest wall compliance. Chest wall escharotomies can improve ventilation substantially in these patients.

Circulation then needs to be assessed. Vital signs and urine output are monitored and intravenous access obtained. The depth and % TBSA burn should be calculated and the need for intravenous resuscitation assessed. In general, burns over 15% TBSA require intravenous fluid resuscitation (Hettiaratchy and Dziewulski, 2004). Several formulae have been used to try and establish the correct amount and type of resuscitative fluid. One of the most commonly used calculations is the Parkland formula which uses lactated Ringers solution at a rate of 3–4 ml/kg body weight/% TBSA burn, which gives the 24 h fluid requirement from the time of burn; half is to be given in the first 8 h post burn, and the remaining half given over the next 16 h. Children require dextrose-containing maintenance fluids in addition when using this formula. The use of colloid versus crystalloid in acute burn resuscitation has been long debated. Proponents of colloid argue that the reduced volumes required minimize the cardiac and electrolyte complications of infusion of large volumes of fluid; however, the benefit of colloid has not been proven in the first 24 h post burn. Regardless of the formula used, the calculation should serve as a general guideline to the amount of fluid needed, and end-points of resuscitation need to be monitored. Some patients may need more fluid and some may need less. Pulse, blood pressure, and urine output are the traditional values monitored (Sheridan, 2000). In children, urine outputs of 1–2 ml/kg/h are desired, while in adults 0.5–1 ml/kg/h is sufficient. Early resuscitation appears to improve outcome.

In full-thickness circumferential burns to the limbs, if there is any impairment to circulation, escharotomies are needed. The incisions should stretch the full range of the burn wound to the edge of normal skin. Generally incisions down each side of the limb are necessary and can usually be performed at the bedside. The fascial compartments should be assessed and, if necessary, also released. In electrical injuries or victims with additional trauma, there should be a lower threshold for fasciotomies. The limbs should be elevated to help reduce further swelling from the resultant edema formation. A secondary survey should be done to assess for any additional injuries, and these treated. Tetanus prophylaxis should be administered if indicated. Early resuscitation and enteral feeding is safe, effective, and important in providing nutrition (Barrow, 2000). Meticulous pulmonary hygiene should be maintained.

For chemical injuries, contaminated clothing should be removed and the area copiously and repeatedly irrigated. Litmus paper may be used to test the pH of the skin to confirm removal of the substance. It is important to know the agent involved, because some chemicals have more specific therapies; for instance, hydrofluoric acid sequesters calcium and calcium gluconate should be applied topically or injected locally. Systemic administration may also be necessary. Eye injuries should also be irrigated copiously and a fluorescein stain done to check for corneal abrasions. If any injury is suspected, the patient should be referred to an ophthalmologist.

Superficial partial-thickness wounds generally do not require operation and are treated topically. A wide variety of dressings are available and suitable for use. The wounds need to be cleaned first and then the dressing applied. Paraffin gauze or hydrocolloid dressings are suitable for clean, superficial wounds. Traditionally, silver-containing ointments and soaks, such as silver sulfadiazine and silver nitrate have also been used. The silver imparts bactericidal properties to the ointments. Biobrane, a bilaminar silicone membrane bonded to a collagen layer, can be applied to these types of wounds because it adheres to the wound, reduces pain and the need for dressing changes, and has good quality healing results. This agent needs to be monitored initially for adherence and infection, and should be removed if not sticking or infected. Human amnion membrane has also been used successfully in treatment of partial-thickness burns, although it carries a potential risk of transmission of infectious diseases (Sheridan, 2000). Numerous other topical dressings and ointments are also available.

Deeper burn wounds require operative treatment. Deep dermal injuries may be treated by debriding the wound tangentially to healthy bleeding tissue. If a significant portion of the dermis is still intact, the wound may be covered temporarily with porcine xenograft or human allograft. If the dermis re-epithelializes, the xeno- or allograft will gradually lift off. If not, it will have to be removed at a later procedure and the area autografted with split-thickness skin grafts taken from the patient's available unburned skin. Full-thickness wounds require complete excision of the dermis. If the subcutaneous tissue underneath is also burned or infected, it may be necessary to excise the wound to the level of fascia. Again, split-thickness autograft is the coverage of choice for these patients. The graft is usually harvested at a depth of 8–12/1000 in. and is not usually meshed for facial burns and, if possible, for hand burns. Otherwise, the graft is usually meshed to allow for greater coverage and drainage of fluid. In large burns, often there is insufficient donor sites to achieve full coverage with autograft in one operation, and multiple debridement and grafting procedures are necessary. The excised wound may be covered temporarily with skin substitutes such as porcine xenograft, human allograft, or synthetic dermal substitutes such as Integra. As the donor sites heal, the burn wounds are autografted serially. Thorough wound care is necessary to reduce the incidence of wound sepsis. Antibiotic therapy should be tailored according to evidence of infection and wound cultures and sensitivities.

It is now possible to use a small sample of unburned skin to culture keratinocytes into epithelial sheets. This approach is most efficacious to cover the patient with very large burns. Problems associated with this approach include fragility of the grafts, delay in obtaining the finished product, and the prohibitive expense for many centers.

Post-operatively, the patient usually requires extensive rehabilitation involving physical therapy to maintain range of motion, the use of splints to prevent joint contractures, and meticulous wound care and scar management. This aspect of therapy is vital and will influence the extent of reconstructive procedures necessary at later stages, such as joint contracture releases. Major burns usually require multiple reconstructive procedures once stable wound coverage has been achieved, including releases of joint contractures and ectropions and reconstruction of destroyed body parts. Moisturization of the healed areas and protection from the sun are also very important.

Outcome

The prognosis for those with thermal injuries has improved over the last 2 decades. Due to advances in techniques of resuscitation, infection control, critical care, and more aggressive surgical management, the mortality for severe burns has decreased markedly. Early fluid resuscitation (commencing within two hours of injury) may have important implications in improving survival and in reducing the incidence of multiorgan failure. The advent of skin substitutes and development of cultured keratinocytes has also improved outcome, because these newer biologic dressings allow better opportunities to achieve wound coverage in large burns. Extremes of age and % TBSA involvement remain important predictors of mortality.

Survival is not the only relevant outcome in thermal injury. Functional outcome, quality of life, participation in society and the work force, and psychologic well-being are all important factors to consider when assessing outcome in the thermally injured patient. Many patients have functional disabilities relating to scar contractures or undergo amputations secondary to burn injuries which impact on activities of daily living and participation in work and school. Patients may become depressed as a result of loss of independence, the necessity to alter their lifestyles, and the alteration in their physical appearances. Psychologic counseling and family and community support are important.

Selected Readings

Atiyeh BS, Gunn SW, Hayek SN (2005) State of the art in burn treatment. World J Surg 29:131–148

Barrow RE, Jeschke MG, Herndon DN (2000) Early fluid resuscitation improves outcomes in severely burned children. Resuscitation 45:91–96

Benson A, Dickson WA, Boyce D (2006) ABC of wound healing. Burns. BMJ 332:649–652

Demling RH (2005) The burn edema process: current concepts. J Burn Care Rehabil 26:207–227

Hettiaratchy S, Dziewulski P (2004) ABC of burns. Pathophysiology and types of burns. BMJ 328:1427–1429

Sheridan RL (2000) Airway management and respiratory care of the burn patient. Int Anesthesiol Clin 38:129–145

Sheridan RL, Tompkins RG (2004) What's new in burns and metabolism. J Am Coll Surg 198:243–263

van Baar M, Essink-Bot ML, Oen IMMH, et al. (2006) Functional outcome after burns: a review. Burns 32:1–9

13 Closed Head Injury

Philip F. Stahel · Wade R. Smith

Pearls and Pitfalls

- Closed head injury represents the leading cause of death in young patients in industrialized countries.
- Patients surviving the initial injury are susceptible to sustaining secondary cerebral insults initiated by the release of endogenous neurotoxic inflammatory mediators.
- Hypoxia and hypotension in the early resuscitative period represents the "key" parameter for induction of secondary brain injury and adverse outcomes.
- The neuroinflammatory response in the injured brain contributes to cerebral edema, increased intracranial pressure (ICP), and decreased cerebral perfusion pressure (CPP).
- ICP monitoring and CPP therapy are recommended as a standard for patients with *severe* closed head injury. The ICP should be kept below 15 mmHg and the CPP above 70 mmHg in order to avoid secondary insults due to cerebral hypoperfusion.
- If a CPP $\geq$ 70 mmHg cannot be achieved by lowering the ICP, the mean arterial pressure (MAP) should be artificially raised by the use of catecholamines (CPP = MAP ICP).
- Arterial "demand" hypertension in head-injured patients should not be lowered therapeutically since this physiological response is aimed at maintaining an adequate CPP once the cerebrovascular autoregulation has failed.

Common Errors of Practice

- Delayed resuscitation from hypotension and hypoxemia.
- Delayed endotracheal intubation in patients with a Glasgow Coma Scale (GCS) score $\leq$ 8.
- Lack of attention to associated injuries (thoracic, abdominal, orthopedic).
- Underestimating magnitude of *mild* or *moderate* head injury, assuming absence of intracranial pathology (patients who "talk and die").
- Underestimating comatose patients with normal computed tomography (CT) scan (diffuse axonal injury).
- Failures in awake patients: (1) Inadequate frequency of neurological examinations; (2) delay in obtaining a CT scan upon neurological deterioration or change in pupil size/reactivity.
- Pharmacological attenuation of increased systemic blood pressure in head-injured patients ("demand hypertension").
- "Blind" therapeutic hyperventilation without keeping the pCO_2 in constant range (3.3–4.7 kPa) and without bedside jugular bulb oxymetry and sequential measurement of the arterio-jugular differences in lactate concentrations.
- Delay in transfer of severely head-injured patients to a facility with neurosurgical capabilities.

Introduction

In industrialized nations, closed head injury represents the leading cause of death and disability in young people. In the USA alone, about 1.5–1.8 million people sustain a traumatic brain injury each year, of which approximately 500,000 require hospital admission. The annual economic burden of direct and indirect costs for traumatic brain injury in the USA is estimated around US$50 billion annually. Despite advances in research and improved neurointensive care in the last decade, the clinical outcome of severely head-injured patients is still poor and the mortality rate remains as high as 35–40%. Research efforts in the past years have highlighted that the intracerebral inflammatory response in the injured brain contributes to the neuropathological sequelae which are, in large part, responsible for the adverse outcome after closed head injury. The extent of residual brain damage is determined by primary and secondary insults. The primary damage results from mechanical forces applied to skull and brain at the time of impact, leading to either focal or diffuse brain injury patterns. Focal brain injury is due to direct concussion/compression forces, while diffuse axonal shearing injuries are usually caused by indirect trauma mechanisms, such as sudden deceleration or rotational acceleration. Secondary brain injury occurs after the initial trauma and is a consequence of complicating processes such as ischemia/reperfusion injuries, cerebral edema, intracranial hemorrhage, and intracranial hypertension. The main risk factors for developing secondary brain injury are hypoxemia and systemic hypotension which occur frequently in the polytraumatized patient. The general surgeon who sees brain-injured patients first, must be skilled in their initial assessment and resuscitation, as a neurosurgeon may not be immediately available. The maintenance of adequate systemic blood pressure and oxygenation is of paramount importance. This chapter provides a concise protocol for the initial assessment and management of patients with closed head injuries.

Clinical Presentation

The diagnosis of closed head injury is established by the history of trauma, by the clinical status, and by CT Scan. Efforts should be made to learn the details of the accident, including the mechanism of trauma. This includes blunt vs. penetrating injury, force of the traumatic impact, condition of the vehicle, and presence of other injured/dead occupants. The condition of the vehicle's interior may reveal potential associated injury patterns, such as a "bull's eye"-break on the windscreen, suggesting direct skull impact with associated shear forces to brain tissue and possibility of associated cervical spine injury, or a bent steering wheel may indicate severe chest trauma leading to hypoxia. The likelihood of serious injuries is significantly increased in patients that have been ejected from the vehicle or in the case of death by another occupant in the same vehicle compartment. It is furthermore important to obtain information about the level of consciousness at the accident scene, the presence of impaired neurologic function, and changes in the level of consciousness until admission to the hospital. Of particular importance is the knowledge of the postresuscitation GCS score, since this parameter represents an important predictor of outcome (❷ *Table 13-1*). Other crucial information includes the presence of anoxia/hypoxia (compromised airways, chest trauma, delayed endotracheal intubation) and the approximate blood loss at the accident scene (massive external bleeding, hemorrhagic shock), as well as the therapy instituted before admission (airway patency, endotracheal intubation, adequate fluid resuscitation).

◘ Table 13-1

Glasgow Coma Scale (GCS) (Teasdale and Jennett, 1974)

Clinical parameter	Points
Eye opening (E)	
Spontaneous	4
To speech	3
To pain	2
None	1
BEST motor response (M)	
Obeys commands	6
Localizes pain	5
Normal flexion (withdrawal)	4
Abnormal flexion (decorticate)	3
Extension (decerebrate)	2
None (flaccid)	1
Verbal response (V)	
Fully oriented	5
Disoriented/confused conversation	4
Inappropriate words	3
Incomprehensible words	2
None	1
GCS score: $\sum$ (E + M + V)	Severity of head injury
14/15 points	Mild
9–13 points	Moderate
3–8 points	Severe

On the accident scene and on hospital admission, all head-injured patients must be systemically assessed and resuscitated according to the American College of Surgeons' "Advanced Trauma Life Support" (ATLS) protocol. The recommendations for the initial management of patients with closed head injury are presented in ❷ Table 13-2. After securing the airway and assuring adequate oxygenation and fluid replacement, concomitant intra-abdominal injuries leading to exsanguinating hemorrhage must be excluded in all head-injured patients with an altered level of consciousness by ultrasonography and/or CT scan. Furthermore, an associated cervical spine injury must be assumed in *all* head-injured patients until proven otherwise, since 5–10% of head-injured patients have concomitant injuries of the cervical spine. The neurologic evaluation is initiated only after vital functions have been stabilized. The level of consciousness is rapidly assessed by the GCS score (❷ Table 13-1). When assessing the GCS, the *best* response post resuscitation is used to calculate the score. In addition to the level of consciousness, the neurologic exam must include the assessment of pupillary size and reactivity, and a brief focused evaluation of peripheral motor function. The clinical exam furthermore includes the inspection of the scalp for lacerations, palpation of the skull for impression fractures, and the search for indirect signs of basilar skull fractures, including periorbital ecchymosis ("racoon eyes"), retroauricular ecchymosis ("Battle's sign"), rhinorrhea/otorrhea due to cerebrospinal fluid (CSF) leakage, and VIIth nerve palsy. The necessity for obtaining a CT scan (❷ Table 13-2) is given under the following circumstances: (1) altered level of consciousness; (2) abnormal neurologic examination; (3) differences in pupil size or reactivity; (4) suspected skull fracture. Furthermore, the CT scan should be repeated whenever there is deterioration in the patient's neurologic status.

◘ Table 13-2

Initial management of head-injured patients *(see text for details and abbreviations)* **(Stahel et al., 2005; The Brain Trauma Foundation, 2006)**

- Initial assessment and resuscitation according to the ATLS protocol. Secure airways and assure adequate oxygenation and fluid replacement. Avoid hypoxemia and hypotension!
- Exclude exsanguinating intra-abdominal injury (focused ultrasonography/"FAST," CT) and other associated systemic injuries.
- Blood alcohol level and urine toxic screening in all head-injured patients.
- *History*:
    - Mechanism and time of injury
    - Loss of consciousness
    - Amnesia (retro-/anterograde)
    - Postresuscitation level of consciousness (GCS)
    - Seizures
    - Presence of headache (mild/moderate/severe)
- *Brief neurologic examination*:
    - Level of consciousness (GCS)
    - Pupillary size and reaction
    - Focal motor deficits
- *Indications for CT scan*:
    - All patients with moderate to severe head injury (GCS < 14).
    - Mild head injury (GCS 14 and 15) in conjunction with one of the following criteria:
        - Presence of skull fracture (clinically or xray)
        - CSF leak (rhinorrhea, otorrhea)
        - Alcohol/drug intoxication
        - Moderate to severe headache
        - Focal neurologic deficits, abnormal pupil size or reactivity
        - Deteriorating level of consciousness (GCS < 14) in the later course
    - Perform a control CT scan before discharge in all patients with moderate to severe head injury (GCS < 14) and in cases of mild head injury (GCS 14 and 15) with pathological initial CT scan.
- *Indications for hospital admission*:
    - All patients with GCS < 15 (observe for at least 24 h, with frequent neurologic examinations)
    - All patients with open head injuries, CSF leak, skull fractures
    - Patients with GCS 15 and one of the following: (1) moderate to severe headache; (2) history of loss of consciousness; (3) amnesia; (4) significant alcohol/drug intoxication; (5) no reliable companion at home for observation; (6) unable to return promptly in case of deterioration.

Classification

Closed head injury may be classified either by morphology, severity, or mechanism of injury. The morphological classification is based on findings in the CT scan according to the guidelines established by Marshall and colleagues (❯ *Table 13-3*). Intracranial CT lesions can be either of focal nature ("evacuated" vs. "non-evacuated" subdural, epidural, or intracerebral hematomas) or diffuse (grade I–IV). The classification by severity according to the GCS score (❯ *Table 13-1*) is clinically relevant, since the postresuscitation score has been shown to significantly correlate with patient outcome. Patients with *mild* head injury (GCS 14 or 15) represent about 80% of all head-trauma patients admitted to the emergency department. These patients usually suffer from a mild cerebral concussion which corresponds to diffuse brain injury with preserved consciousness but a certain degree of temporary neurologic dysfunction. In contrast, a "classic" cerebral concussion results in a reversible

◘ Table 13-3

Morphological classification by CT scan. The classification of intracranial pathology by CT scan according to Marshall et al. correlates significantly with the outcome after closed head injury (Marshall et al., 1992)

CT classification	Definition	Mortality
Diffuse injury (DI) I	Normal CT scan (clinical diagnosis)	
Diffuse injury (DI) II	Open basal cisterns, midline shift 0-5 mm, high- or mixed-density lesions < 25 cc.	15%
Diffuse injury (DI) III	Compressed or absent basal cisterns, midline shift 0-5 mm, high- or mixed-density lesions < 25 cc	
Diffuse injury (DI) IV	Absent basal cisterns, midline shift > 5 mm, high- or mixed-density lesions < 25 cc	
Evacuated mass lesion (EML)	Any surgically evacuated intracranial lesions	
Non-evacuated mass lesion (NEML)	High- or mixed-density lesion > 25 cc, not surgically evacuated	55%

loss of consciousness, which is always accompanied by posttraumatic amnesia. It is important to keep in mind that approximately 3% of patients with *mild* head injury will have a potentially fatal intracranial hemorrhage. Thus, all patients with closed head injury should be admitted to the hospital according to the recommendations outlined in ❷ *Table 13-2*. *Pitfall:* Patients who "talk and die" comprise those who have a GCS > 8 on admission and suddenly deteriorate due to an intracranial mass lesion, typically an acute epidural hematoma (EDH).

Moderate head injury corresponds to a GCS score between 9 and 13 and is associated with an increased risk for intracranial pathology compared to patients with *mild* head injury. As outlined in ❷ *Table 13-2*, a CT scan must be performed in all patients with *moderate* head injury, and all of these patients should be admitted to the hospital for observation. A GCS score ≤ 8 corresponds to a comatose patient, as defined by the inability to open the eyes, to obey commands, and to respond verbally. Thus, *severe* head injury is defined as a GCS score of 3–8. The initial assessment and management of these severely injured patients is described in the following section.

Emergency Room Management

The immediate goal in the management of head-injured patients is the prevention of secondary brain damage by rapid correction of hypoxemia, hypotension, hypercarbia, and hypoglycemia. For airway protection, an oropharyngeal or nasopharyngeal airway may be adequate in drowsy patients with sufficient breathing, while endotracheal intubation by "rapid sequence induction" is indicated in comatose patients (GCS ≤ 8) or in cases of apnea, hypoventilation, risk of upper airway obstruction (maxillofacial fractures, laryngeal injury), and aspiration (vomiting, bleeding). Adequate volume resuscitation is crucial, including the control of external and internal hemorrhages. According to the ATLS guidelines, the initial fluid therapy should be an isotonic electrolyte solution, such as Ringer's

■ Box 13-1

Relationship between CPP, ICP and MAP[a]

CPP = MAP – ICP

[a]CPP, cerebral perfusion pressure; ICP, intracranial pressure; MAP, mean arterial pressure.

lactate, with an initial bolus dose of 1,000–2,000 ml in adults and 20 ml/kg in children. Measurement of the urinary output represents a "prime monitor" for the patients' response to resuscitation, and should be about 0.5 ml/kg/h in adults and 1–2 ml/kg/h in pediatric patients. *Pitfall*: Increased urinary output in head-injured patients due to syndrome of inappropriate ADH secretion (SIADH). A detailed neurologic evaluation should only be initiated after the vital systems have been stabilized. Furthermore, associated injuries, such as a cervical spine injury, blunt chest trauma, intra-abdominal injuries, pelvic ring disruptions, and open fractures must receive adequate attention, as all of these injuries can potentiate the extent of secondary brain damage. According to the ATLS algorithm for early care of severely injured patients, the "A-B-C-D-E" priorities mandate that only hemodynamically stable patients should undergo further diagnostics, such as a craniocerebral CT scan. All head-injured patients with presence of hypoxia and/or hypotension must be fully resuscitated, if required by surgical measures, before CT diagnostics are performed.

The main priority in the early management of head-trauma patients is the maintenance of an adequate CPP above 70–80 mmHg. According to the "Monro-Kellie doctrine," the total intracranial volume remains constant, implying that expanding mass lesions will result in a reduced CPP, thus contributing to secondary brain injury. Due to the interrelation between CPP and MAP (❍ *Box 13-1*), an increased systemic blood pressure must never be therapeutically lowered in head-injured patients unless continuous ICP-monitoring is available ("demand" hypertension!). Standardized therapeutic approaches are aimed at lowering the ICP in order to keep the CPP at a sufficient level. Among the therapeutic modalities are the reduction of mass lesions by surgical evacuation of intracranial hematomas (ICHs), the reduction of brain swelling with osmotic drugs, e.g., mannitol, and therapeutic CSF drainage through intraventricular catheters.

Osmotic Therapy (Mannitol)

When given as a bolus, mannitol augments the intravascular volume, resulting in a transient increase in MAP and CPP. Mannitol also causes an increase in cerebral blood flow (CBF) in cases of impaired cerebrovascular autoregulation, where CBF is directly dependent on systemic arterial pressure. Furthermore, mannitol can induce a cerebral vasoconstriction, resulting in a diminished intracranial volume.

Indications:

- Clinical signs of transtentorial herniation (i.e., loss of consciousness, decerebrate rigidity, ipsilateral pupil dilatation, contralateral hemiparesis), or progressive neurological deterioration, not attributable to systemic pathology.
- Bilaterally dilated and nonreactive pupils.
- Regimen: mannitol (20%), 0.25–1 g/kg IV in 5 min.

Pitfalls:

- Hypovolemia must be avoided by adequate fluid replacement.
- Serum osmolarity must be kept <315 mOsm/l, since hyperosmolarity may induce acute renal failure.

The use of *glucocorticoids* is not recommended for attenuating the neuroinflammatory response in severely head-injured patients. In contrast, based on the devastating results from the prospective multicenter "CRASH" trial on 10,008 head-injured patients randomized for high-dose methylprednis-olone vs. placebo, steroids are now considered harmful for patients with closed head injury as they are associated with a significant increase in posttraumatic mortality. *Barbiturates* are effective in reducing ICP; however, their use is restricted for intensive care therapy with continuous EEG monitoring.

Indications for evacuation of intracranial hematomas:

- Generally, an ICH causing neurological deterioration or >5 mm midline shift in CT scan should be evacuated as soon as possible
- Evacuation of acute subdural hematomas (aSDH) of >3 mm thickness
- Evacuation of aSDH < 3 mm in comatose patients with severe parenchymal injuries and mass effect
- For EDH, surgical evacuation is generally indicated, except in clinically stable patients with a small EDH and minimal pathological findings (GCS 14 or 15)
- Evacuation of large ICH in patients with focal neurological deficits and/or a midline shift in CT scan
- Depressed skull fractures: Indication for operative elevation if the extent of depression is thicker than the adjacent skull in CT scan
- Apart from the evacuation of ICHs, all open head injuries represent an indication for neurosurgical intervention

Indications for continuous ICP-monitoring:

- Patients with severe head injury (postresuscitation GCS ≤ 8) and *abnormal* admission CT scan
- Patients with severe head injury (GCS ≤ 8) and *normal* initial CT scan, but with a prolonged coma > 6 h
- Patients requiring evacuation of ICHs
- Neurological deterioration (GCS ≤ 8) in patients with initially mild or moderate head injury
- Head-injured patients requiring prolonged mechanical ventilation, e.g., due to operations for extracranial injuries, unless the initial CT scan is normal

Intraoperative Management

Craniotomy

One third of patients with severe closed head injury need immediate craniotomy for evacuation of mass lesions, most commonly for aSDH. There is a clear benefit to early evacuation of significant intracranial mass lesions. In patients with clinically *mild* or *moderate* brain injury, craniotomy is performed for depressed skull fractures or for "stable" hematomas on a less urgent basis. The timing of surgery depends on the clinical condition of the patient, in particular on the neurologic exam and CT findings. A comatose patient with a significant intracerebral hematoma causing hemispheric shifting should be taken immediately to surgery. Three types of ICH are encountered as surgical removable mass lesions: (1) aSDH from tearing of a bridging vein from the cortex to the venous sinuses or a cortical artery; (2) EDH from laceration of the middle meningeal artery or from the edges of a skull fracture; and (3) ICH from bleeding within the brain parenchyma. A standard craniotomy is performed with the patient supine and the head turned to the appropriate side and fixed in a Mayfield clamp. The incision is started just anterior to the ear and extended superiorly, 2 cm lateral and parallel to the midline, in the shape of a large question mark. A burr hole is made above the ear, which marks the bottom part of the temporal fossa, to allow immediate evacuation in case of EDH, or evacuation of SDH following incision of the dura. Additional burr holes have to be placed approximately 1.5 cm off the midline to avoid injury to major venous structures, such as the sinus sagittalis. Depending on the type of hematoma, a sufficiently large bone flap is performed for adequate exposure. An EDH is removed after elevation of the bone flap and the lacerated vessel has to be identified and cauterized. SDHs and ICHs can be approached after opening of the dura, which has to be lifted off the underlying cortex carefully. The hematoma is then gently evacuated by suction, irrigation, or other mechanical means. The origin of the hematoma must be identified and cauterized. If necessary, parts of contused brain can be debrided. Complete hemostasis must be achieved prior to closure of the dura. If this is not possible, a tamponade may be performed by the use of topical hemostatic agents (e.g., FloSeal) or by autologous muscle interponates. A Valsalva maneuver may be helpful for verification of secure hemostasis. The dura must be sealed tightly, which can be achieved by the use of an artificial dura patch. Dural tack-up sutures are placed around the periphery of the bony exposure and in the center of the flap. Epidural drains are put in place, after which the bone flap is refixed. In cases of expected postoperative brain swelling, it is advisable to postpone the implantation of the bone flap to a later time-point. Under these circumstances, the resected skull can be stored safely at $-80°C$ or else implanted subcutaneously into the abdominal wall of the patient. Finally, the temporal fascia, galea, and skin are closed.

   Note: Small lesions in the temporal or in the posterior fossa may cause compression to the brainstem and/or obstruction of the CSF flow, therefore early surgical intervention is warranted. For removal of hematomas in the posterior fossa the patient is operated in a prone position.

Emergency Burr Holes

In areas where neuroradiologic imaging (CT scan) or neurosurgical intervention are not readily available, general surgeons should be knowledgeable about the option of placing cranial burr holes for evacuation of ICHs. *Indication*: Rapidly deteriorating neurologic status, not responsive to osmotic therapy (mannitol); e.g., patients with suspected EDH whose level of consciousness or focal neurologic deficit is acutely worsening. The patient is positioned as described above for a craniotomy. A burr hole is placed on the side of the pupillary dilatation or contralateral to the side of the motor deficit. An incision anterior to the ear is taken down to the os zygomaticum, which marks the bottom of the temporal fossa. The hole may be enlarged for evacuation of an EDH or an SDH, the latter after incision of the dura. If necessary, a complete craniotomy can be performed as an enlargement of this approach.

Pitfalls:

- The majority of comatose patients do not have an ICH which needs to be evacuated
- A burr hole may miss the hematoma or drain it insufficiently
- A burr hole may itself induce intracranial bleeding
- Placing a burr hole may consume as much time as transferring the patient to a center with neurosurgical capabilities

Management in the ICU

Postoperatively, patients are transferred to intensive care unit (ICU) and treated according to standardized protocols. The goals of ICU therapy are:

- Achievement and maintenance of adequate gas exchange and circulatory stability by means of endotracheal intubation, mechanical ventilation, adequate volume resuscitation, and administration of vasoactive drugs, if required, as well as prevention of hypoxemia and hypercarbia. The goal is to keep $PaO_2 > 13$ kPa and $PaCO_2$ between 3.3 and 4.5 kPa. No "blind" prophylactic hyperventilation, due to the risk of inducing focal ischemic insults. Aggressive circulatory stabilization: MAP > 80 mmHg, normovolemia, hematocrit $\geq$ 30%.

Note: No antihypertensive therapy up to MAP of 130 mmHg ("demand" hypertension!).

- Repeated, scheduled CT scans for detection of delayed secondary intracranial pathology which may have to be surgically evacuated.
- Profound but easily reversible sedation and analgesia to avoid stress and pain, which may result in increases of ICP and the cerebral metabolic rate.
- Achievement and maintenance of optimal CPP (> 70 mmHg) and cerebral oxygen balance, allowing recovery of damaged brain areas and prevention of secondary brain damage. Here, the monitoring tools include (1) frequent blood gas analyses, (2) continuous ICP registration, (3) jugular bulb oximetry, (4) assessment of arterio-jugular difference in lactate concentrations, (5) transcranial Doppler sonography for assessment of CBF/vasospasms, and (6) repeated or continuous EEG registration. Administration of nimodipine in patients with signs of vasospasm detected by Doppler sonography.
- Avoidance of hyperthermia ($< 38°C$).
- Prevention of hyperglycemia and hyponatremia.
- No routinely performed head elevation (attenuation of CPP!).
- Prevention of stress ulcers and maintenance of gut mucosal integrity by early administration of enteral nutrition.
- Prophylaxis for complicating factors, e.g., pneumonia or meningitis; repeated bacteriological sampling (including CSF through ventricular catheters) and anti-infectious treatment, if necessary.

Therapy in the event of elevated ICP (>15 mmHg, >5 min), after exclusion of surgically removable intracranial mass lesions (step-by-step regimen):

1. Deepening of sedation, analgesia, muscle relaxation.
   - CSF drainage through ventricular catheters, where applicable
   - Moderate hyperventilation, as long as: (a) jugular bulb oxygenation > 60%, (b) arterio-jugular difference in lactate < 0.2 mmol/l, (c) an ICP-lowering effect can be achieved by hyperventilation
2. Osmotherapy: mannitol (20%) bolus IV in steps of 25 – 50 – 100 ml, as long as serum osmolarity < 315 mOsm/l.
3. Moderate hypothermia ($\pm$ 34°C).
4. Barbiturate coma (thiopental IV) under continuous EEG registration. Goal: Burst suppression pattern of 6 bursts/min and a burst suppression relationship of 1:1.

Complications

General complications of severe head injury:

- Cerebral edema may lead to supratentorial swelling and *herniation of the brain* through the dural hiatuses and the foramen magnum.
- *Ischemic brain injury*, following brain herniation or focal cerebral vasospasms.
- *Posttraumatic immunosuppression*, leading to increased susceptibility to pulmonary infections, sepsis, and multi-organ failure.
- *Neurogenic pulmonary edema.* Definition: Pulmonary edema after head injury in the absence of cardial or pulmonary disorders or hypervolemia. *Pitfall*: Fluid overload in brain-injured patients.
- *Syndrome of inappropriate ADH secretion (SIADH)*, characterized by hyponatremia, hypoosmo-larity, and urinary sodium > 25 mEq/l. After hemodynamic stabilization, these patients should be treated by restriction of fluid intake to about 800–1,000 ml/day, using isotonic intravenous fluids (e.g., Ringer's lactate).
- *Disseminated intravascular coagulation (DIC).* The damaged brain tissue represents a powerful activator of the coagulation cascade and may cause a severe consumptive coagulopathy.
- *Gastrointestinal bleeding.* Ulcers of the esophagus, stomach, and duodenum are frequent in comatose head-trauma patients. Prophylaxis: Early enteral nutrition, antacids, and proton pump inhibitors.
- *Heterotopic ossification.* Definition: Late complication of brain injury with unclear etiology, characterized by bone formation in tissues that do not normally ossify. The incidence has been reported in 10–86% of patients with severe head-trauma or spinal cord injury, and represents a major source of morbidity and persisting disability in the course of rehabilitation.

Postoperative complications:

- Incomplete evacuation of intracranial mass lesions
- Reoccurrence of intracranial bleeding
- Surgical infections, e.g., meningitis, meningoencephalitis, brain abscess

Complications of ICU therapy:

- *Cerebral vasospasm* after therapeutic hyperventilation. Prophylaxis: Keeping pCO_2 in constant range (3.3–4.5 kPa) and monitoring of arterio-jugular lactate concentrations, jugular bulb oxymetry, and frequent transcranial Doppler sonography.
- *Complications of Barbiturate coma*: Cardiovascular depression, hepatotoxicity, immunosuppression, and increased incidence of pulmonary infections.

Outcome

The GCS, although originally not intended as a prognostic index, is a strong indicator of outcome after closed head injury. Prospective data from the Traumatic Coma Data Bank (TCDB) in the 1980s revealed that patients with *severe* head injury (GCS score ≤ 8) had an overall mortality rate of 36% at 6 months post injury. Among these, an initial GCS score of 3 was associated with the highest mortality (76%), compared to patients with a score of 6–8 (18%). Patients with *moderate* head injury (GCS score 9–13) are at particular risk of intracranial complications, and their overall mortality is about 7%. Interestingly, patients who "talk" at admission (GCS score > 8) and then deteriorate have a significantly higher mortality than patients with an initial score ≤ 8. While mortality represents a parameter of outcome which is easy to define, the residual impairment in terms of neurological, cognitive, or behavioral deficits is more difficult to assess. Numerous tests and scores offer different approaches for determining the posttraumatic neurological and neuropsychological impairment. For example, the Disability Rating Scale (DRS) and the Glasgow Outcome Scale (GOS; ❷ *Table 13-4*) represent traditional measures of global outcome which provide a basis for comparing the results of treatment in different centers. When analyzed using the GOS, only about 60% of patients with *moderate* head injury have an overall good recovery by 6 months after trauma (GOS score 5), whereas a moderate (GOS score 4) to severe disability (GOS score 3) is described in 26% and 7%, respectively. Analysis of the outcome after *mild* head injury (GCS score 14 or 15) revealed that these patients frequently have posttraumatic neuropsychological sequelae. The likelihood of postconcussional symptoms 1 week after trauma ranged from 80% to 93%, and follow-up studies revealed that up to 60% of patients had residual neurobehavioral deficits after 3 months. However, long-term neurological deficits are rare in patients with *mild* head injury.

◻ Table 13-4

Glasgow Outcome Scale (GOS) (Jennett and Bond, 1975)

Outcome (assessed 3 or 6 months after head injury)	Characteristics	Score
Good recovery	Reintegrated	5
Moderate disability	Independent but disabled	4
Severe disability	Conscious but dependent	3
Persistent vegetative state	Wakefulness without awareness	2
Death		1

Selected Readings

Bayir H, Clark RS, Kochanek PM (2003) Promising strategies to minimize secondary brain injury after head trauma. Crit Care Med 31:S112–S117

Finfer SR, Cohen J (2001) Severe traumatic brain injury. Resuscitation 48:77–90

Gaetz M (2004) The neurophysiology of brain injury. Clin Neurophysiol 115:4–18

Jennett B, Bond M (1975) Assessment of outcome after severe brain damage. Lancet 1 (7905):480–484

Marshall LF, Marshall SB, Klauber MR, et al. (1992) The diagnosis of head injury requires a classification based on computed axial tomography. J Neurotrauma 9 (Suppl. 1): S287–S292

McArthur DL, Chute DJ, Villablanca JP (2004) Moderate and severe traumatic brain injury: epidemiologic, imaging and neuropathologic perspectives. Brain Pathol 14:185–194

Narayan RK, Michel ME, Ansell B, et al. (2002) Clinical trials in head injury. J Neurotrauma 19:503–557

Roberts I, Yates D, Sandercock P, et al. (2004) Effect of intravenous corticosteroids on death within 14 days in 10,008 adults with clinically significant head injury (MRC CRASH trial): randomised placebo-controlled trial. Lancet 364:1321–1328

Schmidt OI, Heyde CE, Ertel W, Stahel PF (2005) Closed head injury: an inflammatory disease? Brain Res Rev 48:388–399

Stahel PF, Heyde CE, Ertel W (2005) Current concepts of polytrauma management. Eur J Trauma 31:200–211

Stover JF, Steiger P, Stocker R (2005) Treating intracranial hypertension in patients with severe traumatic brain injury during neurointensive care: new features of old problems? Eur J Trauma 31:308–330

Teasdale G, Jennett B (1974) Assessment of coma and impaired consciousness: a practical scale. Lancet 2:81–84

The Brain Trauma Foundation (2006) Guidelines for the management of severe traumatic brain injury, 3rd edn. http://www.braintrauma.org

14   Spinal Trauma

Fritz U. Niethard · Markus Weißkopf

Pearls and Pitfalls

- Principles for the treatment of spinal injuries include **reduction** of the traumatic spinal disloca-tion. With reduction, most of the dislocated osteoligamentous tissue is realigned by the ligamen-tous axis. Additional **decompression** may thereafter be performed. Finally, the reduced injured tissue is held in place by **stabilization**.
- The fracture classification for spinal injuries proposed by Magerl et al. is generally accepted for the lower cervical and thoracolumbar spine. This classification is based primarily on both pathologic and morphologic aspects. Three mechanisms of trauma are differentiated: **compression**, **distrac-tion**, and **rotation**.
- Current surgical concepts utilizing state-of-the-art implants enable stability of the injured spine to be regained fully with minor surgical trauma and minimal permanent loss of segmental mobility.
- Overdistraction during reduction maneuvers can lead to additional compromise of neural tissue in cases of spinal cord injury (SCI).
- Fractures of the cervicothoracic junction may be missed in patients in whom appropriate traction is not applied on the shoulder girdle.
- In complete SCI, prognosis for recovery of physiologic motor capabilities remains poor.

Introduction

The spine must serve various functions. In addition to its static function in maintaining upright posture, the spine facilitates motion of both the head in relation to the chest and the chest in relation to the pelvis. It also serves a protective function for the spinal cord. Injury of the spine will result in the loss of these combined functions. A treatment concept for the restoration of the traumatized spine will thus have to address the **reduction** of dislocated structures, the **decompression** of compromised neural tissue, and the **stabilization** of the affected segments to prevent further injury.

Epidemiology and Socioeconomic Impact

Spinal fractures comprise between 0.5% and 2% of all fractures. L1 and Th12 are the most common site of fractures. The thoracolumbar transition is affected in more than 50% of patients.

In 10–15% of spine injuries, more than one level is affected. Spinal trauma is accompanied in 50–60% of cases by other injuries, and in 25–30% it is combined with polytrauma. In a fall from great height, spinal injuries can be associated with calcaneal and hip fractures. Spinal injuries are often caused by traffic accidents (50%) followed by occupational injuries (20%). The increasing number of high-risk sporting activities (such as hang gliding and parachuting) accounts for 10–15% of spinal injuries. In 6% of cases, spinal trauma is a consequence of attempted suicide. The annual reported incidence rate for spinal cord injury (SCI) varies from 25 to 93 per 1 million in populations in the Western world, which is an increase in recent years. In most cases, SCI is the sequelae of a motor vehicle accident or a fall from great height. In a Dutch study, the direct costs for patients with unstable fractures associated with neurologic deficits were calculated at an average of €31,900. This cost does not include the expenses that arise out of rehabilitation programs, which are exceptionally high in paraplegic patients.

Initial Treatment

The prognosis of spinal injury is affected frequently by the initial management of the area of trauma. Because of the high coincidence with other injuries, spinal trauma must always be taken into consideration on the initial assessment. Contusion, hematoma, skin abrasions, gibbus formation, and irregular alignment of the spinous processes might serve as external indicators for spinal injuries. Both the report of pain and the provocation of pain on percussion or compression of the spine also point to violation of the spine. An initial neurologic examination provides information about the level of injury. During the resuscitation of the patient, continuous traction should be applied to the spine. Multilevel support is provided by forklift handling in order to warrant an en bloc carriage (❷ *Fig. 14-1*). The victim is transported on a vacuum mattress, and the C-spine is immobilized in a hard cervical collar (stiff neck). Reduction maneuvers should be avoided outside the hospital. In case of suspected SCI, administration of high-dose methylprednisolone should be initiated outside the hospital.

Corticosteroid Therapy

The effect of high-dose administration of corticosteroids on acute spinal injury was investigated in a randomized, multicenter study. Patients treated with corticosteroids had a significantly better recovery in incomplete spinal injury if the medication was administered immediately after the trauma (within the first 8 h). In more recent reports, the positive effect of the corticosteroid therapy was not confirmed in incomplete cervical SCI; however, administering the dosage regimen is generally recommended, which is given in ❷ *Table 14-1* in incomplete SCI or in any case of neurologic deterioration.

Diagnostics

During the initial assessment of the patient, it is most important to take a detailed history, because the exact analysis of the mechanism of trauma might be suggestive of associated spinal trauma. On physical

◘ Figure 14-1

Initial axis-stable salvage of the trauma victim is performed by an even strain on the various parts of the spine provided by several man support

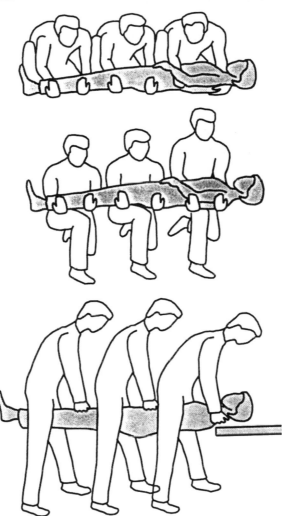

◘ Table 14-1

Corticosteroid dosage for acute spinal cord injuries

Dosage	Time interval
30 mg/kg body weight	During 15 min
Pause	For 45 min
5.4 mg/ kg body weight	During 23 h

examination, the origin of pain origin and external signs of trauma are evaluated in order to localize the injury more precisely. The precise neurologic workup is helpful in determining the exact level of trauma. Early detection of neurologic deficits is of utmost importance, because immediate decompression of the neural structures is the only chance for recovery.

Diagnostic Imaging

Conventional Radiographs

In polytraumatized patients, it is generally recommended to perform x-rays of the C-spine in two planes in addition to anterior–posterior (AP) images of the chest and the pelvis. During the acquisition of the C-spine images, traction is applied to the arms in order to visualize completely the seventh cervical vertebrae. For the assessment of the facet joints, a 15° oblique view, and for the depiction of the neural foramen, a 45° oblique view of the C-spine are performed. The odontoid process can be demonstrated clearly by means of a transorally focused image. The exact course of an odontoid process fracture line can be determined on computed tomography (CT) with films that include sagittal reformations or conventional tomography. Besides traumatization of the bony structures, attention must be directed toward signs of discoligamentous injury, such as:

- Step formation or irregularities in the posterior alignment of the vertebrae
- Altered height of the disk space
- Unequivalent distance of the spinous processes
- Prevertebral shadow formation

Discoligamentous injuries can be displayed more distinctively on functional flexion/extension x-rays. This investigation depends on the patient's compliance and thus may be difficult to carry out in an acutely injured patient with altered mental status. The guided motion is performed by the physician in order to exclude muscle contraction during the maneuver. The standard, conventional radiographic investigation in the region of the thoracic and lumbar spine consists of AP and lateral images. Besides the aspects that refer to the C-spine, the following criteria should be recognized for the thoracic and lumbar spine:

- Angle of the end plates
- Comparison of the anterior and posterior wall height
- Broadening of the vertebrae
- Irregularities or asymmetries of the pedicles
- Misalignment of the vertebrae's axis

Traumatic spondylolysis can be depicted best on oblique views (45°) of the lumbar spine, where the fracture line is visualized in the interarticular portion of the vertebral arch.

Computed Tomography

CT is now part of diagnostic standard in the workup of the spinal trauma patient, particularly those suspected of having spinal injury. CT is of special importance in the assessment of the spinal canal, the stability of the posterior wall, the integrity of the vertebral arch, and the congruence of the facet joints. For a better visualization of rotational spine injuries, the acquired data can be illustrated in 2D and 3D reformations. Currently, it is possible to reduce the data acquisition time with modern scanners to less than 1 min for the whole lumbar spine. Thus, CT is well-suited for the initial acute diagnostic steps.

Magnetic Resonance Imaging

The main advantage of magnetic resonance imaging (MRI) is the optimal illustration of soft tissue structures. Because MRI weighs the water content of different tissues, traumatized tissue will have altered signals because of the edema. In the T2-weighted sequences, edematous tissues appear as an increased signal. Edema, hematomas, and ruptures in the spinal marrow, the intervertebral disk, the longitudinal ligaments, and muscle structures can be demonstrated most sensitively. The T1 sequences illustrate the exact anatomic relationships. For example, the extent of a disk protrusion can be better evaluated using these sequences. Because of the relatively long data acquisition time, this diagnostic media is reserved for the period after vital signs are stabilized.

Biomechanics and Classification of Spinal Injuries

Proper treatment of spinal injuries is initiated based on classification of injury in order to assess the severity of the trauma and thus the resulting instability. Because both rotational and translational motions along the ordinate axis are physiologic, a subtle analysis of the direction of pathologic instability has to be performed. According to biomechanical aspects which are considered in the current classifications, the spine is subdivided into an anterior and a posterior column. The anterior column consists of the vertebral body, the intervertebral disks, and the anterior longitudinal spinal ligament. The posterior column consists of the vertebral arch, the adjacent processes, and all the ligaments including the posterior longitudinal spinal ligament. Compressive load is carried mainly by the anterior column (80%), while the posterior column absorbs 20% of the weight forces. The posterior column has predominately a tension-banding effect, which is maintained by the ligaments and paravertebral muscles. The integrity of the posterior wall of the vertebral bodies has a central importance for the stability of the fracture, because it acts as a fulcrum for the posterior tensile forces. It is of utmost importance to consider these biomechanical relationships in the treatment of spinal injuries, because the decision on whether operative treatment is necessary depends primarily on the stability of the anterior column. In the assessment of the injury direction, the extent and the nature of the instability (i.e., bone and/or soft tissue trauma) has to be defined.

Due to anatomic and functionally different features of the upper and lower C-spine, the classification of the upper C-spine has to be discerned from rest of the spine. There are multiple injury classification schemes published for the upper C-spine addressing the occipito-atlantal and the atlanto-axial joint complex including the concerned vertebrae. Their description would be beyond the scope of this textbook; however, the fracture classification of Anderson and D'Alonso addressing the odontoid process is reported, because this injury is the most common traumatic lesion of the upper spine. Their classification is subdivided into three different types according to the location of the fracture line (❯ *Fig. 14-2*). Type-II injury is unstable and must be fixed operatively in order to prevent pseudarthrosis, whereas the other fractures can be treated conservatively after closed reduction. In the mid-1990s, a comprehensive fracture classification for the thoracolumbar spine was proposed by Magerl et al. This classification was adopted later for the lower C-spine because of similarities in the functional and biomechanical aspects.

The Magerl classification is based on both pathologic and morphologic criteria with regard to the main mechanism of injury. Spinal trauma is divided into three main groups (A, B, and C)

◾ Figure 14-2
Odontoid process fracture classification according to Anderson and D'Alonzo

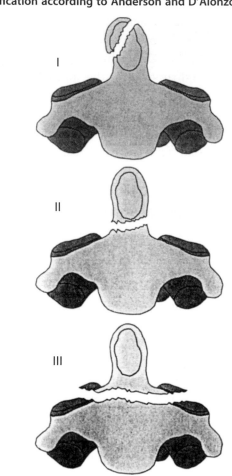

according to their severity. Type-C injury is most unstable. Compression injuries of the vertebral body are classified as Type-A lesions. Type-B injuries are lesions where distraction acts on the anterior and posterior elements of the spine. Spinal trauma where the main force is the axial torque leading to rotational injuries is also rated as a Type-C injury (❯ *Fig. 14-3*). Further subdivision of these injuries is given in ❯ *Table 14-2*.

Treatment

The general treatment strategy consists of three steps:

- Reduction
- Decompression
- Stabilization

◘ Figure 14-3
Various sketches of the Magerl fracture classification for injuries of the thoracolumbar spine

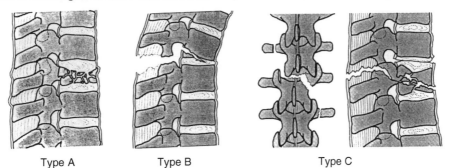

| Type A | Type B | Type C |

◘ Table 14-2
Classification of spinal injuries after Magerl et al

Type A: vertebral body compression	Type B: anterior and posterior element injuries with distraction	Type C: anterior and posterior element injuries with rotation
A1: Impaction fracture	B1: Posterior disruption predominantly ligamentous	C1: Type-A injury with rotation
A2: Split fracture	B2: Posterior disruption predominantly osseus	C2: Type-B injury with rotation
A3: Burst fracture	B3: Anterior disruption through the disc	C3: Rotational-shear injuries

Reduction may be performed as a closed maneuver after the injury is analyzed and classified exactly. According to the instability of the trauma or a possible neurologic deficit, it has to be decided whether a surgical decompression and stabilization is necessary.

Conservative Treatment

Stable injuries of the C-spine generally need no operative intervention. Neck distortions, isolated fracture of the transverse spinous process, or fractures of the apex of the odontoid process (Type I after Anderson and D'Alonso) can be managed as stable injuries and can be treated with a collar. Certain fractures of the base of the odontoid process (Type III after Anderson and D'Alonso) and isolated minor dislocated fractures of the vertebral arch remain stable under tension and compression. In contrast, these fractures are unstable under translational and rotational forces and thus require external stabilization that can be applied by a halo body vest. This brace fixates the head externally against the chest and thus prevents C-spine rotation along the ordinate axes.

In the thoracic and lumbar spine, the integrity of the posterior wall is a crucial indicator for stability of the fracture. The fracture can be addressed as bony stable if the vertebral body's posterior wall is intact. Functional mobilization featuring lordosing physiotherapy will be sufficient in compression injuries (Type A1), where the kyphosis of the end plates is less than 15°. In stable fractures with a greater degree of kyphosis, external stabilization is recommended after closed reduction is performed. Both the Boston Brace and a body cast will be sufficient in retaining the lordosis, if the principle of three-point support is applied. Anteriorly, the brace is supported over the sternum and the symphysis, while the posterior counterpoint is located at the level of the fracture.

Surgical Therapy

An absolute indication for operative intervention includes:

- Neurologic deficit
- High-grade instability
- Severe dislocation
- Failed closed reduction of spine dislocation
- Open spinal trauma

In patients with of neurologic deficit, especially with progressive deterioration, operative decompression must be performed on an emergency basis. Controversy exists as to whether an initially complete paraplegic patient will benefit from emergency decompression, because recovery is by definition impossible; however, we recommend initially treating these patients surgically, if instability, dislocation, or hematoma are detected, because it cannot be discerned in the early phase whether spinal shock mimics complete paraplegia.

Cervical Spine

In the upper C-spine, fractures of the odontoid process are most common. Operative treatment consists of an anterior screw fixation. In case of failed conservative treatment with formation of an odontoid process pseudarthrosis, posterior fixation may be indicated. The posterior atlanto-axial fusion technique was first described by Gallie, where sublaminar wiring is combined with a bone block that is attached onto the lamina. Magerl later described the transarticular screw fixation, where screws are passed through the articular mass between the course of the vertebral artery and the spinal canal. Harms recently described a technique in which polyaxial screws are driven into the lateral masses of both the atlas and the axis. This technique leaves the joint surfaces intact and thus is a motion-preserving technique when applied temporarily. In the lower C-spine, posterior fixation can be obtained by screw and rod systems, where the screws are either anchored in the lateral masses or transpedicularly (● *Fig. 14-4*).

In general, anterior trauma (i.e., compression fracture of the vertebral body or discoligamentous lesion) is addressed by anterior approaches. Here the approach is chosen medial to the vascular sheath while the thyroid gland, larynx, and esophagus are retracted to the contralateral side. Stability is regained by insertion of a tricortical bone or a cage that is set under compression by anterior plating.

Thoracic and Lumbar Spine

During the preoperative planning, a decision must be made as to which approach is best suited to reduce, decompress, and stabilize the fracture. In addition, the patient's general condition must be

☐ Figure 14-4
Stable instrumented fixation of a Type-C1 cervical fracture

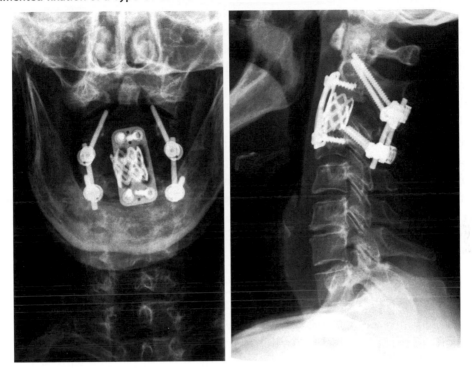

evaluated. Operating time should be limited to the minimum in the polytraumatized patient in the early posttraumatic phase. In general, a posterior approach is recommended, through which reduction of the fracture and decompression can be achieved. In order to reconstruct a vertebral compression, stabilization of the anterior spine followed by insertion of tricortical bone or cage can be carried out via an anterior approach. In order to achieve the physiologic posterior tension, banding compression is applied to the posterior instrumentation. According to the individual situation of the patient, an initial anterior approach or a two-stage approach may be preferred.

The principles of surgical therapy are:

- Complete decompression of neural structures
- Reconstruction of a compression-stable anterior column
- Limitation of the fusion to the injured motion segment

Posterior procedures: The transpedicular screw anchorage introduced by Roy Camille and the further development of the internal fixator in which the screws are attached to rods in an angled stable construct have become the gold standard for the reduction and stabilization of spinal trauma. Because of the high pullout forces, there is no other fixation system available currently that offers similar stability. Depending on the surgeon's experience, the implant insertion may be aided by fluoroscopy or computerized navigation systems. A disadvantage of the open posterior approach is the resulting trauma to the paravertebral muscles. Thus, percutaneous internal fixators which offer both a minimal invasive insertion and reduction capacity are under clinical investigation currently; however, these instruments can only be used in cases where no open posterior decompression is necessary.

Anterior procedures: A stable reconstruction of the anterior column is necessary for all fractures of the thoracolumbar spine except some true distraction injuries (Type B2) of the thoracic spine.

Approaches: The thoracic spine may be approached via a thoracotomy either from the left or the right side depending on the extent of the fracture. The course of the approach via the intercostal space with opening of the pleura is quite painful in the postoperative course. This disadvantage led to the development of endoscopic techniques that may be applied if the reduction of the fracture was complete after the posterior instrumentation.

In the thoracolumbar junction, the diaphragm must be split in order to access the spine. Because both the abdominal and chest cavities are open, this approach is the most invasive access to the spine. The lower lumbar spine can be reached with a retroperitoneal or transperitoneal approach via lumbotomy or a transrectal incision. For access to L4 and L5, special care should be taken during the dissection of prevertebral large abdominal vessels.

In general, both tricortical bone crest and cages can be utilized as implants. The use of pressure stable cages, however, is recommended in the lumbar spine, because the size of the bone graft would result in remarkable donor site morbidity.

Complications

Because the spine features a unique proximity of osseus, neural, and vascular structures, there is a high potential for complications during the insertion of transpedicular screws. Decompression of the spinal canal might result in additional trauma of neural structures. In patients with SCI, the reduction maneuver with the internal fixator can worsen the neurologic situation. General medical complications include thrombosis, embolism, and pneumonia.

Postoperative Treatment and Prognosis

The advantage of the surgical treatment is the restoration of biomechanical stability. Thus patients can be mobilized en bloc immediately postoperatively. Depending on the quality of the bone stock and the resulting stability of the instrumentation, an external brace with a three-point support is prescribed for a period of 12 weeks. Implant removal of the posterior instrumentation may be carried out after 6 months.

Full physical activity is regained after 6 months depending on the bony fusion as evaluated radiologically. Accelerated degeneration of the adjacent segments might occur in the long term as reported as a late sequel of fusion surgery. The long-term prognosis of paraplegic patients often depends on the quality of the rehabilitation. Modern comprehensive care is a multidisciplinary approach comprising orthopedic surgeons, neurologists, physiotherapists, occupational therapists, and nursing specialists.

Evidence-Based Medicine

The treatment of spinal injuries has changed over the past decades. Due to the clinical implementation of Advanced Trauma Life Support (ATLS), spinal trauma is treated adequately in the early stages of trauma care. With the introduction of newer surgical techniques (anterior column spacers, posterior screw rod systems), great advances have been achieved in stable instrumentation of the injured spine for immediate postoperative mobilization. Criticism has been given, however, that many technical and material advances were adopted frequently without scientific evidence. Evidence-based medicine (EBM) not only assesses objective measures but also takes patient-focused outcomes such as self-reported questionnaires into account.

Controversy persists about the value of high-dose administration of corticosteroids. Since the publication of the National Acute Spinal Cord Injury Study (NASCIS-II), there has been an increase in the administration of methylprednisolone in patients with spinal cord trauma. Recent studies have not proven unequivocally better results in the final assessment of patients who received corticosteroids. More research is needed in order to evaluate precisely which kind of SCI benefits from the anti-inflammatory medication.

Also it is not clear that early surgical decompression leads to more favorable results in patients with SCI. While animal studies show an excellent recovery of neural function after immediate decompression, it has been difficult to acquire evidence in the clinical scenario. Currently, there is a prospective observational study underway (Surgical Treatment of Acute Spinal Cord Injury Study – STASCIS) in order to provide better evidence toward optimal timing of surgical intervention. In contrast, there seems to be a consensus that early surgical stabilization is indicated in neurologically intact patients for reduction of complications resulting from immobilization.

Selected Readings

Anderson LD, D'Alonzo RT (1974) Fractures of the odontoid process of the axis. J Bone J Surg 56A:663

Bracken MB, Shepard MJ, Collins WF, et al. (1990) A randomized controlled trial of methyl-prednisolone or naloxone in the treatment of acute spinal cord injury. N Engl J Med 322:1406

Magerl F, Aebi M, Gertzbein SD, et al. (1994) A comprehensive classification of thoracic and lumbar injuries. Eur Spine J 3:184

Pickett GE, Campos-Benitez M, Keller JL, Dugall N (2006) Epidemiology of traumatic spinal cord injury in Canada. Spine 31:799

Roy-Camille R, Saillant G, Berteaux D, Marie-Anne S (1979) Early management of spinal injuries. In: McKibbin B (ed) Recent advances in orthopaedics 3. Churchill Livingstone, Edinburgh, pp 57–87

Whitesides TE Jr (1977) Traumatic kyphosis of the thoracolumbar spine. Clin Orthop 128:78

15 Abdominal Compartment Syndrome

Hanns-Peter Knaebel

Pearls and Pitfalls

- Abdominal compartment syndrome (ACS) is a life-threatening disease.
- Primary, secondary, and tertiary ACS are being recognized recently.
- Primary ACS is associated with abdominal trauma.
- Secondary ACS is a condition caused mostly by ischemia and reperfusion.
- Tertiary ACS is the condition of persistent intra-abdominal hypertension.
- Clinical diagnosis and imaging of ACS is difficult. Early diagnosis is crucial.
- The gold standard of diagnosis remains the measurement of intra-abdominal pressure.
- The critical value of abdominal pressure is between 15 and 20 mmHg.
- Conservative options are extremely important, but conservative treatment of intra abdominal pressures >25 mmHg is usually not effective.
- Decompressive laparotomy is the ultimate therapeutic option to reduce mortality.

Introduction

For many years, abdominal compartment syndrome (ACS) seemed like a forgotten entity or at least a medical condition that physicians and especially surgeons refrained from discussing. In recent years, there has been a substantial increase in knowledge and interest relating to ACS. This chapter will outline some recent developments.

Definitions

In December 2004, the World Congress on the Abdominal Compartment Syndrome was held, with 170 leaders from around the world setting the stage for future understanding of this complex physiologic phenomenon and developing common definitions to facilitate concise academic exchange.

Intra-Abdominal Pressure

Intra-abdominal pressure (IAP) is the pressure within the abdominal cavity. IAP varies with respiration. Normal IAP is approximately 5 mmHg, but it can be increased non-pathologically in obese patients. IAP should be expressed in mmHg (1 mmHg = 1.36 cm H_2O) and measured at end-expiration with the patient in the supine position; abdominal muscle contractions should be absent. The transducer should be zeroed at the level of the midaxillary line. The most accurate method for direct, invasive IAP measurement is direct needle puncture and transduction of the pressure within the abdominal cavity (e.g., during peritoneal dialysis or laparoscopy), but the gold standard for intermittent, indirect, non-invasive IAP measurement is transduction of the pressure within the bladder. The reference method for continuous indirect IAP measurement is a balloon-tipped catheter in the stomach or a continuous bladder irrigation method. The relevant value to be calculated is the abdominal perfusion pressure = mean arterial pressure – IAP.

Intra-Abdominal Hypertension

Intra-abdominal hypertension (IAH) is defined by either one or both of the following: (1) an IAP of 12 mmHg or greater, recorded by a minimum of three standardized measurements conducted 4–6 h apart; (2) an abdominal perfusion pressure of 60 mmHg or less, recorded by a minimum of two standardized measurements conducted 1–6 h apart.

Abdominal Compartment Syndrome

Abdominal compartment syndrome is defined as the presence of an IAP of 20 mmHg or greater with or without abdominal perfusion pressure below 50 mmHg, recorded by a minimum of three standardized measurements conducted 1–6 h apart and single or multiple organ system failure that was not present previously. In contrast to IAH, ACS should not be graded, because it is an all-or-nothing phenomenon leading to immediate therapeutic consequences. IAH is graded as shown in ❷ *Table 15-1*.

Prevalence of Intra-Abdominal Hypertension and Abdominal Compartment Syndrome

The prevalence of IAH in the literature is variable, depending on the threshold used to define IAH and the population studied. A recent multi-center group performed a prospective study of IAH in a

◻ Table 15-1

Proposed grading system for abdominal compartment syndrome based on intra-abdominal pressure

Grade	IAP (mmHg)	Associated signs	Treatment
I	10–15	No signs of ACS	Maintain normovolemia
II	16–25	May have increased PAWP* and oliguria	Hypervolemic resuscitation may be employed but could have drawbacks
III	26–35	Anuria, decreased cardiac output, raised PAWP	Consider abdominal decompression
IV	>35	Anuria, decreased cardiac output, raised PAWP	Abdominal decompression and re-exploration (cave tertiary ACS: avoid primary abdominal wall closure)

*PAWP: pulmonary artery wedge pressure

mixed intensive care unit (ICU) population. In this study, 265 consecutive patients (mean Acute Physiology and Chronic Health Evaluation II (APACHE II) score 17.4) admitted for more than 24 h in one of the 14 participating ICUs were monitored until death, until hospital discharge, or for a maximum of 28 days. Medical patients accounted for 47% of all study patients, whereas elective surgery, emergency surgery, and trauma patients accounted for 28%, 17%, and 9%, respectively. IAH was present when the mean value of the two daily IAP measurements was greater than 12 mmHg. ACS was diagnosed when an IAP above 20 mmHg was associated with at least one organ failure.

On admission, 32% of the population had IAH, and 4% had ACS. Importantly, unlike the occurrence of IAH at day 1, the occurrence of IAH during ICU stay was an independent predictor of mortality. Independent predictors of IAH at day 1 were liver dysfunction, abdominal surgery, fluid resuscitation with more than 3,500 ml during the 24 h before inclusion, and ileus. Previously, we showed that grade 2 IAH (16–20 mmHg) occurs in more than 30% of patients undergoing emergency surgery. Despite increasing reporting of ACS and IAH in the literature, the importance of IAH is often ignored.

Thus, it needs to be noted that the true prevalence of the disease as well as the predisposing risk factors are not completely known and understood (see ❯ *Table 15-2*). Regardless of the uncertainties, it is extremely important to appreciate the severity of the disease because mortality ranges from 29% to 100%.

New Trends in Monitoring Intra-Abdominal Pressure Measurement

There have been significant developments in IAP monitoring. Balogh et al. validated prospectively the technique of continuous IAP monitoring and showed that this new method has almost a perfect agreement with the reference standard of Kron et al. of intermittent measurements of intra-vesical IAP. There are many obvious advantages of the described continuous IAP monitoring. First, it does not

■ Table 15-2

Risk factors, etiology and definitions of abdominal compartment syndrome (ACS)

Primary ACS	Secondary ACS	Tertiary ACS
Blunt or penetrating abdominal trauma with hemorrhage	Extensive fluid resuscitation following major trauma	Recurrent or persistent ACS following prophylactic or therapeutic surgical or medical treatment of ACS (e.g., persistence after decompressive laparotomy, new ACS after definite abdominal wall closure)
Abdomino-pelvic trauma/injury and retroperitoneal hemorrhage	Forced abdominal wall closure (AWC) following peritonitis, ileus or intra-abdominal abscess	
Ruptured aortic aneurysm	Laparoscopy and Pneumoperitoneum	
Ascites formation due to liver cirrhosis, malignoma or pregnancy	Abdominal packing following hemorrhage	
Any other condition that requires early surgical or angio-radiologic intervention (e.g., secondary peritonitis)	Any other condition not originating from an abdominal disease (e.g., sepsis or major burns)	

require a major change in the present practice apart from the use of three-way urinary catheters. This method abandons the cumbersome steps of draining, clamping of the catheter, and filling with 50 ml of normal saline. The monitoring is continuous and does not interfere with the urinary flow through the drainage port of the catheter. Continuous IAP monitoring is less labor intensive and time consuming compared with the standard intermittent measuring technique. These factors will lead to a greater acceptance of IAP monitoring in patients at risk. The indications for monitoring IAP are presented in ❏ *Table 15-3*.

Continuous IAP measurement has several potential advantages. Increasingly, Signal Interpretation and Monitoring will become a more powerful tool for physiologic monitoring. Continuous measurement of the IAP facilitates monitoring the abdominal perfusion pressure both intermittently and continuously.

Pathophysiology

Intra-abdominal pressure is determined primarily by the volume of the viscera and the intra-compartmental fluid load. The pressure-volume curve of the abdominal cavity has been studied in animals. Post-mortem evaluation of human pressure-volume curves may not be reliable because of the post-mortem loss of abdominal wall compliance. In general, the abdominal cavity has a great tolerance to fluctuating volumes, with little increase in IAP. The compliance of the abdominal cavity can be seen at laparoscopy, wherein it is possible to instill as much as 5 l of CO_2 into the peritoneal cavity without exerting any marked influence on IAP. In a previous evaluation of IAP during laparoscopy, we found that the mean volume of gas required to generate a pressure of 20 mmHg was 8.8 ± 4.3 l. Adaptation can occur over time, and this is seen clinically in patients with ascites, large ovarian tumors, and, of course, pregnancy. Chronic ACS occurs in some morbidly obese patients with significantly increased IAP predisposing to chronic venous stasis, urinary incontinence, incisional hernia, and intracranial hypertension. Definitions and etiology of ACS is shown in ❏ *Table 15-2*.

Effect of Increased Intra-Abdominal Pressure on Individual Organ Function

Whereas intra-abdominal hypertension has a global affect on the body, increasing intraabdominal pressure leading to ACS tends to affect one system first, usually the renal or gastrointestinal system. The selective affects of IAH will be discussed in the following section.

❏ Table 15-3

Indications for monitoring of intra-abdominal pressure (IAP)

Indication
Postoperative patients after extensive abdominal surgery
Patients with open or blunt abdominal trauma
Mechanically ventilated ICU patients with other organ dysfunction as assessed by daily Sequential Organ Failure Assessment score (SOFA score)
Patients with a distended abdomen and signs and symptoms consistent with abdominal compartment syndrome: oliguria, hypoxia, hypotension, unexplained acidosis, mesenteric ischemia, elevated ventilating pressure, elevated intracranial pressure

Renal

Renal dysfunction in association with increased IAP has been recognized for more than 100 years, but only recently have its effects on large series of patients been reported. In 1945 in a study of 17 volunteers, there was a reduction in renal plasma flow and glomerular filtration rate in association with increased IAP. In an animal experiment, as IAP increased from 0 to 20 mmHg in dogs, the glomerular filtration rate decreased by 25%. At 40 mmHg, the dogs were resuscitated, and their cardiac output returned to normal; however their glomerular filtration rate and renal blood flow did not improve, indicating a local effect on renal blood flow. The situation in seriously ill patients may, however, be different, and the exact cause of renal dysfunction in the ICU is not clear because of the complexity of critical illness.

The most likely direct effect of increased IAP is an increase in the renal vascular resistance, combined with a moderate resultant decrease in cardiac output. Pressure on the ureter can be excluded as a cause, because investigators placing ureteric stents observed no improvement in renal function and urinary excretion. Other factors contributing to renal dysfunction may include humeral factors and intraparenchymal renal pressures. The concept of renal decapsulation, on the basis of increased intrarenal pressure, was popular some decades ago but now is practiced rarely because it is of no proven benefit.

The absolute value of IAP required to cause renal impairment has not been established. Some authors have suggested that 10–15 mmHg is a critical cut-off value. Maintaining adequate cardiovascular filling pressures in the presence of increased IAP also seems to be of importance.

Cardiovascular

Increased IAP decreases cardiac output as well as increasing central venous pressure, systemic vascular resistance, pulmonary artery pressure, and pulmonary artery wedge pressure. It should be kept in mind that because of the associated increase in intra-pleural pressure, some of the increases in central venous pressure may not reflect the intravascular volume and may be misleading when the patient's volume status is assessed. Cardiac output is affected mainly by a decrease in stroke volume secondary to a decrease in preload and an increase in afterload which is further aggravated by hypovolemia. Paradoxically, in the presence of hypovolemia, an increase in IAP can be associated temporarily with an increase in cardiac output. The normal left atrial/right atrial pressure gradient may be reversed during increased IAP. Venous stasis occurs in the legs of patients with abdominal pressures above 12 mmHg. In addition, studies in patients undergoing laparoscopic cholecystectomy show up to a fourfold increase in renin and aldosterone levels.

Respiration

Animal as well as human experiments have demonstrated that IAP exerts a marked effect on pulmonary function. In conjunction with increased IAP, there is diaphragmatic stenting, exerting a restrictive effect on the lungs with a resultant decrease in ventilation and lung compliance, an increase in airway pressures, and a reduction in tidal volumes. These changes can be seen occasionally during laparoscopy, where lung compliance has been shown to decrease once the IAP exceeds 16 mmHg. Respiratory changes related to increased IAP are aggravated by increased obesity and other physiologic conditions such as severe hemorrhage. There is also some adverse effect on the efficiency of gas exchange. Often patients with increased IAP are acidotic, and whereas this acidosis may initially be metabolic in origin, the effect of increased IAP adds a component complicating respiration.

In critically ill patients receiving ventilation, the effect on the respiratory system can be clinically important, resulting in decreased lung volumes, impaired gas exchange, and high ventilatory pressures. Hypercarbia can occur, and the resulting acidosis can be exacerbated by simultaneous cardiovascular depression as a result of increased IAP. The effects of increased IAP on the respiratory system in the ICU can sometimes be life-threatening, and require urgent abdominal decompression (see ❯ *Figs. 15-1* and ❯ *15-2*). In patients with true ACS undergoing abdominal decompression, there is a remarkable change in intra-operative vital signs. Fortunately, these patients represent the minority rather than a majority of patients with increased IAP and ACS. Frankly, patients should never be allowed to get to this stage. Monitoring of vital signs and acid-base status is vital in this patient population.

Visceral Perfusion

Interest in visceral perfusion has increased with the popularization of gastric tonometry, and there is an association between IAP and visceral perfusion as measured by gastric pH (intestinal pH = pHi – Value).

◻ Figure 15-1
ACS due to SIRS following total pancreatectomy immediately after emergency decompressive laparotomy on the surgical ICU. Due to extremely increased ventilation pressures, the patient could not be transported to the operating room. The impaired perfusion of the small bowel is striking

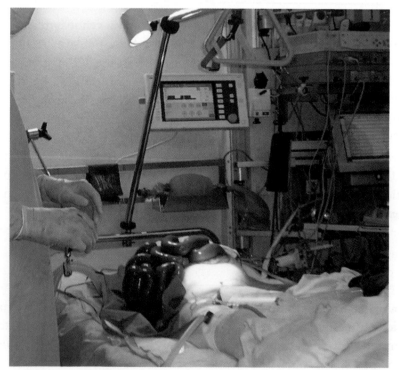

◘ Figure 15-2
Same patient as in ❷ *Fig. 15-1*, 15 min after laparotomy. The small bowel is distended grossly due a paralytic ileus, however the perfusion recovered. Next steps were decompression of the small bowel via intraluminal suction and vacuum-assisted wound closure to avoid tertiary ACS

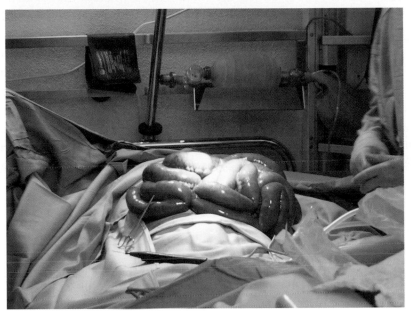

This observation was confirmed in 18 patients undergoing laparoscopy in whom a reduction of 15–54% in blood flow occured in the duodenum and stomach, respectively, at an IAP of 15 mmHg. Animal studies suggest that reduction in visceral perfusion is selective, affecting intestinal blood flow before adrenal blood flow. In a study of 73 post laparotomy patients, IAP and pHi were associated strongly, suggesting that early decreases in visceral perfusion are related to levels of IAP as low as 15 mmHg. Increasing IAP may result in visceral hypoperfusion and subsequently in secondary bacterial translocation as well as affecting wound healing. Both abnormal pHi and IAP predicted the same adverse outcome with increased risk of hypotension, intra-abdominal sepsis, renal impairment, need for re-laparotomy, and fatal outcome. It is important to measure IAP to increase awareness of its potential adverse effects on the gut. The indications for IAP monitoring are shown in ❷ *Table 15-3*.

Conservative Treatment Options

The precise management of IAP remains somewhat clouded by many published anecdotal reports and uncontrolled case series. Aggressive, non-operative intensive care support is critical to prevent the establishment of and the complications of ACS. This approach involves careful monitoring of the cardio-respiratory system and aggressive intravascular fluid replacement, especially if this is associated with hemorrhage. In contrast, excessive fluid resuscitation will add to the problem. Simple measures such as naso-gastric decompression are mandatory. In ❷ *Table 15-4* some of the possible non-surgical options are shown which all have the intention of preventing the full clinical symptoms of ACS.

◼ Table 15-4

Non-surgical therapeutic options for the treatment of intra-abdominal hypertension (IAH) and for the prevention of abdominal compartment syndrome (ACS)

Conservative therapy
Paracentesis
Naso-gastric tubes with gastric suctioning
Gastricprokinetics (metoclopramide, erythromycin, etc.)
Rectal enemas and suctioning
Colonicprokinetics (prostigmine)
Furosemide either alone or in combination with human albumin 20%
Continuous venovenous hemo(dia)filtration with aggressive ultrafiltration
Continuous negative abdominal pressure
Sedation and muscle relaxation
Upright (sitting) body positioning (pilot seat)

Surgical Management

As yet, there are few guidelines for when surgical decompression is required in the presence of increased IAP. Some studies have stated that abdominal decompression is the only treatment and that it should be performed early to prevent ACS. This is an overstatement not supported by level 1 evidence.

The accepted indications for abdominal decompression are related to correcting pathophysiologic abnormalities as much as achieving a precise and optimum IAP. If gas exchange is increasingly compromised with collapse of the lung bases or ventilatory pressures are increasing, abdominal decompression should be considered strongly. Similarly, if cardiovascular or renal function is compromised and increased IAP is suspected, then decompression should be considered early. Unfortunately, visceral hypoperfusion is very difficult to predict apart from gastric tonometry, and guidelines for operative intervention would have to rely on levels of IAP that have been shown to correlate with visceral ischemia.

The approaches to abdominal decompression also vary. Temporary abdominal closure (TAC) has been popularized as a mechanism to avoid many of the consequences of increased IAP. The theoretic benefits of abdominal decompression and TAC are therefore attractive, and some authors have advocated the prophylactic use of TAC to decrease postoperative complications and facilitate planned re-laparotomy (see ❯ *Fig. 15-3*); however, this approach may be hard to justify until a subgroup of high-risk patients can be identified more accurately. Burch et al. have stated that abdominal decompression can reverse the sequelae of the ACS. IAP levels have been advocated as a guide to closure of the abdominal wall, especially in children, but the existing literature currently has few prospective studies. Wittman et al. in two separate studies in 1990 and 1994 evaluated prospectively the outcomes in 157 and 95 patients, respectively. A multi-institutional study of 95 patients concluded that a staged approach to abdominal closure with TAC was superior to conventional techniques for dealing with intra-abdominal sepsis. Rock-hard evidence, however, is still missing.

The common indications for performing TAC include the following: abdominal decompression both prophylactic and therapeutic; to facilitate re-exploration in abdominal sepsis; and inability to close the abdomen. One must remember, however, that the open abdomen is not without its morbidity, needs intensive wound care and attention, and should be re-constructed whenever possible and feasible (see ❯ *Fig. 15-4*).

◘ Figure 15-3
Temporary abdominal wound closure ("zipper") after necrotizing pancreatitis and ACS to facilitate repeated laparotomy and to avoid tertiary ACS

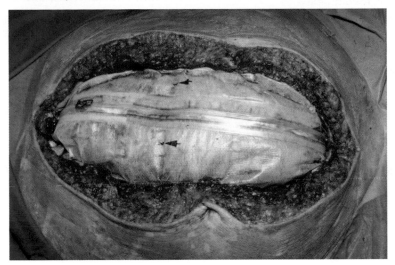

◘ Figure 15-4
Same patient as in❯ *Figs. 15-1* **and❯** *15-2* **after vacuum-assisted wound conditioning prior to plastic reconstruction of the abdominal wall. The small bowel is covered nicely with granulation tissue**

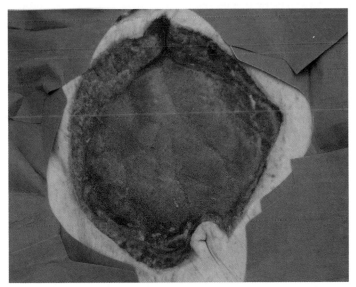

Conclusion

Increasingly, intra-abdominal hypertension (IAH) and abdominal compartment syndrome (ACS) are being recognized and diagnosed and are no longer considered a curiosity or a "forgotten entity." The challenge lies not in identifying predictors of ACS but in optimizing conservative, early-onset treatment as well the operative treatment options, including identifying when and in whom abdominal decompression is necessary. Thus, it seems reasonable that the newly formed Society of the Abdominal Compartment Syndrome will act as a portal for discussion, clinical trials, and research to enhance understanding and optimize patient care.

Selected Readings

Balogh Z, Moore FA (2005) Intra-abdominal hypertension: not just a surgical critical care curiosity. Crit Care Med 33:447–449

Balogh Z, McKinley BA, Cocanour CS, et al. (2003) Supranormal trauma resuscitation causes more cases of abdominal compartment syndrome. Arch Surg 138:637–642; discussion 642–633

Balogh Z, Jones F, D'Amours S, et al. (2004) Continuous intra-abdominal pressure measurement technique. Am J Surg 188:679–684

Burch J, Moore E, Moore F, Franciose R (1996) The abdominal compartment syndrome. Surg Clin North Am 76:833–842

Caldwell CB, Ricotta JJ (1987) Changes in visceral blood flow with elevated intra-abdominal pressure. J Surg Res 43:14–20

Harman KP, Kron IL, McLachlan DH (1982) Elevated intra-abdominal pressure and renal function. Ann Surg 196:594–597

Kron IL, Harman PK, Nolan SP (1984) The measurement of intraabdominal pressure as a criterion for abdominal re-exploration. Ann Surg 196:594–597

Malbrain ML (2004) Different techniques to measure intraabdominal pressure (IAP): time for a critical reappraisal. Intensive Care Med 30:357–371

Malbrain ML, Chiumello D, Pelosi P, et al. (2005) Incidence and prognosis of intraabdominal hypertension in a mixed population of critically ill patients: a multiple-center epidemiological study. Crit Care Med 33:315–322

Pusajo J, Bumaschny E, Agurrola A, et al. (1994) Postoperative intra-abdominal pressure: its relation to splanchnic perfusion, sepsis, multiple organ failure and surgical intervention. Intensive Crit Care Digest 13:2–7

World Society of the Abdominal Compartment Syndrome. www.wsacs.org

Critical Care

16 Acute Renal Failure

Paul E. Bankey

Pearls and Pitfalls

- Post-operative acute renal failure (ARF) is often linked to the diagnosis and resolution of an evolving complication. An aggressive approach to potentially surgically correctable complications causing ARF is warranted.
- An anastomotic leak or intraabdominal abscess can cause ARF with or without systemic infection and should be ruled out early in the setting of oliguria and a rising creatinine.
- Prerenal ARF results from loss of effective circulating volume without direct parenchymal damage to the kidney unless the hypoperfusion is unrecognized or under-treated resulting in progression to ATN. The initial goal in the management of the perioperative ARF is the optimization of the patient's hemodynamic and volume status and by inference renal perfusion. Aggressive volume expansion and maintenance of a MAP > 70 is recommended early in the course of oliguric ARF.
- In patients who are still producing urine, a loop diuretic, such as furosemide, administered in combination with a thiazide (cortical collecting tubule) diuretic, such as hydrochlorothiazide or metolazone, may sustain and improve urine output converting oliguric ARF to high-output ARF and an improved outcome.
- Aminoglycoside nephrotoxicity occurs in a startling 5–15% of patients treated with these drugs. In the setting of concurrent risk factors it is recommended to utilize equally effective non-nephrotoxic antibiotics such as extended spectrum penicillins, cephalosporins, carbapenems, or monobactams.
- Low dose dopamine (1–3 µg/kg/min) has been used to increase renal blood flow in disease processes associated with renal vasoconstriction such as sepsis or liver failure. Recent literature suggests that this practice should be abandoned. Dopamine has not been shown to prevent nor alter the course or outcome of ARF. Dopamine has been shown to have significant adverse effects on the heart, lungs, gastrointestinal tract, endocrine, and immunologic function when the dose is increased for use as a vasopressor.
- Patients with myoglobinuria require additional specific therapy in addition to the optimization of renal perfusion and diuresis to minimize the extent of ARF. Urine output should be maintained at > 150 ml/h through the initial phases of treatment to dilute and clear precipitated and free myoglobin from the tubules.
- Urine pH should be increased above 7 since myoglobin precipitation is lower at alkaline pHs. The overall goal is to produce a high-output *alkaline diuresis*.
- In patients with acute abdominal compartment syndrome, therapy is directed at relieving the intra-abdominal hypertension (>25–30 mmHg). This is most readily accomplished by laparotomy. Standard medical therapy of ARF with volume loading and inotropes usually is ineffective

in this setting; however, the response to abdominal decompression is usually dramatic and life-saving.

- Nutritional support in the setting of acute renal failure should have the same goals of caloric and nitrogen equilibrium as the surgical patient without ARF. Protein support should not be withheld in fear of causing uremic complications, as this will exacerbate wasting of lean body mass and vital organs.

- The primary indications for continuous renal replacement therapy for ARF patients are refractory volume overload, the need for large amounts of blood products, and intolerance to intermittent hemodialysis due to hypotension or arrhythmias.

Introduction

Acute renal failure continues to be an important factor contributing to perioperative and post-traumatic morbidity and mortality. As an isolated organ system failure, ARF has an associated mortality of 8%; however, acute renal failure (ARF) in association with septic shock and multiple organ dysfunction syndrome has a mortality that has remained significantly higher (70–80%). In most clinical series the mortality rate from ARF continues to average 50% depending on the precipitating event, severity of comorbid conditions, and number of complications. The most cost-effective intervention in acute renal failure is its *prevention*, and the most effective means of prevention are to ensure an adequate circulating intravascular volume, avoidance of nephrotoxic agents, and to rapidly treat surgically reversible contributing causes.

There is no consensus definition of acute renal failure in critically ill patients. Recently, a classification of renal dysfunction has been proposed based on serum creatinine and urine output (❷ *Table 16-1*). The classification defines a continuum of kidney dysfunction from risk to injury, and finally to renal failure.

It is rare for the general surgery patient to require direct operation on the kidney, renal vasculature, or urinary tract for treatment of acute renal failure; however, it is not infrequent that deteriorating renal function is a harbinger of a perioperative complication requiring surgical management by the general surgeon.

◻ Table 16-1

Proposed classification for acute renal failure (ARF)

	GFR criteria	Urine output criteria	
Risk	Increased SCr × 1.5 GFR decrease > 25%	UO < 0.5 ml/kg/h for 6 h	High sensitivity
Injury	Increased SCr × 2 GFR decrease > 50%	UO < 0.5 ml/kg/h for 12 h	High sensitivity
Failure	Increased SCr × 3 GFR decrease > 75% or SCr > 4 mg/dl	UO < 0.3 ml/kg/h for 24 h Anuria for 12 h Oliguria	High specificity
Loss	Persistent ARF for > 4 weeks		High specificity
Eskd	End stage kidney disease > 3 months		

GFR: glomerular filtration rate; Scr: serum creatinine; UO: urine output.

Clinical Presentation

The incidence of ARF is reportedly 2–5% in hospitalized patients and medical intervention frequently contributes to the problem. The three most common causes of ARF are: (1) volume depletion or hypotension; (2) aminoglycoside antibiotics; and (3) radio-contrast exposure.

Glomerular filtration rate (GFR) is the most direct indicator of renal function; however, it is difficult to measure directly in clinical practice. Serum concentrations of blood urea nitrogen (BUN) and creatinine (Cr) are more commonly used to assess renal function. The serum creatinine in most instances is an excellent barometer of renal function because a steady-state relationship exists between serum creatinine and GFR. The clinical significance is that an increase in a patient's Cr from 1 to 2 mg/dl signifies a 50% reduction in GFR and from 1 to 4 mg/dl, a 75% reduction. The correlation between Cr and GFR depends upon the assumption that it is delivered to the serum from tissue at a constant rate, which is not always the case. Patients with hypercatabolic states such as trauma or sepsis and patients with diminished muscle mass have conditions that alter the rate of Cr production, reducing the correlation of their serum concentration with renal function. Nomograms are available that accurately correlate age, ideal body weight, and Cr with GFR.

Patients with ARF may be classified based on their urine output. Oliguria is defined as urine output of <0.3 ml/kg/h for 24 h or <400 ml/day (❷ *Table 16-1*). This volume represents the minimum amount of urine in which a normal daily solute load of 500 mOsm can be excreted if the kidney is maximally concentrating urine to 1,200 mOsm/kg of water. Non-oliguric ARF is defined as lack of homeostasis (electrolyte imbalance or azotemia) despite >400 ml/day of urine production. High-output ARF is defined as renal insufficiency with urine outputs >1,000 ml/day and frequently are several liters per day. The clinical relevance of this classification is that non-oliguric renal failure patients have a better prognosis then oliguric or anuric failure; therefore, management should be directed at preventing progression of non-oliguric renal failure to oliguric or anuric ARF.

The etiology of acute renal failure is often divided into three categories (see ❷ *Table 16-2*). *Prerenal* ARF is defined as a reversible rise in serum Cr caused by renal hypoperfusion. In prerenal ARF there is no frank renal parenchymal damage and the reduction in GFR merely reflects a drop in glomerular perfusion. Restoration of renal perfusion rapidly restores GFR and normal serum Cr levels.

Renal perfusion and GFR can be maintained at moderate levels of hypovolemia largely through the actions of sympathetic stimulation and activation of the renin-angiotensin system (autoregulation). Angiotensin II activity results in constriction of the glomerular *efferent* arteriole producing increased *efferent* arteriolar resistance. This increases hydrostatic pressure in the glomerular capillary. Eventually hypoperfusion overwhelms these compensatory mechanisms resulting in progression to renal ischemia and acute tubular necrosis (ATN). The use of Non-Steroidal Anti-Inflammatory Drugs (NSAIDs), which block synthesis of prostaglandins and are frequently used in the perioperative management of pain, are particularly hazardous in the setting of prerenal hypovolemia. Another class of drugs to avoid in the setting of prerenal hypovolemia is the Angiotensin Converting Enzyme (ACE) inhibitors that block production of angiotensin II. Both of these agents interfere with glomerular autoregulatory mechanisms and may precipitate severe renal hypoperfusion and ATN.

Intrinsic or *Intrarenal* ARF reflects direct injury to the renal parenchyma. Acute Tubular Necrosis (ATN) is the most common form of intrarenal ARF and may be caused by a variety of insults such as ischemia or nephrotoxins that lead to necrosis of the tubular epithelia (❷ *Table 16-2*).

◘ Table 16-2

Major causes of acute renal failure

Prerenal	Intrarenal	Postrenal

Intravascular volume depletion
1. Hemorrhage
2. Vomiting
3. Third-spacing
4. Burns
5. Fever
6. Diarrhea
	Ischemic ATN
	1. Shock
	  (i) Septic
	  (ii) Cardiogenic
	  (iii) Hypovolemic
		Neoplasm
		1. Prostate
		2. Cervix
		3. Colorectal

Decreased cardiac output
  1. Congestive failure
  2. Pulmonary hypertension
  3. Myocardial ischemia
	Nephrotoxic ATN
	  1. Aminoglycosides
	  2. Radiocontrast agents
	  3. Myoglobinuria
	  4. Hemoglobinuria
	  5. Chemotherapeutic agents
	  6. Amphotericin B
		Dysfunctional bladder
		  1. Anticholinergic drugs
		  2. Catheter obstruction
		  3. Prostatic enlargement

Decreased renal perfusion with normal or high cardiac output
  1. Sepsis
  2. Cirrhosis
	Glomerulonephritis
	  1. Immune complex mediated
	    (i) Postinfectious
	  2. Vasculitis
		Nephrolithiasis

Drugs
  1. Nonsteriodal anti-inflammatory agents
  2. Angiotensin converting enzyme inhibitors
	Tubulointerstitial disease
	  1. Allergic interstitial nephritis
		Papillary necrosis

	Other vascular
	  1. Thrombotic microangiopathy
	  2. Vascular trauma
	  3. Cholesterol embolization
		Abdominal compartment syndrome

In the surgical setting ATN is frequently encountered following episodes of hypotension, commonly following resuscitation of septic or hemorrhagic shock. It may also occur post-operatively; however, many factors contribute to post-operative ATN in addition to hypotension as evidenced by the observation that in 50% of cases no hypotension is documented. In severe renal hypoperfusion, renal tubular epithelial cells develop hypoxia and necrose especially in areas where metabolic rate is high (proximal tubule and the medullary thick ascending loop of Henle). Even in the presence of relatively adequate renal blood flow severe hypoxia of tubular epithelium can develop. Ischemic epithelia slough into and obstruct the tubular lumen, producing clinically diagnostic granular casts and increased tubular backpressure, exacerbating renal ischemia by further intensifying intrarenal vasoconstriction and decreasing GFR.

Ischemic ATN secondary to renal artery occlusion is a rare cause of ARF that the general surgeon encounters primarily in the setting of blunt or penetrating trauma. The diagnosis is suggested by nonvisualization of the kidney on CT evaluation or hematuria. Irreversible renal injury develops rapidly in the setting of warm ischemia and revascularization within 6 h is the treatment goal. Controversy exists regarding the role of revascularization when the diagnosis of renal artery thrombosis is made beyond 4–6 h and overall renal salvage is low (<10%); however, case reports indicate salvage in kidneys revascularized up to 12 h after injury. Endovascular approaches to renal reperfusion may improve kidney salvage rates. Furthermore, in situations where a patient's solitary kidney is at risk, harvesting, cooling, and autotransplantation has been successfully performed.

A number of pharmacologic agents frequently used or encountered in the care of surgery patients can result in nephrotoxic ATN (❍ *Table 16-2*). Antimicrobial agents commonly used in surgical patients reported to cause ATN include aminoglycosides and amphotericin B. Aminoglycoside nephrotoxicity occurs in 5–15% of patients treated with these drugs. In the setting of renal insufficiency aminoglycosides also cause ototoxicity. Recognition of injury is delayed from its onset since creatinine does not begin to increase until 7–10 days later. Aminoglycoside ARF is dose-dependent and nephrotoxicity is related to the serum concentration, particularly trough levels. Clinical guidelines have been developed for the drug concentration monitoring and dosing of aminoglycosides including both peak and trough levels, typically for gentamicin. Improved understanding of the pharmacodynamics and toxicity of aminoglycoside antibiotics has resulted in the study of once-daily dosing regimens. Although studies have suggested a therapeutic advantage and possibly a decrease in toxicity with once-daily administration, these effects have been modest. Further data are needed to clarify the role of once-daily dosing in critically ill general surgery patients. Aminoglycoside nephrotoxicity is enhanced by the interaction of NSAIDs, endotoxin, cyclosporin A, and amphotericin B and electrolyte disorders such as hypercalcemia, hypomagnesemia, hypokalemia, and metabolic acidosis. Increased nephrotoxicity is also reported in patients receiving concurrent antimicrobial therapy with cephalosporins. In the setting of concurrent risk factors it is recommended to utilize equally effective non-nephrotoxic antibiotics such as extended spectrum penicillins, cephalosporins, carbapenems, or monobactams.

Amphotericin B used for systemic fungal infections causes nephrotoxicity, in most patients. It is strongly bound to cellular membranes and alters permeability. This effect on the renal tubular epithelium leads to failure of hydrogen ion excretion and urinary loss of potassium resulting in the development of a distal type of renal tubular acidosis with hypokalemia. Loss of renal function is proportional to the dose of amphotericin and irreversible renal failure occurs at high doses (>2 g). Saline loading at the time of administration may reduce toxicity. Encapsulation of amphotericin B in liposomes or complexing of the compound with other lipid carriers brings about a major reduction in toxicity and these formulations are being utilized with increasing frequency. Newer agents such as the echinocandins are available for most common fungal infections and have reduced nephrotoxicity, replacing amphotericin B as first line agents.

Another drug related form of intrarenal ARF is interstitial nephritis, which has been classically reported following methicillin use; however, it has also been observed with other antibiotics and medications (sulfamethoxazole, rifampin). Drug-induced interstitial nephritis is considered to be of allergic origin and is often associated with a skin rash and eosinophilia.

Radiocontrast-associated ARF is relatively common because of the ubiquitous use in diagnostic and interventional treatment of general surgery patients. Contrast induced ARF usually presents within 48 h of exposure with the serum Cr peaking at 3–5 days. Frequently these patients have under appreciated preexisting intrinsic renal insufficiency concurrently with other risk factors such as advanced age, diabetes mellitus, volume depletion, or a large dye load. Hospitalized patients with a serum creatinine greater than 1.5 mg/dl have up to a 30–40% incidence of renal dysfunction after intravenous or intra-arterial contrast injection. Limiting the volume of the contrast load can reduce the risk of contrast-associated ARF. The maximum dose of contrast medium that can be safely administered has traditionally been calculated according to the formula: 5ml × kg of body wt (maximum 300 ml)/serum creatinine. The use of nonionic, low osmolal, monomeric, contrast agents have a reduced risk and can be given in larger doses. (1.5 times ionic agents) It is recommended to avoid contrast doses without a 72 h window to allow the kidney to recover. The administration of intravenous saline to insure a replete intravascular volume prior to exposure is also recommended. Prophylactic options are summarized in ❯ *Table 16-3.*

Myoglobinuria is a frequent cause of nephrotoxic ARF in the surgical population. Patients with crush injuries, electrical burns, necrotizing soft-tissue infections, ischemia-reperfusion syndromes such as after revascularization, or who develop compartment syndromes are at high risk for rhabdomyolysis and myoglobinuria. Myoglobin is filtered and precipitates in the renal tubules, obstructing fluid flow, while the heme-molecule causes direct toxicity to the tubular epithelium. Patients with myoglobinuria will present with dark port-wine or tea-colored urine, which may be confused with gross hematuria initially. Serum levels of creatine phosphokinase (CPK) will characteristically be high, greater than 10,000 U/ml and at times greater than 100,000 U/ml in patients with the full-blown disease.

Postrenal ARF results from obstruction of the urinary collection system at one of several levels. Obstruction is usually prolonged and bilateral to result in ARF and prognosis for recovery is dependent on the duration of obstruction. A palpable bladder on exam indicates greater than 500 ml of retained urine consistent with obstruction. In the peri-operative or post-injury patient, it is important to demonstrate that indwelling bladder catheters are patent and within the bladder.

The acute development of abdominal compartment syndrome is increasingly being recognized as a cause of ARF that requires intervention by the general surgeon. Surgical patients can develop this syndrome following large volume resuscitation, placement of intra-abdominal packing for control of hemorrhage, prolonged operation with "tight" abdominal fascial closure, and diffuse peritonitis. The diagnosis is made clinically in a patient with high peak inspiratory pressures and CO_2 retention on the ventilator, progressive

❑ Table 16-3

Prophylaxis of contrast media-induced ARF

Accurate history	Discontinue concomitant risks	Correction of hypovolemia
Major risk factors 1. Pre-existing impairment 2. Dehydration 3. Hypovolemia	Potentially nephrotoxic drugs 1. NSAIDs 2. Aminoglycosides 3. Amphotericin B 4. Vancomycin 5. Diuretics 6. ACE-inhibitors 7. Angiotensin receptor antagonists	Isotonic saline load Half-isotonic saline Sodium bicarbonate soln
Minor risk factors 1. Advanced age 2. Diabetes mellitus 3. Congestive heart failure	Minimize risk if diagnostic or interventional procedure with contrast medium is required 1. Low-osmolal or iso-osmolal contrast medium (iohexol, iopamidol, ioxaglate) 2. Low amount of contrast medium 3. Wait a few days between two contrast administrations if possible	Antioxidant agents N-acetylcysteine pre-treatment
Perform alternative diagnostic procedures in high-risk patients as able		

oliguria, and abdominal rigidity. Bladder pressures are measured in complex cases to confirm the clinical diagnosis with >20–30 mmHg considered significant enough, to warrant abdominal decompression, although no absolute level of intra-abdominal hypertension is considered 100% diagnostic. The cause of acute renal failure in the setting of acute abdominal compartment syndrome is multifactorial and includes reduced cardiac output secondary to decreased venous return from the vena cava, increased pressure on the renal parenchyma causing reduced renal blood flow, and increased renal venous pressure.

Diagnostic Evaluation

The evaluation of the patient with ARF has two major goals: to determine the cause and potential therapy; and to assess the extent of complications and institute supportive care.

Evaluation of volume status is critical in the setting of low urine output and rising BUN and Cr. Accumulated fluid balance is useful. Direct measurement of central venous pressure or pulmonary capillary occlusion pressure is recommended to assist in the determination of intravascular volume status and to optimize renal perfusion in the perioperative or post-injury patient.

Serum and urine chemistries can assist the clinician in the diagnosis and management of the patient with oliguria (see ❯ *Table 16-4*). The fractional excretion of sodium (FENa) and urine sodium are useful measurements of how actively the kidney is resorbing sodium and reflect renal perfusion and intravascular volume status. In prerenal ARF, the kidney is hypoperfused; therefore, it actively resorbs Na and both the urine Na and FENa are *low*. In contrast, renal parenchymal damage results in loss of resorption of Na and the urine Na and FENa are *high*. The urine sediment is also useful in establishing a diagnosis. Muddy brown coarse granular casts in the urine sediment are the classic finding in ATN while white cell casts with eosinophiluria are seen in interstitial nephritis. Urine which dips positive for blood in the absence of red blood cells (RBCs/HPF) on microscopic examination suggests hemoglobinuria or myoglobinuria is present. This combination suggests that rhabdomyolysis or hemolysis as the cause of ARF.

Renal ultrasound imaging should be considered early to rule out obstruction in ARF. It documents that both kidneys are present and may identify other pathology while duplex scanning can demonstrate renal blood flow. Renal ultrasound also allows determination of kidney size with the finding of small kidneys indicating a chronic condition with superimposed acute deterioration.

❑ Table 16-4

Indices that distinguish prerenal ARF from ATN

Measurement	Prerenal ARF	ATN
Specific gravity	>1.020	< or ~1.010
FENa	<0.1–1%	> 1% preferably >3%
Urine osmolality	>500	<350 or ~300
Urine sodium	<20	>40
Serum BUN/Cr	>20	<15 or 10–15
Microscopic sediment	Hyaline casts	Brown granular casts

FENa = fractional excretion of sodium (%) = 100 × (urine Na × serum Cr)/(urine Cr × serum Na).

BUN/Cr = blood urea nitrogen-to-creatinine ratio.

CrCl = creatinine clearance = urine Cr × [timed urine volume (ml/min)]/serum Cr.

Therapy

Therapeutic options for ARF depend on its cause. Prerenal ARF is diagnosed and treated by restoration of renal perfusion. Postrenal ARF frequently requires mechanical intervention, which may be as simple as placement of a Foley catheter or require abdominal decompression. *There is no known therapy to modify the course of Acute Tubular Necrosis (ATN) once established.* The clinician must strive to remove the cause of the disease and provide supportive care until the return of adequate renal function.

Restoration of intravascular volume. Even in patients that are clinically suspected of having ATN, intravascular volume should be normalized as assessed by clinical findings and the monitoring of arterial blood pressure and cardiac filling pressures (preload) utilizing either central venous pressure (>12 mmHg) or pulmonary capillary occlusion pressure (>15 mmHg). If the patient does not respond appropriately to volume loading with increased central venous pressure and increased urine output, a pulmonary artery catheter should be utilized to measure cardiac output and oxygen delivery. Even if hemodynamic parameters appear adequate a trial of fluid is recommended early in the course of oliguric ARF.

Diuretics. If renal function does not improve significantly after optimization of intravascular volume a trial of furosemide (40–320 mg IV in increasing doses) or mannitol (12.5–25 g IV) is recommended. These agents help convert oliguric ARF to non-oliguric ARF. If the urine output does not respond to the initial dose of mannitol, it should be stopped since the intravascular osmotic load can cause exacerbation of fluid overload and pulmonary or cerebral edema. If urine output does not respond to furosemide, then it should be combined with metolazone (5–10 mg orally) or chlorothiazide (500 mg IV). Care must be exercised in avoiding repeated doses of furosemide in the setting of anuria as complications including deafness and allergic interstitial nephritis are reported. In patients that respond to diuretics an individual agent or combination furosemide/mannitol drip can be used and titrated to response (a common recipe is 250 ml of D5W, 200 mg of furosemide, and 12.5 g of mannitol).

Vasopressors. Once intravascular volume has been restored, some patients remain hypotensive (mean arterial pressure < 70). In these patients autoregulation of renal blood flow may be lost. Restoration of MAP to near normal levels is likely to increase GFR. In patients with chronic hypertension or renovascular disease a MAP of 75–80 mmHg may still be inadequate. No vasoactive agent has proven advantageous over another in the management of hypotension and oliguria. In patients with septic shock, profound hypotension, and oliguria, vasopressor therapy with norepinephrine may actually *improve* renal function by enhancing renal perfusion pressure to a greater extent then its vasoconstriction effects. The agent of choice likely will reflect the underlying pathophysiology (sepsis – norepinephrine; heart failure – dobutamine or milrinone). While a renal vasodilator dose of dopamine (1–3 µg/kg/min) may stimulate urine volume, it does not improve GFR, shorten the duration of ARF, or decrease the requirement for dialysis. In addition, dopamine may induce significant arrhythmias and possibly intestinal ischemia. Recent studies involving low-dose dopamine have been meta-analyzed and the results are that low-dose dopamine is not different from placebo in its effects on GFR.

Specific therapies. Patients with myoglobinuria require additional specific therapy: first, it is necessary to push urine output much higher than is necessary for fluid and electrolyte balance. Urine output should be maintained at > 150 ml/h through the initial phases of treatment so as to dilute and clear precipitated and free myoglobin from the tubules. Although neither has been shown to be beneficial in controlled trials, it is recommended that the normovolemic patient with ongoing IV fluid resuscitation receive mannitol (1 g/kg initially) to further induce an osmotic diuresis and perhaps for an anti-oxidant effect. Second, urine pH should be increased above 7 since myoglobin precipitation is lower at alkaline pHs. This is accomplished by adding sodium bicarbonate to the IV fluids, monitoring urine pH at frequent intervals, and utilizing diuretics that promote an alkaline urine such as the carbonic anhydrase-inhibitor acetazolamide rather than furosemide, which tends to create an acidic urine. The overall goal is to produce a high-output *alkaline diuresis*.

In patients with acute abdominal compartment syndrome, therapy is directed at relieving the intra-abdominal hypertension. This is most readily accomplished by laparotomy. Standard medical therapy of ARF with volume loading and inotropes usually is ineffective in this setting; however, the response to abdominal decompression is usually dramatic and life-saving. The remaining wound is covered with an impermeable plastic drape to reduce fluid losses through the temporary abdominal wall hernia.

Complications

The mainstay of therapy for ARF is to control complications until return of adequate renal function (*Table 16-5*). Initial complications reflect the kidney's role as the primary regulator of volume and mineral balance. Subsequently, patients develop uremic symptoms, reflecting the importance of the kidney in excretion of nitrogenous waste.

In oliguric patients, fluid intake must be rigorously monitored. A reasonable goal is for input = output, or the volume of maintenance fluids to equal measured fluid losses (urine, gastrointestinal fluid, surgical drains) plus insensible losses, which can be estimated at 600 ml/day (higher if patient is febrile). Nutritional support in the setting of acute renal failure should have the same goals of caloric and nitrogen equilibrium as the surgical patient without ARF.

Potassium should almost never be administered to an oliguric patient. A particularly deceptive and dangerous situation is the patient with high-output ATN in which potentially large volumes of urine

Table 16-5

Complications of acute renal failure

Complication	Clinical consequence	Therapy
Volume overload	Pulmonary edema Respiratory failure	Fluid and sodium restriction Diuretics
Hyperkalemia	Arrhythmia Ventricular tachycardia Heart block	Potassium restriction Calcium gluconate (10%) Glucose (D50) and insulin Sodium bicarbonate (7.5%) Cation-exchange resin
Metabolic acidosis	Hyperventilation	Sodium bicarbonate for <15 meq/l
Hyponatremia	Water imbalance	Fluid restriction
Hypocalcemia Hyperphosphatemia Hypermagnesemia	Carpopedal spasm Arrhythmia	Phosphate binding antacids Avoid magnesium antacids Supplemental calcium
Uremic syndrome	Nausea and vomiting Pericarditis or pleuritis Mental status changes Anemia Platelet dysfunction	Renal replacement therapy Hemodialysis Hemofiltration

are produced but potassium is not excreted. Hyperkalemia can develop rapidly in this situation if normal urine losses are assumed and electrolyte replacement is performed empirically. Another worrisome situation for rapid development of hyperkalemia is clinical rhabdomyolysis. Here the muscle necrosis releases large amounts of potassium and phosphorus frequently resulting in the need for aggressive therapy and not infrequently, early dialysis. The first and immediate treatment for symptomatic hyperkalemia (K + >6.5 or significant EKG findings of peaked T-waves, widening of QRS complex) is 10% Calcium Gluconate (5–10 ml IV over 2 min) which antagonizes the cardiac and neuromuscular effects. Glucose (50 ml of D50), Insulin (5–10 units regular IV over 5 min), and Sodium Bicarbonate (50 ml IV over 5 min) have an onset of 30–60 min and work primarily by shifting potassium into cells. Binding resins (15–30 g of resin in 50–100 ml of 20% sorbitol p.o. or by enema Q4 h) have an onset of several hours and exchange potassium for sodium.

Renal replacement. Several approaches to renal replacement therapy are available for the surgical patient in ARF. Intermittent hemodialysis has the greatest experience and established efficacy; however, over the last decade the availability of highly permeable membranes has allowed development of continuous renal replacement therapy (CRRT) which gradually removes fluids and solutes, resulting in better hemodynamic stability, and fluid and solute control (see ❷ *Table 16-6*). Dialysis therapy is indicated when the level of waste products in the blood is toxic or when fluid balance cannot be maintained with the use of medication or restriction. There is no evidence that dialysis shortens the course of ARF and because of potential complications of this therapy it should be reserved for well documented complications of ARF. These are listed in ❷ *Table 16-6* and include volume overload, acidosis, hyperkalemia, coma or seizure, uremic bleeding, and pericarditis. Absolute levels of BUN or Cr are not as important a factor in the decision to start dialysis as the patient's overall condition.

Regular dialysis 3× weekly for 4 h at a blood flow rate of 200 ml/min gives the patient the equivalent of an average weekly glomerular filtration rate (GFR) of 10–15 ml/min. Unfortunately, intermittent hemodialysis in the ICU setting is frequently associated with hypotension, hypoxemia, and cardiac arrhythmias which limit the actual time for solute and fluid removal.

Patients that will not tolerate intermittent hemodialysis can be provided renal replacement through the use of a variety of continuous, lower flow techniques that differ in the access utilized and in the principal method of solute clearance. The simplest is slow continuous ultrafiltration (SCUF) which uses mean arterial pressure as the driving force. A dialysate solution can be added to the

❑ Table 16-6

Comparison of continuous renal replacement therapy techniques (CRRT)

	SCUF	CAVH	CVVH	CAVHD	CVVHD
Access	A-V	A-V	V-V	A-V	V-V
Pump	No	No	Yes	No	Yes
Filtrate (ml/h)	100	600	1,000	300	300
Filtrate (l/day)	2.4	14.4	24	7.2	7.2
Dialysate flow (l/h)	0	0	0	1	1
Replacement fluid (l/day)	0	12	21.6	4.8	4.8
Urea clearance (ml/min)	1.7	10	16.7	21.7	21.7
Simplicity	1	2	3	2	3

Simplicity ranked 1–3: 1 = most simple, 3 = most difficult.
SCUF, slow continuous ultra-filtration; CAVH, continuous arterio-venous hemofiltration; CVVH, continuous veno-venous hemofiltration; CAVHD, continuous arterio-venous hemodialysis; CVVHD, continuous veno-venous hemodialysis.

hemofiltration to assist solute removal. This is termed continuous arteriovenous hemodialysis (CAVHD). If mean arterial pressure is inadequate (MAP < 70–80), use of a pump within a veno-venous circuit can be utilized as an alternative. This is termed continuous veno-venous hemofiltration or hemodialysis (CVVH or CVVHD). The advantages of continuous techniques are that they are well tolerated in hypotension and allow a greater volume of fluid removal, facilitating nutritional support, compared to intermittent hemodialysis. Disadvantages of this approach are the need for anticoagulation and the high volume of replacement fluid that must be closely monitored.

Selected Readings

Bellomo R, Ronco C, Kellum J, et al., and the ADQI workgroup (2004) Acute renal failure – definition, outcome measures, animal models, fluid therapy and information technology needs: the Second International Consensus Conference of the ADQI Group. Crit Care 8: R204–212

Better O, Stein J (1990) Early management of shock and prophylaxis of acute renal failure in traumatic rhabdomyolysis. NEJM 322:825–829

Kellum J, Angus D, Johnson J, et al. (2002) Continuous versus intermittent renal replacement therapy: a meta-analysis. Intensive Care Med 28:29–37

McNelis J, Marini C, Simms H (2003) Abdominal compartment syndrome: clinical manifestations and predictive factors. Curr Opin Crit Care 9:133–136

Meschi M, Detrenis S, Musini S, et al. (2006) Facts and fallacies concerning the prevention of contrast medium-induced nephropathy. Crit Care Med 34:2060–2068

Mindell J, Chertow G (1997) A practical approach to acute renal failure. Med Clin North Am 81:731–748

Schenarts P, Sagraves S, Bard M, et al. (2006) Low-dose dopamine: a physiologically based review. Curr Surg 63:219–225

Swan S (1997) Aminoglycoside nephrotoxicity. Semin Nephrol 17:27–33

17 Monitoring of Respiratory Function and Weaning from Mechanical Ventilation

Philip S. Barie · Soumitra R. Eachempati

Pearls and Pitfalls

- The most common reason for mechanical ventilation is to decrease the work of breathing, but other goals include improved gas exchange, resting of respiratory muscles, and prevention of deconditioning.
- Modes of mechanical, machine-delivered breaths triggered by the patient's own inspiratory efforts are preferred.
- Oxygen toxicity should be minimized by using a F_IO_2 which keeps arterial oxygen tension (PaO_2) > 60 mmHg or oxygen saturation > 88%.
- Ideal tidal volumes are about 6 ml/kg and plateau airway pressures should be <35 cm H_2O.
- Use of 5 cm PEEP restores functional residual capacity.
- Although most conscious patients require some form of sedation during mechanical ventilation, sedation should be minimized with daily sedation "holidays" of spontaneous breathing.
- The concept of a "ventilator bundle" optimizes mechanical ventilation and includes 30 degree elevation of the head of the bed, prophylaxis against deep vein thrombosis and gastric stress ulceration, and daily sedation holiday.
- Pulse oximetry measures oxygen saturation very accurately above 70% but requires pulsatile flow; hypothermia, hypotension, peripheral vascular disease, and the use of vasoconstrictor medications will interfere with readings from a pulse oximeter.
- Several newer non-invasive methods of monitoring cardiac output include thoracic bioimpedance, esophageal Doppler measurements, and near-infrared spectroscopy; these techniques are not available universally and have their own disadvantages and disadvantages.
- For arterial monitoring of blood gases or blood pressure, the brachial artery and the femoral artery should be avoided whenever possible.
- Pulmonary artery catheters are used to measure cardiac output, mixed venous oxygen saturation, and preload; the latter is estimated from the wedge pressure which approximates left atrial pressure, in indication of left ventricular end-diastolic pressure.
- Methods of weaning include the trial of spontaneous breathing, combination of SIMV (synchronized intermittent mechanical ventilation), and pressure support. Measurements of maximal negative inspiratory pressure, vital capacity, and minute volume help identify appropriate candidates.

- When weaning a patient from mechanical ventilation, intolerance is evident by increase in respiratory rate, decrease in tidal volume, and increased work of breathing (oxygen requirements), which can lead to decreased oxygen delivery, CO_2 retention, and increased cardiac stress.

Increasing patient acuity requires sophisticated methods to monitor and support these critically ill patients. Mechanical ventilation, a mainstay of modern ICU care, may be required to manage airway patency and support acute respiratory failure. New technology provides several modes of ventilation, with the goals of improved gas exchange, better patient comfort, and ultimately, rapid liberation from the ventilator. During acute respiratory failure, the work of breathing necessary to initiate a breath increases four- to six-fold. The most common reason to initiate mechanical ventilation is to decrease the patient's work of breathing. Additional goals include improved gas exchange, enhanced coordination between support and the patients' own efforts, resting of respiratory muscles, prevention of de-conditioning, and prevention of iatrogenic, ventilator-induced lung injury while promoting healing.

Nearly all ventilators can be set to allow full patient support or periods of exercise (i.e., periods promoting the work of breathing). Thus, choice of ventilator settings is often a matter of physician preference, modifying how positive airway pressure is applied and the interplay between mechanical support and the patients' own efforts. Unless appropriate settings are chosen to synchronize with the patient's own efforts, mechanical ventilation can cause increased work of breathing. Complete suppression of spontaneous breathing leads rapidly to respiratory muscle atrophy, therefore modes of mechanical ventilation are preferred wherein machine-delivered breaths are triggered by the patients' own inspiratory efforts, so as to maintain readiness for the patient to resume the work of breathing once the acute episode resolves, facilitating weaning and liberation from the ventilator.

Routine Ventilator Settings

Ventilator settings are based on the patient's ideal body mass and medical condition, manipulating, at minimum, respiratory rate, tidal volume (V_T), and fraction of inspired oxygen (F_IO_2). The risk of oxygen toxicity is minimized by using the lowest F_IO_2 that can oxygenate arterial blood satisfactorily to maintain arterial oxygen tension (PaO_2) > 60 mmHg or oxygen saturation (SaO_2) > 88%.

Although normal lungs may be ventilated safely with V_T 8–10 ml/kg for prolonged periods, convincing data indicate that a lesser V_T (6 ml/kg) prevents alveolar overdistention in acute lung injury and acute respiratory distress syndrome (ARDS); a lesser V_T helps to decrease endothelial, epithelial, and basement membrane injuries associated with ventilator-induced lung injury. Plateau airway pressure (P_{plat}), measured in a relaxed patient by occluding the ventilator circuit briefly at end-inspiration, should be kept ≤35 cm H_2O. Low V_T ventilation may lead to an increase in $PaCO_2$. Acceptance of an increased $PaCO_2$ in exchange for controlled alveolar pressure is termed *permissive hypercapnia*. It is important to focus on pH rather than $PaCO_2$ during permissive hypercapnia. If the pH decreases to <7.25, respirator rates should be increased or $NaHCO_3$ can be administered.

The respirator rate set on the ventilator depends on the mode. With conventional, assist-control ventilation (ACV), the backup rate should be about four breaths/min less than the patient's spontaneous rate to ensure that the ventilator will continue to supply adequate minute ventilation should the patient have a sudden decrease in spontaneous breathing. With synchronized, intermittent mandatory ventilation (SIMV), the respiratory rate is typically set high at first and then decreased gradually in accordance with patient tolerance.

An inspiratory gas flow rate of 60 l/min is used with most patients during ACV and SIMV. If the flow rate is insufficient to meet the patient's requirements, the patient will strain against his/her own pulmonary impedance and that of the ventilator, with a consequent increase in work of breathing (and thus oxygen/energy consumption).

In the ACV and SIMV modes, the patient must lower airway pressure below a preset threshold (usually minus 1–2 cm H_2O) in order to trigger the ventilator to deliver a tidal breath. Pressure support is an accepted method of assisting spontaneous breathing in a ventilated patient, either partially or fully. The patient triggers the ventilator, which delivers a flow of gas in response up to a preset pressure limit (e.g., 10 cm H_2O) depending on the desired minute ventilation. The gas flow then cycles off when a certain percentage of peak inspiratory flow (usually 25%) is reached. Tidal volumes may vary, just as they do spontaneously.

Positive end-expiratory pressure (PEEP), also referred to as continuous positive airway pressure (CPAP), is added to restore functional residual capacity (FRC) to normal for the patient (usually 5 cm H_2O, absent acute respiratory failure requiring higher therapeutic PEEP). When lung volumes are low, the work of breathing during early inhalation is decreased. Non-compliant lungs require higher intrapleural pressures to inflate to a normal tidal volume, even with CPAP. Addition of pressure support assists the patient to move up the pressure-volume curve (larger changes in volume for a given applied pressure for patients with increased lung compliance). Pressure support ventilation describes the combination of pressure support and PEEP (or CPAP). Although useful in the patient breathing spontaneously, pressure support may also be used to assist spontaneous breaths in SIMV. Weaning may be facilitated using this combination, as the backup (SIMV) rate is weaned initially, and then the pressure support.

Sedation

Most patients who require mechanical ventilation will require sedation, but only a minority (~10%) will also require neuromuscular blockade. Multiple pharmacologic agents are available for sedation (❂ *Table 17-1*), so the choice of agent can be individualized for the patient, but caution must be used to assure that patients are not over-sedated. Titration of sedation to patient comfort is facilitated by providing sedation titrated to a sedation score of 3–4 points on the Ramsay or Riker scale (❂ *Table 17-2*). Intermittent doses of sedatives are often preferred to continuous infusions in an attempt to minimize the amount of sedation. Neuromuscular blockade should be avoided whenever possible because of patient discomfort, worry of ventilator failure or disconnection, and muscular deconditioning.

Prolonged or excessive sedation increases the duration of mechanical ventilation and increases the likelihood of ventilator-associated pneumonia and the need for tracheostomy. Protocolized weaning of sedative medications and daily sedation "holidays" to permit trials of spontaneous breathing help to lessen the duration of mechanical ventilation and decrease the risk of pneumonia and other complications.

☐ Table 17-1

Selected formulary for analgesia, anesthesia, and sedation in the ICU

Agent	Initial IV adult dose
Induction agents	
Etomidate	6 mg or more
Ketamine	1–2 mg/kg
Propofol	1.5–2.5 mg/kg
Intravenous sedatives/analgesics	
Midazolam	0.5–4 mg
Lorazepam	1–4 mg
Morphine	2–10 mg
Hydromorphone	0.5–2.0 mg
Fentanyl	50–100 mcg
Neuromuscular blocking agents	
Succinylcholine	0.75–1.5 mg/kg
Atracurium	0.2–0.5 mg/kg
Cisatracurium	0.2–0.5 mg/kg
Pancuronium	0.05–0.1 mg
Vecuronium	0.08–0.10 mg/kg
Miscellaneous agents	
Dexmedetomidine	1 mcg/kg load, then 0.2–0.7 mcg/kg/h
Haloperidol	2–5 mg
Ketorolac	0.5–1.0 mg/kg
Reversal agents	
Flumazenil	0.1–0.2 mg
Naloxone	up to 0.4 mg
Edrophonium *with*	0.5–1.0 mg/kg
Atropine	0.007–0.014 mg/kg
Neostigmine *with*	0.5–2.0 mg
Glycopyrrolate	0.1–0.2 mg

Dosages should be adjusted as appropriate for renal or hepatic insufficiency.

☐ Table 17-2

Sedation scales in common usage

	Value	Clinical correlate
Ramsey sedation score		
Awake scores 1–3	1	Anxious, agitated, or restless
	2	Cooperative, oriented, tranquil
	3	Responsive to commands
Asleep scores 4–6	4	Brisk response to stimulus[a]
	5	Sluggish response to stimulus
	6	No response to stimulus
Riker sedation-agitation scale		
Dangerous agitation	7	Pulling at catheters, striking staff
Very agitated	6	Does not calm to voice, requires restraint
Agitated	5	Anxious, responds to verbal cues
Calm and cooperative	4	Calm, awakens easily, follows commands
Sedated	3	Awakens to stimulus
Very sedated	2	Arouses to stimulus, does not follow commands
Unarousable	1	Minimal or no response to noxious stimulus

[a]Stimulus: light glabellar tap or loud auditory stimulus.

Ventilator Bundle

Care of the patient on mechanical ventilation is more than just providing ventilation and oxygenation. Such patients are at risk for numerous complications, not all of which are related directly to acute respiratory failure or the actual mechanical ventilation. The clinician must bear in mind the total patient. Prolonged bed rest increases deconditioning, venous thromboembolic complications, and development of pressure ulcers. Neurologic compromise from disease or sedative/analgesic drugs may impair the sensorium, increasing the risk of pulmonary aspiration of gastric contents. Over-sedation may contribute directly to the need for prolonged mechanical ventilation, which is a definite risk factor for ventilator-associated pneumonia (incidence ~2%/day of ventilation). Prolonged ventilation (>48 h) also increases the risk of stress-related gastric mucosal hemorrhage.

Several "best practices" have been combined into a *ventilator bundle* to optimize the outcomes of mechanical ventilation, including four maneuvers: keeping the head of the bed up at least 30 degrees from level at all times unless contraindicated medically, prophylaxis against venous thromboembolic disease, prophylaxis against stress-related gastric mucosal hemorrhage, and a daily "sedation holiday" to assess for readiness to liberate from mechanical ventilation through assessment by a trial of spontaneous breathing. Careful adoption and adherence to all facets of this "ventilator bundle" can decrease the risk of pneumonia along with other maneuvers, such as adherence to the principles of infection control.

Monitoring of Mechanical Ventilation

Blood Gas Monitoring

Blood gas analyzers measure blood pO_2, pCO_2, and pH. Hemoglobin saturation is calculated from pO_2 using the oxyhemoglobin dissociation curve, assuming a normal P_{50} (the pO_2 at which SaO_2 is 50%, normally 26.6 mmHg), and normal hemoglobin structure. Blood gas analyzers with a co-oximeter measure the various forms of hemoglobin directly, including oxyhemoglobin, total hemoglobin, carboxyhemoglobin, and methemoglobin. The bicarbonate, standard bicarbonate, and base excess, however, are calculated from the pH and pCO_2.

A fresh, heparinized, bubble-free arterial blood sample is required. Heparin is acidic; if present in excess, pCO_2 and HCO_3 are decreased spuriously. Delay in obtaining these measurements from an arterial blood sample allows continued metabolism by erythrocytes which decrease the pH and pO_2 and increase the pCO_2. An iced specimen can be assayed accurately for up to 1 h. Air bubbles decrease pCO_2 and increase pO_2.

The solubility of all gases in blood increases with a decrease in temperature, thus hypothermia causes pO_2 and pCO_2 to decrease and pH to increase. Analysis at 37°C of a sample taken from a hypothermic patient will cause a somewhat spurious increase in pO_2 and pCO_2, but the error is usually not meaningful.

Non-invasive Monitoring

Pulse oximetry: Pulse oximetry detects even slight decreases in SaO_2 with only about a 60-s delay. The device calculates SaO_2 by estimating the difference in signal intensity between oxygenated and deoxygenated blood from red (660 nm) and near-infrared (940 nm) light. Pulse oximetry requires pulsatile blood flow to be accurate (● *Table 17-3*), but all things being equal, data can be obtained from a detector on the finger, earlobe, or forehead. Pulse oximetry is very accurate ($\pm 2\%$) for SaO_2 from 70% to 100%, but less so below 70%.

Several aspects of the technology and patient physiology limit the accuracy of pulse oximetry. If the device cannot detect pulsatile flow, the waveform will be dampened. Consequently, pulse oximetry may be inaccurate in patients with hypothermia, hypotension, hypovolemia, or peripheral vascular disease, or in patients being treated with vasoconstrictor medications. Additionally, an increased carboxyhemoglobin concentration will lead to a falsely increased SaO_2, because its reflected light is absorbed at the same wavelength as oxyhemoglobin. Other causes of inaccurate pulse oximetry include ambient light and motion artifact.

Capnography: Capnography measures the concentration of CO_2 in expired gas. This technique is most reliable in ventilated patients and employs either mass spectroscopy or infrared light absorption to detect CO_2. The peak CO_2 concentration occurs at end-exhalation and is regarded as the patient's "end-tidal CO_2" ($ETCO_2$), which approximates the alveolar gas concentration (● *Fig. 17-1*). Capnography is useful to assess the success of airway intubation, weaning from mechanical ventilation, and resuscitation (● *Table 17-4*). Detection of hypercarbia during ventilator weaning can diminish the need for blood gas determinations. Used with pulse oximetry, many patients can be liberated from mechanical ventilation without reliance on blood gases or invasive monitoring.

The characteristics of the waveform provides information about the patient's pulmonary status and in particular whether obstructive disease or inadequate ventilation is present. A sudden decrease or even disappearance of $ETCO_2$ can be correlated with potentially serious pathology or events, such as a low cardiac output state, disconnection from the ventilator, or pulmonary thromboembolism

◘ Table 17-3

Sources of error in pulse oximetry

False depression of SaO_2
Methemoglobinemia (reads at 85%)
Methylene blue dye
Indocyanine green dye
Non-pulsatile blood flow (no reading may be appreciable at all)
Vasoconstriction
Hypotension
Hypothermia
Hypovolemia
Venous congestion with exaggerated venous pulsation
Peripheral edema
Nail polish
Fluorescent lighting
Use of electrocautery (electrical interference)
Severe anemia (Hemoglobin concentration 3–4 g/dl)
Shivering (may cause mechanical loss of signal)
False elevation of SaO_2
Carboxyhemoglobin
No effect
Fatal hemoglobin
Hyperbilirubinemia

Figure 17-1

A normal capnograph tracing

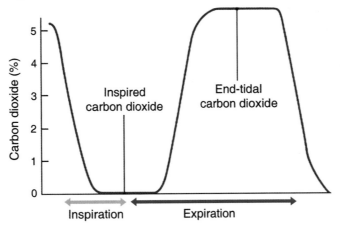

Table 17-4

Changes in end-tidal CO_2 (ETCO$_2$)

Increased ETCO$_2$
Decreased alveolar ventilation
Reduced respiratory rate
Reduced tidal volume
Increased equipment dead space
Increased CO$_2$ production
Fever
Hypercatabolic state
Excess feeding with carbohydrate
Increased inspired CO$_2$ concentration
CO$_2$ absorber exhausted
Increased CO$_2$ in inspired gas
Rebreathing of expired gas
Decreased ETCO$_2$
Increased alveolar ventilation
Increased respiratory rate
Increased tidal volume
Decreased CO$_2$ production
Hypothermia
Hypocatabolic state
Increased alveolar dead space
Decreased cardiac output
Pulmonary embolism (clot, air, fat)
High positive end-expiratory pressure (PEEP)
Sampling error
Air in sample line (no or diminished signal)
Water in sample line (no or diminished signal)
Inadequate tidal volume (no or diminished signal)
Disconnection of monitor from tubing (no signal)
Artificial airway not in trachea (e.g., esophageal intubation) (no signal)

◨ Table 17-5

Indications and contraindications for central venous pressure monitoring and pulmonary artery catheterization

Central venous pressure monitoring
Indications
Major operative procedures involving large fluid shifts or blood loss
Hypovolemia or shock
Intravascular volume assessment when urine output is not reliable or unavailable (e.g., renal failure)
Major trauma
Surgical procedures with a high risk of air embolism, such as sitting-position craniotomy or major liver resection
Frequent venous blood sampling
Venous access for vasoactive or irritating drugs
Chronic drug administration
Inadequate peripheral IV access
Rapid infusion of IV fluids (using large cannulae)
Parenteral nutrition
Insertion of other devices
PA catheters
Transvenous pacing wires
Access for renal replacement therapy
Contraindications
Absolute
Infection at the site of insertion
Large tricuspid valve vegetations
Superior vena cava syndrome
Tumor or thrombus in the right atrium
Relative
Anticoagulant therapy
Coagulopathy
Contralateral diaphragm dysfunction (risk of recurrent nerve injury with internal jugular cannulation)
Newly-inserted pacemaker wires
Presence of carotid disease
Recent cannulation of the internal jugular vein
Thyromegaly or prior neck surgery (especially ipsilateral carotid endarterectomy)
Pulmonary artery catheterization
Indications
Cardiac surgery
Poor left ventricular function (ejection fraction <0.4; end-diastolic pressure >18 mmHg)
Recent myocardial infarction
Complications of myocardial infarction (e.g., mitral insufficiency, ventricular septal defect, ventricular aneurysm)
Combined lesions, e.g., coronary artery disease with mitral insufficiency or aortic stenosis
Asymmetric septal hypertrophy
Intraaortic balloon pump
Non-cardiac indications
Shock of any cause
Severe pulmonary disease
Complicated surgical procedures
Multiple trauma
Hepatic transplantation
Aortic surgery
Contraindications
The same contraindications for central venous catheterization apply here. Additionally
Absolute
Tricuspid or pulmonary valvular stenosis
Right ventricular masses (tumor or thrombus)
Tetralogy of Fallot
Relative
Ventricular arrhythmia

(◉ *Table 17-5*). A gradual increase of ETCO$_2$ can be seen with hypoventilation; the converse is also true. Another cause of a gradually decreasing ETCO$_2$ is hypovolemia.

Non-invasive Cardiac Output

Thoracic bioimpedance: Thoracic bioimpedance determines cardiac output by deriving information from topical electrodes placed on the anterior chest and neck, estimating the left ventricular systolic time interval from time 1/μ-derivative bioimpedance signals. The lag time for the system to provide data is approximately 2–5 min from initial lead placement and activation. The main drawback of thoracic bioimpedance is that it is susceptible to any alteration of the electrode contact or positioning on the patient.

Esophageal Doppler: The esophageal Doppler monitor (EDM) device is a soft, 6 mm catheter placed noninvasively into the esophagus. A Doppler flow probe at its tip allows continuous monitoring of cardiac output and stroke volume. A 4-MHz continuous wave ultrasound frequency is reflected to produce a waveform, representing the change in blood flow in the descending aorta (about 80% of cardiac output) with each pulsation. EDM may be more accurate than a pulmonary artery catheter (see below) in patients with cardiac valvular lesions, septal defects, arrhythmias, or pulmonary hypertension. The primary disadvantage of EDM is loss of waveform with only slight positional changes, leading to dampened, inaccurate readings.

Near-infrared spectroscopy: Near-infrared spectroscopy measures tissue O$_2$ tension non-invasively in close to real time. Near-infrared light of four calibrated wavelengths penetrates tissue to a depth of approximately 15 mm below the sensor, which is placed usually on the thenar eminence. Analysis of reflected light produces an absolute measurement of tissue oxygenation (StO$_2$) in the skeletal muscle microcirculation, which has been evaluated in a wide range of experimental conditions. Skeletal muscle StO$_2$ has been found to correlate with O$_2$ delivery, base deficit, and serum lactate concentration in experimental and clinical hemorrhagic shock. Detection is possible over a StO$_2$ range of 1–99% but is most accurate for StO$_2$ > 70%.

In a recent multicenter trial of 383 patients with major trauma who required blood transfusion, 50 of whom eventually developed multiple organ dysfunction syndrome, the monitoring with near-infrared spectroscopy was begun within 30 min of arrival in the emergency department and continued for 24 h. A StO$_2$ > 75% maintained during the first hour of monitoring indicated adequate tissue perfusion with affected patients having an 88% survival. In contrast, an StO$_2$ < 75% in the first hour was predictive of development of multiple organ dysfunction syndrome (78%); 91% of those patients died.

Invasive Hemodynamic Monitoring

Arterial catheterization: Measurement of arterial blood pressure is the most reproducible method of evaluating hemodynamics. For stable patients, automated non-invasive blood pressure cuff devices can measure blood pressure accurately and precisely (error, ±2%), as often as every 5 min. Blood pressure will be overestimated if the cuff is too small and if systolic blood pressure is less than 60 mmHg. Arrhythmias such as atrial fibrillation degrade accuracy. If blood pressure fluctuates more frequently than intermittent measurements can capture, continuous monitoring is needed via an indwelling arterial catheter.

Indications for invasive arterial monitoring include prolonged operations (>4 h in duration), unstable hemodynamics, substantial blood loss, frequent blood sampling, or a need for precise control of blood pressure (e.g., neurosurgical patients and patients on cardiopulmonary bypass). Patients on mechanical ventilation or inotropic support often benefit from arterial catheterization. Although there is morbidity from the insertion and the indwelling catheter, there is also morbidity from repetitive arterial punctures; the risk: benefit analysis is a matter of clinical judgment for "less unstable" patients.

Arterial catheters may be placed in any of several locations. The radial artery at the wrist is used most commonly; the ulnar artery is usually larger but is relatively inaccessible to percutaneous access. To minimize the possibility of hand ischemia from arterial occlusion or embolization of debris or clot from the catheter tip, careful confirmation of the patency of the collateral circulation of the hand is mandatory before arterial cannulation at the wrist. Alternative sites include the umbilical artery (in neonates) and the axillary and superficial femoral arteries in adults; the latter is not a location of choice because the burden of plaque (and therefore risk of distal embolization) is higher, as is the infection rate. The brachial artery should be avoided; the collateral circulation around the elbow is poor, and the risk of ischemia of the hand or forearm is too great.

Because the arterial waveform may be damped by severe peripheral vasoconstriction during vasopressor therapy, it may be necessary to use a longer catheter at a more central location (e.g., axillary, femoral) to position the catheter tip into an unaffected artery in the torso. Nosocomial infection of arterial catheters is unusual provided basic tenets of infection control are honored, and femoral artery catheterization is avoided. Other complications from arterial catheterization include bleeding, hematoma, and pseudoaneurysm formation.

Central venous pressure monitoring: The central venous pressure (CVP) is an interplay of the circulating blood volume, venous tone, and right ventricular function. By measuring the filling pressure of the right ventricle, the CVP provides an estimate of the status of the intravascular volume. Indications for cannulation of a central vein are numerous, and the contraindications are relatively few (❯ *Table 17-5*). Strict adherence to asepsis, full barrier precautions, and adherence to the principles of infection control are crucial to avoid the potentially life-threatening complication of catheter-related blood stream infection. Central venous access can be obtained at several body sites, including the basilic, femoral, external jugular, internal jugular, or subclavian vein. The internal jugular, subclavian, and femoral veins are used most often, listed in decreasing frequency. The internal jugular vein is most popular site because of ease of accessibility, a high technical success rate, and a low complication rate, although the infection rate is higher than for subclavian vein catheters, allegedly because of more movement at the insertion site. The subclavian site is the most technically demanding for placement and has the highest rate of pneumothorax (1.5–3%), but the infection rate is the lowest of the three. The femoral vein site is least preferred, despite the relative ease of catheter placement. The femoral site is particularly prone to infection, and the risks of arterial puncture (9–15%) and venous thromboembolic complications are much higher than for jugular or subclavian venipuncture. Overall complications are comparable for internal jugular and subclavian vein cannulation (6–12%), and higher for femoral vein cannulation (13–19%).

Pulmonary artery catheterization: A pulmonary artery (Swan Ganz) catheter is a balloon-tipped, flow-directed catheter that is usually inserted percutaneously via a central vein; the balloon tip is then "floated" through the right side of the heart and into the pulmonary artery. This catheter typically contains several ports for pressure monitoring or fluid administration. Some pulmonary artery catheters include a sensor to measure central (mixed) venous oxygen saturation or right ventricular volume. Data from these catheters are used mainly to determine cardiac output and preload, which is estimated most commonly by the pulmonary artery occlusion pressure (PAOP), so-called wedge pressure.

Normally, PAOP approximates left atrial pressure, which in turn approximates left ventricular end-diastolic pressure, itself a reflection of left ventricular end-diastolic volume, which represents preload, the actual target parameter. Many factors cause PAOP to reflect inaccurately the left ventricular end diastolic volume, including mitral stenosis, high levels of PEEP (>10 cm H_2O), and changes in left ventricular compliance (e.g., due to myocardial infarction, pericardial effusion, or increased afterload). Inaccurate readings may result from balloon overinflation, improper catheter position, alveolar pressure exceeding pulmonary venous pressure (as with high pressures of PEEP ventilation), or severe pulmonary hypertension. Increased PAOP occurs in left-sided heart failure, whereas decreased PAOP occurs with hypovolemia or decreased preload.

A desirable feature of pulmonary artery catheterization is the ability to measure central mixed venous oxygen saturation, although sampling from the superior vena cava via a CVP catheter may be comparable. Some catheters have embedded fiberoptic sensors that measure oxygen saturation directly. Causes of low central mixed venous oxygen saturation include anemia, pulmonary disease, carboxyhemoglobinemia, low cardiac output, and increased tissue oxygen demand. Ideally, the pulmonary mixed venous oxygen tension should be 35–40 mmHg, with a central mixed venous oxygen saturation of about 70%. Values of pulmonary mixed venous oxygen tension < 30 mmHg are critically low.

No studies have demonstrated unequivocally that use of pulmonary artery catheters decreases morbidity or mortality; some retrospective data even suggest that they are associated with excess mortality. Critically ill patients who require one or more inotropic agents, despite resuscitation with large volumes of fluid, may benefit from such monitoring, both in the operating room and the ICU, but lack of demonstrable benefit has decreased the use of pulmonary artery catheters substantially.

Newer pulmonary artery catheters allow continuous monitoring of cardiac output and central mixed venous oxygen saturation. Continuous data may be useful when O_2 transport is marginal, such as patients with ARDS on high levels of PEEP. A recent large multicenter trial, however, conducted by the ARDSnet investigators, showed no benefit of pulmonary artery monitoring versus CVP monitoring of fluid administration for patients with ARDS. Complications of pulmonary arterial catheterizations include infection (2–5%), hemo- or pneumothorax (2–5%), migration (5–10%), patient discomfort, arrhythmia (10–15%), and hemorrhage (0.2%). Rare complications include catheter knotting in the right ventricle (especially in patients with heart failure, cardiomyopathy, or pulmonary hypertension), pulmonary infarction, pulmonary artery or cardiac perforation, valvular injury, and endocarditis. Pulmonary artery rupture occurs in fewer than 0.1% of patients with pulmonary artery catheters and is generally fatal. Distal migration of the PAC within the pulmonary artery increases the risk dramatically of pulmonary artery rupture and is one of the few indications for routine daily bedside chest radiography for all patients with acute respiratory failure.

Liberation from Mechanical Ventilation

Objective measures and proactive strategies can hasten the liberation of patients from the ventilator. The stakes are high; each day of mechanical ventilation (e.g., endotracheal or tracheostomy tube) increases the need for sedation, which may postpone "liberation day." Moreover, each day of mechanical ventilation increases the risk of ventilator-associated pneumonia.

Failure to separate from the ventilator may be due to disease- or therapy-related reasons. Most clinical cases of failed liberation from the ventilator are multifactorial, but respiratory muscle fatigue is a common factor, in that the load on the respiratory system exceeds the capacity to breathe (❯ *Table 17-6*). The increased load may take the form of a demand for increased minute ventilation or increased work of breathing. Increased minute ventilation may result from increased CO_2 production, increased dead space ventilation, or increased ventilatory drive. Increased CO_2 production may be caused by a catabolic state or overfeeding with carbohydrate. Increased dead space (ventilation of un- or under-perfused lung) may be caused by decreased cardiac output, pulmonary embolism, pulmonary hypertension, severe acute lung injury, or iatrogenically from ventilator-associated lung injury. Increased ventilatory drive may occur from muscle fatigue or failure, stimulation of pulmonary J receptors (usually by lung inflammation or parenchymal hemorrhage), or lesions of the central nervous system. Psychologic stress is also an important factor that may manifest itself as tachypnea, hypoxemia, agitation, or delirium. Stress may be caused by inadequate analgesia, sedation, or untreated delirium. Acute alcohol or drug withdrawal is a major factor in some patients.

Increased work of breathing results from either increased airflow resistance or decreased thoracic compliance. Airway obstruction can result from reversible small airways disease (e.g., bronchospasm), tracheal stenosis, tracheomalacia, glottic edema or dysfunction, mucus plugging, or muscle weakness. Muscle dysfunction may be caused by nutritional or metabolic causes (including hypocalcemia, hypokalemia, or hypophosphatemia). The critical illness polyneuropathy syndrome has a poorly understood pathophysiology but is associated with sepsis and often diagnosed when sought specifically by electromyography. Other potential causes of muscular failure or weakness include hypoxemia, hypercarbia, and possibly anemia.

Patients who "fight" the ventilator technically have the syndrome of patient-ventilator dyssynchrony. The cause must be sought; sedating the patient more deeply (or administering neuromuscular blockade) before a correctable cause is identified and remedied may be catastrophic if an unstable airway is the cause. A systematic approach to evaluation is advocated. Recognizing that patient and ventilator are supposed to be working in concert facilitates understanding that the problem may be the patient or the ventilator. The cause may be found anywhere on the continuum from the alveolus to the power outlet or the source of respiratory gases (❯ *Table 17-7*). The first step is always to ensure that the patient has a properly positioned, patent airway.

◘ **Table 17-6**

Load on the respiratory system

Demand for increased minute ventilation
Increased carbon dioxide production
Increased dead space ventilation
Increased ventilatory drive
Increased work of breathing
Airway obstruction
Decreased respiratory system compliance
Decreased respiratory system capacity
Impaired central drive to breathe
Integrity of phrenic nerve transmission
Impaired respiratory muscle force generation

■ Table 17-7

Therapies to reverse ventilatory failure

Improve muscular function
    Treat sepsis-avoid aminoglycosides
    Nutritional support without overfeeding (follow indirect calorimetry)
    Replete electrolytes to normal
    Assure periods of rest-do not exhaust the patient
    Limit neuromuscular blockade
    Avoid oversedation
    Identify/correct hypothyroidism
Reduce respiratory load
    Airway resistance
        Ensure airway patency/adequate caliber
    Compliance (elastance)
        Treat pneumonia
        Treat pulmonary edema
        Identify/reduce intrinsic PEEP (auto-PEEP)
        Drain large pleural effusions
        Evacuate pneumothorax
        Treat ileus (promotility agents)
        Decompress abdominal distention/treat abdominal compartment syndrome
        Position patient 30° head-up
    Minute ventilation
        Treat sepsis
        Antipyresis (T > 40°C?)
        Avoid overfeeding
        Correct metabolic acidosis
        Identify/reduce intrinsic PEEP (auto-PEEP)
        Bronchodilators
        Maintain least possible PEEP
        Resuscitate shock/correct hypovolemia
        Identify and treat pulmonary embolism

Liberation from mechanical ventilation may be easy to accomplish after short-term support. As many as 25% of all ventilated patients will experience respiratory distress during the initial weaning attempt, such that mechanical ventilation has to be reinstituted; patients recovering from acute respiratory failure, pneumonia, or major torso trauma can be especially challenging. Patients who cannot be weaned have a characteristic response to spontaneous breathing trials, including an almost-immediate increase in respiratory rate and decrease in tidal volume. As the trial continues over 30–60 min, work of breathing increases substantially by four- to sevenfold. Increased O_2 demand is met by increased O_2 extraction, which eventually causes decreased O_2 delivery and hypoxemia. Pulmonary compliance decreases, and the rapid, shallow breathing pattern causes CO_2 retention. There is considerable cardiovascular stress also, with increased afterload on both ventricles from the large changes in intrathoracic pressure generated by the struggling patient.

Timing is important; if weaning is delayed unnecessarily, the patient remains at risk for a host of ventilator-associated complications. If premature, weaning failure may lead to cardiopulmonary decompensation and need for prolonged ventilation. In general, discontinuation of mechanical ventilation is not attempted with unstable hemodynamics or if $PaO_2 < 60$ mmHg with $F_1O_2 \geq 0.60$.

Of note, adequate oxygenation alone does not predict successful weaning; more important is the ability of respiratory muscles to perform increased work. Decisions based solely on clinical judgment are frequently in error. Parameters gathered traditionally, including the maximal negative inspiratory pressure, the vital capacity, and the minute volume, have limited predictive accuracy. Respiratory frequency $(f)/V_T$ during 1 min of spontaneous breathing (the Rapid Shallow Breathing Index) is more accurate (95% probability of success) if $f/V_T < 80$ after a 30-min trial of spontaneous breathing.

The process of weaning begins by determining patient readiness (❯ *Table 17-8*). Patients should be screened carefully for hemodynamic stability, cooperative mental status, respiratory muscle strength, consistent and adequate wakefulness, ability to manage secretions, nutritional repletion, normalization of acid-base and electrolyte status, and an artificial airway of adequate size. If the aforementioned conditions are addressed, weaning may be attempted.

There are four methods of weaning. Simplest is to perform a trial of spontaneous breathing each day with a T-piece circuit providing oxygen-enriched gas. Initially brief (5–10 min), the trial can be increased in frequency and duration until the patient can breathe spontaneously for several hours. Alternatively, a single trial of up to 2 h in duration is undertaken; if successful, the patient is extubated; if not, the next attempt is made on the following day. More common (and popular) are SIMV and pressure support ventilation, which are often combined. Support is decreased gradually by decreasing respiratory rate or pressure support. When combined, minimum respiratory rate is set to zero before pressure support is decreased. Pressure support of 5–8 cm H_2O is used widely to compensate for the resistance inherent in the ventilator circuit; patients who can breathe comfortably at that level should be able to be extubated. Prospective trials indicate that weaning takes up to three times longer when IMV is used rather than a spontaneous breathing trial. Approximately 10–20% of patients require re-intubation, and affected patients have mortality that is six-fold higher. Use of non-invasive ventilation after extubation may improve the likelihood of successful extubation.

Special Airway Considerations

Unplanned extubation: Patient self-extubation is a morbid event that occurs in approximately 10% of patients undergoing mechanical ventilation. Risk factors include chronic respiratory failure, poor fixation of the airway device, orotracheal intubation (which is decidedly uncomfortable), and inadequate sedation. The associated complications include re-intubation (required in one-half of such patients), ventilator-associated pneumonia, vocal cord trauma, and rarely loss of the airway with attendant cardiovascular and neurologic complications. Re-intubation is more likely in the setting of accidental intubation, decreased mentation, occurrence outside a process of active weaning, and $PaO_2:F_IO_2 < 200$. The risk of unplanned extubation can be decreased by appropriate sedation, vigilance during positioning of the patient and during bedside procedures, proper fixation of the airway device, and daily screening and assessment of patient readiness for liberation from the ventilator.

Re-intubation: Approximately 20% of patients require re-intubation, even if protocols are followed, and the patient meets all criteria for extubation. The rate varies widely among units; a rate that is "too low" may imply that patients are not being weaned aggressively enough, whereas a rate that is "too high" may reflect a high proportion of patients with neurologic impairment who are at highest risk. Paradoxically, use of weaning protocols, which liberate patients from mechanical ventilation sooner are associated with lesser rates of re-intubation. Re-intubation may reflect severity of illness

◘ **Table 17-8**

Cornell protocol for liberation from mechanical ventilation

Screening (performed at least once daily, usually in early AM, by respiratory therapist, nurse, or physician, according to local protocol)

  Resolution of the underlying disease process

  No vasopressors or sedative infusions (except propofol or dexmedetomidine). No neuromuscular blocking agents. Intermittent doses of sedatives are permissible

  No active myocardial ischemia or cardiac rhythm disturbances

  $V_E < 15$ l/min

  $P_aO_2{:}F_IO_2 > 120$ on $F_IO_2 < 0.55$

  $PaCO_2 < 50$ mmHg

  Physiologic pH (7.30–7.50)

  PEEP < 8 cm H_2O

  Pressure support < 8 cm H_2O

  Adequate cough/clearance of secretions

             ↓

        YES/NO → Return to screening

             ↓

Proceed with spontaneous breathing trial-turn off enteral feedings and monitor serum glucose concentration closely, especially if on continuous infusion of insulin

  Spontaneous breathing trial

  Calculate RSBI; target <105

             ↓

      YES/NO → Return to screening −treat to reduce respiratoty load

             ↓

  Continue spontaneous breathing trial

    CPAP with flow-by trigger, no change in CPAP or F_IO_2 over course of 1-h trial

    Failure criteria

      RR > 35 breaths/min for 5 min

      $SaO_2 < 90\%$ for 30 s or more

      HR > 140 beats/min, or sustained D $> 20\%$ in either direction

      $BP_{syst} > 180$ mmHg or < 90 mmHg

      Increased anxiety, agitation, or diaphoresis

          ↓

      PASS/FAIL → Return to screening

          ↓

    Does not require suctioning more than 4 h/day

    President evidence of ability to protect airway (cough, gag reflex)

    No evidence of upper airway obstruction in previous 48 h

    No history of reintubation for excessive tracheal secretions in previous 48 h

       ↓

    T − piecetrail(optional)

       ↓

    PASS/FAIL → Return to screening

       ↓

    EXTUBATE

with substantially increased risks of pneumonia and death. The cause may be either airway compromise or failure of lung/chest wall mechanics (weaning failure).

Tracheostomy: It is challenging to identify patients who will not be able to be removed from the ventilator. Possible reasons include airway obstruction, anxiety or agitation (requiring heavy doses of sedatives), aspiration syndromes, alkalosis, bronchospasm, chronic obstructive pulmonary disease, critical illness polyneuropathy or other forms of neuromuscular disease, electrolyte abnormalities, heart disease, hypothyroidism, morbid obesity, nutrition (over- or under-feeding), opioids, pleural effusion (if large), pulmonary edema, and sepsis.

The timing of tracheostomy remains controversial. There is no consensus definition of when a tracheostomy is "early" (<10 days?) or "late" (>21 days?), although trends are toward earlier performance, with decreased sedation requirements and risk of ventilator-associated pneumonia, greater patient comfort, and facilitated weaning thereafter. The shorter tube decreases airway resistance and work of breathing and facilitates pulmonary toilet by suctioning. Percutaneous tracheostomy has decreased the morbidity of tracheostomy substantially. In addition, modern high-volume, low-pressure cuffs on endotracheal tubes permit translaryngeal intubation for several weeks with relative safety. Patients who are unstable hemodynamically, coagulopathic, or on high levels of PEEP may benefit from having tracheostomy postponed until they are more stable.

Selected Readings

ARDS Network (2000) Ventilation with lower tidal volumes as compared with traditional tidal volumes for acute lung injury and the acute respiratory distress syndrome. N Engl J Med 342:1301–1308

Arroliga A, Frutos-Vivar F, Hall J, et al. (2005) International Mechanical Ventilation Study Group. Use of sedatives and neuromuscular blockers in a cohort of patients receiving mechanical ventilation. Chest 128:496–506

Brochard L, Rauss A, Benito S, et al. (1994) Comparison of three methods of gradual withdrawal from ventilatory support during weaning from mechanical ventilation. Am J Respir Crit Care Med 150:896–903

Dodek P, Keenen S, Cook D, et al. (2004) for the Canadian Clinical Trials Group and the Canadian Critical Care Society. Evidence-based clinical guideline for the prevention of ventilator-associated pneumonia. Ann Intern Med 141:305–313

Eachempati SR, Young C, Alexander J, et al. (1999) The clinical use of an esophageal Doppler monitor for hemodynamic monitoring in sepsis. J Clin Monitor Comp 15:223–225

Kollef MH, Shapiro SD, Silver P, et al. (1997) A randomized, controlled trial of protocol-directed versus physician-directed weaning from mechanical ventilation. Crit Care Med 25:567–574

MacIntyre NR, Cook DJ, Ely EW Jr, et al. (2001) Evidence-based guidelines for weaning and discontinuing ventilatory support: a collective task force facilitated by the American College of Chest Physicians, the American Association for Respiratory Care, and the American College of Critical Care Medicine. Chest 120:375S–395S

National Heart, Lung, and Blood Institute Acute Respiratory Distress Syndrome (ARDS) Clinical Trials Network; Wheeler AP, Bernard GP, Thompson BT, et al. (2006) Pulmonary-artery versus central venous catheter to guide treatment of acute lung injury. N Engl J Med 354:2213–2224

Pinsky MR (2003) Hemodynamic monitoring in the intensive care unit. Clin Chest Med 24:549–560

Yang KL, Tobin MJ (1991) A prospective study of indexes predicting the outcome of trials of weaning from mechanical ventilation. N Engl J Med 324:1445–1450

18 Coma and Altered Mental Status in the Surgical Critical Care Setting; Brain Death

Joshua M. Levine · M. Sean Grady

Pearls and Pitfalls

- Altered consciousness results from dysfunction of either the upper brainstem/diencephalon, or both cerebral hemispheres. Unilateral brain lesions do not cause coma except with shift of midline structures.
- Etiologies of coma may be divided into primary brain disorders – which may be either structural or nonstructural – and systemic causes, such as toxic, metabolic, and infectious encephalopathies.
- Etiologies of coma that mandate emergent diagnosis and treatment to prevent life- or brain-threatening injury include: seizures, brain infections, acute hydrocephalus, herniation, ischemic and hemorrhagic strokes, subarachnoid hemorrhage, cerebral venous sinus thrombosis, hypertensive encephalopathy, and traumatic brain injury (TBI).
- Beware of coma mimics, especially the "locked-in" syndrome, in which the patient is awake and aware of their surroundings but is paralyzed and unable to communicate.
- Neurological examination of the coma patient focuses on four elements: (1) determination of the patient's level of arousal (wakefulness), (2) examination of the eyes, (3) elicitation of motor responses and abnormal reflexes, and (4) observation of breathing patterns.
- Focal neurological signs or abnormalities of the pupillary light reflex suggest a structural cause of coma.
- Induced hypothermia should be considered in patients who are comatose after cardiac arrest.
- Prognosis of coma is based on etiology, clinical signs, and ancillary tests including electrophysiological, neuroimaging, and biochemical studies. However, determining prognosis in any given patient remains a significant challenge.
- Brain death refers to irreversible cessation of whole-brain activity and is a clinical diagnosis.
- The three cardinal features of brain death are: (1) coma, (2) absence of brainstem reflexes, and (3) apnea.

Coma and other disorders of consciousness are common in the surgical intensive care unit (ICU) and indicate a severe disturbance of cerebral function. Management of patients with disturbed consciousness is frequently difficult because there are a myriad of possible causes, many of which require urgent intervention in order to prevent irreversible brain damage. Altered mental status is a medical emergency and mandates a prompt, systematic evaluation to diagnose and treat life- or brain-threatening disorders. Brain death is defined in the USA as irreversible cessation of whole-brain activity and is discussed at the end of this chapter.

States of consciousness fall along a spectrum, with coma at one end and normal consciousness at the other. Patients who are in coma do not respond to external stimuli in a "purposeful" manner but may demonstrate reflexive behavior. Their eyes are closed and sleep–wake cycles are absent. Coma is usually prolonged – lasting for at least hours to days, but rarely permanent – progressing either to death or to a higher level of consciousness. Deterioration of normal consciousness is often designated by terms such as "confusion" or "delirium," "stupor," and "coma." These labels are imprecise and have been defined inconsistently from study to study, and even occasionally within a given study. Attempts have been made to codify criteria for coma, vegetative state, minimally conscious state, delirium, etc. These attempts, while laudable, have not yet led to universal adoption of standard terminology. For practical purposes of the ICU physician, it is therefore advisable to use descriptive terminology and validated scales, such as the Glasgow Coma Scale (GCS).

Anatomy and Pathophysiology of Altered Mental Status

The anatomic basis of consciousness is poorly understood. At a minimum, arousal is dependent on integrity of the ascending reticular activating system, a diffuse network of neurons which originate in the pons and midbrain and project to the diencephalon (thalamus and hypothalamus) and cortex. The cerebral cortex and its subcortical connections are also necessary for normal consciousness. Disturbed consciousness is therefore produced by dysfunction of the upper brainstem/diencephalon, or by global dysfunction of the cerebral hemispheres. A unilateral hemispheric lesion does not produce coma unless either it is large enough to produce significant mass-effect on the contralateral hemisphere, or there is a preexisting contralateral lesion.

Etiologies of Coma

Causes of altered mental status and coma are protean, and are divided into primary brain disorders and systemic derangements that secondarily impact brain function. Primary brain disorders may be structural abnormalities – e.g., brain infarction, hemorrhage, hydrocephalus, contusion, herniation – or they may be nonstructural disturbances, such as seizures. Systemic disturbances that cause encephalopathy include metabolic derangements, exposure to toxins, and systemic infections.

The most common causes of coma are traumatic brain injury (TBI), hypoxic-ischemic encephalopathy (HIE), drug overdose, ischemic and hemorrhagic strokes, central nervous system infections, and brain herniation from space-occupying lesions. ❯ *Table 18-1* lists causes of altered mental status. A detailed discussion of these conditions is beyond the scope of this chapter; however, a few warrant special mention because rapid diagnosis and urgent treatment are essential in order to limit permanent brain injury. These include seizures, brain infections, acute hydrocephalus, herniation, ischemic and hemorrhagic strokes, subarachnoid hemorrhage, cerebral venous sinus thrombosis, hypertensive encephalopathy, and TBI.

◘ Table 18-1

A partial list of the etiologies of coma and altered mental status (Adapted from Stevens and Bhardwaj, 2006)

I. Primary brain disorders
  (a) Structural lesions
    (i) Traumatic brain injury
      1. Diffuse axonal injury
      2. Contusions
      3. Subdural hematomas
      4. Epidural hematomas
    (ii) Cerebrovascular disorders
      1. Ischemic strokes
      2. Spontaneous intracerebral hemorrhage
      3. Subarachnoid hemorrhage
      4. Hypoxic-ischemic encephalopathy
      5. Cerebral venous sinus thrombosis
    (iii) Malignant disease
      1. Brain tumors
    (iv) Infectious diseases
      1. Brain abscesses
    (v) Demyelinating disease
      1. Acute disseminated encephalomyelitis
      2. Central pontine myelinolysis
    (vi) Hydrocephalus
  (b) Nonstructural disorders
    (i) Infectious diseases
      1. Bacterial meningoencephalitis
      2. Carcinomatous or lymphomatous meningitis
      3. Viral encephalitis
    (ii) Generalized seizures, status epilepticus
    (iii) Basilar migraines
II. Systemic disorders
  (a) Toxic encephalopathies
    (i) Medication overdose
      1. Opioids, benzodiazepines, barbiturates, tricyclics, etc.
    (ii) Illicit drug exposure
      1. Opioids, alcohols, amphetamines, etc.
    (iii) Environmental toxin exposure
      1. Carbon monoxide
      2. Heavy metals
      3. Pesticides
  (b) Metabolic encephalopathies
    (i) Hypoglycemia, hyperglycemia
    (ii) Hyponatremia, hypernatremia
    (iii) Hypercalcemia
    (iv) Hepatic encephalopathy
    (v) Uremia
    (vi) Vitamin deficiencies (thiamine, niacin)
    (vii) Hypothermia, severe hyperthermia
    (viii) Hypothyroidism, hyperthyroidism
    (ix) Urea cycle disorders
  (c) Infections
    (i) Urinary tract infections
    (ii) Pneumonia
    (iii) Sepsis

Differential Diagnosis (Mimics) of Coma and the Vegetative State

Patients may become unresponsive from conditions that mimic coma or a vegetative state. In the *locked-in syndrome*, destruction of the ventral pons leaves the patient quadriplegic and mute. Patients are often aware of their surroundings and may communicate only through vertical eye movements and blinking, which are spared. With more rostral pontine lesions, vertical eye movements and blinking are lost. In this state, akin to receiving a neuromuscular blocking agent without a sedative, the patient has no means of communication. Severe *Guillain-Barre syndrome, botulism,* and *critical illness neuropathy* may similarly result in complete de-efferentation. *Catatonia* is a manifestation of severe psychiatric illness in which patients open their eyes, do not speak or follow commands, and may exhibit waxy flexibility. The remainder of the neurological exam and the electroencephalogram (EEG) are normal. *Akinetic mutism*, due to bilateral medial frontal lobe injury, is a profound form of abulia (lack of motivation), in which patients are unable to speak or to move but open their eyes and may track visual stimuli.

Clinical Approach to the Comatose Patient

Overview

Evaluation and management of the comatose patient requires an emergent and structured approach (❂ *Fig. 18-1*). As with all medical emergencies, attention is first directed toward patient resuscitation and stabilization. Respiratory and hemodynamic parameters are rapidly assessed and normalized. A history is obtained and a focused neurological examination is performed. Laboratory tests are sent to evaluate for infection and for severe metabolic and toxic derangements. Supplemental oxygen, thiamine, intravenous (IV) glucose, and naloxone are empirically administered. If a benzodiazepine overdose is suspected, then flumazenil may be administered. If meningitis or encephalitis is suspected, then antibiotics are immediately administered. Noncontrast cranial computed tomography (CT) is obtained to further confirm or exclude a structural lesion, and to look for signs of increased intracranial pressure (ICP). Based on the imaging findings, a more thorough history is obtained and a more detailed clinical examination is performed. Further tests such as magnetic resonance imaging (MRI), electroencephalography, lumbar puncture (LP), and angiographic imaging are performed as indicated.

Initial Resuscitation

Airway

Comatose patients are at increased risk of aspiration due to loss of airway-protective mechanisms such as cough and gag reflexes, and diminished airway tone. Prompt endotracheal intubation is therefore advisable. If there is a known or suspected history of neck trauma, then the cervical spine must be stabilized prior to intubation.

Breathing

Hypercapnic and hypoxemic respiratory failure frequently accompany coma and should be treated with prompt mechanical ventilation. Injuries to the brain stem and spinal cord may cause abnormal

□ Figure 18-1
Algorithm for initial approach to the comatose patient (Adapted from Stevens and Bhardwaj, 2006)

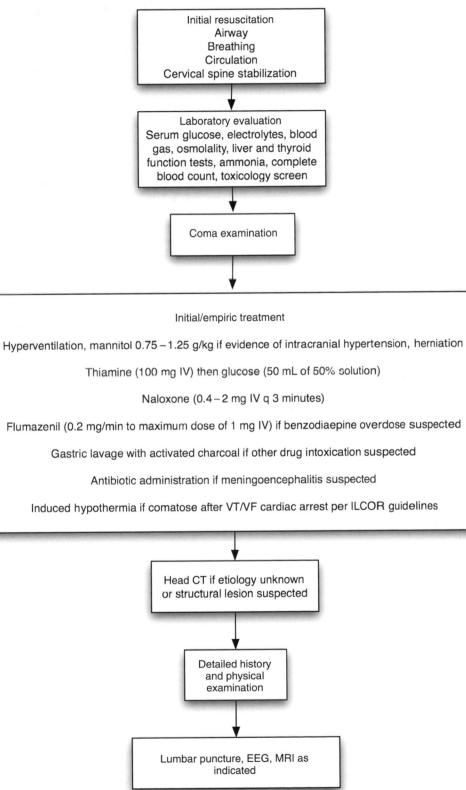

respiratory patterns or complete loss of respiratory drive. Aspiration of gastric contents and prolonged ventilatory failure are common causes of hypoxemia. On occasion, hypoxemia results from neurogenic pulmonary edema.

Circulation

Cardiac arrhythmias may be seen when coma occurs from global ischemia in the setting of myocardial infarction, or pulmonary or fat embolism. Rarely, arrhythmias may result from primary neurological injury. Arrhythmias should be treated according to standard advanced cardiac life support (ACLS) protocols.

Severe hypertension frequently accompanies coma. When coma is accompanied by reduced cerebral blood flow, as occurs with increased ICP or basilar artery thrombosis, hypertension is a compensatory response aimed at restoration of cerebral perfusion pressure. In this situation, aggressive lowering of blood pressure may precipitate cerebral infarction. If, however, coma is the result of severe hypertension, as in hypertensive encephalopathy, then blood pressure must be lowered emergently. It is difficult to distinguish on clinical grounds whether hypertension is the cause or an effect of the underlying problem. In either case, blood pressure should only be lowered if there is clear evidence of end-organ damage (heart failure, kidney failure, hypertensive encephalopathy). IV agents such as labetolol or nicardipine should be titrated to lower the mean arterial pressure by no more than 20%. Nitroprusside may increase ICP and should be used with caution. It is imperative to monitor neurological function for signs of ischemia while blood pressure is being lowered.

Hypotension in the setting of coma is usually due to systemic causes, such as cardiac dysfunction, sepsis, or hemorrhage. Blood pressure should be restored to baseline with isotonic IV fluids and, if necessary, pressors. Hypertonic fluids may be used for volume resuscitation in patients with hypovolemic shock and TBI. Hypotonic fluids may exacerbate brain edema by lowering serum osmolarity and should not be administered. The cause of the hypotension should be sought and rapidly corrected.

History

In many cases, for example, after trauma or cardiac arrest, the cause of the coma is evident. In other cases, clues must be sought from the history. Family members and witnesses must be interviewed about the time course of the illness, preexisting medical conditions, medication history, suicidal behavior, and illicit drug use.

Neurological Assessment

By allowing the examiner to localize the lesion, the initial neurological examination helps to narrow the list of etiological possibilities. For example, integrity of brainstem function and absence of focal signs suggests a toxic or metabolic disorder. In contrast, asymmetric findings and brainstem dysfunction are more consistent with a structural etiology. The exam is also used to exclude conditions which mimic coma. Serial examinations of the comatose patient over time are essential and provide information about efficacy of treatment, worsening of the primary process, and prognosis.

The coma examination is focused on four elements: (1) determination of the patient's level of arousal (wakefulness), (2) examination of the eyes, (3) elicitation of motor responses and abnormal reflexes, and (4) observation of breathing patterns.

1. *Level of Consciousness*

   First, the patient should be observed. Patients who exhibit spontaneous eyes opening, verbalization attempts, moaning, tossing, reaching, leg crossing, yawning, coughing, or swallowing have a higher level of consciousness than those who do not. The examiner should next assess the patient's response to a series of stimuli which escalate in intensity. The patient's name should be called loudly. If there is no response, the examiner should stimulate the patient by gently shaking him. If this produces no response, the examiner must use a noxious stimulus, such as pressure to the supraorbital ridge, nail beds, or sternum, or nasal tickle with a cotton wisp. Responses such as grimacing, eye opening, grunting, or verbalization should be documented. Motor responses provide information not only about sensation and limb strength, but also about level of consciousness. The examiner should note whether stimuli produce "purposeful" or non-stereotyped limb movements – such as reaching toward the site of stimulation ("localization"). This implies a degree of intact cortical function. Stereotyped limb movements are generally mediated by brain and spinal reflexes and do not require cortical input. Examples include extension and internal rotation of the limbs (decerebrate posturing), upper extremity flexion (decorticate posturing), and flexion at the ankle, knee, and hip ("triple-flexion").

2. *Eye Examination*

   In coma, the neuro-ophthalmological examination focuses on (a) the pupils, (b) resting eye position and eye movements, (c) appearance of the retina, and (d) the corneal reflex.

   (a) *Pupillary examination*: Pupillary size, shape, and reactivity to light should be assessed. In general, abnormalities of the pupillary light reflex suggest a structural abnormality. However, certain drugs may also affect the pupillary light reflex. Metabolic causes of coma typically do not affect the pupils. The pupils are normally round, have equal diameters, and briskly constrict when illuminated. When unequal pupils (anisocoria) are observed, it is important to establish whether it is the larger or the smaller pupil that is abnormal. This is accomplished by examining the eyes both in the light and in the dark. When the lights are extinguished, an abnormally small pupil will fail to dilate fully and the degree of anisocoria will increase. In contrast, when the abnormal pupil is the larger one, the degree of anisocoria will be maximal under full illumination when the larger pupil fails to constrict fully. In the ICU, the most important causes of a unilaterally dilated pupil are compressive lesions of the oculomotor nerve complex, such as uncal herniation and intracranial aneurysms. A complete third nerve palsy results in ipsilateral mydriasis, inferolateral deviation of the eye, and a severe ipsilateral ptosis. The most important cause of unilateral small pupil is the Horner's syndrome, which consists of miosis and mild ipsilateral ptosis. Depending on the location of the lesion, ipsilateral facial anhidrosis may also be present. Bilaterally fixed and dilated pupils are seen in the terminal stages of brain death but also with anticholinergic medications, such as atropine. Hyperadrenergic states (e.g., pain, anxiety, cocaine intoxication) produce bilaterally large and reactive pupils. Reactive pinpoint (<1 mm) pupils are observed with opiate and barbiturate intoxication, and after extensive pontine injury.

(b) *Resting eye position and eye movements*: Eye position and spontaneous movements should be noted. Horizontal or vertical misalignment of the eyes as well as spontaneous roving or rhythmic and repetitive vertical movements should be documented. The frontal lobe cortex (frontal eye fields) mediates conjugate deviation of the eyes toward the contralateral side. Lateral deviation of both eyes therefore indicates a destructive lesion in the ipsilateral frontal lobe or an excitatory focus (seizure) in the contralateral hemisphere. A destructive unilateral pontine lesion, and rarely, a thalamic lesion, will cause conjugate deviation to the contralateral side. Downward deviation of the eyes is caused by dysfunction of the dorsal midbrain and is seen with hydrocephalus, tumors, and strokes. Dysconjugate gaze is frequently seen in sedated patients and usually represents unmasking of a latent esophoria or exophoria. Roving, or slow to-and-fro eye movements, implies functional integrity of the brainstem. Ocular bobbing – fast conjugate downward gaze followed by a slow upward correction to midposition – implies extensive pontine injury. Ocular dipping – slow conjugate down gaze followed by fast upward gaze – also localizes to the pons. With a skew deviation, one eye is higher than the other, and the lesion is usually in the midbrain on the side of the higher eye, or in the pontomedullary junction on side of the lower eye. In the critically ill comatose patients, there is a high incidence of nonconvulsive seizures and jerking movements of the eyes may be the only evidence of seizure activity.

If spontaneous eye movements are absent, then an oculocephalic response ("doll's eyes") should be sought by turning the head horizontally and vertically. This maneuver should not be performed on trauma patients with known or suspected cervical spine instability. Normally the eyes move opposite to the direction of head turning. Testing the oculocephalic response may uncover a vertical gaze paresis, a skew deviation, or a sixth nerve palsy that was not otherwise obvious.

If an oculocephalic response cannot be elicited, then an oculovestibular ("cold-caloric") response is sought. First, the tympanic membrane should be visualized to ensure that it is intact and unobstructed. The head of the bed should be set at 30° to align the patient's horizontal semicircular canals perpendicular to the floor. Then, using an angiocatheter or a butterfly catheter without the needle, 30–60 ml of ice-cold water is instilled into the external auditory canal against the tympanic membrane. This inhibits the ipsilateral vestibular system and normally causes the eyes first to move slowly toward the ipsilateral ear and then to jerk quickly toward the contralateral ear. The initial slow response is mediated by the unopposed contralateral vestibular system in the brainstem, and the subsequent corrective nystagmus is mediated by the frontal eye fields. With bilateral cortical dysfunction and an intact brainstem, slow tonic deviation of the eyes toward the ipsilateral ear is observed and is not followed by contralateral nystagmus. In early metabolic coma, the oculocephalic and oculovestibular responses are preserved. Absent responses indicate diffuse brainstem dysfunction and are seen in primary brainstem injury, late transtentorial herniation, barbiturate intoxication, and brain death.

(c) *Retinal examination*: A fundoscopic examination should be performed to look for signs of intracranial hypertension. Papilledema is swelling of the optic nerve head from elevated ICP. It is almost always bilateral and may be accompanied by retinal hemorrhages, exudates, cotton wool spots, and ultimately by enlargement of the optic cup. Papilledema develops over hours to days. Its absence, therefore, does not imply normal ICP, especially in the acute setting. Pulsatility of the retinal veins strongly suggests normal ICP. Terson's syndrome is vitreous, subhyaloid, or retinal hemorrhage associated with subarachnoid hemorrhage.

(d) *The corneal reflex:* The corneal reflex is tested by gently touching the cornea of each eye with a drop of saline or a cotton wisp and observing for eyelid closure. Failure of unilateral eyelid closure suggests facial nerve dysfunction on that side. Failure of bilateral eyelid closure with stimulation of one cornea, but not the other, implies trigeminal nerve dysfunction on the stimulated side. Failure of bilateral eyelid closure upon stimulation of either cornea usually implies pontine dysfunction.

Motor Responses and Abnormal Reflexes

The symmetry of motor responses and reflexes, and the presence of abnormal movements often allow discrimination between structural and systemic etiologies of altered mental status. First, the patient should be observed for any abnormal or spontaneous movements. Asterixis implies a metabolic disturbance such as uremia or hepatic encephalopathy. Twitching or jerking of the face or limbs, even if subtle, raises the suspicion for seizures. Asymmetry of resting-limb position is frequently a subtle sign of weakness. For example, a paretic leg will lie externally rotated. Next, the patient is stimulated and the examiner must search for asymmetry in the patient's face (grimace) and appendicular motor responses. A less vigorous response on one side of the body indicates a contralateral structural lesion involving the motor pathways above the level of the caudal medulla. Paraparesis and quadriparesis raise the possibility of spinal cord injury, especially in the setting of trauma.

Breathing Patterns

A variety of breathing patterns may be observed in coma. Although these may yield clues regarding the location of the intracranial lesion, in clinical practice, breathing patterns are often obscured by the use of sedatives, paralytics, and mechanical ventilation. *Apneustic* respirations are characterized by a prolonged end-inspiratory pause. This pattern may be seen after focal injury to the dorsal lower half of the pons (e.g., stroke), but may also be observed with meningitis, hypoxia, and hypoglycemia. *Cluster breathing* consists of several rapid, shallow breaths followed by a prolonged pause, and localizes to the upper medulla. *Ataxic respirations*, or *Biot's breathing*, is a chaotic pattern in which the length and depth of the inspiratory and expiratory phases are irregular. It may occur after injury to the respiratory centers in the lower medulla. Apnea may be seen in a variety of neurological and non-neurological disorders and is of no localizing value. *Kussmaul respirations* are rapid, deep breaths that usually signal metabolic acidosis, but also may be observed with pontomesencephalic lesions. *Cheyne-Stokes respiration* refers to alternating spells of apnea and crescendo–decrescendo hyperpnea. It has minimal value in localization and is seen with diffuse cerebral injury, hypoxia, hypocapnea, and congestive heart failure. *Agonal gasps* reflect bilateral lower medullary injury and are seen in the terminal stages of brain injury.

◘ Table 18-2

Glasgow Coma Scale (Adapted from Teasdale and Jennett, 1974. Copyright 1974, with permission from Elsevier)

Motor response	
Follows commands	6
Localizes pain	5
Withdraws to pain	4
Flexion	3
Extension	2
None	1
Verbal response	
Oriented	5
Confused speech	4
Inappropriate words	3
Incomprehensible	2
None	1
Eye opening	
Spontaneous	4
To command	3
To pain	2
None	1

The Glasgow Coma Scale

The GCS (❷ *Table 18-2*) is a useful tool for the initial neurological survey. It was initially intended for use in TBI; however, it is now a widely accepted tool for evaluation of consciousness in the general critically ill population. It may be performed quickly and reliably at the bedside. GCS score predicts survival and neurological outcome in TBI, nontraumatic coma, ischemic stroke, intracerebral hemorrhage, subarachnoid hemorrhage, and meningitis. It also predicts mortality in the general critical-care patient. The GCS has limitations. It is a relatively crude instrument that is insensitive to subtle variations in mental status. A given score in the mid-range (6–12) may be assigned to patients with significantly different degrees of impaired consciousness through different combinations of scores in each of the three categories. The GCS has limited utility in patients with aphasia, significant facial trauma, or in those who are sedated or intubated. Despite its limitations, the GCS is a mainstay of clinical assessment that aids in communication, prognostication, and research. The Full Outline of UnResponsiveness (FOUR) score is a new coma scale that incorporates brainstem reflexes and breathing patterns (❷ *Fig. 18-2*). It is simple, recognizes brain death, uncal herniation, and the locked-in state, and has comparable inter-rater reliability to the GCS. Whether this scale gains widespread acceptance remains to be seen.

Laboratory Investigations

Metabolic and toxic encephalopathies account for a significant proportion of altered mental status. Commonly encountered metabolic disturbances include severe hypernatremia and hyponatremia, hypercalcemia, elevated blood urea nitrogen, hyperammonemia, hypoglycemia and hyperglycemia, hypercarbia, hypoxemia, and severe hyperthyroidism and hypothyroidism. A toxicology screen detects exposure to common drugs and toxins. Plasma osmolality should be measured so that the plasma osmolal gap may be determined. The osmolal gap is the difference between the calculated osmolarity ($2[Na] + [BUN]/2.8 + [glucose]/18$) and the measured osmolality. The osmolal gap is elevated with intoxication from alcohols, such as methanol, and ethylene glycol. A complete blood count should be obtained to help assess for an infectious cause of encephalopathy.

Initial Therapy

Initial therapy of the comatose patient is often empiric. If signs or symptoms of increased ICP or herniation are detected, mannitol is administered as a 1 gm/kg IV bolus. Hyperventilation causes cerebral vasoconstriction, which reduces cerebral blood volume and hence lowers ICP. While extremely effective, the effect on ICP is short-lived and hyperventilation may cause cerebral ischemia. Hyperventilation should therefore only be used emergently for a short period of time as a bridge to more definitive (usually surgical) therapy. Rarely, thiamine deficiency may cause profound alterations in consciousness and all patients should receive IV thiamine. Glucose is administered if serum glucose is less than 60 mg/dl or cannot immediately be measured. In patients with very low thiamine stores, glucose administration may theoretically precipitate acute thiamine deficiency.

◻ Figure 18-2

The FOUR score. Instructions for the assessment of the individual categories of the FOUR (Full Outline of UnResponsiveness) score. (a) For eye response (e), grade the best possible response after at least three trials in an attempt to elicit the best level of alertness. A score of E4 indicates at least three voluntary excursions. If eyelids are closed, the examiner should open them and examine tracking of a finger or object. Tracking with the opening of one eyelid will suffice in cases of eyelid edema or facial trauma. If tracking is absent horizontally, examine vertical tracking. Alternatively, two blinks on command should be documented. This will recognize a locked-in syndrome (patient is fully aware). A score of E3 indicates the absence of voluntary tracking with open eyes. A score of E2 indicates eyelids opening to a loud voice. A score of E1 indicates eyelids open to pain stimulus. A score of E0 indicates no eyelid opening to pain. (b) For motor response (M), grade the best possible response of the arms. A score of M4 indicates that the patient demonstrated at least one of three hand positions (thumbs-up, fist, or peace sign) with either hand. A score of M3 (localization) indicates that the patient touched the examiner's hand after a painful stimulus compressing the temporomandibular joint or supraorbital nerve. A score of M2 indicates any flexion movement of the upper limbs. A score of M1 indicates extensor response to pain. A score of M0 indicates no motor response to pain, or myoclonus status epilepticus. (c) For brainstem reflexes (b), grade the best possible response. Examine pupillary and corneal reflexes. Preferably, corneal reflexes are tested by instilling two to three drops sterile saline on the cornea from a distance of 4–6 in. (this minimizes corneal trauma from repeated examinations). Sterile cotton swabs can also be used. The cough reflex to tracheal suctioning is tested only when both of these reflexes are absent. A score of B4 indicates pupil and corneal reflexes are present. A score of B3 indicates one pupil wide and fixed. A score of B2 indicates either pupil or cornea reflexes are absent. A score of B1 indicates both pupil and cornea reflexes are absent. A score of B0 indicates pupil, cornea, and cough reflex (using tracheal suctioning) are absent. (d) For respiration (R), determine spontaneous breathing pattern in a nonintubated patient and grade simply as regular (R_4), or irregular (R_2), Cheyne-Stokes (R_3) breathing. In mechanically ventilated patients, assess the pressure waveform of spontaneous respiratory pattern or the patient triggering of the ventilator (R_1). The ventilator monitor displaying respiratory patterns can be used to identify the patient-generated breaths on the ventilator. No adjustments are made to the ventilator while the patient is graded, but grading is done preferably with $PaCO_2$ within normal limits. A standard apnea (oxygen-diffusion) test may be needed when patient breathes at ventilator rate (R_0) (Reprinted from Wijdicks et al., 2005. With permission)

◘ Figure 18-2 (Continued)

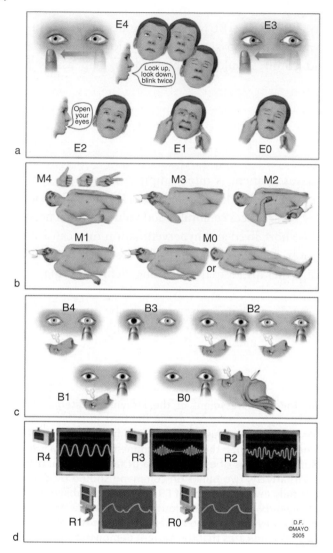

Therefore, glucose should be administered after thiamine. Naloxone is empirically given to reverse opiate intoxication. Routine empiric administration of flumazenil is controversial and should be given only when the history suggests a benzodiazepine overdose. If another toxic ingestion is suspected, then gastric lavage with activated charcoal is appropriate. Bacterial meningitis and herpes simplex encephalitis are associated with high mortality rates if not treated expeditiously. When brain infection is suspected, treatment with antibiotics should occur right away. If a head CT and LP cannot be performed immediately, then antibiotic administration should precede these diagnostic tests. Convincing evidence suggests that patients who are comatose after resuscitation from out-of-hospital cardiac arrest due to ventricular fibrillation (VF) should be cooled to 32–34°C for 12–24 h. It is reasonable to generalize this strategy to patients with in-hospital cardiac arrest and to those with pulseless electrical activity.

Neuroimaging Studies

Noncontrast cranial CT is indicated in all new cases of unexplained coma and is the test of first choice. CT rapidly identifies intra- and extra-axial cerebral hemorrhages, brain herniation, cerebral edema, and hydrocephalus. MRI is indicated in patients whose coma remains unexplained after CT. MRI has a higher sensitivity than CT for acute ischemic stroke, intracerebral hemorrhage, inflammatory conditions, brain abscesses, brain tumors, cerebral edema, cerebral venous sinus thrombosis, and diffuse axonal injury. MRI is less widely available than CT, is more time-consuming, and requires non-ferromagnetic equipment, making it less feasible for many critically ill patients. The risks of transporting patients to the CT or MRI scanner, and the time it takes to complete the studies must be weighed against the benefit of the information they may yield.

Prognosis of the Comatose Patient

Coma, by definition, is self-limited. Survivors may recover to a persistent vegetative state, to complete neurological recovery, or to an intermediate state of neurological disability. The Glasgow Outcome Scale (GOS) is an established metric of recovery (❷ *Table 18-3*). Although it fails to capture the full breadth of possible neurological outcomes, it is widely used by clinical investigators for traumatic and nontraumatic coma.

Determining the prognosis of comatose patients poses a significant challenge. Studies that have addressed the prognosis of coma are plagued by numerous problems that limit their clinical applicability. First, coma has been defined inconsistently across studies. Second, virtually all studies involved patients in whom care was intentionally limited, leading to a "self-fulfilling prophecy" bias. Third, most studies were performed prior to major advances in intensive care, such as induced hypothermia and intensive insulin therapy, which have been shown to improve outcome in certain patient populations. Last, studies have not yet systematically addressed the impact of clinical confounders such as metabolic disturbances, sedative and paralytic medications, and shock.

Prognosis of coma is based on etiology, clinical signs, and ancillary tests including electrophysiological, neuroimaging, and biochemical studies. As a general rule, coma due to closed head injury has a

❑ Table 18-3

The Glasgow Outcome Scale (Adapted from Jennett and Bond, 1975. Copyright 1975, with permission from Elsevier)

1	Death	
2	Persistent vegetative state	Patient exhibits no obvious cortical function
3	Severe disability	(Conscious but disabled) Patient depends on others for daily support due to mental or physical disability or both
4	Moderate disability	(Disabled but independent). Patient is independent as far as daily life is concerned; the disabilities found include varying degrees of dysphagia, hemiparesis, or ataxia, as well as intellectual and memory deficits and personality changes
5	Good recovery	Resumption of normal activities even though there may be minor neurological or psychological deficits

better prognosis than nontraumatic coma. Coma due to penetrating head injury is associated with a poor prognosis. It is probably also true that in cases of nontraumatic coma, nonstructural etiologies are associated with a better prognosis than structural etiologies.

For nontraumatic coma, the best evidence regarding the utility of clinical signs and ancillary tests for prognosis comes from studies of survivors of cardiac arrest. These data are summarized in a practice parameter that was recently issued by the Quality Standards Subcommittee of the American Academy of Neurology. Based on their findings, clinical signs that most accurately portend poor prognosis include myoclonic status epilepticus within the first 24 h after primary circulatory arrest, absence of pupillary responses within days 1–3 after cardiopulmonary resuscitation (CPR), absence of corneal reflexes within days 1–3 after CPR, and absence of extensor motor responses after day 3. Although certain electroencephalographic patterns, such as burst suppression and generalized epileptiform discharges are associated with poor prognosis, EEG lacks sufficient prognostic accuracy and is not recommended as a tool for predicting outcome. Somatosensory evoked potentials (SSEPs) are more useful for prognostication. SSEP is less susceptible than EEG to the confounding effects of drugs and metabolic derangement. Bilateral absence of the N20 component of the SSEP with median nerve stimulation after day 1 most accurately predicts poor prognosis. Numerous serum and cerebrospinal fluid (CSF) biomarkers have been studied for their prognostic value. To date, the only marker with sufficient prognostic accuracy to be recommended is neuron-specific enolase (NSE). Serum NSE levels of >33 µg/l on days 1–3 strongly predict poor outcome; however, this test is not yet widely available. Ongoing studies are addressing the prognostic role of cranial CT, MRI, and magnetic resonance spectroscopy.

Studies to determine prognosis of traumatic coma are inherently difficult. Closed head injury affects a heterogeneous patient population, encompasses a variety of structural brain lesions, and is often accompanied by systemic trauma and major systemic derangements. A handful of factors have been identified that are associated with poor prognosis. These include advanced age, a low initial GCS score, the presence of diffuse axonal injury on neuroimaging studies, and the presence of hypoxia or hypotension. Genetic markers may ultimately prove useful in determining prognosis. Recently, investigators determined that patients possessing the apoE4 allele have a worse outcome after TBI.

Brain Death

Brain death refers to irreversible cessation of whole-brain activity. The concept of brain death was established in the 1950s and diagnostic criteria were first published in 1968. The idea that brain death is legally equivalent to cardiac death has since gained widespread acceptance in the USA and in many Western countries and has greatly facilitated organ donation.

Brain death is a clinical diagnosis that rests on the demonstration of (1) deep coma, (2) absence of brainstem reflexes, and (3) apnea. In an attempt to standardize diagnostic criteria, the American Academy of Neurology published a practice parameter in 1995. However, variations in practice exist across institutions, and physicians who determine brain death must be familiar with the specific protocol used in their hospital.

Prior to the determination of brain death, the physician should establish an irreversible cause of brain failure based on clinical and/or neuroimaging evidence. Medical conditions which might confound the neurological exam – such as hypothermia, severe metabolic or endocrine derangements, hypotension, and drug intoxication – must be excluded or corrected. In general, two clinical examinations, separated by a period of hours, are performed, followed by an apnea test. Coma is demonstrated by the lack of cerebral motor responses to pain in all four extremities. Patients should not grimace to pain. The following brainstem reflexes must be absent: pupillary light reflex, oculocephalic reflex (tested only in patients without cervical spine trauma); oculovestibular reflex, corneal reflex; cough with deep tracheal suctioning; and gag. Prior to apnea testing, the partial pressures of arterial oxygen and carbon dioxide (pCO_2) should be normalized. The patient is disconnected from the ventilator for at least 8 min and observed for respiratory movements. pCO_2 is then measured and the patient is reconnected to the ventilator. Absence of respiratory movements and either a $pCO_2 > 60$ mmHg or a rise in $pCO_2 > 20$ mmHg above baseline constitutes a positive test (consistent with brain death). The apnea test should be terminated immediately if hemodynamic instability or hypoxemia occurs.

Ancillary tests to confirm brain death need not be performed on a routine basis and are used when conditions exist that interfere with the clinical assessment, such as severe facial trauma, preexisting pupillary abnormalities, and toxic levels of certain medications. These tests fall into two categories, electrophysiological tests – EEG and SSEP, and cerebral blood flow studies – including conventional angiography, transcranial Doppler ultrasonography, and technetium-99 m nuclear blood flow scans. Guidelines exist for the performance and interpretation of each type of study.

Conclusions

Altered mental status and coma occur commonly in the surgical ICU. Physicians should develop an efficient diagnostic approach that facilitates rapid treatment in order to minimize additional brain injury. The clinical exam, laboratory tests, and neuroimaging studies are powerful tools that help to determine whether a structural or systemic abnormality exists, thus narrowing the differential diagnosis. Currently there are few widely available means of reliably determining prognosis in comatose patients. Genetic and metabolic markers and advanced neuroimaging modalities may ultimately prove helpful.

Selected Readings

Bernard SA, Gray TW, Buist MD, et al. (2002) Treatment of comatose survivors of out-of-hospital cardiac arrest with induced hypothermia. New Engl J Med 346:557–563

Jennett B, Bond M (1975) Assessment of outcome after severe brain damage. Lancet 1:480–484

The Hypothermia After Cardiac Arrest (HACA) study group (2002) Mild therapeutic hypothermia to improve the neurologic outcome after cardiac arrest. New Engl J Med 346:549–556

Levy DE, Caronna JJ, Singer BH, et al. (1985) Predicting outcome from hypoxic-ischemic coma. JAMA 253:1420–1426

Nolan JP, Morley PT, Vanden Hoek TL, et al. (2003) Therapeutic hypothermia after cardiac arrest. An advisory statement by the Advanced Life Support Task Force of the International Liaison Committee on Ressuscitation. Circulation 108:118–121

Plum F, Posner JB (1980) The diagnosis of stupor and coma, 3rd edn. FA Davis, Philadelphia, PA

Report of the Quality Standards Subcommittee of the American Academy of Neurology (1995) Practice parameters for determining brain death in adults (Summary statement). Neurology 45(5):1012–1014

Stevens RD, Bhardwaj A (2006) Approach to the comatose patient. Crit Care Med 34(1):31–41

Teasdale G, Jennett B (1974) Assessment of coma and impaired consciousness. A practical scale. Lancet 2:81–84

Wijdicks EF, Bamlet WR, Maramattom BV, et al. (2005) Validation of a new coma scale: the FOUR score. Annals Neurol 58:585–593

Wijdicks EF, Hijdra A, Young GB, et al. (2006) Practice parameter: prediction of outcome in comatose survivors after cardiopulmonary resuscitation (an evidence-based review). Neurology 67:203–210

Wijdicks EF, Kokmen E, O'Brien PC (1998) Measurement of impaired consciousness in the neurological intensive care unit: a new test. J Neurol, Neurosurg Psychiatr 64:117–119

19 Management of Cardiac Arrhythmias

Rebecca C. Britt · L. D. Britt

Pearls and Pitfalls

- All arrhythmias are caused by abnormal automaticity, reentry, or a combination of both.
- Narrow complex tachyarrhythmia is defined by a heart rate greater than 100 beats/min with a QRS duration of 120 ms or less as demonstrated on EKG or monitor.
- Wide complex tachyarrhythmia is defined by a heart rate greater than 100 beats/min with a prolonged QRS complex of greater than 120 ms and originates from either a supraventricular or ventricular focus.
- For tachyarrhythmias in the hemodynamically unstable patient, direct current (DC) cardioversion is the treatment option of choice to restore sinus rhythm.
- In the hemodynamically stable patient with atrial fibrillation, treatment strategies include rate control, termination of the atrial fibrillation with maintenance of sinus rhythm, and antiembolic therapy.
- Patients with unstable ventricular tachycardia and ventricular fibrillation should be treated with defibrillation.
- Amiodarone 150 mg IV bolus is the treatment of choice for hemodynamically stable patients with monomorphic ventricular tachycardia.

Introduction

Cardiac arrhythmias are common in the general population and occur frequently in the early postoperative period. While the majority are not clinically significant, transient arrhythmias in the perioperative period are reported as frequently as 60% of the time. A study of 4,181 patients who were in sinus rhythm at the time of initial preoperative evaluation, found perioperative supraventricular arrhythmias in about 8% of patients. These perioperative arrhythmias were associated with a 33% increase in duration of stay.

Anatomy and Physiology

The sinoatrial (SA) node, which lies beneath the junction of the superior vena cava and the right atrial appendage, is supplied by the sinus node artery, which arises from the right or circumflex coronary artery. The atrioventricular (AV) node, which sits on the right atrial side of the AV septum, receives its blood supply from the posterior descending coronary artery. No specific conduction path has been identified from the SA to the AV node. The bundle of His begins at the AV node and usually descends on the left side of the ventricular septum and branches into the left and right bundles just below the aortic valve. The left bundle branch supplies the ventricular septum as well as the anteroseptal and posteromedial papillary muscles. The right bundle supplies the medial papillary muscle as well as the right ventricular wall.

The SA and AV nodes both exhibit automaticity and fire spontaneously. Normal heartbeats originate in the SA node and lead to depolarization through the right and left atria followed by atrial contraction. This impulse stimulates the AV node and the bundle of His, thereby transmitting depolarization waves to the right and left His-Purkinje fibers and thus depolarizes the ventricular wall, leading to ventricular contraction.

All arrhythmias are caused by either abnormal automaticity, reentry, or a combination of both. Abnormal automaticity occurs when pathologic conditions move the resting membrane potential towards threshold, allowing for hyperexcitable, "irritable" cardiac muscle. Normal cardiac muscle has a long refractory period such that few myocytes remain excitable at the end of a beat. Myocardial ischemia, fibrosis, and necrosis lead to slowing of myocardial conduction, such that surrounding fibers may be past the refractory period when the impulse leaves the damages area, which leads to abnormal impulse stimulation with formation of a reentrant circuit.

Etiology

Risk factors for development of supraventricular arrhythmias include age greater than 70 years, preoperative congestive heart failure, and performance of abdominal, thoracic, or major vascular operations. Perioperative ventricular arrhythmias are increased in patients with preoperative ventricular ectopy, congestive heart failure, and smoking. Hypoxia, hypercarbia, hypokalemia, acid-base disorders, acute volume depletion, and myocardial infarction also contribute to the development of arrhythmias.

Clinical Presentation

Continuous electrocardiographic monitoring in the perioperative period leads to the detection of many arrhythmias. Bradycardia, defined by a heart rate less than 60 beats/min, can be normal or abnormal. Tachyarrhythmias, defined by a heart rate greater than 100 beats/min, are divided further into narrow and wide QRS complex tachyarrhythmias. Patients will complain frequently of palpitations and a sense that their heart is racing in the setting of a tachyarrhythmia. Hemodynamic instability may be associated with these arrhythmia.

Narrow complex tachyarrhythmia is defined by a heart rate of greater than 100 beats/min with a QRS duration of 120 ms or less. The site of origin for narrow complex tachycardias is supraventricular with normal conduction through the bundle of His and Purkinje fibers. Examples include sinus tachycardia, supraventricular tachycardia, atrial fibrillation, and atrial flutter.

Wide complex tachyarrhythmia, defined by a heart rate of greater than 100 beats/min with a prolonged QRS complex greater than 120 ms, originates from either a supraventricular or ventricular focus. The accurate diagnosis of wide complex tachyarrhythmias is crucial, because immediate treatment is required frequently; delayed or inappropriate treatment can be dangerous. Examples of wide complex arrhythmias include ventricular tachycardia (VT), Torsades de Pointes, and ventricular fibrillation.

Diagnosis

The initial approach to a patient with arrhythmia is to determine whether the patient is experiencing signs and symptoms related to the rapid heart rate. Symptoms include hypotension, shock, shortness of breath, chest pain, and decreased level of consciousness. If the patient has clinically significant hemodynamic instability, an attempt at cardioversion should be made. Important history should include whether the patient has a history of cardiac arrhythmia as well as whether the patient has a history of structural heart disease, especially previous myocardial infarction. Also important is whether the patient is taking any medicines, and whether the patient has a pacemaker or internal cardiac defibrillator in place. Initial studies should include an electrocardiogram (ECG) and laboratory values, including serum potassium, magnesium, and cardiac enzymes.

Analysis of the 12 lead ECG is critical to determine the etiology of the arrhythmia. Assessment of the ECG includes evaluation of the regularity of the rhythm, the atrial rate, the P wave morphology, and the relationship between atrial and ventricular rates. Sinus tachycardia is characterized by a 1:1 relationship between atrial and ventricular rates with normal P waves and a heart rate between 100 and 180 beats/min. Atrial tachycardia is characterized by an atrial rate of 100–250 beats/min, but with abnormal P wave morphology and long PR intervals. Atrial flutter has an atrial rate usually of 300 beats/min and a ventricular rate one half to one third the atrial rate. Atrial flutter will present classically with a regular ventricular rate of 150 beats/min (2-to-1 block), but may vary between 3-to-1 and 4-to-1 block (regular heart rates of 100 and 75 beats/min). In contrast, atrial fibrillation (❯ *Fig. 19-1*) is characterized by a lack of organized atrial activity, with no clear P waves between QRS complexes, and a irregular ventricular response.

Wide complex tachycardia is most often ventricular tachycardia (VT) (❯ *Fig. 19-2*). The most common algorithm for the diagnosis of wide complex tachycardia is the Brugada criteria, which consists of four steps. The first step is to evaluate for absence of an RS complex in all precordial leads (V1–V6), which is diagnostic of VT with 100% specificity. If an RS complex is present, the RS interval is measured; if the interval is greater than 100 ms, then VT can be diagnosed with 98% specificity. The third step involves looking for evidence of AV dissociation of less than 100 ms in the RS interval, which has a high specificity but a low sensitivity. The final step involves consideration of the morphology of the QRS complex, which has a lower specificity and sensitivity. Torsades de pointes is a polymorphic VT with variability in both the amplitude and polarity, causing the complexes to appear as if they are twisting around the isoelectric line. A prerequisite for the development of Torsades is prolongation of the QT interval. The ECG in ventricular fibrillation (❯ *Fig. 19-3*) shows complexes that are grossly irregular without P waves or clear QRS morphology.

Treatment

Narrow Complex Arrhythmias

The underlying cause of the arrhythmia should be sought and reversed at the onset if possible. A hemodynamically unstable patient or a patient with acute angina with a narrow complex tachyarrhythmia should be treated expeditiously with DC cardioversion. In the clinically and hemodynamically stable patient, an attempt should be made to determine the rhythm. Sinus tachycardia is the most

◘ Figure 19-1
ECG demonstrating atrial fibrillation

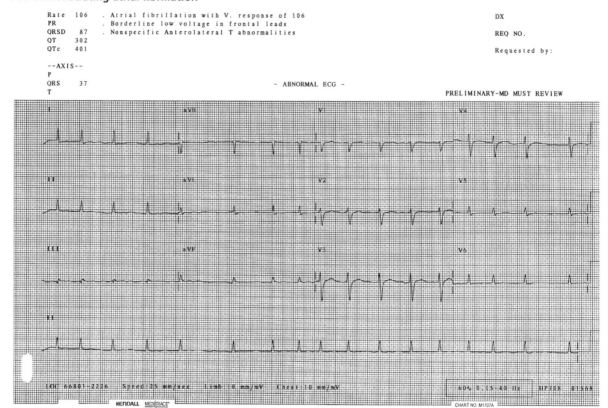

```
Rate   106    . Atrial fibrillation with V. response of 106          DX
PR            . Borderline low voltage in frontal leads
QRSD    87    . Nonspecific Anterolateral T abnormalities              REQ NO.
QT     302
QTc    401                                                            Requested by:

--AXIS--
P
QRS     37                          - ABNORMAL ECG -
T                                                            PRELIMINARY-MD MUST REVIEW
```

common tachycardia and is managed by treating the underlying disorder. Atrial flutter, an inherently unstable rhythm, will usually convert acutely to either normal sinus rhythm or to atrial fibrillation. In a stable patient with atrial flutter, control of the ventricular response rate can be achieved with calcium channel blocker, beta blockers, or digoxin. Narrow complex supraventricular tachycardia can be treated with vagal maneuvers, adenosine, or rate control with beta blockade or calcium channel blockers.

The management of atrial fibrillation (❯ *Fig. 19-4*) is based on the hemodynamic stability of the patient. If the patient is hemodynamically unstable, direct current (DC) cardioversion is the treatment option of choice to restore sinus rhythm. In the hemodynamically stable patient, acute treatment strategies include rate control, termination of the atrial fibrillation with maintenance of sinus rhythm, and antiembolic therapy, depending on whether there is a history of atrial fibrillation in the patient. If atrial fibrillation has been present for more than 48 h, appropriate anticoagulation should be started prior to medical or electrical cardioversion due to the risk of embolic disease from clot in the atrium. Early cardioversion may be considered after appropriate intravenous heparinization and transesophageal echocardiography to rule out atrial thrombus. After cardioversion, management should be followed by 4 weeks of anticoagulation. If clot is present, delayed cardioversion may be performed after several weeks of anticoagulation therapy, which again should be continued for a period of weeks after the cardioversion.

Spontaneous conversion rates are as high as 50–70% in the first 24 h after the onset of atrial fibrillation. Beta blockers and calcium channel blockers used to control the ventricular response rate in

■ Figure 19-2
ECG demonstrating ventricular tachycardia

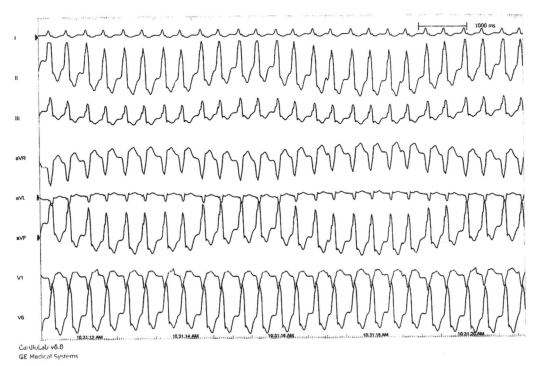

6/29/2006 10:31:11 AM(Speed: 25 mm/s)
87-96-31

CardioLab v6.0
GE Medical Systems

■ Figure 19-3
ECG demonstrating ventricular fibrillation

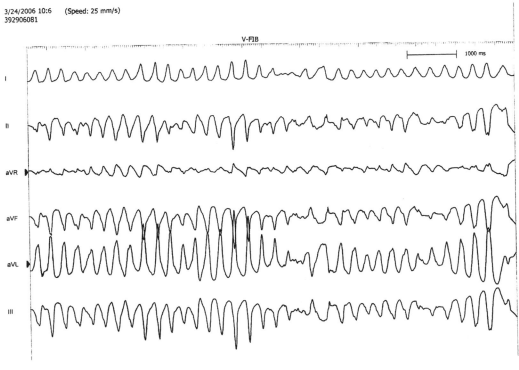

3/24/2006 10:6   (Speed: 25 mm/s)
392906081

V-FIB

◻ Figure 19-4
Algorithm for the management of atrial fibrillation

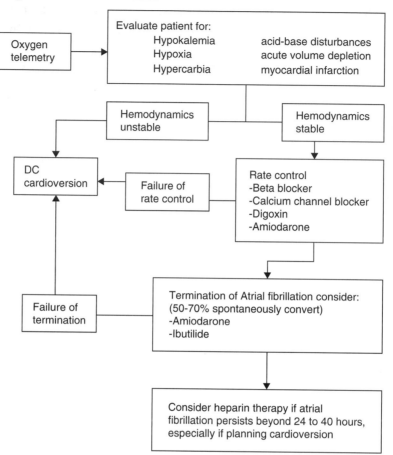

atrial fibrillation rarely will terminate the rhythm. Digoxin is used as an add-on to either calcium channel blockers or beta blockers to control the ventricular rate and is a good choice in the patient with decompensated heart failure because of the positive inotropic effect. Ibutilide is an antiarrhythmic agent that has efficacy in terminating recent onset atrial fibrillation and atrial flutter[3] and also increases the success rate for electrical conversion. Amiodarone is useful to prolong the AV refractoriness and slow the ventricular response, with a conversion rate of 60%, similar to placebo at 24 h. Because of its long half-life, oral amiodarone leads to effective prolongation of atrial refractoriness and is useful for medical cardioversion; 25% of patients with persistent atrial fibrillation convert to sinus rhythm within 4–6 weeks. Electrical DC cardioversion is another option for conversion to a sinus rhythm, with care taken to anticoagulate the patient appropriately who has been in atrial fibrillation for longer than 48 h to decrease the risk of emboli.

Wide Complex Arrhythmias

Asymptomatic, premature ventricular contractions are common and do not require treatment. No medical therapy is indicated for patients with asymptomatic, hemodynamically stable, non-sustained

VT. Underlying abnormalities, such as electrolyte disturbances, hypoxia, structural heart disease, and acute myocardial ischemia, should be ruled out in the setting of non-sustained VT. Patients with sustained VT or ventricular fibrillation should be treated according to ACLS protocols.

The treatment of stable, monomorphic VT depends on the ventricular function. For patients with preserved ventricular function, cardioversion, amiodarone (150 mg IV bolus over 10 min) or procainamide (17 mg/kg load using 20 mg/min followed by 1–4 mg/min IV drip) are acceptable options. For patients with low ejection fractions, amiodarone (150 mg IV bolus) is the treatment of choice. Lidocaine is now considered a secondary agent, because it has limited effect in non-ischemic tissue.

The management of stable, polymorphic VT depends on the duration of the QT interval. Cardioversion is recommended for polymorphic VT with a normal QT interval, because this rhythm is associated often with instability. Electrolyte abnormalities should be corrected, and evidence of ischemia should be sought and treated. Medical therapy for polymorphic VT with normal QT interval includes amiodarone, procainamide, and lidocaine as a secondary agent. Treatment for polymorphic VT with a prolonged QT interval (Torsades) includes IV magnesium and correction of all electrolyte abnormalities. Temporary pacing or IV isoproterenol increases the underlying heart rate and shortens the QT interval, which halts the torsades.

Unstable patients with wide complex tachycardia of any type should be cardioverted. Patients with unstable VT and ventricular fibrillation (VF) are treated with acute cardioversion. If a defibrillator is not immediately available, a precordial thump can be performed immediately after demonstrating pulselessness. Shock is administered first as 200 J, followed by 300 J, then 360 J. If the patient has persistent VT/VF, either epinephrine (1 mg IV) or vasopressin (40 units IV) are given. Amiodarone (300 mg IV) should be given if the patient fails to cardiovert after three rounds of defibrillation.

Selected Readings

Brugada P, Brugada J, Mont L, et al. (1991) A new approach to the differential diagnosis of a regular tachycardia with a wide QRS complex. Circulation 83:1649–1659

Cummins RO (2004) ACLS provider manual, 3rd edn. American Heart Association, Dallas, TX

Naccerelli G, Wolbrette D, Khan M, et al. (2003) Old and new antiarrhythmic drugs for converting and maintaining sinus rhythm in atrial fibrillation: comparative efficacy and results of trials. Am J Cardiol 91:15D–26D

Polanczyc C, Goldman L, Marcantonio E, et al. (1998) Supraventricular arrhythmia in patients having non-cardiac surgery. Ann Int Med 129:279–285

Tielman R, Gosselink A, Crijns H, et al. (1997) Efficacy, safety, and determinants of conversion of atrial fibrillation and flutter with oral amiodarone. Am J Cardiol 79:1054–1059

20 Do Not Resuscitate, Do Not Treat

Laurence B. McCullough · James W. Jones

Pearls and Pitfalls

- Ethics represents an essential component of the modern practice of surgery.
- The tools of ethics include the analysis of concepts and the use of concepts to establish measures regarding surgical management and diagnosis.
- "Do-not-Resuscitate" orders should be negotiated with patients, or the surrogates of patients who cannot participate in decision-making of the informed consent process.
- The living will or directive to physicians is an advance directive that patients use to instruct physicians about the administration of life-sustaining treatment when the patient becomes terminally ill and has lost decision-making capacity.
- A directive to physicians serves as the basis for DNR orders for terminally ill patients who cannot participate in decision making, because such an advance directive provides documentation of the patient's decision about the administration of life-sustaining treatment.
- A Durable Power of Attorney for Health Care or Medical Power of Attorney is a written advance directive by which a patient appoints someone to act as the patient's surrogate decision maker when the patient has lost decision-making capacity.
- It is ethically justified for DNR orders to be suspended in the OR for patients with terminal conditions and may be re-instated when clinical judgment supports the view that life-threatening events will be owed to the patient's underlying terminal condition rather than anesthesia, surgery, and their side-effects.
- A DNR order does not imply that the patient should not be treated. Appropriate pain management, maintenance of dignity, and assuring the comfort of patients who will be allowed to die is ethically required.

Introduction

Ethics is an essential component of the modern practice of surgery. Ethics uses two tools, analysis of concepts and arguments that use these concepts to reach reasoned conclusions, to guide surgeons in making judgments about beliefs and behaviors. Surgeons are familiar with the clinical utility of ethics, inasmuch as it shapes the informed consent process between surgeons and patients about the surgical management of patients' diseases and injuries. It is worth noting that surgeons pioneered the practice of informed consent, starting with simple consent for surgery in seventeenth-century England leading to a sophisticated form of informed consent already in the nineteenth-century United States, well before the development of the doctrine of informed consent in the common and statutory law in the United States and other countries during the twentieth century. DNR orders are based on informed consent. They formalize agreement between physician and patient/surrogates assuring that resuscitation will be limited at critical junctures in a patient's illness.

History Of Ethical Debate About DNR In The OR

Challenging ethical issues arise in the clinical management of patients with serious illness, i.e., diagnoses with a high probability of death even with aggressive clinical intervention. Especially challenging is the place of do-not-resuscitate (DNR) orders in the operating room for patients with advance directives. Advance directives are legal instruments through which a patient makes decisions about life-sustaining treatment that are to be respected and implemented when the patient is, in the attending physician's clinical judgment, no longer able to make decisions for himself or herself. The living will or directive to physicians is used to instruct physicians about the administration or withholding of life-sustaining treatment when the patient has lost decision-making capacity and has a terminal condition (as defined in applicable statutory law). The durable power of attorney for health care or the medical power of attorney is used to appoint someone of the patient's choice, known as an agent or proxy, to make decisions for the patient when the patient is no longer able to do so. Either through a directive to physicians or through a medical power of attorney, a surgeon may be validly instructed in advance by a patient with a terminal condition that he or she does not want life-sustaining treatment administered, including resuscitation. Nevertheless, it is sometimes the case that a terminally ill patient can benefit clinically from surgical management of his or her condition or problem.

When this issue first surfaced about 15 years ago, some argued that DNR orders should be applicable in the operating room as they are anywhere else in the hospital. The argument in support of this position appeals to the ethical principle of respect for autonomy. This principle was understood to mean that the informed preferences of patients regarding end of life care should guide physicians' clinical judgment, decision making, and behavior in all clinical settings. Otherwise, advance directives would have little force or meaning if surgeons could simply override directives at the surgeon's discretion.

Others argued that DNR orders should be suspended in all cases when a patient was taken to surgery. Anesthesiologists and surgeons quite reasonably took the view that intraoperative arrest of a seriously or terminally ill patients should be regarded as a correctable side-effect of anesthesia and not a function of the patient's underlying disease or injury. Moreover, intraoperative resuscitation maintains homeostasis and patients usually recover, in sharp contrast to the overall all low success rate of resuscitation elsewhere in the hospital. It seems inconsistent with professional integrity of surgical clinical judgment and practice to withhold intervention that is effective in achieving the goals of surgery. Seriously or terminally ill patients who consent to surgery can reasonable be presumed to want its functional improvements and palliative effects, but they will not experience these outcomes if an intervention that is usually effective in helping to achieve them is withheld. In short, a strong case can be made on both clinical grounds and on the basis of a reasonable assumption about patients' preferences that DNR orders should be suspended during surgery for seriously ill or terminally ill patients.

Critical Assessment Of Positions On DNR In The OR

When these two positions and the arguments in support of them are subjected to close scrutiny, a major problem with the autonomy-based approach, i.e., routinely implementing DNR orders in the OR, suffers from a serious misconception of the role of the patient's autonomy in the ethics of informed consent and, by extension, advance directives. The first step of the informed consent process is for the surgeon to identify the medically reasonable alternatives for managing the patient's condition or problem, i.e., those that are reliably expected to result in a greater balance of clinical goods over harms for the patient. For patients who are otherwise expected to survive a surgical procedure, death cannot be reasonably construed as a benefit. Thus, continuing DNR status intraoperatively is not medically reasonable. This conclusion is buttressed by the consideration above that maintaining DNR status in the OR is not consistent with professional integrity. If the patient preferred the benefits of an earlier timing of death from a terminal condition, then the patient should refuse surgery, including palliative surgery. The patient, however, does not get to define what is medically reasonable or to require surgeons to act in ways that are not consistent with professional integrity.

Ethical Consensus Concerning DNR In The OR

There has emerged a consensus that it is ethically justified for DNR orders to be suspended in the OR for patients with terminal conditions, including patients who have completed an advance directive that refuses life-sustaining treatment. It is not enough, however, to take the view that DNR orders should be suspended in the OR, because this position does not address the important ethical question of when DNR should be re-instated post operatively. There has emerged a consensus view that DNR status should be restored when life-threatening events are reliably judged to be owed to the patient's underlying terminal condition rather than to anesthesia, surgery, and their side-effects.

What is not mentioned is the fact that although active treatment of problems, from an anesthetic or a procedure, is similar to cardiopulmonary resuscitation, they almost always precede full-blown cardio-pulmonary arrest. As such they are therapies to reverse arrhythmias, hypotension, or hypoxia before the conditions result in cardiopulmonary arrest.

Surgeons should take a preventive ethics approach to DNR in the OR, by talking frankly with patients who remain able to make decisions, or their surrogate decision maker, for patients who do not about the role of DNR in patient care and why DNR status is not medically reasonable intraoperatively. A clear plan should be presented for the timing of a discussion about the re-instatement of DNR status and the surgeon should adhere to this plan. This preventive ethics approach protects both professional integrity and the autonomy of the patient, either as directly exercised by the patient or as indirectly exercised by the patient's surrogate decision maker.

DNR Does Not Mean Do Not Treat

Surgical management of the clinical problems of seriously or terminally ill patients has become an important component of effective palliative care for such patients. Surgeons should keep this larger context in mind, because it helps them to focus on the overall goal of providing appropriate clinical care for terminally ill patients, especially in their last days and hours. Surgeons have a heavily vested interest in providing definitive therapy; as a major part of the surgical persona and the modern armamentarium available emphasizes that role. Hospital mortality rates of individual surgeons are figured into many databases for various purposes. But aside from these distractions, there are many times where relief of bowel obstruction, a tracheotomy, stabilization of a fracture, placement of a supra-pubic cystostomy tube, or the like may bring comfort from torment, which is after all the foundational purpose of medicine.

Selected Readings

Faden RR, Beauchamp TL (1986) A history and theory of informed consent. Oxford University Press, New York

Halevy A, Baldwin JC (1998) Poor surgical risk patients. In: McCullough LB, Jones JW, Brody BA (eds) Surgical ethics. Oxford University Press, New York, pp 152–170

McCullough LB, Jones JW, Brody BA (eds) (1998) Surgical ethics. Oxford University Press, New York

McCullough LB, Jones JW, Brody BA (1998) Informed consent: autonomous decision making and the surgical patient. In: McCullough LB, Jones JW, Brody BA (eds) Surgical ethics. Oxford University Press, New York, pp 15–37

McCullough LB, Coverdale JH, Chervenak FA (2004) Argument-based ethics: a formal tool for critically appraising the normative medical ethics literature. Am J Obstet Gynecol 191:1097–1102

Powderly KE (2000) Patient consent and negotiation in the Brooklyn gynecological practice of Alexander J. C. Skene: 1863–1900. J Med Philos 25:12–27

Walter RM (1991) DNR in the OR: resuscitation as an operative risk. JAMA 266:2407–2412

Wear A (1993) Medical ethics in early modern England. In: Wear A, Geyer-Kordesch J, French R (eds) Doctors and ethics: the earlier historical setting of professional ethics. Rodopi, Amsterdam, The Netherlands, pp 98–130

Wear S, Milch R, Weaver LW (1998) Care of dying patients. In: McCullough LB, Jones JW, Brody BA (eds) Surgical ethics. Oxford University Press, New York, pp 171–197

Youngner SJ, Shuck JM (1998) Advance directives and the determination of death. In McCullough LB, Jones JW, Brody BA (eds) Surgical ethics. Oxford University Press, New York, pp 57–77

21 Multiple Organ Dysfunction: The Systemic Host Response to Critical Surgical Illness

John C. Marshall

Pearls and Pitfalls

- Fluid resuscitation and hemodynamic stabilization is the first priority in the management of a patient with sepsis or SIRS.
- Resuscitation can be expedited and optimized through the use of a resuscitation algorithm.
- Adequate volume resuscitation may compromise respiratory function, and necessitate intubation and mechanical ventilation.
- SIRS is a symptom complex, not a diagnosis and many, but not all, patients may have underlying infection as the cause.
- A presumptive source and bacteriologic diagnosis of infection should be established, and appropriate broad spectrum systemic antibiotics administered.
- Antibiotics should be discontinued within 3 days if no infection is identified, and be only rarely given for a period longer than 7 days.
- A focus of infection amenable to source control measures should be sought, and appropriate interventions performed.
- Patients with significant organ dysfunction should be managed in an intensive care unit (ICU).
- Optimal ICU management requires full attention to the potential harm resulting from critical care interventions.
- The Multiple Organ Dysfunction Syndrome is the outcome of systemic homeostatic changes of SIRS, and the de novo injury associated with ICU intervention.

Introduction

The Multiple Organ Dysfunction Syndrome or MODS is the leading cause of death for critically ill patients admitted to an intensive care unit. This snippet of epidemiologic data — intuitively evident to any clinician who has taken care of the multiply injured, hemodynamically unstable, or overwhelmingly infected patient — belies an intimidating complex mélange of pathologic insights that have emerged in parallel with our capacity to sustain the lives of patients who previously would have died of natural causes. Organ dysfunction, and the intimidating complex innate immune mechanisms that give rise to it, have only emerged as important mechanisms of disease as modern medicine has acquired the capacity to treat entities such as shock and infection, which in an earlier era, were rapidly lethal. Moreover, the injury complex that characterizes MODS is an amalgam created not only by the initial life-threatening insult, but even more importantly by the innate host response to that insult, and by the consequences of the therapeutic interventions that the clinician uses to sustain vital organ dysfunction. MODS is the quintessential iatrogenic disorder; it arises because modern medicine is capable of subverting previously lethal processes, but evolves as a direct consequence of the interventions used to sustain life.

The Acute Response to Danger: An Overview

Complex organisms — humans included — have evolved multiple, frequently overlapping mechanisms to respond to threats that pose a risk to life and limb. Blood, for example, is a liquid suspension that circulates under pressure within the vascular tree. In the absence of the coagulation cascade, the most trivial injury would result in exsanguinations and death. However, uncontrolled coagulation also poses a threat, since it arrests blood flow, and so prevents oxygen delivery to tissues. The complexities of normal coagulation and fibrinolysis reflect the twin biologic imperatives of adequately responding to the danger of bleeding, while minimizing the attendant harm of coagulation.

If the biology of the coagulation cascade is discouragingly complex, that of the innate immune response to infection or other external threats is many magnitudes more so. Indeed coagulation and anti-coagulation comprise part of a larger network of innate host defenses, for it is activation of the coagulation cascade and deposition of fibrin that creates an abscess, and activation of anticoagulant mechanisms that permit its resolution.

A comprehensive discussion of the biology of inflammation is far beyond the scope of this chapter. In general terms, it involves multiple biochemical cascades, each with its own counter-regulatory mechanisms that are activated when cells of the host innate immune system perceive danger. For example, activation of the coagulation cascade by microbial products results in the engagement of complement receptors on neutrophils, priming them for amplified production of reactive oxygen species in response to conserved microbial products. It is instructive, however, to review one of the most important of these — the toll-like receptor pathway — for insights it provides into the clinical expression of sepsis.

Toll-like Receptors (TLR) and the Innate Host Response to Danger

Cells of the innate immune system — monocytes, macrophages, and neutrophils in particular — are genetically programmed to recognize danger, and so can respond rapidly, but non-specifically, to a broad spectrum of potentially lethal threats in the local environment. These threats may be invading micro-organisms such as bacteria, fungi, or viruses, but might equally be products released from injured or dying cells in the local environment. Remarkably, this capacity rests with the ability of a family of ten proteins expressed on the surface of these cells to bind, and respond to a broad array of such signals. These cellular receptors are called toll-like receptors or TLRs — not because they extract a toll, but because they are remarkably similar to a very intriguing protein found in the fruit fly that determines which aspect of the fly is the front and which the back. All in all, that role is quite cool, and "toll" is German for "cool."

TLR4, for example, is the receptor that recognizes and binds endotoxin or lipopolysaccharide — a major component of the cell wall of all Gram-negative bacteria. When TLR4 binds endotoxin, a cascade of intracellular events is activated, that ultimately leads to altered expression of no fewer than 3,147 genes in humans — roughly an eighth of all the genes in the entire human genome (❯ *Fig. 21-1*). Multiple intracellular proteins participate in the intracellular cascade that evokes this genetic response, and so are potentially attractive targets for therapy in the future. But for our purposes, it is sufficient to appreciate that the immediate response to TLR engagement is increased production of key early protein mediators or cytokines, predominant amongst which are tumor necrosis factor (TNF) and interleukin-1 (IL-1). These mediators, in turn, activate other cells, triggering the changes in capillary permeability, vascular reactivity, and intravascular coagulation that result in the clinical picture of sepsis. For example, cytokine-induced increased activity of inducible nitric oxide synthase results in increased generation of nitric oxide, a potent vasodilator that is responsible for the diffuse vasodilatation that is characteristic of resuscitated sepsis. Cytokine-induced increases in the expression of tissue factor on endothelial cells triggers intravascular activation of the coagulation cascade, while the cytokine interleukin-6 triggers the altered pattern of liver protein synthesis that is known as the acute phase response.

■ **Figure 21-1**
Schematic representation of the cellular response to danger. Endotoxin from the cell wall of Gram-negative bacteria binds to a cell surface receptor, TLR4, resulting in the aggregation of a number of adapter proteins that associate with the intracellular tail of the receptor. This process initiates an enzymatic cascade, mediated through the addition or removal of phosphate groups from intracellular proteins. Enzymes that add phosphate groups are called kinases, whereas those that remove them are known as phosphatases. The process promotes the passage of transcription factors such as NFκB to the nucleus; these transcription factors bind to DNA, promoting its transcription to RNA, which in turn leads to the synthesis of new proteins. The initial response results in the synthesis of early inflammatory cytokines such as TNF and IL-1; these, in turn, can act on the cell to induce the expression of a large number of genes involved in the acute response to danger. For example, expression of tissue factor initiates the coagulation cascade, while upregulation of inducible nitric oxide synthase leads to the generation of nitric oxide, a potent vasodilator. The consequences of these processes is intravascular thrombosis, maldistribution of tissue blood flow, and cell death, through necrosis or apoptosis, and hence the clinical presentation of organ dysfunction

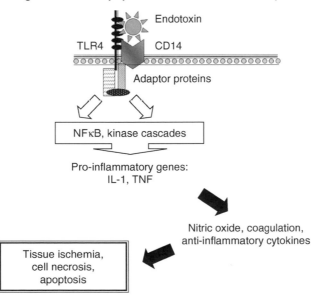

The activation of an innate immune response results in profound and generalized changes in systemic homeostasis that can be equally characterized as pro-inflammatory and anti-inflammatory, and the disappointing results of clinical trials of immunomodulatory therapy for sepsis underline the fact that the therapeutic challenge is much more complex than simply blunting an exaggerated inflammatory response, or augmenting a state of immunosuppression.

Systemic Inflammation: The Clinical Syndrome

Systemic activation of an inflammatory response results in a characteristic series of clinical manifestations. A combination of reduced vascular tone and increased capillary permeability results in a reduction in the intravascular fluid volume, producing hypotension and a reflex tachycardia, with a reduced urine output. Fluid resuscitation will often correct the hypotension, but increased capillary permeability leads to interstitial edema; this edema in the lung leads to tachypnea and hypoxia. Confusion presents – as a result of multiple factors including the altered metabolic state, hypoxia, and cerebral edema. The core temperature is typically increased, but may be low; laboratory manifestations reflect a state of systemic inflammation with leukocytosis (or leucopenia in the early stages), hyperglycemia, and evidence of the activation of an acute phase response (hypoalbuminemia and increased levels of C-reactive protein). Several other manifestations of altered organ function may also be present. Indeed, the clinical syndrome is the systemic equivalent of the cardinal manifestations of local inflammation described by Galen and Celsus 2,000 years ago: *rubor* (vasodilatation), *calor* (fever), *tumor* (increased capillary permeability with edema), *dolor* (malaise and confusion), and *functio laesa* (organ dysfunction).

While clinical features may vary from one patient to the next, the resultant syndrome is known as the Systemic Inflammatory Response Syndrome (SIRS) (❷ *Table 21-1*). When invasive infection is the cause of SIRS, sepsis is present; however SIRS may be present in the absence of infection, and, equally, infection present in the absence of SIRS (❷ *Fig. 21-2*). The syndrome reflects a spectrum of severity. Severe sepsis is sepsis in association with organ dysfunction, while septic shock is present when the process is of sufficient gravity that cardiovascular collapse is present. Increasing severity is associated with increased risk of mortality; the mortality of septic shock is typically 35–40% or higher.

The mortality risk of sepsis arises both from the presence of uncontrolled infection, and from the consequences of the host response to that infection. In fact the host response, rather than the infection that elicited it, is the most important determinant of survival (❷ *Fig. 21-3*).

MODS

The homeostatic changes associated with systemic inflammation can evoke alterations in the function of virtually every organ system. However, six systems predominate: the respiratory, cardiovascular, hematological, gastrointestinal, renal, and central nervous systems. Respiratory dysfunction is also commonly described as the Acute Respiratory Distress Syndrome (ARDS). MODS can be defined as the development of acute and potentially reversible derangements in the function of two or more organ systems. The mortality risk increases with both the *number* of failing organ systems and the *severity* of dysfunction within each system, giving rise to a number of scoring systems such as

◘ Table 21-1

Terminology and definitions

SIRS

A clinical syndrome resulting from the disseminated activation of an acute inflammatory response, and characterized by two or more of:

    Tachycardia (heart rate >90 beats/min)

    Tachypnea (respiratory rate >20 breaths/min, $PaCO_2$ <32 mmHg or mechanical ventilation)

    Hyper- or hypothermia (temperature >38°C or <36°C)

    Leukocytosis or leukopenia (white cell count >11,000 cells/mm^3 or <4,000 cells/mm^3, or >10% band forms)

Infection

The presence of micro-organisms invading normally sterile host tissues

Sepsis

The systemic host response to invasive infection

Severe sepsis

Sepsis in association with organ dysfunction

Septic shock

Sepsis in association with refractory hypotension despite adequate fluid resuscitation

◘ Figure 21-2

The relationship between invasive infection and the host response to that process. Note that infection may exist without significant systemic manifestations, and conversely, that a syndrome of systemic inflammation may arise in the absence of infection. When SIRS results from infection, sepsis is said to be present (Data from Bone et al., 1992)

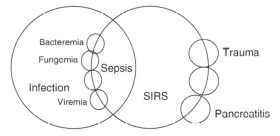

◘ Figure 21-3

The severity of the host response, rather than the stimulus that initiated it, is the primary determinant of outcome in critical illness. In a study of 211 critically ill surgical patients, we found that when patients were stratified by infectious status (either primary infection, or infection acquired within the ICU), non-survivors had significantly higher sepsis scores than survivors, indicating a greater degree of clinical response. On the other hand, when patients with elevated sepsis scores were evaluated, no infectio-related variables could be found that discriminated survivors from non-survivors (Data from Marshall and Sweeney, 1990)

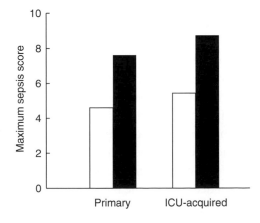

■ Table 21-2

The Multiple Organ Dysfunction (MOD) score

Organ system	0	1	2	3	4
Respiratory[a]					
(PO$_2$/FIO$_2$ ratio)	>300	226–300	151–225	76–150	≤75
Renal[b]					
(Serum creatinine)	≤100	101–200	201–350	351–500	>500
Hepatic[c]					
(Serum bilirubin)	≤20	21–60	61–120	121–240	>240
Cardiovascular[d]					
(Pressure-adjusted Heart rate – PAR)	≤10	10.1–15	15.1–20	20.1–30	>30
Hematologic[e]					
(Platelet count)	>120	81–120	51–80	21–50	≤20
Neurologic[f]					
(Glasgow coma score)	15	13–14	10–12	7–9	≤6

[a]The PO$_2$/FIO$_2$ ratio is calculated without reference to the use or mode of mechanical ventilation, and without reference to the use or level of PEEP.

[b]The serum creatinine level is measured in μmol/l, without reference to the use of dialysis.

[c]The serum bilirubin level is measured in μmol/l.

[d]The pressure-adjusted heart rate (PAR) is calculated as the product of the heart rate and right atrial (central venous) pressure, divided by the mean arterial pressure:

$$PAR = \frac{Heart\ rate \times CVP}{MAP}$$

[e]The platelet count is measured in platelets/ml 10^{-3}.

[f]The glasgow coma score is preferably calculated by the patient's nurse, and is scored conservatively (for the patient receiving sedation or muscle relaxants, normal function is assumed unless there is evidence of intrinsically altered mentation).

the Multiple Organ Dysfunction (MOD) and the Sequential Organ Failure Assessment (SOFA) scores (❍ *Table 21-2*).

MODS is a complex process, reflecting both the physiologic consequences of systemic inflammation, and further injury resulting from interventions used to sustain life. For example, overdistention of the lung during mechanical ventilation can exacerbate acute lung injury, and transfusion and a variety of medications can induce renal and hepatic dysfunction. By promoting the emergence of resistant organisms, systemic antibiotics can increase the risk of nosocomial infection and further organ dysfunction. MODS is a fundamentally iatrogenic disorder: it only arises because the clinician has intervened in an otherwise lethal process, but those interventions themselves can cause further injury.

Clinical Management of the Septic Patient

The development of SIRS or sepsis in the surgical patient is a potentially life-threatening situation, and urgent and appropriate intervention is essential to minimize the mortality risk.

The initial priority is resuscitation and hemodynamic support. Fluid resuscitation can be accomplished with either sodium-containing crystalloids such as normal saline or Ringer's lactate, or with colloids such as albumin; there are no convincing data to support the superiority of one over the other, and as the cheaper option, crystalloids are often the resuscitative fluid of choice. Effective volume losses may be substantial. The patient should receive an initial bolus infusion of 500 ml to a liter of fluid, followed by additional boluses as needed to raise the blood pressure, reduce the heart rate, and restore urine output to more than 30 ml/h. Often many liters of fluid will be required to accomplish these objectives. Optimal resuscitation can be further facilitated by the insertion of a central venous catheter to permit monitoring of central venous pressure and oxygen saturation (ScVO$_2$). A central venous pressure of at least 8 cm H$_2$O should be targeted, although often higher levels are needed to improve heart rate and blood pressure. An ScVO$_2$ of 70 or more should be targeted. When the blood pressure fails to respond to volume challenge (a CVP of more than 8) alone, a vasopressor such as norepinephrine should be added. Similarly, an inotropic agent such as dobutamine, or transfusion of packed red cells, should be considered if the ScVO$_2$ fails to respond to volume challenge alone. Used at the time of initial presentation, this resuscitative algorithm — termed goal-directed resuscitation — has been shown to increase the survival of patients with severe sepsis by as much as 16% (❷ *Fig. 21-4*).

Cultures of blood and other potential infectious foci should be drawn as part of the initial phases of resuscitation, followed by administration of systemic broad spectrum empiric antibiotics — selected on the basis of the presumptive site of infection, and of knowledge of local patterns of bacterial resistance. Comprehensive broad spectrum therapy is provided until culture and sensitivity data are available. The antibiotic spectrum should be narrowed on the basis of these data, and if cultures are negative after 72 h, antibiotics should be discontinued unless there are compelling reasons to suspect undiagnosed infection.

An inciting focus of infection should be sought for each patient with clinical manifestations of sepsis, and once a focus has been identified, appropriate source control measures should be undertaken. Source control interventions can be broadly classified as drainage, debridement and device removal, and definitive management. The need for source control can usually be established on the basis of the clinical presentation, augmented by the findings of radiological examinations such as computed tomography or ultrasonography. As a general principle, the best source control measure is one that accomplishes the source control objective, with the minimal physiologic upset to the patient. Thus percutaneous drainage is preferable to operative drainage of localized collections, and delayed debridement of pancreatic necrosis results in improved survival when compared to early, more aggressive intervention. When a more definitive intervention such as a bowel resection for perforated diverticulitis is performed, careful consideration of subsequent needs for reconstruction can minimize the global morbidity of the intervention. Stomas, if created, should be constructed with a view to

❑ Figure 21-4
Goal-directed resuscitation of the patient with septic shock. Intravenous fluid is first administered to increase the CVP to 8 cm H$_2$O or higher. If this fails to raise the mean arterial pressure to at least 65 mmHg, vasopressors are added, and if the oxygen saturation of blood drawn from the superior vena cava (ScVO$_2$) through the central line is less than 70%, inotropes and blood transfusion are administered (Data from Rivers et al., 2001)

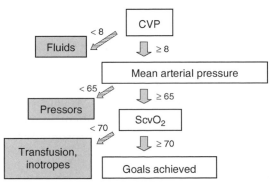

simplifying their closure, by creating a proximal diverting loop stoma, or by bringing both ends of the divided bowel out through the same orifice.

After hemodynamic resuscitation, and treatment of the inciting infection (if any), the management of systemic inflammatory response syndrome is supportive — the goal being to support failing vital organ function while minimizing the inevitable harm associated with life support. The goal of mechanical ventilation, for example, is to ensure adequate gas exchange in the lungs to permit oxygen delivery to the tissues, but to do so without further exacerbating acute lung injury. These potentially competing imperatives can be accomplished by careful consideration of the benefits and harms of intervention. Hemodynamic resuscitation of the septic patient often results in respiratory insufficiency because of increased capillary permeability in the lung. Mechanical ventilation with low tidal volumes (6 ml/kg) can minimize the trauma resulting from the ventilator, and the use of positive end-expiratory pressure (PEEP) keeps lung units open to facilitate gas exchange at low tidal volumes. Provided that oxygen delivery is satisfactory, the fraction of inspired oxygen (FIO_2) delivered by the ventilator can be set at a level adequate to result in oxygen saturation of the arterial blood (SaO_2) to a level of 92–95%. Finally, it is important to remember that the objective is to liberate the patient from the ventilator, and that daily weaning trials can reduce the duration of mechanical ventilation, and so reduce the associated risks.

Nutritional support should be provided, using the enteral route if at all possible. The benefits of formulae supplemented with anti-oxidants or other immunonutrients are unclear. Strict control of blood sugar levels has shown benefit in populations of critically ill surgical patients, though it remains unclear how tight this control should be. Infection prevention is grounded in efforts to remove unneeded invasive devices, to ensure optimal antiseptic care of those that are needed, and to reduce or eliminate unnecessary antibiotic exposure.

An evidence-based overview of the optimal management of the septic patient is beyond the scope of this brief review, but can be found in the guidelines of the Surviving Sepsis Campaign (www.survivingsepsis.org).

Adjuvant Treatments for Sepsis

Evolving insights into the complex biology of the septic response hold the promise of new modes of adjuvant therapy for a process with a mortality of 30% or higher despite adequate conventional management. Currently however, the options, are limited.

Activated protein C (APC or drotrecogin alpha activated) is an endogenous anticoagulant molecule whose levels are significantly reduced during sepsis. In addition to an anticoagulant activity in limiting microvascular thrombosis, APC can bind to cell receptors, reducing levels of inflammatory cytokines and limiting neutrophil activation. In a multicenter randomized trial of drotrecogin alpha in patients with severe sepsis, treatment was associated with a 20% relative improvement in survival, although the effects were seen only in the more severely ill patients. Controversy regarding the identification of the appropriate population of patients to treat, and the substantial cost of the agent, has limited its use in clinical practice. However, it should be considered in the more severely ill patient with sepsis, and in particular, when coagulopathy is a prominent component of the symptom complex.

Pharmacological doses of corticosteroids (50 mg hydrocortisone four times daily) have shown benefit in several small studies of patients with refractory septic shock, and in one larger multicenter French trial of patients with septic shock and non-responsiveness to an ACTH stimulation test. A more recent European trial has failed to replicate this finding, and so the role of adjuvant corticosteroids remains controversial. Given their low cost, and relatively low adverse event rate (they are, however, associated with prolonged neuromuscular weakness following ICU discharge), their use should be considered in patients with septic shock who remain vasopressor-dependent, despite adequate volume resuscitation.

Other therapeutic approaches remain unproven. A few, such as intravenous immunoglobulin, antithrombin, interferon-gamma, or G-CSF – represent commercially available agents that have shown some promise of efficacy in small studies. Others, such as anti-TNF antibodies or the interleukin-1 receptor antagonist, demonstrate efficacy when the results of clinical trials are pooled, but are not commercially available. Presently, the therapeutic benefit is sufficiently small, the appropriate population for therapy sufficiently undefined, and the therapies themselves sufficiently costly, that they must be considered experimental.

Conclusions

MODS is both a clinical syndrome, and a metaphor for a process of care. The syndrome arises through the activation of a systemic host response to a threat to life — infection, injury, ischemia, for example. The physiologic derangements resulting from that process can be corrected by aggressive and timely intervention aimed at rapidly restoring hemodynamic homeostasis. Infection can be treated with antibiotics and surgical source control, and injury can be repaired. Moreover we are on the edge of a new therapeutic approach, based on modulating the complex changes in innate immune function that underlie the clinical syndrome.

On other hand, MODS reflects not only the successes of critical care, but also its limitations. Prolonged support of failing organ system function does not necessarily lead to its reversal and may, indeed, aggravate existing dysfunction, or induce new injury. The line between extraordinary successes of technological medicine, and inappropriate meddling in the natural process of dying is a remarkably fine one.

Selected Readings

Bone RC, Balk RA, Cerra FB, et al. (1992) ACCP/SCCM Consensus Conference. Definitions for sepsis and organ failure and guidelines for the use of innovative therapies in sepsis. Chest 101:1644–1655

Dellinger RP, Carlet JM, Masur H, et al. (2004) Surviving sepsis campaign guidelines for management of severe sepsis and septic shock. Crit Care Med 32:858–873

Levy MM, Fink M, Marshall JC, et al. (2003) 2001 SCCM/ESICM/ACCP/ATS/SIS international sepsis definitions conference. Crit Care Med 34:1250–1256

Marshall JC, Sweeney D (1990) Microbial infection and the septic response in critical surgical illness. Arch Surg 125:17–23

Marshall JC (2003) Such stuff as dreams are made on: mediator-targeted therapy in sepsis. Nature Rev Drug Disc 2:391–405

Marshall JC, Cook DJ, Christou NV, et al. (1995) Multiple organ dysfunction score: a reliable descriptor of a complex clinical outcome. Crit Care Med 23:1638–1652

Rivers E, Nguyen B, Havstad S, et al. (2001) Early goal-directed therapy in the treatment of severe sepsis and septic shock. N Engl J Med 345:1368–1377

22 Hepatic Failure

Patrick K. Kim · Clifford S. Deutschman

Pearls and Pitfalls

- Hepatic failure affects nearly every organ system: neurologic, cardiovascular, gastrointestinal, renal, hematologic, endocrine, and immune.
- Although there are many causes of hepatic failure, few have specific treatments.
- The most common causes of death are cerebral edema, sepsis, and multisystem organ failure.
- Liver transplantation is often the only durable therapy.

The liver plays a central role in substrate and toxin metabolism, protein synthesis, and both innate and acquired immunity. This makes hepatic failure in the surgical patient an extraordinary management challenge. Acetaminophen toxicity is the most common etiology of fulminant hepatic failure in the United States and United Kingdom, but a variety of etiologies can cause hepatic failure (❷ *Table 22-1*). Untreated hepatic failure is highly lethal and, with a few exceptions, much of the current treatment of hepatic failure is supportive. The most common causes of death after liver failure are cerebral edema and sepsis/multisystem organ failure. Survival after hepatic failure depends upon rapid diagnosis, initiation of supportive measures, and prompt evaluation by a liver transplant team. Liver transplantation is often the only curative therapy.

Pathogenesis and Pathophysiology

While hepatic dysfunction adversely affects nearly every organ system (❷ *Fig. 22-1*), the primary defect is an intrinsic failure of hepatocellular synthesis. Simply put, liver cells fail to manufacture the essential products that are required for proper function. This leads to most of the organ dysfunction characteristic of fulminant hepatic failure of chronic cirrhosis. For example, failure to synthesize bile acid and organic anion transporters leads to an inability to clear toxins from the portal and systemic blood. This is reflected in jaundice. Failure to clear byproducts of nitrogen metabolism results in elevations of ammonia and false neurotransmitters. These contribute to encephalopathy, impaired blood-brain barrier and altered cerebrovascular autoregulation. Alterations in hepatic regulation of renal salt handling lead to hyponatremia and total body sodium overload. This may be the basis for the hepato-renal syndrome. The combination of blood-brain barrier dysfunction, hyponatremia and low oncotic pressure from defective albumin synthesis can cause cerebral edema and perhaps coma. Failure of hepatic synthetic function also leads to deficiencies of fibrinogen and coagulation factors II, V, VII, IX, and X. In conjunction with both quantitative and qualitative platelet abnormalities, this results in a profound coagulopathy. The result may be a state of disseminated intravascular coagulation.

◘ Table 22-1

Etiologies of hepatic failure

Drugs and toxins	Halothane
Acetaminophen	Isoniazid
Amanita phalloides mushroom	Rifampicin
Methyldioxymethamphetamine	Valproic acid
("Ecstasy")	Disulfiram
Herbal remedies	Nonsteroidal antiinflammatory drugs
Carbon tetrachloride	
Yellow phosphorus	*Cardiovascular*
Sulfonamides	Right heart failure
Tetracycline	Budd-Chiari syndrome
	Veno-occlusive disease
Viruses	Shock liver
Hepatitis A virus	
Hepatitis B virus	*Metabolic*
Hepatitis D virus	Acute fatty liver of pregnancy
Hepatitis E virus	Wilson's disease
Herpes simplex virus	
Cytomegalovirus	*Others*
Epstein-Barr virus	Sepsis
Varicella zoster virus	Autoimmune hepatitis
Adenovirus	Hepatic infiltration by malignancy
Idiosyncratic	

◘ Figure 22-1

Pathophysiology of systemic derangements in hepatic failure. NO, nitric oxide; DIC, disseminated intravascular coagulation

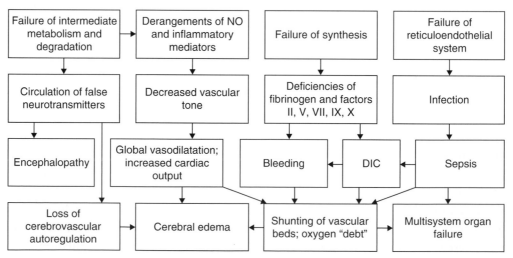

Derangements in the metabolism of nitric oxide and inflammatory cytokines cause vasodilatation, hypotension, low systemic vascular resistance and high cardiac output. This hyperdynamic circulation is similar to sepsis. Like sepsis, the combination of metabolic dysfunction and the DIC-induced microvascular thrombosis lead to poor end organ oxygen extraction and oxygen "debt" despite seemingly adequate oxygen delivery. An initial state of hyperglycemia reflects hormonal tone and high levels of substrate delivery, but masks an intrinsic failure of gluconeogenesis. Ultimately, this defect will cause hypoglycemia. Finally, failure of the reticuloendothelial system predisposes the host to the other major causes of death in hepatic failure: infection, overwhelming sepsis, and multisystem organ failure.

Diagnosis

The diagnosis of hepatic failure is based on history, physical examination, and laboratory studies. The symptoms and signs are largely nonspecific and include malaise, fatigue, anorexia, nausea, abdominal pain, fever, and jaundice. The hallmarks of liver failure are encephalopathy, hyperbilirubinemia, and coagulopathy. The severity of each of these predicts poor outcome. Hepatic failure is further classified based on the interval between onset of jaundice and onset of encephalopathy:

Fulminant	< 2 weeks
Subfulminant	2 weeks – 3 weeks
Late-onset	8 weeks – 24 weeks

If ascites is present, the serum-to-ascites albumin gradient aids in determining the etiology of ascites (❖ *Table 22-2*).

Management

Management of the patient begins with assessment of the patient's ability to maintain airway and breathing. Encephalopathy should be characterized (❖ *Table 22-3*). Endotracheal intubation and

❑ Table 22-2

Serum-to-ascites albumin gradient (SAAG) and differential diagnosis of etiology of ascites

SAAG > 1.1	SAAG < 1.1
Cirrhosis	Malignancy
Budd-Chiari syndrome	Pancreatic disease
Cardiac disease	Bile leak
Portal vein thrombosis	Infection
Myxedema	Nephrotic syndrome
Liver metastasis	

❑ Table 22-3

West Haven staging of hepatic encephalopathy

Grade	Description
0	Detectable only by neuropsychological testing
1	Lack of awareness, euphoria or anxiety, shortened attention span, impaired addition or subtraction
2	Lethargy, minimal disorientation to time, personality change, inappropriate behavior
3	Somnolence but responsive to verbal stimuli, confusion, gross disorientation, bizarre behavior
4	Comatose

mechanical ventilation should be considered for stages 3 and 4 encephalopathy. As with any patient at risk for life-threatening hemorrhage, the patient should have large-bore intravenous access, preferably peripheral, regardless of whether a central catheter is required for monitoring or for infusion of vasopressors. The blood bank must always have an active type and crossmatch specimen. Serum electrolytes should be monitored frequently for abnormalities of serum sodium and potassium. Blood glucose should be monitored frequently for both hyperglycemia and hypoglycemia. Hematologic and coagulation profiles should be checked serially for trends in hemoglobin/hematocrit, platelet count, prothrombin time, international normalized ratio (INR), and partial thromboplastin time. Liver function tests and serum ammonia are frequently obtained, but contribute little to decision-making in the acute setting.

The intravascular volume should be assessed carefully. Intravascular deficits should be repleted and fluid status reassessed frequently. Fluid resuscitation should start with isotonic solutions. Hypotonic solutions should be avoided, especially with preexisting hyponatremia. Fluid resuscitation should be aggressive in intensity, not necessarily in volume. Fluid overload may lead to complications such as heart failure, pulmonary edema, and abdominal compartment syndrome. Fluid resuscitation should favor colloids such as albumin, given the low oncotic pressure typically encountered. Plasma has the benefit of correcting INR while expanding intravascular volume, but in the patient who is not actively bleeding its routine administration is controversial. Plasma transfusion simply to correct an abnormal INR in the absence of active bleeding is not warranted.

Endpoints of resuscitation should be individualized and chosen carefully. A priori, a reasonable target for mean arterial pressure (MAP) is approximately 65 mmHg, at which point end organ perfusion should be assessed. From an intravascular volume standpoint, central monitoring may be necessary after initial fluid resuscitation, as it is often difficult to clinically gauge intravascular volume status. There are few evidence-based guidelines for the use of central venous pressure or pulmonary artery catheters. The decision to use either catheter remains at the discretion of the treating physician.

The thresholds for transfusion of blood and platelets should be individualized. There are no evidence based guidelines for transfusion triggers in patients with hepatic failure. Given the underlying propensity to hemorrhage, at present it seems prudent to set a transfusion trigger around 8 mg/dl, weighing benefits of transfusion with risks of transfusion reactions, immunosuppression, and predisposition to infection. The classic threshold for platelet transfusion is 50,000/mm^3 if an invasive procedure is being planned and 20,000/mm^3 absolute, at which point spontaneous bleeding may occur. In small studies, recombinant factor VIIa has shown promise in correcting clinical coagulopathy and decreasing transfusion requirement. Further study is warranted.

Diagnosis and treatment of cerebral edema is of paramount importance. Cerebral edema is a life-threatening complication and, if allowed to persist, may exclude the possibility of liver transplantation. Unfortunately, cerebral edema is insidious and diagnosis is clinically difficult. The neurologic exam is usually confounded by encephalopathy or obtundation from medications or other causes. Clinical findings such as decerebrate rigidity, disconjugate gaze, loss of pupillary reflexes, and the Cushing reflex (hypertension with bradycardia) are manifestations of cerebral herniation, a late sequela of cerebral edema, and a grave sign. In the patient with abnormal mental status, computed tomography and magnetic resonance imaging may exclude other diagnoses, but neither modality is sufficiently sensitive to diagnose and quantify cerebral edema. The most accurate (and invasive) method is direct monitoring of intracranial pressure (ICP). The benefits of monitoring of the intracranial pressure must be weighed against the increased risks of bleeding and infection that accompany hepatic failure. Compared to intraparenchymal monitors, extradural monitors have the lowest complication rate and are thus preferred. Intracranial hypertension is present when intracranial pressure is >18–22 mmHg. Cerebral perfusion pressure (CPP) is defined as the difference between mean arterial pressure (MAP) and ICP. Target CPP should be approximately 60 mmHg. The cornerstone of ICP management is mannitol, an osmotic diuretic. The recommended dose range is 0.75–1.25 mg/kg body weight, given every 6–8 h. However, studies in head injury demonstrate that mannitol becomes less effective with each dose and as the total cumulative dose increases. This agent may be administered until serum osmolality reaches 320 mOsmol/kg and/or the osmolar gap (the difference between measures and calculated osmoles) is >55 mOsmol/kg. Hypertonic saline has been shown to decrease ICP in patients with traumatic brain injury, but experience in hepatic cerebral edema is limited and the use of this agent cannot be recommended at this time. Vasopressor therapy should be initiated when hypotension persists, despite correction of hypovolemia or when CPP is impaired. Based on the underlying pathophysiologic derangements, the pressor of choice is norepinephrine. Epinephrine, dobutamine, and dopamine are *not* considered first-line drugs to increase MAP. Hyperventilation, which decreases ICP on the basis of selective cerebral vasoconstriction, is useful acutely. It should not be used persistently because vasoconstriction decreases cerebral blood flow and impairs oxygen delivery. Neither barbiturate nor thiopental coma has proven beneficial in hepatic encephalopathy. Propofol is under investigation. Jugular venous bulb oximetry may provide insight into cerebral oxygen consumption-delivery relationship, but it is unclear from these data whether oximetry improves outcomes. The suggested endpoint is O_2 saturation between 65% and 80%. Mild hypothermia has been studied experimentally and is promising. This approach has been shown to decrease ICP by decreasing brain metabolic demand. Studies also suggest that mild hypothermia does not increase bleeding risk. Further study is needed before this therapy can be recommended.

Regarding hepatic encephalopathy, lactulose is the mainstay of therapy. Lactulose acidifies the gut lumen, promoting ammonium ion formation (ammonium ion is not absorbed from the lumen). Lactulose also induces osmotic diarrhea, which removes ammonium from the body. Gut decontamination with metronidazole and oral neomycin theoretically decreases the count of urea-splitting bacteria in the lumen, but it is unclear if this significantly decreases ammonia production. Modified nutritional formulas rich in branched chain and deficient in aromatic amino acids have been studied extensively. They have been shown to improve encephalopathy score, but do not appear to alter outcome.

Bacterial infection occurs in about 80% of patients with hepatic failure, and patients with infection who subsequently develop sepsis are at high-risk for mortality. Although there is debate about which specific regimen is most appropriate, a broad-spectrum antibiotic coverage, most often a 4th generation cephalosporin, probably is warranted. The appropriate duration of prophylactic antibiotic therapy is unclear. Fungal infection occurs in about one-third of patients and similarly portends a poor outcome. At present, it is unclear whether empiric antifungal therapy should be initiated routinely. In patients with suspected infection or sepsis, it is imperative to obtain appropriate cultures immediately, administer broad-spectrum antibiotics, and pursue goal-directed therapy as described for other patients with suspected sepsis.

Renal failure occurs in up to half of patients with hepatic failure and is associated with increased mortality. There is no benefit to infusions of furosemide or dopamine. *Hepatorenal syndrome* is defined as renal dysfunction (serum creatinine > 1.5 mg/dl or creatinine clearance < 40 ml/min) with hepatic

◻ Table 22-4

Etiologies of hepatic failure with specific treatments

Etiology of hepatic failure	Treatment
Acetaminophen toxicity	*N*-acetylcysteine
Herpes simplex hepatitis	Acyclovir
Acute fatty liver of pregnancy	Delivery of fetus
Wilson's disease	Copper chelating agents
Amanita mushroom poisoning	Penicillin and silibinin

failure in the absence of prerenal, intrinsic renal, and postrenal etiologies of renal failure (e.g., hypovolemia, shock, nephrotoxin, significant proteinuria, obstructive uropathy). The treatment of renal dysfunction is supportive, with judicious fluid resuscitation and avoidance of nephrotoxic agents. Renal dysfunction may progress to frank renal failure. In such cases, the choice of renal replacement modality depends on hemodynamic stability. In the hemodynamically unstable patient, continuous renal replacement therapy (e.g., continuous veno-venous hemodiafiltration) is superior to intermittent hemodialysis in its ability to maintain mean arterial pressure.

Hepatic failure is associated with portal hypertension. Formation of porto-systemic collaterals leads to the development of esophageal varices. Variceal bleeding is a grave sign. Although half of variceal bleeding stops spontaneously, over half of these patients have recurrence within 48 h. Blood and blood products should be rapidly transfused. While at one time vasopressin was the preferred approach to variceal bleeding, this agent has been replaced by octreotide. An octreotide infusion of 250 mcg/h IV × 48 h is as effective as a vasopressin infusion in halting variceal bleeding and is associated with a lower incidence of cardiac and gastrointestinal ischemic complications. Endoscopic band ligation and/or sclerotherapy may be useful. For refractory bleeding, transjugular intrahepatic porto-systemic shunt (TIPS) should be considered, with the caveat that the procedure worsens encephalopathy and acutely increases venous return to the heart. Thus, TIPS is relatively contraindicated in patients with pre-existing encephalopathy and cardiac dysfunction. Balloon tamponade may be valuable to consider as a last resort. A variety of balloon tamponade catheters are available. All are based on the same concept: After elective endotracheal intubation and mechanical ventilation, the tube is inserted by the orogastric route. The stomach balloon is inflated and traction is applied to the tube. If bleeding persists, the esophageal balloon is inflated. The balloons are deflated periodically to reduce the risk of pressure necrosis.

As mentioned previously, much of the care is supportive. There are only a few etiologies of hepatic failure with specific therapies (◉ *Table 22-4*). For many cases of hepatic failure, liver transplantation is the only durable therapy.

Prognosis and Outcome Prediction

The King's College Criteria for Liver Transplantation, initially described in 1980, is widely used for evaluating severity of hepatic failure (◉ *Table 22-5*). There is significant experience in its application both for acetaminophen and non-acetaminophen etiologies of hepatic failure. The criteria are quite sensitive in patients with acetaminophen toxicity; those patients who fulfill the criteria have poor outcomes. However, the criteria have poor specificity and negative predictive value for both acetaminophen

◘ Table 22-5

King's College criteria for liver transplantation

Acetaminophen toxicity	Non-acetaminophen etiologies
pH < 7.3	PT > 100 s (INR > 6.5)
*or **all** of the following*	*or **any three** of the following*
Grade III–IV encephalopathy	Age <10 or >40 Years
PT > 100 s (INR > 6.5)	PT > 50 s (INR > 3.5)
Serum creatinine >3.4 mg/dl	Serum bilirubin >17.5 mg/dl
	Period of jaundice to encephalopathy >7 days
	Etiology is non-A, non-B hepatitis, halothane toxicity, idiosyncratic drug reaction, or Wilson's disease

PT, prothrombin time; INR, international normalized ratio.

◘ Table 22-6

Child-Turcotte-Pugh Score

Criteria	Points 1	2	3
Ascites	None	Slight	Moderate
Bilirubin	≤2	2–3	>3
Albumin	>3.5	2.8–3.5	<2.8
INR	<1.7	1.8–2.3	>2.3
Encephalopathy	None	Grades 1 or 2	Grades 3 or 4

Score	Grade	1-Year survival (%)	2-Year survival (%)
5–6	A	100	85
7–9	B	80	60
10–15	C	45	35

INR, international normalized ratio.

◘ Fig. 22-2

Calculation of Model for End-stage Liver Disease (MELD) score. Cr, creatinine; INR, international normalized ratio

$$R = 9.6 \times \log_e(\text{serum Cr, mg/dL}) + 3.8 \times \log_e(\text{serum bilirubin, mg/dL}) + 11.20 \times \log_e(\text{INR}) + 6.4$$

toxicity and non-acetaminophen causes. That is, many patients who do not fulfill the criteria have poor outcomes.

More recently, the Model for End-Stage Liver Disease (MELD) score has been used to stratify degree of hepatic failure. In contrast to the Child-Turcotte-Pugh score (❖ *Table 22-6*) the MELD score does not incorporate evaluation of ascites and encephalopathy, which are somewhat subjective. Rather, the MELD score is determined solely by three ubiquitous laboratory studies: serum creatinine, serum bilirubin, and INR (❖ *Fig. 22-2*).

Treatment: Transplantation and Alternatives

The MELD score, originally developed to predict short-term survival after TIPS procedures, has been validated statistically and has been used since 2002 by the United Network for Organ Sharing (UNOS) for allocation of livers for transplantation. The key to successful transplantation is early evaluation by a dedicated transplant team. If not already in one, the patient should be transferred promptly to a liver transplant center. General contraindications to liver transplantation include extrahepatic malignancy, uncontrolled sepsis, multiple organ failure, and intractable cerebral edema (e.g., sustained ICP >50 mmHg or CPP <40 mmHg).

A variety of short-term alternatives to orthotopic liver transplantation have been proposed. Among the treatments that have been studied are total hepatectomy with portacaval shunting, bioartificial liver, heterotopic liver transplantation, and xenotransplantation. Unfortunately, none has been sufficiently successful to be used clinically.

Conclusion

In summary, hepatic failure is one of the most challenging clinical problems to manage. Nearly every organ system is affected by hepatic failure: neurologic, cardiovascular, gastrointestinal, renal, hematologic, endocrine, and immune. Rapid diagnosis and treatment is essential and early referral to a transplant center is imperative. Cerebral edema, sepsis, and multisystem organ failure are the most common causes of mortality.

Selected Readings

Eghtesad B, Kadry Z, Fung J (2005) Technical considerations in liver transplantation: what a hepatologist needs to know (and every surgeon should practice). Liver Transpl 11:861–871

Jalan R (2003) Intracranial hypertension in acute liver failure: pathophysiological basis of rational management. Semin Liver Dis 23:271–282

Jalan R (2005) Acute liver failure: current management and future prospects. J Hepatol 42:S115–S123

Kamath PS, Wiesner RH, Malinchoc M, et al. (2001) A model to predict survival in patients with end-stage liver disease. Hepatology 33:464–470

O'Grady JG, Alexander GJ, Hayllar KM, Williams R (1989) Early indicators of prognosis in fulminant hepatic failure. Gastroenterology 97:439–445

Sass DA, Shakil AO (2005) Fulminant hepatic failure. Liver Transpl 11:594–605

23 General Principles of Sepsis

Gordon L. Carlson · Paul M. Dark

Pearls and Pitfalls

- Sepsis is a mediator disease, characterized by the host immune and inflammatory response to an infection.
- The outcome of sepsis is critically dependent upon eradicating its source – other aspects of therapy are supportive in nature.
- Prompt recognition and intervention is essential to avoid the development of severe sepsis and septic shock, for which prognosis remains poor.
- Early signs of sepsis in surgical patients may be subtle and easily overlooked and a high degree of suspicion is warranted, especially in the postoperative patient.
- Blood cultures are frequently negative or misleading.
- Radiological management may permit drainage of infected fluid collections, but surgical management is essential in the presence of necrotic tissue and may be the only effective means of establishing adequate source control.

Epidemiology of Sepsis

Infection remains a major cause of morbidity and mortality in general surgical practice, despite advances in perioperative care and refinements in antimicrobial chemotherapy. Ever more complex surgical procedures are being undertaken on an increasingly aged, frail, and comorbid patient population, with specific risk factors for infective complications, including diabetes, malignant disease, and implantation of prosthetic material. Recent estimates in the USA suggest that septic shock accounts for approximately 100,000 deaths each year, is the 13th most common cause of death and, despite the investment of many billions of dollars in novel antimicrobial chemotherapeutic agents, refinements in techniques for organ support, and immunotherapy, there has been little, if any, significant improvement in the outcome of treatment for septic shock for 2 decades. Overall, mortality rates following admission to the intensive care unit (ICU) with septic shock remain approximately 50%. Sepsis syndrome occurs in 400,000 patients per annum in the USA, with surgical patients accounting for almost one third of cases.

Definitions

Sepsis is a disease characterized by the host mediator response to an infection. Many of the clinical and biochemical features that characterize sepsis are related to the release of endogenous mediators, in response to microbial products, including pro-inflammatory cytokines such as tumor necrosis factor

◻ **Table 23-1**

Definitions in sepsis

Systemic inflammatory response syndrome
Two or more of the following:
• Temperature > 38°C or < 36°C
• Heart rate > 90 beats/min
• Respiratory rate > 20 breaths/min
• White blood cell count > 12,000/mm^3, < 4,000/mm^3, or > 10% of immature cells
Sepsis
SIRS plus a documented infection (positive culture)
If culture negative, suspected infection and one of the following:
• Significant edema or positive fluid balance (20 ml/kg over 20 h)
• Hyperglycemia (plasma glucose > 120 mg/dl) in the absence of diabetes
• Inflammatory variables: plasma C-reactive protein > 2 SD above the normal value or plasma procalcitonin > 2 SD above the normal value
• Mixed venous oxygen saturation (SVO$_2$) > 70%
• Cardiac index > 3.5 l/min/M^{23}
Severe sepsis
Sepsis associated with organ dysfunction, hypoperfusion abnormalities, or hypotension
Hypoperfusion abnormalities include, but are not limited to:
• Arterial hypoxemia (PaO$_2$/fraction of inspired oxygen (FiO$_2$) ration of < 300 torr)
• Acute oliguria (urine output < 0.5 ml/kg/h or 45 mmol/l for at least 2 h)
• Creatinine > 2.0 mg/dl
• Coagulation abnormalities (international normalized ratio > 1.5 or activated partial thromboplastin time > 60 s)
• Thrombocytopenia (platelet count < 100,000)
• Hyperbilirubinemia (plasma total bilirubin > 2 mg/dl or 35 mmol/l)
• Tissue-perfusion variable: hyperlactatemia (>2 mmol/l)
• Hemodynamic variables: arterial hypotension (systolic blood < 90 mmHg, mean arterial pressure < 70 mmHg, or a systolic blood pressure decrease > 40 mmHg).
Septic shock
Sepsis-induced hypotension despite fluid resuscitation plus hypoperfusion abnormalities

alpha and interleukins 1 and 6. Release of these mediators can also be induced, however, by noninfective stimuli, including extensive tissue injury, massive blood transfusion, and sterile inflammation, for example, in acute severe pancreatitis. An international consensus has enabled a logical approach to this spectrum of illness, by recognizing that the clinical consequences of endogenous mediator release comprise the systemic inflammatory response syndrome (SIRS), and that sepsis is defined as the development of SIRS as a consequence of infection (❷ *Table 23-1*). In addition to these definitions of sepsis, the classification takes into account sepsis severity, including sepsis syndrome (severe sepsis), which is characterized by sepsis with evidence of deleterious consequences of the host response with respect to organ perfusion and/or function, and septic shock, in which sepsis syndrome is associated with hypotension, which persists despite apparently adequate fluid resuscitation.

Pathophysiology of Sepsis

The complex pathological processes underlying sepsis and its progression to septic shock result primarily from host immune dysregulation associated with widespread cellular injury and associated tissue and organ dysfunction – invading microorganisms appear to act as initiators, but may rapidly become bystanders as maladaptive systemic immune responses develop. Why some surgical patients produce prompt protective immunological responses to microbial invasion while others develop overwhelming and refractory septic shock remains unclear.

Regulated innate immune activation involves early recognition of the pathogenic microorganism by an array of immunocompetent cells such as macrophages, dendritic cells, lymphocytes, neutrophils, and endothelial cells. Toll-like receptors are a class of pattern-recognition molecules variably expressed on these cells which are able to bind with whole subsets of pathogens or their breakdown products (pathogen-associated molecular patterns). The Toll-like receptor family is evolutionarily conserved, representing a phylogenetically ancient defense mechanism in multicellular organisms which, unlike acquired immune function, does not rely on previous pathogen exposure in the host. Toll-like receptors mediate cell-signaling mechanisms that control the release of cytokines from cells exposed to pathogens or their products. Cytokines are soluble, low-molecular weight glycoproteins that regulate innate and acquired immune responses to pathogens. They act pleiotropically on multiple target cells, having both paracrine and endocrine effects depending on levels of production. Cytokines are traditionally classified into those that produce pro-inflammatory effects (e.g., TNFα, IL-1, and IL-8) and those that are anti-inflammatory (e.g., IL-10 and TGFβ). Regulated inflammation, local to the site of pathogen invasion, involves release and amplification of pro-inflammatory mediators that promote activation and tissue recruitment of cells, such as circulating neutrophils that have the capacity to destroy invading pathogens (and surrounding tissue) by release of chemicals such as oxygen radicals. Local activation of other inflammatory systems such as complement, coagulation, and kinin-cascades aids in the effective destruction of pathogens and facilitates an appropriate concentration of the inflammatory processes locally. A careful balanced regulation of pro- and anti-inflammatory cytokines, both temporally and spatially, is thought to limit these processes to the tissue site(s) of invasion, limit tissue injury, and promote healing and resolution. The potential for extensive systemic tissue injury and organ dysfunction is clear if this process becomes severely dysregulated.

The prevailing "canonical" theory of sepsis refers to an uncontrolled systemic inflammatory response to overwhelming infection; death from sepsis is attributable to an overstimulated immune system that produces widespread tissue injury and organ dysfunction. However, most of the evidence for this notion is from rigid animal models of sepsis that do not seem to reflect the veracity of human responses to infection. Indeed, in many animal models of endotoxemia or polymicrobial sepsis, organ dysfunction and/or death is often associated with an early and pronounced pro-inflammatory "cytokine storm," and compounds that block the mediators in these models improve survival. The patterns of systemic cytokine levels in surgical patients with sepsis syndromes suggest that "cytokine storm" is unusual and numerous clinical trials of inflammatory cascade blockade with agents, such as corticosteroids, anti-endotoxin antibodies, TNF antagonism, IL-1 receptor antagonists, and other compounds, have failed to make a significant impact on adult human sepsis syndromes. Observational studies in patients suggest that a dysregulated systemic balance between pro- and anti-inflammatory responses may be more important in terms of the pathogenesis of sepsis rather than the magnitude and character of the initial pro-inflammatory status.

Mapping the inflammatory responses onto the clinical manifestations is troublesome, uncovering our inadequate knowledge of basic mechanisms and the nonspecific diagnostic criteria for clinical recognition of sepsis syndromes. However, the SIRS, or sepsis when infection-related, can be associated with an early systemic pro-inflammatory phenotype usually lasting over a number of days, followed by the development of a counter-regulatory anti-inflammatory syndrome (CARS) characterized by immunosuppression (delayed hypersensitivity, an inability to clear infection, and a predisposition to nosocomial infection). Numerous factors have been implicated in the development of immunosuppression in sepsis including unbalanced anti-inflammatory cytokine production, T-cell anergy and apoptosis-induced loss of adaptive immune system. It is unclear why these events occur and how they are related to initial triggering of immune responses to pathogens. Furthermore, in the critically ill surgical patient, it is also unclear how a complex environment (e.g., surgical tissue injury, anesthesia, blood transfusions, nutritional status, and coexisting medical disease) in association with host genetic factors (e.g. polymorphisms in cytokine genes) may determine the mechanisms of responses to an invading pathogen. However, in the practice of surgical critical care, it is unusual for patients to die from overwhelming SIRS/sepsis resulting from the first infection "hit," but the development of CARS during prolonged critical care is associated with a predisposition to secondary "hits" from nosocomial infection, which is closely associated with the development of "multiorgan dysfunction syndrome" (MODS) and a high chance of death.

Sepsis-Related Organ Dysfunction

During sepsis, the development of organ dysfunction distant from the infection site helps define clinical severity (❯ *Table 23-1*) and is related to outcome. Dysfunction refers to a phenomenon where organ function is not capable of maintaining homeostasis. When more than one organ system is involved it is characterized as MODS, with outcome being directly related to the number and duration of dysfunctional systems. Sepsis-related MODS is the leading cause of death in non-coronary ICUs. Curiously, survival from septic shock is associated with recovery of organ function to baseline. In addition, postmortem examination of surgical patients dying from septic shock uncovers discordance between histological findings and the degree of organ dysfunction. Alongside emerging evidence for mitochondrial dysfunction associated with sepsis and MODS, this clinical evidence suggests cells may develop a "hibernation" phenomenon in response to progressive sepsis, akin to cell stunning following myocardial ischemia.

While any organ can contribute to sepsis-related MODS, the cardiovascular system is commonly implicated and provides an example of how developing organ dysfunction can drive a vicious cycle of systemic immune activation and tissue injury. Cardiac dysfunction is characterized globally by biventricular myocardial dilatation with persisting tachycardia following fluid resuscitation. Despite a normal to high cardiac output, up to a third of patients with sepsis will have myocardial dysfunction as evidenced at the bedside by decreased responsiveness to fluid resuscitation and catecholamine stimulation. Circulating depressant factors, including TNFα and IL-1β, act in synergy on myocytes through nitric oxide dependent and independent pathways, whereas myocardial hypoperfusion is not associated with this phenomenon. Sepsis is also associated with arteriolar vasodilatation and dysregulation of microcirculatory blood flow, mediated via local nitric oxide production, which can become refractory to therapy. Systemic endothelial activation and barrier dysfunction can result in tissue edema formation. In the absence of early adequate resuscitation in combination with increased insensible fluid losses and with myocardial and vascular dysfunction, maldistribution of perfusion to tissues occurs with the threat of ischemic injury and further organ dysfunction. Widespread fibrin deposition in the microcirculation is associated with the early pro-inflammatory phenotype, producing combined fibrin, platelet, neutrophil, and red blood cell microaggregates, which can promote further tissue ischemia. When fibrin deposition is severe, a state of disseminated intravascular coagulation (DIC) can develop and is associated with increased mortality.

The splanchnic circulation is particularly vulnerable to hypoperfusion in the inadequately resuscitated septic patient. Splanchnic hypoperfusion is associated with gut mucosal ischemia, changes in barrier function, and the potential for translocation of enteric flora into gut mucosal cells and gut-associated lymphoid tissue. There is a potential for the hypoperfused gut to generate a localized inflammatory response to these events and when reperfused can contribute further to systemic inflammatory responses and distant organ injury via drainage from the portal circulation and/or mesenteric lymph channels. Experimental evidence and clinical observation in surgical critical care has not been conclusive in this regard, although there is a consensus that gut ischemia-reperfusion may be an important source of systemic pro-inflammation and is clearly associated with the development of nosocomial second "hit" sepsis during subsequent immunosuppression.

Causes of Sepsis in Surgical Patients

Surgical patients may develop sepsis as a consequence of nosocomial infection, or as a feature of diseases that require surgical treatment. A great deal of acute general surgical practice relates to the management of sepsis due to infection within the peritoneal cavity associated with disease and/or perforation of the gastrointestinal tract, whereas nosocomial sepsis in surgical patients most commonly relates to surgical site infection (SSI), including wounds, pneumonia, urinary tract infections, and blood stream infection, which is frequently (though not necessarily) associated with the use of intravascular devices. The incidence of SSI is regarded as a marker of the quality of surgical care, with national surveillance programs collecting data concerning infection rates, clinical outcome, and causative organisms. The vast majority of sepsis in surgical patients relates to infection with gram-positive (60%) or gram-negative (30%) bacteria, and a small, but an increasingly important proportion of cases relates to infection with opportunist pathogens such as fungi, notably *Candida* sp. The most common gram-positive organisms isolated from surgical patients with sepsis are *Staphylococcus* (*epidermidis* and *aureus*) and *Enterococcus* sp. (notably *Enterococcus faecalis*); Hospital-acquired infection, particularly from strains exhibiting multiple antibiotic resistance, such as MRSA (Methicillin-resistant *Staphylococcus aureus*), or VRE (Vanomycin-resistant *Enterococci*) may be particularly difficult to treat. Common gram-negative organisms isolated from surgical patients with sepsis include *Escherichia coli*, *Klebsiella pneumoniae*, and *Pseudomonas aeruginosa*, while gram-negative sepsis in surgical patients in the ICU may also be due to less invasive opportunist organisms, including *Acinetobacter* and *Enterobacter* sp.

Recognition and Diagnosis of Sepsis

Characteristic features of sepsis include fever (hypothermia occasionally occurs in severe sepsis), tachycardia, and tachypnea, accompanied by leukocytosis (leukopenia is occasionally observed in severe sepsis). Rigors are characteristic of episodic bacteremia, typically seen in intravascular catheter infection, or when infection of a duct system is accompanied by mechanical obstruction, for example, in ascending cholangitis or pyelonephritis. In addition to these nonspecific manifestations of systemic inflammation, there may be features indicative of the site of infection, including signs of peritoneal irritation, urinary tract infection a productive cough, or radiological signs of pulmonary consolidation, or, in the case of soft tissue infection, evidence of cellulitis, erythema, swelling, or even discharge of purulent material from a wound site. In some patients with postoperative abdominal infection, including pelvic and subphrenic abscess, sepsis may develop insidiously, unaccompanied by some or even all of the classical signs of infection. In such cases, patients may present instead with failure to make postoperative progress, jaundice, hypoalbuminemia, hyponatremia, and progressive wasting and catabolism, despite apparently satisfactory nutritional support.

It is important to recognize that aerobic and anaerobic blood cultures, though obligatory in the assessment of the septic patient, are likely to be positive on only approximately 20% of occasions. Overall, less than 50% of patients with severe sepsis have a pathogenic organism identified in blood cultures. Diagnosis in many cases is based, at least initially, on clinical suspicion, with antimicrobial chemotherapy initiated on the basis of an assessment of likely pathogens and modified on the basis of culture of samples taken from the site of infection, and, in the case of surgical infections, from pus especially.

Management of Sepsis — Supportive Medical Therapy

Despite half a century of the establishment and refinement of surgical critical care, mortality from severe sepsis and septic shock has not changed, but the incidence of sepsis is increasing in most countries. However, over the past few years a number of unexpected yet important clinical breakthroughs in adjuvant medical therapy have arisen and have been tested in randomized controlled trials. Many of these advances are currently being adopted by the international critical care community in association with coordinated efforts to assess clinical effectiveness.

Cardiovascular Support

Cardiovascular resuscitation with early goal-directed therapy (EGDT) has been shown to improve survival for emergency department patients presenting with severe sepsis and septic shock. Resuscitation aimed at achieving predetermined values of central venous pressure (CVP) and mean arterial pressure (MAP), urine output and central venous (superior vena cava) oxygen saturation ($\geq$70%) for the initial 6 h period was able to reduce 28-day mortality, with a number needed to treat (NNT) of six patients. Central venous oxygen saturation was used as a pragmatic surrogate of tissue perfusion and oxygen utilization, with rising values above 70% representing adequate hemodynamic resuscitation. If the threshold value was not achieved with fluid resuscitation to a predetermined CVP, then packed red blood cell transfusions to achieve an hematocrit of at least 30% and/or dobutamine infusion (up to 20 µg/kg/min) were titrated to achieve the central venous oxygen saturation goal.

Modification of the Inflammatory Response

Recombinant activated protein C (rhAPC) infusion (24 µg/kg/h) over 96 h has been shown to be effective in improving 28-day survival in patients at high risk of death (sepsis-induced organ dysfunction) and a low risk of bleeding at inception; NNT of 13 with a minimum of two organ dysfunction. It may be important to define more fully those patients most likely to benefit from rhAPC infusion and patients with single organ dysfunction (however severe), who are within 30 days of surgery, and may be most likely to develop complications of treatment and have substantially reduced clinical benefit. The inflammatory response to sepsis is pro-coagulant in the early stages, with the potential for microcirculatory perfusion abnormalities. rhAPC has endogenous anticoagulant and anti-inflammatory properties, which may explain its efficacy in early severe sepsis and septic shock (❷ *Fig. 23-1*). Taken together, EGDT in the first 6 h of diagnosis, followed by careful consideration for rhAPC therapy, constitutes an effective global reperfusion strategy for high-risk sepsis and should have a similar priority in critical care as reperfusing the myocardium after acute coronary artery thrombosis. For these approaches to work effectively, emergency medical systems must develop strategies for early recognition of the patient with, or at risk of developing, severe sepsis and septic shock. Unfortunately, the diagnosis of sepsis in critical care is rather nonspecific, particularly as culture-positive sepsis is frequently lacking. The need for specific and sensitive biomarkers of sepsis, and its severity, has never been more urgent and constitutes a significant scientific challenge.

Administering large-dose intravenous corticosteroids (>300 mg/day of hydrocortisone or equivalent) has been a popular intervention for attempted reversal of refractory hypotension resulting from sepsis, until a more recent meta-analysis reported a worsened prognosis following such interventions; with some notable exceptions in pediatric (meningitis) and adult (severe typhoid and PCP in AIDS) infectious diseases. However, a recent multicenter-randomized controlled trial with patients in severe septic shock showed a significant shock reversal and reduction of 28-day mortality (NNT = 10) when

◻ Figure 23-1
The Protein C pathway (Reprinted from Macias et al., 2005. With permission)

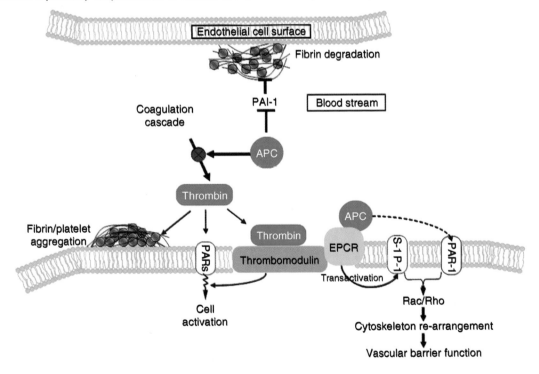

patients with relative adrenal insufficiency (defined as post-ACTH cortisol rise ≥9 μg/dl) received lower-dose "replacement" steroids. Routine low-dose steroids cannot be recommended at this time for sepsis until a number of important questions that were raised by this study are addressed: how is adrenal insufficiency diagnosed in sepsis, what constitutes "low-dose" steroids, and what are the results of a study in patients with sepsis in extremis generalizable to a broader population of critically ill septic patients? These questions are being addressed currently by the international community and further guidance is awaited.

Metabolic and Nutritional Support

A large single-center trial of "tight glycemia" control in postoperative surgical critical care patients (predominantly cardiac surgery) showed improved 28-day survival (NNT = 11) and significant reductions in sepsis-related complications. In the intervention, blood glucose was maintained in the range 80–110 mg/dl (4.4–6.1 mmol/l) using a titrated continuous intravenous insulin infusion. The control of blood sugar appeared to be more important than the amount of infused insulin, but this remains to be formally tested. In addition, other metabolic effects such as a change in circulating lipid profiles may be significant. There is a potential for hypoglycemia, although careful and repeated glucose monitoring in a well-staffed critical care unit, alongside a nutrition protocol that promotes early continuous feeding, can limit these events and ameliorate any potential adverse risk to the patient. Studies aimed at determining the efficacy of less intensive glycemia control may help further reduce any risk of insulin infusions. Another large study at the same center has recently extended the "tight glycemia" approach to medical intensive care and did not replicate the survival advantage in the intervention group on an intention-to-treat basis. At present, the concept and scientific basis for "tight glycemia" control is in evolution and should probably be reserved for critically ill surgical patients in the ICU.

Sepsis is a catabolic state, associated with profound resistance to the anabolic effects of insulin and muscle wasting, despite aggressive nutritional support. Attempts to modify the hormonal environment to promote anabolism using recombinant human growth hormone (rhGH), while attractive in theory, were abandoned when it became clear that this approach resulted in increased mortality, possibly because of GH-induced insulin resistance and the resulting hyperglycemia and increased risk of sepsis. While there has been considerable debate concerning the optimal route for nutritional support in patients with sepsis and the controversial role of immune-enhancing feeds, pragmatic trials have shown that the route of feeding is probably less important than ensuring adequate (but not excessive) provision of calories and nitrogen in a safe manner, tailored to the patient's individual requirements and the ability of their gastrointestinal tract to cope with enteral feeding. Nutritional support should not be expected to reverse catabolism in the presence of ongoing sepsis and dealing with the source of sepsis is one of the most valuable interventions from the nutritional perspective.

Antimicrobial Chemotherapy

Appropriate antibiotic use in sepsis provides a major challenge to the surgeon, critical care physician, and microbiologist because scientific evidence for any particular approach is lacking. In many cases, early use of broad-spectrum antibiotics guided by surveillance-driven local policy against the suspected pathogen(s) in a given clinical sepsis scenario would be considered best practice. Continued laboratory and clinical surveillance should then allow de-escalation and fine-tuning of antimicrobial therapies in order to maximize efficacy and limit drug-induced organ injury and superinfection with multiresistant pathogens. However, in recent years, evidence for adjuvant selective gut decontamination of critically ill patients in intensive care has been growing. There are now two meta-analyses which confirm survival advantage by providing a combination of topical and parenteral broad-spectrum antibiotics aimed at early gut microflora eradication, thereby limiting the role of the gut as a pro-inflammatory organ and source of second "hit" infection during critical care. Despite the compelling evidence for efficacy, early selective gut decontamination in critical illness has not been universally adopted, primarily because of concerns for the development of antimicrobial resistance — evidence for which has not arisen in the meta-analyses. It remains to be seen if the international community reconsiders its approach to the gut microflora which is carried into ICUs by the host.

Management of Sepsis — Principles of Surgical Therapy

In many surgical patients, prompt surgical intervention is of paramount importance in treating sepsis. Although aggressive resuscitation and antimicrobial chemotherapy are essential, a successful outcome of treatment is unlikely unless source control is achieved. Devitalized or necrotic tissue should be removed, the pus drained and sent for culture, and the results used to modify further antibiotic therapy, if appropriate (see above). In many cases of abdominal infection, this can be achieved by percutaneous drainage, under ultrasound guidance without exposing the patient to the additional risk of multiple organ failure syndrome (MOFS) associated with the second "hit" of further surgery. Where source control, however, requires resection or removal of the focus of infection (e.g., a perforated viscus or a leaking anastomosis), this is better accomplished by surgical means. Studies of patients with intra-abdominal sepsis have shown, for example, that ability to eradicate the abdominal septic focus is the single most important determinant of survival, and failure to do so on the first occasion is associated with a significantly increased mortality, which increases stepwise with each successive trip to the theater, and that the prognosis is especially poor if septic shock develops prior to treatment.

The general principles of surgical intervention are to establish adequate drainage of infection and to excise necrotic or devitalized tissue. Obstruction to the biliary or urinary tract must be relieved by radiological, endoscopic, or surgical means. Leakage from the gastrointestinal tract should be dealt with by exteriorization wherever possible. In patients with severe abdominal sepsis, up to 30% of patients exhibit continuing evidence of infection after aggressive surgical intervention, typified by intra-abdominal abscess formation, often with multiple small abscesses between loops of small intestine (tertiary peritonitis). The role of planned relaparotomy, as opposed to laparotomy on demand (in relation to deterioration in oxygenation, organ function, and inotrope requirements), in such cases remains controversial, but case–control studies have shown that planned relaparotomy does not appear to reduce mortality significantly and may increase secondary complications, including the incidence of intestinal fistula. In severe cases of tertiary peritonitis, where sepsis frequently coexists with abdominal hypertension, management may necessitate leaving the abdomen open (laparostomy) to facilitate drainage of the septic focus and planned, staged reconstructive surgery of the gastrointestinal tract and abdominal wall after recovery.

Selected Readings

Bone RC, Balk RA, Cerra FB (1992) Definitions for sepsis and organ failure and guidelines for the use of innovative therapies in sepsis. The ACCP/SCCM consensus conference committee. Chest 101:1644–55

Carlson GL, Irving MH (1997) Infection: recognition and management of infection in surgical patients. In: Hanson G (ed.) Critical care of the surgical patient — a companion to Bailey and Loves' surgery. Chapman & Hall, London, pp. 273–290

Dellinger RP, Carlet JM, Masur H, et al. (2004) Surviving Sepsis Campaign guidelines for management of severe sepsis and septic shock. Crit Care Med 32(3):858–873

Hotchkiss RS, Karl IE (2003) The pathophysiology and treatment of sepsis. N Engl J Med 348(2):138–150

Levy MM, Fink MP, Marshall JC, et al. (2003) 2001 SCCM/ESICM/ACCP/ATS/SIS International Sepsis Definitions Conference. Crit Care Med 31(4):1250–1256

Macias WL, Yan SB, Williams MD, et al. (2005) New insights into the protein C pathway: potential implications for the biological activities of Drotrecogin alfa (activated). Crit Care 9 (Suppl 4):S38–S45

National nosocomial infection surveillance (1998) Systems report, data. Summary from October 1986–April 1998, issued June 1998. Am J Infect Control 26:522–533

Rivers E, Nguyen B, Havstad S, et al. (2001) Early goal-directed therapy in the treatment of severe sepsis and septic shock. N Engl J Med 345(19):1368–1377

Singer M, De Santis V, Vitale D, Jeffcoate W (2004) Multi-organ failure is an adaptive, endocrine-mediated, metabolic response to overwhelming systemic inflammation. Lancet 364(9433):545–548

van den Berghe G, Wouters P, Weekers F, et al. (2001) Intensive insulin therapy in critically ill patients. N Engl J Med 345(19):1359–1367

24 Neurologic Physiology: The Brain and Its Response to Injury

Mamerhi O. Okor · James M. Markert

Pearls and Pitfalls

- Early clinical recognition and radiographic diagnosis are key initial steps in the management of head injury.
- Once a surgical lesion has been ruled out in a severely head-injured patient, aggressive medical management should be instituted. Medical management primarily constitutes supportive therapy aimed at preventing secondary insults to the brain, which should include the detection and treatment of raised intracranial pressure (ICP).
- In the event that first-line therapy for the management of elevated ICPs is unsuccessful, "second-tier" therapy may be cautiously applied.
- Lack of an aggressive initial approach to the head-injured patient can lead to an exacerbation of the initial injury due to potentially avoidable secondary injury—an inadequate resuscitation can lead to superimposed hypoxic or ischemic injury, and delayed institution of measures to combat increased ICP can result in increases in local tissue pressures and local ischemia, or even avoidable herniation syndromes.
- A poor neurologic exam in the setting of an initially normal-appearing computed tomography (CT) scan may be due to toxic/metabolic issues, but also can be a result of a hypoxic injury or diffuse axonal injury (DAI).
- An early accurate neurologic assessment can prevent the clinician from delaying the diagnosis of an intracranial mass lesion that may require immediate operative intervention, particularly if a unilateral fixed and dilated pupil is present, or a patient has a marked hemiparesis.
- Patients in whom such an exam is not possible due to pharmacologic paralysis before such an assessment can be undertaken, require an urgent head CT to avoid missing such a diagnosis.
- Overuse of hyperventilation (prolonged periods of $PaCO_2$ of 25 mmHg or less) can result in rebound intracranial hypertension; $PaCO_2$ should generally be kept in the 30–35 mmHg range. Serum osmolarity should be maintained below 310–320 to minimize the risk of renal injury in the setting of prolonged mannitol administration, and switching to hyperosmolar saline use in these patients can decrease this risk.
- Avoidable use of pharmacologic paralysis can lead to sepsis, pneumonia, and increased ICU stays.

Classification of Brain Injury

Closed head injury can be classified based on severity (mild, moderate, or severe) which is determined largely by Glasgow Coma Scale scoring; mechanism (missile or blunt); and pathology (primary or secondary). A prompt and thorough initial neurologic assessment is crucial in determining the nature of a patient's injury and instituting the appropriate treatment protocol.

Missile Injuries

Missile injuries can be classified as depressed, penetrating, or perforating. In *depressed injuries*, the missile fails to penetrate the skull but produces a depressed skull fracture and/or causes a contusional injury to the underlying brain. Brain damage is therefore focal, and consciousness is rarely altered for long. In *penetrating injuries*, the missile enters the cranial cavity but does not leave it. If the object is small and sharp, and penetration is limited, little direct injury to the skull and brain may occur. The damage is focal, and the patient seldom loses consciousness. However, the missile may penetrate deeply enough to damage vital structures. Penetration through multiple lobes, both hemispheres, the ventricular system, or posterior fossa involvement by the missile will all produce more extensive damage. Even simple penetrating head injuries may allow infection, meningitis, or cerebral abscesses to develop. In a penetrating injury, the missile (usually a bullet) passes and exits the brain but does not leave the skull, resulting in a penetrating brain wound. If the bullet exits the head, the injury is called a *perforating head injury*. The exit wound in the skull is characteristically larger than the entry wound. Low-velocity missiles rarely exit the skull, although they often produce multiple destructive tracts through the brain in which there may be bone fragments, soft tissues, and clothing. Although a high-velocity bullet may pass through the head without causing impairment of consciousness, brain damage in these circumstances tend to be severe and extensive, likely due to the shockwaves generated by the missile. Any missile injury can result in the formation of a hematoma, which can further complicate injury management and patient outcome.

Blunt Injuries

Blunt injuries frequently result in scalp lacerations, skull fractures, contusions, subdural hematomas (SDHs), epidural hematomas (EDHs), and axonal shear injuries. *Scalp lacerations* can be of considerable importance as sources of blood loss and indications of the site of injury. If there is an associated depressed skull fracture, scalp lacerations represent a potential avenue for intracranial infection.

Skull fractures may involve the cranial vault or skull base and may be classified as linear or depressed. The frequency of skull fractures appears to correlate with the severity of head injury. Patients with a fracture have a much higher incidence of intracranial hematoma than patients without a fracture. A depressed skull fracture is considered to be compound if an associated scalp laceration extending through the pericranium is present, and penetrating if a dural laceration exists. Depressed fractures are more likely to provide potential routes for intracranial infections than linear fractures, and are associated with an increased incidence of post-traumatic epilepsy. Skull base fractures may also be complicated by intracranial infections, as organisms may spread from the air sinuses or the middle ear, especially in the setting of an undiagnosed or untreated cerebrospinal fluid (CSF) fistula (CSF rhinorrhea or otorrhea).

Intracranial hemorrhage is a common complication of head injury and is the most common cause of clinical deterioration and death in patients who experienced a lucid interval after injury. Intracranial injury may be subdivided into extra-axial hematomas, which include EDHs, SDHs, subarachnoid hemorrhages, and intracerebral hematomas which arise within the parenchyma of the brain. Although intracranial hematomas can be identified on initial CT evaluation, the severity of its clinical manifestations along with the potential for delayed neurologic deterioration are due in large part to the time it takes for the hematoma to attain a size sufficient to cause brain distortion and herniation, as well as the development of associated edema. Expanding hematomas should be distinguished from delayed hematomas, which are described as lesions that occur more than 24 h after the time of injury that are not evident on initial imaging studies.

Most intracranial hematomas develop within the first 48 h after injury, but SDHs may also be subacute (2–14 days after injury) or chronic (more than 14 days after injury).

Epidural hematomas or EDHs (❯ *Fig. 24-1*) often result from hemorrhage from a meningeal artery, most often a branch of the middle meningeal artery, and are associated with overlying skull fractures in 90% of adult patients. The incidence of skull fractures is lower in children with EDHs. EDHs occur most often in the temporal region but 25% occur elsewhere, such as in the frontal and parietal regions or within the posterior fossa, where they may occur as a result of venous sinus injury. Occasionally, these hematomas are multiple. As the hematoma enlarges, it strips the dural from the skull, forming an elliptical mass that is limited by the dural investment into the calvarial sutures. In patients who experience a lucid interval, there is often little evidence of other types of brain injury. If however, the patient has been in a coma from the time of the original injury, other types of brain injury are likely to

◻ **Figure 24-1**
Epidural hematoma. Note the lentiform nature and the significant mass effect on the ventricular system, with left to right shift. Most of these lesions arise from damage to the middle meningeal artery or other dural vessels, and are often associated with skull fractures

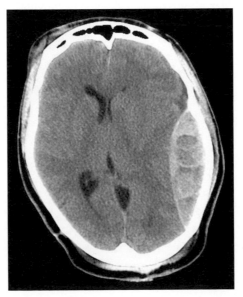

be present. Isolated EDHs of <30 ml in volume infrequently cause an alteration in the level of consciousness or a focal neurologic deficit.

Subdural hematomas or SDHs (❯ *Fig. 24-2*) are brought on by the rupture of the bridging veins that connect cortical veins to dural venous sinuses or from a laceration in a cortical artery. Subdural veins are sensitive to the rate at which they are deformed by acceleration (strain-sensitive). The general morbidity and mortality rates are greater for subdural hematomas than for EDHs because of the higher incidence of concurrent brain damage. SDHs are classified by their appearance, classically on CT imaging, as follows: acute when the hematoma is composed of clotted blood that appears hyperdense to brain tissue on noncontrast head CT; subacute when composed of a mixture of clotted and fluid blood that appears isodense to brain tissue; or chronic when composed purely of liquefied blood and proteins mixed with CSF that appears hypodense to brain tissue. The clotted blood remains for at least 48 h and sometimes several days. The transition to a more fluid blood is largely due to the action of fibrinolytic enzymes that dissolve the clot. These enzymes start this dissolution within 72–96 h after clot formation. After about 3 weeks, no clot remains. In about 25% of patients who undergo evacuation of an acute SDH, acute brain edema occurs in the hemisphere underlying the clot and portends a poor prognosis.

Cerebral contusions have long since been considered the hallmark of head injury. Contusions occur characteristically in the frontal and temporal poles and on the inferior surfaces of the frontal and temporal lobes where the brain tissue comes in contact with the protuberances at the skull base. In early stages, they are hemorrhagic and swollen, but with time they evolve into shrunken gliotic scars. Because the damage is focal, patients with severe contusions may have an uneventful recovery from head injury, provided that they do not develop complications leading to other types of brain damage and that they do not sustain diffuse axonal injury (DAI) at the time of original injury. Contusions can be further subdivided into fracture contusions, coup contusions, contra-coup contusions, and herniation contusions. Fracture contusions occur at the site of a fracture and are particularly severe in the frontal lobe. Coup contusions occur at the site of injury in the absence of a fracture. Contra-coup contusions

❑ Figure 24-2

Subdural hematoma (SDH). Note the convex shape of the lesion. SDHs are usually associated with acute underlying brain injury and generally have a worse prognosis than epidural hematomas (EDHs)

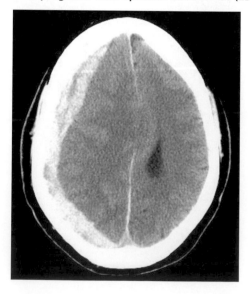

in the brain occur diametrically opposed to the point of injury as a result of brain movement within the calvarium. Herniation contusions occur when the medial parts of the temporal lobes are impacted against the edge of the tentorium, or the cerebellar tonsils are impacted against the foramen magnum at the site of the injury.

Intracerebral hematomas (● *Fig. 24-3*) are found in approximately 15% of all patients who sustain fatal head injuries. These hematomas may be single or multiple, and occur primarily in the frontal and temporal regions. They most likely result from a direct rupture of intrinsic cerebral blood vessel in relation to contusions at the time of injury.

Diffuse axonal injury, or DAI, occurs when the head and brain are subject to severe rotational forces, and is characterized by the shearing of nerve fibers at the moment of injury. The clinical presentation of DAI remains varied. Patients may present with brief periods of altered consciousness or may remain in a coma for extended periods of time. In severe cases, patients with DAI are left in a persistent vegetative state or may expire depending on the severity of concurrent secondary injury. Patients with DAI have a statistically lower incidence of lucid intervals, skull fractures, cerebral contusions, intracerebral hematomas, and evidence of elevated intracranial pressures (ICPs). In the absence of magnetic resonance imaging (MRI) or characteristic CT findings, the diagnosis of DAI is largely exclusionary, encompassing a spectrum of patients with severe closed head injury and a paucity of findings on noncontrast head CT. In its most severe form, DAI is characterized by focal lesions in the corpus callosum, focal lesions in the dorsolateral aspect of the rostral brainstem, and evidence of diffuse injury to axons. These focal lesions may be evident as petechial hemorrhages on a noncontrast CT scan. Since the advent of the MRI with its high sensitivity for parenchymal injury, the definition of DAI has been expanded to include patients with nonhemorrhagic areas of T2 signal within the white matter or at the gray–white junction.

■ Figure 24-3

Multiple intraparenchymal hematomas. These lesions arise within the parenchyma of the brain itself and indicate a significant injury to the brain itself. They can produce mass effect and also may evolve over the days post-injury to produce edema, which may produce increases in ICP if the hematoma is not evacuated surgically

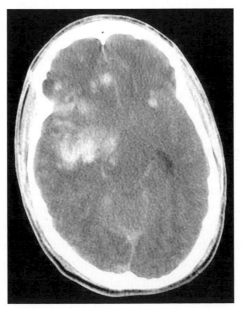

Secondary Brain Injury

An increase in the volume of all or part of the brain is common in patients who sustain severe blunt head injury. The resultant edema may be severe enough to raise the ICP and cause death from brain shift, herniation, and secondary damage to the brainstem. The brain swelling is largely due to an increase in cerebral blood volume (congestive brain swelling) or water content of the brain tissue (cerebral edema). Brain swelling can be classified into three types: swelling adjacent to contusions, diffuse swelling of one cerebral hemisphere, and diffuse swelling of both cerebral hemispheres.

Swelling of the brain adjacent to contusions is common and is due to physical disruption of the tissue with damage to the blood brain barrier and loss of normal physiologic autoregulation of arterioles. Water and electrolytes leak into the brain tissue and spread into the adjacent white matter.

Diffuse swelling of one cerebral hemisphere is most often seen in association with an ipsilateral acute SDH. When the hematoma is evacuated, the brain simply expands to fill the space created. This is attributed to engorgement of a nonreactive vascular bed with regional loss of normal autoregulation and can be accompanied by superimposed ischemia. The initiation of swelling results from cerebral vasodilatation followed by a breakdown of the blood brain barrier, leading to cerebral edema. Some authorities have suggested that in a patient in whom a SDH is not clinically apparent until 2–3 days after the injury, the progressive development of brain swelling is more likely the cause of clinical deterioration and elevated ICP than hematoma expansion.

Diffuse swelling of both cerebral hemispheres tends to occur in young patients. The pathogenesis of this type of brain damage is unclear, but in the pediatric population, dysfunctional autoregulation leading to a loss of vasomotor tone and consequent vasodilatation may contribute to the swelling. If the vasodilatation persists, the blood brain barrier may become defective and true edema may result.

Superimposed ischemic and hypoxic brain damage is common in patients that sustain severe blunt traumatic head injury. It is significantly more common in patients who sustain a clinical episode of hypotension or hypoxia (systolic blood pressure (SBP) < 80 mmHg for at least 15 min, or a PaO_2 < 50 mmHg at some time after injury) than in those who do not. Such damage is also more common in patients who experience high ICPs. A significant correlation also exists between ischemic brain damage in patients who sustain blunt head injury and arterial spasm. The presence of ischemic damage in arterial watershed areas suggests that the patient may sustain a period of cerebral perfusion failure due to an episode of hypotension. Ischemic damage is thus another potential cause of traumatic coma in the absence of an intracranial mass lesion. Such damage is also a frequent finding in patients who remain vegetative or severely disabled after sustaining a head injury.

Evaluation and Management of Severe Closed Head Injury

Early clinical recognition and radiographic diagnosis are key initial steps in the management of head injury. Also important is the need for serial clinical and radiographic assessment of the head-injured patient as the primary thrust of management should be geared towards determining whether the patient has a lesion that requires urgent neurosurgical attention. The initial neurologic assessment of a head-injured patient should be prompt and aimed at evaluating the patient's level of consciousness, as well as symmetry of neurologic function from head to toe. This should include a determination of the patient's Glasgow Coma Scale (GCS) score, a cranial nerve exam that evaluates pupillary function, extraocular movements, facial symmetry, and vital cranial nerve reflexes, as well as a good motor exam. A thorough motor examination, however, may be difficult owing to the presence of other systemic injury, other ongoing diagnostic and therapeutic maneuvers, and lack of patient cooperation. The data acquired are an important indicator of the significance and severity of possible cerebral and brainstem compression. In a pharmacologically paralyzed patient, the pupillary exam encompasses the entirety of the neurologic examination and must be performed in an accurate and serial fashion.

A prompt radiographic evaluation with a noncontrast head CT scan should follow the neurologic assessment, but may be delayed depending on the patient's resuscitative needs and the resources of the treating facility. The identification of a mass lesion or significant alteration in GCS should prompt an urgent neurosurgical consultation.

Surgical Management

In 2006, the Congress of Neurologic Surgeons formed guidelines for the surgical management of traumatic brain injury (TBI). The guidelines are briefly summarized as follows:

- EDHs > 30 ml in volume should be surgically evacuated regardless of the patient's GCS score. Patients with an acute EDH in coma (GCS < 9) with pupillary asymmetry should undergo surgical evacuation as soon as possible.
- An acute SDH with thickness > 10 mm or a midline shift > 5 mm on CT scan should be surgically evacuated regardless of GCS score. All patients with acute SDH in coma should undergo ICP monitoring. A comatose patient with an SDH < 10 mm thickness and a midline shift < 5 mm should undergo surgical evacuation if the GCS score decreases between the time of injury and hospital admission by two or more points, and/or the patient presents with asymmetric or fixed and dilated pupils, and/or the ICP exceeds 20 mmHg.
- Patients with parenchymal mass lesions (contusions and intracerebral hematomas) and signs of progressive neurological deterioration referable to the lesion, medically refractory intracranial hypertension, or signs of mass effect on CT scan should be treated operatively. Patients' GCS scores of 6–8 with frontal or temporal lesions < 20 ml in volume with a midline shift of at least 5 mm and/or cisternal compression on CT scan, and patients with any lesion > 50 cc in volume should be treated operatively.

Medical Management

In the absence of a surgical lesion, rapid and aggressive medical management should be instituted. The medical management of the head-injured patient is directed largely at supportive therapy, as well as the prevention and treatment of the secondary effects of traumatic head injury which manifest primarily as raised ICP.

We tend to err on the side of initiating aggressive treatment of patients with presumed severe TBI (GCS < 8) before a radiographic diagnosis is made because we believe that the rapid initiation of therapeutic measures is paramount in preventing insults that may result from the secondary effects of traumatic head injury. Our treatment strategy is based largely on guidelines set forth by the Brain

Trauma Foundation and Joint Section on Neurotrauma and Critical Care of the AANS in 2000 entitled Management and Prognosis of Severe Traumatic Brain Injury, and is summarized below. While much of this summary comes directly from these guidelines, we have indicated our favored management approaches wherever appropriate.

General Care and Supportive Measures

Hypotension (SBP < 90 mmHg) and hypoxia (apnea, cyanosis, and oxygen (O_2) saturation < 90% in the field or a PaO_2 < 60 mmHg) must be monitored, and avoided if possible or corrected immediately in severe TBI patients. The mean arterial pressure (MAP) should be maintained above 90 mmHg through the infusion of fluids, and judicious use of vasopressors if necessary. Patients who are unable to maintain their airway or remain hypoxemic despite supplemental O_2, must have their airway secured, preferably by endotracheal intubation. Central venous pressure and invasive blood pressure monitoring are mandatory. A Swan-Ganz catheter should be considered strongly in patients with cardiopulmonary disease or those requiring extensive vasopressor therapy. Red blood cell rheology, as well as the oxygen-carrying capacity of blood, should be optimized by maintaining a hematocrit between 30% and 34%. All efforts should be made to avoid hyperglycemia as this can be common in head-injured patients, and may aggravate cerebral edema and secondary injury. Strict glycemic control with frequent blood glucose checks and treatment of elevated levels (<150 mg/dl) with subcutaneous or IV insulin is strongly encouraged. As a treatment option, anticonvulsants may be used to prevent early post-traumatic seizures (seizures occurring within 7 days of the initial injury) in patients at high risk for seizures following head injury. Prophylactic therapy should last no longer than 7 days. Phenytoin and carbamazepine have been shown to be effective in preventing early post-traumatic seizures. However, there is not sufficient evidence to demonstrate that the prevention of early post-traumatic seizures improves outcome following head injury. The use of steroids is not recommended for improving outcome or reducing ICP in patients with severe TBI, as it has not been shown to improve outcome and results in increased complication rates.

Intracranial Pressure Monitoring

ICP monitoring is appropriate in patients with GCS scores of 3–8 after adequate cardiopulmonary resuscitation and abnormal head CT that reveals hematomas, edema, contusions, or compressed basal cisterns. It is appropriate in patients with GCS scores of 3–8 with normal head CT if two or more of the following are noted on admission: age > 40 years, unilateral or bilateral posturing, SBP < 90 mmHg. It is not routinely indicated in patients with mild (GCS 13–15) to moderate (GCS 9–12) head injury; however, a physician may choose to monitor ICP in certain conscious patients with traumatic mass lesions. In the current state of technology, the ventricular catheter connected to an external strain gauge is the most accurate, low-cost, and reliable method of monitoring ICP. It also allows therapeutic CSF drainage. Parenchymal ICP monitoring is similar to ventricular ICP monitoring, but has the potential for measurement drift. Subarachnoid, subdural, and epidural monitors are currently less accurate. The authors' monitor of choice is the ventricular catheter for reasons expressed above. However, in patients with small ventricles, we elect to place a parenchymal monitor if attempts at ventricular cannulation are unsuccessful.

Management of Elevated Intracranial Pressure

Elevations in ICP are tolerated poorly in head injury patients compared with normal individuals because of concomitant dysfunctional autoregulation, brain swelling, and underlying hypoxic ischemic damage (❯ *Table 24-1*). The intracranial cavity consists of CSF, blood, and brain parenchyma. Following head injury, several mechanisms are set in motion in an attempt to counteract ICP elevations in accordance with the Monroe-Kellie doctrine. Initially, CSF volume is reduced by displacement of CSF from the intracranial to the spinal compartment, as well as increased CSF resorption. Continued increases in ICP are compensated for by decreases in the intracranial volume by venous compression. If the ICP continues to rise, however, compensatory mechanisms are exhausted, intracranial compliance decreases, and, as a result, smaller changes in volume lead to larger elevations of ICP. ICP treatment should be initiated at an upper threshold of 20 mmHg. Interpretation and treatment of ICP based on any threshold should be corroborated by frequent clinical examination and cerebral perfusion pressure (CPP) data, which is determined by calculating the difference between the MAP and the ICP. CPP should be maintained at a minimum of 60 mmHg. It remains a crude but rapid estimation of blood flow to the brain. If available, more sophisticated determinants of cerebral blood flow (CBF) may be employed. It is important to note that ICP elevations above 20 mmHg are more deleterious to head trauma patients than decreases in CPP below 60 mmHg, and higher CPPs are not as protective in patients with elevated ICPs. Thus every effort should be made to keep the ICP below 20 mmHg.

Elevations in ICP are initially treated with elevation of the patient's head to 30°, mild hyperventilation maintaining the $PaCO_2$ between 30 and 35 mmHg, CSF drainage, hyperosmolar therapy with mannitol or 3% sodium chloride, sedation with diprivan (Propofol), lorazepam (Ativan), midazolam (Versed) and/or morphine, and chemical paralysis. The elevation of the patient's head of bed up to 30–45° while keeping the neck straight and avoiding any constricting devices around the cervical region, helps facilitate venous drainage without compromising the arterial blood supply. Mild hyperventilation results in a decrease in $PaCO_2$, which ultimately leads to cerebral vasoconstriction and a decrease in CBF followed by a decrease in ICP. Mild hyperventilation therapy ($PaCO_2$ between 30 and 35 mmHg) may be useful during long periods of refractory intracranial hypertension. In the presence of increased ICPs, prolonged aggressive hyperventilation therapy ($PaCO_2 < 25$ mmHg) should be avoided in severe TBI given its effects on cerebral perfusion and potential for cerebral ischemia, especially in the first 24 h following injury when cerebral blood flows. For the same reason, prophylactic hyperventilation therapy should be avoided if possible. However, more aggressive hyperventilation therapy ($PaCO_2 < 30$ mmHg) may be necessary for brief periods when there is acute neurologic deterioration.

Mannitol is effective for control of raised ICP after severe TBI. Effective doses range from 0.25 to 1 g/kg body weight. The indications for use of mannitol *prior to* ICP monitoring are signs of transtentorial herniation or progressive neurologic deterioration not attributable to extracranial complaints. The patient's fluid status must be monitored closely, especially when there is concomitant use of diuretics to ensure the avoidance of hypovolemia and hypotension. Mannitol increases the osmolality of blood acutely, which helps withdraw water from the brain into the bloodstream. It is effective only with an intact blood brain barrier, however, and a delayed rebound phenomenon of elevated ICP can occur secondary to the entry of mannitol into the brain. It also functions as a free radical scavenger and decreases blood viscosity, which transiently increases CBF and triggers cerebral vasoconstriction, which in turn acutely lowers ICP. Serum osmolarity should be kept below 320 mOsm due to concerns for renal failure. Intermittent boluses may be more effective than a continuous

◼ Table 24-1

Outline of management strategy to treat elevated ICP

First-line therapy	*Positional changes*
	Maintain head of bed at 30–45°
	Keep neck straight
	Avoid constrictive devices about cervical spine
	Control PaCO$_2$
	Mild hyperventilation
	(maintain PaCO$_2$ between 30–35 mmHg)
	Hyperosmolar therapy
	Mannitol
	Hypertonic saline
	Sedation
	Diprivan (Propofol)
	Lorazepam (Ativan)
	Midazolam (Versed)
	Chemical paralysis
Second-line therapy	*Aggressive hyperventilation*
	(maintain PaCO$_2$ < 30 mmHg; short duration only)
	High-dose barbiturate therapy
	Decompressive craniectomy

infusion of mannitol. Hypertonic saline (3% or 7.5% NaCl; some investigators use even higher concentrations) is an accepted alternative to mannitol. Like mannitol, it is effective in treating elevated ICP, and has favorable effects of cerebral perfusion and red blood cell rheology. However, it has a more favorable side-effect profile and is the authors' preferred choice for hyperosmolar therapy in the setting of prolonged (> 3–5 days) intracranial hypertension.

Precipitous spikes in ICP should be evaluated with a noncontrast head CT scan. This is aimed at detecting a surgical lesion before it contributes to refractory intracranial hypertension.

"Second-Line" Therapy for Persistent Elevated Intracranial Pressure

In the event that the above-described measures are unsuccessful in addressing elevated ICPs, "second-line" therapy may be instituted. These measures are so named because they are either effective therapies with significant risks or are unproven in terms of benefit on outcome. They include aggressive hyperventilation, high-dose barbiturate therapy, hypothermia, and decompressive craniectomy.

High-dose barbiturate therapy may be considered in hemodynamically salvageable, severe TBI patients with intracranial hypertension refractory to maximum medical and surgical ICP-lowering therapy. The benefits of barbiturates stem from vasoconstriction in normal areas (shunting blood to ischemic brain tissue), decreased metabolic demand for oxygen (CMRO2) with accompanying reduction of CBF, free radical scavenging, reduced intracellular calcium, and lysosomal stabilization. The primary side effect is hypotension due to barbiturate-induced direct myocardial depression and reduction of sympathetic tone, which leads to peripheral vasodilatation.

Induced hypothermia carries many systemic side effects including pneumonia, thrombocytopenia, pancreatitis, renal failure, and myocardial depression. Whole-body temperature reductions are slowly giving way to focal cerebral hypothermia, which appears to have a lower side-effect profile.

Decompressive craniectomy involves the removal of a portion of the calvaria with or without the resection of large areas of contused brain. This measure remains controversial, as results of clinical studies to date have been inconsistent and remain under investigation.

Selected Readings

Bullock MR, et al. (2000) Guidelines for the management of severe traumatic brain injury. American Association of Neurologic Surgeons, Joint Section on Neurotrauma and Critical Care & Traumatic Brain Trauma Foundation, New York

Bullock MR, et al. (2006) Guidelines for the surgical management of traumatic brain injury. Neurosurgery 58(Suppl 3):S2–vi

Lyons MK, Meyer FB (1990) Cerebrospinal fluid physiology and the management of increased intracranial pressure. Mayo Clinic Proc 65:684–707

Rea GL, Rockwold GL (1983) Barbiturate therapy in uncontrolled intracranial hypertension. Neurosurgery; 12:401–404

Tindall GT, Cooper PR, Barrow DL (1996) The practice of neurosurgery, Vol 2. William & Wilkins, Baltimore, MD, pp 1385–1425

Wilkins RH, Rengachary SS (eds) (1996) Neurosurgery, 2nd edn 3 vols. McGraw-Hill, New York, pp 2624–2634

25 Pulmonary Embolism

Lisa K. McIntyre · Lorrie A. Langdale

Pearls and Pitfalls

- Clinical presentation is variable.
- Hypoxemia, respiratory alkalosis, and tachypnea are common but not diagnostic.
- Assessment of clinical risk is crucial to determine the degree of diagnostic testing.
- Spiral CT angiogram of the chest is a cost-effective and accurate initial diagnostic study.
- Ventilation-perfusion scanning is an acceptable study for patients with a contraindication to CT.
- The finding of a DVT with duplex scanning can confirm the diagnosis of PE when the clinical presentation and other diagnostic tests are indeterminate; a negative duplex, however, is insufficient to rule out the diagnosis of PE.
- Initial treatment depends on the degree of physiologic compromise:
  - In hemodynamically stable patients, anticoagulation with unfractionated or low molecular weight heparin is the treatment of choice.
  - In hemodynamically unstable patients, thrombolysis or embolectomy should be considered.
- Vena cava filters are indicated for patients with contraindications for anticoagulation or failure of anticoagulation.
- Prevention and prophylaxis strategies are dependent on individual risk factors.

Introduction

Despite heightened awareness and advances in technology, the nonspecific clinical presentation of pulmonary embolism continues to pose a diagnostic and management challenge. In autopsy studies by Legere and co-authors, pulmonary emboli (PE) were detected in more than 25% of deaths; 70% of these cases were not clinically apparent prior to the patient's demise. Overall, PE complicates the course of approximately 10% of patients with deep venous system thrombosis (DVT). Thrombi involving the lower extremities proximal to the popliteal fossa present the highest risk. More distal clots are associated with emboli in up to 13% of patients, but as many as 50% of those with documented PE have no leg symptoms or identifiable source of clot. In addition, approximately 10% of upper extremity thrombi embolize to the pulmonary vasculature, an incidence that is further increased when thrombi are associated with central venous catheters. Although the majority of emboli do not result in death, fatalities most often occur within hours of the initial event, emphasizing the need for early diagnosis and intervention.

Physiologically, PE is defined primarily as a ventilation/perfusion (*V/Q*) abnormality in which areas of ventilated lung are not perfused. It is rare for this to be purely a perfusion defect.

Incomplete redistribution of regional blood flow without changes in ventilation, right-to-left shunting of deoxygenated blood, resistance-induced decreases in regional capillary transit time, increased oxygen extraction (secondary to decreased cardiac output), and release of vasoactive mediators from platelets within thrombi and damaged endothelium, each contribute to the varying degrees of shunt and V/Q mismatch that underlie the broad spectrum of clinical presentation. Small emboli that pass through the pulmonary vasculature and lodge in the periphery of the lung are often asymptomatic. The more classic symptoms of pleuritic chest pain, hemoptysis, and dyspnea are only observed when emboli are associated with pulmonary infarction. Moderate-sized emboli, trapped in proximal segmental pulmonary vasculature, are associated with more severe dyspnea and hypoxemia. Larger emboli obstructing the pulmonary outflow tract are responsible for hemodynamic instability and sudden death.

Although hypoxemia, respiratory alkalosis, and tachycardia are common features and trigger the clinical suspicion of pulmonary embolism, these characteristics are neither universal nor specific. Infectious diseases, cardiogenic and noncardiogenic pulmonary edema, traumatic lung injuries, and other forms of respiratory distress, are often associated with a similar constellation of symptoms. On the other hand, while the degree of hypoxemia does correlate with the severity of the clinical PE syndrome, a normal A-a gradient and a normal $PaCO_2$ in a patient breathing room air are insufficient evidence to *rule out* the diagnosis. As many as 10% of patients with documented PE may have normal findings on measurement of blood gases. The spectrum of clinical presentation emphasizes the need for sensitive and specific means of distinguishing pulmonary embolism from other etiologies of respiratory distress.

Risk stratification for individual patients is a critical component to the development of a cost-effective diagnostic and management strategy. Well-recognized independent risk factors for development of DVT and subsequent PE include a history of previous DVT, older age, obesity, malignancy, inherited or acquired hypercoagulability states, recent trauma, and immobility (❯ *Table 25-1*). These same risk

◼ Table 25-1

Major general risk factors for venous thromboembolism (VTE) (Reprinted from Geerts et al., 2004. With permission)

Surgery
Trauma
Immobility, paresis
Malignancy
Cancer therapy
Previous VTE
Increasing age
Pregnancy and postpartum period
Estrogen-containing contraceptives or hormonal replacement therapy
Selective estrogen receptor modulators
Acute medical illness
Heart or respiratory failure
Inflammatory bowel disease
Nephrotic syndrome
Myeloproliferative disease
Paroxysmal nocturnal hemoglobinuria
Obesity
Smoking
Varicose veins
Central venous catheterization
Inherited or acquired hypercoagulability

factors also have a cumulative effect on the risk of DVT/PE. Geerts used a prospective cohort design to stratify surgical patients for their risk of DVT/PE based on age, presence of major or minor risk factors, and clinical setting (● *Table 25-2*). This formula for assessment of risk can be particularly helpful for surgical patients in the perioperative period. Outside the perioperative period, a validated clinical decision tree, such as the Wells Criteria for Assessment of Pre-test Probability of Pulmonary Embolism (● *Table 25-3*), offers an objective way to stratify risk. A point-scoring method correlates data from the

◼ Table 25-2

Stratification of surgical patients according to VTE risk without prophylaxis (Reprinted from Geerts et al., 2004. With permission)

Category	Definition	Calf DVT (%)	Proximal DVT (%)	Clinical PE (%)	Fatal PE (%)
Low risk	Age <40 years, no risk factor, minor surgery	2	0.4	0.2	<0.01
Moderate risk	Presence of only one of the following: Age 40–60 years Major surgery Risk factor present	10–20	2–4	1–2	0.1–0.4
High risk	Age >60 years Age >40 years + major surgery + risk factor present	20–40	4–8	2–4	0.4–1.0
Highest risk	Age >40 years + major surgery and: Previous VTE, cancer, or hypercoagulable condition Major trauma Spinal cord injury Hip/knee arthroplasty Hip surgery	40–80	10–20	4–10	0.2–5

DVT, deep vein thrombosis; PE, pulmonary embolism; VTE, venous thromboembolism.

◼ Table 25-3

Wells criteria for assessment of pre-test probability of pulmonary embolism (Data from Wells et al., 2000)

Criteria	Points
1. Suspected PE	3.0
2. An alternative diagnosis is less likely than PE	3.0
3. Heart rate > 100 beats/min	1.5
4. Immobilization or surgery in previous 4 weeks	1.5
5. Previous DVT/PE	1.5
6. Hemoptysis	1.0
7. Malignancy (on treatment or treated within past 6 months)	1.0

Score	Mean probability of PE	% of Patients with this score	Risk
<2	3.6	40	low
2–6	20.5%	53	medium
>6	66.7%	7	high

history and physical with the probability of PE for any individual patient. Once the risk of PE is calculated, this pre-test probability guides the subsequent work-up and leads to a post-test probability if the diagnosis is not definitive.

Diagnostic Tools

While an integral part of the assessment of respiratory distress, chest radiography is usually of little value in confirming the presence of PE. Increased lucency of a lung field (due to occlusion of the central pulmonary artery), atelectasis, small pleural effusions, or pleural-based wedge defects secondary to pulmonary infarctions are considered to be classic radiographic abnormalities, but they are absent in the majority of patients. As many as 40% of patients with PE have a normal study. The primary value of chest radiography is to rule out other etiologies of pulmonary dysfunction and to provide correlation for matching defects identified on *V/Q* scan.

Pulmonary angiography used to be the reference standard for the diagnosis of PE. Due to a small but significant rate of complications, as well as limited availability in many communities, pulmonary angiography has largely been supplanted by spiral CT angiogram of the chest (CTA). Recent studies confirm that the CTA is a cost-effective diagnostic modality with sensitivity and specificity rates of 90% and 94%, respectively, compared to conventional angiogram. For patients who have a contraindication for CT (e.g., contrast allergy or pregnancy), ventilation-perfusion scanning remains the generally accepted initial procedure of choice. Areas of mismatch, characterized by an absence of perfusion in the presence of normal ventilation, suggest PE. Areas of matching ventilation and perfusion deficits are more consistent with intrinsic lung disease. The sensitivity and specificity of *V/Q* scanning are such that a high probability scan coupled with a high pre-test risk probability yields a true positive diagnosis in 85–96% of cases. Fewer than 5% of patients for whom there is a low clinical suspicion of PE and a low probability scan are ultimately determined to have a thromboembolism and therefore may be safely managed without anticoagulation. The large percentage of patients with suspected PE and indeterminate probability scan, however, remain problematic. Further work-up, guided by their risk stratification and pre-test probability, should precede initiation of therapy.

Diagnostic Strategies

Several decision-analysis strategies combining noninvasive studies have been proposed to maximize diagnostic acumen if a definitive study such as CTA is not available. When the clinical presentation, chest radiography, and *V/Q* scanning suggest an intermediate probability of PE, Doppler examination of the upper or lower extremities can help to "rule in" the diagnosis of PE, if the presence of a DVT is accepted as an accurate surrogate to confirm the diagnosis of PE. Although the sensitivity of color Doppler ultrasonography in symptomatic patients has been reported to be as high as 98%, diagnosis of asymptomatic venous thrombosis, even in high-risk patients, has shown a disappointingly high degree of variability, ranging from 38% to 83%. In addition, since 56–67% of patients with angiographic evidence of PE also have negative lower extremity Doppler ultrasonographic examinations, the absence of ultrasonic evidence of DVT does not eliminate the possibility that PE has already occurred. Contrast-enhanced venography, impedance plethysmography, and radioisotope techniques have not been widely adopted in clinical practice owing to limitations in availability and sensitivity.

Another decision-analysis strategy, which has been tested in critically ill, ventilated patients at risk for a variety of respiratory complications, incorporates additional physiologic alterations associated with PE into the overall assessment of clinical probability. Since pulmonary emboli result in obstruction of perfusion without a change in airway patency, physiologic dead space is typically increased with significant thromboembolism. Physiologic dead space may be calculated by measuring end-tidal carbon dioxide. An abnormal result is typically considered to be >20% and is consistent with, though not diagnostic of, PE. D-dimer is a fibrin degradation product formed by the enzymatic activity of cross-linked fibrin polymers. Although always present in patients with thromboembolic states, D-dimer can also be detected in other physiologic states, such as malignancy, post-injury, and pregnancy. A negative D-dimer assay, therefore, can safely rule out the diagnosis of PE in patients with a low pre-test probability, but a positive assay necessitates further testing. Although neither calculation of a high physiologic dead space nor a positive D-dimer test is specific to the diagnosis of PE, their combination does provide some predictive value in that a normal D-dimer and alveolar-dead space percentage carries a false-negative rate of <1%. The positive predictive value of these tests, however, is less certain.

Treatment Strategies

For the majority of patients, anticoagulation with unfractionated heparin remains the therapeutic mainstay for pulmonary embolism. In addition to minimizing the recurrence of PE, anticoagulation limits the long-term sequelae of lower extremity venous stasis associated with an underlying phlebitic obstruction. The immediate goal is to prevent further clot formation. Clot dissolution proceeds through venous fibrinolysis and is largely unaffected by heparin. Therapeutic anticoagulation, as measured by an activated partial thromboplastin time (PTT) of 1.5–2.5 times control values, should be achieved as rapidly as possible since mortality increases in direct proportion to delays in treatment. Patients with excessive levels of heparin-binding proteins will require more than the typical loading dose of 100–200 U/kg, followed by continuous 30,000 U per 24 h infusion of unfractionated heparin to achieve effective anticoagulation. Side effects of heparin include bleeding, hyperkalemia, and thrombocytopenia. Heparin-induced thrombocytopenia and the associated thrombosis syndrome occur in approximately 3% of patients treated with unfractionated heparin and are the result of antibodies to heparin-platelet factor 4 complexes.

In light of these potential complications and following successful trials demonstrating efficacy in DVT prophylaxis, low molecular weight heparins (LMWHs) have been proposed as therapeutic alternatives to unfractionated heparin for the treatment of PE. To date, investigations comparing LMWH to intravenous heparin have shown similar PE recurrence rates, mortality, and bleeding complications. Because these drugs have longer half-lives, LMWHs do offer the benefit of single dose, subcutaneous administration without the need for vigilant monitoring of clotting times. As a result, patients can be treated as an outpatient with LMWHs while awaiting therapeutic anticoagulation with warfarin. However, LMWHs are more difficult to reverse than unfractionated heparin, which poses a potentially significant problem should bleeding complications occur, especially in a post-surgical or post-trauma patient. Conversion to oral warfarin should be started within 3 days of beginning heparin. A transient hypercoagulable state is paradoxically associated with the initiation of warfarin; thus, treatment should overlap intravenous therapy until the international normalized ratio (INR) stabilizes in the therapeutic range (2–3) for at least 48 h.

The choice of initial treatment depends on the severity of physiologic compromise. For patients with *hemodynamic instability*, right-heart failure secondary to massive thromboembolism in the pulmonary outflow tract is usually fatal unless aggressive interventions to relieve the acute obstruction can be employed. In patients for whom there is a high suspicion and probability of PE and no contraindication to therapy, initiation of anticoagulation before imaging studies to confirm the diagnosis should be strongly considered. Supplemental oxygen, mechanical ventilation, invasive hemodynamic monitoring, and inotropic support all have a place in management. If there is no compelling contraindication, early thrombolysis is recommended, as there is clear evidence of improved mortality rates in patients with hemodynamic instability due to PE. Thrombolysis with streptokinase, urokinase, or recombinant tissue-type plasminogen activator (rt-PA) has been advocated as a means of relieving acute pulmonary hypertension and right-heart failure. Unlike heparin, thrombolytics are also effective for the dissolution of established thrombi, and thus may also be useful in the management of patients who present late in their clinical course (up to 14 days after PE).

Debate remains as to the most effective thrombolytic agent. Confounding variables include allergic reactions to streptokinase and urokinase, local versus systemic administration, and the relative balance of clot resolution with the frequency of bleeding complications. While directed thrombolysis offers an effective means for improving pulmonary outflow, the unavoidable systemic effects of clot dissolution pose a significant relative contraindication to its use in the post-trauma or post-surgical patient with coincident massive PE. Surgical embolectomy (Trendelenburg procedure) and catheter embolectomy are safe alternatives in these hemodynamically unstable patients for whom thrombolytic therapy presents an equally life-threatening, potential risk of bleeding. Surgical pulmonary embolectomy may be life-saving, but it is not readily available in most centers. Transvenous catheter pulmonary embolectomy, on the other hand, can be performed in conjunction with diagnostic pulmonary arteriography, avoiding median sternotomy and the potential need for cardiopulmonary bypass. Massive thrombi may be disrupted or extracted (aspirated) in as many as 76% of cases with significant reductions in pulmonary artery pressure and improvement in cardiac function. Treatment should be followed by anticoagulation with standard unfractionated heparin or warfarin therapy. To date, no formal clinical trials comparing directed thrombolysis with embolectomy have been conducted. However, nonrandomized trials comparing catheter embolectomy and heparin to surgical embolectomy and vena cava clipping show similar survival rates.

The placement of a vena cava filter is an appropriate alternative in hemodynamically stable patients with an absolute contradiction to anticoagulant therapy (e.g., head trauma), complications requiring cessation of anticoagulation, or recurrent embolism in the setting of appropriate therapy. In recent years, the use of temporary, retrievable filters have grown in use and are attractive as a "bridge to therapy" when the clinical condition may permit eventual anticoagulation.

Outcomes

Resolution of DVT and respiratory compromise associated with primary and recurrent PE depends on the clinical treatment strategy. Although recanalization occurs in 99% of leg vein segments after anticoagulation therapy, a single episode of DVT increases the risk of developing chronic lower extremity valvular incompetence by a factor of 10. The post-phlebitic syndrome, characterized by stasis ulcerations and limitations to ambulation, carries the added personal and economic costs of poor wound healing and limitations to activity with secondary work restrictions.

The duration of warfarin anticoagulation to treat DVT complicated by PE is the subject of ongoing debate. Indeed, the duration of therapy is dependent on a patient's underlying risk factors for developing DVT and whether these risk factors are temporary (e.g., post-surgical), permanent (e.g., in the setting of coagulation disorders), or idiopathic. The risks of bleeding should also be considered for patients who need long-term or lifelong anticoagulation. Three months of anticoagulation is usually adequate for patients who have an identifiable and temporary risk factor for DVT; the recurrence rate in this population is low. Recommendations for patients with underlying coagulation disorders have not been established with clinical trials. However, patients with an associated malignancy; factor V Leiden defect; deficiencies of plasminogen, plasminogen activator, anti-thrombin III, or protein C or S; myeloproliferative disorders, including polycythemia vera; systemic lupus erythematosus; homocystinuria; and those with "idiopathic" causes for DVT, should probably remain on anticoagulants for at least 6 months, if not indefinitely, after a single episode of venous thrombosis.

A small percentage of patients develop chronic thromboembolic pulmonary hypertension (CTEPH) after PE despite appropriate anticoagulation therapy. This frequently underdiagnosed syndrome is surgically correctable, but must be distinguished from primary pulmonary hypertension complicated by right-sided heart failure. These patients present with gradual onset of worsening exertional dyspnea, hypoxemia, and right-sided heart failure after an asymptomatic period. The early clues to the diagnosis include disproportionately severe symptoms that are unexplained by spirometric measurements and the presence of flow murmurs over the lung field. Pulmonary and hemodynamic signs and symptoms progress without evidence of new perfusion defects on serial V/Q scans, suggesting the involvement of smaller, peripheral pulmonary vessels in the presence of a partially recanalized, proximal pulmonary vasculature. A modest degree of resting pulmonary hypertension, which may be demonstrated with echocardiography, is markedly worsened by exercise. Right-sided heart catheterization in addition to pulmonary angiography is essential to quantify the degree of pulmonary hypertension, rule out competing diagnoses, and define the surgical accessibility of the obstructing thrombotic lesions. This procedure should be delayed for several months after an acute embolic event to allow for maximal resolution and organization of the embolus and avoid an interruption of anticoagulant therapy. Regardless of whether surgical intervention is entertained, patients with demonstrated CTEPH should receive lifelong anticoagulation with a goal INR between 2 and 3.

Surgical treatment of chronic pulmonary thromboembolism is appropriate for symptomatic patients but requires a multidisciplinary approach for diagnosis and management. Careful selection, especially with respect to comorbidities, is mandatory because of the procedural morbidity and mortality, as well as the observation that not all patients with CTEPH benefit from surgery. For those patients not considered surgical candidates, treatment with sildenafil (phosphodiesterase-5 inhibitor) and bosentan (endothelin receptor antagonist) have shown promising preliminary results but have yet to be tested in controlled trials.

Prevention

Clearly, if improved clinical outcomes are to be realized and the complications of PE avoided, practitioners should focus on prevention. The high incidence and potentially devastating consequences of venous thromboembolism mandate the use of DVT prophylaxis in patients at risk. Well-controlled clinical trials have documented the positive impact of prophylactic pharmacologic regimens and intermittent pneumatic compression devices in patients with two or more significant risk factors. Despite wide acceptance of these data, preventive measures are often omitted from routine medical practice.

In addition to serving as a guide to diagnostic testing, assessment of clinical risk is crucial to appropriate prevention strategies. The majority of controlled trials delineating the risk of thromboembolism have focused on surgical patients. Available data, however, suggest that relative risk reductions in the incidence of DVT are comparable between medical and surgical patients. The risk stratification scheme proposed by Geerts offers prophylaxis guidelines based on risk. These guidelines are recommended by the American College of Chest Physicians and were developed after extensive review of the literature and expert consensus (❷ *Table 25-4*).

Many studies have proposed the use of vena cava filters as primary prophylaxis in certain patient populations. Studies assessing the long-term effects of permanent vena cava filters have demonstrated a decreased risk of PE but no difference in mortality and an increase in the risk of recurrent DVT. The use of retrievable filters is an attractive option in those patients where the contraindication to anticoagulation is thought to be temporary. After filter removal, these patients need anticoagulation for only a defined period of time and thus avoid the long-term complications of a permanent filter and prolonged anticoagulation. However, reports vary widely (15–87%) as to the actual rate of successful retrieval of these temporary filters. Furthermore, since most retrievable filters are relatively new, there are no data as to their long-term performance if they are not retrieved.

❑ Table 25-4

Guidelines for prophylaxis of venous thromboembolism in surgical patients according to risk category (Data from Geerts et al., 2004)

Category	Definition	Prevention strategy
Low risk	Age <40 years, no RF, minor surgery	Aggressive and early mobilization
Moderate risk	Presence of only one of the following: Age 40–60 years Major surgery RF present	LDUH every 12 h, LMWH, or GCS/IPC (if bleeding risk)
High risk	Age >60 years Age >40 + major surgery + RF present	LDUH every 8 h, LMWH, or IPC (if bleeding risk)
Highest risk	Age >40 + major surgery and: Previous VTE, cancer, or hypercoagulable condition Major trauma Spinal cord injury Hip/knee arthroplasty Hip surgery	LMWH (trauma, spinal cord injury) LDUH every 8 h + GCS/IPC or LMWH + GCS/IPC Consider extended prophylaxis for cancer or spinal cord injury

GCS, graduated compression stockings; IPC, intermittent pneumatic compression; LDUH, low-dose unfractionated heparin; LMWH, low-molecular weight heparin; VTE, venous thromboembolism, RF, Risk factor.

Selected Readings

Ansell J (2005) Vena cava filters: do we know all that we need to know? Circulation 112:298–299

Geerts WH, Pineo GF, Heit JA, et al. (2004) Prevention of venous thromboembolism: the Seventh ACCP Conference on Antithrombotic and Thrombolytic Therapy. Chest 126(Suppl 3):338S–400S. Review

Hoeper MM, Mayer E, Simonneau G, et al. (2006) Chronic thromboembolic pulmonary hypertension. Circulation 113:2011–2020. Review

Jerges-Sanches C, Ramirez-Rivera A, de Lourdes Garcia M, et al. (1995) Streptokinase and heparin versus heparin alone in massive pulmonary embolism: a randomized controlled trial. J Thromb Thrombolysis 2:227–229

Kline JA, Israel EG, Michelson EA, et al. (2001) Diagnostic accuracy of a bedside D-dimer assay and alveolar dead-space measurement for rapid exclusion of pulmonary embolism: a multicenter study. JAMA 285:761–768

Legere B, Dweik R, Arroliga A (1999) Venous thromboembolism in the intensive care unit. Clin Chest Med 20:367–384, ix. Review

Perrier A, Bounameaux H, Morabia A, et al. (1996) Diagnosis of pulmonary embolism by a decision analysis-based strategy including clinical probability, D-dimer levels, and ultrasonography: a management study. Arch Intern Med 156:531–536

Qanadli SD, Hajjam ME, Mesurolle B, et al. (2000) Pulmonary embolism detection: prospective evaluation of dual-section helical CT versus selective pulmonary arteriography in 157 patients. Radiology 217:447–455

van Erkel AR, van Rossum AB, Bloem JL, et al. (1996) Spiral CT angiography for suspected pulmonary embolism: a cost-effectiveness analysis. Radiology 201:29–36

Wells PS, Anderson DR, Ginsberg J (2000) Assessment of deep vein thrombosis or pulmonary embolism by the combined use of clinical model and noninvasive diagnostic tests. Semin Thromb Hemost 26:643–656. Review

Wells PS, Anderson DR, Rodger M, et al. (2000) Derivation of a simple clinical model to categorize patients probability of pulmonary embolism: increasing the models utility with the SimpliRED D-dimer. Thromb Haemost 83:416–420

26 Right Ventricular Failure and Cardiogenic Shock

James K. Kirklin · Ayesha S. Bryant

Pearls and Pitfalls

- The most common presentation of acute right ventricular failure includes in the setting of inferior myocardial infarction, usually following acute proximal occlusion of a dominant right coronary artery.
- A key modality for diagnosis of isolated right ventricular failure includes transthoracic echocardiography.
- In the presence of acute right ventricular failure, invasive hemodynamic monitoring with a pulmonary artery catheter facilitates diagnostic and therapeutic decisions.
- Initial therapy of right ventricular failure includes inotropic support (usually with milrinone or dobutamine) and administration of colloid or crystallized solutions to a targeted central venous pressure of 18–22 mmHg in order to provide adequate left ventricular filling.
- The administration of agents such as nitric oxide which directly reduce pulmonary vascular resistance is a key component of therapy for right ventricular failure.
- Cardiogenic shock is the leading cause of in-hospital mortality following acute myocardial infarction.
- Despite recent advancements in therapy, hospital mortality approaches 50% when acute myocardial infarction is complicated by cardiogenic shock.
- In profound shock, compensatory mechanisms to support cardiac output such as sympathetic stimulation and peripheral vasoconstriction become maladaptive and contribute to mortality.
- Cardiogenic shock is accompanied by a systemic inflammatory response that potentiates end organ damage.
- Once the clinical syndrome of shock is identified, transthoracic echocardiographic evaluation is essential for identification of a cardiac etiology.
- The current ACC/AHA recommendations for acute MI complicated by cardiogenic shock include early invasive reperfusion for patients less than 75 years of age.
- Intra-aortic balloon pump support and/or mechanical circulatory support should be considered for stabilization of deteriorating hemodynamics and preservation of end-organ function in the presence of cardiogenic shock.
- Despite the high hospital mortality, survivors of myocardial infarction complicated by shock have a favorable long-term outcome.

Right Ventricular Failure

Introduction

Right ventricular failure forms an important subset of congestive heart failure, which affects more than 4.5 million Americans, with over 500,000 new cases diagnosed each year. More prevalent in the elderly, this condition affects approximately 10% of patients over 75 years of age. Furthermore, congestive heart failure is the leading hospital discharge diagnosis in individuals over age 65 years. The pathophysiology of and clinical conditions leading to heart failure provides insights into unique differences between the right and left ventricles, both in normal as well as pathological states.

Pathophysiology of Right Ventricular Failure

The right ventricle consists of two anatomically and functionally distinct cavities (the sinus portion and the outlet chamber or infundibulum). During right ventricular contraction, pressure is generated in the sinus portion with a systolic motion beginning at the apex and moving towards the infundibulum. Due to the compliance of the infundibulum and the relatively thin walled right ventricle, the peak pressure is reduced and prolonged. The right ventricle normally has sustained ejection during pressure development, and this prolonged low-pressure emptying makes the right ventricle very sensitive to changes in afterload. During states of chronically increased afterload, the right ventricle compensates by dilating to maintain stroke volume, though the ejection fraction is reduced and the synchronized contraction of right ventricular components is lost. With increased afterload, the isovolumic contraction phase and ejection time are prolonged, which increases myocardial oxygen consumption.

The right ventricle is primarily perfused by the right coronary artery, with the supply of some regions via the left anterior descending artery. In contrast to left ventricular perfusion, which continues predominantly during diastole, right coronary artery blood flow continues during both systole and diastole. In the presence of important pulmonary artery hypertension, the coronary perfusion gradient is less favorable during systole, and right coronary artery flow occurs mainly during diastole, reducing oxygen supply in the presence of increased demand.

Both the right ventricular free wall (supplied by the right coronary artery) and the interventricular septum (supplied by the posterior descending artery and branches of the left anterior descending artery) importantly contribute to right ventricular contraction. Thus, decreases in perfusion pressure to the right coronary artery have an important adverse affect on free wall contraction, and left ventricular dysfunction involving the interventricular septum adversely affects the septal contribution to right ventricular function.

A major contributor to the clinical sequelae of right ventricular failure is tricuspid regurgitation, which is a common component of the failing right ventricle. The tricuspid valve is anatomically more vulnerable to regurgitation induced by ventricular dilatation than the systemic mitral valve, since the tricuspid valve is crescentic in shape (unlike the circular mitral orifice) and the papillary muscles of the right ventricle are multiple and small (compared to the two large papillary muscles of the mitral valve).

Right ventricular ejection fraction is determined by intrinsic right ventricular contractile function and by right ventricular preload and afterload. The deleterious effects of functional derangements of one ventricle on the performance of the other is termed **ventricular interdependence**. Thus, left ventricular failure, with the resultant increase in pulmonary capillary wedge pressure and pulmonary artery pressure, increases right ventricular afterload and subsequent right ventricular dysfunction. When right ventricular end diastolic volume is increased secondary to chronic increases in right ventricular afterload, the resultant shift of the interventricular septum towards the left ventricular cavity during diastole (contributed to in part by the restrictive effect of the pericardium on the right ventricular free wall) results in impairment of left ventricular filling. Septal displacement of the failing left ventricle increases right ventricular end diastolic pressure, promotes right ventricular dilatation, and increases the tendency for tricuspid regurgitation.

Clinical Presentation of Right Ventricular Failure

Right ventricular failure can present either acutely or as a chronic manifestation of heart failure. The most common presentation of acute right ventricular failure is in the setting of **inferior myocardial infarction**. The typical situation is acute proximal occlusion of a dominant right coronary artery resulting in extensive right ventricular infarction. When the left coronary circulation is dominant (posterior descending artery arising from the distal circumflex), acute occlusion of the left circumflex coronary artery may result in right ventricular infarction. Marked reduction in right ventricular systolic function with inadequate left ventricular filling produces low cardiac output and hypotension, while the alterations in right ventricular compliance promote increased right atrial and central venous pressure.

Acute right ventricular failure/dysfunction is an important complication following certain **cardiac operations**, in particular cardiac transplantation, mitral valve disease with pulmonary hypertension, certain forms of congenital heart disease, and ischemic heart disease. The transplanted right ventricle is very sensitive to increased afterload, and the right ventricle is more susceptible than the left ventricle to inadequate myocardial preservation, particularly in the setting of moderate or marked increases in post transplant vascular resistance. In operations for congenital heart disease, such as in repair of tetralogy of Fallot, direct surgical procedures on or within the right ventricle predispose to right ventricular dysfunction secondary to myocardial injury or creation of pulmonary insufficiency by placement of a transannular patch when there is important obstruction at the level of the pulmonary annulus. In the setting of ischemic heart disease or mitral valve disease with pulmonary hypertension, the presence of important left ventricular dysfunction following operation (with the accompanying marked elevation of left atrial pressure) can induce severe pulmonary hypertension in a reactive pulmonary vasculature. Right ventricular failure may ensue, particularly if the right ventricle is already compromised.

Right ventricular failure secondary to **chronic pulmonary hypertension** (whether the primary etiology is chronic left ventricular failure, chronic lung disease, primary pulmonary hypertension, or pulmonary thromboembolic disease) results from chronic pressure overload and associated volume overload when tricuspid regurgitation becomes severe. In this setting, ascites and lower extremity edema may accompany signs and symptoms of low cardiac output.

Diagnosis

The major modality for diagnosis of right ventricular failure is transthoracic echocardiography. Typical findings include marked depression of right ventricular systolic function, dilatation of the right ventricle, and frequently, moderate to severe tricuspid insufficiency. The echocardiogram provides useful information to distinguish right ventricular dysfunction from other conditions which can induce marked right atrial hypertension including constrictive pericarditis, pericardial effusion with tamponade, and severe tricuspid stenosis.

In the presence of true acute right ventricular failure (as opposed to dysfunction), invasive hemodynamic monitoring with a pulmonary artery catheter capable of measuring thermodilution cardiac output greatly facilitates diagnostic and therapeutic decisions. Whether right ventricular failure occurs secondary to acute myocardial infarction, following cardiac surgery, or from other causes, the hallmark of isolated right ventricular failure is the marked discrepancy between right atrial (or central venous) pressure and pulmonary capillary wedge (or left atrial) pressure. Right atrial pressure is nearly always greater than 15 mmHg in the presence of a normal left atrial or capillary wedge pressure (12 mmHg or less). Depending on the severity of right ventricular failure, cardiac index is reduced (usually 2.0 l/min/m^2 or less). The presence or absence of pulmonary artery hypertension critically influences the selection of therapeutic modalities for augmentation of right ventricular function.

Treatment

Therapy for right ventricular failure focuses on treatment of the underlying etiology if specific therapy is available (such as in treatment of acute myocardial infarction) plus interventions directed at preload adjustment, augmentation of right ventricular contractility, and reduction of right ventricular afterload.

Augmentation of Preload

Volume administration is required when right ventricular failure is severe enough that left ventricular filling is inadequate to generate sufficient cardiac output for adequate organ perfusion. This frequently involves infusion of crystalloid or colloid solutions to a targeted central venous pressure of 18–22 mmHg. When right ventricular failure responds to augmentation of contractility or afterload reduction (see below), the lowest right atrial pressure consistent with adequate cardiac output is desirable. This underscores the importance of direct measurement of right atrial and pulmonary artery pressures as well as cardiac output during the first 48–72 h of therapy. Whole blood or packed red blood cells are initially infused to achieve a hematocrit of 36–40. Once the targeted hematocrit is achieved, additional infusions should consist of colloid (albumin or fresh frozen plasma), although compelling evidence is lacking for the superiority of colloid solutions over saline.

Drugs to Increase Contractility

The most desirable inotropes for right ventricular support are those which increase cardiac contractility, while at the same time reducing pulmonary vascular resistance. Milrinone, dobutamine, and isoproterenol produce a variable reduction in pulmonary vascular resistance and are the most commonly employed inotropic agents for right ventricular failure in the presence of normal or nearly normal systemic blood pressure. Milrinone differs from sympathomimetic agents in that it is in the class of phosphodiesterase inhibitors, which do not act through direct stimulation of adrenergic receptors. Instead, their inotropic effects are exerted through inhibition of phosphodiesterase F-3 (a membrane-based enzyme responsible for the breakdown of cyclic-AMP), resulting in increases in calcium influx. In the presence of systemic hypotension combined with right ventricular failure, combination inotropic therapy is often advisable, with agents such as dopamine and milrinone or dopamine and dobutamine. The recommended dosages of various inotropic agents are discussed in the section on *Treatment of Cardiogenic Shock*.

In the presence of systemic hypotension, vasopressin is a particularly effective agent in that it increases systemic blood pressure, and thereby, may indirectly increase right ventricular perfusion and right ventricular contractility even though it does not have direct positive inotropic effects itself. In addition, vasopressin has a direct pulmonary vasodilator effects. When administered in doses of 0.01–0.04 units/kg/min, vasopressin increases systemic vascular resistance while potentially dilating the coronary and pulmonary arterial circulation.

Reduction of Right Ventricular Afterload

As noted in the previous section, inotropic agents such as milrinone, isoproterenol (⊙ *Table 26-1*), and dobutamine, as well as vasopressin may directly reduce pulmonary vascular resistance. Although a number of direct pulmonary vasodilating agents (without inotropic effects) have been utilized in the past, these have been largely supplanted by inhaled nitric oxide, which has profound pulmonary vasodilator effects. Inhaled nitric oxide can be administered via an endotracheal tube when the patient is mechanically ventilated or via face mask administration. Nitric oxide is generally initiated at 20–40 parts per million in the presence of pulmonary hypertension. When right ventricular function improves and a target pulmonary artery pressure of 35–40 mmHg systolic pressure is achieved, gradual tapering of nitric oxide is initiated. When nitric oxide is reduced to less than about 10 parts per million, very slow weaning should be accomplished because of the potential for rebound pulmonary hypertension following abrupt nitric oxide withdrawal. Recently, inhaled prostacyclin has proved useful in the treatment of right heart failure following cardiac surgery.

In the presence of coexisting severe left ventricular dysfunction and elevated left atrial pressure (particularly in the setting of myocardial ischemia), intravenous nitroglycerin (dose 0.5–2 μg/kg/min) is a useful agent to lower left atrial pressure (via a direct coronary vasodilator effect and through increasing systemic venous capacitance) and secondarily neutralize reactive pulmonary hypertension.

◻ Table 26-1

Properties of vasodilator agents (Adapted from Kirklin et al., 2004)

	Systemic arterial vasodilation	Pulmonary arterial vasodilation	Positive inotropic effect	Increase in systemic venous capacitance
Isoproterenol	++	+++	++++	0
Milrinone	+++	+++	+++	0
Nitroprusside	++++	+++	0	0
Nitroglycerin	++	++	0	+++
Prostaglandin E1	+++	+++	0	0
Prostacyclin	++	+++	0	0
Nitric oxide	0	++++	0	0

Additional Therapeutic Strategies

In the setting of acute inferior myocardial infarction secondary to right coronary artery or circumflex occlusion, **emergent revascularization** with thrombolytic agents, angioplasty, or surgical revascularization is advisable. Since approximately one-half of overall right ventricular function is derived from the right ventricular free wall and half from the intraventricular septum, revascularization of these areas may include consideration of right ventricular marginal arteries in the revascularization plan.

In the presence of decompensated heart failure secondary to progressive right ventricular dysfunction, administration of **nesiritide**, a synthetic form of B-type (brain) natriuretic peptide, may facilitate fluid removal when other diuretics have been unsuccessful. This hormone increases sodium and water excretion and decreases renin and aldosterone secretion without activation of the sympathetic nervous system, thus promoting reduction in preload, pulmonary artery pressure, right atrial pressure and systemic vascular resistance. Nesiritide is usually combined with loop diuretic therapy using a planned continuous infusion for 2–3 days. The generally recommended dose includes a 0.3 µg bolus followed by an infusion of 0.015–0.03 µg/kg/min.

When the measures noted above are inadequate in providing effective systemic perfusion, consideration should be given to **mechanical circulatory support** of the right ventricle. The **Abiomed BVS 5000** (Danvers, Mass) is a short term (1–4 weeks) extracorporeal pulsatile pump that can be used for right, left, or biventricular support. The **Thoratec** (Pleasanton, CA) pneumatic paracorporeal ventricular assist device is a longer-term ventricular assist device which has been utilized for right-, left-, or bi-ventricular support in the United States for over 20 years. Anticoagulation with Warfarin and antiplatelet agents is necessary for prevention of thromboembolism. For smaller patients, the Berlin Heart (Berlin, Germany) (approved in Europe but not yet FDA-approved in the United States) provides similar univentricular or biventricular support with a variety of pump sizes down to 10 ml (for infants) (❯ *Fig. 26-1*).

More recently, percutaneous technology that can be applied in the cath lab includes right ventricular support with the Tandem heart (Pittsburgh, PA), which withdraws blood from the right atrium and infuses it directly into the pulmonary artery.

◘ Figure 26-1

The Berlin Heart paracorporeal ventricular assist device is available in a range of pump sizes from 10 to 80 ml (Courtesy of Berlin Heart AG, Berlin, Germany) (Reprinted from International Heart and Lung Transplantation Monograph Series, vol. 1: mechanical circulatory support, copyright 2006. With permission from the International Society for Heart and Lung Transplantation)

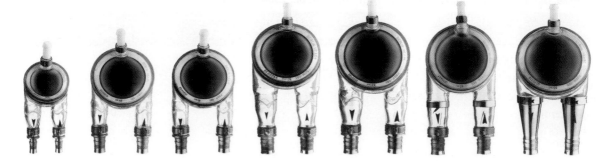

Outcomes

In patients with chronic heart failure the presence of severe right ventricular dysfunction is a powerful predictor of mortality in both dilated cardiomyopathy and in ischemic heart disease. Acute right ventricular failure in the setting of inferior myocardial infarction is associated with approximately a threefold increase in hospital mortality. A dramatic reduction in hospital mortality has been documented with successful primary angioplasty of the coronary vessel causing right ventricular compromise. When acute right ventricular failure complicates cardiac operations, the prognosis is generally favorable when left ventricular function is good and effective cardiac output is restored at a right atrial pressure less than 20 mmHg (without mechanical support) within about 48 h.

Cardiogenic Shock

Introduction

Cardiogenic shock may be defined as inadequate perfusion of the microcirculation to sustain viability of vital organs secondary to a primary cardiac etiology which, if uncorrected, results in death. Cardiogenic shock due to primary pump failure is the leading cause of in-hospital mortality following acute myocardial infarction. Despite numerous advances in the care of patients with myocardial infarction including early revascularization, the mortality remains high, in the range of 50–80% depending upon the specific patient risk profile. With improved understanding of the potential reversibility of stunned or hibernating myocardium following restoration of blood flow, there is a current major emphasis on prompt revascularization. Survivability of cardiogenic shock from other etiologies depends on prompt inotropic and/or mechanical circulatory support of the failing heart.

Pathophysiology

The brain and heart are the two human organs with an absolute aerobic requirement. In an adult at rest, the coronary circulation supplies about 70–80 ml blood/100 g of myocardial tissue/min, from which the myocardium extracts 8–10 ml of O_2/100 g/min. Thus, myocardial mitochondria generate enormous quantities of ATP to meet the cellular ATP demand. During anaerobic metabolism secondary to acute coronary artery occlusion, inadequate ATP generation for surface membrane ion pumps results in marked cellular swelling, which if progressive causes cell death.

In the absence of a mechanical complication of myocardial infarction (such as papillary muscle rupture, ventricular septal defect, or ventricular rupture), an estimated 40% loss of left ventricular myocardium due to severe ischemia or necrosis is required to produce sufficient reduction in stroke volume (and overall cardiac output) to induce cardiogenic shock. Areas of ischemic but not infarcted myocardium are further compromised by the vicious cycle of decreased systolic and increased ventricular diastolic blood pressure, both of which reduce myocardial perfusion pressure (the gradient between coronary diastolic and left ventricular diastolic pressures). In the setting of markedly reduced coronary blood flow secondary to acute vessel occlusion, increasing diastolic pressures associated with pump failure act to increase wall stress, which elevates myocardial oxygen requirements and promotes further ischemia. The metabolic byproducts of reduced organ perfusion, such as lactic acidosis, further depress myocardial function. Compensatory mechanisms to support cardiac output, including sympathetic stimulation to increase heart rate and contractility, produce vasoconstriction which, when severe, reduces renal blood flow and increases left ventricular afterload. These compensatory mechanisms may eventually have a more deleterious than beneficial effect and become *maladaptive,* hastening the spiral toward death.

Another maladaptive response to the development of cardiogenic shock is a systemic inflammatory state which may potentiate end organ damage. Local tissue ischemia and necrosis stimulates the innate immune system, activating complement and leukocytes which increase local capillary permeability, resulting in further tissue damage. Nitric oxide (NO) likely augments the inflammatory response to cardiogenic shock. NO is normally synthesized by endothelial NO synthase and has cardioprotective effects at normal physiologic levels. Cardiogenic shock induces an upregulation of nitric oxide synthase, mediated by Interleukin-6 and possibly other cytokines. At high pathologic levels, NO suppresses mitochondrial respiration and reduces contractility in non-ischemic myocardium. High NO levels also reduce the myocardial inotropic response to β-adrenergic stimulants and cause systemic vasodilation, further promoting the hypotensive state of shock.

Diagnosis

Various criteria have been used to describe the severity of cardiac derangement that constitutes shock. In general, systolic blood pressure is 90 or less in the absence of vasoactive drugs, cardiac index is less than 2.0 l/m/m^2, and there is clinical evidence of end-organ hypoperfusion as indicated by decreased urine output, cool and constricted extremities, and often depressed sensorium. The general clinical features that distinguish cardiac from non-cardiac causes of shock are listed in ❯ *Table 26-2*. Appropriate evaluation for acute myocardial infarction is of the greatest urgency, since emergent revascularization or correction of a mechanical complication of myocardial infarction offers the best chance for survival. Other causes of cardiogenic shock are listed in ❯ *Table 26-3*. Transthoracic-echocardiography is the best modality for the prompt diagnosis of mitral insufficiency or ruptured ventricular septum and assessment of the degree of depression of overall left and right ventricular systolic function. Accumulation of fluid or clot within the pericardial space suggests the possibility of ventricular rupture.

Hemodynamic monitoring with a Swan-Ganz catheter is necessary to quantify the severity of depressed cardiac output and the response to therapy. Large "V" waves on the capillary wedge tracing indicates severe mitral insufficiency and a step-up in oxygen saturation from the right atrium to the pulmonary artery suggests a ruptured interventricular septum. Prompt coronary angiography in the presence of acute myocardial infarction and shock offers the opportunity for prompt revascularization through either angioplasty or emergency surgery.

When cardiogenic shock develops in the absence of acute myocardial infarction, echocardiographic assessment is the cornerstone of diagnosis once the clinical syndrome is identified. Determination of the presence and the severity of ventricular dysfunction is often the most rapid method of distinguishing cardiogenic shock from non-cardiac causes.

◘ Table 26-2

Rapid formulation of a working diagnosis for the cause of shock (Reprinted from Holmes et al., 2003, copyright 2003. With permission from Elsevier)

Diagnostic issue	High-output hypotension: vasodilatory shock	Low cardiac-output hypotension: cardiogenic and hypovolemic shock
Is cardiac output reduced?	No	Yes
Pulse pressure	Wide	Narrow
Diastolic pressure	Extremely low	Low
Extremities, digits	Warm	Cool
Nailbed return	Rapid	Slow
Heart sounds	Crisp	Muffled
Temperature	Abnormally high or low	Normal
White blood cell count	Abnormally high or low	Normal
Site of infection	Present	Absent
	Reduced pump function: cardiogenic shock	Reduced venous return: hypovolemic shock
Is the heart too full?	Yes	No
Symptoms, clinical context	Angina, abnormal ECG	Blood loss, volume depletion
Jugular venous pressure	High	Low
Gallop rhythm	Present	Absent
Respiratory examinations	Crepitations	Normal
Chest radiograph	Large heart, pulmonary edema	Normal
What does not fit?		
Overlapping causes	High right atrial pressure hypotension	Nonresponsive hypovolemia
Septic cardiogenic	High right sided pressure, clear lungs	Adrenal insufficiency
Septic hypovolemic	Pulmonary embolus	Anaphylaxis
Cardiogenic hypovolemic	Right ventricular infarction	Neurogenic shock
	Cardiac tamponade	

◘ Table 26-3

Causes of left ventricular dysfunction in the etiology of cardiogenic shock

Systolic dysfunction
   Myocardial infarction
   Ischemia and global hypoxemia
   Cardiomyopathy
   Myocardial drugs
      Beta-blocker overdose
      Calcium channel blockers
   Myocardial contusion
   Respiratory acidosis
   Metabolic derangements: acidosis, hypophosphatemia, hypocalcemia
Diastolic dysfunction
   Ischemia and global hypoxemia
   Ventricular hypertrophy
   Restrictive cardiomyopathy
   Ventricular interdependence
Greatly increased afterload
   Critical aortic stenosis
   Critical fixed or dynamic left ventricular outflow tract obstruction

Treatment

Initial Management

Initial management includes supplemental oxygen and rapid assessment of circulatory status. In the presence of depressed oxygen saturation despite supplemental oxygen (saturation less than about 90%), if increased work of breathing occurs, or if profound low cardiac output is present, intubation and mechanical ventilation is necessary. Correction of electrolyte abnormalities, detection and treatment of arrhythmias, and management of pain and anxiety should be implemented. The importance of placement of a pulmonary artery catheter is underscored by the frequency of low pulmonary capillary wedge pressure in the face of low cardiac output, indicating the need for fluid administration while accurately monitoring pulmonary artery and central venous pressures.

Inotropic Support

Appropriate selection of inotropic support is a key component of therapy for cardiogenic shock. After initial support with dopamine, norepinephrine, or other alpha adrenergic agents, refinement of inotropic support is directed by the circulatory state, measurements obtained from the pulmonary artery catheter, renal function (and urine output), right and left ventricular function, and the etiology of cardiogenic shock. The specific action and doses of individual inotropes are listed in ❷ *Tables 26-4* and ❷ *26-5*.

◼ Table 26-4

Adrenergic receptor activity and other properties of sympathomimetic amines (Adapted from Kirklin et al., 2004)

	Alpha (peripheral vasoconstriction)	Beta$_1$ (cardiac contractility)	Beta$_2$ (peripheral vasoconstriction)	Chronotropic effect	Arrhythmia risk
Norepinephrine	++++	+++	0	+	+
Epinephrine	+++	++++	+	++	+++
Dopamine[a]	++	+++	+	+	+
Dobutamine	0	+++	++	+	+
Isoproterenol	0	++++	+++	++++	++++
Phenylephrine	++++	0	0	0	0

[a]May cause renal arteriolar dilatation at low doses by stimulating dopaminergic receptors, moderate diuretic effect.

◼ Table 26-5

Standard inotropic doses (Adapted from Kirklin et al., 2004)

Drug	Starting dose (μg/kg/min)	Dosing range (μg/kg/min)
Dopamine	2.5	2.5–20
Dobutamine	2.5	2.5–20
Milrinone	0.2–0.3	0.2–1.0
Epinephrine	0.025	0.025–0.1
Norepinephrine	0.025	0.025–0.1
Isoproterenol	0.025	0.025–0.1

Emergent Revascularization after Acute Myocardial Infarction

Percutaneous angioplasty and stenting of the infarct-related vessel is a cornerstone of current therapy for acute myocardial infarction with shock. Guidelines are less clear about stenoses in non-infarcted-related arteries, but angioplasty can be beneficial if applied to high grade stenoses in vessels which supply a major portion of non-infarcted myocardium.

When emergent catheterization and possible angioplasty are not available, fibrinolytic therapy is recommended for ST-elevation myocardial infarction in patients with cardiogenic shock when there is no contraindication to fibrinolysis.

In the presence of extensive three-vessel coronary artery disease and post-infarction shock, emergency coronary artery bypass surgery is advisable in most instances. Time until revascularization is an important determinant of survival, in that mortality for patients undergoing coronary artery bypass grafting within 18 h of the onset of shock is about 40%, with a significant increase in mortality for longer intervals. ACC/AHA Guidelines indicate that emergency coronary bypass surgery should be considered in patients with cardiogenic shock who have significant left main or severe three vessel disease without major renal or pulmonary comorbidity.

Surgical Therapy for Complications of Acute Myocardial Infarction

In the setting of myocardial infarction complicated by rupture of the interventricular septum or rupture of a papillary muscle with severe mitral regurgitation, early emergent operation with mitral valve repair or replacement and/or surgical closure of the ventricular septal defect is mandatory. All such patients should be treated with intra-aortic balloon support prior to operation. These operations should be undertaken emergently, since the interval between diagnosis and operations is a critical determinant of survival.

Mechanical Circulatory Support

When shock persists despite standard measures including intra-aortic balloon support, inotropic agents and emergency angioplasty, more complex forms of mechanical circulatory support should be considered. Extra-corporeal membrane oxygenator (**ECMO**) support can be rapidly initiated in the intensive care unit setting via percutaneous femoral arterial and venous cannulation. This carries the advantage of rapid percutaneous cardiac support when intra-aortic balloon pumping and other standard interventions are not successful in reversing the shock syndrome. The major disadvantage of ECMO support is the lack of direct decompression of the left atrium with the potential for worsening pulmonary edema, particularly if diffuse capillary leakage (associated with the generalized inflammatory state) is accompanied by persistent elevation of left atrial pressure.

Other standard options for emergent mechanical circulatory support have been described in the earlier section on right ventricular mechanical support, and can provide right, left, or biventricular support. A variety of more chronic implantable volume-displacement or rotary ventricular assist devices are available, but paracorporeal devices are generally preferable in the setting of profound cardiogenic shock of rapid onset. More recently, European centers have reported experience with micro-axial blood pumps, such as the **Impella** (Abiomed – Danvers, MA), which can be inserted through the femoral artery or via a transthoracic approach.

Outcomes

When cardiogenic shock complicates myocardial infarction, the mortality remains excessive. Hospital mortality was approximately 90% during the 1970s and has improved in recent years with aggressive strategies for early reperfusion. Despite these improvements, current hospital mortality is still about 50%. The SHOCK study examined the hypothesis that emergency revascularization for cardiogenic shock due to myocardial infarction results in reduction of 30 day mortality compared with initial medical stabilization and delayed revascularization. Although 30 day mortality between the two groups was not statistically different, the survival at 6 and 12 months was significantly greater in the emergency revascularization group. The benefit of early revascularization was most evident among patients less than 75 years of age. With an aggressive approach to the treatment of post infarction shock, aggressive early revascularization in patients under 75 years of age has reduced overall mortality to about 35%. The rewards of a strategy of aggressive early revascularization (in the cath lab or surgically) are underscored by the very favorable long-term survival of patients who survive to hospital discharge. Among shock patients who survive the first post-infarct year, annual mortality is less than 5%, similar to the general acute infarction population.

Based on the SHOCK trial, the ACC/AHA published a Class 1A recommendation for early invasive reperfusion in acute myocardial infarction complicated by cardiogenic shock for patients younger than 75 years of age; for patients over age 75 invasive intervention was recommended for those with good prior functional status. Current data suggests that an early aggressive invasive approach to myocardial support and revascularization should be the standard of care when acute myocardial infarction is complicated by cardiogenic shock. ACC/AHA Guidelines suggest that intra-aortic balloon pump support and/or ventricular assist devices should be considered for stabilization of deteriorating hemodynamics in preparation for emergent revascularization.

Selected Readings

Antman E, Anbe D, Armstrong P (2004) ACC/AHA guidelines for the management of patients with ST-elevation myocardial infarction-executive summary. A report of the American College of Cardiology/American Heart Association Task Force on Practice Guidelines (Writing Committee to Revise the 1999 Guidelines for the Management of Patients with Acute Myocardial Infarction). J Am Coll Cardiol 44:671–719

Babaev A, Frederick P, Pasta D (2005) Trends in management and outcomes of patients with acute myocardial infarction complicated by cardiogenic shock. JAMA 294:448–454

Blume E, Duncan B (2006) Pediatric mechanical circulatory support in ISHLT monograph series. In: Frazier O, Kirklin J (eds) ISHLT monograph series: mechanical circulatory support. Elsevier, Philadelphia

Cinch J, Ryan T (1994) Current concepts: right ventricular infarction. N Engl Med 330:1211–1217

Hochman J, Sleeper L, Webb J (1999) Should we emergently revascularize occluded coronaries for cardiogenic shock (SHOCK) investigators. Early revascularization in acute myocardial infarction complicated by cardiogenic shock. N Engl Med 341:625–634

Hollenberg S (2004) Recognition and treatment of cardiogenic shock. Semin Respir Crit Care Med 25:661–671

Holmes C, Walley K (2003) The evaluation and management of shock. Clin Chest Med 24:775–789

Kirklin J, Young J, McGiffin D (2004) Heart transplantation, 1st edn. Churchill Livingstone, New York

Mehta S, Eikelboom J, Natarajan M (2001) Impact of right ventricular involvement on mortality and morbidity in patients with inferior myocardial infarction. J Am Coll Cardiol 37:37–43

Sharp R, Gregory A, Mowdy M, Sirajuddin R (2004) Nesiritide for treatment of heart failure due to right ventricular dysfunction. Pharmacotherapy 24:1236–1240

Vida V, Mack R, Castaneda A (2005) The role of vasopressin in treating systemic inflammatory syndrome complicated by right ventricular failure. Cardiol Young 15:88–90

White H, Assmann S, Sanborn T (2005) Comparison of percutaneous coronary intervention and coronary artery bypass grafting after acute myocardial infarction complicated by cardiogenic shock: results from the Should We Emergently Revascularize Occluded Coronaries for Cardiogenic Shock (shock) trial. Circulation 112:1992–2001

27 Nosocomial Pneumonia

Priya Sampathkumar

Pearls and Pitfalls

- Nosocomial pneumonia is the second most common nosocomial infection (after urinary tract infections) and represents the leading cause of nosocomial morbidity and mortality.
- Patients on mechanical ventilation have the highest risk of nosocomial pneumonia. Other patient populations at increased risk of pneumonia include burn, trauma, and cardiothoracic surgery patients.
- The term nosocomial pneumonia includes hospital-acquired pneumonia, ventilator-associated pneumonia, and health care-associated pneumonia. **Health care-associated pneumonia** is a newly described subset of nosocomial pneumonia that develops in patients who are not in the hospital at the time of onset but have had contact with the health care system up to 90 days prior to onset of pneumonia.
- Bacteria cause the majority of nosocomial pneumonia. Fungi are very uncommon causes of nosocomial pneumonia but can occur in immunocompromised hosts. Viruses, such as influenza, also may also cause nosocomial outbreaks.
- Aspiration of micro-organisms from the oropharynx or leakage of organisms around the cuff of the endotracheal tube is the primary mode of entry of bacteria into the lung. Pneumonia develops when host defenses against these organisms are overwhelmed.
- Early hospital-acquired pneumonia and early ventilator-associated pneumonia are likely to be caused by Pneumococcus, Hemophilus, and sensitive gram negative bacilli. In contrast, Pneumonia that occurs later in hospital stay is more likely to be due to multi-drug resistant organisms.
- Congestive heart failure, adult respiratory distress syndrome, and pulmonary contusions can mimic the appearance of pneumonia.
- Culture of lower respiratory tract secretions is the most useful diagnostic test in guiding therapy. Blood and pleural cultures may be helpful in selected situations.
- When treating pneumonia, treat early and aggressively with antibiotics. Target the most likely pathogens. Do not delay administration of antibiotics to obtain cultures.
- Re-evaluate when more data are available; focus phramacologic therapy as soon as possible. Eight days of therapy is probably adequate for most nosocomial pneumonia *except* Pseudomonas pneumonia, where a minimum of 2 weeks is recommended.

Introduction

Nosocomial pneumonia has been defined traditionally as pneumonia that develops more than 48 h after admission to a health care facility, which was not present or developing at the time of admission.

This definition includes the subset of ventilator-associated pneumonia (VAP), which is defined as pneumonia developing >48 h after the onset of mechanical ventilation.

Recently, a new entity has been included in the nosocomial category: *health care-associated pneumonia (HCAP)*, which refers to pneumonia developing in persons who have had contact with the health care system in one or more of the following ways:

1. Received home intravenous antibiotic therapy, chemotherapy, wound care, or hemodialysis within 30 days of onset of pneumonia
2. Resided in a long term care facility or nursing home within 30 days of onset of pneumonia
3. Hospitalized in an acute care hospital for 2 or more days within 90 days of the onset of pneumonia

The reason for the inclusion of HCAP under the nosocomial umbrella is that, although the onset may occur while the patient is in the community, HCAP is usually caused by antibiotic-resistant organisms similar to those seen in hospitalized patients. In addition, the severity, outcome, and recommended treatments resemble those for nosocomial pneumonia rather than for community-acquired pneumonia.

Thus nosocomial pneumonia now represents hospital-acquired pneumonia (HAP), ventilator-associated pneumonia (VAP), and HCAP.

Epidemiology

Nosocomial pneumonia is the second most common nosocomial infection in the United States and is associated with considerable mortality and morbidity. Pneumonia represents the leading cause of deaths due to nosocomial infections, increases hospital duration of stay by an average of 7–10 days, and results in an excess cost of more than US$40,000 per patient. Available data suggest that nosocomial pneumonia occurs at a rate of 5–10 cases per 1,000 hospital admissions, and the incidence increases 6- to 20-fold in mechanically ventilated patients. The risk of VAP is greater in surgical patients compared with medical patients; patients undergoing cardio-thoracic surgery have the highest risk.

The majority of nosocomial pneumonia is caused by bacteria. Occasionally, influenza and respiratory syncytial viruses cause outbreaks of nosocomial pneumonia in high risk patients such as children, the elderly, and immunosuppressed patients. Aspergillus pneumonia can occur in severely immunosuppressed patients, but overall, fungi and viruses are not important causes of nosocomial pneumonia.

Pathogenesis

For nosocomial pneumonia to occur, microbial pathogens first need to gain entry to the lower respiratory tract and then overwhelm normal host defense mechanisms.

Aspiration of micro-organisms from the **oropharynx** or leakage of organisms around the cuff of the endotracheal tube is the primary mode of entry of bacteria into the trachea. Inhalation of microorganisms from contaminated aerosols, hematogenous spread from bloodstream infections, or translocation from the gastrointestinal tract appear to be rare causes of pneumonia. Colonization of the lumen of the endotracheal tube with bacteria encased in a biofilm may play a role in the pathogenesis of VAP.

Factors that increase ease of entry of micro-organisms to the lower respiratory tract (intubation, bronchoscopy, supine positioning) and conditions that predispose to aspiration, such as sedation, altered mental status, tracheoesophageal fistula, gastro esophageal reflux, esophageal stricture, and neuromuscular disorders, increase the risk of pneumonia.

Factors that affect normal host defenses also promote pneumonia. Intubation, pain from surgical incisions, and paralysis impair the cough reflex which is the first line of defense against bacterial entry. Older age, malnutrition, metabolic acidosis, persistent hyperglycemia, and immunosuppressive medications impair both humoral and cell-mediated immunity and the ability of the lungs to clear aspirated micro-organisms. Prolonged antibiotic use and gastric acid suppression make it more likely that the oropharynx and upper airway will be colonized with resistant microorganisms that are more difficult for the body to fight off. Finally, lack of attention to practices of infection control could mean that health care workers carry multi-drug resistant organisms from one patient to another either via contaminated hands or equipment. The above risk factors can also be classified as patient-related, intervention-related, and infection control-related risk factors (❯ *Table 27-1*). Most of the patient-related factors cannot be modified, whereas most of the risk factors in the other two categories can be modified successfully by an educational program.

Etiology: The time of onset of pneumonia is an important predictor of specific causative pathogens. Early onset VAP and HAP, defined as pneumonia occurring within 4 days of hospitalization or intubation usually carry a better prognosis and are more likely to be caused by antibiotic-sensitive bacteria. The organisms most commonly causing pneumonia in this group include *Streptococcus pneumoniae*, *Hemophilus influenzae*, and antibiotic-sensitive gram negative bacilli such as *Klebsiella* and *Enterobacter* species. Late onset HAP and VAP, defined as pneumonia occurring after 5 or more

◻ Table 27-1
Risk factors for nosocomial pneumonia

Patient-related factors
Age >70 years
Severe underlying illness
Malnutrition
Altered mental status
Metabolic acidosis
Hyperglycemia
Intervention-related factors
Intubation and mechanical ventilation
Immunosuppressive medications
Gastric acid suppression
Prolonged antibiotic use
Supine positioning
Surgical procedures on the chest and abdomen
Sedation
Infection control factors
Lack of appropriate hand hygiene by staff
Contaminated respiratory care equipment

days of hospitalization or intubation, tend to be caused by multi-drug resistant pathogens and are associated with poorer outcomes (see ❯ *Table 27-2*). Patients with HCAP who reside in long term care facilities or who have had recent exposure to antibiotics tend to have a spectrum of pathogens that resembles those seen in late onset HAP and VAP.

Pneumonia due to *Staphylococcus aureus* is more common in patients with diabetes, head trauma, patients in intensive care units and those with a recent history of influenza.

Nosocomial pneumonia due to fungi such as *Aspergillus fumigatus* may occur in solid organ or bone marrow/stem cell recipients or in otherwise severely immunocompromised patients. Nosocomial aspergillus infections should prompt a search for an environmental source of fungal spores, such as contaminated air ducts or the dust stirred up by hospital renovation or construction. *Candida* and *Aspergillus* species often colonize the airway of hospitalized patients; however, in the absence of severe immunosuppression, **those fungal species do not cause pneumonia** and do not require treatment. Influenza A can be the cause of nosocomial outbreaks during the influenza season (typically fall and winter). Respiratory syncytial virus (RSV) outbreaks are common in pediatric settings but can also occur in adult patients, especially those with hematologic malignancies.

Diagnosis

Diagnostic tests are important for two reasons: to decide whether pneumonia is the explanation for the patient's signs and symptoms and, second, to determine the etiologic pathogen. The best strategy to make the diagnosis of nosocomial pneumonia remains controversial. In most patients who are not intubated and who are immunocompetent, the diagnosis is made clinically based on presence of a new lung infiltrate plus clinical evidence that the infiltrate is of infectious origin. This evidence includes:

1. New onset of fever >38°C
2. Purulent sputum
3. Leukocytosis or leucopenia
4. Decrease in oxygenation

◻ Table 27-2

Likely pathogens in early and late nosocomial pneumonia

Condition	Most likely pathogens
Early VAP or HAP	• *Streptococcus Pneumoniae*
	• *Hemophilus influenzae*
	• Methicillin sensitive *Staphylococcus aureus (MSSA)*
	• Antibiotic-sensitive gram-negative bacilli
	Klebsiella pneumoniae
	Enterobacter species
Late VAP or HAP, HCAP[a]	• *Pseudomonas aeruginosa*
	• *Resistant Klebsiella*
	• *Acinetobacter*
	• Methicillin resistant *staphylococcus aureus (MRSA)*
	• *Legionella pneumophila*

[a]Often multi-drug resistant organisms.

Although these criteria should raise suspicion of pneumonia, confirmation of the diagnosis of pneumonia is difficult, especially in intubated ICU patients, who may have many reasons to have one or more of these findings. Thus, using clinical criteria alone to diagnose VAP may result in over diagnosis and unnecessary use of antibiotics. Another drawback to using clinical criteria alone is that this method does not identify the etiologic agent.

The diagnosis of the etiologic agent requires generally a lower respiratory tract culture, which can include cultures of endotracheal aspirates, bronchoalveolar lavage (BAL) fluid, or protected specimen brush. Endotracheal cultures are easy to obtain and will usually contain the pathogens found by more invasive cultures. Colonization of the trachea, however, is very common, and a positive culture does not distinguish a pathogen from a colonizing organism. A tracheal aspirate is most useful when negative, as pneumonia is very unlikely in a patient with a negative culture of a tracheal aspirate provided that the patient has not had recent (in the last 72 h) change in antibiotics.

Quantitative cultures of lower respiratory tract specimens can also be used to guide therapy. For BAL fluid obtained either bronchoscopically or by blind suctioning, growth of more than 10^4 colony forming units (cfu)/ milliliter (ml) of fluid is suggestive of pneumonia. For specimens obtained using a protected specimen brush a threshold of 10^3 cfu/ml is used. The main problems with these approaches are that these tests are more invasive, are costly, have poor reproducibility, and require specialized laboratory and clinical skills. False negative results occur, especially in patients who have received antibiotic therapy before the sample is obtained; however, the specificity of these tests is greater than that of sputum/endotracheal aspirate cultures. When positive cultures above the diagnostic threshold are obtained by one of these techniques, they provide strong evidence that the patient has pneumonia with that organism.

Postmortem studies of VAP have demonstrated several characteristics pertinent to diagnostic testing. The process is often multifocal, frequently involving both lungs, and generally in the posterior and lower segments. VAP is often in multiple different phases of evolution at different sites at the same time. Prior antibiotic therapy can influence the number of bacteria found in lung tissue. The multifocal nature of VAP suggests that BAL and endotracheal aspirates can provide more representative samples than the protected specimen brush, which samples only a single bronchial segment. Because of the diffuse bilateral nature of VAP and predominance in dependent lung segments, "blind" BAL and use of a protected specimen brush may be as accurate as bronchoscopic sampling.

Many biologic markers have been studied in an effort to improve the diagnosis of pneumonia. Among critically ill patients, measurements of serum C-reactive protein and procalcitonin have not proven helpful in diagnosing pneumonia. Another biomarker-triggering receptor expressed on myeloid cells (TREM-1) appears promising. TREM-1 is a recently identified molecule involved in the inflammatory response to infection. Neutrophils and monocytes expressing high levels of TREM-1 infiltrate tissues infected with bacteria and fungi. TREM-1 is shed by the membrane of activated phagocytes and can be found in the soluble form (sTREM-1) in body fluids. Presence of sTREM-1 in BAL fluid can be detected rapidly using an immunoblot technique, is a strong predictor of pneumonia. This test may be helpful in distinguishing pulmonary infiltrates due to infectious causes from those from non-infectious causes, when it becomes commercially available.

Blood cultures are helpful when positive, but overall less than 25% of pneumonias are associated with bacteremia. Pleural fluid cultures are rarely necessary to make the diagnosis of pneumonia, but pleural fluid analysis may be helpful, in patients who do not respond to appropriate antibiotic therapy, to identify empyema which may need additional interventions such as a chest tube.

Treatment

Once the decision is made to initiate antibiotic therapy for nosocomial pneumonia, it is important to pick initial antimicrobial coverage that targets the most likely pathogens. Delayed or inappropriate antibiotic therapy is associated with poorer outcome. General principles of treatment are outlined in ❯ *Table 27-3*. The key decision in initial empiric antibiotic therapy is whether the patient has risk factors for multi-drug resistant organisms (MDR). These risk factors are summarized in ❯ *Table 27-4*. Patients deemed at risk of MDR organisms should receive broad spectrum coverage with antibiotics directed against these organisms. The specific choice of agents should be based on local patterns of antibiotic resistance and should also take into account antibiotics that the patient has received within the preceding 2 weeks. Whenever possible, antibiotics chosen for empiric treatment of the pneumonia should include antibiotics from drug classes to which the patient has not been exposed recently. For low risk patients, i.e., early onset VAP and HAP in patients without any of the risk factors for multi-drug resistant organisms, therapy should be targeted against common community-acquired pathogens in addition to *S. aureus* and *Enterobacter* species. An appropriate choice would be a respiratory quinolone (levofloxacin or moxifloxacin), a β-lactam/β-lactamase inhibitor combination (ampicillin-sulbactam), a non-pseudomonal cephalosporin (Ceftriaxone), or a limited spectrum carbapenem (Ertapenem).

Patients who have any risk factors for MDR pathogens should receive combination antibiotic therapy directed against these MDR organisms, including *Pseudomonas* and other resistant gram negatives. This combination should include an anti-pseudomonal cephalosporin (cefepime or ceftazidime) or carbepenem (Imipenem or Meropenem) or an anti-pseudomonal β-lactam/β-lactamase

◻ Table 27-3

Principles of antibiotic therapy for nosocomial pneumonia

- If patient at risk for multi-drug resistant organisms, use combination antibiotic therapy
- Use intravenous antibiotics initially, switch to oral/enteral antibiotics in selected patients with good clinical response and functioning GI tract
- If patient has had recent exposure to antibiotics, choose antibiotics for pneumonia from different antibiotic classes
- Use local resistance patterns to guide choice of antibiotic
- If patient received an initial appropriate regimen, short course therapy i.e. 7–8 days is adequate provided patient has a good clinical response and the pathogen being targeted is **not** *Pseudomonas*

◻ Table 27-4

Risk factors for nosocomial pneumonia caused by multidrug resistant pathogens

- Immunosuppression
- Current hospitalization of 5 days or more
- Presence of known antibiotic resistance in the community or in the specific hospital unit
- Risk factors for HCAP
  - Chronic hemodialysis
  - Residence in a long term care facility
  - Receipt of home infusion therapy or wound care within 30 days of onset of pneumonia
  - Hospitalization in an acute care facility for 2 or more days within 90 days of onset of pneumonia

inhibitor combination (piperacillin/tazobactam) plus a second antipseudomonal drug – either a quinolone (ciprofloxacin or levofloxacin) or an aminoglycoside (amikacin, gentamicin or tobramycin). Because aminoglycosides have poor penetration into respiratory secretions and carry the risk of nephrotoxicity, especially in critically patients, we prefer a quinolone instead of an aminoglycoside whenever possible. Vancomycin or linezolid should be added to this regimen in patients known to be colonized with methicillin-resistant *S. aureus* (MRSA) and in hospital units with a high prevalence of MRSA (❯ *Fig. 27-1*).

Initial therapy should be administered intravenously in all patients with a switch to oral/enteral therapy in selected patients who have a good clinical response and a functioning gastrointestinal tract. Dosing should be adjusted based on the patient's renal function. MDR strains of *Pseudomonas* and *Acinetobacter* resistant to all the commonly used antipseudomonal agents are being reported increasingly worldwide. Colistin, a drug in the polymyxin antibiotic class that fell out of favor several years ago because of its renal toxicity and the emergence of other effective antibiotics, is now regaining importance as the only current drug effective against these strains. Like the aminoglycosides, it is can be administered intravenously or as an aerosol. The aerosol route minimizes the risks of drug toxicity but generally should be used in addition to, not as a substitute for, a systemic agent.

Response to therapy: Clinical improvement usually becomes apparent after 48–72 h of onset of appropriate therapy. This improvement may be evidenced by decrease in white blood cell count and increased oxygenation with resolution of fever. Chest radiographs will not show improvement for several days and may actually get slightly worse in the first few days of treatment. All patients should be re-assessed at day 3 to decide whether the initial diagnosis of nosocomial pneumonia was correct and to assess whether antibiotic therapy needs to be modified based on available culture data. For patients who are deteriorating or not responding to initial therapy, it may be necessary to broaden antibiotic coverage while simultaneously pursuing further diagnostic testing (❯ *Fig. 27-2*), including repeating cultures of lower respiratory tract specimens and searching for an alternative site of infection, such as urinary tract or blood stream infection, surgical site infection, sinusitis, or a complication of pneumonia such as empyema. If the work up for other sites of infection/alternative diagnoses is negative and the patient remains febrile with pulmonary infiltrates, an open lung biopsy should be considered to diagnose infection with an unusual pathogen or a non infectious illness that mimics pneumonia.

Prevention

General measures to reduce the incidence of nosocomial pneumonia include effective infection control measures such as staff education, emphasis on appropriate hand hygiene, isolation of patients with MDR organisms, and vaccination against influenza and *S. pneumoniae* in those patients at risk.

Intubation and mechanical ventilation are the most important risk factors for pneumonia and should be avoided if possible. If intubation is unavoidable, use of orotracheal intubation instead of nasotracheal intubation may reduce the risk of nosocomial sinusitis and subsequent VAP. Continuous aspiration of sub-glottic secretions, maintaining endotracheal cuff pressure at greater than 20 cm of water, and keeping patients in the semi-recumbent position, i.e., elevating the head of bed to 30–45° all reduce the leakage of bacterial pathogens around the cuff into the lower respiratory tract. Minimizing the duration of mechanical ventilation may prevent VAP and can be achieved via protocols to improve the use of sedation, to accelerate weaning from the ventilator, and to reduce the risk of pulmonary

■ **Figure 27-1**
Treatment strategy for nosocomial pneumonia

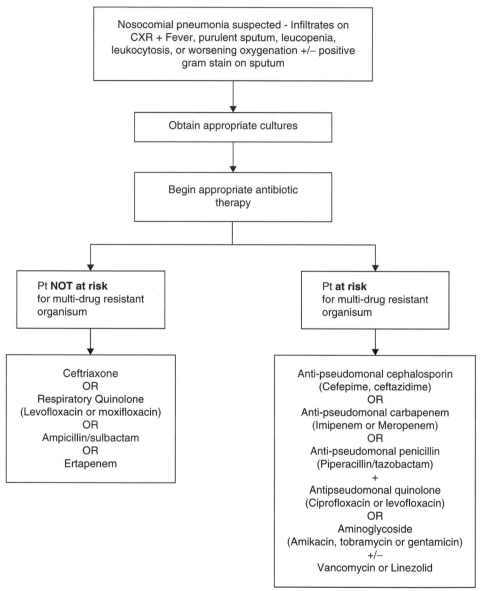

embolism. The use of acid-suppressive medications and antacids, both of which decrease gastric acidity, have been associated with an increased risk of nosocomial pneumonia. Sucralfate, an alternative agent for prophylaxis against stress ulcer, has been associated with lower pneumonia risk but with an increased risk of GI bleeding; hence, we suggest that the decision about the best strategy to use for stress ulcer prophylaxis be tailored to the individual patient.

Many institutions have adopted "bundles" by which several of these interventions are implemented together rather than individually. For instance, the VAP bundle promoted by the Institute for Healthcare Improvement in the US recommends all of the following interventions be implemented: the

◘ Figure 27-2
Re-evaluation 48–72 h after starting antibiotic therapy for suspected nosocomial pneumonia (Adapted from the American Thoracic Society and Infectious Diseases Society of America)

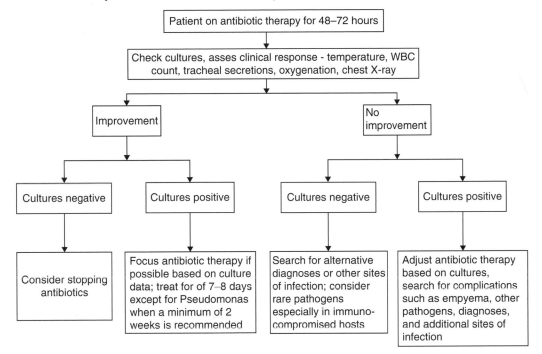

head of bed be raised to >30°, daily sedation holiday along with regular assessment of readiness for weaning, and prophylaxis against stress ulcer and deep vein thrombosis. The Hospital Infection Control Practices Advisory Committee (HICPAC) of the Centers for Disease Control and Prevention has also published comprehensive recommendations for the prevention of nosocomial pneumonia.

Selected Readings

Adair CG, Gorman SP, Feron BM, et al. (1999) Implications of endotracheal tube biofilm for ventilator-associated pneumonia. Int Care Med 25:1072–1076

Collard HR, Saint S, Matthay MA (2003) Prevention of ventilator-associated pneumonia: an evidence-based systematic review. Ann Int Med 138:494–501

Fagon JY, Chastre J, Wolff M, et al. (2000) Invasive and noninvasive strategies for management of suspected ventilator-associated pneumonia. A randomized trial. [Comment]. Ann Int Med 132:621–630

Gibot S, Cravoisy A, Levy B, et al. (2004) Soluble triggering receptor expressed on myeloid cells and the diagnosis of pneumonia. N Engl J Med 350:451–458

Guidelines for the management of adults with hospital-acquired, ventilator-associated, and healthcare-associated pneumonia (2005) American Thoracic Society and Infectious Diseases Society of America. Am J Resp Crit Care Med 171: 388–416

Hoffken G, Niederman MS (2002) Nosocomial pneumonia: the importance of a de-escalating strategy for antibiotic treatment of pneumonia in the ICU. Chest 122:2183–2196

Kollef MH, Shorr A, Tabak YP, et al. (2005) Epidemiology and outcomes of health-care-associated pneumonia: results from a large US database of culture-positive pneumonia. Chest 128:3854–3862

Tablan OC, Anderson LJ, Besser R, et al. (2004) Guidelines for preventing health-care–associated pneumonia, 2003: recommendations of CDC and the Healthcare Infection Control Practices Advisory Committee. Morbidity & Mortality Weekly Report Recommendations & Reports 53(RR-3):1–36

28 Pericardial Tamponade

Gary A. Vercruysse · S. Rob Todd · Frederick A. Moore

Pearls and Pitfalls

- All wounds between the nipples along the length of the sternum have potential to cause pericardial tamponade.
- Treat all potential intrapericardial injuries as an emergency.
- The Focused Assessment for the Sonographic Examination of the Trauma Patient (FAST) is an excellent tool for diagnosis of pericardial effusion.
- Pericardiocentesis is now less often necessary in a trauma center.
- Clamshell Thoracotomy will decompress both a tension pneumothorax and pericardial tamponade.
- A pericardial window should rarely, if ever, be done outside the operating room.
- A pericardial window is easiest to perform through the midline, tendonous portion of the diaphragm.
- If the abdomen is open, cardiac access is easiest through a median sternotomy.
- If the abdomen is closed, and the patient is in extremis, cardiac access is easiest through a clamshell thoracotomy.

Introduction

Life-threatening pericardial tamponade is seen most commonly after penetrating trauma, and occasionally after blunt trauma. Chronic medical conditions may also lead to this phenomenon. Survival is greater in those sustaining knife rather than missile wounds. This observation is intuitive, given the fact that gunshot wounds cause cavitary injury as well as direct injury. Anatomically speaking, atrial injuries are more survivable than ventricular injuries. The low pressure atrium tends to bleed less rapidly than the ventricle, and thus does not lead to rapid, high volume accumulation of pericardial blood. The resulting low pressure tamponade is difficult to diagnose and may not manifest until aggressive volume loading increases accumulation of blood within the pericardium. This chapter will focus on traumatic pericardial tamponade. Specifically, we will discuss its pathophysiology and clinical presentations, diagnostic modalities, and management options.

Pathophysiology and Clinical Presentation

Pericardial tamponade is categorized into two phases: well compensated and poorly compensated. Initially when a patient suffers an injury that leads to pericardial tamponade, the heart chambers are being compressed by blood collecting within the relatively nondistendable pericardium. Volume-loading augments cardiac preload; thus an increase in cardiac filling pressures and resultant increase in Starling forces allow cardiac output to be maintained. This situation represents well-compensated pericardial tamponade. In contrast, as pressure around the heart increases because of ongoing bleeding into the pericardium, preload cannot compensate for the added pressure, and cardiac output suffers. This situation is poorly compensated tamponade and is characterized by tachycardia and a narrowed pulse pressure. The time frame during which this progression occurs is variable, and depends on numerous factors, including underlying medical conditions, cardiac reserve, and the extent of the injury.

Pericardial tamponade after trauma can be seen immediately, as with penetrating injuries to the heart or great vessels, or may present in a delayed fashion. Typically, the delayed presentation is seen days to weeks after the inciting injury. Delayed presentation of pericardial tamponade may occur do to eventual rupture of an injured atrial or ventricular wall, with perforation occurring at the site of a focal contusion. More often, delayed presentation of pericardial tamponade occurs without cardiac rupture. Typically, these patients have suffered blunt chest trauma and may have been coagulopathic at the time of presentation. Presumably, a small amount of blood from a myocardial contusion allows for the gradual exudative accumulation of fluid with pericardium. An alternate cause is the post-cardiac injury syndrome, which is associated with fever and either a pleural or pericardial effusion.

Diagnosis

Clinical

Classically, Beck's triad is used to describe pericardial tamponade. This triad consists of distended neck veins, muffled heart sounds, and hypotension. In the best of circumstances it is only seen in about 25% of patients; however, we acknowledge that in a noisy trauma bay, Beck's triad is identified rarely. Were an electrocardiogram to be performed at this point, it would be of relatively low voltage compared with normal. As intrapericardial pressure increases, diastolic volume decreases, and a compensatory tachycardia occurs, allowing for maintenance of cardiac output. As more fluid accumulates around the heart, tamponade becomes critical, and equalization of atrial and ventricular pressures occurs. Pulses paradoxus, another phenomenon seen in pericardial tamponade, is the decrease of arterial pressure by 10 mmHg or greater during inspiration. This finding is seen in critical tamponade when a marked shift of the ventricular septum into the left ventricle as right heart filling occurs with inspiration, which leads to a decrease in left ventricular end-diastolic volume and stroke volume. Eventually, as diastolic filling time becomes shortened, myocardial perfusion is compromised, and subendocardial ischemia and a lethal arrhythmia lead to sudden death.

Chest Radiograph

The typical, portable, recumbent trauma chest radiograph is suggestive of pericardial tamponade to varying degrees, depending on the degree of tamponade present at the time the film is acquired. These films are more sensitive in detecting rib or sternal fractures, tension pneumothorax, and tension

☐ Figure 28-1
A chest radiograph typical of that seen with massive pericardial tamponade. Notice the shifted trachea and very enlarged cardiac silhouette

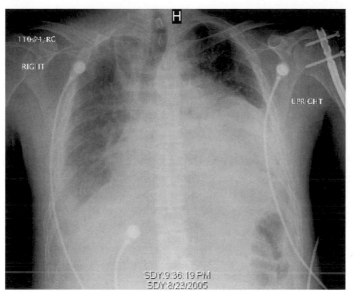

hemothorax, but these chest radiographs can be useful tools nonetheless. A trauma radiograph typical of massive pericardial tamponade is shown in ❯ *Fig. 28-1*. If time permits, diagnosis of tamponade should be correlated with ultrasonography, or physical signs and symptoms prior to undergoing pericardiocentesis or pericardial window, because a large heart can confuse the picture and lead to unnecessary and at times harmful procedures.

FAST Examination

The (FAST) examination is used to diagnose rapidly the presence of free intra abdominal and pericardial fluid. It is used classically in situations of hemodynamic instability after blunt trauma. The FAST examination has four windows, one of which is the pericardial window. This window is sensitive for the detection of intrapericardial fluid and has become very useful in the workup of both blunt and penetrating trauma. The examination can be done with portable equipment in only a couple of minutes and yields very important data. In a classic paper by Rozycki and colleagues in Atlanta, the accuracy of the pericardial view of the FAST examination was studied in patients with truncal trauma without an immediate indication for operative intervention. Of 247 patients examined, 236 FAST exams were true negative examinations, and 10 were true positive examinations. There were no false negative or false positive examinations. Mean duration of the examination was 48 s. The mean time from FAST exam to operation was 12.1 min, and there were no related mortalities. A positive exam is based on three findings: (1) separation of the pericardial layers with an anechoic area, (2) a decrease in the motion of the parietal pericardium, and (3) identification of the swinging motion of the heart within the pericardial sac. It is important to note that this examination is not static and depends on visualizing both the lack of motion of the pericardium and the extra motion of the "ballotable" heart within the pericardium. An example of a positive pericardial window is seen in ❯ *Fig. 28-2*. Although

◻ Figure 28-2
FAST examination showing a positive pericardial view

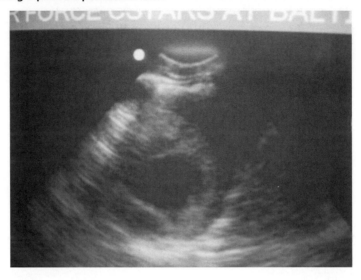

this study was done at an institution where FAST has become second nature to those performing the exam, with adequate training and practice, this is the easiest and least invasive maneuver for diagnosing pericardial tamponade.

Computed Tomography

Computed tomography (CT) is becoming ever more useful to the trauma surgeon in the evaluation of stable trauma patients. With the advent of multi detector, helical, CT, a full body scan can be completed in only a few minutes. It should be stressed however, the hemodynamically unstable patient is not a candidate for CT.

Occasionally, delayed pericardial tamponade can be diagnosed with CT. ❯ *Fig. 28-3* depicts one such example. This patient required endotracheal intubation for respiratory distress 15 days after bilateral long bone and pelvic fractures, as well as multiple rib fractures and pulmonary contusion. He underwent thoracic CT-angiography to exclude pulmonary embolus. Cardiac tamponade was diagnosed, and he was taken to the operating suite immediately for a pericardial window that drained 1.9 l of serosanguineous fluid. This patient was coagulopathic due to a combination of relative malnutrition (vitamin K deficiency) and use of prophylactic low molecular weight heparin, and likely sequestered the fluid secondary to the osmotic load of the old blood and his hypoalbuminemia. He recovered without further sequelae.

Central Venous Catheter

Initial volume loading of the hypotensive trauma patient is standard of care per the Advanced Trauma Life Support course (ATLS). The response to this empiric intervention can help differentiate the type of shock affecting the patient. Patients who respond to fluid loading are most likely hypovolemic, and

□ Figure 28-3
Computed tomographic image showing massive pericardial tamponade

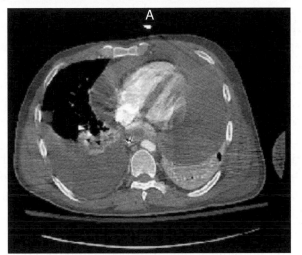

attention should be directed at identifying the source of bleeding. Patients who do not respond are either in severe hypovolemic shock, cardiogenic shock or neurogenic shock. Because most patients tolerate neurogenic shock, it is imperative to differentiate ongoing hypovolemia from cardiogenic shock.

When inserted while the patient is in the trauma bay, the central venous catheter can be used to help facilitate resuscitation and to diagnose pericardial tamponade. When measuring pressures, a central venous pressure >20 mmHg suggests either tension pneumothorax or, if there is a trend of increasing central venous pressure and decreasing systolic blood pressure, then cardiogenic shock or tamponade. A pressure <5 mmHg suggests hypovolemia.

Pulmonary Artery Catheter

In experienced hands, a pulmonary artery catheter (PAC) is very helpful in the resuscitation of critically ill trauma patient who is not responding to ongoing volume loading. In addition to directing resuscitation, a PAC can be useful in the diagnosis of pericardial tamponade. This mode of diagnosis will most likely be used in the setting of delayed tamponade as these catheters are not normally placed in the trauma bay. A PAC showing increased and equal right atrial, right ventricular end diastolic, and pulmonary artery end diastolic pressures is pathognomonic of pericardial tamponade.

Management

Patients arriving with decompensated pericardial tamponade appear ill and are in obvious distress. In this situation, one needs to avoid the reflex of early intubation as this may precipitate cardiac arrest. These patients are extremely dependent on preload to maintain cardiac filling and are maintaining mean arterial pressure by intense vasoconstriction. Pharmacologic agents used in intubation cause vasodilatation and positive airway pressure decreases preload. The combination can precipitate sudden and fatal pulseless electrical activity.

In penetrating thoraco-abdominal trauma, while the airway is assessed and vascular access is obtained, a chest radiograph and FAST examination are both essential in ruling out not only pericardial tamponade but also hemopneumothoraces. If the patient is hypotensive or extremely tachycardiac, and a positive pericardial view is obtained on FAST examination, a pericardiocentesis may be performed to drain temporarily the pericardium. When performing pericardiocentesis, if a central line kit is used, a catheter may be left in the pericardial space to facilitate further drainage while quickly transporting the patient to the operating room. This is the only situation in which we advocate pericardiocentesis.

If the patient is stable and has a positive pericardial view, time should not be spent performing a pericardiocentesis as this may do more harm than good. The best option in this situation is a controlled subxyphoid pericardial window performed in an expectant manner, in a sterile environment where the equipment necessary for cardiac and/or major vascular repair is located. As long as the patient is stable, pericardial window should not be attempted in the trauma bay, as a positive window leads inevitably to median sternotomy and major vascular or cardiac repair, neither of which can be facilitated in this location. After transport to the operating room, the patient should be prepped and draped prior to the induction of general anesthesia, because positive pressure ventilation, vasodilatory drugs, and the cardio-depressant effects of anesthesia may lead to acute decompensation and cardiovascular collapse on induction. If the patient is in the operating room for another reason and celiotomy has already been performed, pericardial window is easiest through the central tendonous portion of the diaphragm and can be accomplished in a matter of seconds and repaired just as quickly.

If the patient is in extremis, a clamshell thoracotomy will facilitate both emergency drainage of the pericardial sac, clamping of the descending aorta if necessary, and cardiopulmonary resuscitation. Cardiac or great vessel injuries will require temporizing measures, often necessitating finger tamponade while moving the patient to a sterile environment with adequate anesthesia support, instrumentation, and lighting for definitive repair (i.e., the operating room); attempts at definitive repair in the trauma bay delay effective repair and are fraught with complications.

Cases of blunt trauma with evidence of immediate pericardial tamponade should be managed in a manner identical to that for penetrating trauma. In these instances, the patient has likely suffered cardiac rupture. For most patients with delayed pericardial tamponade without cardiac rupture, treatment is a subxyphoid pericardial window with closed tube drainage. Less invasive modalities or pericardiocentesis with catheter drainage may also be employed in this situation.

Asystole in the Field

This problem involves a subset of patients in which pericardial tamponade may occur and immediate intervention may be lifesaving. In the case of lost vital signs in the field, the question has been raised repeatedly as to whether or not emergency department (ED) thoracotomy is indicated. A recent study by Moore and colleagues out of Denver found that if a penetrating trauma victim lost vital signs for less than 15 min or a blunt trauma victim for less than 5 min, immediate ED thoracotomy can be lifesaving. In their study, five of the patients were in asystole (narrow complex pulseless electrical activity) at the time of ED thoracotomy, all had pericardial tamponade from ventricular stab wounds, four of the five patients had good neurologic outcomes. Unfortunately, in their study, outcomes in victims of blunt trauma were uniformly bad. Although they had no functional survivors in their blunt trauma cohort, they recommend ED thoracotomy for patients who received cardiopulmonary resuscitation (CPR) for less than 5 min given the fact that case reports are published showing satisfactory outcomes in patients who loose vital signs immediately prior to ED arrival.

Summary

Pericardial tamponade is a surgical emergency. In the field of trauma surgery, many patients will die prior to arrival at the trauma center secondary to acute tamponade. Both physical examination and chest radiography may suggest tamponade. The FAST examination in combination with a good physical examination and chest radiograph is diagnostic in the majority of patients with cardiac tamponade. Pericardial window and ultimately cardiorrhaphy or vascular repair can be lifesaving. When evaluating a trauma patient, do not loose sight of the basics. Diagnosis of pericardial tamponade is not a diagnostic tour de force, but delay in its treatment may have lethal consequences.

Selected Readings

Gabram S, Devanney J, Jones D, et al. (1992) Delayed hemorrhagic pericardial effusion: case reports of a complication from severe blunt chest trauma. J Trauma 32:794–800

Mangram A, Kozar R, Gregoric I, et al. (2003) Blunt cardiac injuries that require operative intervention: an unsuspected injury. J Trauma 54:286–288

Powell DW, Moore EE, Cothren CC, et al. (2004) Is emergency department resuscitative thoracotomy futile care for the critically injured patient requiring prehospital cardiopulmonary resuscitation? J Am Coll Surg 199:211–215

Rozycki GS, Feliciano DV, Schmidt JA, et al. (1996) The role of surgeon-performed ultrasound in patients with possible cardiac wounds. Ann Surg 223:737–746

Solomon D (1991) Delayed cardiac tamponade after blunt chest trauma: case report. J Trauma 31:1322–1324

29 Gastrointestinal Failure

Lena M. Napolitano

Pearls and Pitfalls

- Early aggressive fluid resuscitation is necessary to treat intestinal mucosal hypoperfusion associated with shock states to avoid non-occlusive mesenteric ischemia.
- Intestinal failure is defined as the reduction of functional gut mass below the minimal amount necessary for digestion and absorption adequate to satisfy the nutrient and fluid requirements for maintenance in adults or growth in children.
- Stress-related mucosal disease (SRMD) is multiple superficial erosions occurring in the proximal stomach involving superficial capillaries secondary to mucosal hypoperfusion.
- SRMD is commonly associated with UGI bleeding, but gastric perforations are rare.
- Mechanical ventilation and coagulopathy are the two greatest risk factors for SRMD.
- Acid suppression therapy should be instituted in all patients at risk for SRMD.
- Acute colonic pseudo-obstruction (ACPO) presents with features of large bowel obstruction, without a mechanical cause and is due to an imbalance in the autonomic control of colonic motility.
- Conservative therapy is the preferred initial management for ACPO while identifying and correcting potentially contributory metabolic, infectious, and pharmacologic factors.
- Active intervention for ACPO is indicated for patients deteriorating during initial management and for those with signs or symptoms of ischemia, perforation, significant pain, fever, leukocytosis, or respiratory compromise, and for those failing conservative therapy.
- Neostigmine is effective pharmacologic therapy in the majority of patients with ACPO but requires close cardiovascular monitoring. If this fails, colonic decompression with more invasive methods (colonoscopic, surgical, or radiologic), should be considered.
- ACPO patients with overt perforation or signs of peritonitis should be managed surgically.
- Intra-abdominal hypertension (intra-abdominal pressure ≥ 12 mmHg) and abdominal compartment syndrome (intra-abdominal pressure ≥ 20 mmHg) can result in intestinal mucosal hyperperfusion.
- Abdominal compartment syndrome is associated with new organ dysfunction or organ failure.
- Intra-abdominal pressure is measured by transduction of intravesicular urinary bladder pressure.
- In patients with acute abdominal pain out of proportion to physical findings, especially with a history of cardiovascular disease, acute intestinal ischemia should be suspected.
- Surgical treatment of acute intestinal ischemia due to arterial occlusion includes revascularization, resection of necrotic bowel, and when appropriate, a "second-look" operation 24 h after revascularization.
- Nonocclusive mesenteric ischemia is acute intestinal ischemia in the absence of fixed arterial obstruction and should be suspected in patients with low flow states or shock.

Gastrointestinal failure may manifest in a number of ways. Critically ill patients in intensive care units (ICUs) commonly develop gastrointestinal tract problems as a result of severe physiologic stress. Among the abnormalities observed in such patients are stress-related mucosal disease which may result in acute upper gastrointestinal hemorrhage, disturbances in gastrointestinal motility, mucosal edema related to hypoalbuminemia which may promote intestinal ileus and abdominal compartment syndrome, intestinal hypoperfusion and ischemia, infectious complications such as *Clostridium difficile* colitis, and ultimately short bowel syndrome and intestinal failure.

Stress-Related Mucosal Disease

Stress-related mucosal disease (SRMD) refers to the development of specific, discrete, gastric mucosal lesions in response to severe stress. Although more common in years past when resuscitation was not as well appreciated, SRMD can still occur and cause considerable morbidity and mortality in critically ill patients. Most (75–100%) critically ill patients demonstrate endoscopic evidence of mucosal damage within 24 h of admission to the ICU. Critically ill patients can manifest SRMD in a continuum ranging from superficial erosions that are usually diffuse to the development of stress ulcers, which are deeper mucosal lesions that tend to be more focal and are at higher risk for bleeding. The mortality rate from SRMD bleeding approaches 50%.

Clinically-evident bleeding – the presence of material with the appearance of coffee grounds in the nasogastric (NG) aspirate, guaiac-positive NG aspirate or stool, hematemesis, melena, or hematochezia – occurs in 5–25% of critically ill patients. *Clinically important* bleeding affects 3–6% of patients, and it is more serious than clinically-evident bleeding, because it involves hemodynamic instability or the need for blood transfusion. Clinically-important bleeding is defined as overt bleeding associated with a decrease in systolic blood pressure of more than 20 mmHg within 24 h after gastrointestinal (GI) bleeding, orthostatic increase in heart rate of 20 beats/min, and a decrease in systolic blood pressure of 10 mmHg when the patient assumes an upright position. Other criteria include a decrease in hemoglobin concentration of 2 g/dl and need for transfusion of two units of packed red blood cells within 24 h after bleeding; in addition, the failure of the hemoglobin concentration to increase after transfusion by at least the number of transfused units minus 2 g/dl is worrisome.

SRMD manifests as multiple superficial erosions occurring in the proximal stomach involving superficial capillaries secondary to mucosal hypoperfusion. SRMD is commonly associated with upper GI bleeding, but gastric perforations are rare. In contrast, peptic ulcer disease is manifest by discrete, deep erosions usually in the duodenum and is secondary to other reasons (drugs, H. pylori, hypersecretory states, etc.). In contrast to SRMD, perforation is common.

Acid suppression therapy should be instituted in all patients at risk for SRMD ($\bullet$ *Fig. 29-1*). Gastric acid and pepsin are both necessary for the development of SRMD. Activated pepsin digests the gastric mucosal lining and is inactivated at a pH > 4. Therefore acid suppression therapy reduces gastric acid concentration, inactivates pepsin, and also stabilizes clot formation by facilitation of platelet activation and aggregation.

Risk factors for SRMD are many, but two strong independent risk factors consistently emerge, including respiratory failure requiring mechanical ventilation (odds ratio 15.6) and coagulopathy (odds ratio 4.3). Other risk factors for SRMD, including organ failure, sepsis, hypoperfusion states, traumatic brain injury, burns, and major surgery, also warrant SRMD prophylaxis. Furthermore, aggressive acid suppression therapy should be instituted promptly in any patient with acute upper GI hemorrhage (❯ *Fig. 29-2*) in addition to endoscopy.

Intestinal Ileus

Intestinal ileus, the disturbance of bowel motility characterized by a lack of coordinated intestinal activity and a substantial overall reduction in peristalsis, is common in postoperative and critically ill

◘ Figure 29-1

Algorithm for stress ulcer prophylaxis and prevention of stress-related mucosal disease (Adapted from ASHP Commission on Therapeutics, 1999. With permission)

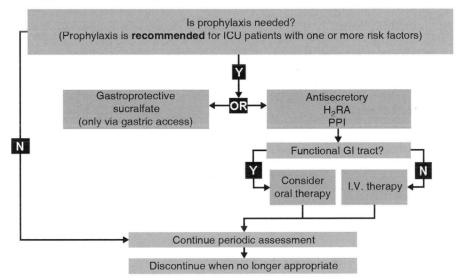

◘ Figure 29-2

Algorithm for acute ulcer bleed. Note: *role of selective second-look endoscopy is unclear (Adapted from Laine and Peterson, 1994. With permission. Copyright 1994 Massachusetts Medical Society. All rights reserved)

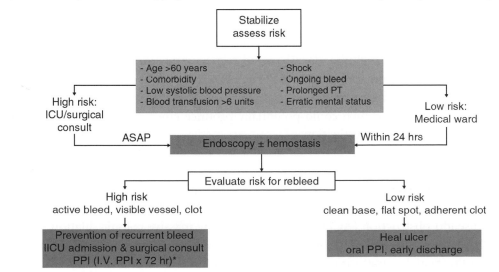

◻ Table 29-1

Prevention and management of postoperative ileus (Adapted from Mattei and Rombeau, 2006. With kind permission of Springer Science and Business Media)

Category	Specific action	Physiologic effect
Pharmacologic	• Minimize opiates • Regional anesthesia techniques • (Prokinetic drugs)* • (μ-agonists)*	• Decreases inhibitory effect of opioids • (Investigational)*
Inflammatory	• Gentle handling of tissues • NSAIDs	• Decreases inflammation
Hormonal	• (Substance P antagonist)* • (VIP antagonist)*	• (Investigational)*
Metabolic	• Maintain electrolyte homeostasis • Maintain acid–base balance • Maintain normothermia	• Decreases inhibitory effects of metabolic derangements
GI physiology	• Early postoperative feedings • Selective use of nasogastric tubes	• Stimulates bowel function
Neurologic	• Thoracic epidural bupivacaine	• Decreases sympathetic nervous activity
Psychologic	• Educate patient regarding expectations of early discharge	• Reduces anxiety

NSAID: nonsteroidal anti-inflammatory drug; VIP: vasointestinal polypeptide; IV: intravenous.
*Refers to investigational drugs under development that are used for their Prokinetic activity, i.e. improving intestinal movement and preventing intestinal ileus.

patients. GI motility is coordinated by several physiologic mechanisms, including the autonomic nervous system, GI hormones, and inflammatory mediators. Anesthesia, surgery, pain control, and fluid resuscitation all alter the activity of one or more of these physiologic controls and can have profound effects on bowel motility.

Traditional regimens that emphasize bowel rest and NG tube decompression for the treatment of ileus do not hasten return of normal bowel function. There is evidence to support several newer concepts in the treatment of ileus (❱ *Table 29-1*). A mandatory period of bowel rest and the routine use of NG tubes are no longer recommended. Early postoperative feeding appears to be safe and may actually stimulate the return of normal bowel function. Minimally invasive surgical techniques, including laparoscopy and other measures to decrease peritoneal inflammation such as gentle tissue handling, seem effective. Reduction or avoidance of opiate analgesics should be considered. The early institution of bowel regimens, including laxatives and rectal suppositories may be helpful, as is early ambulation. Excessive hydration should be avoided as intestinal edema may contribute to ileus. New pharmacologic agents, including μ-receptor antagonists that selectively inhibit the effect of opioids on the gut or μ-receptor agonists which could potentially produce effective analgesia without intestinal effects, are undergoing clinical investigation.

Acute Colonic Pseudo-Obstruction

Acute colonic pseudo-obstruction (ACPO) is characterized by massive colonic dilation in the absence of mechanical obstruction; synonyms include acute colonic ileus and Ogilvie's syndrome. Ischemia or perforation are the feared complications; spontaneous perforation has been reported in 3–15% of patients and carries a mortality of 50% or higher. The rate of perforation and/or ischemia increases rapidly with cecal diameters >10–12 cm and when the duration of distention exceeds 6 days. The pathogenesis is not completely understood but likely results from an imbalance in the autonomic regulation of colonic motor function; excessive parasympathetic suppression results in colonic atony and dilatation.

Early recognition and appropriate management are critical to minimizing morbidity and mortality. In evaluating a patient with signs or symptoms of suspected acute colonic dilation, mechanical obstruction must first be excluded, because surgical management otherwise may be required (❯ *Fig. 29-3*). Although initial conservative management for mechanical obstruction overlays with the initial management of ACPO (e.g., nothing by mouth, intravenous fluids, nasogastric suction), the possibility of mechanical obstruction must always be considered, particularly if there is no response to conservative management. If there is any suspicion of mechanical obstruction, a water-soluble contrast enema of the rectum and distal colon should be obtained.

◻ Figure 29-3
Algorithm for management of acute colonic distention (Reprinted from Saunders and Kimmey, 2005. With the permission of Blackwell Publishing)

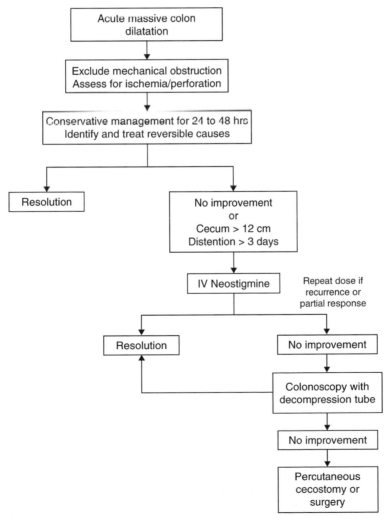

■ Table 29-2

Causes and predisposing factors associated with acute colonic pseudo-obstruction

Postsurgical
• Intra-abdominal operations
• Other operative procedures
• Lumbar/spinal and other orthopedic, gynecologic, urologic surgery
• Renal transplantation
Trauma
• Retroperitoneal trauma
• Spinal cord injury
Medical
• Age
• Sepsis
• Neurologic disorders
• Hypothyroidism
• Viral infection (herpes, varicella zoster)
• Cardiac/respiratory disorders
• Electrolyte imbalances (hypokalemia, hypocalcemia, hypomagnesemia)
• Medications (narcotics, tricyclic anti-depressants, phenothiazides, anti-Parkinsonian drugs, anesthetic agents among others)
• Renal insufficiency

The causes of and predisposing factors are multiple (❷ *Table 29-2*) and often more than one of these factors are present. Most commonly, this syndrome is associated with intraperitoneal or extra-peritoneal surgery, particularly pelvic and lumbar spine surgery. Based on LaPlace's law, increasing diameters accelerate the increase in tension within the colon wall. Although risk increases with expanding dimensions, there is only a poor association with absolute diameters. Some data suggest critical thresholds of 9 cm for the transverse colon and 12 cm for the cecum; however, many patients present with dimensions greater than this without sequelae. The acuity of onset and duration of persistent distention likely correlate more strongly with risk. Approximately 10% of patients have some degree of ischemia in the right colon at the time of colonoscopy. Spontaneous perforation has been estimated to occur in 3–15% of patients.

Conservative Therapy

The initial step in management of ACPO is to initiate therapy for potential contributing factors, including first evaluation for electrolyte and metabolic abnormalities (potassium, phosphorous, magnesium, calcium, and thyroid functions). Blood cultures and empiric antibiotics are indicated if sepsis is suspected clinically. Bowel rest with nasogastric decompression should be initiated. Objective evidence of progress can be monitored radiographically by serial measurement of cecal diameter as often as every 8–12 h. Management includes discontinuation of narcotics, anticholinergic agents, and any other possible offending medications, exclusion of abdominal infection, mobilization out of bed if feasible, and appropriate medical and surgical management for significant concurrent illnesses. The direct benefits of any individual component of care are unknown, because these recommendations have not been studied as single interventions. A trial of conservative measures alone is appropriate in the subset of patients who lack significant abdominal pain, signs of peritonitis, and who have one or more potential underlying factors that are reversible.

Conservative management usually includes NG tube for gut decompression, aggressive use of optimal body positioning, and often, placement of a rectal tube with or without use of low-volume enemas. The prone position with hips elevated on a pillow or the knee chest position with the hips held high often aids the spontaneous evacuation of flatus. These positions should be alternated with right and left lateral decubitus positions regularly each hour, when feasible. When there is no pain and distention is not extreme (<12 cm), conservative measures can be used for 24–48 h before considering other medical or endoscopic intervention, particularly when reversible contributory factors are identified. During this interval, serial physical examinations for tenderness or signs of peritonitis should be performed and plain abdominal radiographs should be obtained every 8–12 h. The reported success of conservative management is variable, with rates from 20% to 92%.

Pharmacologic Therapy

The only consistently positive results have been with neostigmine. Neostigmine is an anticholinesterase, parasympathomimetic agent used for postoperative reversal of nondepolarizing neuromuscular blockade and in the treatment of myasthenia gravis and postoperative urinary retention. The belief that parasympathetic suppression, resulting in decreased colonic motility, plays a central role in ACPO is further supported by successful treatment of ACPO with intravenous neostigmine. Because such parasympathetic stimulation can induce bradycardia, asystole, hypotension, restlessness, seizures, tremor, miosis, bronchoconstriction, hyperperistalsis, nausea, vomiting, salivation, diarrhea, and sweating, administration must be accompanied by close cardiorespiratory monitoring. Toxicity is treated with atropine. Contraindications to use of neostigmine include known hypersensitivity and mechanical urinary or intestinal obstruction. Recent myocardial infarction, acidosis, asthma, bradycardia, peptic ulcer disease, and therapy with beta-blockers are relative contraindications to neostigmine therapy.

Endoscopic and Surgical Therapy

Approaches to mechanical decompression have included passage of decompression tubes under fluoroscopic guidance and colonoscopic decompression with or without placement of an indwelling, transanal decompression tube. Among the invasive therapeutic options, colonoscopic decompression is preferred, and success at the initial procedure, with or without tube placement varied from 61% to 78%, recurrence from 18% to 33%, almost all among patients without tube placement, and ultimate clinical success after one or more procedures was 73–88%. Complications occurred in 4% of patients and in-hospital, but unrelated, mortality rates were 13–32%. It remains unclear whether ischemia is an absolute contraindication to proceeding with decompression. The efficacy of colonoscopic decompression has not been established in randomized clinical trials. Also, perforations have been described in up to 3% of patients undergoing colonoscopic decompression.

Because operative management with colectomy or cecostomy carries greater morbidity than endoscopic decompression, it is therefore reserved for patients who fail endoscopic and pharmacologic efforts and for those in whom exploration of the peritoneal cavity might otherwise be indicated. Primary operative therapy is indicated for patients with predisposing intra-abdominal processes as well as those with suspected or evident free or contained perforation or peritonitis. Percutaneous cecostomy is also an option.

C. Difficile-Associated Disease

Clostridium difficile is a gram-positive, anaerobic, spore-forming bacillus that can cause pseudomembranous colitis and other *C. difficile*-associated diseases (CDAD). Two toxins, A and B, are involved in the pathogenesis of CDAD. Transmission occurs primarily in healthcare facilities, where exposure to antimicrobial drugs (the major risk factor for CDAD) and environmental contamination by *C. difficile* spores are more common.

About 3% of healthy adults and 20–40% of hospitalized patients are colonized with *C. difficile*, which in healthy persons is metabolically inactive in the spore form. The assumption is that perturbation of the competing flora promotes a conversion to vegetative forms that replicate and produce toxins. The characteristic clinical expression is watery diarrhea and cramps, and the characteristic pathologic finding is pseudomembranous colitis.

Early diagnosis and prompt aggressive treatment are critical in the management of CDAD (❯ *Fig. 29-4*). The most common confirmatory study is an enzyme immunoassay for the *C. difficile* A and B toxins (sensitivity 93–100%, sensitivity 63–99%); results are available in 2–4 h. In severe cases, flexible sigmoidoscopy can provide an immediate diagnosis. Treatment consists of the prompt discontinuation of the implicated antimicrobial agent and the administration of oral metronidazole; for severely ill patients and those who do not have a prompt response to metronidazole, oral vancomycin should be considered. Prevention efforts should include fastidious use of barrier precautions, isolation of the patient, environmental cleaning with sporicidal agents active against *C. difficile*, and meticulous hand hygiene.

Both the rate and severity of CDAD is increasing in healthcare facilities worldwide. An increased severity of CDAD has been reported, with resulting admission to ICUs, need for colectomies, and deaths. A new epidemic strain of *C. difficile* has also been identified (BI/NAP1) which carries virulence properties and antibiotic resistance patterns of the European strain ribotype 027. These data have major implications for clinical care. Some institutions, in an effort to limit nosocomial spread, have instituted new practices. If a patient has clinically important diarrhea, he or she is started on oral metronidazole treatment immediately and placed on contact precautions, prior to obtaining the confirmatory test results.

These findings, in conjunction with the emergence of methicillin-resistant *Staphylococcus aureus* (MRSA) and vancomycin-resistant enterococcus (VRE), emphasize the need for all healthcare providers to prescribe antimicrobial agents judiciously and to comply with infection-control measures. The most important of these measures consists of meticulous hand hygiene. Increasing the use of alcohol-based waterless sanitizers has been an important method of increasing hand hygiene compliance among healthcare providers. It is important, however, to continue to encourage hand washing with soap and water when organisms that are resistant to alcohol-based cleaners, such as the potential spore-forming organism *C. difficile*, are identified in the local environment.

Intestinal Hypoperfusion and Ischemia

Ischemia of the intestine may manifest with different clinical features, each requiring a specific diagnosis and treatment approach. Patients with acute abdominal pain out of proportion to physical findings and who have a history of cardiovascular disease should be suspected of having acute intestinal ischemia.

◘ Figure 29-4

Algorithm for the treatment of *C. difficile*-associated diarrhea (Adapted from Viswanath and Griffiths, 1998. Reproduced from the BMJ Publishing Group. With permission)

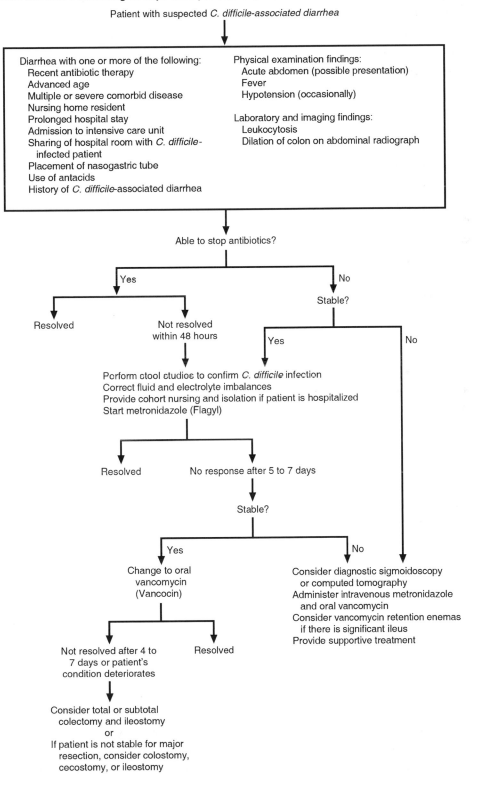

Early identification and treatment of acute mesenteric ischemia is crucial to improve prognosis. Operative treatment of acute obstructive intestinal ischemia includes revascularization, resection of necrotic bowel, and when appropriate, a "second-look" operation 24 h after revascularization. Percutaneous interventions (including transcatheter lytic therapy, balloon angioplasty, and stenting) are appropriate in selected patients with acute intestinal ischemia caused by mechanical arterial obstructions. Patients so treated may still require laparotomy.

Acute intestinal ischemia sufficient to produce infarction also occurs in the absence of fixed arterial obstruction. Nonocclusive mesenteric ischemia (NOMI) should be suspected in patients with low flow states or shock, especially cardiogenic shock, who develop abdominal pain, in patients receiving vasoconstrictor agents, and after revascularization for intestinal ischemia caused by arterial obstruction. Treatment of the underlying shock state is the most important initial step in treatment of NOMI. Arteriography is indicated in patients suspected of NOMI whose condition does not improve rapidly with treatment of their underlying disease. Transcatheter administration of vasodilator medications into the area of vasospasm is indicated in patients with NOMI who do not respond to systemic supportive treatment and in those with intestinal ischemia due to cocaine or ergot poisoning. Laparotomy and resection of nonviable bowel is necessary in patients with NOMI who have persistent symptoms despite treatment.

Acute mesenteric ischemia remains a morbid condition with poor short-term and long-term survival rates. The contemporary management with revascularization with surgical or angiographic techniques, resection of non-viable bowel, and liberal use of second-look procedures can result in the early survival of two thirds of patients with embolisms and thrombosis. Variables independently associated with worse survival include age > 60 years, bowel resection at first-look or second-look laparotomy and previous surgery.

Ischemic colitis, another form of intestinal ischemia, usually affects either just the right or just the left colon and may resolve spontaneously. Bowel rest, IV fluids, and antibiotics are the standard treatment. Initially, operative intervention is indicated for patients with peritonitis, massive bleeding, or fulminant colitis, or those who do not improve after 2–3 weeks of treatment, those evolving to sepsis, or those presenting late with colonic stricture or persistent chronic colitis. Chronic mesenteric ischemia has to be considered in elderly patients or those with risk factors presenting with postprandial abdominal pain and weight loss. Treatment may be performed either by operative revascularization or angioplasty with or without stent placement according to patient conditions and surgical risk.

Abdominal Compartment Syndrome

Intra-abdominal hypertension and abdominal compartment syndrome are being recognized increasingly in the critically ill. Intra-abdominal hypertension is defined by a sustained or repeated pathologic increase in intra-abdominal pressure ≥ 12 mmHg; it is at this pressure that reduction in intestinal microcirculatory blood flow occurs. Normal intra-abdominal pressure is approximately 5–7 mmHg in critically ill adults. Abdominal compartment syndrome is defined as a sustained intra-abdominal pressure ≥ 20 mmHg (with or without an abdominal perfusion pressure < 60 mmHg) that is associated with new organ dysfunction or failure.

Measurement of intra-abdominal pressure is accomplished by indirect means by transduction of intravesicular or "urinary bladder" pressure via the Foley catheter. Intra-abdominal pressure should be measured at end-expiration in the supine position after ensuring that abdominal muscle contractions are absent and with the transducer zeroed at the level of the mid-axillary line, and with a maximal instillation volume of 25 ml of sterile saline into the bladder.

Analogous to the widely accepted and clinically utilized concept of cerebral perfusion pressure, abdominal perfusion pressure is calculated as mean arterial pressure minus intra-abdominal pressure. Abdominal perfusion pressure has been proposed as a more accurate predictor of visceral perfusion and a potential endpoint for resuscitation. A target abdominal perfusion pressure of at least 60 mmHg correlates with improved survival from syndromes of increased intra-abdominal pressures.

Primary abdominal compartment syndrome is associated with injury or disease in the abdomino-pelvic region that frequently requires early surgical or interventional radiologic intervention. *Secondary abdominal compartment syndrome* refers to conditions that do not originate from the abdominopelvic region, and is commonly caused by massive volume resuscitation in a patient with no prior abdominal pathology, i.e., burn patient. *Recurrent abdominal compartment syndrome* (formerly termed tertiary abdominal compartment syndrome) refers to the condition in which abdominal compartment syndrome re-develops after treatment of primary or secondary abdominal compartment syndrome.

Prevention, early recognition, and treatment of abdominal compartment syndrome are of great importance in the prevention of intestinal mucosal hypoperfusion. If abdominal compartment syndrome is related to the development of tense ascites, paracentesis can be considered. In contrast, if abdominal compartment syndrome is related to intestinal and visceral edema, medical management with diuretic therapy or decompressive celiotomy must be considered. In patients at risk for abdominal compartment syndrome postoperatively, such as those where fascial closure would be difficult due to tension, delay in primary fascial closure using an open abdomen approach with delayed fascial closure may be considered. Serial monitoring of intra-abdominal pressure should be considered in all patients at risk.

Short Bowel Syndrome and Intestinal Failure

Intestinal failure can be defined as a decrease in functional gut mass below the minimal amount necessary for digestion and absorption adequate to satisfy the nutrient and fluid requirements for maintenance in adults or growth in children. Intestinal failure occurs when the body is unable to sustain its energy and fluid requirements without nutritional support, due to loss of functional small bowel. In developed countries, intestinal failure mainly includes individuals with the congenital or early onset of conditions requiring protracted or indefinite parenteral nutrition. Short bowel syndrome was the first commonly recognized cause of protracted intestinal failure.

The normal physiologic process of intestinal adaptation after extensive resection usually allows for recovery of sufficient intestinal function within weeks to months. Intestinal adaptation occurs when the remaining gut goes through functional and morphologic changes increasing its absorptive capacity. Factors such as intraluminal nutrients, gastrointestinal secretions, and GI hormones facilitate adaptation. Enteral feeds are a potent stimulant to adaptation and should be started as soon as the clinical situation permits. Some drugs thought to increase intestinal adaptation include glutamine, growth hormone, and glucagon like peptide-2, but there is a paucity of data to guide their use. During this time of intestinal adaptation, patients are sustained on parenteral nutrition. Non-transplant surgery, including small bowel tapering and lengthening to increase absorptive surface area, may allow weaning from parenteral nutrition in some patients. Congenital diseases of enterocyte development, such as microvillus inclusion disease or intestinal epithelial dysplasia, cause permanent intestinal failure for which no curative medical treatment is available. Severe and extensive motility disorders, such as total or subtotal intestinal aganglionosis (long segment Hirschsprung disease) or chronic intestinal pseudo-obstruction syndrome, may also cause permanent intestinal failure.

Prolonged intestinal failure due to short bowel syndrome occurs predictably after extensive intestinal resection and other problems (❯ *Table 29-3*). Short bowel syndrome can be treated with bowel rehabilitation, parenteral nutrition, or intestinal transplantation. The mainstay of management is parenteral nutrition, which is costly and may be associated with the well-recognized problems of liver disease and catheter-related sepsis. Cessation of parenteral nutrition at the earliest possible stage is desirable, but for this, enteral autonomy has to be achieved first. When prolonged parenteral nutrition is unsustainable or associated with unacceptable side effects, small bowel transplantation should be considered as a treatment option (❯ *Fig. 29-5*).

Studies on the outcome of short bowel syndrome show a clear correlation to intestinal anatomy, notably remaining jejuno-ileal length, presence of the ileocecal value, and the colon in continuity with the small bowel. Classification of patients with short bowel syndrome is therefore based on etiology and anatomic characteristics. Anatomic classification of short bowel syndrome, however, poses several difficulties because there is a marked variation in intestinal length in adults, and an even greater variation in children as a result of growth.

The normal length of the small bowel in adulthood has a mean of 550 cm with a wide range of 350–700 cm depending on race, body weight, and the size of the patient. It follows that exact anatomic quantification of the remnant intestinal length necessary to maintain intestinal autonomy is difficult. Individuals with healthy intestinal mucosa may be expected to regain or maintain intestinal autonomy with a jejuno-ileal length of 50–70 cm in the presence of an intact colon, or 150–200 cc in its absence. The determining factor remains the critical mass of residual functional intestinal absorptive epithelia. Therefore, there is a great need for a specific marker of functional epithelial mass and adaptive response, but no such markers have been widely identified.

◻ Table 29-3

Etiology of short bowel syndrome (Adapted from Goulet and Ruemmele, 2006. With permission from the American Gastroenterological Association)

Prenatal	Neonatal	Postnatal
Atresia (unique or multiple)	Midgut volvulus (midgut or segmental)	Midgut volvulus
	Necrotizing enterocolitis	Arterial thrombosis
Midgut volvulus (malrotation)	Arterial thrombosis	Inflammatory bowel disease
Segmental volvulus	Venous thrombosis	Post-trauma resection
Abdominal wall defects		Extensive angioma
Gastroschisis > omphalocele		Non-occlusive mesenteric ischemia
Extensive Hirschsprung's disease		Multiple operations for intestinal obstruction
Apple peel syndrome		Multiple operations for intestinal and enterocutaneous fistulae

◘ **Figure 29-5**

Management of intestinal failure (Reprinted from Goulet et al., 2004. With the permission of Lippincott Williams & Wilkins)

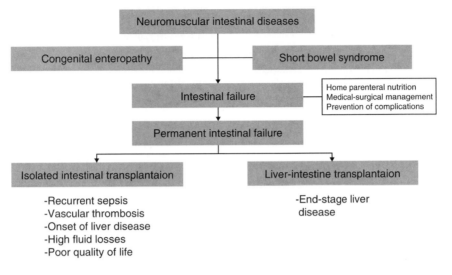

New scientific advances, including the recent identification that a newly identified human protein (R-spondin1) increases dramatically the proliferation and growth of the small and large intestines in mice, are of great interest for the possible eventual treatment of intestinal disorders such as short bowel syndrome and intestinal failure.

Selected Readings

Abraham C, Cho JH (2005) Inducing intestinal growth. N Engl J Med 353(21):2297–2299

American Gastroenterological Association Clinical Practice and Practice Economics Committee (2000) AGA Technical Review on Intestinal Ischemia. Gastroenterology 118:954–968

ASHP Commission on Therapeutics (1999) ASHP report: stress ulcer prophylaxis. Am J Health Sys Pharm 56:347–379

Bartlett JG (2006) Narrative review: the new epidemic of *Clostridium difficile*-associated enteric disease. Ann Intern Med 145:758–764

Berman L, Carling T, Fitzgerald TN, Bell RL, Duffy AJ, Longo WE, Roberts KE (2008) Defining surgical therapy for pseudomembranous colitis with toxic megacolon. J clin Gastroenterol 42(5):476–580

Byrn JC, Maun DC, Gingold DS, Baril DT, Ozao JJ, Divino CM (2008) Predictors of mortality after colectomy for fulminant Clostridium difficile colitis. Arch Surg 143(2):150–154; discussion 155

Fennerty MB (2002) Pathophysiology of the upper gastrointestinal tract in the critically ill patient: rationale for the therapeutic benefits of acid suppression. Crit Care Med 2002(Suppl 30):S351–S355

Goulet O, Ruemmele F (2006) Causes and management of intestinal failure in children. Gastroenterology 130:S16–S28

Goulet O, Ruemmele F, Lacaille F, Colomb V (2004) Irreversible intestinal failure. J Pediatr Gastroenterol Nutr 38:250–269

Gupte GL, Beath SV, Kelly DA, et al. (2006) Current issues in the management of intestinal failure. Arch Dis Child 91:259–264

Hirsch AT, Haskal ZJ, Hertzer NR, et al. (2006) ACC/AHA 2005 Practice guidelines for the management of patients with peripheral arterial disease (lower extremity, renal, mesenteric, and abdominal aortic): a collaborative report from the American Association for Vascular Surgery/ Society for Vascular Surgery, Society for Cardiovascular Angiography and Interventions, Society for Vascular Medicine and biology, Society of Interventional Radiology, and the ACC/AHA Task Force on Practice Guidelines; endorsed by the American Association of

Cardiovascular and Pulmonary Rehabilitation; national Heart, Lung and Blood Institute, Society for Vascular Nursing, Trans Atlantic Inter-Society Consensus; and Vascular Disease Foundation. Circulation 113:463–654

Laine L, Peterson WL (1994) Medical progress: bleeding peptic ulcer. N Engl J Med 331:717–727

Malbrain ML, Cheatham ML, Kirkpatrick A, et al. (2006) Results from the International Conference of Experts on Intra-abdominal Hypertension and Abdominal Compartment Syndrome. I. Definitions. Intensive Care Med 32:1722–1732

Mattei P, Rombeau JL (2006) Review of the pathophysiology and management of postoperative ileus. World J Surg 30:1382–1391

Saunders MD, Kimmey MB (2005) Systematic review: acute colonic pseudo-obstruction. Aliment Pharmacol Ther 15(22):917–925

Zerey M, Paton BL, Lincourt AE, Gersin KS, Kercher KW, Heniford BT (2007) The burden of Clostridium difficile in surgical patients in theUnited States. Surg Infect (Larchmt) 8(6):557–566

30 Diabetes Mellitus and Diabetes Insipidus

Martin D. Smith · Jacobus S. Vermaak

Pearls and Pitfalls

The Latin terms *diabetes* means "a siphon" or "passer through". *Insipidus* implies "tasteless", and *mellitus* "honeyed".

Diabetes Mellitus

- Diabetes mellitus (DM) is a systemic disease; the presenting surgical complaint should not overshadow the global approach needed in evaluating a patient with DM.
- The diabetic emergency can be challenging, and the surgical practitioner should have a clear approach to these very ill patients.
- Glycemic control (irrespective of whether the patient has diabetes mellitus or not) is important in the critically ill patient.
- Avoid complacency in patients thought to have only "mild" diabetes.
- Ultimately, there is no substitute for good patient education to decrease long-term diabetic complications.

Diabetes Insipidus

- The clinician must make the distinction from other causes of polyuria.
- Central and nephrogenic diabetes insipidus (DI) have different clinical and management implications.
- Prevention of hypernatremic dehydration is of critical importance, particularly in patients unable to regulate their own fluid requirements (e.g. the critically ill, the comatose patient, and small infants).

Diabetes Mellitus

Diabetes mellitus (DM) is the most frequent endocrine abnormality encountered by the surgeon. An increased serum glucose concentration is encountered commonly in surgical practice. This finding has ramifications for both the diabetic and non-diabetic patient. DM can present to the surgeon as either:

1. Co-morbidity, e.g. the diabetic patient requiring an inguinal hernia repair
2. A primary surgical pathology:
   (a) Acute complications of diabetes mellitus (e.g. diabetic ketoacidosis (DKA) presenting with a surgical abdomen)
   (b) Chronic complications of diabetes mellitus (e.g. diabetic foot)

Diagnosis

Non-diabetic patients often demonstrate an increased serum glucose concentration during periods of physiologic stress due to activation of the hypothalamic pituitary axis, catecholamine release, and peripheral resistance to insulin. Anxiety to venipuncture in itself can increase the serum glucose concentration. It is thus clear that, although an increased glucose concentration is specific for the diagnosis of DM, it lacks sensitivity.

Timely analysis of the serum glucose specimen is essential as continual glycolysis in the cells renders unpredictably lower values. Whole blood glucose values are up to 15% lower and arterial values up to 7% higher than corresponding plasma values. Capillary whole blood, used in bedside monitoring and serum plasma glucose levels are nearly equivalent. For the purposes of the chapter, we will refer to serum glucose levels only.

Diabetes Mellitus can be diagnosed easily in patients with unequivocal hyperglycemia and the classic DM symptoms of polydipsia, polyuria, DKA, hyperosmolar non-ketotic diabetic coma (HONK), or complications of prolonged exposure to hyperglycemia, with resultant end-organ damage.

For patients without classic symptoms but in whom DM is suspected, an oral glucose tolerance test (OGTT) should be performed: 75 g of anhydrous glucose is given orally (in children 1.75 g/kg up to a dose of 75 g). Glucose values are taken before glucose administration (after an overnight fast of 8–14 h) and 2 h after the glucose load. See ❷ *Table 30-1* for diagnostic values. We recommend that the diagnosis of diabetes mellitus never be made on a single serum glucose value in the asymptomatic patient.

◻ Table 30-1

Serum glucose values for the diagnosis of diabetes mellitus and glucose intolerance (Adapted from the WHO recommendations (World Health Organization, 1985))

	Serum glucose level mmol/l (mg/dl)
Diabetes mellitus	
Fasting level, *or*	Gluc ≥7 (126 mg/dl)
2 h post glucose load, *or both*	Gluc ≥11.1 (200 mg/dl)
Impaired glucose tolerance	
Fasting level, *and*	Gluc <7.0 (126 mg/dl)
2 h post glucose load	7.8 (140) ≤ Gluc < 11.1 (200 mg/dl)

When the diabetic patient presents to the surgeon, the following needs consideration:

1. The type or classification of DM
2. Duration of exposure to hyperglycemia
3. Systemic effects of DM
4. Diabetic emergencies
5. Long-term management of the patient

Classification of DM

Some clinicians use the terms "type 1" DM and "type 2" DM as synonyms for insulin-dependent diabetes mellitus (IDDM) and non-insulin-dependent diabetes mellitus (NIDDM) respectively. It is correct to reserve the term "type 1" diabetes for the immune-mediated DM, and the term "type 2" for the non-immune-mediated DM.

Diabetes mellitus can be classified as follows:

Primary

1. *Type 1 DM* may be diagnosed at any age but is most frequently diagnosed before the age of 30. The primary pathology is the autoimmune destruction of pancreatic beta-cells. Patients are prone to develop DKA and usually will require insulin for glycemic control.
2. *Type 2 DM* is more common and is diagnosed usually after the age of 40 in obese patients due to a decreased peripheral utilization of insulin with insulin "resistance." Patients are more prone to develop hyperosmolar, non-ketotic diabetic coma, and the majority of patients can be controlled on oral hypoglycemic agents. Some patients may have to be controlled on insulin if oral hypoglycemic agents are unsuccessful.
3. MODY (maturity-onset diabetes of young people) is a "non-insulin-dependent diabetes" that has an atypical clinical pattern in that it presents in young adults who are frequently not obese. There is an autosomal dominant inheritance.

Secondary

1. Pancreatic disease. This form of acquired diabetes includes conditions that affect the exocrine pancreas: chronic pancreatitis, pancreatectomy, cystic fibrosis, and pancreatic trauma. Extensive destruction of the pancreas must occur before the reduction in beta cell mass is sufficient enough to ensure diabetes. The exception is pancreatic malignancy, notably adenocarcinoma, which is often associated with new onset diabetes. Unfortunately, this condition cannot be used as a screening test for pancreatic cancer because of its non-specificity and decreased sensitivity.
2. Medication (N-3-pyridylmethyl-N'-p-nitrophenyl urea, the rodenticide Vacor, which is irreversibly cytotoxic to beta cells).

3. Genetic syndromes (e.g. the lipodystrophies).
4. Hormonal induced (e.g. Cushing's disease and pheochromocytoma).
5. Pregnancy (gestational diabetes).

Glucose intolerance itself is not formally classified as diabetes but is predictive for progression to established diabetes.

Duration of DM

Preoperative evaluation of glucose control is important, because prolonged exposure to hyperglycemia poses a risk of serious systemic complications. Especially important is identification of a "brittle diabetic" with erratic glucose control. Certain proteins, notably the B-chain of hemoglobin A and albumin, become glycated. The glycated fraction hemoglobin (measured as HBA1c) normally represents less than 6% of the total hemoglobin; an abnormally high value provides a representation of glucose control over the preceding 3 months. Similarly, glycated albumin (measured as fructosamine) retains the half-life of albumin (21 days) and can provide an estimate of glycemic control for the preceding 3 weeks.

The Systemic Effects of DM

Retinopathy

Most diabetic patients have some degree of retinopathy which is dependent on the duration of disease. Retinopathy is a sensitive predictor of end organ damage. Progressive changes can be seen on fundoscopy. Initially microaneurysms, dot and blot hemorrhages and hard exudates (collectively referred to as "background retinopathy", or nonproliferative retinopathy) occur between 3 and 5 years after the onset of diabetes. When abnormal vessels become occluded, cotton wool exudates are seen (preproliferative retinopathy). The ischemic response stimulates neovascularization (proliferative retinopathy) and then finally fibroproliferative changes which can lead to retinal traction and detachment.

Nephropathy

About a third of patients with diabetes will develop nephropathy. Patients with IDDM are more likely to develop nephropathy than those with NIDDM. The first clinically detectable sign of diabetic nephropathy is microalbuminuria (30–300 mg of albumin/24 h). Microalbuminuria is not detectable by standard urine reagent sticks which generally only detect proteinuria greater than 550 mg/dl. Microalbuminuria is a strong predictor for progression to nephrotic syndrome, hypertension, and eventual end-stage renal disease. Interestingly, persistent microalbuminuria also appears to be predictive for cardiovascular mortality in DM.

Neuropathy

A symmetrical, sensory, peripheral neuropathy is the most common disease pattern. A minority of patients have a painful, peripheral neuropathy. The motor nerves may be involved with focal neuropathies, mononeuritis multiplex, and radiculopathies. Autonomic neuropathy may affect vascular tone, cardiac function, gastric motility, bladder emptying, and erectile function. The autonomic neuropathy may present as a resting tachycardia, abnormal diaphoresis, or postural hypotension alone. Autonomic neuropathy is important to the anesthesiologist, but it affects anesthesia due to increased hemodynamic instability and aspiration due to gastroparesis.

Macrovascular Complications

Accelerated atherosclerotic disease of large vessels is responsible for major morbidity and mortality in DM. More than 75% of diabetic patients will succumb due to complications of diabetic vascular disease, such as coronary artery disease, hypertensive disease, stroke, heart failure, and peripheral vascular disease. In addition, 7% of deaths are attributable to renal failure. The reason why diabetic patients experience accelerated atherosclerosis is unclear, but glycation of lipoproteins and increased platelet adhesion through various means are some of the proposed mechanisms.

The "diabetic foot" is the culmination of multiple systemic effects of diabetes. Peripheral neuropathy results in loss of sensation and altered foot architecture (secondary to motor neuropathy) which increases the risk of unrecognized trauma. Chronic ulceration and poor wound healing is perpetuated by the increased risk of infection, poor nutritional status, and deprived blood. In addition, the hyperglycemia is associated with impaired leukocyte function: chemotaxis, phagocytic capabilities, intracellular killing, and abnormal respiratory burst and superoxide formation. Uncontrolled diabetes puts the patient into a state of malnutrition by producing a relative state of constant catabolism, because the modulating effect of insulin on proteolysis, lipolysis, and glycogenolysis is lost. Because no convincing evidence supports the concept that malnourishment causes diabetes, the term "malnutrition-related diabetes" (MRDM) is obsolete. A previous subtype of MRDM, Fibrocalculous Pancreatic Diabetes (FCDM) is now classified as a disease of the exocrine pancreas which leads to DM.

In the preoperative evaluation of the diabetic patient a thorough investigation is required to identify the above complications.

Diabetic Emergencies

Medical Emergencies

1. Diabetic ketoacidosis (DKA). DKA occurs due to the loss of the modulating effect of insulin on free fatty acid metabolism. The result is ketone-formation and severe fluid deficit. The patient has altered consciousness, ketotic breath, and acidotic breathing. Metabolically, patients have hyperglycemia, a metabolic acidosis, and frequently severe pre-renal azotemia and dehydration

secondary to the osmotic diuresis of the extreme hyperglycemia. Serum amylase activity is commonly increased, but it is rare to have concurrent pancreatitis. Even though the serum potassium is in the normal range (3.5–4.5 mEq/l) because of the acidosis, the total body potassium is severely depleted and should be replaced actively despite an ostensibly normal serum concentration. A septic focus is often present and should be sought actively: e.g. pneumonia, urinary tract infection, etc.

2. Hyperosmolar non-ketotic diabetic coma (HONK). HONK occurs in diabetic patients secondary to the dehydration associated with hyperglycemic osmotic diuresis. This serious condition carries a mortality in excess of 50%. In contrast to DKA, these patients are more prone to seizures, have higher plasma glucose levels (frequently more than 40 mmol/l), and have an even larger fluid deficit. Serum osmolality commonly exceeds 350 mOsm/kg.

3. Other medical emergencies also need consideration, notably the diabetic patient's propensity for "silent" myocardial infarction; diabetic patients might not experience pain or are more prone to present with atypical pain when having a myocardial infarction.

Surgical Emergencies

An aggressive approach must be adopted for the management of diabetic sepsis. Glycemic control may not be achieved if the source of sepsis is not addressed. Life-threatening surgical infections must always be excluded in the diabetic who presents in DKA, specifically wet gangrene, necrotizing fasciitis, emphysematous cholecystitis, and mucormycosis.

Pre-operative Preparation

Elective Procedures (The Diabetic Patient Admitted for Unrelated Pathology)

The approach to these patients includes assessment of recent glycemic control and the systemic complications of diabetes. Patients should be counselled about of the effects of long-term glycemic exposure with regard to nutritional status, surgical fitness, and wound healing.

Patients on oral hypoglycemic agents with good glycemic control may not have to stop their medication for minor procedures. When major operations are planned, oral hypoglycemic agents with a long duration of action should be stopped 24 h prior to operation, while those with short duration of action should be discontinued on the day of operation. Long acting insulin is replaced by short acting insulin. The patient should then be placed on an insulin sliding scale and 5% dextrose/ water infusion to prevent hypoglycemia. The exact protocol should be determined by unit policy and the specific needs of the patient. Whether intermittent insulin administration or continuous infusions are used depends largely on the intensity of the available nursing care (intensive care vs. a normal day care ward). Although preferred, a continuous insulin infusion requires close supervision, and hypoglycemia has dire consequences. Regular glucose monitoring is essential during the procedure. Oral hypoglycemic agents may be restarted with normalization of enteric feeding. In the postoperative period, patients may become insulin-resistant temporarily, and the oral hypoglycemic agents might not attain good glycemic control. Strong evidence exists with regard to the benefits of tight glucose control in the postoperative period. The benefits relate mainly to a decrease in infection-related complications and a modulating effect on the release of inflammatory mediators.

Emergency Procedures

With rare exception, no patient with DKA or HONK should be taken directly to the operating room. The physiologic stress of operation coupled with the immense fluid deficit and metabolic derangement carry a high mortality rate. While it is true that glycemic control is difficult in a diabetic patient with a septic focus, one should address the metabolic derangement and demonstrate a trend toward reversal before undertaking an operation. Insulin and fluids are continued during the procedure.

Although DKA can mimic an acute abdomen, an intra-abdominal septic focus (such as appendicitis) can initiate the ketotic process. The surgeon's priority should be to correct the underlying metabolic derangement and employ non-invasive diagnostic tests to aid the diagnosis. At the other end of the spectrum, diabetic patients may not present with classic signs of peritonitis due to the neuropathy.

The Management of DKA

The patient should be admitted to a high care facility. The mainstay of management is to administer insulin to arrest ketogenesis with replacement of fluid and potassium loss. Infusion of large volumes of crystalloid is recommended. Potassium is replaced expectantly, even if serum values are normal. Insulin should preferably be administered intravenously, but intramuscular administration can be considered while venous access is being established. Although phosphate levels also decrease during resuscitation, it is recommended to treat this expectantly. The use of sodium bicarbonate is not recommended unless the pH is less than 6.9 because of side effects such as hypernatremia, hypokalemia, and a relative cerebrospinal fluid acidosis – despite an increase in serum pH. The end-point of the intervention is not normalization of serum glucose level but rather normalization of ketotic acidosis, because the patient can still be in DKA with a normal serum glucose concentration. When the serum glucose approaches levels less than 15 mmol/l, fluid resuscitation should continue, but with 5% dextrose water to counteract the hypoglycemic effects of the insulin infusion. Although the end point of treatment is reversal of the ketoacidosis, the risk-benefit ratio needs to be considered seriously for the patient who requires an urgent operative procedure.

Glycemic Control in the Critically Ill Patient

New onset hyperglycemia is common in critically ill patients, and tight glucose control is recommended, because hyperglycemia in critically ill patients has been shown to be an independent risk factor for poor outcome. Whether the beneficial effects of tight glucose control come from the actual administration of insulin or from the normalization of glycemia remains unknown. Several groups have postulated that insulin per se could be responsible for the benefits observed through its anabolic effects.

Long-Term Management of the Diabetic Patient

A multidisciplinary approach is essential; involvement of the primary care practitioner, the family, a dietician, the podiatrist, and specialist physicians are essential. Weight control and dietary measures might be the only requirements for glycemic control in the patient with NIDDM. Cessation of smoking and regular exercise should be encouraged. The family should be involved and be informed of the warning signs of hypoglycemia. The patient should wear a bracelet identifying him or her as a diabetic. Education is indispensable, and counseling at every encounter with a health care worker is essential.

Due to the high sensitivity of a fasting plasma glucose level, screening programs can be implemented to avoid the long-term complications of diabetes mellitus.

Diabetes Insipidus

Diabetes insipidus (DI) is a collective term used to describe impairment of renal conservation of water related either to impaired vasopressin secretion or to an abnormal renal response to vasopressin. Diabetes insipidus that develops due to decreased vasopressin secretion from the neurohypophysis is referred to as "central DI" and is usually the consequence of head trauma or a post-operative effect of neurosurgical procedures. A decrease in the renal response to vasopressin is referred to as "nephrogenic DI" related to nephropathy. See ❯ *Table 30-2*.

The Diagnosis of DI

In the absence of other factors, large volumes of dilute urine, as much as 3–6 ml/kg/day, with an osmolality of less than 200 mOsm/kg, is virtually diagnostic. As a response to polydipsia, conscious

◻ Table 30-2

Comparing central and nephrogenic diabetes insipidus (DI)

	Central DI	Nephrogenic DI
Pathophysiology	↓Circulating vasopressin	↓Renal response to vasopressin
Etiology	Head injury	Polycystic kidney
	Hypothalamic neoplasms	Nephrotic syndrome
	Cerebral aneurysms	Amyloidosis
	Stroke	Sjögren's syndrome
	Meningitis	Myeloma
	Idiopathic	Lithium
		Normal aging process
Genetics	Autosomal dominant	X-linked
		Autosomal recessive
Management	Adequate fluid management	Adequate fluid management
	Address the cause, if possible	Address the cause, if possible
	DDAVP	Indomethacin
	Vasopressin	Amiloride
	Clofibrate	Thiazide diuretics
	Carbamazepine	

patients are able to maintain their own fluid balance. In contrast, in the intensive care scenario, where the patient's autonomy for self-regulation of fluid balance is limited, or when managing small infants who are unable to communicate thirst, prevention of hypernatremic dehydration is a priority.

The diagnosis of DI is established when a patient is unable to reduce their urine output and increase urine osmolality after a period of controlled fluid deprivation. Central versus nephrogenic DI can be distinguished by the patient's ability to increase urine osmolality after the administration of DDAVP (1-deamino-8-D-arginine vasopressin) in central DI.

Diabetes insipidus needs to be differentiated from other causes of polyuria, such as primary polydipsia, metabolic disease (diabetes mellitus, hypercalcemia), systemic illness (myeloma, sickle cell disease, resolving acute tubular necrosis), and medications (diuretics, etc.).

Physiology and Pharmacology of DI

Vasopressin is synthesized in the supraoptic and paraventricular nuclei of the hypothalamus and stored in the posterior lobe of the pituitary gland. Circulating vasopressin binds to vasopressin receptors found in vascular tree, many areas of the central nervous system, the adrenal glands, and platelets. The drug vasopressin has an enhanced clinical effect on V_1 receptors causing vasoconstriction, platelet aggregation, and decreased splanchnic perfusion and has benefit in the resuscitative scenarios of cardiac arrest and upper gastrointestinal bleeds. V_2 receptors are concentrated in the renal collecting ducts. Stimulating V_2 receptors allow water channel proteins, called aquaporins, to increase water extraction from the renal collecting ducts in order to concentrate urine. The synthetic analogue of vasopressin 1-deamino-8-D-arginine vasopressin (DDAVP, or desmopressin) can be administered intravenously or intranasally with equal effect and differs from vasopressin in being longer-acting and having its clinical effect primarily on V_2 receptors without producing vasoconstriction. DDAVP stimulates endothelial cells to release Factor VIII, a property with clinical application in Hemophilia A and Von Willebrand's disease.

Treatment of DI

Both types of diabetes insipidus need attention to fluid management and especially so when the patient's autonomy is diminished. Prevention of hypernatremic dehydration by consciously increasing fluid intake is essential. The underlying cause needs to be addressed.

Central DI: The abnormality with central DI is a decreased circulating vasopressin, and thus, treatment with DDAVP is appropriate. Vasopressin, however, has side-effects, such as vasoconstriction, reduced splanchnic perfusion, and platelet aggregation, as well as ACTH release and increased glycogenolysis, each of which limits its potential usefulness in central DI. Other medications to potentiate the effects of a low circulating endogenous vasopressin level can also be considered, including clofibrate, used in hyperlipidemia, carbamazepine, an anti-epileptic drug, and chlorpropamide, a dangerous sulfonylurea with a long half-life and associated prolonged hypoglycemia; this latter drug is generally not recommended.

Nephrogenic DI: Certain medications can be used as an adjunct to fluid management to increase the renal response to circulating vasopressin, including NSAIDs, in particular, indomethacin, which seems to enhance the antidiuretic response to vasopressin, and amiloride, useful in lithium-induced nephrogenic DI. Amiloride blocks the uptake of lithium by the sodium channels in the collecting ducts. Ironically, a thiazide diuretic can be effective for the management of nephrogenic DI, although its mechanism of action in DI is uncertain.

The management challenge in DI relates to controlling the patients fluid and electrolyte status, particularly in the intensive care setting. Prognosis is related to the underlying cause, and medication can be used to decrease the morbidity associated with polyuria and polydipsia.

Selected Readings

Butler SO, Btaiche IF, Alaniz C (2005) Relationship between hyperglycemia and infection in critically ill patients. Pharmacotherapy 25:963–976

Coursin DB, Connery LE, Ketzler JT (2004) Perioperative diabetic and hyperglycaemic management issues. Crit Care Med 32(Suppl):S116–S125

The Expert Committee on the Diagnosis and Classification of Diabetes Mellitus (1997) Report of the Expert Committee on the Diagnosis and Classification of Diabetes Mellitus. Diabetes Care 20:1183–1197

Falanga V (2005) Wound healing and its impairment in the diabetic foot. Lancet 366:1736–1743

Jackson EK (1996) Vasopressin and other agents affecting renal conservation of water. In: Hardman JG, Limbird LE, Molinoff PB, et al. (eds) Goodman and Gilman's the pharmacological basis of therapeutics, 9th edn. McGraw-Hill, New York, pp 715–731

Montori VM, Bistrian BR, McMahon MM (2002) Hyperglycemia in acutely ill patients. JAMA 288:2167–2169

Nathan DM (1993) Long-term complications of diabetes mellitus. N Engl J Med 328:1676–1685

World Health Organization (1985) Diabetes mellitus: report of a WHO Study Group. Technical Report Series 727. WHO, Geneva

Section 4

Head and Neck

31 Incidence, Etiology, Diagnosis, and Staging of Head and Neck Cancer

Kepal N. Patel · Jatin P. Shah

Pearls and Pitfalls

- Head and neck cancer encompasses a broad spectrum of diseases, including epithelial malignancies of the upper aerodigestive tract, malignancies of the skin, paranasal sinuses, salivary glands, the thyroid and parathyroid glands, as well as less common tumors originating from soft tissue, bone and neurovascular structures of the head and neck.
- Head and neck squamous cell cancer (oral cavity/pharyngeal and laryngeal cancer) accounts for approximately 3% of all new cancers and 2% of all cancer deaths in the United States annually.
- Worldwide, head and neck squamous cell carcinoma is the fifth most common cancer and accounts for 6% of all new cancer cases and 5.2% of all cancer deaths.
- The large geographic variability in the incidence of head and neck cancer is secondary to different customs and practices.
- Tobacco and alcohol are the major risk factors for head and neck cancer; this effect is synergistic and multiplicative.
- Viral agents such as Epstein-Barr virus and human papilloma virus have been associated with an increased risk of developing nasopharyngeal and oropharyngeal cancer.
- Other risk factors for head and neck cancer include nutritional, occupational (nickel, wood dust, solvents), prior history of head and neck radiation, immunosuppression and predisposing conditions.
- Mucosal changes leading to field cancerization are common; leukoplakia and erythroplakia are premalignant lesions.
- Every patient with cancer of the head and neck requires a comprehensive evaluation by a multidisciplinary team, including the head and neck surgeon, radiation oncologist, medical oncologist, nutritionist, speech pathologist, and social worker.
- When eliciting history, questions should address symptoms that might be expected if anatomic structures adjacent to the primary site were invaded.
- Patients who present with symptoms suggestive of head and neck cancer should be evaluated by a physician experienced in performing thorough head and neck examination, with attention to the local and regional extent of the disease and possible cervical lymph node metastases.
- Fiberoptic endoscopy should be part of the office examination in evaluating the upper aerodigestive tract in patients with suspected head and neck cancer.
- Approximately 5% of patients with head and neck cancer will have a second primary squamous cell carcinoma of the head and neck, esophagus or lung.

- Appropriate diagnostic and functional imaging can help evaluate the extent of local tumor involvement and regional and distant metastasis, which is critical in staging, treatment planning and prognosis.
- Fine needle aspiration biopsy is the preferred technique to obtain a tissue diagnosis from a neck node.
- Cancer staging is an essential method of categorizing patients for the rapid communication of disease extent, the planning of treatment strategies, the comparison of results after treatment, and the provision of prognostic information to patients. Head and neck cancers are staged according to the TNM system of the AJCC and UICC.

The term head and neck cancer encompasses a broad spectrum of diseases, often linked to a wide variety of causative agents. The majority of these are malignancies of the upper aerodigestive tract, however malignancies of the skin, paranasal sinuses, salivary glands, and the thyroid and parathyroid glands are also included in this category, as well as less common tumors originating from soft tissue, bone and neurovascular structures of the head and neck. With the exception of primary glandular neoplasms, the majority of head and neck cancers are of epithelial origin and theoretically begin as superficial lesions. For the purpose of this chapter, head and neck cancer will refer to squamous cell carcinoma of the upper aerodigestive tract, which includes the oral cavity, pharynx (nasopharynx, oropharynx and hypopharynx) and larynx. The focus of this chapter is on the incidence, etiology, diagnosis, and current staging of head and neck cancer.

Incidence

The American Cancer Society has projected that approximately 47560 new cases of head and neck cancer will be diagnosed in the United States and 11260 deaths will result from head and neck malignancies in 2008. This accounts for approximately 3.3% of all new cancers and 2% of all cancer deaths in the United States annually. The patterns of head and neck cancer development are influenced by a variety of demographic factors, including gender, race, age and geographic location.

Gender differences reveal a significantly higher prevalence of head and neck cancer in men than in women. Incidence in men is double that in women for oral cavity/pharyngeal cancers and these tumors have the eighth highest incidence (3%) of all malignancies in males in the United States. Likewise, the incidence rates in men are approximately four times higher than in women for laryngeal cancer in the United States, and worldwide laryngeal cancer is approximately seven times more common in men than in women, the highest gender ratio of any cancer site.

Race-based differences in the incidence of head and neck cancers also exist. Black women and white women have similar rates of oral cavity/pharyngeal cancer, however black men have a 30% higher rate of oral cavity/pharyngeal cancer than white men. Black men and black women both have double the rate of laryngeal cancer than that of white men and white women, respectively.

The median age of patients with head and neck squamous cell carcinoma is approximately 60 years. However, the incidence of these cancers in young adults (age <40 years) appears to be increasing. Carcinoma of the tongue appears to account for the majority of this increased incidence.

While head and neck cancer is relatively rare in the United States, it is the fifth most common cancer worldwide. The combined worldwide incidence of oral cavity/pharyngeal and laryngeal cancer was approximately 643,869 new cases in 2002, or 6% of all new cancer cases. The worldwide mortality from these malignancies was estimated to be 351,740, representing 5.2% of all cancer deaths. It should be stressed that head and neck cancer refers to malignant tumors of the oral cavity, pharynx (nasopharynx, oropharynx and hypopharynx) and larynx. Other sites (i.e., cutaneous, paranasal sinus, salivary gland and thyroid) are not included in these data.

In some parts of the world, head and neck cancers represent the most common malignancies found in men. For example, Melanesia, a group of islands in the Pacific, has the highest worldwide incidence of oral cavity carcinoma (31.5 per 100,000 in men and 20.2 per 100,000 in women). Rates are also high in south Asia, western Europe, southern Africa, Australia/New Zealand and southern Europe. These patterns reflect prevalence of specific risk factors such as tobacco/alcohol use in western Europe, southern Europe and southern Africa, and the chewing of betel quid in southcentral Asia and Melanesia. The high rate of oral cancer in Australia is due to lip cancer (related to solar irradiation).

There is a large geographic variability in the incidence of laryngeal cancer. High risk countries are in southern Europe (France, Italy, Spain), eastern Europe (Russia, Ukraine), western Europe, western Asia (Turkey, Iraq) and South America (Uruguay, Argentina). In western Asia, larynx cancer accounts for 4.7% of cancers in men. The risk of larynx cancer is greatly increased by tobacco smoking and alcohol consumption, an effect which is multiplicative. Populations at high risk are therefore those where both habits are common.

Nasopharyngeal cancer (NPC) is relatively rare on a world scale (80,000 new cases per year, 0.7% of all cancers with an age-standardized incidence rate generally <1 per 100,000). However, NPC has a very distinctive geographic distribution. The rate of NPC is very high in populations living in or originating from southern China. Populations elsewhere in China, southeast Asia, northeast India, North Africa, and the Inuits (Eskimos) of Canada and Alaska have moderately elevated rates. Risk factors include a strong genetic component, an association with human leukocyte antigen profile, infection with Epstein-Barr virus, and the consumption of certain salted, preserved or fermented dietary items. This may be the consequence of the raised nitrosamine content of such items. Fresh vegetables and fruits have been found to be protective.

Other demographic factors related to an increased incidence of head and neck cancer include low socioeconomic status. These patients often have poor dental hygiene and present with advanced stage disease.

Etiology

Tobacco and Alcohol Exposure

More than 75% of all head and neck cancers can be attributed to tobacco and alcohol consumption. Cigarette smoking is the single most important risk factor in head and neck cancer. Tobacco is a carcinogen that initiates a linear dose response carcinogenic effect in which duration is more important than the intensity of exposure. In heavy smokers 15 years must pass after quitting before the risk approximates the level of nonsmokers. Tobacco contains over 30 known carcinogens. The majority of these are polycyclic aromatic hydrocarbons and nitrosamines. The major carcinogenic activity of cigarette smoke resides in the particulate (tar) fraction, which contains a complex mixture of interacting cancer initiators, promoters and co-carcinogens.

Alcohol is an equally important promoter of carcinogenesis and a major synergistic contributing factor to the development of head and neck cancer. Studies attempting to correlate the type of alcoholic beverage with specific cancer risks have been conflicting. Most investigators believe that ethanol is the main causative factor. The mechanisms by which alcoholic use contributes to the risk of head and neck cancer are not clearly defined. Theories suggest that alcohol may (1) contain other carcinogenic compounds, (2) act as a solvent that enhances the penetration of tobacco or other carcinogens into tissues, (3) generate metabolites that are carcinogenic, (4) enhance nutritional deficiencies, and (5) catalyze the activation of other compounds into carcinogens. The association between alcohol and head and neck cancer is stronger for pharyngeal cancer than for other head and neck sites. Drinkers carry an increased risk of developing head and neck cancer at sites that come in direct contact with the alcohol (oral cavity/pharynx). This suggests that the carcinogenic effects of alcohol act through topical exposure. An association between the use of ethanol containing mouthwash and head and neck cancer supports this idea. The risk of developing oral cavity/pharyngeal cancer in chronic mouthwash users is 40% greater in males and 60% greater in females after adjusting for alcohol and tobacco consumption. This risk increases in proportion to the duration and the frequency of mouthwash use.

Alcohol appears to have an effect on the risk of head and neck cancer independent of tobacco, but these effects are consistently significant only at the higher level of alcohol consumption (>4 oz. daily). The major clinical significance is that it potentiates the carcinogenic effect of tobacco at every level of tobacco use. The causative effect is most striking at the highest exposure levels to both. The magnitude of the effect is synergistic rather than simply additive. Non-smoking males who consume more than four alcoholic drinks per day have a six-fold increase in the risk of developing oral cavity/pharyngeal cancer, and non-drinking males who smoke more than two packs of cigarettes per day have greater than a seven-fold increase in risk. In males who consume more than four drinks and two packs of cigarettes per day, the risk increases more than 37 times, reflecting a multiplicative rather than an additive effect of the two factors combined.

Other methods of tobacco consumption, such as cigar and pipe smoking, are also clearly associated with an increased risk of head and neck cancer. The pooling of saliva containing carcinogens in gravity dependent regions may account for the frequent location of oral carcinomas along the lateral and ventral surfaces of the tongue and in the floor of the mouth. Smokeless tobacco (snuff and chewing) has been associated with increased risk of oral cavity cancer. Smokeless tobacco users and pipe smokers who have a habitual position for the quid or pipe stem often develop carcinomas and dysplasias of the specific site of use (lip, buccal mucosa, gum). Furthermore, cultural and customary practices of various geographic areas may increase the carcinogenic potential of the tobacco. For example, in southeast Asia, reverse smoking (in which the lighted end of the cigarette is held within the mouth) is a common practice. This custom promotes carcinogenesis and contributes to the high incidence of oral cavity cancer in this region.

Field Cancerization

Slaughter et al. proposed that long term exposure to tobacco and alcohol results in diffuse molecular and clinical changes to the mucosa of the upper aerodigestive tract. This condemned mucosa is prone to the development of multifocal cancers. Clinically, this is evidenced by an increased risk of multiple primary carcinomas. Active smokers experience a four-fold increased risk of developing second primary lesions compared with non-smokers or former smokers. These findings suggest that the continued exposure of the upper aerodigestive tract to carcinogens results in a gradual accumulation of genetic alterations. These changes lead to premalignant lesions, index squamous cell carcinomas and ultimately second primary malignancies. This results in the progression of normal mucosa to hyperplasia, atypia, dysplasia, carcinoma in-situ and eventually invasive carcinoma. This genetic progression model correlates well with the theory of field cancerization and with the fact that head and neck cancers tend to arise from previously existing precancerous lesions such as leukoplakia or erythroplakia.

Infectious Agents

Viral agents have been implicated in the pathogenesis of head and neck cancer. The human papillomavirus (HPV) is a well established cause of benign recurrent oral, nasal and respiratory papillomas. Increasing data have emerged supporting a role for HPV in the pathogenesis of a subset of head and neck carcinomas, particularly those that arise from the lingual and palatine tonsils within the oropharynx. High risk HPV-16 is identified in the overwhelming majority of HPV-positive tumors, which have molecular-genetic alterations indicative of viral oncogene function. HPV infection may be altering the demographics of head and neck cancer patients, as these patients tend to be younger, non-smokers and non-drinkers. There is sufficient evidence to conclude that a diagnosis of HPV-positive head and neck cancer has significant prognostic implications; these patients have at least half the risk of death from head and neck cancer when compared with the HPV-negative patient. The HPV etiology of these tumors may have future clinical implications for the diagnosis, therapy, screening, and prevention of head and neck cancer.

There is a strong epidemiological link between Epstein-Barr virus (EBV) and nasopharyngeal carcinoma. The association appears strongest with non-keratinizing undifferentiated NPC, World Health Organization (WHO) types II and III. Recently EBV has also been detected in well differentiated type I carcinomas. EBV is currently being studied as a serologic and mucosal marker to enhance the screening of NPC in endemic areas. Evidence of EBV DNA in cervical lymph node metastases of unknown primary origin has been used to identify a nasopharyngeal primary, and recently studies detecting EBV DNA in peripheral blood has demonstrated prognostic significance for predicting survival and distant metastases. Other agents such as Herpes simplex virus and Helicobacter pylori have been suggested as risk factors for oral cavity and laryngeal carcinoma respectively. Studies to confirm these findings are still in progress.

Nutritional Considerations

Diet and nutrition have also been shown to affect the incidence of head and neck cancer. Consumption of dry, salted fish has been implicated in the development of NPC in southeastern China, a region where this malignancy has a particularly high incidence. The volatile carcinogen dimethylnitrosamine, found in salted fish, may be responsible for this association. The increased risk of carcinoma of the post-cricoid area in elderly female patients with iron deficiency anemia and esophageal webs, known as

Plummer-Vinson syndrome, is also well established. Recent studies have shown that the consumption of fresh fruits and vegetables may decrease the risk of oral and pharyngeal cancer in women.

Occupational Exposure

Occupational exposures probably play a minor role in the development of squamous cell carcinoma in most head and neck sites. However, they are major risk factors for malignancies of the sinonasal region. There is a strong association between sinonasal squamous cell carcinoma and nickel exposure. There is a similar relationship between exposure to wood dust particles and sinonasal adenocarcinoma. Other occupational exposures such as asbestos, coal products, welding fumes, leather tanning solvents, and radium may confer an increased risk of NPC or sinonasal malignancies.

Other

Previous exposure of the head and neck to radiation is associated with an increased risk of malignancy. However, these malignancies are usually not squamous cell carcinomas. Children and young adults who received therapeutic radiation to the head and neck are at increased risk of developing sarcomas of the head and neck, and thyroid and salivary malignancies.

Poor dentition and poor oral hygiene have been correlated with lower socioeconomic status and higher incidence of oral cavity cancer. Marijuana smoke has a four times higher tar burden and 50% higher concentration of benzopyrene and aromatic hydrocarbons than tobacco smoke. It has been suggested that marijuana is a risk factor for head and neck cancer, however direct evidence of marijuana as an etiologic factor does not exist because most users are also exposed to tobacco and alcohol.

In India and parts of Asia, oral tobacco is commonly consumed in a preparation known as "pan", which combines tobacco with betel leaf, slaked lime and areca nut. These betel quid are associated with an increased risk of oral cavity cancer. This risk increases in a dose dependent manner, with the number of betel quid per day and years of betel quid use. It has also been shown to act synergistically with tobacco and alcohol.

Gastroesophageal reflux disease has been suggested to be a risk factor for cancers of the pharynx and larynx. Immunosuppressed individuals and patients with certain predisposing conditions such as Li-Fraumeni syndrome, Fanconi's anemia, Bloom syndrome and ataxia-telangiectasia are at increased risk for developing head and neck cancer.

The etiology of head and neck cancer is multifactorial. Improvements in our understanding of the molecular events involved in malignant transformation may offer new treatment options for patients with head and neck cancer.

Diagnosis

Every patient with cancer of the head and neck requires a comprehensive evaluation by a multi-disciplinary team, including the head and neck surgeon, radiation oncologist, medical oncologist, nutritionist, speech pathologist, and social worker.

History

A thorough history and physical examination are essential in directing the examiner toward the site of disease and possible extent of disease. Symptoms such as pain, numbness, odynophagia, dysphagia, trismus, hoarseness, dyspnea, epistaxis, otalgia, nasal obstruction, change in vision, headache, vertigo, tinnitus, weight loss and other constitutional symptoms should be elicited. Symptoms related to the tumor often suggest a specific anatomic site. For example, hoarseness indicates probable laryngeal involvement. Questions should address symptoms that might be expected if anatomic structures adjacent to the primary site were invaded. This will help ascertain the limits of the tumor. The severity of disease is determined by the duration, type, and rapidity of progression of symptoms and the functional impairment experienced by the patient. Symptoms of systemic disease, such as bone pain, necessitate a metastatic workup.

A social history establishes risk factors for head and neck cancer. Tobacco and alcohol use should be quantified. Note that patients often underestimate the quantity of alcohol that they consume. Other risk factors should be elicited, such as occupational exposure, radiation exposure, dentition problems, sun exposure, and family history. Certain head and neck tumors (i.e., medullary thyroid cancer) may have a familial pattern of transmission and may warrant a detailed family history.

Psychosocial assessment is often overlooked in the evaluation of patients with head and neck cancer. Patients are more psychologically invested in the head and neck than in other parts of the body. Unlike other cancer patients, head and neck cancer patients are often unable to conceal their affliction from public view. Dysfunction and disfigurement of the structures of the head and neck can lead to social isolation. The quality of life for these patients is often very poor. This can be a difficult challenge for the patient and the physician. Preoperative counseling should be offered to help reduce uncertainty and anxiety. Meeting with speech therapists, nutritionists and support groups can be very beneficial. The clinician should provide appropriate pre-treatment counseling and encourage patient participation.

A careful history generates a complete differential diagnosis, ensuring that all diagnostic possibilities are considered prior to the establishment of a definitive diagnosis.

Physical Examination

General

The overall appearance of the patient is assessed with an immediate overview of the functional status, level of comfort, obvious deformities, nutritional status, and respiratory status.

Face, Ears, and Eyes

All facial, scalp and neck skin lesions are inspected. The postauricular and preauricular regions are palpated. The pinna and external auditory canal are examined. The tympanic membrane and middle ear are evaluated with an otoscope. The eyes are examined for extraocular motility, visual acuity, pupil reactivity and globe position.

Key findings in the examination of the face, ears and eyes:

1. Facial asymmetry and/or weakness – facial nerve involvement
2. Facial numbness, change in sensation – trigeminal nerve involvement
3. Serous otitis media – Eustachian tube obstruction from nasopharyngeal or paranasal sinus tumor
4. Diplopia, restriction in mobility or a displaced globe – mass compression from a paranasal sinus or orbital tumor

Nasal Cavity, Paranasal Sinuses, and Nasopharynx

Examination of the nasal cavity and nasopharynx is best performed endoscopically. Flexible and rigid endoscopy in the awake patient will allow inspection of the entire nasal mucosal lining. Within the nasopharynx, special attention is paid to Rosenmuller's fossa, a recess posterior to the Eustachian tube orifice that is a common site of origin for nasopharyngeal carcinoma. Paranasal sinus masses can be difficult to evaluate on physical examination (❷ *Fig. 31-1*). Inspection of the dentition, hard palate, and the alveolar ridge in the oral cavity may reveal signs of an inferior maxillary sinus mass.

Key findings in the examination of the nasal cavity, paranasal sinuses, and nasopharynx:

1. Fullness of the external cheek – an underlying mass
2. Cheek numbness – involvement of the infraorbital nerve
3. Trismus – extension of the tumor into the pterygoid musculature
4. Globe displacement, restriction of extraocular movement, and loss of vision – orbital involvement

Oral Cavity and Oropharynx

Examination of the oral cavity and oropharynx consists of careful inspection and palpation of all subsites (❷ *Fig. 31-2*). The surface characteristics of the mucosa are evaluated for any irregularities. Bimanual palpation is particularly helpful in the assessment of masses of the floor of mouth, as well as submental, submandibular and buccal masses. Appropriate visualization and evaluation of the base of tongue with either a mirror exam or flexible fiberoptic office endoscopy is essential.

Key findings in the examination of the oral cavity and oropharynx:

1. Mandibular involvement – important for both staging and treatment planning
2. Tongue deviation – hypoglossal nerve weakness on the side to which the tongue deviates
3. Restriction of tongue motion – deep invasion with infiltration of the extrinsic and intrinsic tongue musculature
4. Impaired sensation of the tongue, lower alveolus, or lower lip – involvement of the mandibular division of the trigeminal nerve

■ Figure 31-1

Anatomy of the paranasal sinuses (Courtesy of the American Society of Clinical Oncology)

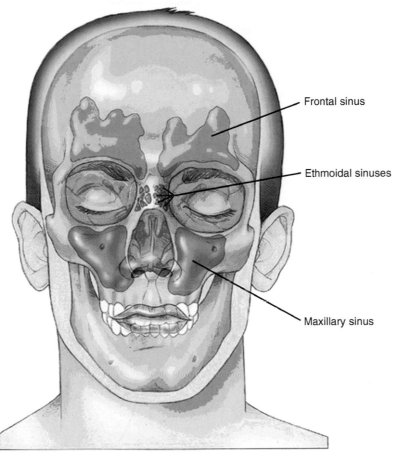

Larynx and Hypopharynx

Appropriate evaluation of all the subsites of the larynx and hypopharynx is essential (❯ *Fig. 31-3*). Flexible fiberoptic endoscopy allows for detailed visualization of the larynx and hypopharynx and is a vital part of the routine head and neck examination in the office. Vocal cord mobility (fully intact, decreased or fixed) and voice quality are noted. The surface characteristics of the mucosa are evaluated for any irregularities.

Key findings in the examination of the larynx and hypopharynx:

1. Sensation of the supraglottis – superior laryngeal nerve function
2. Dysphagia – pyriform sinus or post cricoid space mass (can be difficult to evaluate – examination under anesthesia may be required)
3. Aspiration, hoarseness – vocal cord mobility

□ Figure 31-2
a. Anatomy of the oral cavity; b. and the oropharynx (Reprinted from Shah and Patel, 2003. With permission from Elsevier)

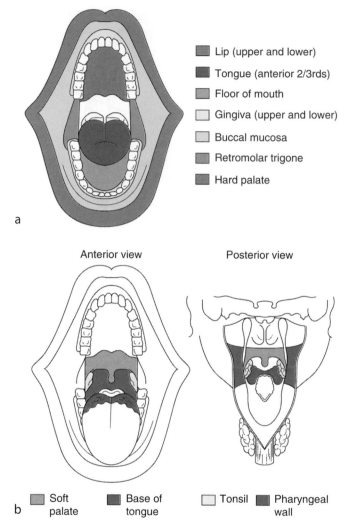

Neck

Squamous cell carcinomas of the upper aerodigestive tract metastasize to the cervical lymph nodes in a predictable pattern (❷ *Fig. 31-4*). Knowledge of these patterns, may help detect the primary tumor location. The neck is palpated with particular attention to the regions at highest risk for regional nodal metastases.

Key findings in the examination of the neck:

1. Palpable masses – assess for size, location, texture, mobility, skin involvement
2. Assess the thyroid and cricoid cartilages, the thyrohyoid and cricothyroid membranes, the thyroid gland and the laryngeal mobility over the prevertebral fascia
3. Shoulder weakness – spinal accessory nerve involvement

◘ Figure 31-3
a. Anatomy of the larynx; b. and the hypopharynx (Reprinted from Shah and Patel, 2003. With permission from Elsevier)

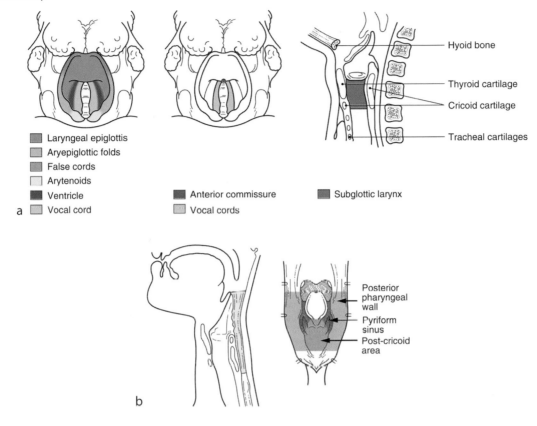

It is imperative that patients who present with symptoms suggestive of head and neck cancer be evaluated by a physician experienced in performing a thorough head and neck examination, including rigid and flexible fiberoptic endoscopy. Mistakes commonly made in the evaluation of patients with head and neck cancer can lead to treatment delays.

Imaging

Appropriate diagnostic imaging of head and neck tumors is crucial. Accurate evaluation of the extent of local tumor involvement and regional and distant metastasis is critical in staging, treatment planning and prognosis. For example, tumors encasing the carotid vessels and invading the prevertebral fascia may not be amenable to surgical resection. Radiologic images can provide valuable information on tumor extension into anatomic spaces or tissue planes, involvement of neurovascular structures, and erosion of bone. Furthermore, diagnostic imaging may help locate the occult primary cancer, and detect cervical metastases that may not be palpable on physical examination.

Computed tomography (CT) and magnetic resonance imaging (MRI) are the predominant imaging modalities used in the head and neck. CT offers superior bone detail, lower cost and

◘ Figure 31-4

a. Cervical nodal basins; b. and patterns of metastases (Reprinted from Shah and Patel, 2003. With permission from Elsevier)

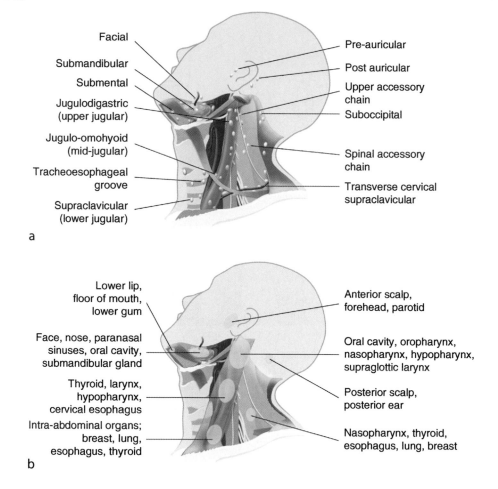

better availability. MRI is better in assessing tumor invasion of nerves, dura, brain, muscle and soft tissues. It is often preferred for evaluation of the nasopharynx and base of tongue. Each modality has its advantages, even within anatomic subsites. For example, CT is useful in detecting bone invasion of the mandible, however MRI can show involvement of the mental nerve and inferior alveolar nerve. The decision to use MRI vs. CT is based on the information needed in a particular case.

Positron emission tomography (PET) using 18F fluorodeoxyglucose is a newer imaging modality that is being used to evaluate patients with head and neck cancer. PET imaging assesses tissue metabolic activity. It has proven useful in distinguishing recurrent tumor from post-treatment fibrosis, evaluating tumor response to non-operative therapies, detecting occult primary lesions, and detecting regional and distant metastases. It has poor spatial resolution, rendering it less suitable for accurate anatomic assessment of tumor extent. Machines that combine PET with CT are therefore preferred.

Conventional angiography or magnetic resonance angiography (MRA) are useful in assessing tumor invasion of major vessels, collateral circulation and patency. Ultrasonography is very useful and widely popular in evaluating thyroid masses, guiding fine needle aspiration biopsies and following indeterminate lymph nodes and cystic lesions.

Biopsy

Once the tumor has been evaluated by physical examination and diagnostic imaging, a tissue specimen is required to establish a pathologic diagnosis. Fine needle aspiration biopsy (FNAB) is the preferred technique for palpable neck masses, lymph nodes, thyroid nodules and parotid lesions. Ultrasound guided or image guided FNAB is appropriate for non-palpable masses. FNAB is highly sensitive and carries few associated risks. The cytopathologist should be well trained in head and neck aspiration cytology. Open biopsy may be indicated when FNAB is non-diagnostic. A general principle is to plan the biopsy in a manner which avoids tumor contamination and facilitates future surgical removal.

Lesions of the oral cavity can be biopsied in the office with local anesthesia. Lesions of the oropharynx, nasopharynx, hypopharynx and larynx usually require biopsy under general anesthesia. This allows for a complete endoscopic examination of the upper aerodigestive tract, including a detailed inspection of the site and extent of the primary tumor and detection of occult second primary tumors. Approximately 5% of patients with head and neck cancer will have a second primary squamous cell carcinoma of the head and neck, esophagus or lung. Esophagoscopy and bronchoscopy should be performed as dictated by the patient's symptoms and when the risk of multiple primary tumors is high. The routine performance of these procedures in all patients with head and neck cancer is of low yield and remains controversial. Directed biopsies of suspicious lesions with intraoperative frozen section analysis is the preferred technique. Highly suspicious lesions warrant multiple biopsies with frozen section analysis until the diagnosis can be more clearly established.

Future Directions

As our understanding of the molecular mechanisms involved in carcinogenesis increases, it is likely that certain findings will be incorporated into clinical practice. Specific tumor markers may help identify patients at risk of treatment failure and recurrence. New molecular targets may allow for novel therapeutic applications. As technology advances, developments in radiographic techniques may prove beneficial to the evaluation of the patient with head and neck cancer.

Staging

The single most important factor in patient assessment, treatment planning, and survival prognostication is accurate staging. It provides a universal measurement of the extent of cancer and allows for communication of disease extent to others. The current staging guidelines in use for head and neck cancer are from the 2002 Cancer Staging Manual of the American Joint Committee on Cancer (❷ *Table 31-1*). Staging involves an accurate assessment of tumor at the primary site (T),

◻ Table 31-1

Staging of head and neck cancer (American Joint Committee on Cancer, 2002. With permission; www.springeronline.com)

T staging for all head and neck sites except the thyroid and major salivary glands	
LIP AND ORAL CAVITY	
Primary tumor (T)	
TX	Primary tumor cannot be assessed
T0	No evidence of primary tumor
Tis	Carcinoma in situ
T1	Tumor 2 cm or less in greatest dimension
T2	Tumor more than 2 cm but not more than 4 cm in greatest dimension
T3	Tumor more than 4 cm in greatest dimension
T4a (lip)	Tumor invades through cortical bone, inferior alveolar nerve, floor of mouth, or skin of face (ie, chin or nose)
T4a (oral cavity)	Tumor invades through cortical bone, into deep [extrinsic] muscle of tongue (genioglossus, hyoglossus, palatoglossus, and styloglossus), maxillary sinus, or skin of face
T4b	Tumor involves masticator space, pterygoid plates, or skull base and/or encases internal carotid artery
Note: Superficial erosion alone of bone/tooth socket by gingival primary is not sufficient to classify as T4	
PHARYNX	
TX	Primary tumor cannot be assessed
T0	No evidence of primary tumor
Tis	Carcinoma in situ
Nasopharynx	
T1	Tumor confined to the nasopharynx
T2	Tumor extends to soft tissues
T2a	Tumor extends to the oropharynx and/or nasal cavity without parapharyngeal extension[a]
T2b	Any tumor with parapharyngeal extension[a]
T3	Tumor involves bony structures and/or paranasal sinuses
T4	Tumor with intracranial extension and/or involvement of cranial nerves, infratemporal fossa, hypopharynx, orbit, or masticator space
Oropharynx	
T1	Tumor 2 cm or less in greatest dimension
T2	Tumor more than 2 cm but not more than 4 cm in greatest dimension
T3	Tumor more than 4 cm in greatest dimension
T4a	Tumor invades the larynx, deep/extrinsic muscle of tongue, medial pterygoid, hard palate, or mandible
T4b	Tumor invades lateral pterygoid muscle, pterygoid plates, lateral nasopharynx, or skull base or encases carotid artery
Hypopharynx	
T1	Tumor limited to 1 subsite of hypopharynx and 2 cm or less in greatest dimension
T2	Tumor invades more than 1 subsite of hypopharynx or an adjacent site, or measures more than 2 cm but not more than 4 cm in greatest diameter without fixation of hemilarynx
T3	Tumor measures more than 4 cm in greatest dimension or with fixation of hemilarynx
T4a	Tumor invades thyroid/cricoid cartilage, hyoid bone, thyroid gland, esophagus, or central compartment soft tissue[b]
T4b	Tumor invades prevertebral fascia, encases carotid artery, or involves mediastinal structures
[a]Parapharyngeal extension denotes posterolateral infiltration beyond the pharyngobasilar fascia.	
[b]Central compartment soft tissue includes prelaryngeal strap muscles and subcutaneous fat.	
LARYNX	
TX	Primary tumor cannot be assessed
T0	No evidence of primary tumor
Tis	Carcinoma in situ
Supraglottis	
T1	Tumor limited to one subsite of supraglottis with normal vocal cord mobility
T2	Tumor invades mucosa of more than one adjacent subsite of supraglottis or glottis or region outside the supraglottis (e.g., mucosa of base of tongue, vallecula, medial wall of pyriform sinus) without fixation of the larynx

■ **Table 31-1 (Continued)**

T3	Tumor limited to larynx with vocal cord fixation and/or invades any of the following: postcricoid area, preepiglottic tissues, paraglottic space, and/or minor thyroid cartilage erosion (e.g., inner cortex)
T4a	Tumor invades through the thyroid cartilage and/or invades tissues beyond the larynx (e.g., trachea, soft tissues of neck including deep extrinsic muscle of the tongue, strap muscles, thyroid, or esophagus)
T4b	Tumor invades prevertebral space, encases carotid artery, or invades mediastinal structures
Glottis	
T1	Tumor limited to the vocal cord(s) (may involve anterior or posterior commissure) with normal mobility
T1a	Tumor limited to one vocal cord
T1b	Tumor involves both vocal cords
T2	Tumor extends to supraglottis and/or subglottis, or with impaired vocal cord mobility
T3	Tumor limited to larynx with vocal cord fixation
T4a	Tumor invades cricoid or thyroid cartilage and/or invades tissues beyond the larynx (e.g., trachea, soft tissues of neck including deep extrinsic muscles of the tongue, strap muscles, thyroid, or esophagus)
T4b	Tumor invades prevertebral space, encases carotid artery or invades mediastinal structures
Subglottis	
T1	Tumor limited to the subglottis
T2	Tumor extends to vocal cord(s) with normal or impaired mobility
T3	Tumor limited to larynx with vocal cord fixation
T4a	Tumor invades cricoid or thyroid cartilage and/or invades tissues beyond the larynx (e.g., trachea, soft tissues of neck including deep extrinsic muscles of the tongue, strap muscles, thyroid, or esophagus)
T4b	Tumor invades prevertebral space, encases carotid artery, or involves mediastinal structures
NASAL CAVITY AND PARANASAL SINUSES	
TX	Primary tumor cannot be assessed
T0	No evidence of primary tumor
Tis	Carcinoma in situ
Maxillary sinus	
T1	Tumor limited to the maxillary sinus mucosa with no erosion or destruction of bone
T2	Tumor causing bone erosion or destruction including extension into the hard palate and/or middle nasal meatus, except extension to posterior wall of maxillary sinus, subcutaneous tissues, floor or medial wall of orbit, pterygoid fossa, ethmoid sinuses
T3	Tumor invades any of the following: bone of the posterior wall of maxillary sinus, subcutaneous tissues, floor or medial wall of orbit, pterygoid fossa, ethmoid sinuses
T4a	Tumor invades anterior orbital contents, skin of cheek, pterygoid plates, infratemporal fossa, cribriform plate, sphenoid or frontal sinuses
T4b	Tumor invades any of the following: orbital apex, dura, brain, middle cranial fossa, cranial nerves other than maxillary division of trigeminal nerve V2, nasopharynx, or clivus
Nasal cavity and ethmoid sinus	
T1	Tumor restricted to any one subsite, with or without bony invasion
T2	Tumor invading two subsites in a single region or extending to involve an adjacent region within the nasoethmoidal complex, with or without bony invasion
T3	Tumor extends to invade the medial wall or floor of the orbit, maxillary sinus, palate, or cribriform plate
T4a	Tumor invades any of the following: anterior orbital contents, skin of nose or cheek, minimal extension to anterior cranial fossa, pterygoid plates, sphenoid or frontal sinuses
T4b	Tumor invades any of the following: orbital apex, brain, middle cranial fossa, cranial nerves other than V2, nasopharynx, or clivus
N Staging for all head and neck sites except the nasopharynx and thyroid	
Nx	Regional lymph nodes cannot be assessed
N0	No regional lymph node metastasis
N1	Metastasis in a single ipsilateral lymph node, 3 cm or less in greatest dimension
N2	Metastasis in a single ipsilateral lymph node, more than 3 cm but not more than 6 cm in greatest dimension; or in multiple ipsilateral lymph nodes, none more than 6 cm in greatest dimension; or in bilateral or contralateral lymph nodes, none more than 6 cm in greatest dimension
N2a	Metastasis in a single ipsilateral lymph node more than 3 cm but not more than 6 cm in greatest dimension

◻ Table 31-1 (Continued)

N2b	Metastasis in multiple ipsilateral lymph nodes, none more than 6 cm in greatest dimension
N2c	Metastasis in bilateral or contralateral lymph nodes, none more than 6 cm in greatest dimension
N3	Metastasis in a lymph more than 6 cm in greatest dimension

N Staging for tumors of the nasopharynx

Nx	Regional lymph nodes cannot be assessed
N0	No regional lymph node metastasis
N1	Unilateral metastasis in lymph node(s), 6 cm or less in greatest dimension, above the supraclavicular fossa[a]
N2	Bilateral metastasis in lymph node(s), 6 cm or less in greatest dimension, above the supraclavicular fossa[a]
N3	Metastasis in a lymph node(s) >6 cm and/or to supraclavicular fossa
N3a	Greater than 6 cm in dimension
N3b	Extension to the supraclavicular fossa[a]

[a]Midline nodes are considered ipsilateral nodes.

M Staging for head and neck tumors

Mx	Distant metastasis cannot be assessed
M0	No distant metastasis
M1	Distant metastasis

Stage grouping for all head and neck sites except the nasopharynx and thyroid

Stage group	T stage	N stage	M stage
0	Tis	N0	M0
I	T1	N0	M0
II	T2	N0	M0
III	T3	N0	M0
	T1	N1	M0
	T2	N1	M0
	T3	N1	M0
IVA	T4a	N0	M0
	T4a	N1	M0
	T1	N2	M0
	T2	N2	M0
	T3	N2	M0
	T4a	N2	M0
IVB	T4b	Any N	M0
	Any T	N3	M0
IVC	Any T	Any N	M1

Stage grouping for tumors of the nasopharynx

Stage group	T stage	N stage	M stage
0	Tis	N0	M0
I	T1	N0	M0
IIA	T2a	N0	M0
IIB	T1	N1	M0
	T2a	N1	M0
	T2b	N0	M0
	T2b	N1	M0
III	T1	N2	M0
	T2a	N2	M0
	T2b	N2	M0
	T3	N0	M0
	T3	N1	M0
	T3	N2	M0
IVA	T4	N0	M0
	T4	N1	M0
	T4	N2	M0
IVB	Any T	N3	M0
IVC	Any T	Any N	M1

regional lymphatic metastases (N), and distant metastases (M). Each primary tumor has a unique propensity for local and regional spread, which must be appreciated when evaluating head and neck cancer patients. Prognosis correlates strongly with the stage at diagnosis. For many head and neck cancer sites, survival exceeds 80% in patients with stage I disease. However, patients with Stage IV disease at diagnosis have a survival rate of less than 40%. Other factors such as co-morbidities, histopathological and molecular features, and imaging have not been incorporated into the current staging system, but may eventually assist in providing more accurate predictions of outcome in the future.

Selected Readings

American Joint Committee on Cancer (2002) AJCC Cancer Staging Manual, 6th edn. Springer, New York

Blot WJ, McLaughlin JK, Winn DM, et al. (1988) Smoking and drinking in relation to oral and pharyngeal cancer. Cancer Res 48:3282–3287

Fakhry C, Gillison ML (2006) Clinical implications of human papillomavirus in head and neck cancers. J Clin Oncol 24:2606–2611

Jemal A, Siegel R, Ward E, et al. (2008) Cancer statistics, 2008. CA Cancer J Clin 58:71–96

Parkin DM, Bray F, Ferlay J, Pisani P (2005) Global cancer statistics, 2002. CA Cancer J Clin 55:74–108

Patel SG, Shah JP (2005) TNM staging of cancers of the head and neck: striving for uniformity among diversity. CA Cancer J Clin 55:242–258; quiz 261–262, 264. Review

Shah JP, Patel SG (2003) Head & neck surgery & oncology, 3rd edn. Mosby, Edinburgh

Slaughter DP, Southwick HW, Smejkal W (1953) Field cancerization in oral stratified squamous epithelium; clinical implications of multicentric origin. Cancer 6:963–968

Winn DM, Blot WJ, McLaughlin JK, et al. (1991) Mouthwash use and oral conditions in the risk of oral and pharyngeal cancer. Cancer Res 51:3044–3047

Winn DM, Ziegler RG, Pickle LW, et al. (1984) Diet in the etiology of oral and pharyngeal cancer among women from the southern United States. Cancer Res 44:1216–1222

32 Cancer of the Oral Cavity and Oropharynx

Richard O. Wein · Randal S. Weber

Pearls and Pitfalls

- Nonhealing ulcers (>2 weeks duration) of the oral cavity and oropharynx, including the lateral tongue may be malignant and require prompt biopsy.
- New-onset otalgia, in a patient without a prior history of ear problems, requires a thorough examination of the upper aerodigestive tract.
- A "chronic" sore throat, cervical lymphadenopathy, and nontraumatic trismus in a smoker should be considered consistent with a neoplastic process until proven otherwise.
- Habitual tobacco use and alcohol abuse are the most significant risk factors for the development of a head and neck squamous cell carcinoma.
- Fine-needle aspiration biopsy should be considered prior to open neck biopsy for neck masses of unknown origin.
- Dental procedures in patients with a history of prior radiation therapy to the head and neck should be performed by individuals experienced in the care of radiated patients.
- Accurate TNM staging is the goal of diagnostic evaluation (clinical and radiographic) and aids in assessing prognosis and treatment planning.

Basic Science

Squamous cell carcinoma is the most common cancer within all sites of the upper aerodigestive tract. Understanding the molecular biological events leading to the development of this cancer has been the focus of a significant quantity of research. Many of the oncogenes, tumor suppressor genes and chromosomal imbalances associated with the development of squamous cell carcinoma have been identified yet benefits such as gene therapy are only starting to become reality. Current nationwide oncology group studies are exploring the efficacy of therapies directed at inhibiting epidermal growth factor receptors and factors associated with angiogenesis.

The habitual use of tobacco and alcohol are considered the most common preventable exposures associated with the development of head and neck cancers. The relationship of the risk factors is synergistic with alcohol serving as a promoter for the carcinogenic effects of tobacco. Smoking alone confers a 2–3-fold increased risk for the development of neoplasia with the risk being directly proportional to the years spent smoking and the number of cigarettes smoked per day. Individuals who smoke more than 40 cigarettes/day and consume more than four alcoholic drinks/day are 35 times more likely to develop an oral or oropharyngeal carcinoma than controls. Induction of specific p53 mutations within upper aerodigestive tract tumors have been noted in patients with a history of tobacco and alcohol use. Additional described risk factors include sun exposure (lip cancer), viruses, smokeless tobacco, and betel quid use.

Clinical Presentation

In 2005, approximately 30,000 Americans were diagnosed with a cancer of the oral cavity or oropharynx. The median age at the time of diagnosis is 63 years. Males have a higher frequency of diagnosis than females (15.5 vs. 6.4 per 100,000). Unfortunately at the time of diagnosis, only one-third of previously untreated patients present with disease confined to their primary site. Over 50% of patients demonstrate evidence of regional metastasis at initial presentation. Approximately 10% of patients are found to have distant metastasis at the time of their initial diagnosis.

Although they represent adjacent anatomical sites located in the head and neck, differ in clinical presentation and treatment philosophy. Both cancers of the oral cavity and oropharynx have several subsites with varying anatomy that have implications for local spread of disease and functional outcome after treatment. The oral cavity is composed of the mucosal lip, buccal mucosa, alveolar ridges, retromolar trigone, floor of the mouth, hard palate and anterior two-thirds of the tongue (❯ *Fig. 32-1*). Posterior to the oral cavity is the oropharynx, which is contiguous with the nasopharynx

◘ Figure 32-1

Oral cavity anatomy. a. Includes locations of the oral tongue, hard palate, retromolar trigone, buccal mucosa, lip, upper and lower alveolar ridge, and floor of the mouth. b. Coronal cross-section demonstrates deep anatomy at risk for spread of oral tongue and floor of the mouth cancers, including neurovascular bundles with CN XII and lingual nerve, deep tongue musculature, and mandible

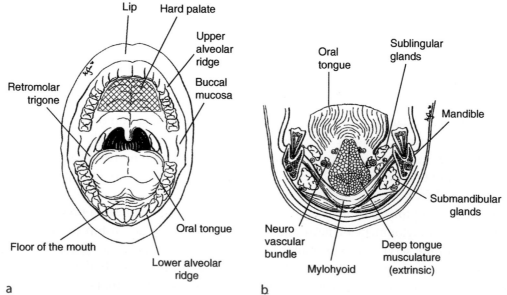

☐ **Figure 32-2**

Oropharynx anatomy. a. Sagittal and coronal cross-section demonstrating the relationship of the oropharynx to the nasopharynx and hypopharynx. b. Oral view demonstrating oropharyngeal anatomy including tonsils, tonsillar arches, soft palate, and base of the tongue. c. Posterior-anterior view demonstrating the transition to the base of the tongue at the circumvallate papilla, tonsils, and relationship to the larynx

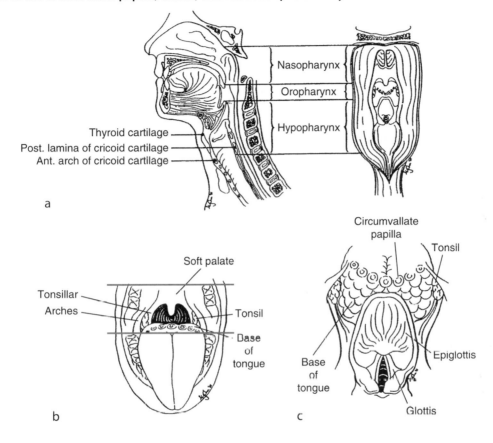

superiorly and hypopharynx inferiorly. The oropharynx includes the soft palate, base of the tongue, anterior/posterior tonsillar pillars, and posterolateral pharyngeal walls (❯ *Fig. 32-2*).

The typical patient with a carcinoma of the oral cavity or oropharynx presents with a series of complaints. They range from having an ill-fitting denture, a non-healing ulcer, bleeding, localized oral pain, otalgia (ear pain), dysphagia (difficulty swallowing), odynophagia (pain with swallowing), or dysphonia (change in vocal quality). The development of regional lymphadenopathy may also be the presenting complaint that leads a patient to evaluation.

The general head and neck physical examination requires evaluation of the patient's general appearance, ears, nose, oral cavity, oropharynx, nasopharynx, larynx, hypopharynx, and neck. The physical examination of the oral cavity requires a headlight and tongue blades to assist in the visualization for premalignant changes (leukoplakia, erythroplakia, lichen planus) and/or exophytic/ulcerative lesions. Bimanual exam of the tongue and floor of the mouth is helpful in determining submucosal spread of disease and may assist in identifying submental and submandibular lymph node spread. An assessment of cranial nerve function (sensory and motor) is important to identify evidence of soft tissue atrophy (such as with cranial nerve XII involvement) or paresthesia (such as lip numbness) associated with tumor spread. The status of a patient's dentition is assessed and frequently requires dental consultation for further evaluation and care. Staging for oral cavity tumors is dependent on size and extent of spread. Tumors less than 2 cm are T1, Tumors greater than 2 cm and less than 4 cm are T2, and tumors greater than 4 cm are considered T3. Tumors that are T4 are divided into T4a (treatable invasive spread) and T4b (unresectable features – carotid encasement, pterygoid plate/skull base spread). Features that make a tumor, independent of size, T4a in status include cortical bone involvement (mandible), deep extrinsic tongue musculature involvement or skin of the face (❯ *Fig. 32-1B*).

The oropharyngeal examination is an extension of the oral cavity exam and requires that attention be directed to the oropharynx for soft tissue asymmetry (such as peritonsillar region and soft palate). Indirect mirror exam and flexible laryngoscopy allow assessment of the base of tongue and adjacent anatomy. These examination techniques allow for an estimation of the primary site's proximity to the midline. This is important in determining the potential risk of lymphatic spread to both sides of the neck. Staging for tumors of the oropharynx parallels that of oral cavity tumors (T1 <2 cm, T2 >2 cm and <4 cm and T3 >4 cm). T4a tumors may involve the larynx (❯ *Fig. 32-2C*), deep tongue musculature, medial pterygoid, hard palate, or mandible. Similar to oral cavity tumors, T4b lesions have unresectable features.

Neck examination requires the sequential assessment of the levels of the neck (I–VI, ❯ *Fig. 32-3*) where lymph nodes reside that may harbor metastatic disease. This assessment aids the surgeon in estimating the extent of neck dissection required if necessary and in performing TNM staging. Neck staging ranges from N1 to N3. N1 disease indicates a single ipsilateral lymph node metastasis less than 3 cm. N2 disease is divided into N2a (single ipsilateral node >3 cm yet <6 cm), N2b (multiple ipsilateral lymph nodes involved), and N2c (ipsilateral and/or contralateral lymph nodes involved). N3 nodal status indicates lymph node metastasis >6 cm in greatest dimension.

Finally, the diagnostic clinical examination may require assessment of the reconstructive options available if a resection requires removal of a significant quantity of soft tissue and/or bone that would impair postoperative speech and swallowing. Typical donor site for head and neck reconstruction include pedicled flaps such as the pectoralis major myocutaneous flap and microvascular options such as the radial forearm or the fibular free flap reconstruction.

The differential diagnosis for malignant lesions of the oral cavity is broad and includes verrucous carcinoma, minor salivary gland carcinomas, and mucosal melanoma. Verrucous carcinoma is a white, exophytic, locally aggressive variant of squamous carcinoma that does not tend to spread to regional lymphatics that are treated with surgical excision. Minor salivary gland carcinomas (adenoid cystic, mucoepidermoid) tend to present as submucosal masses along the posterolateral aspect of the hard palate. They require surgical excision of a portion of the maxilla, palatal rehabilitation (obturator versus surgical reconstruction), and may necessitate postoperative radiation. Mucosal melanoma is associated with a poor long-term prognosis because of a proclivity for distant metastases.

Diagnosis

The diagnosis of an oral cavity or oropharyngeal cancer starts with a biopsy. For accessible oral lesions, a punch biopsy or cup forceps can frequently be performed in the office setting. For individuals

⬛ Figure 32-3

Lymphatic zones of the neck. Level I – submental and submandibular triangles, level II – upper jugular lymphatics, level III – mid-jugular lymphatics, level IV –lower jugular lymphatics, level V – posterior cervical triangle, level VI – central compartment lymphatics, level VII – superior mediastinal lymphatics (American Joint Committee on Cancer (AJCC), 2002. With permission; www.springeronline.com)

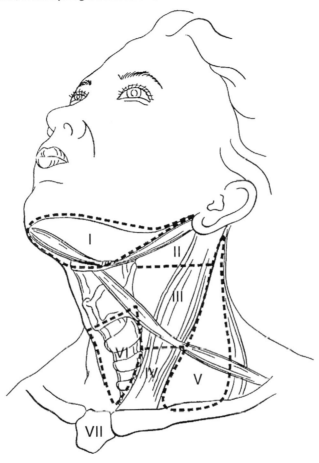

presenting with lesions inappropriate for office-based biopsy and cervical lymphadenopathy, fine needle aspiration offers an excellent means to establishing diagnosis.

Operative direct laryngoscopy and biopsy is required to establish diagnosis in patients with tongue base lesions and allows the surgeon to gauge the extent and spread of a lesion while the patient's airway is secure. Additionally, it can allow for the assessment of potential synchronous aerodigestive tract lesions. After establishing the histopathologic diagnosis, imaging is frequently necessary to further assess extension and involvement of associated anatomy and the presence of regional lymphadenopathy. Obtaining CT scans with contrast of the primary site and neck are an excellent means of assessing these diagnostic issues. MRI offers good soft tissue differentiation and may be desirable in assessing oral tongue and tongue base lesions. Panorex, in addition to CT scan, is typically performed to assess mandibular invasion. PET scanning and/or CT examination of the chest allows for assessment of distant spread of disease which is most frequently to the lungs.

The goal of clinical, operative, and radiographic assessment should be to allow accurate staging of the tumor and to allow the physician to best decide the appropriate treatment for the patient's cancer. The clinical exam and imaging should generate a T (primary site), N (regional lymphatics), and M (distant metastasis) stage that aid in assessing prognosis. The best prognosis is associated with early stage disease (Stage I – T1N0M0, Stage II – T2N0M0) as opposed to advanced stage disease (Stage III – T1–3N1M0, Stage IVa/IVb – Any T, N2/3, M0). In general, the presence of regional metastases decreases prognosis by 50%. Patients with distant metastases are considered candidates for palliative care.

Treatment

As a general rule, many early-stage (T1, selected T2) head and neck cancers can be treated with monomodality therapy (surgery or radiation), while advanced-stage lesions (T3, T4) typically require combination therapy, such as surgery followed by postoperative radiation therapy. The primary treatment philosophies differ for oral cavity and oropharyngeal carcinomas. Most oral carcinomas, early- and advanced-stage, are treated initially with surgical intervention. For oropharyngeal carcinoma, the primary treatment of choice varies between institutions and includes chemoradiation versus surgery with postoperative radiation therapy.

Prior to the start of treatment, particularly in patients who may require radiotherapy, dental preservation is required to determine if dental extraction is necessary. Patients requiring radiation therapy require lifelong dental follow up because of the risk of osteoradionecrosis.

In patients presenting with dysphagia associated with pretreatment weight loss or in whom significant dysphagia is anticipated with treatment (surgery or chemoradiation), percutaneous enteral gastrostomy (PEG) tube may be necessary. For patients with borderline airways (e.g. large base of tongue cancers) or in whom surgical resection and reconstruction will result in an initially unstable airway, temporary tracheotomy may be necessary.

For small oral cavity carcinomas (T1, selected T2) of the tongue and floor of the mouth, a transoral approach to wide local excision may be possible. A 2 cm margin around the macroscopic extent of tumor is typically employed at the start of resection. Intraoperative frozen assessment of the operative margins can aid the surgeon in identifying those patients with microscopic extension prior to closure or reconstruction of the operative site. For many subsites within the oral cavity, healing by secondary intent can produce equivalent results to primary closure when the operative defect is of limited size. Split-thickness skin grafting can be utilized effectively for slightly larger defects when scar contracture is anticipated to affect oral rehabilitation. Local tissue flaps such as tongue flaps are discouraged because of the impact that restriction of tongue mobility can have on speech and swallowing.

In lesions that approach the alveolar aspect on the mandible without evidence (radiographic or clinical) of gross bony invasion, limited resections of the bone such as with marginal mandibulectomy can be performed. For extensive cancers with gross mandibular extension, segmental resection is necessary to completely excise the tumor. Resections requiring removal of the anterior mandible (symphysis) mandate reconstruction of bone and soft tissue components to avoid a postoperative result that requires lifelong tracheostomy and PEG tube dependence with cosmetic results referred to as the "Andy Gump" deformity. Lesions of the posterolateral mandible, in particular in older patients without dentition, may not require bony reconstruction and can have acceptable speech and swallowing function with a "mandibular swing."

For oral lesions extending posteriorly, approaches that increase operative exposure such as mandibulotomy (division and retraction of the mandible) allow the surgeon to gain access and more easily resect and reconstruct a tumor. Another option is the pull-through technique, utilized in resecting extensive oral (oral tongue and floor of the mouth) and oropharyngeal lesions (tongue base) without mandible involvement, such that the oral contents are mobilized from the mandible and delivered to the neck in the submental/submandibular region for resection.

Reconstruction of oral defects focuses on obtaining maximal postoperative function such that patients have the best possible speech, swallowing (allowing removal of a PEG tube after the completion of treatment), and airway (allowing decannulation of a tracheotomy), while allowing the patient to heal in an appropriate timeframe. The workhorse flaps for oral soft tissue reconstruction include the anterolateral (myocutaneous, cutaneous) thigh and radial forearm (fasciocutaneous) free flap. For composite defects, the fibular (osteocutaneous) flap allows for the reconstruction of mandible and oral soft tissue components.

As opposed to oral cavity tumors, oropharyngeal carcinoma can be treated with either radiation-based protocols or with surgery with planned postoperative radiation therapy. In the setting of early-staged lesions (T1, selected T2), "radiation-alone" protocols can be considered. The development of techniques such as intensity-modulated radiation therapy (IMRT) have allowed for more precise control of radiation to a region of tumor while reducing associated tissue toxicity. Protocols utilizing concomitant boost radiotherapy have resulted in a reduction of overall treatment time (through delivery of a second daily fraction of radiation) while achieving favorable local and regional control rates. Referred to as organ preservation therapy, protocols utilizing induction chemotherapy and concurrent chemoradiation have been advocated for T2/T3 oropharyngeal cancers. Surgery is reserved in this setting for salvage (after chemoradiation) for selected patients with persistent disease.

In patients with resectable advanced disease (extensive T3, T4) where chemoradiation is less likely to result in a complete response (such as with mandible involvement), surgical resection with reconstruction and postoperative radiation is utilized. Functional outcome in this setting can be poor and necessitate prolonged use of both a tracheotomy and PEG-based nutrition.

Neck dissection is performed for both therapeutic and elective indications. The aggressiveness of neck dissection varies from the radical neck dissection, removing lymph node levels I–V, spinal accessory nerve, internal jugular vein, and sternocleidomastoid muscle, to the modified radical and selective neck dissections that address only specific lymph node basins (e.g. supraomohyoid neck dissection – lymph node levels I–III). Neck dissection is performed to address the regional lymphatic spread of the primary carcinoma.

Elective neck dissection is performed in patients with a primary site cancer without clinical evidence of regional metastasis who have a risk of occult spread that exceeds 20%. Almost every presentation of cancer within the oral cavity and oropharynx, including early-stage lesions, has a risk of occult spread to the ipsilateral regional lymphatics that exceeds this threshold with the exception of small lip and hard palate tumors. Selective neck dissection is performed in early-stage neck disease (N0, N1, selected N2a), while more extensive neck dissections are performed when multiple lymph node metastases exist or a suspicion of extracapsular lymph node spread is noted on preoperative imaging. When carotid encasement or deep neck musculature is noted, curative treatment of regional metastases is not considered possible. In patients with an oropharyngeal carcinoma undergoing primary chemoradiation therapy that experience an incomplete response in the neck, completion neck dissection is necessary.

Outcome

The overall 5-year survival rate for all patients with oral and oropharyngeal carcinomas from 1995–2001 as calculated by SEER NCI data was 59.4%. Observed survival statistics by stage for oral cavity and oropharyngeal carcinoma are provided in ❍ *Figs. 32-4* and ❍ *32-5*. Prognosis for head and neck cancers is linked to pretreatment staging. The most significant impact on survival is seen with neck metastasis. The 5-year relative survival rate falls from 81.3% in patients without regional spread to 51.7% when metastatic lymphadenopathy is present.

Delays in the initiation of postoperative radiotherapy, and breaks in any radiotherapy course (postoperative or primary treatment intent), can significantly impact locoregional control and survival.

Functional outcome after treatment is dependent upon the initial stage at the time of presentation and the therapies required to treat the primary site and regional lymphatics. Dysphagia and xerostomia are common side effects for individuals requiring radiation therapy. Scar contracture and lymphedema can slow the return to normal oral intake of nutrition and prevent immediate tracheostomy decannulation.

Long-term follow-up is required in these patients to monitor for local, regional, and distant recurrence of disease. Clinic visits (in the post-treatment setting) require assessment of the patient's ability to speak and swallow, weight loss or gain, onset of referred otalgia, and discussion of tobacco

◻ **Figure 32-4**
Five-year, observed survival by "combined" AJCC stage for squamous cell carcinoma of the oral cavity, 1985–1991. *95% confidence intervals correspond to year-5 survival rates (American Joint Committee on Cancer (AJCC), 2002. With permission; www.springeronline.com)

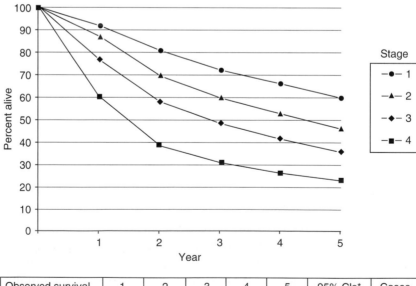

Observed survival by stage	1	2	3	4	5	95% CIs*	Cases
1	91.6	80.6	72.0	66.1	59.8	57.7 – 61.8	2511
2	87.0	69.6	59.7	53.0	46.3	43.8 – 48.7	1839
3	76.7	58.1	48.7	41.6	36.3	33.6 – 38.9	1431
4	60.2	38.4	30.9	26.5	23.3	21.5 – 25.0	2433

◘ Figure 32-5

Five-year, observed survival by "combined" AJCC stage for squamous cell carcinoma of the oropharynx, 1985–1991. *95% confidence intervals correspond to year-5 survival rates (American Joint Committee on Cancer (AJCC), 2002. With permission; www.springeronline.com)

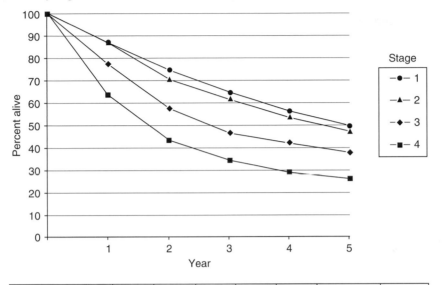

Observed survival by stage	1	2	3	4	5	95% CIs*	Cases
1	87.0	74.4	64.6	56.5	50.0	46.7 – 53.4	980
2	86.6	70.4	61.8	53.9	47.5	44.3 – 50.6	1107
3	77.1	57.0	46.7	42.2	37.9	35.3 – 40.4	1520
4	63.6	43.5	34.2	28.9	26.1	24.5 – 27.6	3419

use. Detailed physical examination is required to assess for the presence of recurrence and the development of complications related to treatment, such as osteoradionecrosis. Techniques including bimanual palpation, mirror exam, and flexible laryngoscopy should be used in assessing patients.

Selected Readings

American Joint Committee on Cancer (2002) AJCC Cancer Staging Manual, 6th edn. Springer-Verlag, New York

Blot WJ, McLaughlin JK, Winn DM, et al. (1988) Smoking and drinking in relation to oral and pharyngeal cancer. Cancer Res 48:3282–3287

Brennan JA, Boyle JO, Koch WM, et al. (1995) Association between cigarette smoking and mutation of the p53 gene in squamous cell carcinoma of the head and neck. N Engl J Med 332:712–717

DeNittis AS, Machtay M, Rosenthal DI, et al. (2001) Advanced oropharyngeal carcinoma treated with surgery and radiotherapy: oncologic outcome and functional assessment. Am J Otolaryngol 22:329–335

Eicher SA, Weber RS (1996) Surgical management of cervical lymph node metastases. Curr Opin Oncol 8:215

Greene FL, Page DL, Fleming ID, et al. (2002) AJCC Cancer Staging Manual, 6th edn.Springer, New York

Gwozdz JT, Morrison WH, Garden AS, et al. (1997) Concomitant boost radiotherapy for squamous carcinoma of the tonsillar fossa. Int J Radiat Oncol Biol Phys 39:127–135

Machtay M, Rosenthal DI, Hershock D, et al. (2002) Organ preservation therapy using induction plus concurrent chemoradiation for advanced resectable oropharyngeal carcinoma: A University of Pennsylvania phase II trial. J Clin Oncol 20:3964–3971

Ries LAG, Harkins D, Krapcho M, (eds) SEER Cancer Statistics Review, 1975–2003, National Cancer Institute, Bethesda, MD, http://seer.cancer.gov/csr/1975_2003

Urken ML, Buchbinder D, Costantino PD, et al. (1998) Oromandibular reconstruction using microvascular composite flaps: report of 210 cases. Arch Otolaryngol Head Neck Surg 124:46–55

Wein RO, Weber RS (2005) Malignant neoplasms of the oral cavity. Chapter 70 in vol 2 of Cummings Otolaryngology-Head and Neck Surgery, 4th edn. Elsevier Mosby, Philadelphia

33 Larynx and Hypopharynx

J. Scott Magnuson · Glenn E. Peters

Pearls and Pitfalls

- Symptoms relating to cancer of the larynx include: hoarseness, dyspnea, hemoptysis, odynophagia, and referred otalgia.
- Cancer of the larynx often presents at an earlier stage.
- Symptoms relating to cancer of the hypopharynx include: dysphagia, odynophagia, and weight loss.
- Cancer of the hypopharynx often presents at a later stage.
- Flexible endoscopy provides an excellent way to evaluate the larynx and hypopharynx.
- Computed tomography is useful to confirm clinical findings, as well as evaluate the pre-epiglottic space, paraglottic space, cartilage invasion, and nodal status.
- A biopsy is required prior to the initiation of treatment.
- Squamous cell carcinoma accounts for greater than 95% of malignancies of the larynx and hypopharynx.
- Conservation therapy provides equivalent outcomes to that seen with non-conservation therapy.
- Early glottic cancers have a cure rate of around 90–100%.
- While radiation therapy may provide similar survival results, significant morbidity may be associated with the treatment.
- Airway management requires a high level of expertise in order to provide a safe airway.
- A gastrostomy tube may be required to support nutritional intake.
- Management of the airway is of primary concern in the postoperative setting.
- Decannulation of the tracheotomy tube is performed after the patient tolerates plugging of the tube and flexible endoscopic examination demonstrates a safe airway.
- Swallowing rehabilitation is performed with the assistance of a speech-language pathologist.
- Swallowing rehabilitation cannot begin until after decannulation of the tracheotomy tube and healing of the stoma.
- Alaryngeal speech is taught by a speech-language pathologist.
- Adjunctive radiation therapy is indicated for advanced disease and prognostically adverse histopathological findings.
- Recurrence is assessed by physical exam and radiological imaging.

Introduction

Malignancies of the larynx and hypopharynx are more commonly found in older men with a history of tobacco exposure. Presentation of these cancers differs by site. Laryngeal cancer often presents at an earlier stage because of symptoms relating to the airway. Visualization of the disease in this location is also relatively simple. Persistent hoarseness and dyspnea may lead to an office examination that demonstrates a neoplasm located in the glottis. Hypopharyngeal cancer may present at a later stage because the symptoms are more discrete. Dysphagia and weight loss may be attributed to other causes while the cancer goes unnoticed. Visualization of the hypopharynx is also more difficult because of the collapse of the tissue in that area.

Treatment for malignancies of the larynx and hypopharynx is based on stage, anatomical considerations, and patient goals. Conservation therapy is directed to patients who may present at an earlier stage, have a cancer in a location amenable to partial resection, or desire organ preservation. Radical resection with or without adjunctive treatment is used for those patients who present with a more advanced neoplasm.

Survival is largely related to stage at presentation. While advances in surgical and non-surgical treatment have not had a tremendous effect on survival, emphasis has been placed on patient quality of life. Improvements in organ preservation treatments, as well as aggressive rehabilitation, have led to evaluation of outcomes outside of survival.

Clinical Presentation

Symptoms relating to malignancies of the larynx include hoarseness, dyspnea, hemoptysis, dysphagia, chronic sore throat, and referred otalgia. Small changes in the anatomy of the larynx produce dramatic effects, leading to early evaluation.

On the other hand, tumors of the hypopharynx may go undetected for a longer period of time, leading to presentation at a later stage. Symptoms of dysphagia, odynophagia, and weight loss may be attributed to other illnesses, delaying the diagnosis of malignancy.

Tumor (T) staging for malignancies of the larynx is based on location and function (❯ Table 33-1). The larynx is divided into three subgroups: supraglottis, glottis, and subglottis. Each site has a unique T-stage that is determined by involvement of specific anatomical areas by the tumor. In addition, vocal cord function affects the T-stage for each subgroup.

T-staging for malignancies of the hypopharynx is based on location, function and size (❯ Table 33-2). There are three subsites named to the hypopharynx: postcricoid area, posterior pharyngeal wall, and the pyriform sinuses. The number of subsites involved, the size of the tumor, and the function, of the larynx determines the T-stage.

Nodal (N) and metastasis (M) staging is the same for both the larynx and hypopharynx (❯ Table 33-3). The size and number of involved lymph node(s) determines the N-stage, while the presence of distant metastasis determines the M-stage.

Evaluation

Evaluation of tumors of the larynx and hypopharynx includes the use of several tools available to the surgeon. Office examination relies on the use of flexible endoscopic equipment for visualization. Palpation of the neck provides information relating to metastatic lymphadenopathy. Imaging assists

◘ Table 33-1

Tumor (T) staging for laryngeal cancer (Wolf, 1991)

Primary tumor
- TX: Primary tumor cannot be assessed
- T0: No evidence of primary tumor
- Tis: Carcinoma in situ

Supraglottis
- T1: Tumor limited to one subsite of supraglottis with normal vocal cord mobility
- T2: Tumor invades mucosa of more than one adjacent subsite outside of supraglottis without fixation of the larynx
- T3: Tumor limited to the larynx with vocal cord fixation and/or invades any of the following: postcricoid area, pre-epiglottic tissue, paraglottic space, or erosion of inner cortex of thyroid cartilage
- T4a: Tumor invades through thyroid cartilage and/or invades tissue beyond the larynx
- T4b: Tumor invades prevertebral space, encases carotid artery, or invades mediastinal structures

Subsites
- False vocal cords
- Arytenoids
- Suprahyoid epiglottis
- Infrahyoid epiglottis
- Aryepiglottic folds

Glottis
- T1: Tumor limited to the vocal cord(s), which may involve the anterior or posterior commissure, with normal mobility
  - T1a: Tumor limited to one vocal cord
  - T1b: Tumor involves both vocal cords
- T2: Tumor extends to the supraglottis and/or subglottis, and/or with impaired vocal cord mobility
- T3: Tumor limited to the larynx with vocal cord fixation and/or invades paraglottic space, and/or erosion of inner cortex of thyroid cartilage
- T4a: Tumor invades through the thyroid cartilage and/or invades tissue beyond the larynx
- T4b: Tumor invades prevertebral space, encases carotid artery, or invades mediastinal structures

Subglottis
- T1: Tumor limited to the subglottis
- T2: Tumor extends to the vocal cords with normal or impaired mobility
- T3: Tumor limited to the larynx with vocal cord fixation
- T4a: Tumor invades cricoid or thyroid cartilage and/or invades tissue beyond the larynx
- T4b: Tumor invades prevertebral space, encases carotid artery, or invades mediastinal structures

in the evaluation by confirming physical findings, as well as further delineating the disease. Finally, a diagnosis is established with a biopsy that is evaluated by a pathologist.

Endoscopy

Traditionally, direct rigid laryngoscopy and esophagoscopy are performed to evaluate, stage, and biopsy neoplasms of the larynx and hypopharynx while the patient is under a general anesthetic. However, the development of the flexible endoscope has improved the ability to closely evaluate the larynx and hypopharynx. With the patient awake, the different anatomical areas of the larynx and hypopharynx can be separately inspected, and the function of the larynx can be recorded. Newer models of the flexible endoscopes contain side ports that allow for the administration of local anesthetics, insufflation of air, and biopsies of the tumor.

▣ Table 33-2

Tumor (T) staging for hypopharyngeal cancer (Wolf, 1991)

Primary tumor
• TX: Primary tumor cannot be assessed
• T0: No evidence of primary tumor
• Tis: Carcinoma in situ
• T1: Tumor limited to one subsite of the hypopharynx and <2 cm in greatest dimension
• T2: Tumor invades more than one subsite of the hypopharynx or an adjacent site, or measures >2 cm but <4 cm in greatest dimension without fixation of the hemilarynx
• T3: Tumor measures >4 cm in greatest dimension or with fixation of the hemilarynx
• T4a: Tumor invades thyroid/cricoid cartilage, hyoid bone, thyroid gland, esophagus, or central compartment soft tissue of the neck
• T4b: Tumor invades prevertebral fascia, encases carotid artery, or involves mediastinal structures
Hypopharyngeal subsites
• Postcricoid area
• Pyriform sinuses
• Posterior pharyngeal wall

▣ Table 33-3

Nodal (N) staging for the neck (Wolf, 1991)

Regional lymph nodes
• NX: Regional lymph nodes cannot be assessed
• N0: No regional lymph node metastasis
• N1: Metastasis in a single ipsilateral lymph node, <3 cm in dimension
• N2: Metastasis in a single ipsilateral lymph node, >3 cm but <6 cm in dimension, or in multiple ipsilateral lymph nodes, 6 cm in dimension, or in bilateral or contralateral lymph nodes, <6 cm in dimension
• N2a: Metastasis in a single ipsilateral lymph node, >3 cm but <6 cm in dimension
• N2b: Metastasis in multiple ipsilateral lymph nodes, <6 cm in dimension
• N2c: Metastasis in bilateral or contralateral lymph nodes, <6 cm in dimension
• N3: Metastasis in a lymph node, >6 cm in dimension

Imaging

Assessment of laryngeal and hypopharyngeal tumors can be further defined with the use of radiographic imaging. Computed tomography (CT) is useful in demonstrating tumor involvement of the preepiglottic space, paraglottic space, and cartilage erosion. This information, while important for treatment planning, is not apparent at the time of examination. In addition, CT and magnetic resonance imaging (MRI) are helpful in identifying suspicious cervical adenopathy.

Chest radiographs are used to evaluate distant metastatic disease or a second primary malignancy. Chest CT is not recommended for every metastatic evaluation, but instead, is reserved for suspicious findings on plain films.

Utilization of positron emission tomography (PET) for assessment of the primary tumor and detection of metastasis is increasing. The usefulness of this imaging technique is still under investigation and the limits of detection are not well understood.

Diagnosis

The diagnosis of a laryngeal or hypopharyngeal malignancy relies on histopathological evaluation. To provide tissue for the diagnosis, a biopsy of the primary tumor is required. Metastatic cervical adenopathy can also be a source of tissue for diagnosis. Fine-needle aspiration of pathologic cervical adenopathy is an effective way of establishing a diagnosis of malignancy. This technique is preferred over open biopsy of lymph nodes in order to avoid violation of the neck. The principles of surgical treatment for metastatic cervical adenopathy are based on a previously unoperated neck. An open biopsy alters the tissue planes used in cervical lymphadenectomy, and therefore, is reserved for only those cases where a diagnosis cannot be established by other means.

Pathology

Squamous cell carcinoma (SCC) accounts for greater than 95% of the malignancies of the larynx and hypopharynx and is the focus of this chapter. Certain benign lesions, such as sarcoidosis, Wegener's granulomatosis, fungal laryngitis, and tuberculosis, present with a similar appearance of SCC, and therefore, must be excluded. In addition, the premalignant lesions of leukoplakia, erythroplakia, and carcinoma *in situ* each require biopsy and appropriate treatment. The biopsy should be deep and wide enough to exclude the diagnosis of invasive carcinoma. In persistent premalignant lesions, repeat biopsies at scheduled intervals should be performed to rule out the progression of invasive carcinoma.

Histological differentiation does not directly correlate with survival. Instead, survival is better predicted by the TNM-staging at the time of presentation.

Treatment Options

Historically, cancer of the larynx and hypopharynx was treated with radical excision to include removal of the larynx and cervical lymph nodes. Treatment philosophies evolved to provide equivalent survival outcomes with the intention of causing less morbidity. This led to the development of treatments aimed at preserving laryngeal and hypopharyngeal function.

Conservation Therapy

Conservation therapy includes both surgical and non-surgical treatment. Organ preservation techniques have allowed for partial removal of the larynx while preserving enough anatomy to allow for function. Additionally, radiation treatment and chemotherapy have provided similar survival rates while maintaining function.

Early glottic cancers have a high cure rate, approaching 100%, despite treatment selection. Johnson et al. reported surgical cure rates of 98% and 94% for T1 and T2 vocal cord tumors, respectively. Endoscopic laser resection of laryngeal tumors also provides excellent cure rates. Steiner reported adjusted 5-year survival rates for endoscopic laser resection to be 100% for T1 and T2 glottic tumors.

Radiation for early glottic cancers provides similar results. However, since management of tumor recurrence following radiation therapy may not include conservation surgery, the patient must be instructed of possible outcomes.

Advanced cancers of the larynx may also be treated with organ-sparing surgical and non-surgical techniques. Partial and near-total laryngectomies still preserve some degree of function and have similar control rates as seen with non-surgical treatment. Wolf compared induction chemotherapy followed by radiation therapy to surgery followed by radiation therapy for patients with advanced laryngeal cancer and found equal 2-year survival rates of 68%. As demonstrated in this study, organ preservation does not always equal organ function. Therefore, discussion with the patient regarding possible outcomes following conservation therapy should be carried out.

Non-Conservation Therapy

Non-conservation therapy is the standard by which other techniques are measured. Total laryngectomy and total laryngopharyngectomy are used for advanced cancers of the larynx and hypopharynx. Cancer of the hypopharynx adds a degree of difficulty when planning surgical treatment. Total laryngopharyngectomy often leaves little pharyngeal mucosa for complete closure of the pharyngeal defect, requiring additional tissue for closure. This tissue may come from regional myocutaneous rotational flaps or distant myocutaneous free flaps.

Additionally, non-conservation therapy is often used for conservation therapy failures. Surgical complication rates are significantly higher for these patients, and this alone may justify non-conservation therapy as the initial treatment.

Intraoperative Management

Management of the airway is of primary concern for patients with tumors of the larynx and hypopharynx. Obstructive lesions complicate obtaining a safe airway during induction of anesthesia. Choices for managing the airway include routine or fiberoptic intubation, awake tracheotomy, or transtracheal jet ventilation.

For patients undergoing biopsy without definitive treatment, consideration should be given to the airway after extubation. Besides the lesion that may obstruct the airway directly, post-biopsy edema may also cause some degree of obstruction. Intraoperative debridement of the airway using either a carbon monoxide laser or laryngeal microdebrider can often provide a safe airway, avoiding the placement of a tracheotomy.

Partial laryngeal surgery may also require the placement of a tracheotomy as a temporary means of providing a safe airway during the immediate postoperative period.

Obstruction from post-surgical edema or increased risk of aspiration following partial laryngeal surgery is improved with the use of a temporary tracheotomy.

Another consideration during surgery is the ability of the patient to maintain adequate nutritional intake following surgery. If significant dysphagia or risk of aspiration is likely, a gastrostomy tube is indicated until the patient is able to rehabilitate.

Postoperative Management

The immediate postoperative management, includes wound care, airway management and swallowing rehabilitation. Soon after the wounds have appropriately healed, decisions regarding postoperative radiation therapy must be made. Routine surveillance for recurrence is carried out for a period of years. Throughout this time, emphasis is placed on rehabilitating the patient to a functional and satisfactory lifestyle.

Hospital Stay Considerations

Regardless of the degree of resection of the larynx and hypopharynx for malignancy, a postoperative hospital stay is likely. Of primary concern is the management of the airway. Procedures not requiring a tracheotomy are observed for the development of airway edema and respiratory distress. Generally, an observation of 24 h is sufficient. When a tracheotomy is performed, a decision regarding the timing of decannulation must be made. In order to assess the ability of the patient to breath without a tracheotomy tube, a standard protocol is followed. First, the tracheotomy tube cuff is deflated around postoperative day 1. Then, the cuffed tracheotomy tube is exchanged for a smaller, uncuffed, non-fenestrated tracheotomy tube around postoperative day 3. On postoperative day 4, the new tracheotomy tube is plugged and remains plugged at the comfort of the patient. If the patient can keep the tracheotomy tube plugged for 24 h, and a flexible endoscopic evaluation demonstrates a safe airway, the tube is decannulated at the bedside. Those patients not tolerating plugging of the tracheotomy tube are discharged with the tube for possible decannulation in the outpatient setting.

In addition to the management of the airway, a plan for swallowing rehabilitation must be made. This decision is made with the assistance of a speech-language pathologist. In general, swallowing rehabilitation is not begun until the tracheotomy tube is removed and the stoma has closed. If this occurs in the hospital, a bedside evaluation by the speech-language pathologist, to also include a modified barium swallow, is performed. Otherwise, swallowing rehabilitation is performed in the outpatient setting.

Total laryngectomy patients do not begin oral intake until postoperative days 5–7. Clear liquids are first introduced to the patient, and the presence or absence of a pharyngocutaneous leak is confirmed. In the absence of a leak, the patient is allowed to begin a full liquid diet and is advanced in the outpatient setting. If a gastrostomy tube is used to provide or supplement the nutritional intake of the patient, teaching is given to the patient and family regarding the proper use of the tube.

The speech-language pathologist also begins speech rehabilitation in the hospital. For patients who receive a total laryngectomy, alaryngeal speech is accomplished with the use of an electromechanical device that is held by the patient and placed on the neck. These vibrations produce a sound that exits the mouth. The speech-language pathologist teaches the patient how to make words with the mechanical sound. Other types of alaryngeal speech are taught in the outpatient setting.

Adjunctive Radiation Therapy

To decrease the chance of recurrence and increase the rate of survival, postoperative radiation therapy may be recommended. Indications for adjunctive radiotherapy are based on tumor size, stage of disease, and histopathological findings. Large tumors with local destruction of surrounding cartilage, bone and muscle have a higher rate of recurrence and therefore benefit from postoperative radiation therapy. Similarly, Stage III and IV disease is more likely to recur. Nodal status also influences the decision for adjunctive radiotherapy. Multiple metastatic lymph nodes (two or more) are more likely to fail only surgical treatment. Microscopically, the presence of extracapsular nodal extension and positive surgical margins indicate the need for postoperative radiation therapy.

Assessment of Recurrence

Surveillance for recurrence is performed by all those involved in the care of the patient. The tools used for the initial evaluation of the patient are also used to evaluate the patient after treatment. The development of recurrence decreases with time and is more likely to occur in the first year. A routine schedule includes return visits every other month in the first year, decreasing each year thereafter. Important indicators suggesting a recurrence include the report of new pain by the patient, a new mass or lesion seen on physical exam or x-ray, or unexplained change in voice, dysphagia, or weight loss.

Conclusion

Efforts in preserving laryngeal function may have improved the quality of life for the patient, but have not improved overall survival. Patients presenting at an earlier stage have a better prognosis than those presenting with more advanced disease. Routine surveillance is key to early detection and early treatment. Care for the patient with laryngeal or hypopharyngeal cancer requires the input of many specialties. Organization for this care is directed by the surgeon.

Selected Readings

American Joint Committee on Cancer (2002) AJCC cancer staging manual, 6th edn. Springer, New York

Ferlito A, Shaha A, et al. (2001) Incidence and sites of distant metastases from head and neck cancer. ORL 63:202

Johnson J, et al. (1993) Outcome of open surgical therapy for glottic carcinoma. Ann Otol Rhinol Laryngol 102:752

Shaha A, Webber C, Marti J (1986) Fine needle aspiration in the diagnosis of cervical adenopathy. Am J Surg 4:420

Steiner W (1993) Results of curative laser microsurgery of laryngeal carcinomas. Am J Otolaryngol 14:116–121

Wolf GT (1991) Induction chemotherapy plus radiation compared with surgery plus radiation in patients with advanced laryngeal cancer. N Engl J Med 324:1685

34 Tumors of the Sinonasal Cavity and Anterior Skull Base

William R. Carroll

Pearls and Pitfalls

- A high index of suspicion is necessary to detect sinonasal malignancies at an early stage when treatment is most effective. Persistent "sinus" symptoms that fail to respond to routine medical therapy should be investigated further.
- The majority of sinonasal malignancies are best treated with surgical resection.
- High-resolution scans documenting the bony and soft tissue extent of the tumor are needed for accurate treatment planning.
- The surgical plan should include three considerations: (1) route of approach, (2) extent of bone resection, and (3) reconstruction of resultant defect.
- Failure to include a multidisciplinary surgical team for lesions approaching the skull base.
- Incomplete resection and failure to achieve clear surgical margins. Adjuvant radiation may not prevent local recurrence, and secondary salvage surgical procedures are much less likely to provide adequate disease control.

Introduction

Tumors of the nasal cavity and paranasal sinuses often grow undetected for many months before becoming symptomatic. Because these lesions are often large and adjacent to the orbit and skull base, treatment may be difficult, disabling and disfiguring. The surgeon's role in early detection and aggressive, appropriate treatment is critical for effective management.

Incidence/Etiology

Neoplasms of the nasal cavity and paranasal sinuses are rare, comprising about 5% of all head and neck malignancies and affecting about 2,000 Americans each year. Sinonasal malignancies are twice as common in men. The majority occur between the ages of 45 and 85. Although rare in the United States, these cancers are clustered in particular geographic regions including Japan and among the Bantu people of South Africa.

Risk factors for sinonasal tumors differ from other sites in the head and neck. Smoking is still a major risk factor but occupational exposure appears to be more important for these cancers than for other sites in the head and neck. Woodworkers, most notably, have higher rates of nasal and paranasal sinus cancer. Occupational exposure to dusts from textiles, leather, flour, glues, formaldehyde, solvents used in furniture and shoe production, nickel and chromium dust, isopropyl alcohol, and radium have all been proposed to increase the risk of nasal and paranasal sinus cancer. Family history does not seem to be an important risk factor. In the United States, many patients with sinonasal malignancies have no identifiable risk factors.

Pathology

The most common disorders of the nasal cavity and paranasal sinuses are inflammatory rather than neoplastic. Acute and chronic bacterial infections, allergic and chronic fungal disease are responsible for a large percentage of adult primary care physician visits. Differentiating these common inflammatory disorders from neoplastic disease is crucial for early detection and effective management (see Clinical Presentation).

Malignant sinonasal tumors may be classified as epithelial or non-epithelial and may be primary or metastatic. Epithelial malignancies are more common and will be the primary focus of this chapter. Squamous cell carcinoma (SCCA) is the most common sinonasal malignancy. In contrast to other head and neck sites, SCCA comprises only 60–70% of sinonasal malignancies. Malignancies of minor salivary glands and the mucus secreting glands including mucoepidermoid carcinoma, adenoid cystic carcinoma, and adenocarcinoma comprise up to 20% of sinonasal malignancies. Olfactory neuroblastoma, also called esthesioneuroblastoma, represents approximately 10% of sinonasal malignancies. This tumor arises from the olfactory nerves at the cribriform plate. Biologic behavior of the disease is closely correlated with histologic differentiation. Poorly differentiated tumors are associated with a poor prognosis. Lymphoma and other lymphoproliferative malignancies comprise about 5% of sinonasal malignancies. A particularly lethal undifferentiated carcinoma of the nasal cavity and paranasal sinuses is sinonasal undifferentiated carcinoma (SNUC). Aggressive bony destruction and early metastases are hallmarks of SNUC. The pathogenesis and optimal treatment of SNUC remain subjects of debate. Mucosal melanoma also occurs in this region and the long-term prognosis is poor.

Clinical Presentation

The early signs and symptoms of sinonasal tumors are subtle and easily mistaken for chronic inflammatory disease. Common presenting symptoms include nasal obstruction, facial pressure or pain, loss of smell or epistaxis. Most patients with these symptoms do not have cancer. However, when these symptoms persist despite adequate therapy, or when the symptoms are unilateral, the physician must have a high index of suspicion for neoplastic disease. Detection of these tumors at an early stage offers the best chance of cure.

Physical findings associated with early-stage sinonasal tumors include intra-nasal mass, bulging of the lateral nasal sidewall, and unilateral drainage originating from the sinus ostia. Signs of more advanced disease include proptosis, visual changes, facial swelling, palate erosion, and altered sensory-motor function, particularly in cranial nerves III–VI.

Sixty to seventy percent of sinonasal tumors occur in the maxillary sinus, 20–30% in the nasal cavity, 10–15% in the ethmoid sinuses, and <5% in the frontal and sphenoid sinuses. The close proximity of the nose and paranasal sinuses to the orbit, skull base, and intracranial contents explains the signs and symptoms of advanced disease. These relationships are illustrated in ❷ *Figs. 34-1* and ❷ *34-2*.

Workup

Diagnostic Work-Up

A high index of suspicion is needed to detect sinonasal malignancies at an early stage. When symptoms of chronic sinus disease fail to respond to reasonable medical intervention, further workup is required to rule out neoplastic disease. Remember, inflammatory disease of the sinuses rarely causes any sign or symptom suggesting extension of the disease process beyond the sinonasal tract (example diplopia). Any symptom suggesting extra-sinus extension warrants immediate investigation. The diagnostic work-up is actually fairly simple and should include a careful intra-nasal exam and radiographic studies. High-resolution CT scans are sufficient in most cases for diagnostic evaluation. A normal intranasal exam coupled with completely negative CT scans of the paranasal region virtually excludes the possibility of sinonasal malignancy.

Biopsy is needed to confirm diagnosis as treatment options differ widely with tumor types. Simple trans-nasal biopsy is often adequate. When an open or endoscopic approach to the sinuses is needed for biopsy, the approach should be planned with subsequent surgical access in mind. Whenever

◻ Figure 34-1
CT scans of normal paranasal sinus anatomy. Note the proximity to the skull base and thin bone separating the sinuses from the orbit and intracranial cavity

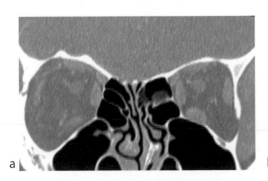
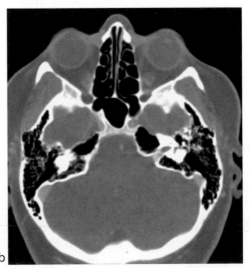

■ Figure 34-2

Primary ethmoid malignancy with extension into orbit, nasal cavity, maxillary sinus, and floor of anterior cranial cavity

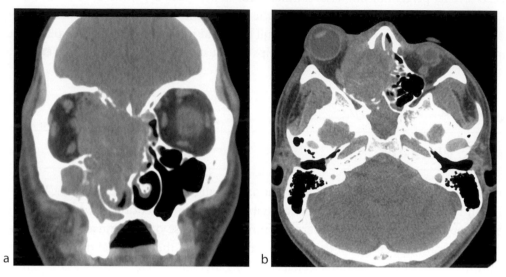

a   b

possible, utilize biopsy sites that can be completely resected without compromising the definitive surgical procedure.

Staging Work-Up

TNM staging of sinonasal tumors is summarized in ❯ *Table 34-1* The TNM staging system does not include the frontal and sphenoid sinuses due to the rarity of these lesions.

The National Comprehensive Cancer Network (NCCN), a consortium of 20 comprehensive cancer centers in North America, publishes guidelines for the workup and treatment of cancers by site, including sinonasal malignancies. For staging work-up, the NCCN recommendations include diagnostic biopsy, CT or MR scanning of the head and neck, and a chest x-ray to exclude pulmonary metastases. For high-grade malignancies of the sinonasal tract, a more extensive metastatic work-up including CT scan of the chest and abdomen or whole body PET imaging may be a reasonable option. There are no data confirming that any additional staging work-up improves survival or treatment outcome, though these studies may spare some patients an aggressive resection in the face of otherwise occult metastatic disease.

Treatment

General

Surgical resection is the mainstay of treatment for sinonasal tumors. Early stage lesions are often treated with surgery alone. Radiation alone may also be effective for early stage disease. Controlled trials comparing efficacy do not exist. Advanced lesions usually require surgery with adjuvant

◘ Table 34-1

TNM staging of nasal cavity and paranasal sinus tumors (American Joint Committee on Cancer, 2002. With permission; www.springeronline.com)

Primary tumor (T)	
TX	Primary tumor cannot be assessed
T0	No evidence of primary tumor
Tis	Carcinoma in situ
Maxillary sinus	
T1	Tumor limited to maxillary sinus mucosa with no erosion or destruction of bone
T2	Tumor causing bone erosion or destruction including extension into the hard palate and/or middle nasal meatus, except extension to posterior wall of maxillary sinus and pterygoid plates
T3	Tumor invades any of the following: bone of the posterior wall of maxillary sinus, subcutaneous tissues, floor or medial wall of orbit, pterygoid fossa, ethmoid sinuses
T4a	Tumor invades anterior orbital contents, skin of cheek, pterygoid plates, infratemporal fossa, cribriform plate, sphenoid or frontal sinuses
T4b	Tumor invades any of the following: orbital apex, dura, brain, middle cranial fossa, cranial nerves other than maxillary division of trigeminal nerve (V_2), nasopharynx, or clivus
Nasal cavity and ethmoid sinus	
T1	Tumor restricted to any one subsite, with or without bony invasion
T2	Tumor invading two subsites in a single region or extending to involve an adjacent region within the nasoethmoidal complex, with or without bony invasion
T3	Tumor extends to invade the medial wall or floor of the orbit, maxillary sinus, palate, or cribriform plate
T4a	Tumor invades any of the following: anterior orbital contents, skin of nose or cheek, minimal extension to anterior cranial fossa, pterygoid plates, sphenoid or frontal sinuses
T4b	Tumor invades any of the following: orbital apex, dura, brain, middle cranial fossa, cranial nerves other than (V_2), nasopharynx, or clivus
Regional lymph nodes (N)	
NX	Regional lymph nodes cannot be assessed
N0	No regional lymph node metastasis
N1	Metastasis in a single ipsilateral lymph node, 3 cm or less in greatest dimension
N2	Metastasis in a single ipsilateral lymph node, more than 3 cm but not more than 6 cm in greatest dimension, or in multiple ipsilateral lymph nodes, none more than 6 cm in greatest dimension, or in bilateral or contralateral lymph nodes, none more than 6 cm in greatest dimension
N2a	Metastasis in a single ipsilateral lymph node, more than 3 cm but not more than 6 cm in greatest dimension
N2b	Metastasis in multiple ipsilateral lymph nodes, none more than 6 cm in greatest dimension
N2c	Metastasis in bilateral or contralateral lymph nodes, none more than 6 cm in greatest dimension
N3	Metastasis in a lymph node, more than 6 cm in greatest dimension
Distant metastasis (M)	
MX	Distant metastasis cannot be assessed
M0	No distant metastasis
M1	Distant metastasis

radiation ± chemotherapy. Studies are underway to evaluate the efficacy of concurrent chemoradiation for primary management of squamous cell carcinoma of this region. To date, however, chemoradiation has unproven efficacy as initial treatment.

Exceptions to this generalization should be noted. Lymphoproliferative disorders are managed non-surgically. Sinonasal tumors with distant metastases are usually managed non-surgically, though rarely, the patient may still benefit from palliative resection of the primary lesion. Pre-operative chemotherapy and/or radiation have been used with olfactory neuroblastoma, neuroendocrine carcinoma, and the very aggressive SNUC. Lesions that are metastatic to the sinonasal region from elsewhere in the body are managed as symptoms dictate. Renal cell carcinoma, for example, may appear as an isolated sinonasal lesion. If bleeding and local tissue destruction are difficult to control, surgical resection may be indicated. More typically, metastatic lesions are managed non-surgically.

In planning treatment for sinonasal malignancies, the surgeon must consider three questions:

1. Which soft-tissue surgical approach will provide optimal exposure?
2. What extent of bony resection is needed?
3. Which method of reconstruction will be used?

Surgical Approach

Sinonasal tumors can be approached endoscopically, trans-facially, or by combined trans-cranial/trans-facial (craniofacial) resection. The route of approach depends on a number of factors including tumor location, tumor type, reconstructive options, and surgeon comfort. A general discussion of each approach follows. A comprehensive review of the indications and techniques for all of the approaches is beyond the scope of this chapter. The suggested readings include excellent sources for more detail on surgical approach.

Trans-Nasal Endoscopic Approach

Trans-nasal endoscopic approaches derive from procedures originally used to treat inflammatory disease of the paranasal sinuses. As optics and 3-D image guidance have improved, these techniques have been adapted for progressively more complex tumor resections. Early-stage lesions of the nasal septum and lateral nasal sidewall can often easily be resected with widely clear margins by trans-nasal approaches. Lesions involving the anterior skull base, such as olfactory neuroblastoma, are now being approached endoscopically when lateral and intracranial extension are minimal. Proponents of endoscopic resection argue that the optics allow wide exposure through a narrow opening and that the oncologic result should be the same with less access-related morbidity. Skeptics question whether the piecemeal resection required to remove larger tumors provides comparable rates of disease control. Data are just beginning to appear that will shed light on the oncologic outcomes of endoscopic approaches.

Trans-Facial Approach to the Sinonasal Cavity

Trans-facial approaches to the nose and paranasal sinuses have been the mainstay of surgical access for all lesions that do not extend to the skull base. Trans-facial approaches either utilize incisions placed in favorable lines through the facial skin or incisions confined to the mouth and nasal cavity which minimize facial scarring.

(a) Mid-facial degloving: Facial degloving approaches utilize sublabial and intra-nasal incisions to lift the facial skin superiorly and off of the midfacial bony structures. Facial degloving provides excellent access to the lower facial skeleton. Medial maxillectomy and inferior maxillectomy are easy to perform through a facial degloving approach. When bone cuts must be placed above the level of the inferior orbital rim, however, visualization may be limited and facial incisions indicated.

(b) Facial incisions: Approaches utilizing facial incisions are illustrated in ❷ *Fig. 34-3A* and ❷ *Fig. 34-3B*. These approaches include the lateral rhinotomy, Weber-Ferguson, and Weber-Ferguson with Diffenbach extension. The lateral rhinotomy incision is useful for smaller lesions of the nasal cavity and medial maxilla. The Weber-Ferguson incision, in contrast, provides wide access for most sinonasal tumors. Complete maxillectomy, ethmoidectomy, and excision of the nasal cavity are routinely completed through the Weber-Ferguson incision. The Diffenbach extension of the Weber-Ferguson incision adds a sub-ciliary or trans-conjunctival extension laterally. This addition allows improved access to the lateral orbit and malar eminence. The authors have used the Diffenbach extension primarily when orbital exenteration is necessary or tumor extends laterally beneath the malar eminence. For most other cases, the standard Weber-Ferguson incision is adequate.

Combined Craniofacial Approach

When sinonasal tumors extend to or through the anterior skull base, the superior margin of resection is shifted intracranially. If the bone of the skull base is intact, dura is preserved. If dura is involved, it too must be included in the resection specimen. In either case, surgical resection becomes a shared effort with the neurosurgical team. Pre-operatively, there needs to be open communication between the multiple surgeons involved with a plan for managing the sinonasal portion of the resection, the intracranial portion of the resection and for reconstruction of the resultant defect. Not uncommonly, three teams of surgeons are involved: head and neck surgeons, neurosurgeons and reconstructive

🔲 **Figure 34-3**
a. Lateral rhinotomy incision following naso-facial crease. b. Weber-Ferguson incision for access to entire maxilla. The lateral rhinotomy noted above is extended through the lip following the philtrum and upper vermillion to the middle of the lip. To create the Diffenbach extension for better lateral exposure (not shown), an extra incision is made from the medial canthal region just below (subciliary) or just inside (trans-conjunctival) the lower eyelid

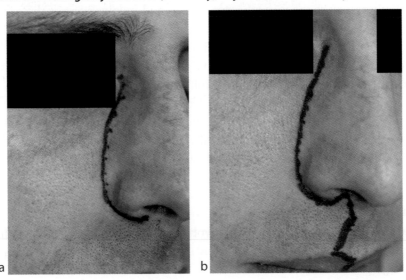

a   b

surgeons. Careful pre-operative planning and imaging should prevent the unfortunate scenario of attempting to resect a sinonasal lesion that is unexpectedly found to involve the skull base intra-operatively.

Craniofacial resection begins with creation of a bi-coronal scalp flap that is elevated below the level of the orbital rims. If the lesion is located at the skull base with limited inferior extension, no further soft tissue access may be needed. Additional trans-facial access is achieved by the addition of a lateral rhinotomy or Weber-Ferguson incision on the more involved side, coupled with a medial orbital incision contralaterally. The combined incisions preserve facial vasculature and provide access to the facial skeleton, orbit, and the cranial cavity.

Extent of Resection

Tumor location and tissue type will determine extent of resection. Bone cuts are planned to allow en-bloc removal of involved structures while preserving adjacent and often vital structures.

Total Maxillectomy

The goal of total maxillectomy is removal of all of the bony walls surrounding the maxillary sinus. Since 60–70% of sinonasal malignancies occur within the maxillary sinus, familiarity with total maxillectomy is essential for management of this group of tumors. Total maxillectomy can be easily altered to accommodate resection of specific subsites as noted in the sections below.

Approach   Classically, maxillectomy has been performed through trans-facial incisions such as the Weber-Ferguson. In selected cases, the midface degloving approach may provide adequate exposure and minimize facial scarring. Lateral rhinotomy and trans-nasal endoscopic approaches are probably inadequate for total maxillectomy.

Resection   Since no two lesions occupy exactly the same space within the maxilla, thin slice maxillo-facial images are extremely useful in operative planning for maxillectomy. The authors prefer multi-planar maxillofacial CT imaging in planning precise placement of bone cuts. MRI is also very helpful in distinguishing inflammatory changes in adjacent sinuses and involvement of the orbit or cranial base.

Five primary bone cuts are required for total maxillectomy (❷ *Fig. 34-4*). These cuts may be performed in any order. Bleeding caused by these bone cuts is difficult to control until the specimen is removed. The sequence described orders the cuts generating the most blood loss last so that the specimen may be quickly removed and bleeding minimized. The five bone cuts include: (1) zygomatico-maxillary suture line, (2) orbital floor and medial orbital wall, (3) naso-maxillary suture line, (4) hard palate, and (5) pterygoid plates. These cuts will require adjustment right-to-left and up-and-down depending on the precise location of the tumor within the maxilla. The procedure can be extended as necessary to include the orbit, the anterior skull base, the opposite nasal cavity and the pterygomax-illary space.

Medial Maxillectomy

Medial maxillectomy is indicated for tumors involving the common wall separating the nasal and maxillary cavities and tumors of the inferior ethmoid sinus region. Most tumors will be earlier stage with

Figure 34-4
Bone cuts for total maxillectomy. See text for description of cuts

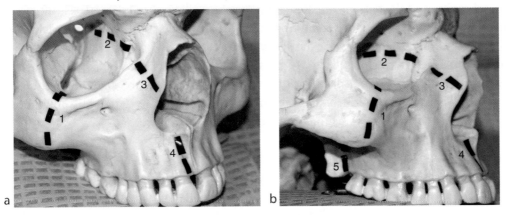

Figure 34-5
Bone cuts for medial maxillectomy. See text for description of cuts

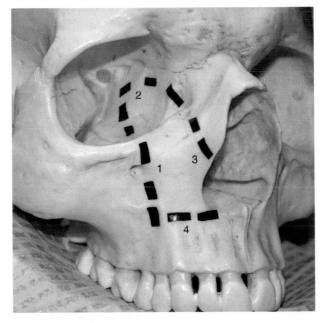

limited involvement beyond the lateral nasal wall. The soft-tissue approach for a medial maxillectomy may be open transfacial, midface degloving, or transnasal endoscopic.

Once adequate exposure is obtained, bone cuts are marked (● *Fig. 34-5*). The bone cuts include: (1) removal of the anterior face of the maxilla medial to the infra-orbital foramen, (2) an orbital cut from the inferior rim carried medially to the lamina papyracea, (3) a nasomaxillary suture line cut extending from cut "2" into the piriform aperture, (4) a cut at the base of the lateral nasal wall near the junction with the palate, and (5) posterior lateral nasal wall cuts behind the level of the turbinates.

Inferior Maxillectomy

Inferior maxillectomy is indicated for tumors involving the inferior portion of the maxillary sinus, the inferior nasal cavity, and the hard palate. Resection may be unilateral or bilateral as is often required for lesions involving the nasal cavity or primary palate. The soft tissue approach for inferior maxillectomy is transoral with midface degloving as extensively as needed.

Bone cuts for the inferior maxillectomy are similar to those for total maxillectomy (❍ *Fig. 34-6*). The difference obviously is the position of the superior cuts. These are made below the orbital rim and when possible, below the infraorbital foramen. The anterior cut is extended through the lateral and posterior walls of the maxillary sinus to complete the superior release.

Craniofacial Resection

Sinonasal tumors originating high in the nasal cavity (such as olfactory neuroblastoma) or high in the ethmoid region often abut the anterior skull base at the cribriform plate or the fovea ethmoidalis. For benign tumors, resection from below via transnasal or transfacial approaches with careful debridement along the bony roof of the nasal and ethmoid cavity may prove adequate. Malignancies require a negative superior margin which may not be obtainable by approaching only from below. When the bony skull base must be resected to achieve a clear superior margin, craniofacial resection is the procedure of choice. The alternative is aggressive tumor removal from below with adjuvant radiation to hopefully eliminate microscopic disease. In most series, however, optimal local-regional control rates are achieved instead with complete surgical resection with clear margins.

Craniofacial resection is a true inter-disciplinary effort, involving a head and neck surgeon and neurosurgeon at a minimum. For large defects of the skull base and those created in previously radiated fields, a reconstructive surgeon may be needed as well for vascularized tissue interposition. Craniofacial resection may be combined with maxillectomy or orbital resection as indicated by tumor extent.

◻ **Figure 34-6**
Bone cuts for inferior maxillectomy

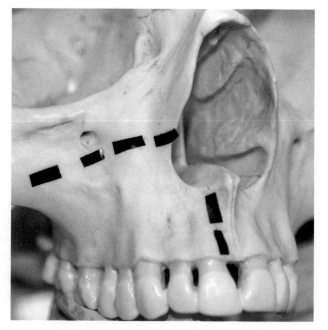

The soft tissue approach from above is a bi-coronal scalp flap. When the primary lesion is located high in the sinonasal cavity, inferior mobilization of the bi-coronal flap may provide adequate soft tissue access for the facial portion of the resection as well. When the primary lesion extends below the midpoint of the orbit, most surgeons also use transfacial or midfacial degloving incisions for improved inferior visualization.

Tumor resection proceeds from both the facial and intracranial aspects. Bone cuts are located to allow en-bloc tumor resection. The lateral cut is usually placed within the superior orbit on the side ipsilateral to the tumor. The posterior cut is the most difficult to visualize and is usually positioned at the planum sphenoidale anterior to the anterior clinoid process. The internal carotid artery, the optic chiasm, and the pituitary fossa are in close proximity, necessitating good visualization and certainty of anatomic position. The dura of the floor of the anterior fossa may be included as a margin with immediate repair.

Reconstruction

Total Maxillectomy

Total maxillectomy creates both a functional and aesthetic defect that should be considered at the time of initial resection. The functional defect results from loss of the palate allowing communication of the oral cavity with the sinonasal tract. This communication makes both speech and oral intake difficult. The barrier between the oral and sinus cavity should be re-established by prosthesis or by flap reconstruction. Packing the cavity at the time of surgery in preparation for delayed prosthetic reconstruction is the simplest option. A prosthodontist may also come to the operating room and insert a temporary obturator that is secured by wire suture. Flap reconstruction has become a widely used alternative. The other functional defect is hyophthalmos and enophthalmos resulting from loss of orbital floor support. This defect is minimized when the orbital septum and soft-tissue sling supporting the globe are not compromised by the resection.

The aesthetic defect created by maxillectomy is flattening of the malar eminence and a retracted or hollow appearance of the lower midface from loss of the alveolar arch. When possible, the malar flattening can be minimized by placing the zygomatico-maxillary bone cut slightly more medially, sparing the malar eminence. The hollow appearance of the lower mid face is corrected by prosthetic reconstruction of the maxillary alveolus and teeth.

Medial Maxillectomy

Reconstruction of the medial maxillectomy defect may be completely unnecessary. The bone loss is typically of no functional or aesthetic consequence. If the medial canthal tendon has been transected, reattachment may improve post-operative appearance, though many surgeons simply allow scar contracture to pull the tendon back into position. If the lacrimal duct has been transected, the remaining portion is typically marsupialized into the nasal cavity. Stenting is recommended by some surgeons.

Inferior Maxillectomy

Reconstructive issues following inferior maxillectomy are similar to total maxillectomy with one exception. The orbital floor should be intact and require no reconstruction. The opening between the mouth and sinonasal cavity may be closed with a maxillary prosthesis or closed with a soft tissue flap.

Craniofacial Resection

Reconstructive concerns following craniofacial resection include: (1) re-establishing a water-tight dural closure to seal and isolate the CSF, (2) placement of a vascularized tissue layer between the sinonasal roof and the intracranial contents, and (3) ensuring adequate rigid support for the floor of the anterior fossa to prevent frontal lobe herniation into the nasal cavity.

Prognosis

A number of factors affect prognosis of sinonasal tumors including tumor type, location, and stage of disease at presentation. This range of variables and the relative rarity of these tumors confound attempts to clearly state prognosis. The overall 5-year survival rate for patients with sinonasal carcinoma is approximately 50%. In general terms, SNUC and mucosal melanoma are locally aggressive and metastasize early. Overall 5-year survival rates are 40% or less. Epithelial malignancies such as squamous cell carcinoma and adenocarcinoma have a better prognosis if detected at a resectable stage. Overall 5-year survival rates average 60–75%. With appropriate therapy, olfactory neuroblastoma should have 5-year survival rates approaching 90%.

As surgeons, we can do little to influence the presenting tumor type or location. We can, however, influence early detection and selection of appropriate, aggressive treatment. All sinonasal malignancies have higher survival rates when detected at an early stage.

Selected Readings

American Joint Committee on Cancer (2002) AJCC Cancer Staging Manual, 6th edn. Springer-Verlag, New York

Hanna EYN, Westfall CT (2003) Cancer of the nasal cavity, paranasal sinuses and orbit, Chapter 9. In: Myers EN, Suen JN, Myers JN, Hanna EY (eds) Cancer of the head and neck. W.B. Saunders, Philadelphia, pp 155–205

Janecka IP (1997) Facial translocation approach, Chapter 6. In: Janecka IP, Tiedemann K (eds) Skull base surgery. Lippincott-Raven, Philadelphia, pp 183–220

MacDonald AJ, Harnsberger HR (2004) Nose and sinus imaging. In: Harnsberger HR et al. (eds) Diagnostic imaging: head and neck. Section II, 2. Amirsys, Salt Lake City

Mehta RP, Ceuva RA, Brown JD (2006) What's new in skull base medicine and surgery: Skull Base Committee Report. Otolaryngol Head Neck Surg 135:620–630

NCCN (National Comprehensive Cancer Network) (2006) Practice Guidelines for Oncology (revised 2006). www.nccn.org

Pearson, BW (1999) Surgical anatomy of the nasal cavity and paranasal sinuses, Chapter 26. In: Thawley SE, Panje WR, Batsakis JG, Lindberg RD (eds) Comprehensive management of head and neck tumors. W.B. Saunders, Philadelphia, pp 540–557

35 Neck Metastasis and Unknown Primary Tumor

Silvio Ghirardo · Jerry Castro · Bhuvanesh Singh

Pearls and Pitfalls

- The presence of a clinically palpable, unilateral, firm, enlarged cervical lymph node in an adult should be considered metastasis until proven otherwise, and should initiate a systemic search for the primary site.
- Despite the advent of new diagnostic studies, a detailed patient history, physical examination, and fine-needle aspiration biopsy are the cornerstones of the evaluation of enlarged cervical nodes.
- Metastases to the cervical lymphatics at presentation constitute the single most important factor determining outcome of patients with head and neck squamous cell carcinoma.
- Regional lymphatic metastases from head and neck neoplasms occur in a predictable and sequential fashion to specific regional lymph nodal groups.
- If the risk of occult metastasis is greater than 10–20%, elective dissection of the neck nodes is recommended.
- Selective neck dissection is used for accurate staging and treatment of the clinically negative neck at risk for harboring micrometastases.
- Outcomes are comparable in patients with nodal metastases that have undergone a classical radical neck dissection or a modified neck dissection preserving the spinal accessory nerve.
- Radical neck dissection is still indicated and utilized for N3 disease and clinical signs of gross extranodal disease.
- Evaluation post-chemoradiation requires a combination of clinical examination and imaging to assess the need for salvage neck dissection.
- PET scanning to assess for residual disease after chemoradiation should not be performed earlier than 10–12 weeks after completion of chemoradiation treatment.

Introduction

Metastasis to the cervical lymph nodes is the single most important factor determining the outcome of patients with head and neck squamous cell carcinoma (HNSCC). Nodal metastasis can occur in one of three clinical settings: known primary tumor with clinically detectable metastasis, known primary tumor with occult metastasis, or unknown primary tumor with clinically detectable metastasis. A better understanding of the patterns of lymph node metastases and prognostic factors has allowed for modifications in the therapeutic approach, resulting in improvements in functional outcome, quality of life, and the evolution of adjuvant treatments that have improved management of the neck in patients with HNSCC.

Basics of Neck Nodal Management

Head and Neck Lymphatic Anatomy

Regional metastasis from head and neck cancer occurs in a predictable, sequential fashion to specific lymph node groups. For a given primary tumor, not all regional lymph node groups are at risk for nodal metastases. In the absence of grossly palpable metastatic lymph nodes, understanding the patterns of neck metastasis can facilitate treatment of the neck. Accordingly, specific nodal groups can be targeted in treatment planning for a given primary site in the head and neck region. Conversely, if lymphatic metastasis has occurred and the primary tumor site is unknown, specific anatomic sites should be investigated for primary tumors.

The neck is divided into four major nodal groups. The Anterior and Lateral Neck Nodal group is further divided into six levels (❯ *Table 35-1*) with biological and clinical significance to describe various methods of selective neck dissection.

Submental (sublevel IA): Central triangular region bounded by the anterior belly of the digastric muscles and the hyoid bone. These nodes are at risk for harboring metastases from the floor of the mouth, anterior oral tongue, anterior mandibular alveolar ridge, and lower lip.

Submandibular (sublevel IB): Lymph nodes within the boundaries of the anterior belly of the digastric muscle, the stylohyoid muscle, and the body of the mandible. The submandibular gland is included in the resection. These nodes are at risk for harboring metastases from the oral cavity, anterior nasal cavity, and soft tissue structures of the midface and submandibular gland.

Upper jugular (sublevels IIA, IIB): Lymph nodes surrounding the upper level of the internal jugular vein and adjacent spinal accessory nerve, extending from the skull base to the level of the hyoid bone. The medial boundary is the stylohyoid muscle, and the lateral boundary is the posterior border of the sternocleidomastoid muscle. Sublevel IIA is located medial to the vertical plane defined by the spinal accessory nerve. Sublevel IIB is located lateral to the vertical plane defined by the spinal accessory nerve. The upper jugular is at risk of harboring metastases from tumors arising from the oral cavity, nasal cavity, nasopharynx, oropharynx, hypopharynx, larynx, and parotid gland.

Middle jugular (level III): Lymph nodes surrounding the middle portion of the internal jugular vein, extending from the hyoid bone to the inferior border of the cricoid cartilage. The medial boundary is the lateral border of the sternohyoid muscle, and the lateral boundary is the posterior border of the sternocleidomastoid muscle. These nodes are at risk for harboring metastases from the oral cavity, nasopharynx, oropharynx, hypopharynx, and larynx.

Lower jugular (level IV): Lymph nodes surrounding the lower-third of the internal jugular vein, extending from the inferior border of the cricoid cartilage to the clavicle. The medial boundary is the lateral border of the sternohyoid muscle, and the lateral boundary is the posterior border of the sternocleidomastoid muscle. These nodes are at risk for harboring metastases from the hypopharynx, thyroid, cervical esophagus, and larynx.

Posterior triangle group (sublevels VA, VB): The superior boundary is the apex formed by convergence of the sternocleidomastoid and the trapezius muscles. The inferior boundary is the clavicle. The

□ Table 35-1

Anatomical structures defining the boundaries of neck levels and sublevels (Reprinted from Robbins et al., 2002. Copyright 2002, American Medical Association. With permission)

Level	Superior	Inferior	Anterior (Medial)	Posterior (Lateral)
IA	Symphysis of mandible	Body of hyoid	Anterior belly of contralateral digastric muscle	Anterior belly of ipsilateral digastric muscle
IB	Body of mandible	Posterior belly of digastric	Anterior belly of digastric	Stylohyoid muscle
IIA	Skull base	Horizontal plane defined by the inferior body of the hyoid bone	Stylohyoid muscle	Vertical plane defined by the spinal accessory nerve
IIB	Skull base	Horizontal plane defined by the inferior body of the hyoid bone	Vertical plane defined by the spinal accessory nerve	Lateral border of the sternocleidomastoid muscle
III	Horizontal plane defined by the inferior body of the hyoid bone	Horizontal plane defined by the inferior border of the cricoid cartilage	Lateral border of the sternohyoid muscle	Lateral border of the sternocleidomastoid muscle or sensory branches of cervical plexus
IV	Horizontal plane defined by the inferior border of the cricoid cartilage	Clavicle	Lateral border of the sternohyoid muscle	Lateral border of the sternocleidomastoid muscle or sensory branches of cervical plexus
VA	Apex of the convergence of the sternocleidomastoid and trapezius muscles	Horizontal plane defined by the lower border of the cricoid cartilage	Posterior border of the sternocleidomastoid muscle or sensory branches of cervical plexus	Anterior border of the trapezius muscle
VB	Horizontal plane defined by the lower border of the cricoid cartilage	Clavicle	Posterior border of the sternocleidomastoid muscle or sensory branches of cervical plexus	Anterior border of the trapezius muscle
VI	Hyoid bone	Suprasternal	Common carotid artery	Common carotid artery

medial boundary is the posterior border of the sternocleidomastoid muscle, and the lateral boundary is the anterior border of the trapezius muscle. Sublevel VA is separated from VB by a horizontal plane marked by the inferior border of the anterior cricoid arch. Thus, sublevel VA includes the spinal accessory nodes, and sublevel VB includes the nodes along the transverse cervical vessel and the supraclavicular nodes, with the exception of Virchow's node which is located at level IV. The posterior triangle nodes are at risk for harboring metastases from the nasopharynx, oropharynx, and cutaneous structures of the posterior scalp, and neck.

Anterior compartment (level VI): Includes the pretracheal, paratracheal, precricoid, and the perithyroidal nodes, including lymph nodes along the recurrent nerves. The superior boundary is the hyoid bone, the inferior boundary is the suprasternal notch, and the lateral boundaries are the common carotid arteries. These nodes are at risk of harboring metastases from the thyroid gland, glottic and subglottic larynx, apex of the pyriform sinus, and cervical esophagus.

Anatomic radiological landmarks have been identified to accurately designate lymph nodes according to the nodal level system (Chung et al., 2004). The inferior border of the hyoid separates levels II and III, and the inferior border of the cricoid separates levels III and IV. A vertical plane along the posterior margin of the submandibular gland sets the limit between levels I and II. The medial margin of the common and internal carotid arteries separates level III and IV (lateral) from level VI (medial) in the lower neck; it also separates level II and III (lateral) from the retropharyngeal nodes (medial) in the upper neck.

Neck Nodal Staging

The factors included in the neck nodal staging system have remained relatively stable over revisions (❷ *Table 35-2*). In the newest (sixth) edition of the AJCC–UICC cancer staging system, neck nodal staging has not changed for squamous cell carcinomas. The outcome of N0 (no detectable metastasis) is far superior to N1 (ipsilateral node ≤3 cm), N2 – single (N2a), multiple ipsilateral (N2b) or bilateral nodes (N2c – >3 cm and ≤6 cm), or N3 (node >6 cm), with anticipated overall survival of 85–95%, 40–60%, 30–40% and > 25%, respectively. Other factors that will be monitored for potential inclusion

■ Table 35-2

AJCC 6th edition neck staging

Neck staging in all sites in head and neck (except thyroid and nasopharynx)	
NX	Regional nodes can not be assessed
N0	No regional node metastasis
N1	Metastasis in a single ipsilateral lymph node, 3 cm or less in greatest dimension
N2	Metastasis in a single ipsilateral lymph node, more than 3 cm but not more than 6 cm in greatest dimension; multiple ipsilateral nodes, not more than 6 cm in greatest dimension; or in bilateral or contralateral lymph nodes, not more than 6 cm in greatest dimension
N2a	Metastasis in a single ipsilateral lymph node, more than 3 cm but not more than 6 cm in greatest dimension
N2b	Metastasis to multiple ipsilateral nodes, not more than 6 cm in greatest dimension
N2c	Metastasis to bilateral or contralateral lymph nodes, not more than 6 cm in greatest dimension
Neck staging for thyroid	
NX	Regional nodes cannot be assessed
N0	No regional node metastasis
N1a	Metastasis to level VI (pretracheal, paratracheal, and prelaryngeal/Delphian lymph nodes
N1b	Metastasis to unilateral, bilateral, or contralateral cervical, or superior mediastinal lymph nodes
Neck staging for nasopharynx	
NX	Regional nodes cannot be assessed
N0	No regional node metastasis
N1	Unilateral metastasis to lymph node(s), 6 cm or less in greatest dimension, above the supraclavicular fossa[a]
N2	Bilateral metastasis to lymph node(s), 6 cm or less in greatest dimension, above the supraclavicular fossa[a]
N3	Metastasis in a lymph node(s)[a] > 6 cm and/or to the supraclavicular fossa
N3a	Greater than 6 cm in dimension
N3b	Extension to supraclavicular fossa[b]

[a]Midline nodes are considered ipsilateral nodes.

[b]Supraclavicular zone or fossa is relevant to the staging of nasopharyngeal carcinoma and is the triangular region originally described by Ho. It is defined by three points: (1) The superior margin of the sternal head of the clavicle, (2) superior margin of the lateral end of the clavicle, (3) the point where the neck meets the shoulder. Note that this would include caudal portions of levels IV and V. All cases with lymph nodes (whole or part) in the fossa are considered N3b.

into future versions of the staging system include the location of the involved lymph node in the upper (designated "U" for above lower border of cricoid) or lower (designated "L" for below lower border of cricoid) and presence of extranodal spread. Key differences in the staging system are present for nasopharynx and thyroid cancers based on differences in behavior. Nodal staging for nasopharyngeal cancers reflects the staging approach used in Ho's classification. N1 represents a single, unilateral node ≤6 cm above the supraclavicular fossa, N2 is bilateral metastasis ≤6 cm that is above the supraclavicular fossa, and N3 for nodes >6 cm (N3a) and/or involved in the supraclavicular fossa (N3b). For thyroid cancer, the nodal stage is either N0 or N1, with N1a being metastasis to pretracheal, paratracheal, and prelaryngeal/Delphian nodes, and N1b to cervical or superior mediastinal nodes.

Management of Known Primary Tumor with Clinically Detectable Metastasis

Over the last two decades, there have been significant changes in the management of nodal metastasis from head and neck primary tumors. These changes are most influenced by an understanding of patterns of nodal spread, the use of adjuvant radiation (and now chemoradiation) after surgery, and the use of definitive chemoradiation treatment to manage nearly all laryngopharyngeal cancers. The approach to management of the neck is primarily dictated by the location and treatment selected for the primary tumor. If the primary is treated with surgery (oral cavity, salivary, thyroid), surgical management of the neck is advocated. Conversely, if the primary is treated with radiation or chemoradiation (laryngopharyngeal cancers), surgery for neck nodal disease is reserved for salvage.

Surgical Management of the Neck

George Crile is credited with the first formal description of a systematic removal of nodal metastasis from head and neck primary tumors. In this operation, all nodal basins at risk for metastasis were removed en bloc together with the sternocleidomastoid muscle, internal jugular vein, and accessory nerve. Although highly effective, this procedure resulted in significant cosmetic and functional morbidity to the patient (❷ Fig. 35-1). An understanding of the patterns and progression of lymphatic metastasis from primary sites in the head and neck region has allowed modifications to the classic radical neck dissection that reduce morbidity while maintaining therapeutic efficacy. These modified radical neck dissections (mRND) involve removal of level I-V lymphatic basins and include three types based on the non-lymphatic structures preserved. The mRND type I includes resection of the sterno-cleidomastoid muscle and internal jugular vein, along with the nodal basin. By preserving the accessory nerve, the mRND type I avoids much of the functional disability seen with radical neck dissection without compromising survival and neck nodal control. It has become the procedure of choice for the surgical management of the neck in the setting of detectable nodal metastasis. The mRND type 2 involves preservation of the sternocleidomastoid and accessory nerve, and the mRND type 3 adds the preservation of the internal jugular vein. The mRND type 3 dissection is the treatment of choice for thyroid cancers.

◘ Figure 35-1

Classical radical neck dissection results in significant cosmetic and functional debility. Effects include cosmetic deformity, adhesive capsulitis, and subluxation of the sternoclavicular joint, trapezius wasting, winging of the scapula, limitation in shoulder abduction, and chronic pain

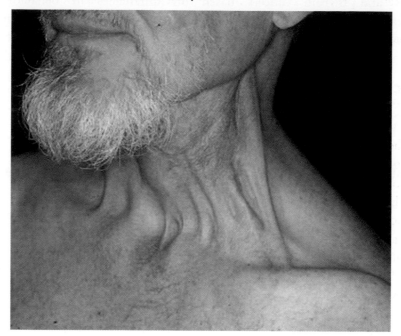

Neck Management in the Post-chemoradiation Setting

The completion of landmark chemoradiation trials has altered the standard of care for tumors of the laryngopharyngeal complex, including the larynx, oropharynx, and hypopharynx. In this setting, the evaluation and management of the neck has become quite challenging. In the past, planned neck dissection was advocated for all patients with N2 or N3 disease at presentation, regardless of response to chemoradiation treatment. More recently, a controversy has developed as to the need for planned neck dissection in all cases. Many now advocate dissection in patients with clinical, radiographic, or functional evidence of residual disease post-chemoradiation treatment. Neck response to chemoradiation treatment should be evaluated at least 10–12 weeks after completion of treatment. This assessment should include a thorough clinical exam and PET-CT study. Elective dissection should be performed if any of the modalities are suspicious for residual nodal involvement. The extent of neck dissection is still a matter of debate. Many advocate radical or modified radical neck dissection; others advocate tailoring the dissection to the site of disease.

Management of Known Primary Tumor with Occult Metastasis

If there is no clinically detectable metastasis, observation may be satisfactory. If the N0 neck progresses to N1 at the time of detection, intervention is warranted. However, studies show that patients with N0 necks that subsequently present with clinical N1 disease in fewer than 70% of cases and pathological

N1 disease in only 30% of cases. This means that 70% of observed patients have pathological N2 or N3 disease at re-presentation with obvious clinical implications. Accordingly, most surgeons advocate evaluation of the regional lymphatics in patients with head and neck cancer, especially if primary surgical management is planned. Effective management of subclinical nodal metastasis requires an understanding of the risk for nodal spread, patterns of metastasis for a given primary site, and tools available for assessment.

Risk for Subclinical Nodal Metastasis

There is no single variable that can predict the presence of occult nodal metastasis from a given primary tumor. The key factors influencing the development of nodal metastasis include the tumor location, T-stage, and histomorphologic characteristics. In general, the risk of metastasis increases from the anterior to the posterior aspect of the upper aerodigestive tract (lips less than 5%; hypopharynx as high as 70%). In the laryngopharyngeal compartment, the risk of metastasis increases from the center to the periphery (vocal cord less than 2%, pharyngeal wall approximately 70%). The risk of metastasis increases in the oral cavity from the superior to the inferior aspect (hard palate less than 5%; floor of the mouth approximately 50%). There is a strong correlation between the T-stage and the risk of metastasis, increasing from <15% for T1 to 15–30% T2, and from 30–45% for T3 to as high as 75% for T4 tumors. Within the oral cavity, the depth of invasion is also correlated to the risk of metastasis. Tumors less than 2 mm in depth have a <10% risk for regional metastasis, while those greater than 2 mm have a significantly higher risk (35–50%). Other factors that have been less convincingly associated with risk for metastasis include tumor differentiation and pattern of invasion at the host tumor interface.

Although not yet established, molecular markers show future promise for predicting the presence of micrometastasis in the clinically negative neck. Early genomic studies have shown the most promising results. In one study, characterization of patients by results from cDNA microarray analysis shows an 80% accuracy in predicting for nodal metastasis when tumor subsite and pathological node status were considered simultaneously. However, there is insufficient evidence to support the use of molecular studies in clinical practice at present.

Evaluation of Subclinical Metastasis

Although it remains the cornerstone for assessment, it is important to understand that physical examination is not accurate in the staging of neck metastasis, having high false-positive (4–42%) and false-negative rates (up to 77%) that vary with the patient's body habitus, location of the lymph node, and the experience of the examiner. CT and MRI improve the accuracy of nodal staging, but still show a relatively high error rate (8–31%). The accuracy of radiographic diagnosis of lymph node metastasis is improved by considering size (>1.5 cm), rim enhancement, central necrosis, and extranodal invasion. Evaluation of a clinically negative neck by FDG-PET offers similar sensitivity. Sentinel lymph node biopsy has shown promising results in detecting occult nodal metastasis from head and neck primary tumors, and is being studied in a multicenter clinical trial. However, at present, sentinel lymph node biopsy should only be used in controlled settings by experienced investigators. Given all of these factors, surgical removal of cervical nodes remains the standard for assessment for occult metastasis. In general, if the risk of occult metastasis is greater than 10–20%, elective dissection of the neck nodes is recommended. As discussed above, metastasis to regional nodal sites occurs in a predictable manner. Accordingly, all nodal basins do not need to be removed to accurately assess for the presence of occult metastasis.

Extent of Neck Dissection for Assessment of Occult Metastasis

An understanding of the nodal basins at risk has led to the modifications in neck dissection to remove only those nodal basins involved. These modifications are termed selective neck dissections, and include the supraomohyoid neck dissection and the lateral (or jugular) neck dissection.

Oral Cavity

In general, the major nodal basins at risk from a primary tumor in the oral cavity are in levels I, II, and III. Based on this, the supraomohyoid neck dissection was devised to include removal of nodal basins at risk. In the setting of a negative supraomohyoid neck dissection, the risk for nodal failure is less than 5–10%, similar to what is seen with more extensive surgery. Byers brought to our attention the presence of "skip metastasis" isolated to level III or IV (16%) nodes or subsequent failure at level 4 after classic supraomohyoid neck dissection including levels I–III (8%). Based on this finding, we routinely include level IV nodes with supraomohyoid dissections. The other factors that merit consideration are the need for dissection of level IIb (the triangle formed by the posterior belly of the digastric, the spinal accessory nerve, and the sternocleidomastoid muscle) in the absence of metastatic disease at level IIa (area anterior to the spinal accessory nerve), which has the potential to severely impact accessory nerve function. Several studies have shown that level IIb only harbors metastatic nodes when level IIa contains metastatic nodes. For lesions located in the floor of the mouth, ventral surface, or midline tongue, a bilateral supraomohyoid neck dissection should be contemplated.

Larynx

The larynx consists of three subsites: supraglottic, glottic, and subglottic (rarely the primary tumor site). These subsites have different embryologic origins and different lymphatic patterns. The supraglottic larynx has a very high propensity for bilateral lymphatic spread. Early-stage glottic tumors rarely metastasize to the neck, therefore elective dissection is not indicated. With any supraglottic, subglottic, or advanced larynx primary treated surgically in the setting of no detectable nodal metastasis, a selective neck dissection removing levels II, III, and IV (lateral neck dissection) is recommended. In the setting of primary site failure in the larynx after definitive chemoradiation, surgical resection of levels II, III, and IV should be contemplated as part of surgical salvage treatment.

Nasopharynx

There is no role for neck dissection as the primary modality of treatment in nasopharyngeal cancers. In these cases, radiation and chemotherapy are the treatment of choice for the primary tumor of the neck. These patients rarely fail.

Oropharynx (Tonsil, Base of the Tongue, Oropharyngeal Wall) and Hypopharynx

Currently these patients are treated with chemoradiotherapy, although surgery has a role in salvaging the primary site and the neck. If primary surgical treatment is contemplated in the absence of clinically detectable metastasis, ipsilateral selective neck dissection should be performed including levels II, III, and IV for lateral tumors, and bilateral dissection contemplated for midline tumors.

Management of Unknown Primary Tumor with Clinically Detectable Metastasis

An unknown primary tumor is defined as the presence of histologic evidence of malignancy in the cervical lymph nodes with no apparent primary site of origin for the metastatic tumor. By definition, these patients present with a mass in the neck as the primary complaint. In this setting, the presence of a clinically palpable, unilateral, firm, enlarged cervical lymph node in an adult should be considered metastatic until proven otherwise, and it should initiate a systematic search for the primary. The entity of branchial cleft carcinoma is often brought up in the discussion of a nodal neck metastasis from an unknown primary tumor, especially in the setting of cystic metastasis. Although they do occur, branchial cleft cyst carcinomas are very rare and should only be considered after a thorough work-up for a primary tumor has been completed.

Assessment of the Metastatic Node

Fine-needle aspiration biopsy (FNAB) is the preferred method to obtain the diagnosis in this setting, the results of which can assist in establishing subsequent management (❯ *Fig. 35-2*). Open biopsy is *only used* in cases where two FNABs fail to establish a diagnosis. If open biopsy is contemplated, the incision should be placed so that it overlaps the incision required for a comprehensive neck dissection.

◻ Figure 35-2

Evaluation of metastasis from unknown primary tumor. Fine-needle aspiration can help guide the evaluation. In the setting of an anaplastic tumor, supplement immunohistochemical and/or molecular studies to help determine the lineage of the tumor. ND = neck dissection; RT = radiation therapy

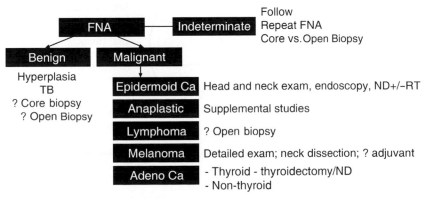

Assessment for the Primary Tumor

The histological content and location of the node is a guide for identifying the primary tumor (❯ *Fig. 35-3*). Squamous cell carcinomas in level I metastasis are typically from oral cavity primaries. Level II, III, and upper level IV are likely to be metastatic from a primary in the laryngopharyngeal complex. Metastasis in level Va should raise concern for a nasopharyngeal or posterior scalp primary. The presence of lower neck and supraclavicular (level IV, Vb) adenopathy should raise concern for the presence of a primary tumor below the clavicle (lung). If metastatic adenocarcinoma is found in the upper neck, a salivary gland primary tumor needs to be considered, while adenocarcinoma in the lower neck is likely from a distant site (lung, breast, GI tract).

The work-up for the identification of a primary tumor starts with a thorough history (including prior skin cancer history) and examination of the head and neck, including the scalp, external auditory canal, and the skin. The physical examination should include palpation of the tonsillar fossae and base of the tongue, and bimanual palpation of the floor of the mouth. The axillae and groin should also be examined to rule out systemic adenopathy. A flexible fiberoptic endoscopic exam of the upper aerodigestive tract should be a routine part of the examination. The impact of fiberoptic examination on detection of the primary tumor is best appreciated in the changing location and rate of subsequent primary detection. In the pre-fiberoptic era, subsequent primaries developed in over 30% of cases, with the most common site for a missed primary being the nasopharynx. With the use of fiberoptic examination (and routine use of adjuvant radiation therapy), the rate of subsequent failure at a primary site is just over 10%, with the base of the tongue being the most common site. PET scanning has played an increasing role in the evaluation of unknown primary cancers. Detection of the unknown head and neck primary with FDG-PET ranges from 5% to 60%. These differences could be attributable to different approaches used in patients with an unknown primary, inclusion criteria, and verification methodology. The current recommendation when using FDG–PET is to obtain this study before a biopsy, because inflammation at the site of biopsy increases the false-positive rate. A positive FDG-PET scan helps guide the physician in performing a biopsy in the operating room.

A key part of the evaluation is examination under anesthesia, including systematic visualization of the laryngopharyngeal complex with guided biopsies. It is important to remember that in 80% of

◻ Figure 35-3
Potential location of primary tumor based on location of lymph node metastasis

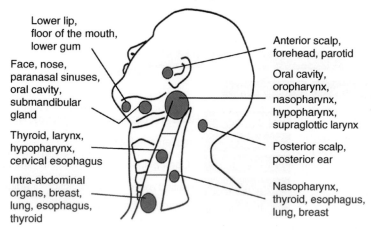

Lower lip, floor of the mouth, lower gum

Face, nose, paranasal sinuses, oral cavity, submandibular gland

Thyroid, larynx, hypopharynx, cervical esophagus

Intra-abdominal organs, breast, lung, esophagus, thyroid

Anterior scalp, forehead, parotid

Oral cavity, oropharynx, nasopharynx, hypopharynx, supraglottic larynx

Posterior scalp, posterior ear

Nasopharynx, thyroid, esophagus, lung, breast

patients presenting with a neck mass, the primary tumor is identified during the office examination and an additional 15% are detected in the operating room. The extent of endoscopy is often an issue of debate, centering on the benefit of routine application of bronchoscopy and esophagoscopy as part of the examination under anesthesia. Most authors agree that there is limited benefit to adding a bronchoscopy, especially in light of negative radiographic findings in the chest. While it is rare to find a primary in the cervical esophagus, advocates of esophagoscopy point to the identification of synchronous second primary tumors as a rationale for the procedure, but this is rare. Tumors are often hidden in the tonsillar crypt and can be missed on surface examination. Accordingly, it has now become routine to perform an ipsilateral tonsillectomy if no other primary is identified.

Management of Unknown Primary Tumor

If the primary tumor remains unidentified after a thorough evaluation, management involves neck dissection followed by adjuvant radiation or chemoradiation treatment. Although there is debate, most physicians include the neck and potential mucosal sites where a primary tumor may remain undetected. In this regard, it is very important to confirm that the nasopharynx is not a likely source for the tumor. Excluding the nasopharynx from the radiation ports significantly reduces morbidity for the treatment. The prognosis will depend on the stage of the neck at presentation.

Adjuvant Treatment for Neck Metastasis After Surgical Resection

The final issue that requires consideration is the need for adjuvant radiation or chemoradiation in the setting of positive nodal involvement. Given the significant influence of the presence of nodal involvement on outcome and the significant improvement in disease control with the use of adjuvant radiation treatment, adjuvant radiation therapy is advocated in all cases with nodal metastasis. Some authors suggest that in selected cases where a single node contains small volume metastasis after mRND or selective neck dissection, the neck can be observed. Moreover, recent studies suggest that the use of chemoradiation in the adjuvant setting for "high-risk" disease, which in the neck includes advanced nodal disease (N2, N3) or the presence of extranodal extension, improves locoregional control and possibly survival.

Selected Readings

Andersen PE, Cambronero E, Shaha AR, Shah JP (1996) The extent of neck disease after regional failure during observation of the N0 neck. Am J Surg 172:689–691

Andersen PE, Warren F, Spiro J, et al. (2002) Results of selective neck dissection in management of the node-positive neck. Arch Otolaryngol Head Neck Surg 128:1180–1184

Chung CH, Parker JS, Karaca G, et al. (2004) Molecular classification of head and neck squamous cell carcinomas using patterns of gene expression. Cancer Cell 5:489–500

Cooper JS, Pajak TF, Forastiere AA, et al. (2004) Postoperative concurrent radiotherapy and chemotherapy for high-risk squamous-cell carcinoma of the head and neck. N Engl J Med 350:1937–1944

Induction chemotherapy plus radiation compared with surgery plus radiation in patients with advanced laryngeal cancer (1991) The Department of Veterans Affairs Laryngeal Cancer Study Group. N Engl J Med 324:1685–1690

Kutler DI, Wong RJ, Schoder H, Kraus DH (2006) The current status of positron-emission tomography scanning in the evaluation and follow-up of patients with head and neck cancer. Curr Opin Otolaryngol Head Neck Surg 14:73–81

Robbins KT, Clayman G, Levine PA, et al. (2002) Neck dissection classification update: revisions proposed by the American Head and Neck Society and the American Academy of Otolaryngology-Head and Neck Surgery. Arch Otolaryngol Head Neck Surg 128:751–758

Ross GL, Soutar DS, Gordon MacDonald D, et al. (2004) Sentinel node biopsy in head and neck cancer: preliminary results of a multicenter trial. Ann Surg Oncol 11:690–696

Shah JP, Medina JE, Shaha AR, et al. (1993) Cervical lymph node metastasis. Curr Probl Surg 30:1–335

Singh B, Balwally AN, Sundaram K, et al. (1998) Branchial cleft cyst carcinoma: myth or reality? Ann Otol Rhinol Laryngol 107:519–524

36 Parotid and Salivary Glands

Alexander C. Vlantis · C. Andrew van Hasselt

Pearls and Pitfalls

- Approximately 25% of parotid, 50% of submandibular and 80% of sublingual/minor salivary gland tumors are malignant.
- The commonest salivary gland tumor is a benign pleomorphic adenoma.
- The commonest malignant parotid tumor is a mucoepidermoid carcinoma.
- The commonest malignant submandibular/sublingual/minor salivary gland tumor is an adenoid cystic carcinoma.
- Most salivary tumors present as a painless swelling of the gland.
- Ultrasonography (US) with guided fine needle aspiration cytology (FNAC) is the initial investigation for all parotid and submandibular gland tumors.
- When FNAC is inconclusive, an excisional, incisional or core biopsy is needed for histological diagnosis.
- An incisional biopsy is used for large intraoral lesions and where the patient is not a surgical candidate.
- MRI or CT is required when clinical, US, or FNAC features suggest malignancy and also for those sites where the rate of malignancy is high, such as the submandibular and sublingual glands.
- FNAC and imaging can never totally exclude a malignant tumor.
- The minimum operation for a tumor of the parotid gland is a superficial parotidectomy with identification and preservation of the facial nerve.
- In rare situations, a partial parotidectomy/lumpectomy may be performed by an experienced parotid surgeon.
- Facial nerve branches should not be sacrificed unless tumor grossly attaches to or surrounds the nerve.
- The primary aim of surgery is to achieve cure and/or a definitive diagnosis which is attained by the complete surgical excision of an operable benign or malignant salivary gland tumor.
- The minimum operation for a submandibular tumor is an extracapsular submandibulectomy/submandibular triangle clearance/level I dissection.
- A neck dissection is only done for clinically positive lymph node metastases.
- Postoperative radiotherapy is indicated for all malignant salivary gland tumors except stage I low grade mucoepidermoid carcinoma and acinic cell carcinomas excised with clear resection margins.

Introduction

General Introduction

The parotid, submandibular and sublingual glands make up the major salivary glands while the minor salivary glands, of which there are about 800, are found within the mucosa of the upper aerodigestive tract. The salivary glands give rise to a heterogeneous group of benign and malignant tumors that account for 3–6% of all head and neck tumors. About 65% occur in the parotid glands, 10% in the submandibular glands and 25% in the sublingual and minor salivary glands. As a general rule, 25% of parotid gland tumors, 50% of submandibular gland tumors, and 80% of sublingual and minor salivary gland tumors are malignant (❖ *Table 36-1*). The palate is the commonest site for minor salivary gland tumors. Overall, the commonest salivary gland tumor is a benign pleomorphic adenoma while the commonest malignant salivary gland tumors are adenoid cystic carcinoma and mucoepidermoid carcinoma (❖ *Table 36-2*). Metastases to regional lymph nodes are uncommon, with a reported overall incidence of about 16%, while distant metastases are found in about 3% of patients at presentation.

Relevant Embryology

The parotid glands develop from ectodermal epithelial buds while the submandibular and sublingual glands develop from endodermal epithelial buds. The submandibular and sublingual glands evolve ahead of the developing lymphatic system while the parotid glands form later. Developing parotid epithelial buds surround divisions of the developed facial nerve and lymphatic system, which explains the presence of intra-glandular lymph nodes within the parotid gland but not within the other major salivary glands.

◘ Table 36-1

Incidence of salivary gland tumors[a] and malignant lesions by site (Spiro, 1986)

	Incidence of tumor[a] by site	% of tumors malignant	Incidence of malignant lesion by site
Parotid	70%	25%	45%
Submandibular	8%	43%	10%
Sublingual	1%	82%	2%
Minor	21%	82%	42%

[a]Benign and malignant.

◘ Table 36-2

Histological distribution of malignant salivary tumors by site (Spiro, 1986)

	Parotid	Submandibular	Minor & Sublingual
Mucoepidermoid carcinoma	44%	30%	25%
Adenoid cystic carcinoma	9%	36%	35%
Adenocarcinoma	10%	7%	29%
Mixed malignant tumor	17%	19%	6%
Acinic cell carcinoma	12%	2%	1%
Squamous cell carcinoma	7%	6%	–
Other	1%	–	4%

Relevant Anatomy

The *superficial cervical fascia* of the neck envelops the platysma and continues onto the face as the *superficial facial fascia* to wrap around the muscles of facial expression. These fasciae and muscles form the superficial musculo-aponeurotic system (SMAS) which is elevated as a myofascial-cutaneous flap during parotidectomy.

The *superficial layer of deep cervical fascia* which envelops the sternocleidomastoid muscles and submandibular glands in the neck, envelopes the parotid glands and masseter muscles as the *parotidomasseteric fascia* in the face. The branches of the facial nerve and the parotid duct remain deep to this fascia such that blunt dissection superficial to the parotidomasseteric fascia will not injure branches of the facial nerve during anterior elevation of the flap.

The *parotid gland* lies in the retromandibular fossa and is divided into a superficial or lateral lobe (80% of the gland) and a deep lobe (20% of the gland) by the traversing branches of the facial nerve. The capsule of the parotid gland is formed by the superficial layer of deep cervical fascia. The parotid duct, or Stensen's duct, crosses the masseter muscle halfway between the zygoma and the oral commissure and pierces the buccinator muscle at the anterior border of masseter to enter the oral cavity opposite the second upper molar tooth. Blood supply is from branches of the maxillary artery. Lymphatics drain to the upper jugular lymph nodes. The facial nerve is the most important of the three nerves relating to the parotid gland. It exits from the skull base through the stylomastoid foramen and enters the posterior portion of the gland where the main trunk divides into an upper zygomatico-temporal division and a lower cervico-facial division. The five terminal branches exit from the anterior border of the gland deep to the parotidomasseteric fascia on the masseter muscle as the temporal, zygomatic, buccal, mandibular and cervical branches. The great auricular nerve originates from the cervical plexus (C2, 3) and crosses the sternocleidomastoid muscle from its posterior border to enter the tail of the parotid where it divides into an anterior and a posterior branch. Preserving the posterior branch at surgery preserves sensation of the lobule and lower half of the concha. The auriculotemporal nerve is a branch of the mandibular division of the trigeminal nerve and carries parasympathetic secretomotor fibres from the otic ganglion to the parotid gland. Innervation of sweat glands by regenerating parasympathetic secretomotor fibres causes Frey's syndrome or gustatory sweating.

The *submandibular gland* lies in the submandibular triangle, deep to platysma, adjacent to the anterior and posterior bellies of digastric. It wraps around the posterior border of the mylohyoid muscle, with a smaller portion deep to and a larger portion superficial to the muscle. The capsule of the gland is formed by the superficial layer of deep cervical fascia. Branches of the facial artery supply the gland which is drained by sublingual, submental and facial veins. The lymphatic drainage is via periglandular and perivascular submandibular lymph nodes to deep upper cervical lymph nodes. Wharton's duct opens at the sublingual papilla in the anterior floor of the mouth. Three nerves relate to the submandibular gland. The marginal mandibular branch of the facial nerve lies just deep to the fascia enveloping platysma, and if the nerve dips below the inferior border of the body of the mandible, it crosses the capsule of the submandibular gland and facial vein in the neck. The lingual nerve supplies parasympathetic secretomotor fibres to the submandibular gland via the submandibular ganglion. At a slightly deeper fascial plane is Wharton's duct, and at an even deeper plane is the hypoglossal nerve.

The *sublingual glands* rest against the sublingual recess of the mandible close to the symphysis on the mylohyoid muscle and are closely related to the lingual and hypoglossal nerves, the submandibular duct and mucosa of the floor of the mouth. Lymphatic drainage is to submandibular lymph nodes.

The gland is composed of a major sublingual gland and 8–30 smaller minor sublingual glands which open either directly onto the floor of the mouth or into the submandibular duct. The nerve supply is similar to that of the submandibular gland.

The *minor salivary glands* lie in the mucosa of the upper aerodigestive tract and are classified according to their site. Their small ducts open individually onto the surface of the mucosa.

Etiology

A relationship between radiation exposure and a salivary gland tumor has been suggested.

Clinical Presentation

History and Examination

Most salivary tumors present as a painless *swelling*. Tumors in the deep parotid lobe may present as medial displacement of the lateral oropharyngeal wall as they enlarge within the parapharyngeal space. Sublingual tumors may present with pain or numbness of the tongue. Minor salivary tumors may ulcerate as they enlarge. *Pain* is due to infection, hemorrhage or cystic degeneration in a benign tumor while in a malignant tumor usually indicates nerve invasion. *Nerve palsy* and *enlarged cervical lymph nodes* suggest that a tumor is malignant. The *duration* of the tumor is not specifically related to malignancy.

A careful clinical examination must estimate the size and mobility of the tumor and determine whether there is fixation to adjacent structures such as skin and bone. Involvement of the facial, hypoglossal, lingual, marginal or other nerves must be assessed and the neck palpated for lymphadenopathy. The oropharynx must be inspected to assess the parapharyngeal space and the intra-oral portion of the submandibular gland palpated through the floor of the mouth. Induration, an irregular surface, fixation, skin or nerve involvement or cervical lymphadenopathy suggest malignancy.

Pre-Operative Evaluation

Fine Needle Aspiration Cytology

Fine needle aspiration cytology (FNAC) is the initial investigation of choice for all salivary gland tumors, with ultrasound used to guide the needle into smaller lesions. Malignant cells may be the only objective evidence of malignancy in an otherwise clinically and radiologically benign salivary gland mass. FNAC is simple to perform and can differentiate correctly between a benign and a malignant tumor in 85% or more of cases. FNAC is also useful in distinguishing between an inflammatory and a benign or malignant mass. Furthermore, the technique helps to exclude other causes of salivary masses, such as a lymphoma, for which surgery is not initially indicated. The result of FNAC gives the surgeon useful information with which to counsel the patient and to plan for surgery.

Biopsy

When FNAC is inconclusive, a biopsy is required for histological diagnosis. An *excisional* biopsy is always performed with curative intent and is appropriate for small intraoral lesions and for small tumors of the parotid (a superficial parotidectomy) and submandibular glands (a submandibulectomy). A small bore *core-needle* biopsy can be performed when an experienced cytologist is not available or when a lymphoma is suspected. This should be done under ultrasound guidance as injury to the facial nerve or glandular artery is possible. An open *incisional* biopsy is used for bigger intraoral lesions and where the patient is not a surgical candidate. The key to establish the malignant nature of a tumor is the demonstration of an infiltrative margin. A transoral incisional biopsy of an oropharyngeal or parapharyngeal mass should not be done as there is a danger of injuring medially displaced nerves or major vessels.

Imaging

Ultrasonography (US), MRI and CT are used to image tumors of the salivary glands. Imaging is used to map the extent of the tumor and attempts to characterize the tumor. There are imaging features that can characterize benign tumors such as pleomorphic adenomas and Warthin's tumors, however imaging can never totally exclude a malignant tumor. Malignant features include poorly defined borders, extension into adjacent structures and metastatic lymphadenopathy.

Ultrasonography with guided FNAC is advocated as the initial investigation for all parotid and submandibular gland tumors. For small (<3 cm) benign appearing tumors in the superficial lobe of the parotid gland, which should undergo a superficial parotidectomy as definitive management, no further imaging is required. However, *MRI or CT* is required when there are clinical, US or FNAC features that suggest malignancy and also for those sites where the rate of malignancy is high, such as the submandibular and sublingual glands. MRI or CT is required to delineate the full extent of large tumors, extension into the deep lobe as seen on US, protrusion into the oral cavity or oropharynx or when involvement of the parapharyngeal space is suspected. Overall, MRI has several advantages over CT in that it can give a better picture of spread into adjacent soft tissues including perineural invasion, and is more sensitive (but less specific) at detecting bone invasion. MRI can often demonstrate the intra-parotid facial nerve.

Histological Classification of Salivary Gland Tumors

The current 1991 WHO and 1996 Armed Forces Institute of Pathology classification of salivary gland tumors is based on morphology and is complex but necessary to provide an accurate histological diagnosis (● *Table 36-3*). The histology has prognostic implications and provides information for treatment optimization. Acinic cell carcinoma and grade I and II mucoepidermoid carcinomas are considered to be low-grade malignancies while grade III mucoepidermoid carcinoma and other carcinomas are considered to be high-grade malignancies. Although tumor grade is important, it must be considered in the context of stage. In general, the size of the tumor is of more prognostic value than the grade of a tumor with larger malignancies having a poor prognosis regardless of their grade, and high grade malignancies having a reasonable prognosis when they are small.

Staging

The T, N and M categories are based on the clinical examination and imaging. Carcinomas of the major salivary glands are classified according to the 2002 unified TNM staging system of the American Joint Committee on Cancer (AJCC) and the International Union Against Cancer (UICC) (❯ *Table 36-4*). Minor salivary gland tumors are classified according to their anatomic site of origin.

◘ Table 36-3

WHO histological classification of salivary gland tumors (Seifert and Sobin, 1992)

Tumor type
Adenomas
Pleomorphic adenoma
Myoepithelioma (Myoepithelial adenoma)
Basal cell adenoma
Warthin tumor (adenolymphoma)
Oncocytoma (oncocytic adenoma)
Canalicular adenoma
Sebaceous adenoma
Ductal papilloma
Cystadenoma
Carcinomas
Acinic cell carcinoma (low grade)
Mucoepidermoid carcinoma grade I and II (low grade)
Mucoepidermoid carcinoma grade III (high grade)
Adenoid cystic carcinoma
Polymorphous low-grade adenocarcinoma (terminal duct carcinoma)
Epithelial-myoepithelial carcinoma
Basal cell adenocarcinoma
Sebaceous carcinoma
Papillary adenocarcinoma
Mucinous adenocarcinoma
Oncocytic carcinoma
Salivary duct carcinoma
Adenocarcinoma
Malignant myoepithelioma (myoepithelial carcinoma)
Carcinoma in pleomorphic adenoma (malignant mixed tumor)
Squamous cell carcinoma
Small cell carcinoma
Undifferentiated carcinoma
Other carcinomas
Nonepithelial tumors
Malignant lymphomas
Unclassified tumors
Tumor-like lesions

◧ Table 36-4

TNM staging of malignant salivary gland tumors (Reprinted from Sobin and Wittekind, 2002. Copyright 2002, Wiley-Liss. With permission)

TNM clinical classification		
T – primary tumor		
TX	Primary tumor cannot be assessed	
T0	No evidence of primary tumor	
T1	Tumor 2 cm or less in greatest dimension without extraparenchymal extension[a]	
T2	Tumor more than 2 cm but not more than 4 cm in greatest dimension without extraparenchymal extension[a]	
T3	Tumor more than 4 cm and/or tumor with extraparenchymal extension[a]	
T4a	Tumor invades skin, mandible, ear canal or facial nerve	
T4b	Tumor invades base of skull, pterygoid plates or encases carotid artery	
N – regional lymph nodes		
Nx	Regional lymph nodes cannot be assessed	
N0	No regional lymph node metastasis	
N1	Metastasis in a single ipsilateral lymph node, 3 cm or less in greatest dimension	
N2a	Metastasis in a single ipsilateral lymph node, more than 3 cm but not more than 6 cm in greatest dimension	
N2b	Metastasis in multiple ipsilateral lymph nodes, none more than 6 cm in greatest dimension	
N2c	Metastasis in bilateral or contralateral lymph nodes, none more than 6 cm in greatest dimension	
N3	Metastasis in a lymph node more than 6 cm in greatest dimension	
M – distant metastases		
Mx	Distant metastasis cannot be assessed	
M0	No distant metastasis	
M1	Distant metastasis	
Stage grouping		
Stage I	T1	N0	M0
Stage II	T2	N0	M0
Stage III	T3	N0	M0
	T1, T2, T3	N1	M0
Stage IVA	T1, T2, T3	N2	M0
	T4a	N0, N1, N2	M0
Stage IVB	T4b	Any N	M0
	Any T	N3	M0
Stage IVC	Any T	Any N	M1

Classification applies to carcinomas of the major salivary glands. Minor salivary gland tumors are classified according to their anatomic site of origin.

Midline nodes are considered ipsilateral nodes.

[a]Extraparenchymal extension is clinical or macroscopic evidence (not microscopic evidence alone) of invasion of soft tissues or nerves, except those listed under T4a and T4b.

Differential Diagnosis

Adenomas

A **pleomorphic adenoma** or **benign mixed tumor** is the commonest salivary gland tumor, accounting for 65% of salivary tumors. They present as slow growing, asymptomatic discrete hard masses which enlarge and become nodular if left untreated. As most pleomorphic adenomas occur in the superficial lobe of the parotid gland, the treatment of choice is a partial or superficial parotidectomy, which aims to excise the tumor with the capsule intact and with a cuff of normal salivary tissue. Rupture of the capsule with tumor spill will increase the risk of recurrence. While a more conservative extracapsular dissection or simple enucleation may be associated with lower rates of facial nerve palsy and Frey's syndrome, protrusions of tumor can extend through the capsule into adjacent parotid parenchyma. Thus an adequate cuff of normal parotid tissue must be taken with the tumor to prevent local recurrence. If left untreated, there is an increasing chance of malignant transformation with time, and so patients should be encouraged to undergo surgery without undue delay.

A **myoepithelioma, myoepithelial adenoma** and **oncocytoma** present in a similar way to a pleomorphic adenoma. A **monomorphic adenoma** is a slow growing and non-aggressive tumor that occurs in minor salivary glands.

A **Warthin's tumor** (also known as an adenolymphoma or papillary cystadenoma lymphomatosum) presents as a painless, slow growing, well demarcated fluctuant cystic mass in the tail of the parotid gland of elderly males and are bilateral in about 10% of cases. They can usually be diagnosed with FNAC. They are the second most common benign salivary and parotid gland tumor and rarely undergo malignant transformation.

Carcinomas

A **mucoepidermoid carcinoma** (MEC) is the commonest malignant salivary gland tumor. It is the commonest malignant parotid tumor and the second most common malignant submandibular gland tumor. It characteristically presents as a painless solitary mass in the parotid or submandibular gland. In a minor salivary gland, it can mimic a benign or inflammatory lesion, and on the palate a mucocoele or dental abscess. An MEC may increase in size after a period of dormancy. They are divided into low- and high-grade tumors which has prognostic significance in terms of survival. However, in the submandibular gland, grading is not a reliable predictor of survival and all submandibular gland MECs should be treated aggressively. An MEC of the submandibular gland has a significantly worse prognosis than those occurring in the parotid gland. Although grading is useful, stage is a better indicator of prognosis. The risk of distant metastases after 10 years is 16%.

An **adenoid cystic carcinoma** (ACC) is the second most common malignant salivary gland tumor after MEC, but is the commonest malignant tumor of the submandibular and minor salivary glands. These tumors present initially as asymptomatic masses, with pain and tenderness developing later in the disease. They grow persistently and relentlessly. Their local extent is almost always greater than can be appreciated clinically or on imaging due to their tendency to be aggressively invasive. ACCs are slow to metastasize and have a prolonged natural history, an unpredictable clinical course and a tendency to recur locally after a symptom-free period. They metastasize to the lungs, but seldom to regional lymph nodes. At the time of diagnosis, half of all cases show evidence of wide local infiltration with early bone involvement and perineural infiltration which is a typical feature of ACC. The 5-year survival is favorable but not the longer term survival. The rate of distant metastases after 10 years is 30–40%. The presence of lung metastases should not alter the treatment of the primary because single and multiple metastases may remain stable for extended periods.

The typical history of a **malignant mixed tumor** (MMT) is of a long standing salivary mass that suddenly increases in size. Approximately 6% of pre-existing pleomorphic adenomas undergo malignant transformation, referred to as *carcinoma ex-pleomorphic adenoma*, and are included with these tumors. An MMT occurs more commonly in the submandibular than parotid gland. They are firm and may be nodular or cystic. MMTs tend to present at an older age than pleomorphic adenomas, 60 vs. 45 years, are usually bigger than pleomorphic adenomas and have been present for almost twice as long. They are difficult to diagnose and are generally aggressive. They carry a poor prognosis and regional and distant metastases are common. Nodal metastases are present in 11% of patients at presentation, and 39% of patients will eventually develop distant metastases.

Acinic cell carcinomas are slow growing low-grade malignant tumors which mainly occur in the parotid gland and seldom metastasize to lymph nodes. They are usually well defined, are more common in females and may rarely be bilateral. A lymph node metastasis is present in about 10% of cases at diagnosis.

Adenocarcinomas not otherwise specified (NOS) are a miscellaneous group of about 10 subtypes of adenocarcinomas that cannot be defined more accurately by conventional microscopy. They mainly occur in the minor salivary glands and are aggressive. Local recurrences and distant metastases are a feature. Those that occur in the submandibular gland carry a worse prognosis than those in the parotid gland. There is a high incidence of regional and distant metastases at presentation.

Polymorphous low grade adenocarcinomas occur almost exclusively in minor salivary glands. They do not always behave as a low grade lesion and are capable of aggressive local destruction and regional metastases. Perineural invasion is a feature.

Primary **squamous cell carcinoma** of the salivary glands is rare. Conversely, metastatic squamous cell carcinoma to the parotid gland and intraparotid lymph nodes is more common and a search for a primary tumor should be made. About 30% have regional neck node metastases at diagnosis and the prognosis is poor.

Nonepithelial Tumors

These include soft tissue sarcomas such as malignant schwannomas and fibrosarcomas, leukemias and myelomas. Malignant lymphomas, mainly non-Hodgkin's type, usually occur in the parotid gland rather than in other glands.

Secondary Tumors

Metastatic tumors include carcinomas and melanomas, mainly from a head and neck primary.

Tumor-like Lesions

A host of conditions including sialadenitis, sialadenosis (including Sjogren's syndrome, Sarcoidosis and Wegener's granulomatosis), oncocytosis, necrotizing sialometaplasia (salivary gland infarction), benign cysts and hemangiomas can mimic tumors. HIV and AIDS associated salivary lesions must routinely be considered in areas of high incidence.

Parapharyngeal Space Tumors

The commonest tumor of the parapharyngeal space is a salivary gland neoplasm which must be differentiated from neurogenic tumors such as a neurilemoma, neurofibroma and paraganglioma.

Surgical Management

Management of the Tumor

Principles: The primary aim of surgery is to achieve cure and/or a definitive diagnosis. This can only be accomplished by the complete surgical excision of an operable benign or malignant salivary gland tumor. Exceptions to this principle are those tumors treated with primary radiotherapy such as lymphomas, myelogenous leukemias and myelomas and inoperable tumors.

Parotid Gland: As the superficial lobe of the parotid gland is the commonest site for benign and low grade malignant lesions, a *superficial parotidectomy* with identification and preservation of the facial nerve is the management of choice. A superficial parotidectomy involves removal of that part of the gland lateral or superficial to the facial nerve. However, small benign lesions can be treated with a *partial parotidectomy* in which the mass, together with an adequate margin of normal parotid tissue, is carefully dissected from the adjacent gland and facial nerve branches.

A *total parotidectomy*, which involves the removal of the superficial lobe, careful mobilization of the intact facial nerve, and then removal of the deep lobe of the parotid gland, should be performed for all other lesions.

A modified Blair incision is most often employed and offers good access with acceptable cosmetic results. Alternatively, a facelift incision can be used in which the skin flap is elevated in a plane just deep to the superficial musculo-aponeurotic system (SMAS) and platysma.

One or more of the following techniques can be used to identify the facial nerve trunk:

- The trunk is 1 cm medial and 1 cm inferior to the tip of the tragal cartilage pointer.
- The tympanomastoid suture runs to the stylomastoid foramen from which the facial nerve emerges.
- The facial nerve trunk shares the same plane as the attachment of the posterior belly of digastric to the mastoid process.
- The third part of the facial nerve is found within the temporal bone.
- A retrograde dissection of a distal branch of the facial nerve, usually the marginal branch, will lead back to the trunk.
- The use of a facial nerve monitor.

A *radical parotidectomy* is performed when a tumor breaches the capsule of the parotid gland necessitating a wide en-bloc excision of all parotid tissue including the facial nerve and any involved adjacent tissue such as bone and muscle.

Consent should include information about the procedure, the potential for a more extensive resection and a neck dissection, and sensory loss in the distribution of the great auricular nerve. Pre-operative discussion should also cover facial nerve weakness which will usually be temporary but may be permanent, the soft tissue defect in the parotid bed, the scar and potential early and late complications.

Parapharyngeal space tumors: Most PPS tumors can be removed via a submandibular approach. This approach involves the removal of the submandibular gland, a superficial parotidectomy in which the branches of the facial nerve are identified, division of the stylomandibular ligament and anterior dislocation and displacement of the mandible.

Submandibular gland: An extracapsular excision of the entire submandibular gland is appropriate management for benign lesions. However, for malignant lesions, the approach depends on the extent of the tumor. Malignant lesions confined to the gland can be treated with an extracapsular excision of the gland and clearance of the submandibular triangle (level 1B), preserving all nerves unless there is evidence of their involvement by tumor. When the tumor extends through the capsule of the gland, resection must include all involved tissue with a view to obtaining clear margins.

Sublingual gland: T1 lesions should be excised together with the submandibular gland as the submandibular duct may be compromised with even a limited excision. For T2 and larger lesions, a more aggressive en-bloc resection and perhaps a pull-through procedure is indicated. Resection of the lingual nerve with frozen section control and a marginal mandibulectomy if the tumor involves the periosteum are often necessary. If there is obvious mandible invasion, a segmental mandibulectomy with a free flap reconstruction is performed.

Minor salivary glands: Surgery depends on the site and extent of the lesion. Complete surgical excision is usually curative for benign lesions. Surgery for malignant lesions can be extensive and may involve a partial maxillectomy or marginal or segmental mandibulectomy. Most patients will require postoperative radiotherapy.

Management of the Facial Nerve

Dissection of the parotid gland from the facial nerve is best undertaken from the main trunk to the peripheral branches. Accidental nerve transection requires immediate microsurgical resuturing or grafting. Facial nerve branches should not be sacrificed unless the tumor is grossly attached to or surrounds the nerve. Conversely, a branch should be sacrificed if attempts to preserve it will lead to rupture of the capsule resulting in tumor spillage. Prior to proceeding with a nerve resection, frozen section pathology can usually distinguish a benign from a malignant lesion. The surgeon's clinical judgment must also dictate whether to save or sacrifice the facial nerve. Facial nerve involvement by tumor requires frozen section examination of the cut ends to ensure negative margins and immediate reconstruction with the great auricular nerve as a cable graft. There is evidence that sacrifice of the facial nerve may not improve the outcome of patients with malignant parotid tumors.

Management of the Neck

Node positive neck (N+): The treatment for a clinically positive or histologically positive neck is an ipsilateral therapeutic neck dissection, generally followed by external beam radiation therapy to the neck and primary site. The extent of the neck dissection depends on the nodes involved and should attempt to spare vital structures.

Node negative neck (N−): The N0 neck is treated when the risk of occult metastases is high. Elective neck dissection and radiation therapy have a similar ability to control occult neck disease, hence the choice of treatment depends on features of the primary tumor, the patient and the surgeon. Features of the primary tumor that place the neck at risk of having occult metastases are often the same as those that increase the risk of local recurrence. These include high-grade tumors (SCC and MEC), histological type (adenocarcinoma, anaplastic carcinoma, undifferentiated Ca, high grade MEC, SCC, salivary duct carcinoma), advanced T stage, tumor size, facial nerve palsy at presentation, extraparenchymal extension and perilymphatic invasion. Two approaches can be taken. If these factors dictate that the patient will receive post-operative radiation therapy, there is no indication to dissect an N0 neck. Alternatively, lymph node sampling of levels I and II at the time of primary surgery, with frozen section analysis for high-grade tumors, can determine the need for further lymph node dissection and therapeutic neck dissection. If metastases are found, the patient is treated as for a positive neck and given postoperative radiation therapy on indication. If frozen section is not available, a level I–III selective supra-omohyoid neck dissection can be performed for suspected malignant parotid, submandibular or sublingual tumors that have a propensity to metastasize.

Other Management

Radiotherapy: Patients with unresectable tumors or those who are unfit to undergo surgery may be treated with primary radiation therapy.

Non-treatment: All salivary gland tumors should be treated once the appropriate investigations are done. If salivary gland tumors are not treated, benign tumors will slowly enlarge with consequential local symptoms and malignant transformation is a risk. Malignant tumors will enlarge and invade local structures and metastasize regionally and distantly. Airway encroachment and obstruction may occur if the tumor is in the upper aerodigestive tract.

Factors Affecting Survival

Clinical stage: At presentation this is the most reliable predictor and critical factor for outcome and survival; tumor size rather than tumor histology. Stage III and IV tumors are unlikely to do well, regardless of their grade. The T-stage predicts for local control, regional control, distant metastases and overall survival.

Grade: Low grade tumors such a low-grade mucoepidermoid carcinomas and acinic cell carcinomas carry a better prognosis than do high-grade tumors such as high-grade mucoepidermoid carcinomas, adenoid cystic carcinomas, adenocarcinomas, malignant mixed tumors and squamous cell carcinomas.

Histological type: The histopathological nature of a submandibular gland tumor is a major prognostic factor and is an independent prognostic factor for distant metastases. MEC of the submandibular gland has a significantly worse prognosis than those occurring in the parotid gland.

Lymph node metastases: This is the leading predictor for regional control, distant metastases and overall survival on multivariate analysis. Extranodal spread is an independent prognostic factor for distant metastases rather than regional control.

Tumor size: Tumors less than 4 cm (T1 or T2) do better than those greater than 4 cm, regardless of histology or grade. They have a better survival and less locoregional recurrence and distant metastases.

Adjuvant radiation therapy offers a survival advantage to tumors greater than 4 cm, but less so to smaller tumors.

Positive margins: A positive margin is an absolute indication for postoperative radiation therapy. The status of the resection margin is an independent prognostic factor for local control.

Facial nerve palsy: A facial nerve palsy is a reliable indicator of malignancy, and is also associated with worse regional control and survival, despite radical resection.

Skin infiltration: Clinical and pathological involvement of the skin is a predictor for poor regional control, distant metastases and overall survival.

Distant metastases: The rate of distant metastases at 10 years for T1 tumors is 13% and for T2 tumors 30%, indicating that a third of high grade tumors fail at distant sites. The rate of distant metastases of adenoid cystic carcinoma after 10 years is 30–40%. The commonest sites of distant metastases are the lung and bone.

Pain: With a known malignant lesion, pain predicts a poor outcome.

Recurrence: Recurrence of a high grade malignancy carries a poor prognosis.

Gender: Males fare worse than females.

Location: The anatomical region is a prognostic factor for local control and overall survival. Parotid malignancies carry a better prognosis than tumors in other salivary glands. The oral cavity carries a relatively favorable prognosis.

Treatment modality: Postoperative radiation therapy improves local and regional control.

Bone invasion by a tumor signifies a poor prognosis.

Overall, local and regional control rates are in the order of 83% and 89% respectively after 5 years and 78% and 87% respectively after 10 years. The most frequent failures are due to distant metastases, which occur in 15–37% of patients after 10 years. Overall disease free survival ranges from 37% to 55%.

Postoperative Management

Complications

Nerve palsy: Occasionally, some degree of postoperative **facial nerve** weakness is encountered even though the facial nerve is anatomically intact. Most facial nerve palsies will recover within 3 months and by a year typically all have recovered. Facial nerve weakness is more common after a total parotidectomy and re-operation than with a superficial parotidectomy. An important factor with facial nerve palsy is protection of the eye. The **marginal branch** is the branch most at risk during parotid and submandibular surgery. The nerve should preferably be identified at the time of submandibular surgery; alternatively an inferiorly divided facial vein can be used to retract the soft tissues surrounding the nerve superiorly ensuring it remains safely out of the surgical field. Paralysis of the marginal branch results in weakness of the depressor of the lower lip. Injury to the **lingual and hypoglossal nerves** can occur during submandibulectomy and sublingual gland excision.

Hemorrhage and hematoma: Intra-operative bleeding should be controlled with bipolar diathermy or ligatures. A suction drain left in the wound at the end of the procedure must function effectively. If a hematoma does occur, it must be evacuated under general anesthesia with care taken to preserve the integrity of the facial nerve. The wound should be washed and closed over a new suction drain and peri-operative antibiotics started or continued for 5 days.

Infection is rare.

Flap necrosis: A good flap design and correct plane of dissection is essential to avoid necrosis of the distal tip of the postauricular skin flap.

A seroma requires repeated aspiration and may require re-insertion of a suction drain, taking care to avoid damaging the facial nerve.

A sialocoele requires repeated aspiration and botulinum toxin injection can be considered if the sialocoele does not settle.

A salivary fistula usually settles with time and a pressure dressing, and rarely needs to be managed by completing the parotidectomy with facial nerve preservation. An alternative non-surgical management option is botulinum toxin injection into the remaining parotid parenchyma under ultrasound guidance.

Frey's syndrome or gustatory sweating occurs postoperatively when postganglionic parasympathetic nerve fibres innervate sweat glands in the overlying skin. Facial sweating, facial moisture or facial flushing occurs during eating. A starch-iodine test can assess the presence and severity of the gustatory sweating and the skin managed with botulinum toxin injection.

Neuroma formation causes localized neck pain and tenderness and is usually prevented by placing a ligature on the cut end of all sensory nerves divided during surgery. A symptomatic neuroma can be carefully excised.

Local recurrence of a benign pleomorphic adenoma is avoided by performing a superficial parotidectomy as a minimum procedure and ensuring that the capsule does not rupture. Recurrence of a pleomorphic adenoma requires excision of the tumor/s with facial nerve preservation. Recurrence of a malignant tumor requires excision of the recurrence, involved adjacent tissues and remaining parotid tissue with preservation of the facial nerve if oncologically possible, all with the aim of achieving clear surgical margins. Local recurrence of a malignant lesion is treated similarly to the disease at initial presentation – complete surgical excision followed by adjuvant RT (external beam or brachytherapy) if possible.

The **surgical scar** usually heals well, but occasionally a hypertrophic or keloid scar may develop.

Radiotherapy

Postoperative radiotherapy (PORT) is indicated for all malignant salivary gland tumors except stage I low grade MEC and acinic cell carcinomas excised with clear resection margins. Close or positive margins of low grade tumors, especially near the facial nerve, are an indication for PORT. Additional indications for PORT include extraparenchymal extension, dermal and perilymphatic invasion, T3 and T4 tumors, tumors larger than 3–4 cm, pre-operative facial nerve palsy, deep lobe involvement, perineural invasion, lymph node metastases, and local recurrence not previously irradiated.

Both local and regional control and survival is significantly improved in patients receiving PORT for stage III and IV tumors. However, other studies have indicated that PORT may not influence distant metastases or improve overall survival.

Follow-up

The follow-up of patients treated for salivary gland malignancies must be longer than for other head and neck tumors. Evaluation of the outcomes of these patients may require a follow-up period of 20 years.

Selected Readings

Ahuja AT, Evans RM, Vlantis AC (2003) Salivary gland cancer. In: Ahuja A, Evans R, King A, van Hasselt CA (eds) Imaging in head and neck cancer: a practical approach. Greenwich Medical Media Limited, London, pp. 115–141

Brandwein MS, Ferlito A, Bradely PJ, et al. (2002) Diagnosis and classification of salivary neoplasms: pathologic challenges and relevance to clinical outcomes. Acta Otolaryngol 122:758–764

Ferlito A, Pellitteri PK, Robbins KT, et al. (2002) Management of the neck in cancer of the major salivary glands, thyroid and parathyroid glands. Acta Otolaryngol 122:673–678

Rinaldo A, Ferlito A, Pellitteri PK, et al. (2003) Management of malignant submandibular gland tumors. Acta Otolaryngol 123:896–904

Rinaldo A, Shaha AR, Pellitteri PK, et al. (2004) Management of malignant sublingual salivary gland tumors. Oral Oncol 40:2–5

Seifert G, Sobin LH (1992) The World Health Organization's histological classification of salivary gland tumors. A commentary on the second edition. Cancer 70:379–385

Sobin LH, Wittekind C (eds) (2002) UICC International Union Against Cancer. TNM classification of malignant tumors, 6th edn. Wiley-Liss, New York, pp. 48–51

Speight PM, Barrett AW (2002) Salivary gland tumors. Oral Dis 8:229–240

Spiro JD, Spiro RH (2003) Cancer of the parotid gland: role of 7th nerve preservation. World J Surg 27:863–867

Spiro RH (1986) Salivary neoplasms: overview of a 35-year experience with 2807 patients. Head Neck Surg 8:177–184

Terhhard CHJ, Lubsen H, van der Tweel I, et al. (2004) Salivary gland carcinoma: independent prognostic factors for locoregional control, distant metastases, and overall survival: results of the Dutch head and neck oncology cooperative group. Head Neck 26:681–693

Wahlberg P, Anderson H, Biörklund A, et al. (2002) Carcinoma of the parotid and submandibular glands – a study of survival in 2465 patients. Oral Oncol 38:706–713

37 Neurovascular and Soft Tissue Neoplasms of the Head and Neck

William I. Wei

Pearls and Pitfalls

- Neurovascular neoplasms include: schwannomas, neurofibromas, paragangliomas, and carotid body tumors (neoplasms).
- Soft tissue neoplasms include: lipomas, fibrosarcomas, rhabdomyosarcomas, malignant fibrous histiocytomas, dermatofibrosarcoma protuberans, osteogenic sarcomas, and leiomyosarcomas.
- Carotid body and glomus jugulare neoplasms are most common; the diagnosis should be suspected strongly by their location; biopsy is contraindicated because of their vascularity.
- The best treatment of neurovascular neoplasms involves resection with sparing of the vasculature (carotid body neoplasms) or nerve (schwannoma) whenever possible.
- Size, shape, consistency, and fixation are important factors to note on physical examination, because these findings tend to correlate with malignant vs. benign histology and therefore with prognosis.
- Imaging of soft tissue masses in the neck is best achieved with magnetic resonance imaging, but computed tomography may also provide anatomic detail. Unless angiographic embolization is planned, angiography has little to offer.
- Therapy is optimally attained with complete resection; one exception might be rhabdomyosarcomas, for which chemoradiation therapy represents the first line therapy.
- Use of postoperative adjuvant chemotherapy and radiation therapy, while used often for sarcomas of the head and neck region, remains of unproven value.
- Radiation-induced sarcomas are best treated by resection.

Neurovascular Neoplasms

Neurogenic and neurovascular neoplasms form a small proportion of all the neoplastic lesions located in the head and neck region. These neoplasms are grouped among soft tissue tumors, but in view of the presentation and the particular investigations to be carried out for therapy, they should be considered separately. Schwannomas and neurofibromas can arise from any part of the head and neck region. In the neck, when they arise from the cranial nerves, they are medially situated, yet when they originate from the cervical plexus, they are located in the more lateral parts of the neck.

Neurovascular paragangliomas are neoplasms arising from the paraganglionic tissue related to the arterial vasculature or the cranial nerves. Carotid body neoplasms account for more than 60% and glomus jugular neoplasms for 30% of all the paragangliomas in the head and neck region. Approximately 10% of these patients have multiple or bilateral neoplasms, and a family history is also present in about 10% of all patients. Around 5% of the paragangliomas are malignant, as demonstrated by metastasis.

Neurogenic Neoplasms

The presentation is usually a mobile mass in the neck that arises in a plane perpendicular to the long axis of the nerve. These neoplasms are not tender or pulsatile. Although they tend to grow slowly, on occasion they exhibit aggressive growth and compress the vasculature in the neck. Occasionally, the patient may present with paralysis of the affected cranial nerve. When the sympathetic trunk is affected, its appearance on magnetic resonance imaging (MRI) will demonstrate the extent of the tumor and its location, situated posteromedial to the carotid artery; when it is located posterolateral to the carotid artery, then it indicating that it arises most likely from the vagus nerve. These neoplasms, however, may arise from any nerves in the neck. Resection of the neoplasm sometimes is done to improve the aesthetic outcome.

Because they arise from the sheath of the nerve, neurilemmoma or schwannoma often can be removed without jeopardizing the affected nerve function. In contrast, neurofibromas are integrated with the nerve, and thus it is not possible to remove the neoplasm without affecting the function of the nerve. Most neurogenic neoplasms, even those located in the parapharyngeal space which extends to the skull base, can be removed through primary operative approaches from the neck. Ordinarily, after complete resection of the tumor, the segment of the nerve will be resected as well, and thus, the patient must be informed preoperatively regarding the functional morbidity after the resection of the nerve with the neoplasm.

Carotid Body Neoplasms

Carotid body neoplasms, also named chemodectomas, are benign neoplasms arising from the chemoreceptor cells in the carotid sheath. These fascinating neoplasms are seen most frequently at the bifurcation of the carotid artery. Patients present typically with a painless, slowly enlarging mass in the upper neck. On clinical examination, the parapharyngeal mass is pulsatile, located in the upper third of the neck, and may push the lateral pharyngeal wall medially. The mass is firm in consistency and more mobile in the transverse direction than vertically.

Once the diagnosis of carotid body neoplasm is suspected, fine needle aspiration cytology should not be obtained, because it may provoke bleeding from this very vascular tumor. Imaging studies should be carried out. Although carotid angiogram would show the pathognomonic finding of the splaying or outward bowing of the internal and external carotid arteries (❷ *Fig. 37-1A*), it has the risk of provoking cerebral ischemia through embolization, and thus enhanced CT or MRI has become the first imaging procedure of choice. Magnetic resonance arteriogram is another safe alternative diagnostic tool (❷ *Fig. 37-1B*). Carotid angiography can be performed preoperatively together with selective embolization of the vascular feeders of the tumor to reduce bleeding at the time of operative resection, although this maneuver is indicated only rarely.

◘ **Figure 37-1**
Carotid body neoplasm. a. Carotid angiogram showing a vascular tumor splaying the internal and external carotid arteries. b. MRI showing the carotid body tumor (T) situated between the external and internal carotid arteries (arrows)

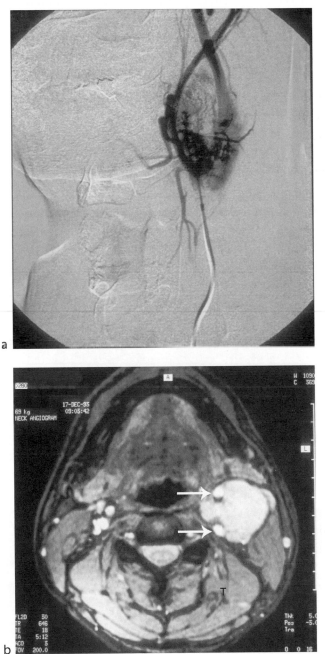

Because carotid body neoplasms arise close to the vagus nerve, hypoglossal nerve, and accessory nerve, an enlarging neoplasm in this region may lead to stretching of these cranial nerves. Multiple cranial nerve palsies have serious functional consequences, and thus it is advisable to remove the tumor when it is small and when the patient's general condition permits.

Operative resection is carried out under general anesthesia with the patient lying supine and the head turned to the opposite side. Preoperative embolization of the tumor is optional, depending on the vascular anatomy and the expertise available. The incision is placed along the skin crease of the neck. The sternomastoid muscle is retracted laterally. Any hyperplastic lymph nodes lying over the surface of the neoplasm are removed to facilitate exposure. The internal jugular vein, the vagus nerve, and the hypoglossal nerve are separated carefully from the tumor. The trunk of the common carotid artery, the distal end of the internal carotid artery, and the branches of the external arteries are freed and controlled. Then the tumor is removed with the dissection plane in the subadventitial plane over the carotid vessels (❯ *Fig. 37-2*). Small bleeding points from the neoplasm are coagulated with the bipolar cautery. Vascular clamps should be available in case the wall of the carotid artery is injured and arterial repair is necessary.

◳ Figure 37-2
a. Dissection of the carotid body neoplasm is carried out along the subadventitial plane at the bifurcation of the carotid artery. b. Complete removal of the carotid body neoplasm, preserving the vessels

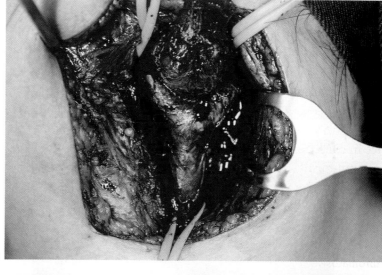

a

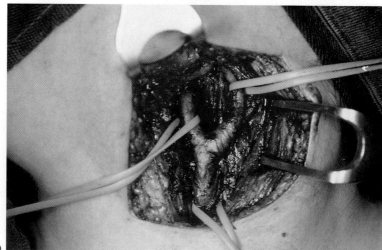

b

Soft Tissue Neoplasms

Soft tissue tumors in the head and neck region are grouped as benign or malignant pathologies that originate from various soft tissues.

Clinical Diagnosis: Malignant neoplasms arising from the soft tissues of the head and neck region are relatively rare and thus are misdiagnosed frequently. These neoplasms have a wide range of histologic types, and their respective behavior further complicates the treatment. In patients with neurofibromatosis, their originally benign neurofibromas have a risk of malignant transformation (❯ *Fig. 37-3*). Patients who have had previous radiation therapy are more prone to the development of fibrosarcoma and osteosarcoma, especially in heavily irradiated areas. Patients with a history of nasopharyngeal carcinoma sarcomas may develop in the paranasal sinuses and the neck. Immunocompromised patients, particularly organ recipients and were treated with immunosuppressive therapy, and patients suffering from HIV infection, have a higher risk of soft tissue neoplasms, especially lymphomas. Children with rapid growing subcutaneous masses also require further investigation.

Clinical Evaluation of Soft Tissue Tumor

Some clinical features of the soft tissue tumor provide information of the pathologic diagnosis as well as prognosis. *Size*: Size alone does not always correlate with the benign or malignant nature of the mass. A rapid increase in size frequently suggests that a tumor is sinister. *Shape*: Sarcomas arising from a nerve usually grow along the long axis of the nerve and appear as a fusiform mass, while liposarcomas or fibrosarcomas often have a round or ovoid configuration and are often immobile. *Consistency*: Detecting a difference in consistency throughout the mass may be subtle, and repeated examination is useful for evaluation. A uniformly firm or hard mass in the soft tissue should be considered malignant

◪ Figure 37-3
A patient with neurofibromatosis with malignant transformation of a neurofibroma

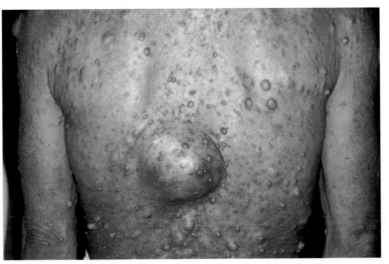

until proven otherwise. *Fixation*: Invasion or infiltration of surrounding tissue, such as vessels, nerves, muscle, or bone, is a sign of an aggressive pathology and portends a poor prognosis.

In children, masses located in the temporal area, the maxillary region, or along the lateral margin of the nose should arouse the suspicion of a rhabdomyosarcoma, while masses in the scalp are usually benign. Sarcomas in the neck in general have a better prognosis than those in the head.

Imaging

Most soft tissue neoplasms in the head and neck region can be assessed adequately by modern imaging modalities. These imaging tests include high-resolution ultrasonography, multislice spiral CT, and MRI. Angiography (digital subtraction/CT or MR angiography) is required occasionally to delineate the full extent of the vascular supply, such as in vascular malformations. Angiography also allows access for selective embolization. Positron emission tomography (PET) is useful in differentiating recurrent or residual soft tissue sarcomas from post-therapy changes and in the detection of distant metastasis.

Imaging of the soft tissue mass aims at differentiating neoplasms from non-neoplastic conditions such as branchial cleft cyst, lymphangioma, or pseudotumoral conditions. Some soft tissue neoplasms have pathognomonic features on imaging that lead to a definitive diagnosis, including lipoma, hemangioma, lymphangioma, neurogenic neoplasms, and paraganglioma. Most malignant soft tissue neoplasms, unfortunately, have non-specific imaging characteristics other than infiltration of surrounding tissues.

Imaging by both CT and ultrasonography can be used to accurately guide biopsy of non-specific soft tissue masses. The determination of the exact location and extent of the tumor contributes to accurate staging. Involvement of surrounding neurovascular bundles, adjacent viscera, and underlying bone, as well as the detection of distant metastases provide important guidelines for therapy.

MRI is the modality of choice for imaging of soft tissue neoplasms, due to the superior quality of soft tissue contrast, the capability of multiplanar imaging, and because ionizing radiation is not involved (◉ *Fig. 37-4*). Moreover, MRI demonstrates the relationship of the lesion with vessels, nerves, tendons, and surrounding structures and provides a roadmap for operative planning. In contrast, although CT involves ionizing radiation, CT is superior to MRI only for detection of cortical bone erosion.

Diagnosis

In view of the therapeutic implications and prognostic factors, it is essential to obtain adequate tissue from the tumor for histologic examination. Biopsy allows determination of the histologic type and grade of the neoplasm. Fine needle aspiration or trucut biopsy often will not provide enough tissue for a pathologic examination to achieve a definite diagnosis. For superficial lesions, an incisional biopsy usually provides adequate amount of tissue, while for deep-seated lesions, this type of biopsy may be insufficient, and, moreover, disrupts the tissue planes. When a sarcoma is suspected, excisional biopsy of the lesion should be carried out if anatomically feasible. The whole resected specimen should undergo pathologic examination to determine the histology.

Sarcomas tend to metastasize by the hematogenous route to distant sites rather than through lymphatics to the regional lymph nodes. Thus, chest radiography is essential before therapy and other imaging modalities such as CT or MRI provide information about the extent of the local disease;

■ Figure 37-4
MRI delineating the extent of a sarcoma(s) in the palate. a. Axial view; b. coronal view; c. sagittal view

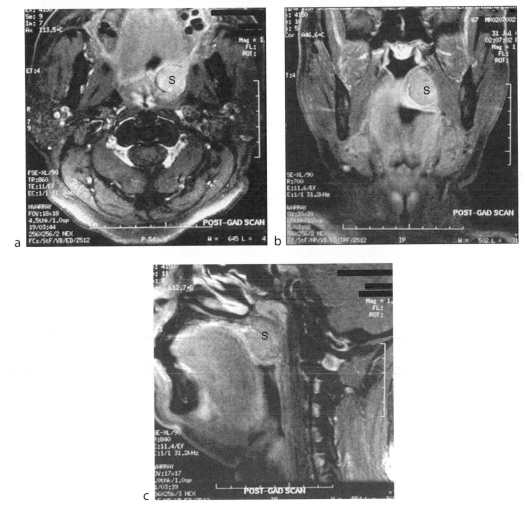

however, because the treatment of sarcomas has become more aggressive, pulmonary metastases do not necessarily preclude resection.

Treatment

The successful management of sarcoma in the head and neck region depends upon a multidisciplinary approach involving radiation oncologists, medical oncologists, pediatricians, pathologists, and surgeons. When diagnosed early, many of the soft tissue sarcomas can be cured, even when metastatic to the lung.

Staging of Soft Tissue Sarcoma

It is difficult to stage precisely the wide varieties of sarcomas. The staging system proposed by the Memorial Sloan-Kettering Cancer Center is based on favorable and unfavorable features of the neoplasm.

Favorable features include size < 5 cm, an anatomically superficial location, and a low histologic grade. *Unfavorable features* involve size > 5 cm, a deeply situated location, and a high grade histology. The stages are:

Stage 0   3 favorable features;
Stage I   2 favorable features;
Stage II   1 unfavorable feature;
Stage III   2 unfavorable features;
Stage IV   3 unfavorable features, distant metastasis

Rhabdomyosarcoma

These often aggressive neoplasms constitute 45% of all sarcomas originating in the head and neck region. The orbit is the most common site, followed by paranasal sinuses, nasal cavity, naso-pharynx, and middle ear. Histologically, rhabdomyosarcoma has four types: embryonal, embryonal with botryoid variation, alveolar, and pleomorphic. Prognosis depends on two factors, first on the histologic type, with the botryoid type being the best, and second on the location of the neoplasm, with those arising in the orbit being most favorable and those in the parameningeal sites the worst. Patients with no macroscopical disease after resection have > 90% cure rate, while the overall cure rate is 55%.

Cross-sectional imaging with CT or MRI is performed to assess the local extent of the neoplasm. The primary treatment is biopsy, followed by radiotherapy and chemotherapy. The current chemotherapeutic agents of choice are Vincristine, Actinomycin D, and Cyclophosphamide given independently or concomitantly with radiotherapy. Radical resection usually is reserved for a salvage procedure.

Fibrosarcoma

Fibrosarcoma constitutes about 10% of all soft tissue sarcomas, of which 20% occur in the head and neck region. This neoplasm presents as a painless and slow growing mass. Because it is radioresistant, treatment is radical operative excision. Radical resection with reconstruction should be performed whenever appropriate.

Malignant Fibrous Histiocytoma

These variants of fibrosarcoma represent the most common soft tissue sarcoma in adults, but only about 3% are located in the head and neck region. There is a male predominance and most arise in patients 50–70 years of age. About 30% of these neoplasms involve the sinonasal tract. The treatment of choice is operative resection of the primary neoplasm, with neck dissection reserved for neck metastases. The overall 5-year survival approaches only 50%. Bad prognostic factors include size greater than 6 cm, older age, and extensive local involvement.

Dermatofibrosarcoma Protuberans

This neoplasm constitutes around 10% of sarcomas of the head and neck region. Dermatofibrosarcoma protuberans usually present as a firm, solitary, elevated, and slowly growing nodule on the scalp or the neck skin. Macroscopically, they appear to be well encapsulated, but microscopically the neoplasm may extend for up to 3 cm from the gross edge. Radical resection with a 3 cm margin gives a 5-year survival of over 90%. They have a high propensity for local recurrence even after a curative resection. Postoperative adjuvant radiotherapy for those neoplasms with a close operative margin reduces local recurrence (❷ *Fig. 37-5*).

Osteogenic Sarcoma

The malignant spindle cells of osteogenic sarcomas produce osteoid or primitive bone. Osteogenic sarcoma in the head and neck region presents most commonly at 20–30 years of age, about a decade later than those in the long bones. They frequently present as a painful mass in the mandible or maxilla and 50% are high-grade neoplasms. The treatment is aggressive operative resection with adequate margins. Pulmonary metastases are present in 30% of patients.

Adjuvant chemotherapy or radiotherapy has no proven value, although for large neoplasms, adjuvant treatments are often given.

■ Figure 37-5
A patient with recurrent dermatofibroma protuberans

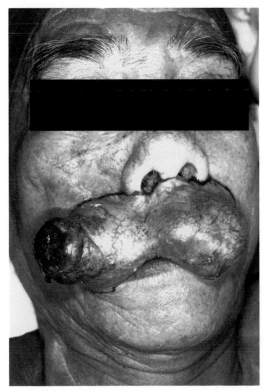

■ Figure 37-6
A patient has a leiomyosarcoma of the floor of mouth

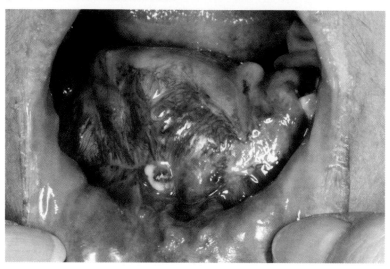

Leiomyosarcoma

These neoplasms usually present in the fifth or sixth decade as a soft tissue mass arising from smooth muscle in the neck. Leiomyosarcomas comprise only 6% of the head and neck sarcomas. The most common site is in the scalp, superficial tissues, and the paranasal sinuses. Leiomyosarcomas are usually well circumscribed, and the potential for metastases is low. Operative excision is the treatment of choice. As postoperative radiotherapy is useful for extremity leiomyosarcoma, it is frequently given for these neoplasms in the head and neck region as well (❷ *Fig. 37-6*).

Radiation-Induced Sarcoma

These sarcomas are an uncommon sequela of radiotherapy; however, these neoplasms are expected to increase over the years as patients survive longer after current modalities of radiation therapy. These sarcomas do not respond to radiation or chemotherapy, and thus resection is the mainstay of management. The overall 5-year survival is around 60%. In the head and neck region, radiation-induced sarcomas occur frequently in the maxilla, mandible, and neck. Adequate operative resection with well-thought-out reconstruction contribute to the most favorable outcome; the often heavily irradiated local environment requires microvacular free tissue transfer for reconstruction.

Selected Readings

Dickens P, Wei WI, Sham JST (1990) Osteosarcoma of the maxilla in Hong Kong Chinese postirradiation for naso-pharyngeal carcinoma. A report of four cases. Cancer 66:1924–1926

Hajdu S, Shiu MH, Brennan MF (1988) The role of the pathologist in the management of soft tissue sarcoma. World J Surg 12:326–331

Maurer HM, Beltangady M, Gehan EA (1988) The intergroup rhabdomyosarcoma study – I: a final report. Cancer 61:209–220

Maurer HM, Gehan EA, Beltangady M (1993) The intergroup rhabdomyosarcoma study – II. Cancer 71:1904–1922

Patel SG, See AC, Williamson PA, et al. (1999) Radiation induced sarcoma of the head and neck. Head Neck 21:346–354

Tran LM, Mark R, Meier R (1992) Sarcomas of the head and neck: prognostic factors and treatment strategies. Cancer 70:169–177

Gastrointestinal

Part 1

Esophagus and Paraesophageal Region: Benign

38 Gastroesophageal Reflux Disease

Owen Korn

Pearls and Pitfalls

- Do not start treatment without a prior endoscopy to assess the esophagus and to exclude pathology of the stomach or duodenum.
- To search for intestinal metaplasia, take biopsies below the squamous-columnar line.
- An anti-reflux operation should not be offered without a complete evaluation, including endoscopy and biopsy, esophageal contrast radiology, esophageal manometry, and 24 h intraesophageal pH monitoring.
- Patients with uncomplicated gastroesophageal reflux disease (GERD) should be followed on a clinical and endoscopic basis yearly or every 2 years.
- Very symptomatic patients who do not respond to medical treatment should be evaluated thoroughly before operation is undertaken.
- Extraesophageal symptoms (asthma, cough, etc.) may be indications for anti-reflux surgery but require a detailed evaluation.
- Hiatal hernia is not synonymous with GERD.
- GERD with dysphagia should be assessed very carefully preoperatively, and the patient should be warned that this symptom may not improve or may even worsen.
- Do not confuse achalasia with GERD, or GERD with achalasia.

Basic Concepts

Lower Esophageal Sphincter

Clinical and manometric studies show a clear sphincteric mechanism at the gastroesophageal junction (GEJ) which constitutes a major barrier against esophageal reflux of gastric content. Despite this, the existence of an anatomic sphincter at this level has been debated for centuries. The main problem until recent years has been to demonstrate a distinct ring of a thickened circular muscle separated from the adjoining muscles by a septum of connective tissue. Such a structure does not exist at GEJ, and many studies support the concept of a "functional" lower esophageal sphincter (LES).

Anatomic studies have demonstrated a particular orientation of the fibers of the internal muscular sheath at the GEJ forming a layer of semicircular fibers or "clasps" oriented transversally. At the GEJ, these "clasp" fibers are inserted firmly into the submucous connective tissue at the margin of contact with the oblique fibers on the opposite side. The oblique fibers replace progressively the short transverse muscle bundles of the esophagus at the greater curvature, and they build a type of muscular

■ Figure 38-1

Schematic representation of the arrangement of the muscular fibers at the gastroesophageal junction. The area within the frame is the high pressure zone or, in other words, the lower esophageal sphincter. a: lateral view; b: oblique view from the lesser curve

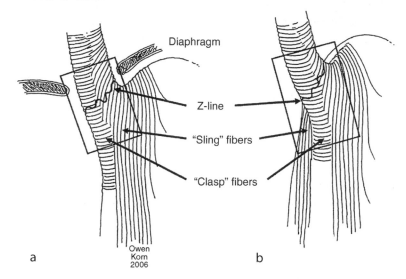

sling structure that covers the end of the esophagus and the anterior and posterior wall of the stomach, the so-called gastric sling fibers. Therefore, the LES is not an annular sphincter but rather formed by two muscle bundles which act in a complementary way: the "clasp" and the "oblique" muscular fibers (❷ *Fig. 38-1*).

Pathophysiology

Gastroesophageal reflux is linked generally to changes in dietary habits, aerophagy, and smoking is associated with many factors, such as motor disturbances of the esophagus, hiatal hernia, short esophagus, acid and/or bile reflux, delayed emptying of the stomach, and obesity, among others. Many of these factors, however, do not cause the reflux but rather are related more closely to the consequences of the reflux. From a mechanical point of view, gastroesophageal reflux in health and disease is related to loss of the barrier that confines the gastric contents to the stomach, either from inappropriate relaxation or incompetence of the LES. Transitory relaxation of the LES not mediated by swallowing, a physiologic phenomenon that allows for the release of gas from the stomach, has been cited as a factor in the majority of normal reflux events, as well as in certain pathologic situations; however, based on manometric evaluation, there is strong evidence supporting a severe mechanical compromise of the LES in patients with GERD.

Mechanical dysfunction of the LES: Mittal has suggested that the initial event in GERD is related most likely to frequent relaxation of the LES with reflux of gastric acid. The presence of acid in the esophagus causes esophagitis, which reduces the sphincter pressure and impairs esophageal contractility. Development of a hiatal hernia enlarges the esophageal hiatus, further impairing the sphincteric function of the crural diaphragm.

In contrast, DeMeester and his group have proposed that GERD may start in the stomach, secondary to gastric distension and delayed gastric emptying. The gastric distension causes unfolding of the LES with exposure of the terminal squamous epithelium within the LES to acid gastric juice. The length of the LES becomes no longer adequate for competency, causing a precipitous decrease in sphincter pressure, loss of the sphincter resistance, and reflux. Repetitive swallowing to clear the refluxed acid causes further gastric distention and initiates a vicious cycle.

A third potential mechanism postulated by Korn et al. involves progressive dilation of the gastroesophageal junction or cardia, probably secondary to esophagitis, which causes an irreversible change in the arrangement of the muscular bands that shape the LES, compromising LES function.

Based on these considerations, the goal of operative therapy is to restore normal competence of the intrinsic sphincter or to create a new, functional sphincter mechanism.

Clinical Presentation

Gastroesophageal reflux is a normal physiologic event occurring generally in the post prandial period. These episodes are short-lasting, the quantity refluxed is usually small, and the refluxate is removed rapidly from the distal esophagus by esophageal clearing without damage to the esophagus. These events go unnoticed by the subject. In contrast, heartburn is the sensation caused usually by the presence of acid in the distal esophagus, while regurgitation is the clinical sensation of ascent of the refluxed material toward the mouth. These are the main two symptoms of gastroesophageal reflux, but their presence does not necessarily mean an incompetent LES, just as the absence of these symptoms does not exclude pathologic gastroesophageal reflux. Occasional heartburn is a common symptom in one of three normal subjects, while in one of ten subjects, heartburn is a common complaint.

In an attempt to establish the diagnosis of gastroesophageal disorder, we have adopted the following definition: presence of chronic symptoms lasting more than 3 months and/or existence of morphologic or functional complications of the esophagus, or well-documented, reflux-induced extra-esophageal complications (asthma, chronic cough, dysphonia, globus pharyngeus, dental deterioration, otitis, and glossitis).

Besides the classic symptoms of heartburn (95%) and regurgitation (70%), some patients complain of dysphagia (30%) or even retrosternal pain that can mimic cardiac pathology. Up to 20% of patients complain of isolated, extra-esophageal symptoms, such as cough, shortness of breath at night, *globus pharingeous*, dental deterioration, otitis, and glossitis.

In daily practice, patients end up in the surgeon's office most commonly referred by their physicians or gastroenterologists. Rarely, patients start with the surgeon, or they become tired of having to rely on medications and/or hear about a minimally invasive approach to operative treatment. Other scenarios involve referrals from otolaryngologists for dysphonia or "posterior laryngitis" or from pulmonologists for chronic cough or nighttime asthma. Finally, the patient with dysphagia must be approached carefully, because dysphagia is an uncommon symptom of GERD unless a complication has occurred, such as a stricture or the development of adenocarcinoma in Barrett's esophagus.

Diagnosis

The approach to diagnosis varies a bit depending on the extent of previous evaluation. If the patient is being seen for the first time, we believe an upper endoscopy is warranted before starting therapy, although we acknowledge the existence of protocols that suggest that when faced with a patient with classic symptoms of GER, therapy can be started and the response assessed later. In contrast, in patients with a long history of "treated" GERD referred for operative treatment, a thorough re-evaluation is in order to be certain that the patient does not have achalasia, another gastroduodenal disorder, or a chronic morphologic change in the esophagus – stricture, esophageal shortening, complicated hiatal hernia, or Barrett's esophagus. Therefore, repeat endoscopy by the treating surgeon or at the least with the surgeon present to observe seems prudent.

Upper endoscopy: Preoperative study should include upper endoscopy to assess the state of the esophagus, investigate for Barrett's, and exclude distal lesions. A contrast radiograph of esophagus, stomach, and duodenum can be useful in the preoperative evaluation in order to detect motility disorders, esophageal stricture (length and internal diameter), anatomic dilation of the gastroesophageal junction or cardia, and presence of a true hiatal hernia, although endoscopy has almost replaced the need for a contrast study.

Endoscopy will reveal patients who have esophagus without mucosal injuries (approximately 50%), others with different degrees of esophagitis (35% of patients), and finally a group of patients with Barrett's esophagus on the first endoscopy (about 15%). The procedure should include taking biopsies above the Z line to look for the existence of chronic esophagitis, supporting the diagnosis of chronic reflux. Moreover, the endoscopist should determine whether there is ascension of the Z line or irregularities or tongues of columnar metaplasia and then should take the necessary multiple biopsies below the Z line to assess the existence of intestinal metaplasia. Besides examining the entire esophagus, the stomach and duodenum should be examined carefully for other disorders, especially for gastric cancer in those geographic areas of the world where gastric cancer has a high prevalence.

Conventional or computerized manometric study: Manometry of the esophagus and LES does not make the diagnosis of GERD but will support the clinical diagnosis if a mechanically incompetent LES is demonstrated (resting LES pressure $\leq$6 mmHg, total length $\leq$20 mm, or LES abdominal length $\leq$10 mm); these findings suggest a severe anatomic and functional abnormality of the sphincter. In addition, the amplitude and coordination of esophageal contractions provide potentially useful information of esophageal function, especially if esophageal contractile activity is diminished markedly; the latter finding may alter the extent of operative fundoplication.

24 h intraesophageal pH-probe monitoring (24 h pH study): This test is actually the "gold standard" to establish the presence of pathologic gastroesophageal reflux, defined as the excessive duration of exposure of the esophageal lumen to gastric juice. The study is performed by placing a small diameter pH electrode, introduced transnasally, 5 cm proximal to the LES, which has been located previously by manometry.

A special, computerized program allows analysis of the stored data and gives a profile of the number, duration, and timing of reflux episodes culminating in a score which combines six different parameters. A combined score $\leq$ 14 is normal. Probably the most useful value is the total time per 24 h during which intraesophageal pH is <4, with normal being $\leq$4% (55 min). In addition, it is important to correlate the relationship between reflux periods and symptoms. This test represents the most objective means to establish presence of a pathologic gastroesophageal reflux, and many surgeons believe that every candidate for an anti-reflux operation should have this test prior to operation.

24 h bilirubin monitoring of the distal esophagus: The importance of duodenal reflux into the esophagus in the pathophysiology of GERD and its complications is also well recognized. Although this test is not a routine procedure for most patients with GERD, it should be considered in patients with suspicion of duodenal reflux, especially in patients with Barrett's esophagus or in patients with symptoms of gastroesophageal reflux but with a normal 24 h pH study.

Impedance study: Recently, impedance technology with the capability of detecting all types of reflux (acid, non-acid, liquid, mixed, and air) has been developed. Recent work has shown that non-acid reflux can be an important clinical problem with over half of the reflux events not detected by pH studies. The additional information provided by impedance technology is likely to have a major impact on our understanding and clinical management of patients with GERD. While experience to date is limited, this technology may prove to be the best assessment of sphincter competency.

Medical Treatment and Operative Indications in GERD

Today, practically all patients with GERD can be managed symptomatically with medical treatment by modifying lifestyle and dietary habits, plus the use of proton pump inhibitors with or without prokinetics. Medical therapy, however, is mainly symptomatic, designed to inhibit acid production, minimize heartburn, and improve esophagitis, but it does not stop the reflux, because it is not able to restore sphincter function. In contrast, reflux of duodenal content is not controlled, and regurgitation of gastric contents during exercise or when recumbent can be very bothersome and persists in spite of complete acid blockade. As medical therapy accomplishes symptomatic well-being in most all patients, it becomes very difficult to accept failure of medical treatment as an indication for operation. Indeed, when the indication for operative intervention is a failure of medical management, the patient requires very careful and comprehensive review.

The ideal candidate for an anti-reflux operation is a patient with typical symptoms of heartburn and/or regurgitation, with pH-proven, pathologic esophageal acid exposure and who is dependent on proton-pump inhibitors for symptomatic relief. A multivariate analysis of the factors predicting a successful outcome after laparoscopic Nissen fundoplication identified these three parameters as the most important preoperative predictive factors: the 24 h pH probe study, typical symptoms of gastro-esophageal reflux, and a good response to medical treatment (❷ *Table 38-1*). Considering the previous statement, we believe that current indications in GERD for an anti-reflux operation are:

1. Recurrent symptomatology appearing early after stopping appropriate medical treatment
2. Dependence or increasing requirements of acid-suppressive drugs
3. Persistent and/or progressive GERD despite active medical treatment
4. Young patients obliged to medical treatment for life

◘ Table 38-1

Predictor of outcome after laparoscopic fundoplication: stepwise logistic regression results in 199 patients* **(Adapted from Campos et al., 1999. With permission of Springer Science + Business Media)**

Predictor	Adjusted odds ratio* (95% confidence intervals)	Wald's *P*-value
24 h pH composite score	5.4 (1.9–15.3)	<0.001
Typical primary symptoms	5.1 (1.9–13.7)	<0.001
Good response to medical therapy	3.3 (1.3–8.7)	<0.03

*Odds ratios and corresponding *P* values are adjusted for all other factors in the model.

5. A mechanically incompetent LES
6. Laryngo-respiratory symptoms secondary to GERD
7. Alterations in esophageal motility
8. True hiatal hernia and GERD
9. Severe abnormal acid reflux on 24 h pH probe study

For all these indications, probably the most difficult indication to define clearly is persistent and/or progressive disease. These patients usually are well-managed with medical therapy; nevertheless, clinical experience suggests that they often end up at the surgeon's door. Characteristically, these patients become dependent on drugs and experience cycles of remission and relapse. The most important issue is to recognize some of the risk factors that seem to define a more severe clinical profile, such as:

1. Severe mechanical defect of the LES established by manometric study
2. Severe erosive esophagitis at endoscopy
3. Supine reflux
4. Mixed reflux
5. Persistent esophageal stricture
6. Barrett's esophagus, especially with any element of dysplasia

In early stages of GERD, it may be very difficult to demonstrate a mechanically incompetent LES according to standard manometric parameters. As the disease progresses and lesions and/or complications become evident, the finding of a mechanically defective sphincter is common, being present in more than 90% of patients with Barrett's esophagus. Although it is argued that damage to the sphincter is either primary or secondary to the esophageal damage, what is clear is that sphincter damage cannot be recovered and is irreversible despite aggressive medical therapy. Anti-reflux surgery can, however, restore or improve lost sphincter function when there is still a remnant of an intrinsic sphincter. In these cases, anti-reflux surgery offers a therapeutic alternative that is more efficient than any medical therapy and eventually may change the natural course of the disease.

Operative Treatment of GERD

The goals of operative intervention and the techniques used to reach that goal are detailed as follows:

- Fundoplication (Nissen) or cardial calibration (Hill-Larraín)
  - Restores or recovers the function of a mechanically incompetent LES and narrows or calibrates the dilated gastroesophageal junction
  - Increases resting LES pressure, decreasing the frequency of reflux
  - Optimizes sphincteric competence
- Posterior Gastropexy
  - Fixes the abdominal esophagus below the diaphragmatic hiatus
  - Maintains the distal esophagus subject to intraabdominal pressure
  - Prevents para-esophagic hiatal hernia

- Closure of the diaphragm pillars
  - Increases resistance to reflux during increases in abdominal pressure
  - Complement sphincteric action
  - Avoids paraesophageal hiatal hernia

According to the majority of experts in anti-reflux surgery, there are no differences in the operative treatment of a patient with acid gastroesophageal reflux with or without esophagitis from that of a patient with Barrett's esophagus. Most anti-reflux procedures employ some type of fundoplication technique, usually the Nissen fundoplication, with satisfactory results. In contrast, we believe that the operative treatment of the patient with acid GERD should differ from that of a patient with long-segment or complicated Barrett's esophagus, because clinically and pathophysiologically they represent different disease processes. The patient with acid GERD usually has a sphincter less damaged mechanically, a not very dilated gastroesophageal junction and diaphragmatic hiatus, a more or less preserved esophageal motility, and a pathologic predominance of acid reflux. In contrast, Barrett's esophagus usually occurs at a later state of chronic gastroesophageal reflux, and many (including the author) believe that reflux of bile should be a major target of the anti-reflux procedure.

In addition, a number of procedures have been developed to treat the "shortened" esophagus, often by a Collis-Nissen technique performed laparoscopically. In our experience, we have never observed the so-called short esophagus of a magnitude described in the literature and never more than 2 cm. Based on our experience, after complete dissection of the esophagogastric junction, we have always found the gastroesophageal sphincter to be in an intraabdominal location. Also, in the case of true hiatal hernias, with the hernia sac and the part of the stomach proximal to the hiatus, it has always been possible to relocate the LES within the abdomen.

Outcome

To be successful, anti-reflux surgery must provide long-term relief of reflux symptoms and not create complications or complaints secondary to the operation. Operative or postoperative complications (splenic injury, hemorrhage, pulmonary complications, temporary dysphagia) occur on average in 8–10% of patients, and the rate of conversion to an open procedure is about 2% in accomplished hands (range 1–10%) Mortality is uncommon, but patients should be warned that they will have some dysphagia for 1–2 months postoperatively. With the use of fundoplicature techniques in patients with non-complicated acid GERD, the results in our group in the long term (5 or 10 years) show 85% good to excellent results, comparable to the data of most authors in the literature. Objective studies have shown that >90% of patients will have negative pH studies 1–3 years after laparoscopic Nissen fundoplication (⊙ *Table 38-2*). It is important to point out that all series of anti-reflux techniques should be assessed in the long range, because in 2–3 years most of the patients with simple reflux are clinically well.

Finally, we should point out that GERD, given its frequency and importance especially with today's possibilities of study and therapy, is at the center of interest of many groups. For that same reason, it has been exposed to the interplay of diverse interests in different medical and surgical fields as well as in the technologic industries. Thus, those treating these patients

◻ Table 38-2

24 h pH studies after laparoscopic Nissen fundoplication (Reprinted from Peters et al., 2000)

Primary author	pH-negative patients	Follow-up (months)
Hinder	21/24 (87%)	3–12
Hunter	49/54 (91%)	12
Watson	42/48 (87%)	3
Peters	26/28 (93%)	21
Csendes	35/45 (77)	40

need to be extremely cautious and critical of all new therapies (operative, endoscopic, etc.) and to maintain a critical attitude based on objective and controlled studies and not based only on impressions.

Selected Readings

Campos GM, Peters JH, DeMeester TR, et al. (1999) Multivariate analysis of factors predicting outcome after laparoscopic Nissen fundoplication. J Gastrointest Surg 3:292–300

Darling G, Deschamps C (2005) Technical controversies in fundoplication surgery. Thorac Surg Clin 15:437–444

Dent J, Holloway RH, Toouli J, Dodds WJ (1988) Mechanisms of lower oesophageal sphincter incompetence in patients with symptomatic gastroesophageal reflux. Gut 29:1020–1028

Kahrilas PJ, Lee TJ (2005) Pathophysiology of gastroesophageal reflux disease. Thorac Surg Clin 15:323–333

Korn O, Stein HJ, Richter T, Liebermann-Meffert D (1997) Gastroesophageal sphincter: a model. Dis Esoph 10:105–109

Peters JH, Hagen JA, DeMeester SR, et al. (2000) Advances in surgical techniques and technology: a decade of laparoscopic Nissen fundoplication. Contemp Surg 56:138–151

Skinner DB (1985) Pathophysiology of gastroesophageal reflux. Ann Surg 202:546–556

Watson TJ, Peters JH (2005) Evaluation of esophageal function for antireflux surgery. Gastrointest Endosc Clin N Am 15:347–360

39 Paraesophageal Hiatus Hernia

Luigi Bonavina

Pearls and Pitfalls

- Paraesophageal (type II) hiatus hernia represents a distinct anatomic and clinic entity requiring a unique therapeutic strategy, and is differentiated from the more common type I (sliding) hiatus hernia.
- All symptomatic patients, in the absence of prohibitive operative risk, should undergo elective repair to prevent life-threatening complications, such as obstruction, strangulation, perforation, and bleeding.
- Extended transmediastinal dissection and complete sac excision are mandatory to reduce the stomach and the distal esophagus safely into the abdomen; a Collis gastroplasty is necessary only infrequently.
- The anterior sac can be left attached to the cardia and used for downward traction; identify and avoid injury to the anterior vagus nerve.
- A retrogastric lipoma is constant and should be excised to enable complete dissection of the diaphragmatic pillars behind the esophagus; identify and avoid injury to the posterior vagus nerve.
- Crural repair with prosthetic patch onlay has the potential to reduce the recurrence rate but insufficient data are available at present to confirm safety, best prosthetic, and long-term effectiveness.
- The addition of a Nissen-or Toupet-fundoplication techniques reduces the incidence of postoperative gastroesophageal reflux.
- The role of a concomitant anterior gastropexy constructed to prevent intraabdominal gastric volvulus and recurrent hernia remains controversial.
- Laparoscopic repair is feasible and remains the approach of choice in patients with paraesophageal hiatus hernia.

Hiatal hernias are heterogeneous anatomic and clinical entities. Classification into four types is widely accepted. Sliding hernia is the result of an upward migration of the esophagogastric junction into the mediastinum (type I hiatus hernia). Paraesophageal hiatus hernia (type II hiatus hernia) occurs as a result of an anterior defect in the diaphragmatic hiatus leading to an upward dislocation of the gastric fundus alongside the cardia. Subsequent progressive enlargement of the hiatus and the hernia sac leads to a mixed paraesophageal and sliding hernia (type III hiatus hernia) which may evolve to the final stage characterized by a complete, intrathoracic, "upside-down" stomach. Therefore, the distinction between type II and type III hernias is somewhat artificial because they are considered a continuous disease spectrum. Infrequently, the colon can migrate into the hernia sac (type IV hiatus hernia).

Approximately 10% of hiatus hernias have a paraesophageal component, and among these patients, 90% have a mixed type III hernia.

The true incidence of paraesophageal hernia in the overall population is unknown because of minimal or even absence of symptoms in many individuals. The majority of patients with paraesophageal hernia are elderly females who often present with multiple comorbidities.

A progressive, structural deterioration of the phrenoesophageal ligament may explain the higher incidence of paraesophageal hernia in the older age group. Anatomic changes involve thinning of the upper fascial layer of the ligament (continuation of the endothoracic fascia) and loss of elasticity of the lower fascial layer (continuation of the transversalis fascia). In a mixed type III hernia, because of continuous stretching in the cranial direction from intra-abdominal pressure, the esophagogastric junction migrates into the mediastinum through the widened hiatus; a portion of the lesser curvature of the stomach accompanies the esophagogastric junction and forms part of the wall of the hernia sac. Consequently, the lower esophageal sphincter lies outside the abdominal cavity and is unaffected by its environmental pressures. As the size of the hernia increases, the greater curvature will roll up along the left side of the esophagogastric junction into the posterior mediastinum. The stomach can become incarcerated above the diaphragm; if a 180° rotation occurs around its longitudinal axis, this forms an organoaxial volvulus or, less commonly, if the rotation occurs around the transverse axis, it is called a mesoaxial volvulus (❷ *Fig. 39-1A, B*). These volvuli can cause a number of mechanical complications resulting in vascular congestion of the gastric mucosa, gastric outlet obstruction, and impairment of pulmonary function due to displacement of the lung (❷ *Table 39-1*).

◘ Figure 39-1
Schematic view of the organo-axial (a) and of the meso-axial gastric volvulus (b)

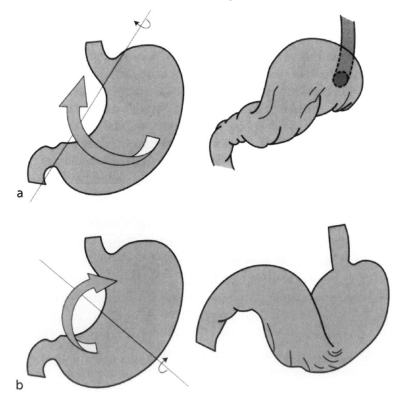

■ Table 39-1

Classification and characteristics of hiatal hernias

Hernia type	Location of EGJ	Hernia contents	Size	Rotation	Spontaneous reducibility	Major complications
I (sliding)	Intra-thoracic	Fundus	1–5 cm	None	Commonly complete	Reflux esophagitis, Barrett's esophagus
II (true paraesophageal)	Intra-abdominal	Fundus	1–5 cm	None or organoaxial	Often fixed	Obstruction, strangulation, perforation, bleeding
III (mixed)	Intra-thoracic	Fundus + body	>50% of stomach	Organoaxial and mesoaxial	Fixed	Obstruction, strangulation, perforation, bleeding
IV (mixed + other contents)	Intra-thoracic	Fundus + body + other	>50% of stomach + colon	Organoaxial and mesoaxial	Fixed	Obstruction, strangulation, perforation, bleeding

Clinical Presentation

Up to 50% of patients with paraesophageal hiatus hernia are asymptomatic or complain of only minor symptoms. Typical chronic symptoms include postprandial distress (epigastric fullness, nausea, intermittent vomiting, chest discomfort, dyspnea), heartburn, regurgitation, dysphagia, and hematemesis. Acute symptoms can mimic an acute myocardial infarction and develop as a consequence of complete gastric outflow obstruction. Anemia secondary to chronic bleeding and lung dysfunction secondary to aspiration are the most typical signs associated with paraesophageal hiatus hernia (❷ Table 39-2). In as many as 20% of patients, the clinical presentation of a massive and incarcerated paraesophageal hernia may be urgent or emergent. Acute distress with chest pain and inability to vomit can occur as a result of complete obstruction, strangulation, or perforation of the intrathoracic stomach.

Diagnosis

A paraesophageal hiatus hernia is often suspected on the basis of an abnormality on an incidental chest x-ray because of a retrocardiac air bubble with or without an air-fluid level on the lateral view (❷ Fig. 39-2). A barium swallow confirms the diagnosis (❷ Fig. 39-3A, B). Computed tomography (CT) of the chest and abdomen are of little value in the diagnosis, but may provide information on surrounding anatomy and will exclude concomitant pathology (❷ Fig. 39-4). Upper gastrointestinal endoscopy is mandatory in all patients to exclude the presence of esophagitis, Barrett's esophagus, or associated adenocarcinoma. A mixed type III hernia can be identified on retroversion of the endoscope by noting a gastric pouch lined with rugal folds above the diaphragm, and the gastroesophageal junction entering about midway up the side of the pouch (❷ Fig. 39-5). In some circumstances, due to the organoaxial rotation of the stomach, it can be difficult to advance the endoscope into the antropyloric region. Preoperative esophageal function studies are typically unnecessary when symptoms are related clearly to gastric outlet obstruction and distension of the intrathoracic stomach. However, if dysphagia is an accompanying symptom, an esophageal manometry should be performed

◘ Table 39-2

Symptoms associated with paraesophageal hiatus hernia in 141 patients (Data from Hiebert, 1995)

Symptoms	%
Epigastric fullness	83
Post-prandial pain	75
Regurgitation	60
Heartburn	57
Nausea/vomiting	41
Aspiration	41
Dysphagia	38
Bleeding	32
Respiratory embarrassment	25
Complete obstruction	13

◘ Figure 39-2

Lateral chest film: retrocardiac air-fluid level is suggestive of paraesophageal hernia

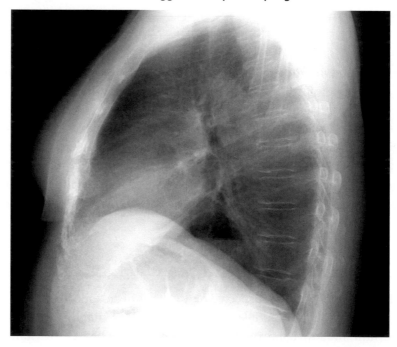

to rule out achalasia. Because many of these patients are elderly, non-invasive cardiac stress testing should also be considered before planning an operation.

Treatment

Operative repair is currently the only effective therapy for paraesophageal hiatus hernia. It has long been advised that any medically fit patient should undergo operative correction irrespective of symptoms or age. This recommendation was based on reports suggesting a 30% risk of developing

◘ Figure 39-3
a, b. Barium swallow study showing a mixed type III paraesophageal hiatus hernia

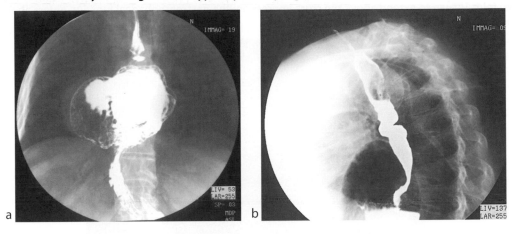

◘ Figure 39-4
Chest CT showing almost complete dislocation of the stomach in the lower mediastinal compartment

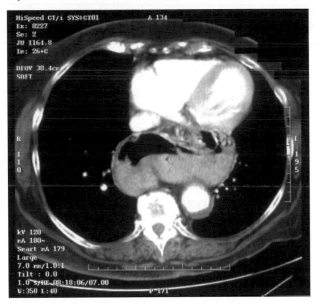

life-threatening complications with these types of hernia, and an associated increased risk of mortality with emergent intervention. Some authors, however, advocate a careful watchful waiting strategy in selected asymptomatic or minimally symptomatic patients based on the apparent reduced morbidity and mortality of urgent/emergent intervention compared with previous estimates.

Traditional repair of paraesophageal hiatus hernia has consisted of left thoracotomy or laparotomy. The minimally invasive laparoscopic approach has gained wide acceptance quickly over the past decade. The main advantages of a laparoscopic approach for patients include less postoperative discomfort, earlier mobilization, reduced perioperative morbidity, and shorter hospital stay and convalescence. It is imperative that the laparoscopic repair follow the same surgical principles adopted in the traditional

◘ Figure 39-5

Typical appearance of a type III paraesophageal hiatus hernia on endoscopic retroversion: a gastric pouch lined with rugal folds is seen to extend above the crura impression; the gastroesophageal junction enters about midway up the side of the pouch

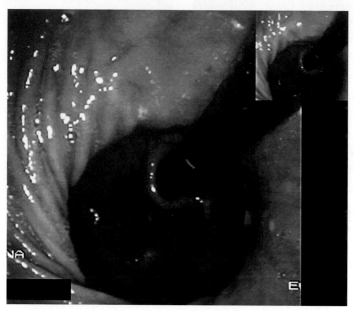

operation, i.e., complete tension-free reduction of the stomach and distal esophagus in the abdominal cavity *en bloc* with the hernia sac, and the appropriate repair of the crura. Even in the laparoscopic era, however, several areas of controversy persist in the management of paraesophageal hiatus hernia. These include the treatment of a short esophagus, the importance of sac excision, the role of a prosthesis in the repair of the crura defect, the need for a fundoplication, and the need for an anterior gastropexy.

Technique of Laparoscopic Repair

The patient is placed in the dorsal lithotomy position using reverse Trendelenburg (20–30°) as needed. The surgeon is positioned between the patient's legs. The pneumoperitoneum is induced by means of a Veress needle placed in the umbilicus or in the left hypochondrium in obese patients and maintained at an average of 13 mmHg; it is wise to lower insufflation pressures to 9 mmHg occasionally to avoid hypercarbia and hypotension in an elderly, frail patient. Five trocars, two 10 mm and three 5 mm ones, are used for the operation. The first 10 mm port is placed in the midline about 15 cm below the xiphoid process and is used for the 30° scope. The second 10 mm port is placed under direct vision higher in the left midclavicular line and is used for the needle-holder, the ultrasonic shears, and the irrigation-aspiration device. A 5 mm port is placed at the same level in the right midclavicular line for the operating grasper. Two additional 5 mm trocars are placed just below the xiphoid process for the liver retractor and in the left midclavicular line at the level of umbilicus for the stomach retractor. A common mistake is to place the ports too low in the abdominal wall, thereby making the mediastinal dissection more difficult. The operation starts by gently pulling the gastric fundus in the caudal direction with atraumatic graspers and dissecting the peritoneum off the free edge of the left crura as far posteriorly as possible. Inserting a rolled-up piece of gauze at the level of the gastrosplenic ligament provides additional retraction and improves visualization of this area. Blunt and sharp dissection is used to tease gently the entire hernia sac out of the mediastinum by entering the avascular plane between the endoabdominal fascia and the muscle body of the left crus. Accurate hemostasis is achieved with the ultrasonic shears. Both the surgeon and the anesthesiologist should be aware of the risk of pneumothorax at this time. The dissection continues anteriorly toward the right crus. The redundant hernia sac is left attached to the anterior aspect of the esophagogastric junction, purposely, because this strong tissue can then be used for effective gastric retraction. The lesser omentum is then opened and the right crus identified. The dissection continues posteriorly where a large lipoma is usually identified and needs to be resected to allow creation of a window behind the esophagus. Working through this window from the right side may help not only to recognize and preserve the posterior vagal nerve, but also to complete the dissection of the left crus and the posterior aspect of the gastric fundus. At this point, the distal esophagus can be encircled with a soft drain. The mediastinal cavity is inspected for hemostasis, and further blunt/sharp dissection is performed to ensure that an adequate length of the esophagus has been reduced into the abdomen without any tension. On rare occasions, a Collis gastroplasty may be necessary. The standard posterior crural repair is performed using 4–6 interrupted sutures of 2-0 polypropylene using extracorporeal knots. Teflon pledgets can be used to buttress these sutures. A synthetic prosthesis can be used to reinforce the crural repair. In selected patients we have used a onlay composite mesh, such as the Crurasoft patch (Bard) and the Parietex composite (Sofradim), fixed to the crura with a few stitches. Others have used a bioprosthesis. A fundoplication is added routinely in these patients regardless of the presence of reflux before the operation. In elderly patients, we prefer to perform a Toupet fundoplication which encompasses the posterior 180–270° of the distal esophagus. The first two stitches fix the apex of the gastric fundus to the left and the right crura, respectively; four more sutures are then placed between the gastric wall and each side of the esophagus. An anterior gastropexy can be added to the repair when the reduced stomach is prone to recurrent torsion. A closed-suction drain is placed in the mediastinum, and another drain under the left liver. All patients undergo an oral soluble contrast study on postoperative day 1, and a clear liquid diet is started. Most patients are discharged on postoperative day 2 or 3.

Outcome

Laparoscopic approach for paraesophageal hiatus hernia is feasible, safe, and effective. Postoperative complications are similar to those seen after conventional antireflux surgery, except for a higher reported incidence of esophageal and gastric injuries. Durability of the repair is still the critical issue. Most series have used primarily symptomatic follow-up and have reported recurrence rates of 0–5%. However, postoperative radiographic studies have found high rates of asymptomatic anatomic recurrence, ranging from 23% to 46%. Dissection of the hernia sac promotes safe mobilization of the esophagus and may improve the short and long-term success rate. It is not clear whether the use of a prosthesis to reinforce the crural repair outweighs the potential risk of visceral erosion, particularly with a synthetic polypropylene mesh. In conclusion, laparoscopic repair remains the approach of choice in patients with paraesophageal hiatus hernia. There is an ongoing need to assess mechanisms of late recurrence and reduce its incidence.

Selected Readings

DeMeester T, Bonavina L (1989) Paraesophageal hiatal hernia. In: Nyhus L, Condon R (eds) Hernia. Lippincott, Philadelphia, pp 684–693

Ferri L, Feldman L, Stanbridge D, et al. (2005) Should laparoscopic paraesophageal hernia repair be abandoned in favor of the open approach? Surg Endosc 19:4–8

Hashemi M, Peters J, DeMeester T, et al. (2000) Laparoscopic repair of large type III hiatal hernia: objective follow-up reveals high recurrence rate. J Am Coll Surg 190:539–547

Hiebert C (1995) Massive incarcerated hiatal hernia. In: Pearson FG et al. (eds) Esophageal surgery. Churchill Livingstone, New York, pp 267–271

Skinner D, Belsey R (1988): Types II, IIA, III, and paraesophageal hiatal heria. In: Management of esophageal disease, Saunders, Philadelphia, pp 631–639

Stylopoulos N, Gazelle G, Rattner D (2002) Paraesophageal hernias: operation or observation? Ann Surg 236: 492–500

Watson D, Davies N, Devitt P, Jamieson G (1999) Importance of dissection of the hernial sac in laparoscopic surgery for large hiatal hernias. Arch Surg 134:1069–1073

Wo J, Branum J, Hunter J, et al. (1996) Clinical features of type III (mixed) paraesophageal hernia. Am J Gastroenterol 91:914–916

40 Barrett's Esophagus

Attila Csendes

Pearls and Pitfalls

- Suspect Barrett's esophagus (BE) in a white, adult, middle-aged patient with a long-standing history of gastroesophageal reflux.
- BE is a frequent histologic finding in the distal esophagus, provided routine biopsy samples are taken.
- BE is a preneoplastic disease with an annual incidence of adenocarcinoma is 0.5–0.8%.
- Adenocarcinoma can appear in patients with short-segment BE.
- Short-segment BE is four times more frequent than long-segment BE.
- Adenocarcinoma of the distal esophagus originating from BE has increased 500% in the last three decades.
- The end-point of medical treatment is the control of symptoms, which is not equivalent to control of acid and duodenal reflux into the distal esophagus.
- Increased experimental evidence shows that the mixture of acid and duodenal juice refluxing into the esophagus is deleterious and carcinogenic.
- Low grade dysplasia is a good index for eventual development of high grade dysplasia or adenocarcinoma.
- Antireflux surgery seems to be superior to medical treatment but does not prevent the appearance of adenocarcinoma.
- Nearly 50% of patients with high grade dysplasia may already have an early localized or multifocal adenocarcinoma.
- In patients with high grade dysplasia, endoscopic ablation is a good alternative to esophagectomy, although residual BE and even adenocarcinoma may develop beneath the new squamous epithelium.
- Nissen fundoplication is an excellent operation for patients with short-segment BE, with regression of intestinal metaplasia in about 50% of patients.
- In patients with long-segment BE, acid suppression and duodenal diversion seems a more appropriate alternative to Nissen fundoplication, producing permanent control of acid and duodenal reflux and a change in the natural history of BE, by eliminating the appearance of adenocarcinoma.

Barrett's esophagus (BE) is an acquired condition in which the distal squamous epithelium of the esophagus is replaced by a columnar mucosa containing intestinal metaplasia due to chronic gastroesophageal reflux disease (GERD). In 1950, Barrett described the presence of a peptic ulcer with a distal tubular segment of intrathoracic stomach, with the presence of a congenitally short esophagus. Others, however, found in this "intrathoracic tubular stomach" the presence of mucosal glands in the submucosa, more typical of the esophagus and not of an intrathoracic stomach, clarifying this as columnar lined epithelium of the esophagus and showed it to be associated with hiatal hernia.

Classically, a diagnosis of BE required that at least 3 cm of the distal esophagus be lined by metaplastic columnar epithelium, which is now called long-segment BE. By contrast, the existence of "short-segment" BE, involving columnar mucosa plus intestinal metaplasia of either circumferential increase (>1 cm) or one or more tongues (>1 cm) or a combination of these findings, but always less than 3 cm in length, is recognized increasingly and is four times more common than "long-segment" BE. The main importance of BE is that it predisposes the development of adenocarcinoma.

Epidemiology

BE is found in 1–2% of unselected normal population undergoing endoscopy and in 6–20% of patients submitted to endoscopic evaluation for symptoms of GERD. Intestinal metaplasia of the cardia, which is the histologic finding of intestinal metaplasia in otherwise normal endoscopy (and therefore not true BE) is found in 12% of patients with GERD, without the endoscopic findings of a BE. Its importance and future behavior have not been evaluated nor clarified (❯ *Fig. 40-1*).

The incidence of BE has increased markedly since 1970, due in part to the increase in endoscopic procedures. Autopsy studies suggest that for each known case of long-segment BE, there are 20 additional unrecognized patients. BE is more frequent among white, Anglo Saxons, Europeans, and the Hispanic population and is much less common among the African and Asian population. In the last 3 decades, there has been a 500% increase in the incidence of adenocarcinoma arising from BE with the majority located at the distal esophagus, while squamous-cell carcinoma has decreased

◻ **Figure 40-1**
Schematic representation of endoscopic histologic and manometric studies in patients with cardia intestinal metaplasia (IM), short-segment Barrett's esophagus, and long-segment Barrett's esophagus. The length and location of the lower esophageal sphincter is established clearly, as well as the oral displacement of the squamo-columnar junction, with a 2 cm "shortening" of the esophagus in patients with long-segment BE

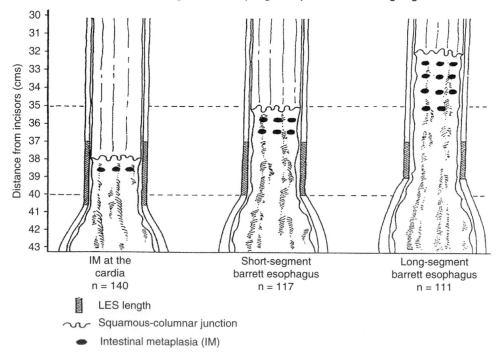

continuously. The reason for this increase in unknown. Epidemiologic studies have identified a variety of risk factors for the development of esophageal adenocarcinoma: the presence of BE is the only clearly recognized risk factor. Severe, long-standing symptoms of reflux, increased body mass index, and dietary and environmental issues (smoking and a diet low in fresh fruit) are also important factors. The precise incidence of adenocarcinoma in patients with BE is uncertain, varying from 1/52 to 1/297 patient-years of follow up. Recent studies suggest that the annual risk is 0.5–0.8%.

Pathogenesis

In most patients, BE develops in the setting of chronic symptomatic GERD, in which two metaplastic events occur (❂ *Fig. 40-2*). The first involves a phenotypic transformation of squamous cells to cardiac mucosa secondary to chronic acid reflux. The second metaplastic change involves the appearance of intestinal goblet cells without the normal absorptive capacity (incomplete intestinal metaplasia), believed secondary to duodeno-esophageal reflux and genetic predisposition. Clinical and endoscopic evidence cannot determine precisely when the condition developed or its extent. Many investigators believe that BE usually develops to its full extent all at once, and that there is no substantial progress in length with time.

BE is associated clearly with a mixture of severe acid reflux and duodenal content refluxing into the distal esophagus. In animal experiments, acid reflux alone is a rare cause of adenocarcinoma of the esophagus, while mixed reflux is associated clearly with development of adenocarcinoma. Bile salts are probably the noxious component in the refluxed duodenal juice, being pH-dependent (❂ *Fig. 40-3*). For bile salts to cause injury, they must be soluble and unionized. A pH less than 2 produces irreversible precipitation; however, at a pH of 3–5, a mixture of bile salt and bile acids is present and can rapidly cross the mucosal cell membrane and destroy the mitochondria. Other abnormalities found in patients with BE are the presence of an incompetent lower esophageal sphincter (LES) and an alteration in esophageal motility producing a disturbance in esophageal clearance.

Three types of columnar epithelia have been described in BE: (1) specialized columnar epithelium (intestinal metaplasia) with a villiform surface and intestinal-type crypts lined by mucus-secreting cells

◘ Figure 40-2
Development of Barrett's esophagus and adenocarcinoma through the occurrence of two metaplastic changes. The first metaplastic change is basically a phenotypic change, while the second metaplastic change is a genotypic change

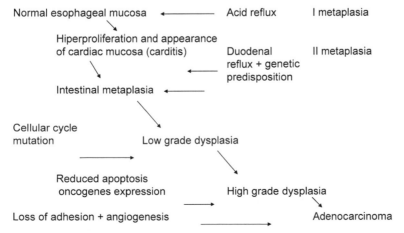

◘ Figure 40-3
Harmful effect of the gastric and duodenal juice to the distal esophagus. Experimentally, gastric juice alone at pH 2 to 4, by activating pepsin, is able to produce only erosive esophagitis. Bile salts present at the gastric lumen are pH dependant and at pH 3 to 5, together with acid, are noxious to esophageal mucosa producing BE and even adenocarcinoma

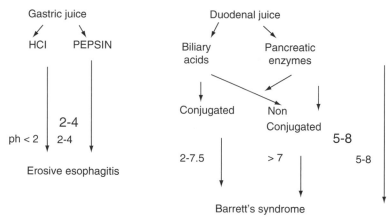

and goblet cells, (2) fundic type epithelium containing chief and parietal cells, and (3) junctional type epithelium with a foveolar surface and mucus-secreting cells. The latter two epithelial cells can be found normally at the cardia or esophagogastric junction (EG). The cell of origin of BE remains unclear, but evidence points to multipotential stem cells as the site of origin of BE. There are some problems in the clear definition of Barrett's esophagus:

- The precise identification of the gastroesophageal junction can be controversial. The anatomic end of the esophagus corresponds to the distal limit of the sling and clasp fibers of the lower esophageal sphincter. Radiologically, it is difficult to locate precisely. To the physiologists, the esophagogastric junction corresponds to the limit of the LES. For the endoscopists, the E-G junction corresponds to the proximal margin of the gastric folds.
- The endoscopic and manometric landmarks may be imprecise due to the constant physiologic movement of the esophago-gastric junction.
- In normal subjects, the squamous-columnar junction is located in the mid-portion of the LES, which means that nearly 15 mm of the final portion of the abdominal esophagus is covered by gastric or columnar mucosa. This squamo-columnar junction is displaced orally with severe reflux.

Clinical Features

It is impossible to confirm the presence or the diagnosis of a BE by only clinical means; endoscopy and biopsy are required. BE is usually discovered in middle aged adults (mean age 55 years old) with a slight male predominance. Symptoms of GERD are present usually for at least 10 or more years; however, 11% of patients with short-segment BE and 2% with long-segment BE are truly asymptomatic and are found only by endoscopic evaluation.

Hiatal hernia, as well as complications such a peptic ulcer of the esophagus or strictures, are more common in patients with long-segment BE compared with patients with short-segment BE. The presence of dysplasia at the metaplastic mucosa is 3–4 times greater in patients with long-segment BE.

Diagnosis

Endoscopic examination with multiple biopsies is required to establish the diagnosis of a BE. Endoscopically, Barrett's mucosa has a salmon-pink appearance almost identical to that of gastric mucosa. The columnar-lined mucosa extends proximally up the esophagus in irregular, finger-like or tongue projections or, less frequently, as a circumferential sheet. There may be isolated or heterotopic islands of gastric mucosa surrounded by squamous epithelium in the distal esophagus. The presence of goblet cells in cardiac mucosa stained with Alcien blue at pH 2.5 confirms the existence of a Barrett's mucosa. Intestinal metaplasia is found in only 1/3 of the patients with "short-segment" BE. The prevalence of intestinal metaplasia increases in parallel with the length of the columnar epithelium, and when BE is >6 cm, practically 100% of patients have intestinal metaplasia. Thus, BE is often suspected at the time of endoscopy but not always confirmed.

What does this mean? At the time of endoscopy, landmarks should be evaluated and defined carefully. If the squamo-columnar junction is 10 mm or more above the level of the esophagogastric junction defined as the proximal margin of gastric folds under partial insufflations, biopsy specimens should be obtained, and if goblet cells are present, the patient is considered to have BE and should be placed under medical treatment and surveillance. The risk of adenocarcinoma is increased to 1/50 to 1/250 patient-years of follow up, which means a risk 30- to 120-fold greater than the general population. The annual incidence of adenocarcinoma varies between 0.5–1% among patients with BE. Other laboratory investigations should be considered in patients with BE, especially in those who are candidates for surgical therapy. The prevalence of a mechanically defective sphincter on manometry is greater in patients with BE and parallels the length of the columnar mucosa. Similarly, poor esophageal contractility also is present often, and clearance of the esophagus may be delayed. Acid reflux and duodenal reflux are also greater in patients with long-segment BE compared with patients with short-segment BE. Therefore, not only acid but bile and pancreatic juice may be present in the refluxed material.

Medical Treatment

The main goal of medical therapy is to maintain patients with BE free of symptoms and to heal esophagitis. Proton pump inhibitors result consistently in relief of symptoms and healing of esophagitis. But symptom control is not necessarily equivalent to normalization of acid or duodenal exposure of the distal esophagus, despite use of high-dose proton pump inhibitors; 15–40% of patients still have pathologic acid reflux while receiving 20 mg of Omeprazole twice daily. The same phenomenon occurs with duodeno-esophageal reflux, which is not controlled at all by proton pump inhibitors. Nevertheless, aggressive and effective acid suppression with high doses of proton pump inhibitors may result in partial or no regression of the BE. Medical treatment, however, does not appear to decrease incidence of adenocarcinoma. In a recent meta-analysis, in the medical group, there were 5.3 cancers per 1,000 patient-years. The only hope to improve the survival rate in these patients is to detect the cancer in an early and potentially curable stage.

One potential strategy to decrease mortality rate of adenocarcinoma is to identify patients at risk by screening patients, especially white men, 50 years or older with long-standing reflux by endoscopy with biopsy. The other way to decrease the incidence of lethal adenocarcinoma is endoscopic surveillance. Adenocarcinomas detected in a surveillance program are found at an earlier stage compared with patients not undergoing routine endoscopic surveillance. Indeed, a 5-year endoscopic surveillance program proved to be the most cost-effective strategy. Endoscopic surveillance, however, has not been evaluated in prospective randomized studies. The technique of surveillance is controversial: the number of biopsy samples, location of the biopsies, pathologic analysis, use of special stains, normal or jumbo biopsy forceps, etc. The intervals of surveillance are also under discussion; suggestions include 2–3 years without dysplasia, 1 year with low grade dysplasia, and every 3 months with high grade dysplasia.

Ablation Therapy

Given the limitations of medical or surgical therapy, a variety of techniques of mucosal ablation have been evaluated based on the theory that after "burning" the abnormal (metaplastic and dysplastic) mucosa, squamous re-epithelization will occur in an environment with decreased or nonexistent acidity. The ablation can be accomplished by a variety of different techniques, such as thermal ablation, photodynamic therapy, and endoscopic mucosal resection.

Thermal ablation is performed by employing Nd:YAG laser or multipolar electro coagulation. Although there is histologic reversal in nearly 80% of patients, adverse effects have been described, such as chest pain, strictures, pleural effusion, and perforation. The follow up of patients is short, and there are some recurrences or maintenance of underlying intestinal metaplasia.

Photodynamic therapy utilizes a light-sensitive drug concentrated in neoplastic tissue. The drug is activated by light, producing toxicity which selectively injuries neoplastic tissues; it is a better therapy for long-segment BE. Although regression in several series varies from 70% to 90%, complete regression of BE is achieved in nearly 50% of patients. Intestinal metaplasia and even adenocarcinoma have been described, however, developing underneath the new squamous epithelium. Strictures may also occur.

These ablation therapies, although feasible, present a number of difficult issues, such as the persistence of intestinal metaplasia, development of adenocarcinoma in buried islands of intestinal metaplasia, and the eventual risks, costs, and maintenance of aggressive acid suppression therapy, either medical or surgical.

Endoscopic mucosal resection has become a potentially therapeutic procedure. It should be used in small (<20 mm), well-differentiated mucosal adenocarcinoma or high grade dysplasia. Complications can occur with subsequent development of high grade dysplasia or cancer. It is an alternative option in patients in whom the surgical risk is prohibitive.

Medical Versus Surgical Therapy

DeMeester has defined the goals of management (medical or surgical) to be:

- To prevent the development of the metaplastic mucosa by stopping reflux early in the disease process.
- To promote or induce healing or regression of the metaplastic epithelium such that intestinal metaplasia is eliminated.
- To induce quiescence of the intestinalized metaplastic epithelium and halt its progression to dysplasia or cancer.

As has been discussed before, the goal of medical treatment of patients with BE is the control of symptoms; however, eradication of symptoms cannot be equated with elimination of reflux, and even after continuous medical treatment, Barrett's mucosa develops in 12% of the patients. Furthermore, during continuous medical treatment, dysplasia and adenocarcinoma have appeared. Therefore, none of the three goals have been shown to be achieved adequately by medical treatment.

Several retrospective nonrandomized studies have compared medical and surgical treatment in patients with BE. Attwood performed a 3-year follow up in patients under medical treatment or who submitted to fundoplication, reporting better results after anti-reflux surgery. McCallum, Katz, and others suggested that anti-reflux surgery prevents the development of dysplasia and adenocarcinoma better than medical treatment.

There are three prospective, randomized studies concerning this aspect. Parrilla and colleagues in Spain found that symptomatic results were similar in both groups, but intestinal metaplasia did not disappear in any patient. There was persistence of acid reflux in 15% of the surgical patients. High grade dysplasia and adenocarcinoma appeared in a similar proportion in both groups. The important finding was that after successful anti-reflux surgery, results seem to be better than after medical treatment, although one patient in the surgical group also developed adenocarcinoma. Spechler also performed a prospective randomized study with a long follow up. At 8–10 years after surgery, outcomes were similar, with the same proportion of patients in each group developing adenocarcinoma and nearly 65% of the surgical group needing antisecretory drugs. This study has seriously challenged the advantages of anti-reflux surgical treatment (fundoplication).

Surgical Treatment

The goals of surgical treatment in patients with BE are outlined in ❯ *Table 40-1*. The results of patients with short-segment BE must be separated from those in patients with long-segment BE. From 1980 to 2005, some 32 articles addressed the surgical treatment of patients with BE, all involving classic anti-reflux procedures, mainly Nissen fundoplication, Hill's posterior gastropexy, or Belsey Mark IV, Collis-Nissen, or Collis-Belsey procedures. Four publications addressed patients with short-segment BE. Unfortunately, as the final results are mixed with patients with long-segment BE, the only specific data are the loss of intestinal metaplasia and the eventual progression to dysplasia or adenocarcinoma. All four publications reported a certain degree of regression of intestinal metaplasia to cardiac mucosa but no progression to adenocarcinoma. Only one patient developed low grade dysplasia. Therefore, patients with short-segment BE can be treated by fundoplication, with very low morbidity or mortality and with good long term results.

◻ **Table 40-1**

Goals of surgical treatment in patients with Barrett's esophagus

1.	Control of symptoms
2.	To stop the reflux of acid and duodenal content to the distal esophagus
3.	To prevent or eliminate the development of complications late after surgery, such as strictures or peptic ulcer
4.	To prevent proximal progression to the BE
5.	To induce regression of intestinal metaplasia to cardiac or fundic mucosa
6.	To induce regression of dysplasia to non dysplastic mucosa
7.	To prevent the progression towards dysplasia or adenocarcinoma

In contrast, the results of anti-reflux surgery in patients with long-segment BE are as follows. Although the follow up is relatively short (80% have a follow up less than 5 years), there is an inverse correlation between clinical success and duration of follow up. The longer the follow up, poor outcomes and recurrence of reflux occur frequently due to the fact that acid reflux is not fully eliminated or stopped with antireflux surgery. In all reports in which there is mention of pH studies after surgery, positive values vary between 9% and 60%. Duodenal reflux has been evaluated in only two reports, and despite lack of symptomatic reflux, bile reflux may persist.

The effect of anti-reflux surgery in obtaining or achieving regression of intestinal metaplasia to cardiac or fundic mucosa in patients with long-segment BE has also been evaluated in 15 studies. Regression of intestinal metaplasia is rare (5%), and, therefore, operated patients require endoscopic surveillance. Classic anti-reflux surgery is unable to prevent development of adenocarcinoma, similar to results after medical treatment. Therefore, in patients with long-segment BE, classic anti-reflux surgery probably cannot be recommended as an anti-neoplastic measure, based on a meta-analysis.

In summary, although anti-reflux surgery effectively alleviates GERD symptoms in patients with long-segment BE, surgical outcome is less optimal, than that encountered in patients with GERD without BE. Complete regression of columnar mucosa is extremely uncommon, and long-term durability remains unanswered. Its role as a adjuvance to ablation therapy is unknown. Therefore, the reported results after anti-reflux surgery suggest that it does not influence markedly the natural history of BE concerning development of dysplasia or adenocarcinoma.

A surgical procedure that we have been using in patients with long-segment BE is the operation of acid suppression and duodenal diversion (❷ *Fig. 40-4*). This procedure involves truncal or selective vagotomy, partial distal gastrectomy, fundoplication, and gastrojejunostomy with a Roux-en-Y limb 70 cm long. While ostensibly aggressive, acid production is decreased (vagotomy-gastrectomy), duodenal reflux is eliminated (Roux-en-Y drainage), and gastroesophageal reflux is diminished (fundoplication).

In patients with long-segment BE in whom there is a chronic and severe reflux not only of acid but also of duodenal content secondary to an incompetent LES, a significant dilation of the esophagogastric junction occurs in association with structural damage of the LES due to loss of the function of the clasp and sling fibers at this level. This phenomenon appears to explain why over long term follow up (10 years or more), the failure rate of classic anti-reflux surgery increases compared with the results seen 2 or 3 years after surgery. We started to employ the technique of acid suppression and duodenal diversion in patients with long-segment BE. The results of 245 patients so treated are shown in ❷ *Table 40-2*. Symptoms of chronic reflux were controlled in 91%. Loss of intestinal metaplasia is 10 times greater when compared with classic anti-reflux surgery (55 vs. 5%). Regression of low grade dysplasia to non dysplastic mucosa is also greater. The most striking point is that after this operation, no adenocarcinoma has developed, and only 1% of patients have progressed to low grade dysplasia.

Our approach currently is the following. Patients with low grade dysplasia should undergo repeated endoscopy with multiple biopsies. If pathologic review shows low grade dysplasia, the patient is treated with aggressive medical therapy for 1 year; if repeat endoscopy still shows low grade dysplasia and if functional studies (24 h pH monitoring and manometry) show that acid reflux is present, surgical therapy is suggested (❷ *Fig. 40-5*). For the patient with short-segment BE and a negative Bilitec study (bile reflux), a laparoscopic Nissen fundoplication is performed. If the Bilitec study is positive or if the patient has a long-segment BE, our policy is to perform the more aggressive procedure of acid suppression and duodenal diversion. In 37 patients with low grade dysplasia submitted to this operation, regression of nondysplastic mucosa was obtained in 91%, while in patients with long-segment BE, this value was 63%.

◘ Figure 40-4
Schematic representation of the proposed surgical treatment for patients with long-segment Barrett's esophagus (Reprinted from Csendes, 2004)

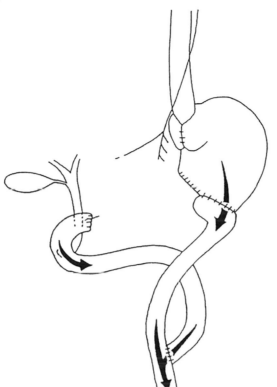

◘ Table 40-2
Results of acid suppression and duodenal diversion, in patients with long-segment Barrett's esophagus (N = 245)

Control of symptoms	91%
Decrease of maximal acid output (PAO)	90%
Percent patients with an abnormal (+) acid reflux	15%
Percent patients with an abnormal (+) duodenal reflux	5%
Regression of intestinal metaplasia to cardiac mucosa	55%
Regression of low grade dysplasia to nondysplastic mucosa	62%
Progression to dysplasia	1%
Progression to adenocarcinoma	0

The optimal treatment for patients with high grade dysplasia is very controversial. DeMeester et al have proposed to treat this issue in a very precise and simple way:

- To determine the probability that adenocarcinoma will develop in a patient with high grade dysplasia over time.
- To determine the real value of all actual techniques to differentiate high grade dysplasia from adenocarcinoma.
- To determine which is the best option for treating these patients.

◧ Figure 40-5

Proposed surgical treatment for patients with cardia intestinal metaplasia or Barrett's esophagus

1. Cardia intestinal metaplasia with symptoms and pathologic acid reflux
    ———————➤ Laparoscopic antireflux surgery
2. Short-segment BE
    ———————➤ Laparoscopic antireflux surgery
3. Complicated long segment BE
    ———————➤ Laparoscopic antireflux surgery
    ———————➤ Vagotomy-gastrectomy with Roux-en-Y anastomosis + fundoplication
4. High grade dysplasia or adenocarcinoma
    ———————➤ Esophagectomy

High-grade dysplasia will progress to adenocarcinoma in about 25% of patients followed for 2–3 years after diagnosis. Although high grade dysplasia without cancer follows a relatively benign course in the majority of patients, others develop cancer. A policy of endoscopic surveillance alone is not advisable, because adenocarcinoma even with lymph node metastasis can develop, and surgical results at that stage of disease should be considered.

Ablation therapy has been employed increasingly, and the results were discussed above. Two recent analyses addressing cost effectiveness of the different procedures in patients with high grade dysplasia have concluded that ablation therapy followed by endoscopic surveillance is a better option compared with esophagectomy, but these were theoretic analyses, and clinical trials should be performed in order to prove this approach.

For many patients, esophagectomy is the treatment of choice among those with high grade dysplasia and suspicion of adenocarcinoma. Obviously, it is mandatory to balance the potential risk of esophagectomy against the benefit of a curative resection. Therefore, esophagectomy should be performed only in a specialized surgical unit with a "high-volume" of esophageal operations. The procedure for restoration of the gastrointestinal tract can be either by colon interposition or a gastric pull up.

Selected Readings

Csendes A (2004) Surgical treament of barrett's esohagus 1980-2003. World J Surg 28:225–231

Csendes A, Burdiles P, Braghetto I, Korn O (2004) Adenocarcinoma appearing very late after antireflux surgery for Barrett's esophagus. Long term follow up, review of the literature and addition of six patients. J Gastrointest Surg 8:434–441

Csendes A, Burdiles P, Braghetto I, Smok G, Castro C, Korn O, Henriquez A (2002) Dysplasia and adenocarcinoma after classic antireflux surgery in patients with Barrett's esophagus. The need for long term subjective and objective follow up. Ann Surg 235:178–185

DeMeester TR (2001) Barrett's esophagus. Curr Probl Surg 38:549–640

Falk GW (2002) Barrett's esophagus. Gastroenterology 122:1569–1591

Nandurkar S, Talley NJ (1999) Barrett's esophagus: the long and the short of it. Am J Gastroent 94:30–40

Parrilla P, Martínez de Haro L, Ortiz A, et al. (2003) Long term results of a randomised prospective study comparing medical and surgical treatment of Barrett's esophagus. Ann Surg 237:291–298

Richter JE (2001) Antireflux surgery and adenocarcinoma of the esophagus. Let the truth be told. Gastroenterology 121:1506–1508

Spechler SJ (1997) The columnar lined esophagus. Gastrointest Clin N Am 26:455–466

41 Achalasia: Chagas' Disease

Ivan Cecconello · Flavio Roberto Takeda · Henrique Walter Pinotti

Pearls and Pitfalls

- Chagas' disease is related etiologically to the protozoan hemoflagellate, *Trypanossoma cruzi* with destruction of Meissner's and Auerbach's plexuses of the esophagus.
- Esophagogram and manometry of the esophagus are fundamental for the diagnosis and allow classification into three stages: incipient, non-advanced, and advanced (end stage).
- Non-operative treatment provides only temporary relief of dysphagia.
- Cardiomyotomy with partial fundoplication is indicated in the non-advanced variant of achalasia and provides relief of dysphagia.
- Motility studies confirm a significant decrease of LES pressure after both types of operation, open or laparoscopic.
- The benefits of minimally invasive surgery include reduction of pain, short hospital stay, and more rapid return to normal activities.
- Advanced achalasia is treated by transhiatal esophagectomy without thoracotomy and cervical gastroplasty.
- The occurrence of Barrett's epithelium in the esophageal stump will prompt annual endoscopic follow-up and resection with disease progression.
- Construction of an elongated gastric tube (instead of the whole stomach) to achieve reduction in gastric acid and pepsin production with the continuous use of PPIs often proves of value with this challenge.
- Coloplasty should not be used due to the frequent association of achalasia and megacolon in Chagas' disease.

Chagas' disease is endemic and caused by the protozoan hemoflagellate, *Trypanossoma cruzi* and may affect multiple organs, particularly the myenteric plexus of the gastrointestinal tract and the heart. The involvement of the esophagus, including its dilatation, occurs in approximately 7–18% of patients in the chronic phases of Chagas' disease.

Different phases may be recognized in the history of chagasic achalasia: (1) occurrence of the disease in ancient South America was evident in pre-Inca and Inca mummies, (2) description of the clinical signs and symptoms of the disease and its geographic distribution (e.g., "choking disease" in Brazil) from the beginning of the 19th century to the first decades of the 20th century, (3) the period from the 2nd to the 7th decade of the 20th century when the morphologic and physiopathologic characteristics of the disease were defined, (4) recognition of the chagasic etiology of the diseases in the 1940s and 1950s, and (5) the current phase with evidence of a decrease in the incidence of the disease. Migration to urban areas, better sanitation, enhanced living conditions for the rural population, and the systematic application of insecticides to the residential dwellings are among principal factors responsible for control of the disease.

Pathogenesis

After the initial inoculation after a bite by the vector – a triatome which mixes its feces with the victim's blood – there is local growth of the trypanosoma. This phase is followed by a transient parasitemia (➲ *Fig. 41-1*) lasting days or weeks, during which the microorganism lodges within various organs, notably, the gastrointestinal tract and the heart. The intensity of the parasitemia and the number of *T. cruzi* that infest different organs is dependent on an immunologic reaction between the parasite and the infected host.

In human Chagas' disease, there is a net loss of neurons from the autonomic system (➲ *Fig. 41-2*). Early studies indicate that sera from over 80% of patients contained anti-neuron autoantibodies. Several groups have identified cross-reactive antibodies between *T. cruzi* and mammalian nervous tissue. A mononuclear inflammatory infiltrate occurs in the submucosal and muscular layer of esophageal wall with a net decrease of CD_4 and T-cells and an inversion of the CD_4/CD_8 peripheral T-cell ratio.

Figure 41-1
T. cruzi in a blood sample

Figure 41-2
Myenteric plexus inflammation with loss of esophageal ganglion cells which were destroyed in the acute phase of disease in a patient with chagasic achalasia

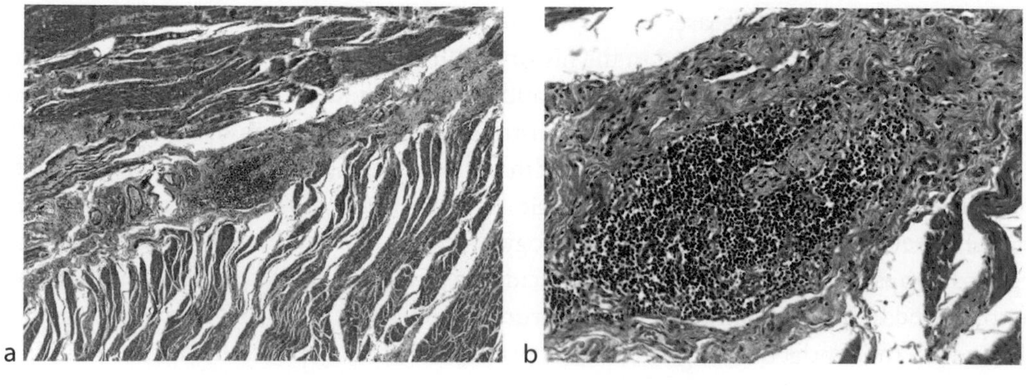

T. cruzi infection may also function as a booster to autoimmunity and inflammatory cytokine production leading to tissue damage in individuals with susceptible genetic profiles.

With achalasia, the intensity of destruction of Meissner's and Auerbach's plexuses account for the subsequent pathophysiologic alterations and symptoms. It is believed that abnormality of motility (as detected by manometric methods) is found when >50% of these cells are destroyed; esophageal dilation occurs only when the destruction affects 90% of the ganglion cells. The major malfunctions detected by manometric studies are an achalasia-like hypertonicity of the lower esophageal sphincter (LES), aperistalsis, and swallowing waves of longer duration.

Diagnosis

The major complaints of patients with achalasia are long-standing dysphagia and regurgitation frequently associated with nutritional depletion. Endoscopy of the upper digestive tract is essential to rule out the concomitant presence of carcinoma. Esophagography and manometry of the esophagus are fundamental for the diagnosis. These exams have enabled us to classify achalasia into three stages:

(a) *Incipient*: without esophageal dilation, but with specific motility disorders (achalasia-like changes and aperistalsis)
(b) *Non-advanced*: moderate dilation, stasis, and manometric findings of hyperactivity of the esophagus or aperistaltic waves with low amplitude and long duration
(c) *Advanced (end stage)*: frank dilation, atony of the body of the esophagus, or important megaesophagus (❷ *Fig. 41-3*).

Treatment

Nonoperative treatment of chagasic achalasia with drugs such as nifedipine has not produced consistent results; at most, these agents provide only temporary relief of dysphagia. Botulin-toxin injection in the LES via endoscopy showed improvement of dysphagia in 58% of patients in a follow-up of 6 months; interestingly there was no significant decrease in the pressure of the LES after the intrasphincteric injection.

Dilatation: Hydrostatic dilation has been employed in many clinics with incipient achalasia. In a prospective randomized clinical study, 40 patients in the initial stage of achalasia managed by hydrostatic dilatation of the cardia (20 patients) or by cardiomyotomy with partial fundoplication (20 patients) were followed for 3 years. Both procedures were performed without substantial morbidity and no mortality. Results were similar regarding ongoing suppression of dysphagia. Radiologically, the methods were equivalent, because they promoted resolution of the stasis and maintenance of the esophageal diameter. Endoscopic follow-up did not show any differences between the procedures in terms of the development of reflux esophagitis, with a rate of only 5% for each group of patients. Manometry demonstrated that the operative treatment produced a greater decrease in LES sphincter pressure compared to manometric dilation, although the latter also decreased ES pressure. As measured by esophageal pH monitoring, dilatation demonstrated a greater propensity for reflux compared to the

◘ **Figure 41-3**
Esophagogram with an advanced disease- megaesophagus

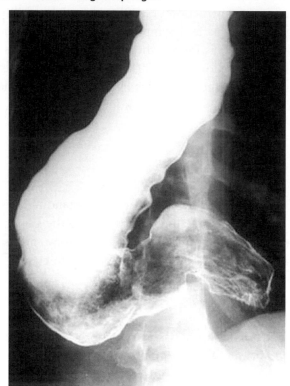

operative approach. It was concluded that both methods offer benefit in the treatment of the initial stage of achalasia; however, esophageal pH monitoring indicated that dilatation was associated with a greater index of esophageal acid exposition time.

Cardiomyotomy with partial fundoplication has been utilized in various clinics in the past 35 years. This technique combines a wide cardiomyotomy with a partial abdominal fundoplication. Initially patients were operated via an upper midline laparotomy; since 1991, the technique is via the laparoscopic approach. The procedure includes an extramucosal cardiomyotomy extending 2 cm below and 5–6 cm above the esophagogastric junction with mobilization of the gastric fundus and the "*vasa breviae*" when necessary. Thereafter, the superior surface of the fundus is sutured to the posterior esophageal wall followed by suturing to the anterior surface of the esophagus along the left and right margins of the myotomy (❷ *Fig. 41-4*). Positioning of operative trocars is similar to that for the treatment of gastroesophageal reflux disease; any injury to the mucosa is sutured with monofilament 4-0 suture and is covered with the gastric fundus.

With this procedure, 1,029 patients were operated on by the authors through laparotomy and 297 with laparoscopic approach. Open surgery had a few intraoperative complications which included splenic injury (3%) corrected by electrocautery or by suturing, and mucosal perforation (4%). Mortality was <0.1% (❷ *Table 41-1*).

In the patients operated on by laparoscopic approach (n = 297), mucosal perforation occurred in 4%, pleural lesions in 1%, with three (1%) conversions to laparotomy. One patient had an esophageal

◘ Figure 41-4

Surgical treatment of achalasia via a laparoscopic approach performing cardiomyotomy and fundoplication. a. extramucosal cardiomyotomy; b. the posterior surface of gastric fundus is sutured to the back of the esophageal wall and anterior surface of the esophagus along the left border of the myotomy; c. final aspect after suture of the stomach to the right border of the myotomy

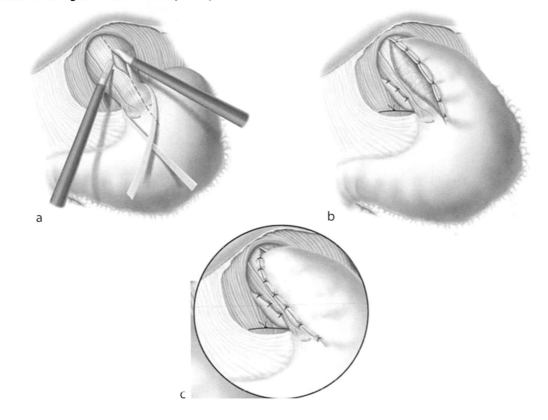

◘ Table 41-1

Cardiomyotomy and fundoplication complications

	Open (%) n = 1029	Laparoscopy (%) n = 297
Splenic lesion	3.0	–
Splenectomy	0.7	–
Mucosa perforation	4.4	4.4
Pleural lesion	–	0.7
Esophageal fistulae	0.02	0.3
Pulmonary embolism	0.01	–
Mortality	0.01	0.7
Conversion to open operation		1.0

fistula necessitating treatment by total parenteral nutrition. Mortality was 0.3% due to postoperative esophageal rupture secondary to regurgitation after feeding.

Relief of dysphagia was accomplished in most of the patients (❷ *Fig. 41-5*). Motility studies confirmed a significant decrease of LES pressure after both types of operation. Decreases in the

■ Figure 41-5
Late follow-up results in patients submitted to cardiomyotomy and partial fundoplication

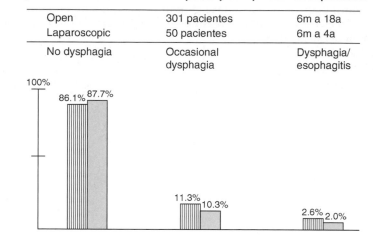

Open	301 pacientes	6m a 18a
Laparoscopic	50 pacientes	6m a 4a
No dysphagia	Occasional dysphagia	Dysphagia/esophagitis

esophageal diameter were observed frequently after the procedure (● *Fig. 41-6*). The benefits of minimally invasive approach include reduction in postoperative pain, shorter hospital stay, and faster return to normal activity.

Associated diseases: Additional (concomitant) involvement of the gastrointestinal tract by Chagas' disease with associated achalasia includes gastroparesis with impairment of gastric emptying, megaduodenum, and cholelithiasis. These conditions are treated concomitant with the achalasia, by pyloroplasty, latero-lateral duodenojejunostomy (with use of the third portion of the duodenum), and cholecystectomy.

When chagasic megacolon is evident, a mild degree of constipation can be treated with laxatives or with periodic rectal enemas. Patients with intractable and recurrent fecal impaction or recurrent sigmoid volvulus must be treated surgically. On rare occasion, the disorder is treated simultaneously with achalasia. In our experience, the treatment of choice is rectosigmoidectomy with immediate, posterior, end-to-side colorectostomy.

Esophagectomy without thoracotomy: In order to avoid thoracotomy and blind dissection, a technique for removing the esophagus under direct vision with wide opening of the diaphragm through the abdominal route was developed by Pinotti and includes:

– Upper median laparotomy with phrenotomy (● *Figs. 41-7A* and *B*);
– Retraction of the pericardium and pleura with cranial dissection of the esophagus. Special types of cauterization and/or clipping can be used for ligating vessels around the esophagus or arising from the aorta
– A second team approaches the cervical esophagus simultaneously via a left transverse cervical incision, 2 cm above the left clavicle. The esophagus is freed distally with special retractors and transected at the level chosen for the anastomosis
– After complete dissection, the esophagus is removed through the abdominal incision
– The stomach is freed preserving the right vascular pedicles and part of the lesser curvature is resected with the esophagus (● *Fig. 41-7C*)

□ Figure 41-6
Esophagogram of a patient with achalasia before and after cardiomyotomy and partial fundoplication

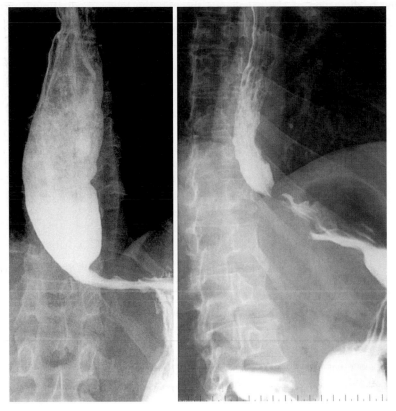

–   The stomach is pulled up through the posterior mediastinum and anastomosed to the cervical esophagus (❷ *Fig. 41-7D*)

Postoperative enteral feeding is maintained for 10 days until radiologic demonstration of an intact anastomosis. Enteral feeding can be prolonged during the period of closure of any eventual anastomotic fistula.

One hundred and sixty-six patients with advanced achalasia were operated utilizing the described technique. The mortality rate for the series was 3.0%. Deaths were attributable to fistulas related to the pyloroplasty, mediastinal hemorrhage, and acute pancreatitis in the immediate postoperative period. Eighty-three patients were followed for an average time of 8 years (3–27 years). All underwent clinical and endoscopic evaluation pre- and post-operatively at 6 months (❷ *Table 41-2*). Dumping and diarrhea occurred primarily early after operation due to the vagotomy during the esophagectomy.

All patients treated with esophagectomy without thoractomy returned to social life and were able to join the work force; mild dysphasia was observed in 6% of the patients. Weight gain was observed in 80%. One patient developed a squamous cell carcinoma in the esophageal stump 13 years after esophagectomy which was resected locally.

Clinical and endoscopic findings confirmed a clinically important increase in heartburn, regurgitation, diffuse gastritis, esophagitis, and Barrett's epithelium in the esophageal stump with time due to

◼ Figure 41-7
Surgical treatment of advanced achalasia through esophagectomy without thoracotomy. a. Upper laparotomy with median phrenotomy; b. dissection of the esophagus through the lower mediastinum; c. mobilization of the stomach; d. pull-up of the stomach to the cervical region with esophagogastric anastomosis

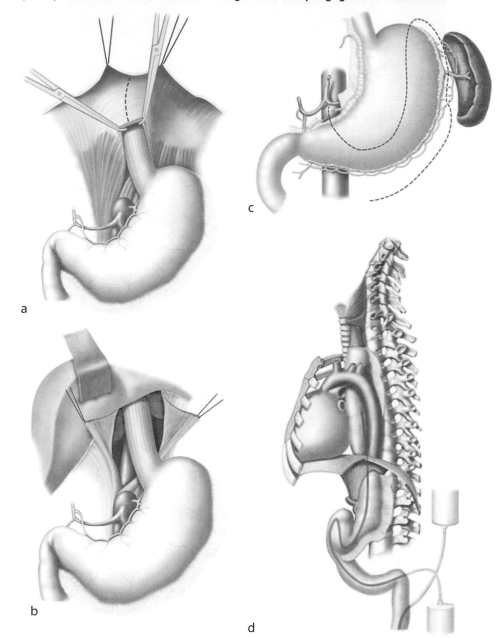

duodeno-gastroesophageal reflux. Continuous use of PPIs (proton-pump inhibitors) was suggested. The presence of Barrett's epithelium in the esophageal stump demands annual endoscopic and histologic follow-up. Employment of an elongated gastric tube (instead of the whole stomach) in order to decrease gastric acid and pepsin production may be of value in this challenge.

◘ **Table 41-2**

Esophagectomy without thoracotomy: late follow-up (83 patients)

	6 m (%)	7 years (%)
Dysphagia	30	6
Regurgitation	34	35
Heartburn	12	45
Weight gain	71	76
Diarrhea	44	2
Dumping	15	1
Esophagitis	20	66
Barrett esophagus	–	27

Esophagectomy with cervical esophagogastrostomy remains an excellent choice for the treatment of end-stage chagasic achalasia. Due to the possible occurrence of simultaneous megacolon, coloplasty is not recommended.

Selected Readings

Bettarello A, Pinotti HW (1976) Oesophageal involvement in Chagas' disease. Clin Gastroentrol 5:103–117

Cecconello I (1998) Long-term evaluation of gastroplasty in achalasia. In: Siewert R, Holsher AH (eds) Diseases of the esophagus. Springer-Verlag, Berlin, pp. 975–978

Cecconello I, Mariano da Rocha J, Zilberstein B, et al. (1993) Reflux esophagitis and development of ectopic columnar epithelium in the esophageal stump after gastric transposition. In: Nabeia K, Hanaoka T, Nogami T (eds) Recent advances in diseases of the esophagus. Springer-Verlag, Berlin

Cunha-Neto E (2001) Understanding the immunopathogenesis of Chagas disease: perspectives for the new millennium. In: Pinotti HW, Cecconello I, Felix VN, Oliveira MA (eds) Recent advances in disease of the esophagus. Manduzzi Editore, Bologna, pp. 197–204

da Silveira AB, Arantes RM, Vago AR, et al. (2005) Comparative study of the presence of Trypanosoma cruzi kDNA, inflammation and denervation in chagasic patients with and without megaesophagus. Parasitology 131:627–634

Felix VN (1998) Achalasia. a prospective results of dilatation and myotomy. Hepatogastroenterol 45:97–108

Meneguelli UF (2001) Chagasic megaesophagus – historical aspects and present situation in South America. In: Pinotti HW, Cecconello I, Felix VN, Oliveira MA (eds) Recent advances in disease of the esophagus. Manduzzi Editore, Bologna, pp. 197–204

Moraes-Filho JP, Bettarello A (1989) Response of the lower esophageal sphincter to pentagastrin on patients with megaesophagus secondary to Chagas' disease. Rev Hosp Clin Fac Med Sao Paulo 44:178–180

Pinotti HW (1964) Contribuição para o estudo de fisiopatologia do megaesôfago. Thesis, Faculdade de Medicina da Universidade de São Paulo

Pinotti HW. (1988) The basis of its treatment. In: Siewert JR, Holscher AH (eds) Diseases of esophagus. Springer-Verlag, Berlin, pp. 17–19

42 Esophageal Perforation

S. Michael Griffin · Jonathan Shenfine

Pearls and Pitfalls

- Esophageal perforation is a rare but hazardous event.
- Iatrogenic damage during upper gastrointestinal endoscopy accounts for the majority of injuries.
- Therapeutic endoscopy carries a 200-fold higher perforation risk than diagnostic endoscopy.
- Clinical features depend on the cause, site and time of injury.
- Severe, sudden chest pain after vomiting associated with subcutaneous emphysema is pathognomic of spontaneous perforation of the esophagus.
- Survival is dependent on rapid control of mediastinal and pleural contamination.
- Surgery is mandatory when gross contamination is present, when there is tissue loss or in perforations associated with caustic injuries.
- Thorough wound debridement, lavage of pleural and mediastinal cavities and drainage are probably more important than any specific repair technique employed in cases where surgery is performed.

Introduction

Esophageal perforation is a rare event, which can occur through a variety of insults and carries a high morbidity and mortality due to difficulty in accessing the esophagus, the unusual blood supply, the lack of a strong serosal layer, and the proximity of vital structures. The limited exposure that clinicians gain often means that few have the knowledge and skills required to deal with these injuries. This lack of experience is compounded by the lack of an evidence base for management, which is directly due to the scarcity of cases and heterogeneous presenting features. As a result, misdiagnosis and inappropriate management are all too common with potentially catastrophic consequences.

This chapter focuses on the diagnosis and management of spontaneous and iatrogenic esophageal perforation, external trauma and caustic perforation.

Etiology

Iatrogenic Perforation of the Esophagus

Iatrogenic damage to the esophagus can occur from within, such as during endoscopic instrumentation, or from without such as by paraesophageal surgery, with the former being far more common. Due to advances in imaging technology and the inherent safety of the procedure with a relatively low risk of esophageal perforation (0.03% of diagnostic procedures), flexible videoendoscopy has almost totally replaced rigid esophagoscopy. However, despite this safety record, a dramatic increase in the number of endoscopic examinations performed and associated instrumentation has led to a rise in the number of iatrogenic injuries with an associated overall mortality rate of 19%. As such, prevention of these injuries by awareness and training is most likely to reduce the rate of morbidity and mortality.

Inappropriate force used to "intubate" the esophagus can easily cause a proximal perforation and this hazard is augmented with hyper-extension of the neck, arthritis of the cervical spine or in the presence of an esophageal diverticulum. However, by far the majority (75–90%) of iatrogenic perforations occur in the distal esophagus often in the presence of an underlying abnormality, such as a benign or malignant stricture, with perforation occurring just above due to formation of a false passage or from within due to splitting of the abnormal esophagus. Therapeutic endoscopy carries a 200-fold higher perforation risk (approximately 5%) than diagnostic endoscopy, both for cancer-related procedures and those carried out for benign conditions. Endoscopic palliation of malignant dysphagia especially where pre-dilatation of malignant strictures has been used accounts for the majority of injuries. The risk is greatest in patients who have received prior radiotherapy or chemotherapy. Pneumatic dilatation for achalasia remains a high-risk procedure due to the high pressures and large diameter balloon involved. Perforation is also possible with variceal ligation and sclerotherapy and these procedures may be associated with delayed perforation due to transmural necrosis.

Non-endoscopic instrumentation of the esophagus can also lead to direct trauma, for example, from nasogastric tube or transesophageal echocardiography probe insertion. It can also be due to from esophageal intubation by an endotracheal tube or indirect trauma from pressure necrosis due to the cuff of a tracheal tube or, even from close lying intercostal chest drains. Paraesophageal surgery, such as anti-reflux surgery, can also inadvertently lead to direct trauma, but the risk is low (0–1.2%).

Spontaneous Perforation of the Esophagus

The rare, eponymous Boerhaave's syndrome is defined as complete disruption of the esophageal wall occurring in the absence of pre-existing pathology. It is characterized by barogenic esophageal injury leading to immediate and gross gastric content contamination of the pleural cavity, with rapid and catastrophic onset of chemical and bacterial mediastinitis. A history of a sudden rise in intra-abdominal pressure is present in 80–90% of cases usually as a result of retching or vomiting but cases have resulted from blunt trauma, weight lifting, parturition, defecation, the Heimlich maneuver or status epilepticus.

Vomiting results from involuntary abdominal and diaphragmatic contraction with pyloric closure and cricopharyngeus relaxation, and raised intra-abdominal pressure leading to reflux of gastric contents through a passive esophagus. Mackler demonstrated in the 1950s that if flow is obstructed, then an increase in intra-luminal pressure suddenly occurs, and a rapid rise of only 5 psi can result in esophageal perforation. However, although vomiting is commonplace, spontaneous perforation of the esophagus is so rare factors that are as yet undetermined, may be of relevance.

Penetrating Injuries of the Esophagus

Sharp, penetrating injuries of the thoracic esophagus are uncommon except with gunshot wounds but the more superficially lying cervical esophagus may be injured by knife wounds to the neck. These injuries often occur in conjunction with other serious injuries to surrounding viscera so are easily missed and the consequent delay greatly increases morbidity and mortality. A high index of suspicion, based on the tract of the injury is therefore of paramount importance.

Blunt Esophageal Trauma

Blunt esophageal trauma is extremely uncommon and usually occurs only in conjunction with high velocity injuries. As such, they are often associated with immediately life threatening airway or cardiopulmonary damage and compromise. In rapid deceleration events, the otherwise well protected thoracic esophagus may be injured by traction laceration, vascular thrombosis or barogenic damage. Blunt cervical esophageal perforation can occur when the neck or upper chest impacts a fixed structure, by extreme "whiplash" flexion-extension or an associated cervical fracture — usually in cases from road traffic accidents.

Caustic Injuries

Serious ingestion of a caustic substance leading to esophageal perforation is uncommon but devastating. Although accidental ingestion in childhood account for the majority of caustic trauma injuries, adult ingestion are more often deliberate with suicidal intent and are therefore usually the more serious in nature. Most caustic substances can be grouped into acids or alkalis and are readily available as cleaners, in batteries and in industrial practice. Acids are unpleasant to swallow and produce a coagulative necrosis and are thus less likely to be penetrative. In contrast, alkalis are marginally more palatable and resultant liquefactive necrosis is rapidly transmural. However, in general, the severity of the injury is related to the concentration, amount, viscosity, and duration of contact between the caustic agent and the esophageal mucosa and the ingestion of any strong caustic agent in sufficient quantity will inflict a potentially fatal esophageal injury.

Clinical Presentation

Clinical features of esophageal perforation depend on the cause, site and duration after injury.

Full-thickness, intrathoracic, iatrogenic perforations are usually recognized and visualized immediately or there is at least a high index of suspicion. They are commonly associated with chest pain, dysphagia and odynophagia, often allied to a sympathetic nervous system response with pallor, sweating, peripheral circulatory shutdown, tachycardia, tachypnea and overt hemodynamic shock. Systemic symptoms are less common with cervical perforations which present with neck pain, dysphonia, cervical dysphagia, hoarseness, and subcutaneous emphysema predominating.

Spontaneous esophageal perforation classically presents with sudden, distressing, retrosternal or epigastric pain following an episode of raised intra-abdominal pressure, usually vomiting, with subsequent subcutaneous emphysema (Mackler's triad). A dramatic sympathetic nervous system response is usually present. Within 24–48 h a systemic inflammatory response gives way to cardiopulmonary collapse and multiorgan failure as a consequence of overwhelming bacterial mediastinitis.

Penetrating esophageal trauma manifests in the same fashion as iatrogenic trauma but a high index of suspicion, based on the tract of the injury is essential for diagnosis; damage should be suspected in any transcervical or transmediastinal wound, especially when gunshot derived.

Blunt esophageal trauma is rare and usually only occurs in high impact events so is frequently associated with more immediately life threatening airway or cardiopulmonary damage. Again a high index of suspicion is necessary and esophageal perforation actively excluded.

Clinical features in patients with caustic esophageal perforation are dependent on the substance and the time course since ingestion. The absence of oral burns or pharyngo-esophageal symptoms does not exclude a significant esophageal injury. However, drooling and hypersalivation are common when oropharyngeal burns are present and together with stridor and hoarseness are the warning signs of potentially life-threatening airway edema. The typical symptoms of esophageal injury are of dysphagia and odynophagia and perforation should be suspected with severe retrosternal or epigastric pain especially if this radiates to the back, and is accompanied by abdominal tenderness, shock, respiratory distress, pleural pain, or subcutaneous emphysema. In contrast to other injuries, a perforation may develop as a delayed phenomenon and intensive observation and re-assessment of these patients is vital.

Investigations

A classical history and thus a high clinical suspicion is the most reliable parameter for the successful diagnosis of esophageal perforation, but atypical symptoms, the similarity to more common cardiore-spiratory disorders and a shocked, confused and distressed patient can misdirect the clinician. As time passes, the critical condition of the patient obscures relevant clinical features and the pursuit of incorrect investigations make the diagnosis even more elusive. The following investigations are the most helpful in establishing the diagnosis.

Plain Radiography

The typical findings of esophageal perforation on a plain chest radiograph are pleural effusion, pneumomediastinum, subcutaneous emphysema, hydropneumothorax, pneumothorax and collapse or consolidation but these findings may be subtle and are dependent on the site, the extent of trauma and the time interval following the insult. ❯ *Figure 42-1* demonstrates the typical appearance of an esophageal perforation causing pneumomediastinum following the dilatation of a benign stricture. In caustic injuries there may be radiographic signs of aspiration.

Contrast Radiography

Oral water soluble contrast radiography (❯ *Fig. 42-2*) is the investigation of choice to confirm perforation and this helps to ascertain the site, degree of containment and degree of drainage and aqueous agents are rapidly absorbed, do not exacerbate inflammation and have minimal tissue effects. False negative results are not uncommon with contrast studies due to the rapid passage of low-viscosity

◘ Figure 42-1
Chest radiograph following esophageal dilatation of a benign stricture demonstrating pneumomediastinum (arrows highlight gas in the left mediastinum)

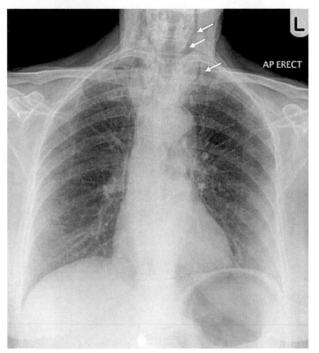

contrast past a small hole closed by edema or due to extravasation of contrast from the tear site parallel to the esophageal shadow. As such, if negative, films should be repeated in the lateral or oblique positions or using barium.

Upper Gastrointestinal Endoscopy

Flexible videoendoscopy is an expert procedure as it carries significant risk in inexperienced hands. ❷ *Figure 42-3* demonstrates the endoscopic appearance of a spontaneous esophageal perforation. Nevertheless, with fluoroscopic guidance it allows crucial assessment of the site, the mucosal trauma, and reveals any underlying pathology facilitating placement of a nasogastric or nasojejunal tube for drainage or feeding. This is especially useful in an "on table" situation where trauma is suspected but where other injuries preclude radiological examination. Similarly, in caustic injuries, endoscopy allows assessment of the stomach for possible reconstruction.

Computed Tomography (CT)

CT is an increasingly useful investigation (❷ *Fig. 42-4*) in those patients stable enough to undergo scanning but the radiology department is a dangerous place for an unstable patient. CT is especially

◘ Figure 42-2
Contrast swallow demonstrating esophageal leak. A naso-jejunal feeding tube has been sited

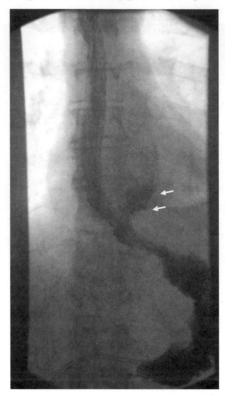

◘ Figure 42-3
Endoscopic view of spontaneous esophageal perforation

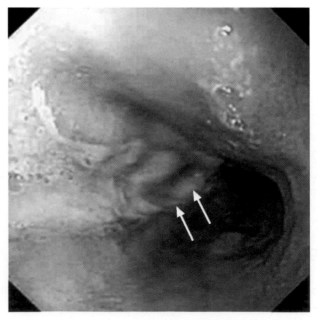

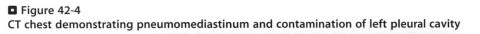

■ Figure 42-4
CT chest demonstrating pneumomediastinum and contamination of left pleural cavity

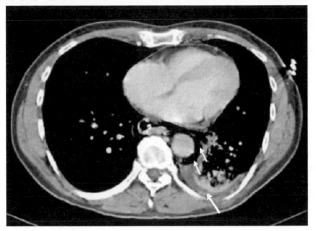

useful in cases of external trauma, caustic injuries and in critically ill patients with an atypical presentation. In combination with interventional radiological techniques, CT has also revolutionized the management of intra-thoracic collections.

Other

Drainage of gastric contents on thoracocentesis is diagnostic and may be aided by measurement of pH, amylase or microscopy for squamous cells. Administration of oral dyes, such as methylene blue, may be a useful adjunct if there is a communicating drain.

Management

All patients with esophageal perforation should be viewed as critically ill. The immediate priorities are the establishment of a secure and adequate airway, the stabilization of cardiovascular status and the relief of pain. The initial resuscitation is documented in ❷ *Table 42-1* and regular re-assessment is obligatory.

The rarity of esophageal injuries and the consequences of incorrect management have limited the ability to evaluate differing treatments. Published case series often span many years, many centers, many surgeons and many techniques. Non-operative treatment has become the standard management of iatrogenic esophageal perforation with a low mortality due to sophisticated respiratory, nutritional and antimicrobial support but this should be viewed as "radical" in other situations. Survival is dependent on avoiding or controlling mediastinal and pleural contamination and surgery remains mandatory when gross contamination is present, and there is loss of tissue or when the perforation has been due to a caustic injury. Where possible, all patients with an esophageal perforation should be managed in specialist units by specialist surgeons with a multi-disciplinary approach to care. Hospitals

◻ Table 42-1

Initial resuscitation following suspected esophageal perforation

Initial resuscitation
• Control of airway
• Administration of oxygen
• Early anesthetic assessment
• Large bore intravenous access
• Intravenous fluid resuscitation
• Central venous access and arterial line monitoring ± inotropic support
• Urethral catheterization
• Fluid balance monitoring
• Intravenous broad spectrum antibiotic and antifungal agents
• Intravenous antisecretory agents (proton pump inhibitors)
• Strict nil by mouth
• Large bore intercostal chest drainage — possibly bilaterally
• Nasogastric tube (only to be placed under endoscopic vision or radiological guidance)

lacking in these specialist facilities or the appropriate and versatile surgical cover necessary to operate on the esophagus by abdominal or left or right thoracic approaches, should transfer the patients at the earliest opportunity after stabilization.

Non-operative Management

With advances in radiological interventional techniques, antibiotics and enteral nutrition, successful non-operative management is possible in selected patients. Two patient groups in particular are suitable for consideration: those diagnosed rapidly with minimal contamination or those with a delayed diagnosis who have demonstrated tolerance to the perforation. Some guidance for patient selection is possible using the criteria detailed in ❯ *Table 42-2*.

◻ Table 42-2

Criteria for non-operative management of esophageal perforation

Criteria for non-operative management of esophageal perforation
• Contained perforation
• Free flow of contrast back into esophagus on contrast swallow
• No symptoms or signs of mediastinitis
• No evidence of solid food contamination of pleural or mediastinal cavities
Other factors to consider
• Perforation is "controlled"
• No underlying esophageal disease or loss of tissue
• Non-caustic injury
• No sepsis
• Availability for intensive observation and access to multi-disciplinary care
• Low threshold for intervention
• Enteral feeding established

Distal Perforation

Patients require intensive observation and should strictly not receive any oral intake. Chest drains are placed where pleural perforation has occurred and contrast radiology, endoscopy and CT performed to monitor the status of the esophageal leak and collections. All patients should be given broad-spectrum, intravenous antibiotics, anti-fungal and anti-secretory agents with a low threshold for drainage of collections and surgical intervention. Enteral feeding may be established using a surgical feeding jejunostomy or a naso-jejunal feeding tube placed under endoscopic and/or radiological assistance together with a nasogastric tube placed to decompress the stomach. Non-operative treatment must not be "conservative" and intervention when required, should be rapid and aggressive.

Removable self-expanding metal stents may help to seal iatrogenic perforations of malignant tumors if deemed unfit for resection but stent insertion cannot be recommended for perforations within a normal esophagus, as expansion of the stent may expand the defect.

Cervical Perforation

Perforations of the cervical esophagus are often managed non-operatively with percutaneous drainage of collections. However, when uncontained, primary closure with prevertebral lavage and drainage using a left lateral incision anterior to the sternocleidomastoid is recommended and is tolerated well by even critically ill patients.

Operative Management

Surgery is appropriate if the patient has overt signs of sepsis, shock, gross contamination, an underlying obstructive pathology, a retained foreign body, a caustic injury or has failed non-operative management. Virtually all gunshot wounds require surgery. The prime objectives are to clear the contamination and then to restore esophageal integrity whilst preventing further soiling. A feeding jejunostomy should be fashioned for enteral feeding. Depending on the perforation site, a right sided (for upper or mid esophagus) or left sided (distal esophagus) postero-lateral thoracotomy is used at an appropriate level. The pleural cavity is cleaned and lavaged, the mediastinal pleura incised to expose the injury and necrotic, and devitalized tissue debrided. In spontaneous perforation, an extended myotomy should be made as the mucosal injury is usually longer than the muscular one. Iatrogenic perforations frequently occur in association with an underlying pathology such as carcinoma, peptic stricture or achalasia. As a result, surgery can have a high mortality rate despite minimal contamination.

Primary Repair

A primary suture repair is the most common surgical technique and may be buttressed with nearby tissues to reinforce the suture line. This repair is associated with a high leak rate so should be reserved for those with demonstrably healthy tissue and limited soiling.

T-Tube Repair

Repair over a T-tube is a viable alternative in view of the high leak rate for primary repair. This diverts swallowed secretions via a controlled esophago-cutaneous fistula allowing healing to occur without ongoing contamination. A 6–10 mm diameter T-tube is placed through the tear with the limbs directed proximally and distally beyond the boundaries of the perforation and the esophageal wall is closed around loosely. The tube is brought out through the chest wall and secured with a further drain placed down to the repair and apical and basal intercostal chest drains. The T-tube is left until a defined tract is established with the majority removed between 3 and 6 weeks.

Exclusion and Diversion

Exclusion of the contaminated mediastinum and diversion of secretions maximizes healing while minimizing risk. Although the techniques used to achieve this are complex and do not appear to achieve any better results than other simpler treatments, it remains in the armamentarium of the esophageal surgeon.

Resection

Esophageal resection is a major undertaking, but in the presence of a diseased esophagus, may be the only solution. Immediate reconstruction can be employed where there is minimal contamination but a delayed approach can also be adopted. Patients with a caustic perforation almost always require an emergency esophago-gastrectomy as the stomach is also usually injured. Immediate reconstruction with a colonic interposition graft can be performed or delayed for 6–8 weeks if there is minimal local contamination. Resection should also be considered in patients with extensive, circumferential mucosal injuries as these can lead to problematic strictures and a significant long term cancer risk. An alternative, if the esophagus is intact and respiratory complications supervene, is defunctioning via a cervical esophagostomy and the formation of a feeding jejunostomy with resection and reconstruction delayed until the patient is stable. The mortality for these injuries is between 13% and 40% with the majority of deaths occurring in the adult suicidal group. Mortality mainly stems from respiratory complications and delay in aggressive surgical treatment of transmural necrosis. There is no place for "conservative" treatment in the case of a severe caustic injury.

Perforation and Cancer

Perforation of an inoperable malignant stricture should be managed non-operatively, in this situation a sealing self-expanding metal stent may be the most appropriate treatment. In patients with less clearly defined operability most authors recommend resection. However, this carries considerably mortality (between 22 and 75%) and long term survival is compromised such that this treatment should be considered palliative. As such, every effort should be made to prevent iatrogenic injury during staging procedures.

Conclusions

The fragility of the esophageal wall, the lack of serosa, the proximity of vital organs, the inaccessibility and the lack of symptoms and signs can mean that even small perforations of the esophagus can be ultimately fatal. Overall mortality for esophageal perforation from any cause is high and the majority of surgeons only deal with a handful of difficult cases in their career. These cases are therefore best managed by specialist units with ancillary staff trained, equipped and experienced to prevent the potentially disastrous consequences of misdiagnosis and inappropriate management. Prevention of iatrogenic injuries through appropriate endoscopic training is the key to improving outcomes.

Selected Readings

Abbott OA, Mansour KA, Logan WD Jr, et al. (1970) Atraumatic so-called "spontaneous" rupture of the esophagus. A review of 47 personal cases with comments on a new method of surgical therapy. J Thorac Cardiovasc Surg 59:67–83

Bufkin BL, Miller JI Jr, Mansour KA (1996) Esophageal perforation: emphasis on management. Ann Thorac Surg 61:1447–1451; discussion 51–2

Derbes VJ, Mitchell RE Jr (1955) Hermann Boerhaave's Atrocis, nec descripti prius, morbi historia, the first translation of the classic case report of rupture of the esophagus, with annotations. Bull Med Libr Assoc 43:217–240

Estrera A, Taylor W, Mills LJ, et al. (1986) Corrosive burns of the esophagus and stomach: a recommendation for an aggressive surgical approach. Ann Thorac Surg 41:276–283

Griffin SM, Lamb PJ, Shenfine J, et al. (2008) Spontaneous rupture of the oesophagus. Br J Surg 95:1432–1439

Jones WG 2nd, Ginsberg RJ (1992) Esophageal perforation: a continuing challenge. Ann Thorac Surg 53:534–543

Mackler S (1952) Spontaneous rupture of the esophagus: an experimental and clinical study. Surg Gynecol Obstet 95:345–356

Zargar SA, Kochhar R, Nagi B, et al. (1992) Ingestion of strong corrosive alkalis: spectrum of injury to upper gastrointestinal tract and natural history. Am J Gastroenterol 87:337–341

43 Esophageal Diverticula

Jörg Hutter · Hubert J. Stein

Pearls and Pitfalls

- Only symptomatic esophageal diverticula require treatment
- Most traction diverticula are asymptomatic
- Pulsion diverticula are due to a distal functional esophageal obstruction (motor disorder)
- Surgical treatment must address the underlying pathogenetic mechanism, i.e. a myotomy at the site of the functional distal obstruction in pulsion diverticula is mandatory
- Minimally invasive (endoscopic, thoracoscopic, laparoscopic) approaches are feasible but still associated with high complication or failure rates

Introduction

A diverticulum is a pouch or sac that protrudes from the gastrointestinal wall and can derive from any tubular organ in the gastrointestinal tract. True diverticula contain all layers of the gastrointestinal wall. Most diverticula of the esophagus consist of mucosa, submucosa, and strands of muscle fibers only and are, therefore, "false" diverticula.

Esophageal diverticula are classified according to their location (cervical vs. midesophageal vs. epiphrenic) and the presumed underlying pathogenetic mechanism (pulsion vs. traction). Pulsion diverticula typically occur proximal to a physiologic sphincter or proximal to areas of functional resistance to food passage and are assumed to be caused by excessive intraluminal pressure on the esophageal wall. Traction diverticula result from traction forces arising from outside the esophageal wall and usually occur in response to periesophageal inflammation such as chronic lymphadenitis.

The most common diverticula in the upper digestive tract are Zenker's diverticula. They are located in the cervical region and originate from the posterior wall of the hypopharynx proximal to the upper esophageal sphincter. These esophageal diverticula should, thus, be more adequately termed hypopharyngeal diverticula. Midesophageal diverticula are those at or close to the level of the tracheal bifurcation while epiphrenic diverticula are located within a few centimeters proximal to the lower esophageal sphincter (❷ *Fig. 43-1*).

Zenker's Diverticulum

A Zenker's diverticulum results from an outpouching in a weak muscular portion at the posterior hypopharyngeal wall immediately proximal to the upper esophageal sphincter, the so-called Killian's

☑ Figure 43-1

Typical location and frequency distribution of esophageal diverticular (Modified from Stein et al., 2006. With permission of Springer Science and Business Media)

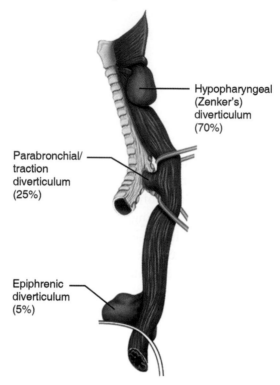

Hypopharyngeal (Zenker's) diverticulum (70%)

Parabronchial/ traction diverticulum (25%)

Epiphrenic diverticulum (5%)

triangle. They are diagnosed typically in persons over the age of 50 years and are more common in males than females. The estimated incidence is 2 per 100,000/year.

The pathogenesis of Zenker's diverticulum is related to a decreased compliance of the cricopharyngeal muscle, the major component of the upper esophageal sphincter. This decreased compliance results in decreased contractility and increased resistance to the passage of a bolus from the hypopharynx into the cervical esophagus. The most widely accepted pathogenic mechanism of these diverticula is related to a dysfunction of the upper esophageal sphincter, e.g. abnormal or inadequate opening of the upper esophageal sphincter on swallowing as a result of a primary myogenic or neurologic disorder. This theory is supported by the observation of an increased intrabolus pressure on hypopharngeal manometry in patients with Zenker's diverticulum. Whether chronic gastroesophageal reflux can also contribute to the formation of a Zenker's diverticulum is still controversial.

Over time, a permanent, narrow-mouthed outpouching of the posterior hypopharyngeal wall develops and enlarges inevitably. As a result, saliva, secretions, liquid, and food will pool dependently in the diverticulum sac and cannot empty easily into the esophagus. In the early phase, patients may complain only of a vague globus sensation, intermittent cough, and excessive salivation. Intermittent dysphagia, regurgitation of undigested foods, and aspiration follow as the disease and the size of the diverticulum progress. A Zenker's diverticulum may become large enough to produce a visible mass in the neck, which may gurgle on palpation (Boyce's sign) or obstruct the esophagus by compression. To aid in swallowing, patients may develop elaborate maneuvers: clearing the throat, coughing, or placing external pressure on the neck. The most serious complication associated with Zenker's diverticulum is aspiration, which can lead to pneumonia or lung abscess. Perforation (sometimes iatrogenic on forceful attempts to access the esophagus with an endoscope or a tube), bleeding, and carcinoma may also complicate Zenker's diverticula.

Small Zenker's diverticula are often missed on endoscopy. Thus, endoscopy is not the method of choice to establish a diagnosis, but it is often used to exclude other upper gastrointestinal disorders. Usually, a Zenker's diverticulum is diagnosed with contrast radiography. Small diverticula can be missed if they are superimposed on the main column of barium in the esophagus. This error can be avoided by rotating the patient during the examination and using high speed video or cinematographic recordings of the pharyngoesophageal phase of swallowing (❯ *Fig. 43-2*). Esophageal manometry is not required typically; however, it may help to illuminate the functional obstruction at the upper esophageal sphincter and the increased intrabolus pressure in the hypopharyngeal region.

Every symptomatic Zenker's diverticulum, irrespective of its size, is considered an indication for operative intervention. Based on its pathogenesis, the treatment of Zenker's diverticulum is aimed at the underlying disorder of the upper esophageal sphincter with the goal of increasing the compliance of the upper esophageal sphincter and facilitating its opening during a swallow. Standard operative treatment, thus, comprises a simple cricopharyngeal myotomy which is adequate treatment for small diverticula. For large diverticula, myotomy with suspension or excision of the diverticulum is indicated (❯ *Fig. 43 3*). Both these procedures provide similar good outcome in more than 90% of patients with a low incidence of complications. Simple excision of the diverticulum without myotomy will result in

▣ Figure 43-2
Radiographic image of a Zenker's diverticulum (Modified from Stein et al., 2006. With permission of Springer Science and Business Media)

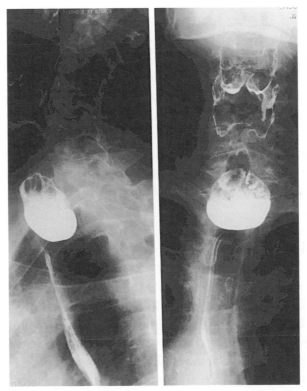

◧ Figure 43-3

Classic open surgical approach to Zenker's diverticulum. a. Access and exposure; b. cricopharyngeal myotomy; c. diverticulectomy; d. status after myotomy and diverticulectomy; e. status after myotomy and pexy of the diverticulum to the prevertebral fascia (Modified from Stein et al., 2006. With permission of Springer Science and Business Media)

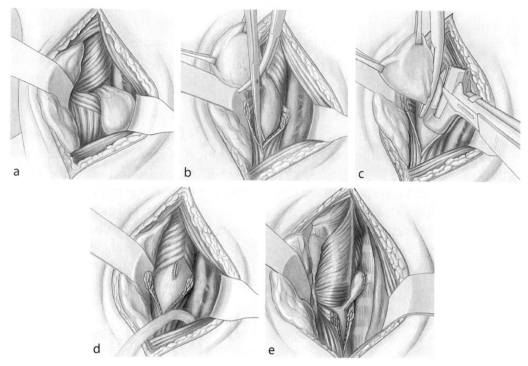

high leakage rates from the diverticulectomy site; on long-term follow up, recurrences of the diverticulum may occur, because the underlying pathogenetic mechanism has not been addressed.

More recently, minimally invasive, transoral endoscopic methods have been described and are used increasingly. These endoscopic techniques include transoral, endoscopic esophagodiverticulostomy using a surgical stapler (❷ *Fig. 43-4*) and transoral division of the bridge between the esophagus and the diverticulum with a diathermic knife, laser, or argon plasma coagulation.

Despite some enthusiastic results from small series employing these techniques, a critical comparison shows that open techniques probably afford better long-term symptomatic relief than endoscopic approaches, especially in patients with small diverticula.

Midesophageal Diverticula

These more unusual diverticula are located in the middle third of the esophagus within 4–5 cm proximal or distal to the level of the carina. Until the late twentieth century, midesophageal diverticula were caused commonly by traction due to mediastinal fibrosis or chronic lymphadenopathy from pulmonary tuberculosis or histoplasmosis. In the past, the majority of mid-esophageal diverticula were diagnosed incidentally in patients who had tuberculosis 20–30 years earlier. Because these diseases are far less common today and rarely progress to cause traction on the esophagus, patients presenting with a

◘ Figure 43-4

Schematic drawing of transoral stapling esophago-diverticulostomy for Zenker's diverticulum (Modified from Stein et al., 2006. With permission of Springer Science and Business Media)

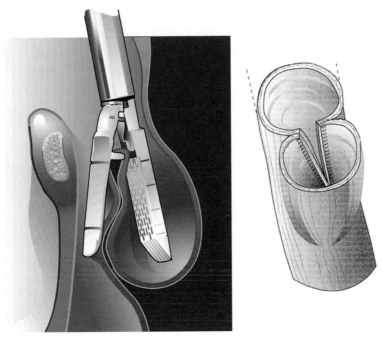

midesophageal diverticulum have become rare and, if no history of tuberculosis exists, should be evaluated for motility disorders of the esophageal body which may cause a pulsion diverticulum in this region.

Patients with midesophageal traction diverticula are usually asymptomatic; only the few with an excessively large diverticulum sack may report dysphagia, retrosternal pain, regurgitation, belching, epigastric pain, heartburn, and weight loss. In patients with a midesophageal pulsion diverticulum, symptoms may also result from an associated or underlying motor disorder or other underlying disease and not from the midthoracic diverticulum. Although complications are unusual, spontaneous rupture, iatrogenic perforation, exsanguination, aspiration, esophagobronchial fistula, and carcinoma have been reported.

Most patients with midesophageal diverticula require no treatment. Only in those with clear symptoms related to the diverticulum surgery is indicated. If no underlying motor disorder or esophageal obstruction is present, a simple resection of the diverticulum is the procedure of choice. Access through the right chest, via thoracotomy or thoracoscopy avoids the aortic arch and provides excellent exposure of the esophagus and airway at the tracheal bifurcation. Placing a bougie in the esophagus before excision of the diverticulum avoids compromise of the esophageal lumen. The diverticulum is resected with a stapling device. The closure may be buttressed with pleura, pleuropericardial fat pad, or omentum. An additional longitudinal myotomy of the esophagus distal to the origin of the diverticulum must be added in those with a pulsion diverticulum due to the underlying motor disorder (see below).

Epiphrenic Diverticula

Epiphrenic diverticula are mucosal outpouchings of the esophageal wall that occur usually in the distal third of the esophagus. They are typically pulsion diverticula, that develop secondary to increased intraesophageal pressure, usually due to distal esophageal and/or lower esophageal sphincter motility disorders (such as achalasia, hypertensive lower esophageal sphincter or diffuse esophageal spasm).

The clinical manifestations of epiphrenic diverticula are variable with little correlation between the severity of symptoms and the size of the diverticulum. Distinguishing between symptoms of the diverticulum and those caused by the underlying motility disorder can be difficult.

A videotaped barium esophagogram best detects the presence of an epiphrenic diverticulum and often also allows characterization of the underlying motility disorder. Many patients show bizarre, non-propulsive tertiary contractions in the distal esophagus and/or a non-relaxing lower esophageal sphincter during the examination. In addition to the fixed, relatively wide-mouthed diverticulum, transient outpouchings can occur proximally in segments where peristalsis is absent. Endoscopy provides little information about diverticula but may be useful to assess associated esophageal problems like reflux disease. Manometry of the esophagus and the lower esophageal sphincter is mandatory to prove and classify the underlying motility disorder.

Only symptomatic epiphrenic diverticula are an indication for operation. Although good outcomes have been reported with diverticulectomy alone by some, the standard operation has become a distal esophageal myotomy (including the lower esophageal sphincter) in combination with a diverticulectomy. The myotomy will address the underlying motor disorder and avoid recurrences. Because myotomy across the lower esophageal sphincter is associated with a destruction of the physiologic antireflux mechanism, the addition of an antireflux procedure to diverticulectomy and myotomy is recommended. To avoid postoperative dysphagia, the added antireflux procedure should by only a partial fundoplication (e.g. a Dor or Toupet fundoplication). The classic approach is through the left chest, because this approach provides optimal access to the lower esophagus and esophagogastric

◧ **Figure 43-5**

Radiographic image of an epiphrenic diverticulum (left) and schematic drawing of a laparoscopic transhiatal approach for diverticulectomy (right) (Modified from Stein et al., 2006. With permission of Springer Science and Business Media)

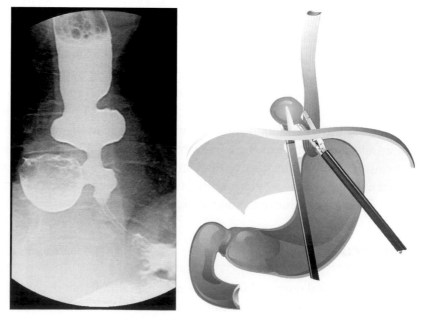

junction. Recently, laparoscopic and thoracoscopic approaches to epiphrenic diverticula have been reported (❯ *Fig. 43-5*). The complication rate of this approach in the few small published series is, however, relatively high, with fistula rates from the site of the diverticulectomy of up to 20%.

Selected Readings

Allen MS (1999) Treatment of epiphrenic diverticula. Semin Thorac Cardiovasc Surg 11:358–362

Bonavina L, Khan NA, DeMeester TR (1985) Pharyngoesophageal dysfunction: the role of cricopharyngeal myotomy. Arch Surg 120:541–549

Fernando HC, Luketich JD, Samphire J, et al. (2005) Minimally invasive operation for esophageal diverticula. Ann Thorac Surg 80:2076–2081

Feussner H (2007) Endoscopic therapy for Zenker diverticulum – the good and the bad. Endoscopy 39:154–155

Gutschow CA, Hamoir M, Rombaux P, et al. (2002) Management of pharyngoesophageal (Zenker's) diverticulum: which technique? Ann Thorac Surg 74:1677–1682

Nehra D, Lord RV, DeMeester TR, et al. (2002) Physiologic basis for the treatment of epiphrenic diverticulum. Ann Surg 235:346–354

Omote K, Feussner H, Stein HJ, Siewert JR (1999) Endoscopic stapling diverticulostomy for Zenker's diverticulum. Surg Endosc 13:535–538

Rosati R, Fumagalli U, Bona S, et al. (1998) Diverticulectomy, myotomy, and fundoplication through laparoscopy: a new option to treat epiphrenic esophageal diverticula? Ann Surg 227:174–178

Stein HJ, Feussner H, von Rahden BHA, et al. (2006) Gutartige Erkrankungen von Ösophagus und Kardia. In: Siewert JR, Rothmund R, Schumpelick V (eds) Praxis der Viszerlachirurgie - Gastroenterologische Chirurgie, 2nd edn. Springer Medizin Verlag, Heidelberg, The Netherlands, pp. 241–294

Thomas ML, Anthony AA, Fosh BG, et al. (2001) Oesophageal diverticula. Br J Surg 88:629–642

Part 2

Esophagus and Paraesophageal Region: Malignant

44 Esophageal Cancer: Diagnosis and Staging

J. Rüdiger Siewert · Marcus Feith

Pearls and Pitfalls

- The aim of any diagnostic procedure is to identify the R0-resectable patient population.
- Topographic-anatomic localization and histologic proof of an esophageal cancer with endoscopy and biopsy is the essential diagnostic step.
- For squamous cell carcinoma of the esophagus, exclusion of a tracheo-bronchial fistula is required by esophageal contrast radiography, spiral computed tomography (CT), or bronchoscopy.
- Exclusion of distant metastases is best achieved with multislice spiral CT and/or positron emission tomography (PET).
- Diagnostic laparoscopy is the standard in advanced adenocarcinoma of the distal esophagus before embarking on multimodal approaches.
- The evaluation of the N-category before therapy remains a difficult and unreliable criteria for evaluation.
- T-category stage in esophageal cancer is best evaluated with endoscopic ultrasonography and is necessary for decision-making for further neoadjuvant, multimodal approaches.
- Synchronous carcinoma of the upper airways is common in squamous cell carcinoma and should be excluded by bronchoscopy and direct laryngoscopy.
- Response prediction with a neoadjuvant therapeutic approach is essential to future therapeutic assessment.
- Quantitative measurements of tumor uptake by PET may allow the evaluation of the response to 2 weeks of neoadjuvant therapy.
- Preoperative risk analysis for patients with esophageal cancer defines factors essential to the planned therapeutic approach.
- With high global risk scores, a risk analysis of organ function related to the esophageal surgery is required.
- Patients with hepatic cirrhosis should be excluded generally from esophageal surgery.
- The composite risk score may be utilized to define the cardiorespiratory function and cervical and abdominal vascular status prior to the planned therapeutic protocol.

Basic Diagnosis

As a consequence of dysphagia or other clinically relevant disorders of swallowing, the first diagnostic attempt is performed frequently by general practitioners or gastroenterologists. This is completed by primary endoscopy which leads directly to a diagnosis and histologic conformation. The x-ray or barium swallow is being used less often in recent years. The primary aim in diagnostic workup is to define the reasons for dysphagia. A more detailed diagnosis can be established subsequently. Thus, a comprehensive approach to diagnosis is necessary, because the questions which need to be answered differ widely. (Primary diagnosis: What is the reason for dysphagia? Secondary diagnosis: Is the tumor resectable? Is there evidence of distant metastases?)

Normally a biopsy is taken at the time of the first endoscopy. The discovery of a malignancy of the esophagus is the reason for sending the patient to the oncologist or surgeon. The best therapeutic approach is to refer the patient to an multidisciplinary center in a hospital with comprehensive experience in the treatment of esophageal malignancies ("High Volume Hospitals"). The secondary diagnostic staging can be performed in such a center and is then completed in a logical order.

Specific Diagnosis

The aim of any diagnostic procedure with therapeutic relevance is to identify the R0-resectable patient population. The major operative aim is to achieve complete macroscopic and microscopic tumor resection (❷ *Table 44-1*). These patients should be included in surgical therapeutic protocols. The following diagnostic information is necessary for an individualized decision formulation.

First Step: Topographic-Anatomic Localization and Histology of the Primary Tumor

The first diagnostic step needed to achieve a specific diagnosis of esophageal carcinoma is a repeat endoscopy with multiple biopsies of the primary cancer. Chromoendoscopy with methylene blue and Lugol iodine will enhance the endoscopic determination of extent, thereby allowing directed

◘ Table 44-1

Independent prognostic factors after resection of esophageal cancer (n = 1285). A multivaríate analysis

	B	SE	Wald	df	Significance	Exp (B)
Adenocarcinoma/squamous cell carcinoma	0.696	0.132	27.641	1	0.000	2.005
Sex	−0.269	0.147	3.324	1	0.068	0.764
Age	0.011	0.045	4.374	1	0.036	1.011
Lymph nodes positive	0.036	0.007	24.07	1	0.000	1.037
Lymph nodes total	−0.011	0.004	7.741	1	0.005	0.989
pN (lymph nodes)	0.573	0.102	31.791	1	0.000	1.773
M (distant metastases)	0.284	0.144	3.908	1	0.048	1.329
R (residual tumor)	0.56	0.094	35.817	1	0.000	1.752
G (grading)	0.071	0.078	0.824	1	0.364	1.073
pT (tumorinfiltration)	0.309	0.06	26.39	1	0.000	1.863
Postoperative complications	0.569	0.101	34.747	1	0.000	1.814

biopsies of macroscopically nonvisible early carcinoma and will enhance the identification of sites of multicentric tumor growth. The biopsy is important for verification of histologic type, tumor differentiation, and subsequent tumor grading; this biopsy specimen may be used for future evaluation of molecular prognostic factors.

From the surgeon's perspective, the main criterion for resectability of squamous cell carcinoma of the esophagus is its anatomic relation to the tracheo-bronchial system. With growth, contact of the primary tumor with the tracheo-bronchial system or with evidence of a tracheo-bronchial fistula suggests that curative surgical resection is not possible. The combined resection of esophagus including parts of the tracheo-bronchial system or even a pneumonectomy is technically possible but prognostically ineffective. These advanced surgical approaches are obsolete in the paradigm of the present oncologic approach to esophageal surgery for esophageal cancer.

Especially problematic are esophageal tumors localized in direct relation to the trachea. The tissue layer between esophagus and trachea is very thin; a complete R0-resection is only possible in early carcinoma (T1/T2 infiltration).

To identify the relation of esophageal carcinoma to the tracheo-bronchial system, use of high resolution, multislice spiral CT for study of the mediastinum is recommended. Also, esophageal contrast radiography identifies the relationship of the primary tumor to the tracheal bifurcation. The contrast radiogram will provide evidence optimally of an existing fistula of the tracheo-bronchial system to the mediastinum. Endoscopic ultrasonography (EUS) is ineffective for the diagnosis of tracheo-bronchial infiltration of esophageal carcinoma because of the reduced ability to visualize the airway system.

Second Step: Exclusion of Distant Metastases

In the presence of distant metastases, a surgical resection, even with palliative intent, is unreasonable. In practice, the authors exclude the presence of liver and pulmonary metastases by CT. The fluorodeoxyglucose-positron emission tomography (FDG-PET) is used increasingly to evaluate for distant tumor spread. The FDG-PET is utilized currently for assessment of therapeutic response for prediction of patient outcome after neoadjuvant therapy; therefore, a pretherapeutic FDG-PET is required.

In our opinion, skeletal scintigraphy (bone scan) is not useful in the primary diagnostic approach. Similarly, a bone marrow biopsy to identify isolated tumor cells is only practicable for use in randomized experimental therapeutic studies.

Use of diagnostic laparoscopy in patients with squamous cell carcinoma of the esophagus is of value only to *exclude hepatic cirrhosis*. In contrast, 30% of patients with adenocarcinoma of the distal esophagus are confirmed with diagnostic laparoscopy to harbor occult liver metastases or the presence of peritoneal carcinomatosis despite the false-negative staging information that results with CT (❷ *Table 44-2*). Diagnostic laparoscopy, thus, remains the standard staging approach for advanced adenocarcinoma of the distal esophagus, i.e. before a multimodal approach.

Third Step (Staging In Detail): T- and N-Category of the Primary Tumor

After exclusion of distant metastases in esophageal carcinoma, the therapeutic approach is influenced by the T-category (❷ *Table 44-3*). The evaluation of the N-category preoperatively is difficult, and data

◻ Table 44-2

Information in diagnostic laparoscopy in squamous cell carcinoma or adenocarcinoma of the esophagus (Stein et al., 1997)

	Liver metastases	Peritoneal carcinosis	Tumor cells in abdominal lavage	Liver cirrhosis
Squamous cell carcinoma of the esophagus				
T1/T2-tumor	0/19 (0%)	0/19 (0%)	0/19 (0%)	2/19 (11%)
T3/T4-tumor	3/36 (8%)	0/36 (0%)	0/36 (0%)	5/36 (14%)
Adenocarcinoma of the distal esophagus				
T1/T2-tumor	1/9 (11%)	0/9 (0%)	0/9 (0%)	0/9 (0%)
T3/T4-tumor	4/16 (25%)	3/16 (19%)	4/16 (25%)	0/16 (0%)

◻ Table 44-3

Prevalence of lymph node metastases in adenocarcinoma or squamous cell carcinoma of the esophagus in relation to the pT-category (resected patients at the department of surgery of the Technical University Munich)

	Squamous cell carcinoma of the esophagus	Adenocarcinoma of the esophagus
pT1-category		
Mucosa pT1a	8	0
Submucosa pT1b	36	20
pT2-category	58	67
pT3-category	74	85
pT4-category	79	89

obtained radiographically may be unreliable. Thus, prediction of tumor infiltration in lymph nodes is based principally on the size of the lymph nodes. Direct biopsy of lymph nodes via medianoscopy, thoracotomy, or CT is ill-advised, because regional lymph node metastases do not represent a contraindication for surgery.

The "gold standard" to evaluate the T-category in esophageal carcinoma is the EUS. The predictive value of the T-category with EUS by experienced examiners exceeds 80%. The presence of stenosis secondary to tumor infiltration is a indication of an advanced tumor stage (T3/T4). Additional information of the topographic anatomy, extraluminal growth characteristics, and relationship to surrounding organs is evident with EUS. Conclusions regarding the N-category and R0-resectability are possible via inference from the T-category. With the new multislice spiral CT, enhanced staging criteria for the T-category have been reported (❷ *Table 44-4*).

Special Diagnostic Aspects

●   Exclusion of synchronous carcinoma of the upper airway in esophageal carcinoma.

Synchronous carcinoma of the upper airways is evident in as many as 10% of patients with squamous cell carcinoma of the esophagus. To exclude synchronous carcinoma, we suggest a bronchoscopy and direct laryngoscopy.

◘ Table 44-4

Diagnostic procedures in esophageal carcinoma

Diagnostic procedure	Question
Obligate diagnostic endoscopy and biopsy	Tumor growth and histology
Multislice spiral computed tomography/ esophageal contrast radiogram	Localization and relation to tracheo-bronchial system
CT scan thorax and abdominal	Exclusion of distant metastases
Additional diagnostic procedures	
Endoscopic ultrasonography	Determination of the T-category
Tracheoscopy and biopsy	By esophageal carcinoma with direct localization to the tracheo-bronchial system: exclusion of infiltration
Diagnostic laparoscopy	By advanced (T3/T4) primary adenocarcinoma: exclusion of liver or peritoneal metastases
Direct laryngoscopy	In squamous cell carcinoma: exclusion of synchronous carcinoma of the upper airways

- Response prediction and response evaluation in neoadjuvant therapeutic approaches.

Because only patients with an objective response to neoadjuvant chemotherapy or combination radiochemotherapy benefit from multimodal therapeutic approaches, response prediction remains a subject of active investigation. Actually, only tumor grading represents a clear "predictor" for the outcome after neoadjuvant therapy. Importantly, the presence of the G4-grading or of small cell tumor components in the pretherapeutic biopsy enhances the success of chemotherapy. In studies, the level of ERCC-1-gene expression and thymidylate-synthase activity of the tumor showed remarkable results for the evaluation of response to neoadjuvant polychemotherapy. Unfortunately, definitive, reliable parameters do not exist for the prediction of clinical response or that expected in conventional imaging for patients after use of neoadjuvant chemotherapy or irradiation treatment.

Thus, the identification of novel parameters that predict response and prognosis are crucial for future therapeutic interventions. Post-therapeutic assessment of tumor response by FDG-PET has been shown to correlate with histopathologic tumor regression and patient survival. Furthermore, quantitative measurements of tumor FDG-uptake may allow an early evaluation of the metabolic response to neoadjuvant therapy after only 2 weeks of therapy.

Risk Analysis

Major risk assessment for patients with esophageal carcinoma must include preservation of organ function related to the esophageal surgery (◉ *Table 44-5*). Global risk scores reported in the literature fail principally to evaluate operative risk. In squamous cell carcinoma of the esophagus, preoperative risk analysis includes factors that influence therapeutic decisions. The epidemiologic correlate of a high incidence of alcohol abuse in patients with squamous cell carcinoma of the esophagus requires the analysis of liver function; the exclusion of more advanced cirrhosis (Childs B or C), with all diagnostic approaches (serum albumin, coagulation tests, aminopyrine breath test) and morphologic examination (ultrasonography, CT), including liver biopsy, may be required. Biochemical, radiologic, and histologic evidence of cirrhosis is a relative contraindication to surgical resection of esophageal carcinoma.

Respiratory function has to be evaluated prior to resection of esophageal carcinoma; however, these results provide only a marginal influence on the surgical approach, because postoperative use of respiratory therapy is routine. A detailed evaluation of cardiac and vascular function is recommended in any patient considered for esophagectomy in whom the history, physical examination, chest radiograph, or standard electrocardiogram show any abnormality.

Establishment of a useful risk analysis especially for patients with squamous cell carcinoma of the esophagus categorizes objectively the general status, compliance, and cooperation of the individual patient for these extended surgical procedures. It is imperative to establish the presence preoperatively of chronic alcohol abuse at the time of surgery; the postoperative morbidity is as great as 50% in chronic alcohol abuse. The diagnosis of alcoholism within standard clinical routine may be difficult; in most cases, the treatment of alcohol-related diseases and complications is protracted.

In summary, the risk of esophagectomy in patients with potentially resectable esophageal cancer can be assessed objectively before operative treatment and quantified by the *composite risk score* (❍ *Table 44-6*). Strict inclusion of the risk score in the preoperative decision-making process decreases the postoperative morbidity and mortality. Patients should only be referred for esophagectomy if the risk score reflects a relatively healthy and cooperative patient. In our own experience, up to 30% of the patient population is excluded because of a negative preoperative composite risk score (❍ *Figs. 44-1* and ❍ *44-2*).

◻ Table 44-5

Selection of the therapeutic approach based on pretherapeutic assessment of the resectability of the tumor and functional analysis

General condition	RO-resection possible	RO-resection questionable	Infiltration tracheo-bronchial and/or distant metastases
Good	Primary resection	Multimodal therapy	Palliation
Compromised	Primary resection	Multimodal therapy or definitive CTx/RCTx	Palliation
Severely impaired	Definitive CTx/RCTx Local access (stent, laser therapy)	Definitive CTx/RCTx Local access (stent, laser therapy)	Palliation

◻ Table 44-6

Composite risk score system (Bartels, 1998)

Parameters	Preoperative classification[a]	Weighting factor	Minimum score	Maximum score
General status	1-2-3	4	4	12
Cardiac function	1-2-3	3	3	9
Liver function	1-2-3	2	2	6
Pulmonary function	1-2-3	2	2	6
Composite score			11	33

[a] Preoperative classification: 1 normal, 2 compromised, 3 severely impaired.

◘ Figure 44-1
Diagnostic flow sheet adenocarcinoma (Barrett carcinoma) of the distal esophagus

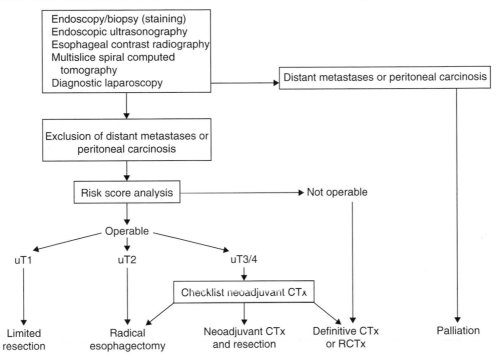

◘ Figure 44-2
Diagnostic flow sheet squamous cell carcinoma of the esophagus

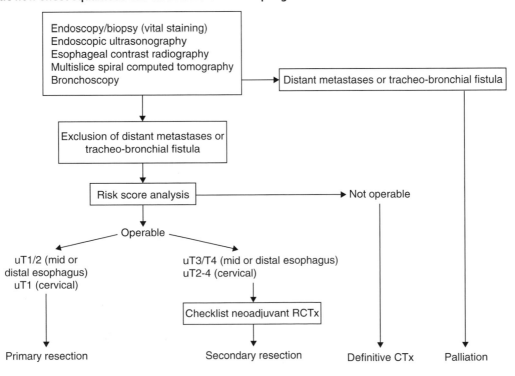

Selected Readings

Bartels H, Stein HJ, Siewert JR (1998) Preoperative risk analysis and postoperative mortality of oesophagectomy for resectable oesophageal cancer. Br J Surg 85:840–844

Dittler HJ, Siewert JR (1993) Role of endoscopic ultrasonography in esophageal carcinoma. Endoscopy 25:156–161

Feith M, Stein HJ, Siewert JR (2006) Adenocarcinoma of the esophagogastric junction: surgical therapy based on 1602 consecutive resected patients. Surg Oncol Clin N Am 15:751–764

Ott K, Weber W, Siewert JR (2006) The importance of PET in the diagnosis and response evaluation of esophageal cancer. Dis Esophagus. 19:433–442

Riedel M, Hauck RW, Stein HJ, et al. (1998) Preoperative bronchoscopic assessment of airway invasion by esophageal cancer: a prospective study. Chest. 113(3):687–695

Siewert JR, Stein HJ, Feith M, et al. (2001) Histologic tumor type is an independent prognostic parameter in esophageal cancer: lessons from more than 1000 consecutive resections at a Single Center in the Western World. Ann Surg 234:360–369

Siewert JR, Stein HJ, Feith M (2003) Surgical approach to invasive adenocarcinoma of the distal esophagus (Barrett's cancer). World J Surg 27:1058–1061

Stein HJ, Feith M (2001) Prognostic factors in cancer of the esophagus. In: Gospodarowicz MK, Henson DE, Hutter RVP, et al. (eds) Prognostic factors in cancer. Wiley-Liss, New York, pp. 237–249

Stein HJ, Kraemer SJ, Feussner H, et al. (1997) Clinical value of diagnostic laparoscopy with laparoscopic ultrasound in patients with cancer of the esophagus or cardia. J Gastrointest Surg 1:167–172

45 Esophageal Cancer: Transhiatal Resection

Hubert J. Stein

Pearls and Pitfalls

- A wide-splitting of the esophageal hiatus and use of special retractors allows good access to the distal esophagus and lower posterior mediastinum.
- Radical resection of the distal esophagus and lymphadenectomy of the lower posterior mediastinum can be achieved transhiatally up to the level of the tracheal bifurcation.
- Transhiatal, distal esophageal resection and transhiatal, subtotal esophageal resection are safer than thoraco-abdominal approaches.
- For most patients with adenocarcinoma of the distal esophagus or esophagogastric junction, transhiatal resection has equivalent outcomes to transthoracic approaches.
- The use of circular stapling devices allows safe construction of esophageal anastomoses through the esophageal hiatus after transhiatal distal esophageal resection.
- The cervical anastomosis remains the "Achilles' heel" of transhiatal subtotal esophagectomy.
- In patients with early esophageal cancer *without* lymph node metastases, a transhiatal resection with preservation of the vagus and undiseased esophagus should be considered as the standard of care.

Introduction

Numerous approaches exist for removing the esophagus in patients with esophageal cancer, most requiring access through the left or right chest in addition to a laparotomy. Removal of the intrathoracic esophagus in a patient with esophageal cancer *without thoracotomy* by employing a transabdominal/transhiatal and transcervical approach was first performed successfully by the British surgeon Turner in the 1930s at a time when thoracotomy was associated with a formidable mortality risk. After the introduction of endotracheal anesthesia and safe techniques of thoracotomy, which permitted transthoracic esophagectomy under direct vision, the technique of transhiatal esophagectomy was almost abandoned for years and used only for removal of a "healthy esophagus" in patients with cervical esophageal cancer, for palliation of incurable esophageal cancer, and for patients with caustic, pharyngo-esophageal strictures. In the 1980s, esophagectomy without thoracotomy was "rediscovered" and perfected and popularized subsequently by Orringer et al. as a safer alternative to abdomino-thoracic or thoraco-abdominal approaches for cancer at virtually every level of the esophagogastric junction and the esophagus. Because the focus of Orringer's approach was clearly to minimize the morbidity of esophagectomy and to palliate malignant dysphagia, others claimed that this approach "ignored" some of the classic principles of cancer surgery (i.e. wide local excision and lymphadenectomy), and therefore the role of transhiatal resection of esophageal cancer as a curative procedure remained controversial.

Clear local resection margins and lymph node status are the dominant prognostic factors after surgical resection in patients with esophageal cancer. The prevalence and patterns of lymphatic spread of esophageal cancer have been shown to be related closely to the depth of invasion, histologic tumor type, and location of the primary neoplasm in the esophagus. Because systematic lymphadenectomy in the upper abdomen and lower posterior mediastinum, but not in the upper mediastinum, is possible with a transhiatal resection, a more differentiated view of the role of the various resection techniques and surgical approaches has emerged recently.

Tumor biology, pattern of lymphatic spread, type of affected patients, and prognosis after surgical resection differs markedly between adenocarcinoma of the esophagogastric junction, adenocarcinoma of the distal esophagus, and squamous cell cancer of the thoracic esophagus. Surgical strategies for treatment of adenocarcinoma arising in the distal esophagus or the vicinity of the esophagogastric junction, therefore, must be planned differently from those for squamous cell cancer of the intrathoracic esophagus. In particular, a subtotal esophagectomy is rarely necessary to achieve a clear proximal margin for a distal esophageal adenocarcinoma or adenocarcinoma of the esophagogastric junction invading the distal esophagus. These concepts are in marked contrast to those in squamous cell esophageal cancer, where extensive submucosal spread and multicentricity within the entire esophagus is not uncommon. Furthermore, in contrast to squamous cell esophageal cancer, lymphatic metastases are found predominantly in the lower posterior mediastinum and upper abdomen in patients with adenocarcinoma of the distal esophagus or esophagogastric junction. While at most centers a transthoracic approach with subtotal esophagectomy and systematic mediastinal lymphadenectomy is considered standard for patients with squamous cell esophageal cancer, a distal esophageal resection with lymphadenectomy of the lower posterior mediastinum and upper abdomen may suffice for many, if not most, patients with adenocarcinoma at or close to the esophagogastric junction.

Based on these data, the surgical approaches to esophageal cancer should be tailored to the required oncologic radicality for complete tumor removal and locoregional lymph node clearance. The perceived benefits of surgical radicality must then be balanced against the risk of the procedure. With this concept, transhiatal approaches to the esophagus have a firm place in the armamentarium of individualized surgical treatment strategies for esophageal cancer, particularly in patients with adenocarcinoma of the distal esophagus or esophagogastric junction.

Three entirely different approaches are referred to as "transhiatal esophageal resection" or "esophageal resection without thoracotomy":

1. Transhiatal resection of the distal esophagus with an anastomosis to the remnant esophagus performed transhiatally in the lower posterior mediastinum
2. Transhiatal subtotal esophagectomy with an anastomosis to the remnant cervical esophagus performed in the neck
3. Limited and vagal-sparing transhiatal esophageal resection for early carcinoma without lymph node metastases

These procedures differ markedly in the extent of esophageal resection and lymphadenectomy and must be differentiated when discussing the merits and risks of "transhiatal resection."

Transhiatal Resection of the Distal Esophagus with Lower Mediastinal Anastomosis

In patients with adenocarcinoma at or in the vicinity of the esophagogastric junction, a subtotal esophagectomy is required only rarely to achieve clear proximal resection margins. Rather, a complete resection of the primary tumor can in most instances also be achieved with clear proximal margins via a transhiatal access through a laparotomy only. Furthermore, lymphatic spread of such neoplasms is directed predominantly toward the lower posterior mediastinum and the upper abdomen. Consequently, in most instances, there is no need to perform a lymphadenectomy of the proximal mediastinum. A wide anterior or left lateral splitting of the esophageal hiatus and insertion of specially designed, extra-long retractors through the hiatus into the mediastinum allows good access up to the level of the tracheal bifurcation and facilitates complete clearance of the lymphatic tissue in the lower posterior mediastinum (❯ *Fig. 45-1*). Resection of up to 10 cm of the distal esophagus together with a lymphadenectomy up to the tracheal bifurcation is possible through this approach. Circular stapler devices allow a safe anastomosis with the remnant esophagus in the lower mediastinum without thoracotomy (❯ *Fig. 45-2*).

In the author's experience, the oncologic results and the long-term outcome of this approach are at least as good as those with the more radical abdomino-thoracic procedures with a two-field or three-field lymphadenectomy, while the surgical procedure was safer and the postoperative course smoother when thoracotomy was avoided. This experience was recently confirmed by a prospective, randomized study from the National Cancer Center in Tokyo. In this study, the abdominothoracic approach was associated with a higher postoperative mortality rate and a significantly higher postoperative overall morbidity as compared to the transhiatal approach. There were no significant differences in long-term survival between the two procedures. Thus, a thoracotomy with subtotal esophagectomy and proximal

◻ **Figure 45-1**
Wide exposure of the distal esophagus and lower posterior mediastinum after splitting of the esophageal hiatus. Left: graphic depiction. Right: intraoperative view. (Left figure modified from Siewert et al., 2006. With kind permission of Springer Science and Business Media)

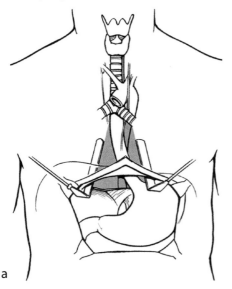
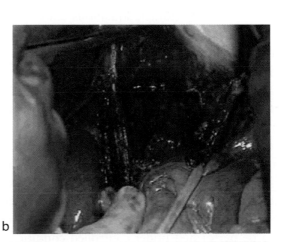

a

b

◘ Figure 45-2

Esophago-intestinal end-to-side anastomosis in the lower posterior mediastinum after transhiatal distal esophageal resection. Left: end-to-side anastomosis with a circular stapler device. Right: graphic depiction of a completed esophagojejunostomy immediately below the level of the tracheal bifurcation after total gastrectomy and transhiatal resection of the distal esophagus

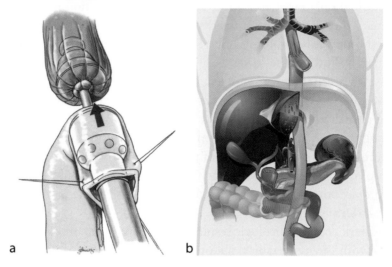

a   b

mediastinal lymphadenectomy is *not* necessary for the vast majority of patients with adenocarcinoma of the gastric cardia or subcardiac region, even when distal esophageal invasion is present. The thoracotomy only adds morbidity without a survival benefit. Rather, a pure transabdominal/transhiatal approach is the access of choice, whenever a clear oral resection margin can be achieved by this procedure.

Transhiatal Subtotal Esophagectomy with Cervical Anastomosis

Transhiatal subtotal esophagectomy with a cervical anastomosis is the procedure popularized by Orringer and colleagues in the early 1980s. Although the principles of surgical oncology for procedures aiming at cure (wide local excision and lymphadenectomy) argue against the use of this procedure for patients with intrathoracic squamous cell cancer, the advantage of this approach for patients with adenocarcinoma of the distal esophagus which cannot be resected completely through an abdominal approach alone. Additionally, another indication for the approach is evident with poor pulmonary function who may not tolerate thoracotomy. The procedure encompasses both an abdominal and transhiatal mobilization and cervical esophago-gastric anastomosis. In modification of Orringer's more palliative viewpoint, a wide splitting of the esophageal hiatus and retraction of the diaphragmatic crura laterally and the heart anteriorly also allows a lymphadenectomy of the lower posterior mediastinum and wide local excision of distal esophageal neoplasms. "En bloc" mobilization of the distal esophagus and all surrounding tissues including both mediastinal pleural sheets is possible under direct vision up to the level of the tracheal bifurcation (❯ *Fig. 45-3*). The "blind" and "blunt" phase of the operation is then restricted to only a few centimeters of the retrotracheal, intrathoracic esophagus (❯ *Fig. 45-4*). With the use of a modified mediastinoscope inserted through the neck incision, this part of the operation may also be performed under controlled conditions and lymph node biopsies in this area becomes

◘ Figure 45-3
Wide local excision of the distal esophagus and surrounding structures with a transhiatal approach (Modified from Siewert et al., 2006. With kind permission of Springer Science and Business Media)

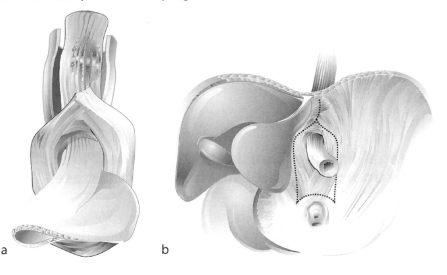

a   b

◘ Figure 45-4
The "blunt" and "blind" phase of transhiatal subtotal esophagectomy via an abdominal and cervical incision. Left: graphic depiction. Right: intraoperative view: two fingers of the left hand of the surgeon mobilize the proximal intrathoracic esophagus from the posterior wall of the trachea. The right hand is inserted into the mediastinum through the hiatus mobilizing the proximal esophagus from below (Left figure modified from Siewert et al., 2006. With kind permission of Springer Science and Business Media)

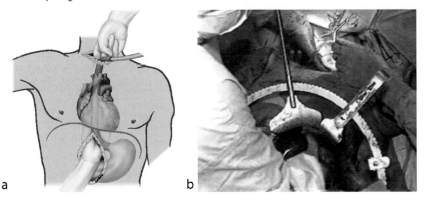

a   b

possible. Nevertheless, even with this technical support, one must realize that a formal lymphadenectomy in the upper mediastinum will not possible with the transhiatal and transcervical access.

The need for a cervical anastomosis remains the major problem of this procedure. Although cervical anastomotic leaks pose a lesser problem during the postoperative course compared with intrathoracic anastomotic leaks, cervical leaks are more common and usually result in strictures requiring repeated dilatations.

Recently, a large, prospective, randomized trial from the Netherlands by Hulscher and colleagues compared transhiatal subtotal esophagectomy with abdominothoracic esophagectomy in patients with adenocarcinoma of the distal esophagus or gastric cardia. Transhiatal subtotal esophagectomy was associated with fewer postoperative complications (in particular pulmonary complications), shorter postoperative mechanical ventilation time, a shorter postoperative stay in an intensive care unit, and a shorter overall hospital stay. Although survival analysis showed a trend toward a prognostic benefit in the patients with a more radical abdominothoracic approach, this difference was not significant on statistical analysis. Compared with abdominothoracic esophagectomy, a transhiatal subtotal esophagectomy has been established to be a less invasive and a safer approach to patients with adenocarcinoma of the distal esophagus or gastric cardia, without a significant loss in long-term prognosis. This technique, therefore, can be advocated for patients with distal esophageal adenocarcinoma particularly if, due to preexisting comorbidity, a thoracotomy is perceived as hazardous or risky, and a transhiatal resection of the distal esophagus alone does not permit complete tumor removal.

Limited and Vagal-Sparing Transhiatal Esophageal Resection for Early Esophageal Carcinoma without Lymph Node Metastases

Due to endoscopic surveillance programs and an increased awareness in industrialized nations, esophageal cancer is diagnosed increasingly at early stages, particularly in patients with known precancerous lesions, e.g. Barrett's esophagus. Large studies indicate that lymph node metastases are virtually absent if the neoplasm is limited to the mucosa. Consequently, systematic lymphadenectomy is not needed in such patients. Many of these patients are treated by endoscopic ablation or endoscopic resection. These endoscopic techniques, however, do not address the underlying precancerous epithelium or the multicentricity of such neoplasms. Recurrences are common after endoscopic intervention for early esophageal cancer. Because no lymphatic spread is anticipated in such patients, more limited, local techniques of resection with lesser morbidity preserve more healthy esophagus and minimize organ dysfunction and are thus suited ideally for these patients. Transhiatal approaches to esophageal resection meet these requirements. Several such procedures have been reported in recent years. In patients with early adenocarcinoma or a high grade intraepithelial neoplasia ("high grade dysplasia") arising in Barrett's esophagus, a limited transhiatal resection of the distal esophageal segment affected with the Barrett's metaplasia and reconstruction with jejunal interposition provides cure and preserves undiseased esophagus (❷ *Fig. 45-5*). Because vagal innervation of the upper gastrointestinal tract and the gastric reservoir function can be preserved, this approach is associated with a very good quality of life. Vagal-sparing, subtotal transhiatal esophagectomy is another alternative in such patients with a reported very good quality of life.

Summary

Transhiatal approaches to esophageal resection have been proven to be safer than abdominothoracic esophagectomy. In patients with adenocarcinoma of the distal esophagus and esophagogastric junction, a transhiatal resection of the distal esophagus in combination with lymphadenectomy of the lower posterior mediastinum is oncologically equivalent to more radical procedures employing thoracotomy and systematic mediastinal lymph node dissection. With modern circular stapling devices, safe anastomoses with the esophageal remnant can be performed transhiatally up to the level of the tracheal bifurcation. The cervical anastomosis remains the "Achilles' heel" of transhiatal subtotal esophagectomy. In patients with early esophageal cancer without lymphatic spread, transhiatal vagal-sparing approaches should be the standard of care.

◘ Figure 45-5
Graphic depiction of a limited transhiatal distal esophageal resection with jejunal interposition

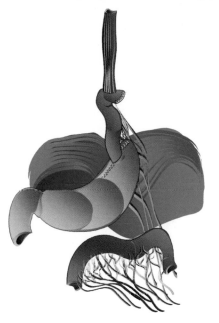

Selected Readings

Banki F, Mason RJ, DeMeester SR, et al. (2002) Vagal-sparing esophagectomy: a more physiologic alternative. Ann Surg 236:324–336

Bumm R, Feussner H, Bartels H, et al. (1997) Radical transhiatal esophagectomy with two-field lymphadenectomy and endodissection for distal esophageal adenocarcinoma. World J Surg 21:822–831

Hulscher JB, van Sandick JW, de Boer AG, et al. (2002) Extended transthoracic resection compared with limited transhiatal resection for adenocarcinoma of the esophagus. N Engl J Med 347:1662–1669

Kitajima M, Kitagawa Y (2002) Surgical treatment of esophageal cancer – the advent of the era of individualization. N Engl J Med 347:1705–1709

Orringer MB, Marshall B, Iannettoni MD (1999) Transhiatal esophagectomy: clinical experience and refinements. Ann Surg 230:392–404

Sasako M, Sano T, Yamamoto S, et al. (2006) Left thoracoabdominal approach versus abdominaltranshiatal approach for gastric cancer of the cardia or subcardia: a randomised controlled trial. Lancet Oncol 7:644–651

Siewert JR, Feith M, Werner M, Stein HJ (2000) Adenocarcinoma of the esophagogastric junction. Results of surgical therapy based on anatomical/topographic classification in 1,002 consecutive patients. Ann Surg 232:353–361

Siewert JR, Stein HJ, Feith M (2006) Ösophaguskarzinom. In: Siewert JR, Rothmun M, Schumpelick V (eds) Praxis der Viszeralchirurgie, Siewert Onkologische Chirurgie, 2nd edn. Springer-Verlag, Heidelberg, pp 403–434

Stein HJ, Feith M, Brücher BLDM, et al. (2005) Early esophageal cancer: pattern of lymphatic spread and prognostic factors for long term survival after surgical resection. Ann Surg 242:566–572

46 Transthoracic Esophagectomy

Toni Lerut · Willy Coosemans · Georges Decker · Paul De Leyn · Philippe Nafteux ·
Dirk Van Raemdonck

Pearls and Pitfalls

- Lymphatic dissemination occurs early in the natural history of cancer of the esophagus and gastroesophageal junction.
- The pattern of lymphatic dissemination is difficult to predict, irrespective of the localization of the primary tumor.
- Intramural "jump-metastases" are common because of an extensive submucosal lymphatic plexus.
- Wide periesophageal "en bloc" resection and extensive two-field lymphadenectomy (three-field lymphadenectomy for middle- and proximal-third carcinomas) offer superior technique to obtain a macroscopic and microscopic complete R0 resection.
- Because of the preferential cephalad lymphatic dissemination, right-sided transthoracic esophagectomy is the preferred approach for supracarinal tumors.
- Distal-third esophageal and gastroesophageal junction cancers often have lymphatic dissemination along the lesser curvature toward the celiac axis. The left thoracoabdominal approach provides excellent exposure to combine radical resection in the chest with a DII lymphadenectomy in the superior abdominal compartment.
- Primary radical esophagectomy results in overall 5-year survival of 30–40% and 20–25% for advanced stage III and IV disease, respectively. These figures are the gold standard to which all other therapeutic modalities should be compared.
- One year following esophagectomy, quality of life scores return to baseline for the majority of patients.
- Minimally invasive thoracoscopic and laparoscopic esophagectomy may evolve to the preferred approach for early (T1) carcinoma of the esophagus and GE junction.

Introduction

The surgical treatment strategy of esophageal carcinoma is complex and the long term outcome of surgical therapy is often disappointing. Surgical resection can be impeded by the contiguous anatomic relations of the esophagus with the trachea, both main-stem bronchi and, more distally, the pericardium, aorta, and diaphragm. A malignancy arising from the esophagus may easily invade these adjacent organs, which makes the tumor surgically unresectable. Additionally, lymphatic dissemination is an early event and has a negative influence on survival. Lymph node metastases are found in less than 5% of intramucosal tumors, but in 30–40% of submucosal tumors. The esophageal wall is characterized by an extensive submucosal lymphatic plexus, which supplies a drainage route for early dissemination and gives rise to "jump-metastases" (i.e. lymph nodes adjacent to the primary tumor are unaffected, but more distant-located lymph nodes contain metastases).

Transmural tumors are showing lymph node involvement in over 80% and the number of involved nodes increases with the volume of the tumor.

Principles of Surgical Treatment

It is generally accepted that surgical resection should only be performed with curative intent. Resection is ill-advised when macroscopically incomplete, due to invasion of adjacent structures and/or non-resectable metastases are to be expected. Absolute contra-indications for esophagectomy include local tumor invasion of non-resectable neighboring structures (T_4), carcinomatosis peritonei, hematogenous parenchymatous metastases involving the liver and non-resectable metastatic lymph nodes.

The pattern of lymphatic dissemination is difficult to predict, but carcinomas of the proximal and middle thirds of the esophagus preferably metastasize to the cervical region, whereas more distal-lying tumors and tumors of the gastro-esophageal junction more commonly metastasize to the lymph nodes around the celiac axis.

Resectable metastatic lymph nodes in the region of the primary tumor, including the celiac trunk and its trifurcation removed with distal third tumors and cervical nodes for middle and proximal tumors, are not necessarily a contra-indication for surgery. The presence of lymph node metastases, however, has a negative influence on survival, even following extensive lymphadenectomy.

Macroscopic as well as microscopic completeness (R_0) of resection is the ultimate goal of esophagectomy. Thus, optimal pre-operative staging is of paramount importance as well as individual case presentation and discussion at the multidisciplinary tumor board.

Optimal staging today includes endoscopy and biopsy, which are followed with echoendoscopy, high resolution CT scan, and PET scan.

Before embarking on major surgery, careful evaluation of medical operability is essential. Indeed many patients present with a history of alcohol and tobacco abuse requiring careful evaluation of cardiovascular, pulmonary, and liver functions.

Early-stage lymphatic dissemination, as well as completeness of tumoral resection (R_0), pose challenges for radical surgical treatment and are still debatable. The concept of extensive en bloc resections was reported in 1963 by Logan, but its associated mortality of more than 20% in the original report, discouraged general acceptance. Skinner and Akiyama reintroduced the concept of en bloc resection combined with extensive lymphadenectomy. Ultimately, they were able to reduce operative mortality to 5%, with 5-year survival rates of 18% and 42%, respectively.

The radical en bloc resection, as opposed to the *standard resection*, aims at performing the wide, radical peritumoral nodal resection of the middle and distal thirds of the posterior mediastinum.

The two-field lymph node dissection. The early lymphatic dissemination, by means of longitudinal spread along the esophagus via the submucosal plexus to the upper mediastinum and abdomen, has advanced the advocacy of Japanese researchers for the two-field lymphadenectomy. This approach provides wide local excision of the primary tumor with lymphadenectomy of the entire posterior mediastinum; this technique includes resection of subcarinal nodes and nodes along the left recurrent nerve and the brachiocephalic trunk. Lymph nodes contiguous with the celiac trunk, common hepatic and splenic arteries, as well as the lymph nodes along the lesser gastric curvature and lesser omentum, are included.

The three-field lymph node dissection. The pattern of lymphatic dissemination is not restricted to the thorax and abdomen. About 20% of the patients with distal tumors present with metastasis in the cervical region. This metastatic pattern initiated consideration of the three-field lymph node dissection. In this operation, besides the already mentioned removal of thoracic and abdominal nodes, the cervical field is dissected, includes the paraesophageal, carotid vessel adenopathy, and supraclavicular nodes.

These considerations on radicality of resection and extent of lymphadenectomy are the rationale that justifies the *transthoracic approach* as opposed to the *transhiatal approach*. The rationale for the transhiatal esophagectomy is merely based on an effort to decrease perioperative morbidity and possibly postoperative mortality. Recent observations indicate that the results of radical esophagectomy are superior to those formerly quoted; contemporary results suggest overall 5-year survival figures that approach 40%.

Technique

Esophageal tumors situated in the proximal and middle thirds of the intrathoracic esophagus are probably best approached via the *right* thoracic cavity. In contrast, distal tumors and tumors of the gastro-esophageal junction are best approached from the *left* side.

When the transthoracic approach is used, double lumen endotracheal intubation with intra-operative deflation of the lung at the operative side greatly facilitates the dissection in the posterior mediastinum.

The most commonly used transthoracic approaches are the Ivor Lewis (two hole) and Mc Keown (three hole) right thoracic approach and the left-sided approach through a left thoracophrenolaparotomy.

Ivor Lewis Procedure (Esophagectomy with Dorsolateral Thoracotomy)

The procedure can be started either by a laparotomy followed by thoracotomy or vice versa (Clark et al., 1994). When the operation is initiated by laparotomy, the procedure is commenced by mobilization of the stomach. The esophagus is mobilized in the hiatus. After resection of the lesser curvature, a gastric tube is fashioned. The abdominal part is completed with a lymphadenectomy of the superior abdominal compartment, i.e. the lymph nodes along the celiac trunk and its branches, the splenic and common hepatic artery (DII lymphadenectomy).

After closure of the laparotomy the patient is repositioned in the left lateral decubitus position and a standard posterolateral right thoracotomy is performed, entering the chest through the fifth intercostal space. This access allows a perfect visualization of the posterior mediastinum. The esophagus is removed en bloc with its adjacent structures and is dissected from the vertebral body to the pericardium (❯ *Fig. 46-1*). The resection includes the removal of all tumor bearing esophagus surrounded by a wide envelope of adjacent tissues. To do so, the azygos vein and its associated nodes are removed with the thoracic duct, subcarinal nodes, para-esophageal nodes, all in continuity with the resected esophagus. The resected specimen also incorporates the mediastinal pleura on both sides. When indicated for middle and proximal third carcinoma, a meticulous dissection of the lymph nodes along the left recurrent nerve and the brachio-cephalic trunk may be performed in the same intervention. The gastric tube which has been

■ Figure 46-1

En bloc esophagectomy. All tissues surrounding the esophagus including azygos vein en thoracic duct are left on the specimen. The aorta shows its ligated intercostals vessels and esophageal bronchial arteries. The subcarinal nodes are removed en bloc with the specimen (Reprinted from Skinner, 1983. Copyright 1983. With permission from the American Association for Thoracic Surgery)

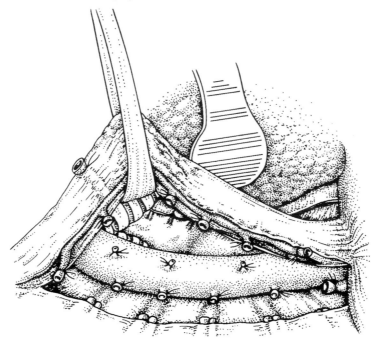

temporarily fixed to the remainder of the lesser curvature is pulled into the chest; an anastomosis is fashioned high in the apex of the chest will complete the procedure.

Mc keown Procedure (Esophagectomy with Anterolateral Thoracotomy and Cervical Anastomosis)

In this procedure the patient is placed in a supine position but with slight elevation of the right side of the chest (Hulscher et al., 2002; ❷ *Fig. 46-2*). This position allows for a synchronous abdominal midline laparotomy. A right anterolateral thoracotomy in the fourth or fifth intercostal space and a cervical incision on either the right or left side. The technique of gastric mobilization, abdominal lymphadenectomy, and transthoracic mobilization of the esophagus is essentially the same as described in the previous operation. The anastomosis is performed via a separate left cervicotomy through which the proximal esophagus and the attached gastric tube are pulled up into the operative field. The main disadvantage of this operation is however that the extent of radicality; lymphadenectomy is more difficult to achieve as compared to the previously described technique.

Left Thoracoabdominal Approach

The left thoracic approach is considered by many authors as the standard approach for carcinoma of the lower esophagus and cardia (❷ *Fig. 46-3*). The operation was popularized by Sweet. The left

McKeown technique. Illustration of the incisions. The intervention can also be performed without having to turn the patient avoiding a need for repeat preparation and draping. The right thoracotomy is usually made in the fourth interspace (Reprinted from Pearson, 1995. Copyright 1995. With permission from Elsevier)

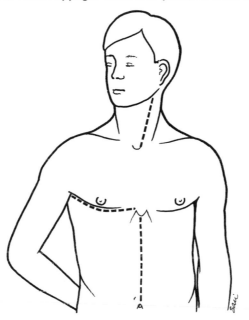

postero-lateral approach may be extended anteriorly across the costal margin as advocated by Belsey. This provides a true thoracoabdominal exposure of both the superior abdominal compartment and posterior mediastinum. With this approach, the chest is entered through the sixth intercostal space. After dividing the costal margin, the diaphragm is incised at its periphery as an inverted T-shape incision, the short limb of the T incising the abdominal wall over a few centimeters. This approach allows an optimal direct vision for both the abdominal and chest cavities via one single incision. As a result, through this incision maximum exposure/resection can be achieved. The entire thoracic esophagus can be dissected through the left-sided approach. The dissection of the esophagus from beneath the aortic arch requires ligation and transection of the bronchial arteries just below the arch. The mobilization is then continued by blunt finger dissection behind the aortic arch and up into the apex of the chest. The mediastinal pleura above the aortic arch is opened. After transecting the esophagus at a level below the cardia, the esophagus is pulled and delivered through the opened mediastinal pleura above the aortic arch and transected. Lymphadenectomy in both the abdomen and posterior mediastinum can be performed. After resecting the esophagus, the gastric tube is brought upward through the hiatus and behind the aortic arch and temporarily fixed to the esophageal stump in the apex of the chest. The incision is then closed and the patient is turned to a supine position. Through a left cervicotomy, the esophageal stump with the attached gastric tube is exteriorized into the operative field and a cervical esophagogastrostomy is performed. This cervical part of the operation can be combined with a bilateral lymphadenectomy (third field) through a U-shape incision in the neck. In the three-field lymphadenectomy, lymph nodes along the trachea and upper esophagus as well as lymph nodes in the lateral compartment (i.e. deep external cervical and deep lateral cervical regions), are removed bilaterally.

◘ Figure 46-3

Left thoracoabdominal approach. The chest is entered through the sixth intercostal space. After dividing the costochondral margin an inverted T shaped incision is made in the diaphragm at its periphery taking care to avoid injury to the phrenic nerve (Reprinted from Lerut and Van Lanschot, 2004)

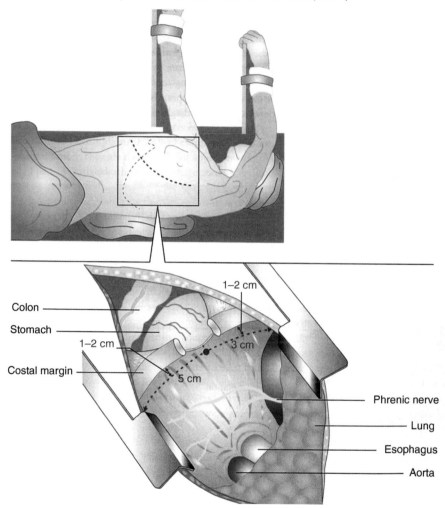

Minimally Invasive Esophagectomy

In an effort to limit the physiologic stress of esophagectomy while preserving the principle of en bloc resection, a minimally invasive approach to esophageal resection allowing the same type of resection compared to the transthoracic approach has been developed (❯ *Fig. 46-4*).

The best indications for minimally invasive esophagectomy (MIE) are Barrett's high grade dysplasia or small tumors (T1a or eventually T1b without suspicious nodes). The patient is intubated with a single lumen tube and positioned supine in the jackknife position. The first port is placed in the right paramedian position after a CO_2 pneumoperitoneum is established to a pressure of 15 mmHg. The remaining four ports are placed under laparoscopic visualization.

The stomach is mobilized using the ultrasonic sheers and clips where necessary. Care is taken during this dissection to preserve the gastroepiploic arcade. With the greater and lesser curves

◘ Figure 46-4
a. Total thoracoscopic – laparoscopic esophagectomy. Position of the trocars. b. Mobilization of the esophagus with division of azygos vein. c. Completed reconstruction (Reprinted from Luketich, 2003 Copyright 2003 with permission of Annals of Surgery)

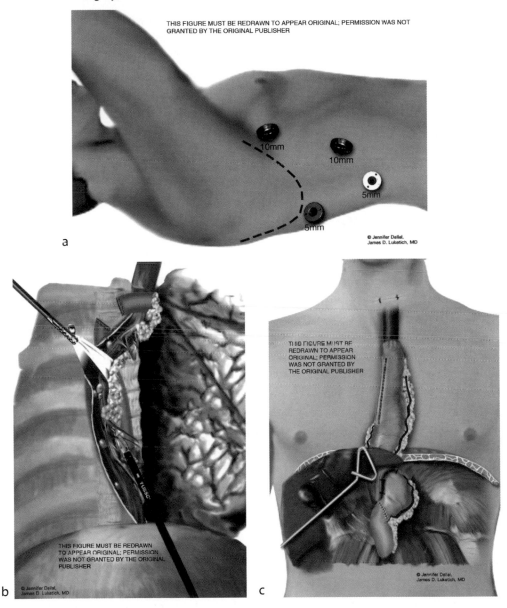

mobilized, the stomach can be retracted superiorly allowing exposure of the left gastric vessels, and dissection of the left gastric and celiac axis lymph nodes. The vascular pedicle is divided with an endovascular stapler, most easily with the lesser curve exposure.

A narrow gastric tube is constructed by dividing the stomach starting at the distal lesser curve, following transection of the right gastric vessels. Careful, atraumatic construction of the gastric tube is critical. Every effort is made to minimize traumatic grasping of the stomach during the dissection. The gastric tube is then sutured to the stomach at the distal resection margin. The next step in the abdominal operation includes dissection of the phrenoesophageal ligament, which opens the plane into the thoracic cavity.

The patient is then intubated with a left-sided double lumen endotracheal tube and positioned in the full left lateral decubitus for right thoracoscopy; the right lung is deflated. Four thoracoscopic ports are introduced into the right hemithorax. The azygos vein is divided with an endovascular stapler. The esophagus is dissected circumferentially. Care is taken to avoid injury to the right or left main stem bronchi as the subcarinal nodes are removed en bloc with the specimen. During mobilization, thoracic duct lymphatic channels and aorto-esophageal vessels should be carefully divided. The dissection is carried superiorly into the thoracic inlet. Dissection of all mediastinal lymphatics including paraesophageal nodes, subcarinal nodes, nodes along the recurrent laryngeal nerve, and nodes along the brachiocephalic trunk up to the lower cervical lymph nodes is possible.

The esophagogastric specimen is then pulled up out through the left cervical incision and the anastomosis is fashioned in a separate cervical incision.

The Debate: Lesser or More Radical Approach

Over the years, controversy remained as to the radicality of resection and extent of lymphadenectomy. Those who believe that lymph node involvement equates to systemic disease will advocate a simple resection and reconstruction, typically via a *transhiatal approach.*

Advocates of more radical surgery suggest that the natural course of the disease may be influenced in a positive way by radical esophagectomy and extensive (two- or three-field) lymphadenectomy typically performed through a transthoracic approach. Although several publications both from Japan and the West seem to indicate a benefit in favor of the more radical approach, definitive proof is lacking. More radical resections seem to result in overall survival rates between 35% to 50% (❯ *Table 46-1A*), whereas transhiatal resection has 5-year survival rates between 15% to 20% (❯ *Table 46-1B*), but these non-randomized data may have been influenced by selection bias.

Hulscher et al. recently published a randomized trial comparing limited transhiatal resection versus transthoracic resection with extended en bloc lymph node dissection for adenocarcinoma of the esophagus and GEJ. Although no statistically significant overall difference was evident, there was

◻ Table 46-1A

Survival after radical surgery

Author		N pat.	3-year survival	5-year survival
Ando	Ann Surg 2000	419	52%	40%
Akiyama	Ann Surg 1994	913	52,6%	42.4%
Isono	Oncology 1991	1,740	42%	34.3%
JCOG9204	JCO 2003	242	65%	52%
Lerut	Ann Surg 2004	174	55%	42%
Collard	Ann Surg 2001	235 R0	65%	49%
		324 R0–R2	50%	35%
Hagen	Ann Surg 2001	100	60%	52%
Altorki	Ann Surg 2001	111	52%	40%
Hulscher	NEJM 2002	114	42%	40%

▢ Table 46-1B

Survival after radical surgery, Stage III (T$_{3-4}$N$_1$)

Author		N pat.	5-year survival
Ando	Ann Surg 2000	201	37,6
Akiyama	Ann Surg 1994	175	27% (2F)/56% (3F)
Baba	Ann Surg 1994	22	30%
Lerut	J Thor Cardiovasc Surg	162	26%
Collard	Ann Surg 2001	98	30%
Hagen	Ann Surg 2001	32	26%
Altorki	JTCVS 1997	33	34.5% (4 year)

a clear long-term trend in favor of the more extensive approach, in particular for adenocarcinoma of the distal esophagus. From the Japanese data and some series in Western centers, it seems that cervical lymphadenectomy (three-field) may offer a survival advantage for patients with supra-carinal tumors. In squamous cell carcinoma, Alkorki reported a 5-year survival of 40% and Lerut obtained for middle-third squamous cell carcinoma a 5-year survival of 28% following three-field lymphadenectomy in patients with positive cervical lymph node. These results definitively question the value of the actual UICC/TNM staging of these tumors in which cervical lymph node involvement is classified as Stage IV disease, and which is generally considered as a non-curable disease. Outcomes data further suggest the influence of hospital volume indicating the potential beneficial effect of centralization of esophagectomy as suggested by an increasing number of publications.

Quality of Life After Operation

The intent of potentially curative resection and reconstruction in symptomatic esophageal cancer patients is improvement in their quality of life, even when the resection is only considered palliative. Both curative and palliative surgery improves food passage. The nature of the operation – transhiatal versus transthoracic, or the position of the proximal anastomosis – high thoracic versus cervical, provides only limited effect on the quality of life. Gastro-esophageal reflux and dumping syndrome are encountered in more than half of the patients. Twenty to 25% of patients also encounter problems ingesting solid food as a result of the relative stenosis of the proximal anastomosis. An anastomosis at the cervical level has a significantly *lower* probability of symptomatic reflux than one positioned within the thorax; however, the thorax anastomosis has a higher probability of leakage and benign stricturing. Global quality scores reveal a significant decrease in physical and role functional scales with an increase in fatigue, nausea, pain, dyspnea, deglutition, and GI symptoms. However, a gradual improvement is noticed over time; one year following resection, patients not suffering from tumor recurrence consider their quality of life comparable to that of their pre-disease state. Ten years after operation two-thirds of the surviving patients appear to maintain satisfactory ability for solid-food ingestion.

A disturbing finding at long term follow-up however is the development of metaplastic columnar mucosa in the cervical esophagus after esophagectomy. This most likely results as a consequence of acid and bile reflux. The true importance and risk for malignant degeneration of this observation is not yet known.

Selected Readings

Akiyama H, Tsurumaru M, Kawamura T, Ono Y (1981) Principles of surgical treatment for carcinoma of the esophagus: analysis of lymph node involvement. Ann Surg 194:438–446

Akiyama H, Tsurumaru M, Udagawa H, Kajiyama Y (1994) Radical lymph node dissection for cancer of the thoracic esophagus. Ann Surg 220:364–373

Altorki N, Kent M, Ferrara C, Port J (2002) Three-field lymph node dissection for squamous cell and adenocarcinoma of the esophagus. Ann Surg 236:177–183

Belsey RH (1988) Surgical exposure of the esophagus. In: Skinner DBJ, Belsey RH (eds) Management of esophageal disorders. W.B. Saunders, Philadelphia, pp. 192–201

Birkmeyer JD, Siewers AE, Finlayson EV, et al. (2002) Hospital volume and surgical mortality in the United States. N Engl J Med 346:1128–1137

Clark GW, Peters JH, Ireland AP et al. (1994) Nodal metastasis and sites of recurrence after en bloc esophagectomy for adenocarcinoma. Ann Thorac Surg 58:646–654

Hulscher JB, van Sandlick JW, de Boer AG, et al. (2002) Extended transthoracic resection compared with limited transhiatal resection for adenocarcinoma of the esophagus. N Engl J Med 347:1662–1669. See also N Engl J Med 2003, 348:1177–1174

Kato H, Watanabe H, Tachimori Y, Iizuka T (1991) Evaluation of neck lymph node dissection for thoracic esophageal carcinoma. Ann Thorac Surg 51:931–935

Lerut T, Nafteux P, Moons J, et al. (2004) Three field lymphadenectomy for carcinoma of the esophagus and gastroesophageal junction in 174 R_0 resections. Impact on staging, disease free survival and outcome. A plea for adaptation of the TNM classification in upperhalf esophageal carcinoma. Ann Surg 240:962–974

Lerut T, Van Lanschot J (2004) Cancer of the esophagus and gastro-esophageal junction: surgical aspects, Chapter 3. In: Van Lanschot J, Gouma D, Jansen P, et al. (eds) Integrated medical and surgical gastroenterology. Bohn Stafleu Van Loghum, Houten, The Netherlands

Lewis I (1946) The surgical treatment of carcinoma of the esophagus with special reference to a new operation for growths of the middle third. Br J Surg 34:18–31

Logan A (1963) The surgical treatment of carcinoma of the esophagus and cardia. J Thorac Cardiovasc Surg 46:150–161

Luketich JD, Alvelo-Rivera M, Buenaventura PO, et al. (2003) Minimally invasive esophagectomy: outcomes in 222 patients. Ann Surg 238:486–494

McKeown KC (1976) Total three-stage esophagectomy for cancer of the esophagus. Br J Surg 63:259–262

McLarthy AJ, Deschamps C, Trastek VF, et al. (1997) Esoophageal resection for cancer of the esophagus: long-term function and quality of life. Ann Thorac Surg 63:1568–1572

Oberg S, Johansson J, Wenner J, Walther B (2002) Metaplastic columnar mucosa in the cervical esophagus after esophagectomy. Ann Surg 235:338–345

Pearson FG (1995) Synchronous combined abdominothoraco-cervical esophagectomy, Chapter 42. In: Pearson FG, Deslauriers J, Ginsberg RJ, et al. (eds) Esophageal surgery. Churchill Livingstone, New York

Skinner DB (1983) En bloc resection for neoplasms of the esophagus and cardia. J Thorac Cardiovasc Surg 65:59–71

Sweet RH (1945) Surgical management of carcinoma of the midthoracic esophagus. Preliminary report. N Engl J Med 433:1–7

Part 3

Stomach: Benign and Malignant

47 Peptic Ulcer Disease and *Helicobacter Pylori*

Kent-Man Chu

Pearls and Pitfalls

- *Helicobacter pylori* plays a prominent role in upper gastrointestinal disease worldwide.
- More than 50% of the world's population is infected with the organism; in those infected individuals, the estimated lifetime risk for ulcer disease and gastric cancer are 15% and 0.5–2%, respectively.
- Whether an individual will develop *H. pylori*-related disease depends on bacterial virulence, host genetic susceptibility, and environmental factors.
- There appears to be a negative association between *H. pylori* infection and gastroesophageal reflux disease.
- *H. pylori*-related duodenal and gastric ulcers are associated with antral-predominant and diffuse gastritis, respectively.
- Twenty percent of patients are asymptomatic until complications develop.
- First-line eradication treatment involves triple therapy with a proton pump inhibitor or ranitidine bismuth citrate, and two antimicrobial agents like clarithromycin, amoxicillin, or metronidazole. Medications are given twice daily for 7–14 days.
- In patients with perforated duodenal ulcer, when present, *H. pylori* is the most important factor associated with subsequent ulcer recurrence; eradication of *H. pylori* colonization is associated with a markedly reduced rate of ulcer recurrence.
- *H. pylori*-negative duodenal ulcer is independently associated with older age, concomitant medical problems, recent operation, underlying sepsis, and NSAID usage.
- *H. pylori*-negative duodenal ulcer presents more commonly with bleeding, with a larger ulcer, or with multiple ulcers.

Introduction

Peptic ulcer disease is a global health problem. It has long been recognized that acid plays an important and necessary role in peptic ulcer disease, and reduction of acid production has been the primary goal in both medical and surgical treatment of the disease. Nevertheless, despite the introduction of potent acid-lowering medications, recurrence of ulcer has been frequent after cessation of medication.

The past two decades have seen profound changes in our understanding of peptic ulcer disease and with this knowledge have come marked changes in our approach toward treatment. There have been two major advances. First, minimally invasive surgical techniques were applied to elective operation for resistant ulcer disease as well as to emergency operation for ulcer perforation. Second, *Helicobacter pylori* was recognized as an important cause of ulcer disease after the bacteria was first described by Warren and Marshall in 1983. It is now possible to cure peptic ulcer disease in many patients by eradicating *H. pylori*.

Today, thanks to the success of ulcer treatment by eradication of *H. pylori* colonization, the need for elective operation of ulcer disease has decreased markedly or virtually disappeared. Nevertheless, ulcer complications and *H. pylori* negative ulcer disease remain prominent clinical problems, especially in our aging population.

Helicobacter Pylori

The Organism

H. pylori infection of the stomach is not a new phenomenon. As early as 1893, the Italian investigator Giulio Bizzozero described spiral organisms in the stomach. In 1915, Rosenow and Sanford described what they believed to be *streptococci* in the margins of gastric and duodenal ulcers. In 1938, Doenges reported finding spirochetes in 103 (43%) of 242 stomachs examined at autopsy, and in 1975, Steer reported gram-negative bacteria over the gastric mucosa in about 80% of patients with gastric ulcer. But it was not until 1983, when Warren and Marshall (both awarded the Nobel Prize in 2005) reported the successful culture of *"Campylobacter" pyloridis*, that the potential importance of this bacterium began to be appreciated. In 1989, the organism was renamed *Helicobacter pylori*. Since then, 18 other *Helicobacter* species have been found, one in man and the remainder in other animals.

H. pylori is a curved or S-shaped, gram-negative rod approximately 0.5 by 3 μm in size that is a microaerophilic, motile organism usually with four to seven sheathed flagella at one pole. The *H. pylori* genome consists of a single circular chromosome encoding about 1,600 genes. The unique characteristic of *H. pylori* is its ability to produce urease.

The natural habitat of *H. pylori* is the human stomach. The bacteria are found particularly on mucus-secreting cells because of strong and specific binding of bacteria to a protein, Trefoil factor 1, expressed by these cells. In an infected stomach, the highest density of *H. pylori* is found in the antrum. In the biopsy-based tests for *H. pylori*, therefore, biopsies should be obtained from the antrum to minimize sampling error. Interestingly, the greatest density of the bacteria will shift to the proximal stomach after treatment with a potent acid inhibitor, like a proton pump inhibitor. The method of transmission or infection with *H. pylori* is not defined clearly, but current evidence is consistent with both oral-oral and fecal-oral transmission. Interpersonal transmission or infection from a single environmental source is suggested by studies showing an increased prevalence among family members of patients with *H. pylori* infection.

Epidemiology

Studies of populations in developing countries suggest that, until the last century, nearly all humans carried *H. pylori* or closely related bacteria in their stomachs. *H. pylori* infection is usually acquired in childhood. With improvements in socio-economic conditions, fewer children are infected with *H. pylori*. Improvement in nutrition and a clean water supply have been proposed for this trend. Alternatively, some investigators have proposed that most transmission is from child to child and that decreasing family size reduces the chance for transmission. Currently, more than 50% of the world's population is infected with the organism. In addition, there is usually an increase in *H. pylori* prevalence with increasing age, suspected to be due to a cohort effect in which the greater prevalence in older individuals is the result of a greater rate of infection earlier in life.

On the whole, the prevalence of *H. pylori* infection is about 30–40% in the developed countries and 80–90% in the developing countries. In Asia, Malaysia has the lowest prevalence rate of about 5%, while most of the other Asian countries have a prevalence rate of about 60%.

Disease Associations

Infection with *H. pylori* causes an element of histologic chronic gastritis in all those infected, but not all individuals with *H. pylori* infection will develop ulcer disease. In fact, the estimated lifetime risk for ulcer disease is only about 15%, a concept still imprecisely understood.

As many as 2% of individuals with *H. pylori* infection may develop gastric cancer. In 1994, *H. pylori* was declared a Group 1 (a definite cause of cancer in humans) carcinogen by the International Agency for Research on Cancer (IARC) based on 13 epidemiologic studies reporting odds ratios between 2.13 and 8.67 of developing gastric cancer if infected by *H. pylori*. Chronic inflammation as a result of *H. pylori* infection can lead to gastric atrophy and intestinal metaplasia, a suspected precursor of gastric cancer. An experimental model of gastric cancer related to *H. pylori* infection has been developed in Mongolian gerbils. *H. pylori* infection also increases the risk of developing gastric mucosa-associated lymphoid tissue (MALT) lymphoma by six-fold; this association is important because the eradication of *H. pylori* alone may lead to regression of low grade MALT lymphomas.

Whether an individual will develop *H. pylori*-related disease appears to depend on three factors: virulence of the strain of *H. pylori*, host genetic susceptibility, and environmental factors such as diet and smoking. The most important bacterial virulence factors are related to the cytotoxin-associated gene (*cag*A) and vacuolating cytotoxin-associated gene (*vac*A). The *cag*A + strains induce more intense inflammation and are associated more commonly with ulcer disease and gastric cancer than are the *cag*A – strains. The high prevalence of *cag*A + strains in China and Japan appears to explain the greater incidence of gastric cancer in these countries. Unlike *cag*A, the *vac*A gene is present in all strains. *vac*A is, however, polymorphic, varying most notably in two regions called the mid- (m1 and m2) and signal (s1 and s2) regions. Among all the combinations, the s1m1 type of *vac*A is associated more commonly with duodenal ulcer and gastric cancer. The inflammatory response to *H. pylori* infection is dependent on the host genetics. Polymorphisms in the host cytokine genes influence the level of cytokine production by cells after contact with *H. pylori*. Polymorphisms in the IL-1β gene cluster are associated with an augmented cytokine response to *H. pylori*, which appears to increase the risk of gastric atrophy, achlorhydria, intestinal metaplasia, gastric ulcer, and gastric cancer.

The role of *H. pylori* infection in the development of gastroesophageal reflux disease (GERD) remains controversial. It appears that *H. pylori* may protect against the development of GERD in some individuals. Reflux esophagitis and esophageal adenocarcinoma are rare in countries where *H. pylori* infection is common. The efficacy of proton pump inhibitors appears to be better in the presence of *H. pylori* infection.

An increasing number of extra-digestive conditions are associated with *H. pylori* infection. Examples include idiopathic thrombocytopenic purpura (ITP), coronary artery disease, bronchiectasis, cerebrovascular disease, growth retardation, diabetes mellitus, and auto-immune thyroiditis. Although an association with *H. pylori* infection has not been fully confirmed, the latest Maastricht Guidelines for *H. pylori* eradication developed by the European *Helicobacter pylori* Study Group (EHSG) recommend *H. pylori* eradication as the first line treatment for patients with ITP who are *H. pylori* positive.

Pathogenesis of Ulcer Disease

Although genetic factors appear to be important from previous epidemiologic studies, it remains unclear how they contribute to the development of ulcer disease. The concordance for ulcer disease among identical twins is approximately 50%. About 40% of patients with duodenal ulcer have a positive family history. It is uncertain whether the apparently greater risk of ulcer disease in first-degree relatives can be explained by the transmission of *H. pylori* within families or by the host genetic susceptibility as explained above.

Although *H. pylori* is very important, no single pathogenic mechanism has been identified for ulcer disease. The pathogenesis of ulcer disease appears to be multifactorial and involves factors like acid secretion, mucosal defense, and environmental factors.

Acid secretion: The Schwarz's dictum "no acid – no ulcer" has been cited in textbooks since its first description in 1910 and appears to still be true. Prior to the discovery of *H. pylori*, three major disturbances in gastric physiology were noted in patients with duodenal ulcer disease: increased basal and stimulated acid secretion, impaired acid inhibition of gastrin release from the antrum, and increased acid load in the duodenum. Patients with duodenal ulcer produce on average twice the amount of gastric acid in response to the same degree of gastrin stimulation as patients who do not have a duodenal ulcer. This relative increase in acid secretion was postulated to be due to an increase in the mass of parietal (acid-secreting) cells in the stomach or to an increased sensitivity to circulating gastrin.

Duodenal ulcer only develops when *H. pylori*-related inflammation occurs predominantly in the antrum. Exactly how antral *H. pylori* leads to ulceration in the duodenal mucosa is not well understood and appears to be multifactorial. *H. pylori* infection of the antral mucosa results in depletion of antral somatostatin and an increased release of gastrin, and thus an increase in acid secretion. As a result of the prolonged exposure to acid, the duodenal mucosa will develop gastric metaplasia. *H. pylori* is able to then colonize this metaplastic mucosa and the resultant inflammation further precipitates duodenal ulcer formation.

Unlike duodenal ulcer, gastric ulcer is also associated with diffuse gastritis. *H. pylori*-related gastric ulcer is found most commonly at the transitional zone between antrum and corpus on the lesser curve. This region has a tendency for dense colonization of *H. pylori*, intense inflammation, and intestinal metaplasia, and the resultant epithelial damage leads directly to ulceration; how and why the ulcer develops here, however, is still not well understood.

Mucosal defense: Mucosal bicarbonate secretion, prostaglandin production, and blood flow are all important for mucosal defense. Although the gastric lumen is highly acidic, the production of mucus and bicarbonate by the mucosal cells maintains an almost neutral pH at the mucosal surface. A lower basal bicarbonate secretion occurs in patients with duodenal ulcer in comparison with normal individuals. Moreover, after instillation of a physiologic amount of hydrochloric acid, the bicarbonate secretion in patients with duodenal ulcer is only about 40% of the normal response. In such individuals, therefore, even if normal amounts of acid are produced, duodenal ulcer can still occur, because the bicarbonate secretion is lower than normal. Consistent with this concept is the observation that duodenal bicarbonate secretion returns to normal after eradication of *H. pylori* in patients with duodenal ulcer. In an animal study, *H. pylori* hinders duodenal nitric oxide synthase activity and subsequent bicarbonate secretion.

Reduction of mucosal prostaglandin production appears to be another contributing factor in ulcer formation. Prostaglandins stimulate the duodenal mucosa to secrete bicarbonate. In patients with duodenal ulcer, gastric mucosal production of prostaglandin E2 and other prostanoids is decreased.

Maintenance of gastric mucosal blood flow enhances mucosal defense. Apart from supplying nutrients and oxygen to the mucosal cells, mucosal blood flow removes protons from the interstitial fluid so as to maintain an almost neutral pH. Gastric mucosal ischemia is believed to contribute to gastric ulcer formation. Patients with gastric ulcer have a lesser mucosal blood flow along the lesser curve of the stomach where gastric ulcers occur. Moreover, blood flow in the base of an ulcer is less than that of the normal mucosa; in contrast, at the edge of a healing ulcer, blood flow is greater. Other factors are known to affect gastric mucosal blood flow. Examples include epidermal growth factor and dopaminergic agonists which have a protective effect on ethanol-induced mucosal injury by the enhancement of gastric blood flow.

Environmental factors: Environmental factors that contribute to development of ulcer disease include cigarette smoking, dietary habits, environmental stress, non-steroidal anti-inflammatory drugs (NSAID), and *H. pylori* infection.

A number of mechanisms have been postulated to explain the harmful effects of cigarette smoking, including stimulation of acid secretion, reduction in prostaglandin synthesis, enhancing pyloric incompetence, increasing duodenogastric bile reflux, and decreasing gastric mucosal blood flow. Cigarette smoking also impairs ulcer healing and increases the risk of ulcer recurrence.

Although dietary habits and environmental stress are thought to be important etiologic factors in ulcer disease, consistent evidence supporting their importance is lacking. Change in dietary habits has not been shown to accelerate ulcer healing.

The mechanisms by which NSAIDs produce mucosal damage are not fully understood but appear to involve both direct topical injury and systemic effects. The direct effects include injury of the gastric mucosal cells by the acidity of NSAIDs, decrease in mucus secretion, inhibition of mucosal production of prostaglandins (and thus mucosal protective function), and interference with cell turnover. The ulcerogenic actions of NSAIDs appear largely to be caused by their systemic effects. Inhibition of cyclooxygenase with a resultant decrease in prostaglandin production, especially PGE1, PGE2, and PGI2, is thought to be the most important cause. NSAIDs inhibit both plasma and mucosal prostaglandin production in man. Because mucosal prostaglandin production plays an important role in normal mucosal defense, reduction in prostaglandin production increases the risk of ulcer formation. The risk of developing an ulcer with NSAID usage appears to be further increased by a past history of peptic ulcer disease, advancing age, increasing NSAID dosage, concurrent intake of corticosteroids, cigarette smoking, and alcohol intake.

Clinical Presentations of Ulcer Disease

Epigastric pain or discomfort is the most frequent symptom of gastroduodenal ulcer disease. Other common but non-specific symptoms include anorexia, weight loss, nausea, fatty food intolerance, bloating, and belching. The mean age of patients with gastric ulcer is older than that for patients with duodenal ulcer. Based on symptoms alone, it is often impossible to distinguish between duodenal and gastric ulcers. There is also considerable overlap of symptoms between ulcer disease and non-ulcer dyspepsia. Moreover, approximately 20% of patients are asymptomatic until the ulcer progresses to complications such as bleeding or perforation.

In view of the non-specific nature of the symptoms of ulcer disease, accurate diagnosis depends on flexible endoscopy, which allows direct inspection and biopsy for histologic examination of gastric ulcer and for *H. pylori* infection. A double-contrast oral barium study is an alternative, but it is impossible to obtain a biopsy for histologic diagnosis during a barium study.

About 15–20% of patients with an active gastric or duodenal ulcer develop gross hemorrhage, and occult blood loss is more common. When an ulcer crater erodes into a major vessel, severe bleeding may occur (see Chapter 50). The most important tool for the investigation of upper gastrointestinal bleeding is flexible endoscopy. Endoscopy allows accurate localization of the site of bleeding as well as assessment of stigmata of recent hemorrhage. Therapeutic intervention with injection of epinephrine or thermocoagulation can be performed during the same procedure.

When an ulcer erodes through the full thickness of the gastric or duodenal wall, it may perforate or penetrate into surrounding structures. Ulcer perforation is less common than hemorrhage but more common than obstruction. Perforation occurs in about 5–10% of patients with active ulcer disease. The patient with ulcer perforation presents typically with sudden onset of severe abdominal pain, marked abdominal tenderness, and ileus. An erect chest radiograph reveals the presence of free air under the diaphragm in the majority of patients with ulcer perforation. The condition is associated with substantial mortality, especially in patients with concurrent medical illness, preoperative shock, or longstanding perforation of more than 24 h.

Gastric outlet obstruction results from impairment of antral motility as a consequence of acute inflammation and edema around an ulcer or more likely from mechanical obstruction due to scarring from a chronic ulcer. The former tends to resolve with conservative treatment, while the latter usually requires operative or endoscopic intervention. Obstruction develops in less than 5% of patients with ulcer disease, and more commonly with duodenal, pyloric, or prepyloric ulcer. The onset is insidious, and patients may present with nausea, vomiting, and abdominal distension.

Diagnosis of *H. Pylori* Infection

A variety of tests are available for the diagnosis of *H. pylori* infection. Such tests can be classified into invasive and non-invasive tests. Invasive tests require endoscopic mucosal biopsies. The traditional invasive tests include histology, rapid urease test, and culture, while the traditional non-invasive tests include urea breath test and serology. Two biopsy specimens are adequate for an accurate histologic diagnosis of *H. pylori* infection. The reported sensitivity and specificity of histology are both about 90%. Histologic examination, however, is expensive and labor-intensive, and the result is not usually available on the same day. For outpatients, it is highly desirable and cost-effective to obtain the *H. pylori* status during the same endoscopy procedure, so that they do not have to return again for future investigation of appropriate treatment. The rapid urease test on gastric biopsy specimens is considered to be the initial test of choice in patients undergoing endoscopy because of its low cost, rapid availability of results, simplicity, and accuracy. This test involves a preparation containing urea and a pH sensitive marker. In the presence of urease produced by H. pylori, urea will be converted to ammonia with a resultant change in pH and thus in color. The CLO test (Delta West Ltd., Perth, Australia), which consists of an agar gel containing urea, phenol red, buffers and a bacteriostatic agent in a sealed plastic slide, was the first urease test to become available commercially. To date, several commercial kits are marketed for urease testing; all have good sensitivities (80–98%) and specificities (94–100%) for the diagnosis of H. pylori infection. A number of locally made, non-commercial preparations have also been described; these preparations are considerably cheaper than the commercial kits but are equally accurate for the diagnosis of H. pylori infection. The use of a rapid urease test to confirm successful eradication of II. pylori is not recommended because of the higher chance of false negative test as a result of a low density of bacteria.

Culture of H. pylori is difficult and accounts for its low sensitivity of 60–90%. Culture, however, is the most specific test (100%) for H. pylori infection. Culture is usually reserved for research studies or for testing of antibiotic sensitivity.

More sophisticated invasive tests include polymerase chain reaction (PCR) and confocal endomicroscopy. PCR will increase the detection rate of H. pylori in histologically negative biopsies. It can also be used to detect bacterial virulence factors like cagA and to assess antibiotics susceptibility. Confocal endomicroscopy allows direct observation of bacteria in the gastric mucosa after topical application of acriflavine stain, but it is more cumbersome and expensive.

The urea breath test (UBT) is considered the best test for H. pylori after eradication therapy when repeated assessment by endoscopy is not necessary. The reported sensitivity and specificity are both about 95%. Two versions of UBT are available, one using non-radioactive 13C-urea and the other using radioactive 14C-urea. In the presence of H. pylori, the bacterial urease will convert the orally ingested labeled urea into ammonia and labeled carbon dioxide. The breath sample is then collected and analyzed. Although a simple test, the radioactive version is not recommended for pregnant women or children. The 13C-UBT requires a mass spectrometer for analysis and is, therefore, more expensive.

Serology is one of the least expensive tests for H. pylori. The sensitivity and specificity vary widely between different preparations. One major disadvantage of serology is its inability to differentiate between prior exposure and active infection. Several commercial stool antigen tests have become available in recent years. The available studies so far indicate that stool antigen tests are inferior to UBT, but they may be an alternative option when UBT is not available.

Treatment of Ulcer Disease

Medical treatment: The earliest forms of medical treatment for ulcer disease involved dietary manipulation. The Sippy regimen introduced in 1915 (hourly feeding of milk and small bland meals), the Winkelstein milk drip introduced in the 1930s, the use of antacids and anticholinergic drugs, and bed rest were all considered standard treatment for ulcer disease until 40 years ago. Carbenoxolone sodium and other mucosal protective agents were introduced in the 1960s and 1970s. Owing to a lack of effective medication, operative treatment was considered the only effective long term means for preventing ulcer recurrence in the 1970s.

In the late 1970s, a large dose of antacid (equivalent to 1,000 mmol/day) was shown to result in healing of about 80% of duodenal ulcer after 4 weeks of treatment, confirming the therapeutic value of acid neutralization in ulcer healing. These large-dose antacid regimens were, however, inconvenient and tolerated poorly by patients.

Because defective mucosal defense was considered important in ulcer formation, mucosal protective agents like sucralfate and bismuth were introduced for the treatment of ulcer disease. In the 1970s, bismuth salts were demonstrated to be effective as a single agent in the healing of ulcer disease.

The discovery of the histamine H2-receptor antagonist cimetidine by Nobel laureate Sir James Black in 1972 marked an important milestone in the medical treatment of ulcer disease. The introduction of cimetidine coincided with the wide availability of flexible endoscopy and the general acceptance of the importance of prospective randomized, double blind, controlled trials for the assessment of treatment efficacy. More H2-receptor antagonists were developed subsequently, including ranitidine, famotidine, and nizatidine. The availability of the H2-receptor antagonists revolutionized the treatment of ulcer disease, and ulcer healing rates of 80–95% were attained after 6–8 weeks of treatment. Owing to their remarkable efficacy, good tolerability, ease of use, and excellent safety, H2-receptor antagonists were considered the standard treatment for ulcer disease throughout the 1980s.

The advent of proton pump inhibitor, omeprazole, achieved an even more powerful acid inhibition. Several other proton pump inhibitors, like esomeprazole, lansoprazole, pantoprazole and rabeprazole, are now available. These very potent acid inhibitors appear to produce more rapid ulcer healing than standard doses of H2-receptor antagonists. The intake of omeprazole 20 mg daily results in a duodenal ulcer healing rate of more than 90% after 4 weeks of treatment. Moreover, in several multi-center, double blind trials, omeprazole achieved significantly greater rates of duodenal ulcer healing at 2 weeks and, in most cases, at 4 weeks than H2-receptor antagonists.

Although the treatment of ulcer disease has been successful with the use of acid inhibitory drugs, ulcer recurrence after cessation of medication remains a problem. In fact, 50% of patients who received ranitidine alone for healing of duodenal or gastric ulcer suffered a relapse within 12 weeks of healing. In the past, either maintenance medical treatment or operative therapy was offered to such patients. Currently, a cure seems to be possible for patients with ulcer disease related to *H. pylori* infection.

Eradication therapy: In 1994, the National Institutes of Health Consensus Development Conference recommended the addition of antimicrobial agents to anti-secretory drugs to treat all patients with *H. pylori*-associated peptic ulcer disease. The development of effective therapies for the eradication of *H. pylori* has been difficult. Although the organism is sensitive to many antibiotics *in vitro*, the *in vivo* sensitivity is much less. In fact, none of the available antibiotics can achieve an eradication rate of more than 50% if given as a single agent. Borody and colleagues first described the "classical" triple therapy which consisted of bismuth, metronidazole, and tetracycline. Despite achieving an eradication rate of approximately 90% in meta-analysis, its success has been hindered by poor compliance, all-too-frequent side effects, and a decrease in efficacy with the development of metronidazole-resistant strains of *H. pylori*.

The first-line regimen today is triple therapy with a proton pump inhibitor or ranitidine bismuth citrate, and two antimicrobial agents like clarithromycin 500 mg, amoxicillin 1 g, or metronidazole 500 mg, all given twice daily for 7–14 days. The reported eradication rates vary owing to the different prevalence of drug-resistant strains among different populations. In general, the eradication rate is about 85–90%. In the case of eradication failure, culture and testing for antibiotics sensitivity should be considered. Quadruple therapy with bismuth 120 mg qid, a proton pump inhibitor bid, tetracycline 500 mg qid, and metronidazole 500 mg tid for 7 days is usually recommended. In a recent meta-analysis, the efficacy of a triple therapy containing levofloxacin for 10 days was superior to the classic quadruple therapy.

Surgical treatment: Historically, before the availability of anti-secretory drugs, the definitive treatment for ulcer disease was an operative anti-ulcer procedure. Theodor Billroth (1829–1894) performed the first successful distal gastrectomy for gastric cancer in 1881, followed shortly by a successful Billroth I gastrectomy by Ludwik Rydygier (1850–1920) for a benign pyloric ulcer. Rydygier also introduced gastrojejunostomy for the treatment of duodenal ulcer in 1884. Eugen Bircher (1882–1956) reported the performance of vagotomy. In 1922, Andre Latarjet (1876–1947) reported the need to add a drainage procedure, namely gastrojejunostomy, after a vagotomy.

During the 1920s, ulcers were generally thought to be due to gastric stasis, and the good results achieved by Latarjet were attributed to the gastrojejunostomy. It was not until the 1940s when Lester Dragstedt (1893–1975) established that a truncal vagotomy helps heal duodenal ulcers, because it decreases gastric secretion. Subsequently, the role of the antrum in gastric physiology became better understood, and vagotomy with antrectomy was recognized to reduce gastric acid secretion the best. In fact, the ulcer recurrence rate after this procedure is as low as 1%.

In the 1960s and 1970s, recognizing the side effects of truncal vagotomy, more selective types of vagotomy (selective vagotomy, proximal gastric vagotomy, and posterior truncal vagotomy with lesser curvature seromyotomy) were introduced. The more selective types of vagotomy, however, were associated with a somewhat higher ulcer recurrence rate of up to 30%.

The advent of laparoscopic surgery in the late 1980s was an important development in the history of ulcer surgery. With its advantages of a shorter and less painful post-operative course, shorter recovery times, earlier return to work, reduced scarring, and preservation of abdominal wall strength, laparoscopy has stimulated interest in transforming previously established open techniques into laparoscopic procedures. Laparoscopic anti-ulcer surgery was no exception. In fact, various laparoscopic acid-reduction procedures have been developed. While there was great excitement about the development of various laparoscopic procedures for peptic ulcer disease, the eradication of *H. pylori* became the established treatment for peptic ulcer disease in the early 1990s. As a result of the effectiveness of medical treatment, including eradication therapy for *H. pylori*, the need for elective operations for peptic ulcer disease have been almost eliminated in the recent decade.

Emergency operations are still required to treat ulcer complications like bleeding or perforation. The introduction of therapeutic endoscopy has diminished dramatically the need for emergency operation to treat bleeding peptic ulcers. Nevertheless, an emergency operation is indicated when endoscopic therapy fails. Currently, such elderly patients are often frail and have multiple medical problems.

H. Pylori and Duodenal Ulcer Perforation

About 5–10% of patients with an untreated active duodenal ulcer will experience an episode of perforation during their lifetime. Closure with an omental patch remains standard treatment in many centers because of simplicity, short operating time, and low morbidity. In the past, simple closure was known to be associated with a very high rate of ulcer recurrence, 30–50%. Therefore, definitive acid reduction operations were advocated for emergency treatment of healthy patients with perforated duodenal ulcer in order to reduce the likelihood of recurrent ulceration. Recent studies, however, have shown that in younger patients with perforated duodenal ulcer, *H. pylori* is an important factor associated with subsequent ulcer recurrence, and its eradication is associated with minimal ulcer recurrence.

Currently, simple closure with an omental patch combined with intense antisecretory therapy for perforated duodenal ulcer is recommended. In the presence of irreversible pyloric stenosis, truncal vagotomy and pyloroplasty should be considered. Post-operatively, antisecretory drugs such as H_2-receptor antagonists should be maintained until the *H. pylori* status is known. Gastroscopic examination should be performed 2 months after operation to both confirm healing of ulceration as well as to obtain antral biopsy specimens for determination of *H. pylori* status. Eradication therapy is recommended for patients who continue to test positive for *H. pylori*.

H. Pylori-Negative Duodenal Ulcer Disease

Previous studies have reported that more than 90% of patients with duodenal ulcers and 60% with gastric ulcers are infected with *H. pylori*. The use of NSAIDs was suggested to be the major cause of duodenal ulcers in patients > 50 years old and in the remaining *H. pylori*-negative ulcer disease. The prevalence of *H. pylori* infection in patients with duodenal ulcer was believed to be so high that confirmatory testing before eradication treatment was considered unnecessary by some centers. Recently, however, the prevalence of *H. pylori*-positive duodenal ulcer was found to be decreasing and was only about 75% in a number of studies. It is therefore important to confirm the *H. pylori* status before prescribing eradication therapy.

H. pylori-negative duodenal ulcer was found to be associated independently with older age, concomitant medical problems, recent operation, underlying sepsis, and NSAID usage. It is noteworthy that *H. pylori*-negative duodenal ulcers present more commonly with bleeding, with a larger ulcer, or with multiple ulcers. In the elderly patient requiring emergency operation for bleeding duodenal ulcer, which is usually large in size, acid-reduction operation should be entertained in view of the likelihood that the ulcer is unrelated to *H. pylori* infection.

Selected Readings

Chu KM, Kwok KF, Law SYK, et al. (1999) *Helicobacter pylori* status and endoscopy follow-up of patients having a past history of perforated duodenal ulcer. Gastrointest Endosc 50:58–62

Chu KM, Kwok KF, Law S, Wong KH (2005) Patients with *Helicobacter pylori* positive and negative duodenal ulcers have distinct clinical characteristics. World J Gastroenterol 11:3518–3522

Marshall B (1983) Unidentified curved bacilli on gastric epithelium in active chronic gastritis. Lancet 1:1273–1275

McColl KEL (1997) Pathophysiology of duodenal ulcer disease. Eur J Gastroenterol Hepatol 9 (Suppl 1):S9–S12

Peterson WL, Fendrick AM, Cave DR, et al. (2000) *Helicobacter pylori*-related disease: guidelines for testing and treatment. Arch Intern Med 160:1285–1291

Walsh JH, Peterson WL (1995) The treatment of *Helicobacter pylori* infection in the management of peptic ulcer disease. N Engl J Med 333:984–991

Warren JR (1983) Unidentified curved bacilli on gastric epithelium in active chronic gastritis. Lancet 1:1273

48 Peptic Ulcer Disease: Perforation

Anja Schaible · Peter Kienle

Pearls and Pitfalls

- The epidemiology of peptic ulcer disease has changed dramatically.
- The medical management of symptomatic peptic ulcer disease has improved.
- There has been no decrease in ulcer perforations over the last decades.
- Two main trends responsible for the unchanged rate of complications (perforation, bleeding)
  - Decrease in prevalence of *Helicobacter pylori*
  - Increase in use of NSAIDs
- Ulcer perforations occur mostly in stomach (60%) or duodenum (40%)
- One third to one half of ulcer perforations are associated with NSAID use
- Clinical presentation tends to occur in 3 phases
  - Phase one: 0–2 h after onset, Initial sudden onset of severe abdominal pain
  - Phase two: 2–12 h after onset, Less abdominal pain
  - Phase three: >12 h after onset, Increasing abdominal extension
- Rapid diagnosis is essential!
- Perforation is largely a clinical diagnosis: abdominal rigidity
- Abdominal x-ray: look for free air; no further examination necessary: this is an indication for surgical exploration
- Basic support involves: intravenous fluid, nasogastric tube, antibiotics
- Further therapy
  - Non operative management is possible in selected patients
  - Normally: surgical exploration, is indicated, possibly laparoscopic
    - Prompt closure or patching with omentum of the site of perforation
    - Lavage with 10–20 l
- Morbidity and mortality have decreased
- Mortality rate for operations after peptic ulcer perforation, however, remains high at 2–8%

Introduction

The epidemiology of peptic ulcer disease continues to change. Ulcer incidence increases with age for both duodenal and gastric ulcers. Duodenal ulcers occur generally two decades earlier than gastric ulcers. All over the world, the incidence of ulcer has decreased over the last decades, more for duodenal ulcers than for gastric ulcers, and the overall frequency of hospitalization and death from peptic ulcer has diminished considerably. Despite dramatic improvements in the medical management (Proton Pump Inhibitors, PPI) and the lower rate of peptic ulcer disease, the incidence of potentially life-threatening ulcer complications such as perforation (and bleeding) has not decreased over the last decades.

Two opposing main trends are responsible for the stable complication rate: first a decrease in the prevalence of *Helicobacter pylori* due to improved socioeconomic conditions, and second, an increase in use of non steroidal antiinflammatory drugs (NSAID). NSAID use, which is an independent risk factor for ulcers, is common especially in elder individuals. These two main trends have resulted in an increase in ulcer complications in older patients and a decline in younger patients. There are not much data regarding the frequency of complications but suggest that complications occur at a rate of 1–2% per ulcer per year. Giant ulcers and pyloric channel ulcers may be associated with a higher rate of complications. The majority of gastric ulcers are located along the lesser curvature and anterior wall especially in the antrum, whereas duodenal ulcers are localized predominantly in the first part of the duodenum, especially on the anterior surface. Seldom, perforations are located on the dorsal wall toward the lesser omentum.

Ulcer perforations due to peptic ulcer disease are located mostly in the stomach or duodenum. Other small intestinal ulcers are defined as defects in the gastrointestinal mucosa extending through the muscularis mucosa and can generally occur in the whole gastrointestinal tract. Other organs are affected only rarely and should be distinguished from peptic (acid-induced) ulcers, e.g. ulcers in the proximal small bowel from drug exposure, or especially after oral potassium chloride tablets, NSAIDs or aspirin, or in the wake of blood flow disturbances or in the postoperative setting. Advanced malignant diseases seldom show free perforation of the tumor. Important causes for peptic ulcers are listed in ❯ *Table 48-1*.

Duodenal and gastric ulcers account for 60% and 40% of perforations due to peptic ulcer disease. One third to one half of perforated ulcers are associated with NSAID use; these usually occur in elderly patients. Low dose aspirin increases the risk of GI complications caused by NSAIDs and selective Cox-2 inhibitors. The association between ulcer perforation and H-pylori remains controversial: some studies found a correlation, while others did not.

Clinical Presentation

Peptic ulcers may present with a wide variety of symptoms. Although many patients complain of upper abdominal discomfort, others are completely asymptomatic, sometimes until perforation occurs. About one third of patients with peptic ulcer disease present with a complication as the first symptom, especially older individuals with NSAID-induced perforation. The majority of patients with peptic ulcer perforation, however, will have a history of ulcer symptoms.

In 1997, Silen described three clinical phases of perforated ulcer (see ❯ *Table 48-2*). In the initial phase (within 2 h of onset), patients develop sudden onset of severe abdominal pain, sometimes even producing syncope. Patients often describe an abrupt pain like a thrust with a stab. Localization is usually epigastric, but it quickly becomes generalized and presents as an acute abdomen. Acid fluid in the peritoneal cavity releases vasoactive mediators causing tachycardia, cool extremities, and a low temperature. The severity of onset depends on how much fluid is released. The stage may last

◘ Table 48-1

Important causes for gastrointestinal ulcers

Note	
Infection	*Helicobacter pylori*
	HSV
	CMV
Drug exposure	NSAIDs
	Aspirin
	Corticosteroids
	Bisphosphonates
	Clopidogrel
	Potassium chloride
	Chemotherapy
Hormonal or mediator-induced	Gastrinoma (Zollinger-Ellison syndrome)
	Systemic mastocytosis
	Antral G cell hyperfunction
Radiation therapy	
Infiltrating disease	Sarcoidosis
	Crohn's disease
Ulcer associated with systemic disease	Stress (ICU) ulcers
	Organ transplantation

only a few minutes up to 2 h. Pain may radiate to the top of the right or both shoulders. Abdominal rigidity then begins to develop.

In the second phase, abdominal pain may lessen and may result in an underestimation of the situation. Patients in this phase often feel that things are getting better. Pain is usually less than in phase one but is now more generalized, often getting worse with movement. Rectal examination is often tender as is palpation of the right lower quadrant due to irritation from inflammatory fluid. The duration of the second phase is usually 2–12 h after primary onset.

The third phase usually begins more than 12 h after onset. Now increasing abdominal distension is noted, but abdominal pain, tenderness, and rigidity may be less evident than in phase one. Temperature and hypovolemia due to third-spacing develop, tachycardia worsens, and hypovolemic shock may occur. The patient now looks very ill clinically, and rapid diagnosis is essential.

Not all patients develop the classic symptoms described above. Especially if patients have had abdominal operations previously with subsequent adhesions, the ulcer may not perforate into the free abdominal cavity but into other organs or be contained by the omentum. Therefore, patients with milder symptoms have to be evaluated carefully in order to exclude a perforation.

Diagnosis

A detailed history should ask for ulcer symptoms in the last weeks such as abdominal pain especially in the epigastrium (❯ *Table 48-3*). Abdominal pain before oral intake is associated with a duodenal ulcer, whereas pain after oral intake is more typical for a gastric ulcer. A prolonged ulcer history is common among patients with complicated ulcers; these patients with a history of complicated ulcer disease are prone to experiencing another complication. A detailed drug history in regard to NSAIDs, aspirin, corticosteroids, potassium chloride, and other drugs is mandatory.

Physical examination reveals exquisite tenderness, abdominal rigidity in all four quadrants perhaps accentuated in the epigastric area, rebound, and loss of bowel sounds. Physical examination provides the essential clues, because perforation is largely a clinical diagnosis.

In the diagnostic pathway, the next step is a blood sample for measuring leucocytes and CRP. An upright abdominal x-ray will show free air beneath the diaphragms (❷ *Fig. 48-1*). If so, no further diagnostic studies are necessary, and an indication for operative exploration is present. In contrast, 10–20% of patients with an ulcer perforation will not have free air. In this situation, leakage of water soluble contrast (Gastrografin) is a useful confirmatory test. A better alternative is a CT with oral contrast in order to detect small amounts of free air or fluid. CT is able to detect both ulcer perforation and other pathologies such as colon perforation.

If the diagnosis remains unclear, an endoscopy of the stomach can help to make the diagnosis of perforation and is not contraindicated in our opinion, although some groups believe so. Furthermore, endoscopy can localize the perforation and influence the operative procedure (laparoscopic or conventional approach).

For differential diagnosis, other etiologies of an acute abdomens have to be considered. First, other areas of potential of perforation must be considered, especially the sigmoid. But if there is free air in the x-ray, the patient usually requires operative intervention anyway, and exploration will show the location of the perforation. In contrast, there are a lot of other diseases which can cause an acute abdomen, such as perforated appendicitis, small bowel ileus or intussusception, acute pancreatitis, mesenterial infarction, and myocardial infarction (❷ *Table 48-4*).

Treatment

Intravenous fluids, stabilization of hemodynamic instability, and nasogastric suction are the first steps of the treatment strategy, which have to be applied earlyon. The further treatment is operative,

◘ Table 48-2

Clinical phases of perforated ulcer

Phase 1	0–2 h after onset, Sudden severe abdominal pain
Phase 2	2–12 h after onset, Less pain than in phase 1
Phase 3	>12 h after onset, Increasing abdominal extension

◘ Table 48-3

Diagnostic pathway

1. Detailed history	Epigastric abdominal pain?
	Drugs (NSAIDs, Aspirin)?
2. Physical examination	Abdominal rigidity?
	Bowel movements?
3. Blood sample	Leucocytes, CRP
4. Abdominal x-ray	Free air?

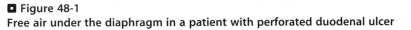

■ Figure 48-1
Free air under the diaphragm in a patient with perforated duodenal ulcer

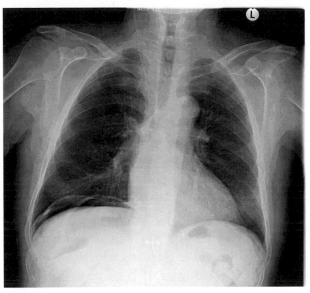

normally. Intravenous antibiotics should be administered prior to incision and when peritonitis is confirmed for upto 5 days postoperatively.

Nonoperative management, including parenteral nutrition and antibiotics, may be successful in well-selected patients. In 1989, Crofts et al. reported a group of 83 patients with a perforated ulcer randomized to initial medical therapy or immediate laparotomy with operative repair. In this study, 70% of the patients randomized to a nonoperative approach avoided operative intervention, while only 11 of 40 patients required surgery. The hospital stay was 35% longer in the group treated conservatively. The authors concluded that an initial period of non operative treatment with careful observation was safe in patients under age 70. When non operative management is considered, one has to be certain that no extravasation of contrast to the abdominal cavity occurs. Another possibility for non operative management is the unusual situation, where perforation is detected several days after the incident. Although some patients will seal their perforated ulcers without an operation, such an approach has been associated with morbidity and mortality, particularly in high-risk patients.

Normally, if clinical examination reveals abdominal rigidity, and free air is detected by x-ray or CT scan, operative intervention is generally required. A delay in intervention will be associated with a subsequent septic complication. The objective of therapy for perforation is prompt closure of the perforation in the duodenum or stomach. In the stomach, ulcers should be excised to rule out a malignancy, while in the duodenum, closure without excision is the usual practice. Usually, sutures placed in seromuscular fashion across the site of perforation are sufficient for secure closure. Some groups tie in a tag of omentum with these sutures to prevent a leakage of the suture line, but there is little evidence for this. Thorough lavage of the peritoneal cavity with 10–20 l fluid is an essential part of the operation.

Laparoscopic repair appears to be a reasonable option for patients with a history less than 24 h, with no hypovolemic shock, and with a perforation not more than 6 mm. In up to 25%, conversion to an open operation is necessary. Morbidity and mortality seem to be comparable in published series, but larger randomized studies are still lacking.

▢ Table 48-4

Differential diagnosis of acute abdomen

Appendicitis, acute or perforated
Small bowel intussusception or ileus
Perforated diverticulitis
Acute or perforated cholecystitis
Acute pancreatitis
Mesenterial infarction
Myocardial infarction

The role of definitive ulcer surgery with an acid-reducing procedure remains unclear without current understanding of ulcer pathogenesis. Most large studies of patients who have undergone definitive ulcer surgery were performed prior to the recognition of the role of *H. pylori* treatment. A recent randomized study showed that 1 year after a prompt closure and consequent *H. pylori* eradication, only 5% of patients developed recurrent ulcers. Therefore, our approach in most perforations is prompt closure with additional removal of the ulcer when localized in the stomach and an extensive lavage of the abdominal cavity. In selected cases of large perforating ulcers of the stomach, more extensive resections such as Billroth I or II resections may become necessary.

Outcome

Morbidity and mortality after peptic ulcer perforation has decreased continuously over the last decades because of better antibiotic therapy. The main risk factors for mortality are the duration of the interval between perforation and operation, the patient's age, and comorbidity factors. In recent studies the mortality rate for operations after peptic ulcer perforation ranged between 2 to 8%.

Selected Readings

Bloom BS, Kroch E (1993) Time trends in peptic ulcer disease and in gastritis and in duodenitis: mortality, utilization and disability in the United States. J Clin Gastoenterol 17:33–342

Crofts TJ, Park KG, Steele RJ, et al. (1989) A randomized trial of non operative treatment for perforated peptic ulcer. N Engl J Med 320:970

El-Serag HB, Sonnenberg A (1998) Opposing time trends of peptic ulcer and reflux disease. Gut 43:327–33

Gunshefski L, Flancbaum L, Brolin RE, Frankel A (1990) Changing patterns in perforated peptic ulcer disease. Am Surg 56:270

Katkhouda N, Mavor E, Mason RJ, et al. (1999) Laparoscopic repair of perforated duodenal ulcers: outcome and efficacy in 30 consecutive patients. Arch Surg 134:845–848

Ng EK, Lam YH, Sung JJ (2000) Eradication of Helicobacter pylori prevents recurrence of ulcer after simple closure of duodenal ulcer perforation: randomized controlled trial. Ann Surg 231:153–158

Silen W (1996) Cope's early diagnosis of the acute abdomen. Oxford University Press, New York

49 Peptic Ulcer Disease: Obstruction

David A. Berg · Daniel T. Dempsey

Pearls and Pitfalls

- The most common cause of gastric outlet obstruction in today's era of histamine receptor blockers, proton pump inhibitors, and effective treatment of *Helicobacter pylori* is malignancy, no longer peptic ulcer disease.
- Over 90% of serious peptic ulcer complications are associated with *Helicobacter pylori* infection, NSAID use, and/or smoking.
- The classic indications for operative intervention for peptic ulcer disease are perforation, bleeding, and obstruction; the latter is the least common.
- The primary symptom of gastric outlet obstruction is postprandial, non-bilious vomiting.
- Volume contraction and persistent vomiting of gastric contents leads to a hypochloremic, hypokalemic metabolic alkalosis in patients with gastric outlet obstruction.
- All patients with gastric outlet obstruction should have flexible upper endoscopy with biopsies of the stenosis and any active ulcer and/or scar. Upper GI contrast radiography often yields complimentary information.
- Gastric outlet obstruction from chronic peptic ulcer disease is unlikely to respond to conservative management and will require either endoscopic and/or operative intervention.
- An acute prepyloric or duodenal ulcer may cause gastric outlet obstruction due to edema and/or motor dysfunction; this usually resolves with gastric decompression and aggressive medical treatment.
- Endoscopic balloon dilation is a non-operative approach that offers excellent initial symptomatic relief in many patients with obstructing peptic ulcer, but the beneficial effect is often transient.
- More than two or three endoscopic dilations over greater than 1 year suggests that an operation should be considered to treat the obstruction from chronic peptic ulcer. Younger, good-risk patients should be considered for operation sooner.
- The operative procedures of choice for obstructing duodenal ulcer are highly selective vagotomy with gastrojejunostomy, and truncal vagotomy and antrectomy. The latter should be avoided in poor-risk or chronically asthenic patients and patients with a difficult duodenum.
- Obstruction associated with gastric ulcer (prepyloric or otherwise) is best treated with resection if this can be done safely. If resection is not performed, intraoperative biopsies should be considered.
- Pyloroplasty should be avoided as a drainage procedure in patients with obstructing peptic ulcer disease.

Introduction

Fifty years ago, peptic ulcer was a surgical disease: operation was the only widely effective curative treatment. Currently, many clinicians view peptic ulcer as a non-operative disease. But this is not entirely accurate because the number of operations performed today for peptic ulcer complications (bleeding, perforation, obstruction) is similar to what it was 50 years ago. Advances in the understanding of peptic ulcer pathophysiology and the development of more effective diagnostic and therapeutic modalities have decreased dramatically the number of operations performed electively for intractable, nonhealing peptic ulcers and for bleeding peptic ulcers. But there persists a subset of patients who develop life-threatening complications of peptic ulcer disease, namely recurrent or persistent bleeding, perforation, or obstruction, who will require operation for definitive treatment. It is essential that the general surgeon be familiar with the surgical options useful for the management of these complications. Herein, we present a brief overview of peptic ulcer disease, focusing specifically on management of gastric outlet obstruction. Approximately 2,000 patients per year will ultimately require operation for obstructing peptic ulcer disease.

Causes of Gastric Outlet Obstruction in the Adult

Today the most common cause of gastric outlet obstruction is cancer, and not peptic ulcer disease. Thus, it is more important than ever for the surgeon not to mistake a malignant gastric outlet obstruction for a benign obstruction associated with peptic ulcer disease. The most likely primary adenocarcinomas presenting with gastric outlet obstruction are pancreatic, gastric, and duodenal in declining order of frequency. Primary lymphoma of the stomach, duodenum, or pancreas may also obstruct the gastric outlet; the same is true for GI stromal neoplasms of the stomach and duodenum. Extrinsic neoplastic obstruction of the gastric outlet may occur from metastatic disease to the porta hepatis. Rarely, recurrent colon cancer at the site of a previous ileocolonic anastomosis can obstruct the gastric outlet by direct extension.

Although several decades ago peptic ulcer disease was the most common cause of gastric outlet obstruction in adults, currently it is less common than obstruction due to cancer of the pancreas, stomach, or duodenum. Patients with obstructing peptic ulcer disease may have a long history of ulcer symptoms, but some have little or no history suggestive of chronic ulcer disease. The site of the primary ulcer may be duodenal, gastric (type 3–prepyloric, not type 1–angularis, or type 4–juxtaesophageal), or both (so called type 2-gastric ulcer). Commonly, there is a discrete stricture in the duodenal bulb, but other patterns are not uncommon, e.g. a prepyloric stricture, a post bulbar stricture, or a long chronic cicatrix extending from the prepyloric to postpyloric region.

Other possible benign causes of gastric outlet obstruction in the adult include entities that usually present in childhood such as duodenal web, duodenal duplication, and hypertrophic pyloric stenosis. Finally, it is important to consider primary gastroparesis or chronic bowel obstruction masquerading clinically as a mechanical gastric outlet obstruction, especially after a previous vagotomy.

Pertinent Pathophysiology

Peptic ulcers form as a result of acid-peptic injury to the gastroduodenal mucosal barrier. *Helicobacter pylori* infection, NSAID use, and smoking are causative factors in the majority of duodenal and gastric ulcers, and over 90% of serious peptic ulcer complications are associated with one or more of these three factors. For the surgeon treating the patient with obstructing peptic ulcer, it is important to keep this in mind for several reasons. First, if the patient has gastric outlet obstruction from an acute edematous process, the blockage (mechanical and/or functional) may resolve with acid suppression and elimination of the causative factors. Although many patients with obstructing peptic ulcer will not have demonstrable *H. pylori* infection (i.e. the tests for helicobacter are negative), we treat this empirically whenever possible in all patients with ulcer disease severe enough to warrant surgical consultation. Second, the likelihood of recurrent or persistent ulcer after an operation for obstruction is dependent on the ability of the clinician and the patient to eliminate the associated causative factors. Thus it may be irrational to do a larger ulcer operation (e.g. vagotomy and antrectomy) in order to minimize the risk of recurrence if the surgeon is confident that the helicobacter, NSAIDs, and/or smoking can be eradicated. Finally, an absence of these causative factors should increase the index of suspicion for cancer or gastrinoma. Regarding the diagnosis of the latter, it is important to remember that antral distention is a stimulus for gastrin secretion. Thus it is not uncommon for the patient with obstructing peptic ulcer to have a somewhat increased serum gastrin level and gastric acid hypersecretion. A secretin stimulation test may be useful to rule out gastrinoma.

Chronic gastric outlet obstruction leads to gastric dilation, muscular hypertrophy, and abnormal gastric motor activity. Although surgical lore has suggested that the motor activity may improve after several days of gastric decompression, in our experience it may take weeks for gastric motor function to improve after operation for obstruction. If gastrojejunostomy is chosen as a surgical option to treat obstructing peptic ulcer, it is important to consider vagotomy, because the aforementioned acid hypersecretion may predispose to marginal ulceration. Motor function of the distal stomach (and therefore gastric emptying) may be better preserved if a highly selective vagotomy is performed rather than a truncal vagotomy. Rarely, gastrojejunostomy alone and lifelong proton pump inhibitors may be acceptable treatment in the selected, elderly but reliable patient. Last, it is important for the operating surgeon to be aware of the degree to which the gastric wall may thicken. Due to this strong consideration should be given to using the larger (i.e. green) stapling cartridges or to hand-sewing anastomosis and oversewing staple lines.

Clinical Presentation of Obstructing Peptic Ulcer Disease

Patients with gastric outlet obstruction often present with a prolonged history of symptoms. The majority of patients complain of nausea relieved frequently by *nonbilious vomiting*. Abdominal distention or bloating, vague epigastric discomfort, early satiety, and/or weight loss are also common. Emesis of undigested food may occur as long as 24–48 h after ingestion. Not uncommonly, patients have eliminated many solid foods from their diets and often do not present to hospital until they are weakened acutely with dehydration. Physical examination may reveal epigastric tenderness, abdominal distension with or without tympany, hypoactive bowel sounds, or visible peristalsis. The classic sign of gastric outlet obstruction, a succussion splash, is present in only 25% of patients. Placing the stethoscope over the epigastrium and gently rocking the supine patient from side to side may elicit this sign. Volume contraction and electrolyte disturbances are common due to a prolonged history of nonbilious vomiting. The classic electrolyte abnormality is hypochloremic, hypokalemic, metabolic alkalosis. In chronic cases, patients may be severely malnourished, and parenteral nutrition should be considered.

Patients with obstructing peptic ulcer disease often report a history of previous ulcers, as well as the use of NSAIDs, antacids, or antisecretory drugs. Over 90% of patients report a recent or remote history of epigastric pain, often non-radiating and burning in character. Heme-positive stool and/or anemia are not uncommon, but the latter may not be apparent until after rehydration.

Diagnosis and Management

Peripheral intravenous access is established and fluid/electrolyte repletion begun with isotonic saline. A Foley catheter is placed. Once there is evidence of adequate renal function, potassium chloride is added to the intravenous solution. Vital signs, urine output, and electrolytes are followed as guides to the adequacy of resuscitation. Placement of a large bore nasogastric tube will decompress the stomach. Ideally, a plain upright x-ray of the chest and abdomen obtained prior to the placement of the tube often shows massive gastric distention with a large air fluid level; the absence of small bowel distention should corroborate the diagnosis of gastric outlet obstruction. The patient is maintained with nothing by mouth on nasogastric suction, and continuous intravenous proton pump inhibitors are administered. NSAIDs are eliminated if possible. Parenteral nutrition may be necessary. Once the patient has been resuscitated adequately and the stomach has been adequately decompressed, upper endoscopy is performed. It is imperative that biopsies of ulcers as well as the site of obstruction are performed to help rule out malignancy. A high index of suspicion for malignancy must exist especially in older patients and those without a known history of peptic ulcer disease. Age greater than 55 and lack of a history of peptic ulcer disease have been identified as independent predictors of malignant gastric outlet obstruction (up to a fivefold increased risk). Biopsies of the antrum are helpful in evaluating the presence of H pylori infection. An upper GI contrast study complements the upper endoscopy and is particularly useful to the surgeon in evaluating the anatomy of the antrum, pylorus, and duodenum. Abdominal CT should be considered if malignancy is suspected.

Numerous diagnostic criteria have been used to define gastric outlet obstruction. These criteria may include any of the following: postcibal gastric volume greater than 300 ml after 4 h, an overnight residual gastric volume greater than 200 ml, a positive saline load test (750 ml test volume with residual greater than 400 ml after 30 min), endoscopy revealing a stenotic pylorus preventing passage of a 9 mm endoscope, or an upper gastrointestinal contrast study with greater than 60% of barium retained in the stomach after 4 h. Most patients with benign gastric outlet obstruction secondary to peptic ulcer disease are managed clinically, with invasive treatment (endoscopic dilation or operation) reserved for patients who cannot tolerate a full liquid diet after about 1 week of intensive pharmacologic treatment and nasogastric decompression. Acute ulcers, often associated with clinically significant obstruction secondary to edema and/or impaired gastric motility, will usually respond to a 3–5 day conservative trial of hydration, decompression, and antisecretory therapy. Due to extensive pyloric scarring and rigidity, chronic gastric outlet obstructions from recurrent peptic ulcers are much less likely to respond to conservative management and will require either endoscopic and/or operative intervention. At least 50% of patients admitted to hospital today with obstructing peptic ulcer will require such intervention.

Endoscopic Balloon Dilation

Endoscopic balloon dilation is a non-operative approach that offers excellent initial symptomatic relief in many patients, but the beneficial effect is often transient. It is most useful in poor risk patients, or as a temporizing measure in patients with other active medical issues that make operation risky (e.g. recent myocardial infarction or active pneumonia). Endoscopic balloon dilation for peptic ulcer strictures has rendered both operative dilation and operative stricturoplasty for this disorder moot.

In studies with longer duration of follow-up, many patients (over 80% in some studies) eventually need repeated dilations, with a substantial proportion of those patients requiring operative treatment. Thus operation should be considered in most good-risk patients who fail conventional medical therapy. To date, large studies examining the long-term effects of endoscopic balloon dilation are lacking. No studies exist with median follow up greater than 4 years and sample size greater than 50 patients. Up to one half of patients requiring repeated dilatation for recurrent obstruction will require an operation ultimately. Factors shown to be predictive of requiring operative treatment are duration of endoscopic treatment greater than 1 year and the need for more than two or three endoscopic dilatations. Prior NSAID use, presence of an acute ulcer, site of obstruction, or gender does not influence the need for operative treatment after endoscopic dilatation.

The role of *Helicobacter pylori* in patients with benign gastric outlet obstruction treated with pneumatic dilatation is poorly defined. It has been speculated that effective treatment of *Helicobacter pylori* in patients with obstructing peptic ulcer disease will improve the outcome of balloon dilatation. Some gastroenterologists suggest that treatment of confirmed *Helicobacter pylori* infection is an important adjunct to endoscopic balloon dilatation if operation is to be avoided. Limited data show that patients negative for *Helicobacter pylori* respond poorly to endoscopic dilatation and should be considered for early surgical referral. Clearly, more data are needed to elucidate further the role that treatment of *Helicobacter pylori* may or may not play in the response to endoscopic balloon dilatation.

Endoscopic balloon dilatation for obstructing peptic ulcer was first reported in the early 1980s. Currently, a through-the-scope technique is used in which balloons of increasing diameters (8 mm through 16 mm) are advanced across the strictured pylorus and inflated sequentially. Procedural variables that have not been standardized or studied include the duration of insufflation, frequency of dilatation, and size of balloons. The main morbidity of this procedure is perforation requiring emergency operation, with reported rates ranging from 0% to 6%. Performing repeated endoscopic balloon dilatations may risk further scarring of the duodenum, which may lead to a complicated duodenal stump closure if subsequent resection is required. Finally, it must be recognized that this treatment may delay the diagnosis of an obstructing cancer.

Operative Management

Operative treatment is indicated for most good risk patients who fail conventional medical treatment for obstructing peptic ulcer. Operative treatment is also indicated for patients who have persistent or recurrent symptoms after two or three endoscopic balloon dilatations. Finally, operative treatment is indicated for perforation (endoscopic or spontaneous), massive bleeding, and suspicion of cancer. Intraoperative options for obstructing duodenal ulcer include truncal vagotomy and antrectomy, truncal vagotomy and drainage, or highly selective vagotomy and gastrojejunostomy. The addition of a feeding jejunostomy tube should be considered in most all of these patients and especially for the severely malnourished patients.

The ideal operation for successful treatment of obstructing peptic ulcer must relieve the obstruction, control the ulcer disease, have low morbidity and mortality rates, and produce few late complications. It should also diagnose and treat adequately the occasional patient with an obstructing carcinoma. Truncal vagotomy and antrectomy (TV/A) is the most definitive operation for obstructing peptic ulcer. This operation has the least ulcer recurrence, but as mentioned above, this resective approach might be a less valuable asset in the modern era when elimination of causative factors should minimize the risk of ulcer recurrence perhaps without the need of a major, extirpative procedure. Another potential advantage of TV/A is in the treatment of type 2 (gastric and duodenal) or 3 (prepyloric) gastric ulcers associated with outlet obstruction. Distal gastric resection remains the procedure of choice for gastric ulcer, both because of the cancer risk and because it eliminates the area where recurrent or persistent gastric ulcer may occur. Vagotomy should be performed, because type 2 and type 3 gastric ulcers tend to behave clinically like duodenal ulcers, and acid hypersecretion is thought to be more important in the pathophysiology of these lesions than in the more common, type 1 gastric ulcers.

There are clearly disadvantages to the routine use of TV/A for obstructing peptic ulcer. The operative mortality is about double that of the other (nonextirpative) procedures mentioned above, and the procedure should be avoided in hemodynamically unstable patients and in debilitated or poor risk patients. Also, after TV/A, a substantial number of patients (5–10%) may develop postgastrectomy problems, e.g. dumping, postvagotomy diarrhea, delayed gastric emptying, and afferent or efferent limb problems. Prior to recommending an elective TV/A, the surgeon should ask his- or herself, "How would this patient look 10 pounds lighter?" If the answer to this question is anything other than "fine," another surgical option should be considered. This consideration is especially pertinent to the asthenic female. Finally, resection should be avoided in patients with extensive inflammation and/or scarring of the proximal duodenum, because a secure anastomosis (Billroth I) or duodenal closure (Billroth II) may be compromised.

Truncal vagotomy and drainage (TV/D) with a gastrojejunostomy is advantageous, because an experienced surgeon can perform this procedure quickly and safely. This operative approach also affords the surgeon the opportunity to biopsy the area of obstruction and can be performed as a minimally invasive or laparoscopic-assisted operation. Finally, in the event that dumping is debilitating, the gastrojejunostomy can be reversed provided there is a patent pyloric channel. The main disadvantages of TV/D are the side effects (10% dumping and/or diarrhea) and a 10% rate of recurrent ulcer. Pyloroplasty should be avoided in patients with obstructing peptic ulcer except for the occasional patient with a discrete juxtapyloric stricture. In most patients with obstructing peptic ulcer, Heinecke-Mikulicz pyloroplasty is difficult or impossible. Jaboulay pyloroplasty has been shown in a small prospective clinical trial to be inferior to resection or gastrojejunostomy. Moreover, because recurrent ulceration after TV/D is a possibility, all types of pyloroplasty may make subsequent distal gastric resection, if necessary, more difficult.

Highly selective vagotomy (also called parietal cell or proximal gastric vagotomy) and gastro-jejunostomy is a good option for many patients requiring operation for obstructing peptic ulcer. It is a low risk procedure that treats both the ulcer diathesis (highly selective vagotomy) and the obstruction (gastrojejunostomy). It can be performed as a laparoscopic-assisted procedure, and the gastrojejunostomy is potentially reversible. Preservation of the vagal innervation to the distal stomach supposedly allows the antral propulsive activity to return to normal once the obstruction is bypassed; this may lead to improved gastric emptying. Marginal ulceration may be more common after this operation than after TV/A or TV/D, but some chronic oral acid suppressive medication can be prescribed easily and safely. Moreover, if causative factors (helicobacter, NSAIDs, smoking) are eliminated, risk of recurrent ulcer should be minimized. If recurrent ulceration develops, a secondary operation (thoracoscopic vagotomy or distal gastrectomy) can be performed in a straightforward manner. The disadvantage of highly selective vagotomy and gastrojejunostomy is the risk of marginal ulceration and the risk of dumping from bypassing the pylorus. There has been one randomized, controlled clinical trial on surgical treatment of obstructing duodenal ulcer. Csendes et al. enrolled 90 patients and compared highly selective vagotomy + gastrojejunostomy, highly selective vagotomy + Jaboulay gastroduodenostomy, and selective vagotomy + antrectomy. Mean follow-up was 98 months. Highly selective vagotomy + gastrojejunostomy and selective vagotomy + antrectomy were found to be better than highly selective vagotomy + Jaboulay gastroduodenostomy in terms of patient symptoms on late follow-up. Based on their findings, the authors recommended highly selective vagotomy + gastrojejunostomy as the treatment of choice for obstructing duodenal ulcers, provided the surgeon has experience performing highly selective vagotomy.

The surgeon treating patients with obstructing peptic ulcer should be ever mindful of the possibility of malignant gastric outlet obstruction. One drawback of the minimally invasive approach to treating obstructing peptic ulcer may be the increased difficulty in appreciating a mass that would be readily apparent by palpation during an open procedure. The surgeon should not hesitate to convert to open operation if the suspicion for cancer is high. Even if the suspicion of cancer is not high, early open reoperation should be considered in the patient who does poorly after TV/D or HSV/GJ.

Conclusion

For many patients with obstructing peptic ulcer, endoscopic balloon dilatation combined with medical therapy is a practical, initial approach; however, long-term follow-up data are sparse, and patients often require repeated dilatations. Most good-risk patients with gastric outlet obstruction from chronic peptic ulcer disease are best served ultimately by operation. A high index of suspicion for carcinoma (the most common cause of gastric outlet obstruction nowadays) must be maintained. Vagotomy and antrectomy, truncal vagotomy and gastrojejunostomy, and highly selective vagotomy and gastrojejunostomy are all reasonable options depending on the circumstances. Resection should be avoided in high-risk patients, those with a chronically thin body habitus, and patients with a difficult duodenum. Highly selective vagotomy (or truncal vagotomy) and gastrojejunostomy is an excellent choice for many patients, and these procedures can often be accomplished with minimally invasive techniques. Highly selective vagotomy has the theoretic advantage of maintaining innervation to the antropyloric muscle and avoiding the occasionally severe postvagotomy syndromes. Diagnosis of an occult cancer may be easier with an open operation. Gastric ulcers are best resected if this can be done safely.

Selected Readings

Awan A, Johnston DE, Jamal MM (1998) Gastric outlet obstruction with benign endoscopic biopsy should be further explored for malignancy. Gastrointest Endosc 48:497–500

Behrman SW (2005) Management of complicated peptic ulcer disease. Arch Surg 140:201–208

Boylan JJ, Gradzka MI (1999) Long-term results of endoscopic balloon dilatation for gastric outlet obstruction. Dig Dis Sci 44:1883–1886

Csendes A, Maluenda F, Braghetto I, et al. (1993) Prospective randomized study comparing three surgical techniques for the treatment of gastric outlet obstruction secondary to duodenal ulcer. Am J Surg 166:45–49

Gibson JB, Behrman SW, Fabian TC, Britt LG (2000) Gastric outlet obstruction resulting from peptic ulcer disease requiring surgical intervention is infrequently associated with helicobacter pylori infection. J Am Coll Surg 191:32–37

Guzzo JL, Duncan M, Bass BL, et al. (2005) Severe and refractory peptic ulcer disease: the diagnostic dilemma. Dig Dis Sci 50:1999–2008

Harbison SP, Dempsey DT (1995) Peptic ulcer disease. Curr Prob Surg 42:335–454

Kochhar R, Sethy PK, Nagi B, Wig JD (2004) Endoscopic balloon dilatation of benign gastric outlet obstruction. J Gastroenterol Hepatol 19:418–422

Millat B, Fingerhut A, Borie F (2000) Surgical treatment of complicated peptic ulcers: controlled trials. World J Surg 24:299–306

Perng C-L, Lin H-J, Lo W-C, et al. (1996) Characteristics of patients with benign gastric outlet obstruction requiring surgery after endoscopic balloon dilation. Am J Gastroenterol 91:987–990

Zittel TT, Jehle EC, Becker HD (2000) Surgical management of peptic ulcer disease today-indication, technique and outcome. Langenbeck's Arch Surg 385:84–96

50 Peptic Ulcer Disease: Hemorrhage

John B. Ammori · Michael W. Mulholland

Pearls and Pitfalls

- Hemorrhage is the most common complication of peptic ulcer disease (PUD).
- The two most common causes of PUD are: infection with *Helicobacter pylori* and the use of nonsteroidal anti-inflammatory drugs (NSAIDs).
- Approximately 80% of bleeding episodes resolve spontaneously.
- Endoscopy is essential for early diagnosis and treatment.
- Eradication of *H. pylori* reduces rebleeding rates.
- Proton pump inhibitors are warranted after therapeutic endoscopy, when endoscopy is unavailable or delayed, and in patients with hemodynamic instability.
- Rebleeding is best treated endoscopically, except in elderly (>60 years) patients and those with clinically significant comorbid disease.
- Operative intervention is indicated for initial bleeding that cannot be controlled endoscopically, rebleeding in an elderly patient or one with clinically significant comorbidities, and after two rebleeding episodes in other patient populations.
- Ulcer excision is performed for gastric ulcers while duodenal ulcers are managed by direct suture of the ulcer bed.

Introduction

Peptic ulcer disease (PUD) remains a worldwide health concern. The three most common complications of PUD are bleeding, perforation, and obstruction. Peptic ulcer bleeding is the most common complication, occurring in 10–15% of patients during the disease course and is responsible for approximately 40% of deaths resulting from peptic ulcer. Peptic ulcer is the most common cause of upper gastrointestinal (UGI) bleeding, accounting for more than half of UGI bleeding. Bleeding occurs more commonly from ulcers in the duodenum rather than the stomach, often due to posterior erosion into the gastroduodenal artery. With the recognition of the importance of *Helicobacter pylori*, medical treatment of PUD has evolved over the past 20 years. In spite of treatment advances, the incidence of complicated disease has not changed. The number of operations for bleeding has decreased dramatically as endoscopy has become mainstay therapy. Despite these factors, the mortality rate (8–10%) has remained stable as a result of the changing demographics of PUD bleeders to an older patient population with more attendant comorbidities. There has also been a shift in the type of operations performed, with an increase in the use of local procedures combined with eradication of *H. pylori*. An aggressive, but rational approach is crucial for safe diagnosis and management.

Basic Science

The most common cause of PUD worldwide is *Helicobacter pylori*. The organism is estimated to infect up to 60% of the world's population and leads to peptic ulceration in 6–20% of the infected population. *H. pylori* infestation is associated with 60–70% of gastric ulcers and 90% of duodenal ulcers. For reasons that are not well understood, infection is 15–20% more prevalent in patients with uncomplicated ulceration relative to those with bleeding ulcers.

H. pylori is a spiral, gram-negative bacterium first described by Warren and Marshall in 1983. After colonization of the gastric lumen, bacterial and host responses are elicited. *H. pylori* produces urease, an enzyme which hydrolyzes urea to produce ammonia, thereby neutralizing gastric acid to provide an optimal microenvironment for survival. Urease production appears to be critical to the pathogenicity of *H. pylori*, because mutant strains of *H. pylori* without urease activity are unable to produce colonization. The bacterium passes through the mucous layer of the stomach and becomes attached to the gastric epithelium. When attached, *H. pylori* causes direct cellular injury and changes gastric secretory physiology. Infected patients have increased levels of circulating gastrin and decreased somatostatin levels. These endocrine alterations lead to increased basal and maximal acid outputs; acid secretory abnormalities return to normal after bacterial eradication. Interestingly, the bacterium does not colonize the duodenal epithelium at sites of ulceration.

The second most common cause of PUD is the use of nonsteroidal anti-inflammatory drugs (NSAIDs). Ulceration occurs by inhibition of prostaglandin production; local prostaglandins normally protect the gastric mucosa by stimulating mucus and bicarbonate production. Approximately 1–4% of chronic NSAID users will develop a peptic ulcer. NSAID use accounts for 25–30% of gastric ulcers and 5–10% of duodenal ulcers. *H. pylori*-positive patients who use NSAIDs have a two-fold increased risk of bleeding compared with *H. pylori*-negative NSAID users.

Initial Presentation and Assessment

Patients with bleeding peptic ulcers present commonly with hematemesis with or without melena. If the bleeding is massive, hematochezia may occur. Nasogastric lavage yielding blood or "coffee-ground" material confirms an UGI bleed. A negative lavage does not exclude an UGI bleeding occurring in the duodenum distal to a closed pylorus.

Initial assessment must include a medication history to determine the use of NSAIDs, anticoagulants, and anti-platelet agents. Vital signs are obtained to document signs of hypovolemia and shock. Resuscitation begins immediately with the infusion of crystalloid fluids through two large bore (14 or 16 Ga) intravenous lines in the antecubital spaces. Patients are transfused with packed red blood cells if vital signs do not normalize after 2 l of crystalloid or if there is evidence of continuing substantive blood loss. Patients who are unable to protect their airway risk aspiration and should be intubated endotracheally.

After vital signs have stabilized, the patient should undergo an esophagogastroduodenoscopy (EGD) as the diagnostic test of choice. Initial endoscopy should be performed emergently in high-risk patients, such as the elderly and those with major comorbidities, and ideally within 24 h in all patients. Thirty to 90 min prior to EGD, 250 mg of erythromycin may be given intravenously to promote gastric emptying and improve visibility of the gastric mucosa. The diagnostic goals of EGD are to localize the bleeding site and determine the risk for rebleeding. The ulcer can be graded by the Forrest classification

◘ Table 50-1

Forrest classification of Bleeding Peptic Ulcer (Modified from Forrest, 1974)

Forrest classification	Description
Ia	Spurting active bleeding
Ib	Nonspurting active bleeding
IIa	Nonbleeding "visible vessel"
IIb	Nonbleeding ulcer with overlying clot
IIc	Nonbleeding ulcer with hematin covered base
III	Clean ulcer base with no signs of bleeding

◘ Table 50-2

Stigmata of ulcer hemorrhage and risk of recurrent bleeding without endoscopic therapy (Adler et al., 2004. Copyright 2004. With permission from the American Society for Gastrointestinal Endoscopy)

Stigmata	Risk of recurrent bleeding without therapy
Active arterial (spurting) bleeding	Approaches 100%
Nonbleeding "visible vessel" ("pigmented protuberance")	Up to 50%
Nonbleeding adherent clot	30–35%
Ulcer oozing (without other stigmata)	10–27%
Flat spots	<8%
Clean-based ulcer	<3%

(❷ *Table 50-1*). The risk of recurrent bleeding can be predicted based on ulcer size (>1 cm) as well as the endoscopic appearance of the ulcer bed (❷ *Table 50-2*). Therapeutic management is dictated by the endoscopic appearance as discussed below.

Because gastric cancer may present as a bleeding ulcer, multiple biopsies are required of all gastric ulcers. Duodenal ulcers are associated rarely with a malignancy, and therefore biopsies are not mandatory unless indicated by the presence of a mass. All patients should undergo testing for *H. pylori* by rapid urease test, though this test may have reduced sensitivity during an active bleed; specificity, however, approaches 100% even during active bleeding. If the rapid urease test is negative, serologic testing for IgG antibody can be performed, as well as histologic assessment of biopsy material taken from the gastric antrum during endoscopy.

Treatment and Outcome

EGD is not only the diagnostic test of choice, but also acts as the potential first line therapeutic option. Approximately 80% of peptic ulcer bleeding resolves spontaneously with medical therapy alone. The indications for therapy are based on the endoscopic appearance of the ulcer. Ulcers associated with actively spurting vessels, non-bleeding "visible vessels," or adherent clot should be treated. Endoscopic therapy is not required for lesions with slow oozing and no other stigmata, flat pigmented spots, or clean-based ulcers.

The three major modalities used during endoscopic therapy are injection therapy, thermocoagulation, and mechanical therapy. Injection therapy acts primarily by tamponade due to the volume effect with a secondary pharmacologic effect dependent on the agent used. Epinephrine secondarily causes vasoconstriction; in contrast, ethanol, ethanolamine, and polidocanol are sclerosants that cause direct tissue injury and thrombosis, while thrombin and fibrin provide a hemostatic seal. Thermocoagulation involves the use of a probe positioned on the bleeding site to provide local tamponade followed by application of heat or electrocoagulation to achieve coagulative coaptation. Mechanical methods include endoclip placement or band ligation. Several trials have compared these methods, as well as treatment with combinations of modalities. One prospective, randomized study showed improvements in rebleeding rates, need for operative intervention, and mortality with combination therapy. With injection of 1–2 ml of epinephrine (1:10,000 dilution) and the addition of either thermocoagulation or endoclip placement, initial hemostasis was achieved in 98% of patients.

After successful endoscopic therapy, aggressive medical management is required to prevent recurrent bleeding. All patients with a positive rapid urease test should be treated aggressively with antibiotic therapy to eradicate *H. pylori* with a planned reevaluation in 6 weeks to confirm eradication of the *H. pylori*. A recent meta-analysis demonstrated a rebleeding rate of only 2% after successful eradication of *H. pylori* colonization, a marked and persistent reduction compared with untreated patients. NSAIDs should be withheld during the acute recovery period and indefinitely, if possible. Short-term intravenous proton pump inhibitors (PPIs) are recommended to reduce rebleeding risk for all patients who required endoscopic treatment, particularly in elderly patients with comorbid diseases. Additionally, PPIs should be considered prior to initial endoscopy for patients who present with hemodynamic instability, need for blood transfusions, or delay in endoscopic evaluation. Initiation of PPI therapy should never delay or supersede endoscopy in an actively bleeding patient. H2-receptor antagonists, however, are often ineffective in preventing rebleeding. Maintenance acid suppression therapy is not required after eradication of *H. pylori*. Patients who are NSAID-dependent should be maintained on chronic PPI therapy, as should the small percentage of patients whose ulcer diathesis is unrelated to NSAID use or *H. pylori* infection.

After initial endoscopic hemostasis, 10–25% of patients will rebleed. Gastric ulcers along the lesser curvature and posterior wall duodenal ulcers have the highest risk of rebleeding. Nearly all rebleeding occurs within 48–96 h of the initial intervention. Some surgeons advocate a second-look endoscopy 24 h after initial treatment for possible re-treatment of the high-risk lesions. This approach remains controversial and cannot be recommended as routine. Recurrent bleeding should be treated with aggressive resuscitation and repeat therapeutic endoscopy, which can control approximately 75% of rebleeding episodes with reduced morbidity and no difference in mortality compared with operative therapy. There is, however, a subset of high-risk patients, defined by age >60 years and the presence of major comorbid conditions, who have improved outcomes with early operative intervention rather than a second endoscopic treatment. These patients are not capable of sustaining either the prolonged hypotension or the episodic anemia related to delayed definitive operative control of the bleeding site.

Emergency operative intervention for bleeding peptic ulcers is required in 10–20% of patients hospitalized for UGI bleeding. Operation is indicated for active hemorrhage that is either refractory or inaccessible to initial therapeutic endoscopy. After successful endoscopic control initially, rebleeding is an indication for operative treatment. Elderly patients and those with severe comorbid conditions should undergo operation after the first bleeding recurrence, while most others should be given a chance at a second therapeutic endoscopy; should this second endoscopic treatment fail or the patient rebleed, operative intervention is recommended.

The primary goal of operative therapy for bleeding PUD is stopping the hemorrhage. Bleeding gastric ulcers should be resected, whenever possible. Resection of the ulcer achieves hemostasis, while also providing tissue to examine for gastric cancer. For ulcers located high on the lesser curve of the stomach near the gastroesophageal junction, resection may be difficult. In this situation, there are several options. One option is direct suture ligature of the ulcer base, as well as multiple biopsies to exclude cancer. Other options include resection with gastroplasty closure, or distal gastrectomy extended along the lesser curve to include the ulcer (Pauchet procedure).

For bleeding duodenal ulcers, a Kocher maneuver provides best access to the duodenum. Through a lateral (usually longitudinal) duodenotomy, four quadrant intraluminal suture ligatures are placed

◘ Figure 50-1
Algorithm for the treatment of patients with upper gastrointestinal bleeding from peptic ulcer disease (Reprinted from Cowles and Mulholland, 2001. With the permission of Lippincott Williams & Wilkins)

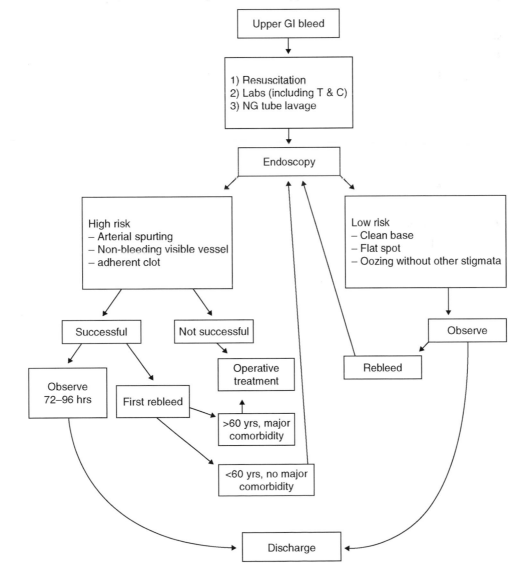

around the bleeding vessel at the base of the ulcer. Extraluminal ligation of the gastroduodenal artery has been described, but generally is unnecessary unless intraluminal ligation fails. Special care should be taken to avoid the common bile duct, which passes behind the first and second portions of the duodenum. ❯ *Figure 50-1* demonstrates a treatment algorithm for UGI bleeding caused by PUD.

Prior to the current appreciation and understanding of the role of *H. pylori* and NSAIDs, a secondary goal of operative treatment was reduction of gastric acid output in order to prevent ulcer recurrence. Acid reduction can be achieved by removal of vagal input (vagotomy) with or without the removal of gastrin-producing G cells of the antrum (antrectomy). Several options are available, which include truncal vagotomy and pyloroplasty, highly selective vagotomy (also called parietal cell or proximal gastric vagotomy), and truncal vagotomy and antrectomy. Studies performed prior to the understanding of the importance of *H. pylori* showed that there was no difference in mortality, but a higher rebleeding rate with local hemorrhage control versus local hemorrhage control plus an anti-ulcer procedure. With effective therapy to eradicate *H. pylori* and avoidance of NSAIDs, 95% of ulcers are cured. In patients who are NSAID-dependent, chronic PPI therapy will decrease ulcer rates. For these reasons, an acid-reducing operation is indicated only rarely. NSAID-dependent patients who are intolerant of PPI therapy may be candidates for a true anti-ulcer procedure.

Selected Readings

Adler DG, Leighton JA, Davila RE, et al. (2004) ASGE guideline: the role of endoscopy in acute non-variceal upper-GI hemorrhage. Gastrointest Endosc 60:497–504

Calvet X, Vergara M, Brullet E, et al. (2004) Addition of a second endoscopic treatment following epinephrine injection improves outcome in high-risk bleeding ulcers. Gastroenterology 126:441–450

Cowles RA, Mulholland MW (2001) Surgical management of peptic ulcer disease in the Helicobacter era-Management of bleeding peptic ulcer. Surg Laparo End Perc Tech 11:2–8

Erstad BL (2001) Proton-pump inhibitors for acute peptic ulcer bleeding. Annals Pharmacol 35:730–740.

Feldman RA, Eccersley AJ, Hardie JM (1998) Epidemiology of *Helicobacter pylori*: acquisition, transmission, population prevalence and disease-to-infection ratio. Brit Med Bull 54:39–53

Forrest JAH (1974) Endoscopy in gastrointestinal bleeding. Lancet 304:394–397

Gisbert JP, Khorrami S, Carballo F, et al. (2004) *H. pylori* eradication therapy vs. antisecretory non-eradication therapy (with or without long-term maintenance antisecretory therapy) for the prevention of recurrent bleeding from peptic ulcer. Cochrane Database of Systematic Reviews 2:CD004062

Lau JY, Sung JJ, Lam YH, et al. (1999) Endoscopic retreatment compared with surgery in patients with recurrent bleeding after initial endoscopic control of bleeding ulcers. New Engl J Med 340:751–756

51 Gastric Ulcer

Cheong J. Lee · Diane M. Simeone

Pearls and Pitfalls

- Gastric ulcers comprise 20% of all peptic ulcer disease and can form in the presence of low to normal acid secretion: *Type I* and *IV* Gastric ulcers are *not* associated with acid hypersecretion, whereas *Types II* and *III* ulcers involve acid hypersecretion.
- All patients with suspected gastric ulcer disease should be evaluated for *H. pylori* infection.
- Endoscopy is the diagnostic modality of choice for evaluating gastric ulcer. Multiple biopsies of an ulcer (at least 7) is required to effectively exclude an underlying neoplasm.
- High suspicion of malignancy should be maintained in older patients with gastric ulcer and those with refractory disease.
- Persistent ulcers after 12 weeks of maximal medical therapy are considered to have refractory disease and require surgical management.
- Choice of operative therapy depends upon the type of gastric ulcer encountered.
- Laparoscopic repair of perforated ulcers have equivalent outcomes when compared with conventional operations.
- Complications of gastric ulcer surgery include: delayed gastric emptying, dumping syndrome, postvagotomy diarrhea, chronic gastroparesis, alkaline reflux gastritis, and afferent or efferent loop syndrome.

Epidemiology and Pathophysiology

Peptic ulcer disease remains a major public health problem, affecting more than 4 million people in the United States. Even with the discovery and elucidation of *Helicobacter pylori*'s role in peptic ulcer formation and subsequent advancement in medical therapy, mortality and complications from peptic ulcer disease still remain substantial as a growing cohort of aging patients with comorbidities seek treatment; ulcer disease is listed as a contributing cause of death in more than 10,000 cases annually. The pathogenesis of peptic ulceration is complex and multifactorial, but often considered an alteration in the balance between acid-peptic secretion and mucosal defense. Luminal secretion of acid is essential to ulcer formation ("no acid – no ulcer"). Unlike duodenal ulcers, gastric ulcers, which comprise about 20% of peptic ulcer disease, may form in the presence of low to normal acid secretion, attesting to the theory that compromised mucosal defense is prerequisite for ulcer formation. Mucosal infection with *Helicobacter pylori* is implicated in the pathogenesis of ulcer formation in most patients. Environmental factors such as ingestion of non steroidal anti-inflammatory drugs (NSAIDS) and cigarette smoking are other important contributors in compromising gastric mucosal defense. A number of rare familial syndromes associated with gastric ulcerations have been described, but there is no clear racial predilection for ulcer development.

Clinical Presentation and Diagnosis

The classic symptom of peptic ulcer disease is epigastric pain. Patients typically complain of burning, gnawing, or stabbing pain of the upper abdomen that is worse in the morning. Ingestion of food or antacids generally provides relief. Physical exam findings are minimal in uncomplicated cases. A number of patients who are asymptomatic may present with microcytic anemia and guaiac-positive stools. Patients with accompanying anorexia, gastric outlet obstruction, and weight loss should be thoroughly evaluated for the presence of malignancy. The differential diagnosis to consider is broad and includes a wide variety of diseases of the upper gastrointestinal tract, including nonulcerative dyspepsia, gastroesophageal reflux disease, gastric neoplasms, along with inflammatory and neoplastic disease encompassing the pancreas, and cholelithiasis. Less commonly, ulcer pain may be mimicked by mesenteric ischemia or coronary artery disease.

All patients with suspected gastric ulcer disease should be evaluated for *H. pylori* infection. Simple noninvasive diagnostic tests such as serologic antibody testing, urea breath testing, and stool antigen screening are available for initial assessment. In younger patients with mild or intermittent symptoms without systemic symptoms or ulcer complications, treatment following non-invasive testing is appropriate, while in older patients, further diagnostic measures should be taken.

Presently, endoscopy has become the preferred method of evaluating patients with suspected ulcer disease. In a controlled trial comparing endoscopy with barium contrast examination, endoscopy was both more sensitive (92% vs 54%) and more specific (100% vs 91%) in its diagnosis. Endoscopy also allows for biopsy of the mucosa, which is critical in confirming the diagnosis, as well as to rule out neoplasm. Obtaining at least seven biopsy samples of the ulcer is required to effectively exclude an underlying neoplasm.

Traditionally, gastric ulcer has been categorized based upon its anatomic location (❯ *Fig. 51-1*). *Type I* ulcers are most common (50%) and occur in the body of the stomach along the lesser curvature at the incisura. Patients with *Type I* ulcers have low to normal acid secretion. *Type II* gastric ulcers (25%) also occur along the lesser curvature, but are associated with a duodenal ulcer component. *Type II* ulcers are associated with acid hypersecretion, as are *Type III* ulcers (20%), which are located in the prepyloric region. *Type IV* ulcers (<10%) occur high along the lesser curvature of the stomach near the gastroesophageal junction. *Type IV* ulcers are associated with low to normal acid secretion (see ❯ *Table 51-1*).

Medical Therapy

Once diagnosis has been confirmed and malignancy ruled out, the goal of the therapy is directed towards elimination of the inciting causes of ulcer formation, eradication of *H. pylori* and reduction of acid secretion. Patients should be questioned regarding the use of ulcerogenic agents, namely non steroidal anti-inflammatory agents or steroids, which should be discontinued or weaned as much as possible. In the absence of treatment, spontaneous healing of *H. pylori* infected ulcers occurs in less

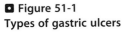

Figure 51-1
Types of gastric ulcers

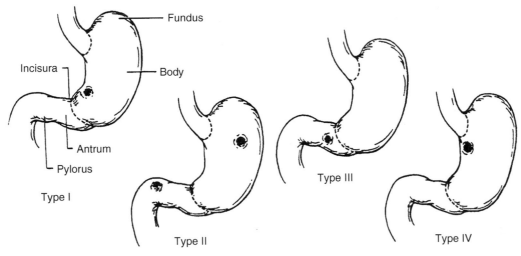

Table 51-1

Types of gastric ulcers and recommended surgical treatment

Gastric ulcer	% incidence	Location	Acid secretion	Recommended surgical management
Type I	50	Body of the stomach along the lesser curvature	Low	Billroth I or II
Type II	25	Body of the stomach along the lesser curvature with duodenal ulcer component	High	Billroth I or II + vagotomy
Type III	20	Prepyloric region	High	Billroth I or II + vagotomy
Type IV	<10	High along the lesser curvature of the stomach near the gastroesophageal junction	Low	Csendes' gastrectomy or Pauchet + Billroth I

than 1% of cases. Most widely used treatment regimens include a combination of an antisecretory drug, commonly the H2 receptor antagonist ranitidine or the proton pump inhibitor omeprazole, along with two antibiotics, clarithromycin and amoxicillin or metronidazole. Most series find triple combination antibiotic therapy to be more effective than a single antimicrobial agent, with treatment of patients with triple therapy for 7–14 days resulting in ulcer healing in greater than 90% of patients after 8 weeks on repeat endoscopy. Those with gastric ulcer unrelated to *H. pylori* infection should stop the inciting agent and be placed on antisecretory therapy. In patients that require long-term NSAID or steroid therapy, elective surgery may be considered in management of their ulcer disease. All patients with a documented gastric ulcer should undergo repeat endoscopy 8–12 weeks after therapy to assess healing. If an ulcer has failed to completely heal after 12 weeks of continuous medical therapy or if the patient has more than one recurrence, then the patient is considered to have intractable disease. The differential diagnosis of a non-healing ulcer includes persistent *H. pylori* infection, Zollinger-Ellison syndrome, NSAID abuse, mesenteric ischemia, and microscopic malignancy. In the presence of a non-healing gastric ulcer, repeat endoscopy with multiple biopsies is recommended to re-evaluate the gastric mucosa for persistent *H. pylori* infection or an occult malignancy. Zollinger-Ellison syndrome should be excluded by examining the patient's basal serum gastrin levels or by performing a secretion stimulation test. Once measures have been taken to rule out occult, treatable causes of intractability, elective surgery can be planned.

Surgical Therapy: Elective

Surgical intervention for ulcer disease is reserved for patients who have failed or cannot comply with medical therapy or for those that present with complications. Generally, ulcers that have failed maximal medical therapy for 12 weeks or the inability to rule out an occult malignancy are criteria for elective surgical intervention. For *Type I* gastric ulcers, a distal gastrectomy with Billroth I or II (❯ *Fig. 51-2*) reconstruction is recommended for most patients, since this approach removes both the ulcer and the diseased antrum. Resection of the diseased segment also allows for more thorough evaluation of a potential underlying malignancy. With antrectomy and reconstruction, acid secretory potential is reduced and gastric drainage is accelerated. Low recurrence rates (0–5%) and excellent symptomatic relief are usually achieved. The operative mortality has been reported to range anywhere from 0% to 6%. Since *Type I* gastric ulcers are rarely associated with acid hypersecretion, the addition of a vagotomy is felt to be unnecessary. This is supported by results from a large series from the Cleveland Clinic reporting on 349 cases of gastric ulcer evaluated from 1950 to 1979. The study found equivalent ulcer recurrence rates following gastric resection for *Type I* gastric ulcer either with or without vagotomy.

Since *Type II* and *III* ulcers are associated with excessive acid secretion, the operative approach includes ulcer excision along with vagotomy. *Type II* gastric ulcers occur synchronously with scarring or ulceration in the duodenum or pyloric channel. They tend to be large, deep ulcers, with poorly defined margins. A truncal vagotomy and antrectomy with Billroth I reconstruction is the preferred surgical option and accomplishes both goals of ulcer excision and decreasing acid secretion. Recurrence rates are less than 5% with an operative mortality rate of about 1%. *Type III* ulcers, which are prepyloric, can also be managed with an antrectomy and vagotomy with Billroth I reconstruction. A Billroth II

◨ **Figure 51-2**

Billroth I and Billroth II reconstruction (Reprinted from Doherty, 2006. With permission of the McGraw-Hill Companies)

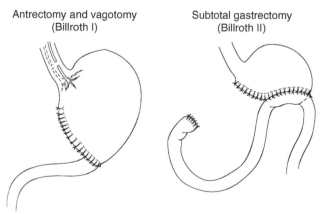

Antrectomy and vagotomy
(Billroth I)

Subtotal gastrectomy
(Billroth II)

reconstruction with creation of a gastrojejunostomy can be performed in either *Type II* or *Type III* ulcers if the more physiologic Billroth I reconstruction becomes technically challenging, such as in cases of excessive scarring or inflammation of the duodenum. Highly selective vagotomy is also an option, but has been associated with poor results for both *Type II* and *Type III* ulcers, with ulcer recurrence rates ranging from 16% to 44% in several series.

Type IV gastric ulcers are uncommon and may be technically challenging due to their anatomic location high along the lesser curvature, close to the gastroesophageal junction. Ulcer size, distance from the gastroesophageal junction, and surrounding inflammation are important determinants of technical approach. Like *Type I* ulcers, *Type IV* ulcers are not associated with acid hypersecretion and a vagotomy is not necessary. Ulcers that are 2–5 cm from the cardia can be managed with a distal gastrectomy, which is extended along the lesser curvature to include the ulcer (the Pauchet procedure) and a Billroth I reconstruction. For ulcers high up near the gastroesophageal junction, a subtotal gastrectomy with a Roux-en-Y jejunal reconstruction (Csendes' procedure) may have to be undertaken (❯ *Fig. 51-3*).

Surgical Therapy: Emergent

Bleeding, perforation, and obstruction are the principal complications of gastric ulcer disease. Because patients with complications from gastric ulcer tend to be elderly and have comorbidities, operation in the emergent setting is associated with high overall mortality, ranging from 10% to 40%. In patients who have bleeding gastric ulcers, indications for emergent operative intervention include: (1) hemo-dynamic instability despite vigorous resuscitation (>3 unit transfusion), (2) failure of endoscopic techniques to arrest hemorrhage, and (3) recurrent hemorrhage after initial stabilization with up to two attempts at obtaining endoscopic hemostasis. Other relative indications for surgery include rare blood type or difficult crossmatch, refusal of transfusion, shock on presentation, and bleeding chronic gastric ulcer. In hemodynamically unstable patients, vessel ligation with oversewing or excision of the ulcer should be expeditiously performed. If unknown, *H. pylori* status can be determined with mucosal biopsy and rapid urease test. Excision alone, however, is associated with rebleeding in as many as 20% of patients.

◘ **Figure 51-3**
Csendes' procedure, used to treat gastric ulcers close to the gastroesophageal junction (Reprinted from Csendes et al., 1978, copyright 1978. With permission from Excerpta Medica, Inc)

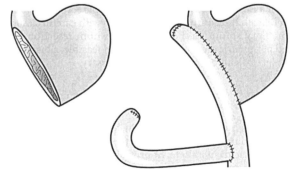

In hemodynamically stable patients, a more definitive approach is undertaken with distal gastrectomy and Billroth I or II reconstruction. Bilateral truncal vagotomy is also performed to address acid hypersecretion in patients with *Type II* and *III* ulcers. Patients who undergo truncal or parietal cell vagotomy in this setting have higher ulcer recurrence rates postoperatively, and their use in the urgent or emergent setting is not recommended. With bleeding *Type IV* ulcers, an antrectomy with extension to include the ulcer is preferred. If, however, this approach becomes technically challenging, an alternative approach is to identify and ligate the left gastric artery and to biopsy and oversew the ulcer through a high anterior gastrotomy.

In patients with a perforated gastric ulcer, hemodynamic stability and medical comorbidities become important factors in surgical decision making. The preferred approach to a patient with a perforated ulcer is definitive antrectomy to include the ulcer and, if indicated, a vagotomy. If the patient is at an unacceptably high risk because of advanced age, comorbid disease, intraoperative instability, or severe peritoneal soilage, omental plication of the perforation with biopsy can be performed. In selected patients with a sealed perforation, nasogastric suction, broad spectrum antibiotics, and supportive therapy can be considered. For patients presenting with perforation as their first presentation of gastric ulcer disease with untreated *H. pylori* infection, non-resectional surgical therapy is a reasonable option with medical treatment of *H. pylori* postoperatively. If *H. pylori* is adequately treated, these select patients will have low ulcer recurrence rates. In this cohort of patients, repeat endoscopy should be performed at about 6 weeks postoperatively to gauge appropriate ulcer healing. Any stable patient with a long standing ulcer history should undergo definitive ulcer surgery with an antrectomy and Billroth I or II reconstruction if they develop a perforation. Likewise, in patients with medication induced gastric ulcers that present with perforation, and those medications are essential, definitive anti-ulcer surgery should be planned.

Gastric outlet obstruction is typically a complication of *Type II* and *III* ulcers. Chronic scarring of the duodenum or acute inflammation and subsequent edema is typically the underlying cause. After correction of fluid and electrolyte abnormalities, operation is generally indicated if obstruction fails to resolve after 72 h with antisecretory therapy and nasogastric tube decompression. In some cases, endoscopic dilatation has been performed successfully; however, the long-term patency rates are not as good as surgical treatment of gastric outlet obstruction. For those patients who undergo surgical intervention, the procedure of choice is an antrectomy with Billroth I or II reconstruction. Placement of a feeding jejunostomy tube at the time of surgery is usually recommended to improve the patient's nutritional status and because the chronic gastric outlet obstruction predisposes delayed postoperative gastric emptying.

Laparoscopic Surgery

In recent years, laparoscopic surgical approaches have gained popularity for the management of peptic ulcer disease. Several series in the literature demonstrate that a laparoscopic approach is a viable option for perforated peptic ulcer, with outcomes comparable to open surgery. There is growing evidence from these series that laparoscopy is associated with less postoperative pain, reduced pulmonary complications, a shorter postoperative hospital stay, and earlier return to normal daily activities than the conventional open repair. Most of these studies have focused on omental repair of perforated duodenal or juxtapyloric ulcers, and limited evidence exists with regards to repair of other types of perforated gastric ulcers. A laparoscopic approach to operative management of refractory gastric ulcers and gastric ulcers complicated by bleeding and gastric outlet obstruction is feasible, but has not been well-studied.

Postoperative Management and Potential Complications

In the postoperative period, low continuous nasogastric suction is continued until the patient has evidence of resolving ileus. The patient is supported with intravenous fluids or parenteral nutrition, if indicated, until they are able to maintain oral intake. Patients with prolonged gastric ileus may require enteric feedings through a feeding tube. A naso-enteric feeding access or a feeding jejunostomy can be established at the time of the operation if prolonged ileus is anticipated. Antibiotic use should be limited to perioperative use unless the patient had peritonitis and contamination from a perforated ulcer, in which case, antibiotic use should be continued postoperatively until the patient has resolution of fever and leukocytosis.

Early complications from gastric ulcer surgery are numerous, including superficial and deep infection, bleeding, delayed gastric emptying, and anastomotic leak. In patients who undergo emergent surgical intervention, postoperative complications may develop related to the patients' preexisting comorbidities such as cardiac and respiratory disease. Late sequelae of gastrectomy are thought to be due more in part to the complications associated with vagotomy rather than gastric resection itself, however, have been referred to collectively as the *postgastrectomy syndromes*. Most patients note a change in their digestive habits postoperatively, and about 20% are significantly affected. Most patients adapt over time with 5% of patients developing lifelong symptoms and 1% of patients severely debilitated by these symptoms. The late complications of gastric ulcer surgery include delayed gastric emptying, dumping syndrome, post vagotomy diarrhea, chronic gastroparesis, alkaline reflux gastritis, and afferent or efferent loop syndrome.

Postvagotomy diarrhea develops in approximately 30% of patients after truncal vagotomy. The condition may be related to the rapid passage of unconjugated bile salts from the denervated biliary tree into the colon, where they stimulate secretion. In most cases, it is self limiting. In persistent cases, cholestyramine administration has been shown to be beneficial.

Dumping syndrome occurs in about 20% of patients after gastrectomy or vagotomy and drainage procedures. Patients experience postprandial gastrointestinal discomfort, which may include nausea, vomiting, diarrhea, and cramps, with vasomotor symptoms such as diaphoresis, palpitations, and flushing. Although the pathogenesis is incompletely understood, the syndrome is frequently attributed to the rapid emptying of hyperosmolar food, particularly carbohydrates, into the small bowel. This causes rapid intraluminal fluid shifts due to the osmotic gradient and may be confounded by the release of one or more vasoactive hormones, such as serotonin and vasoactive intestinal polypeptide. Patients may complain of the same constellation of symptoms hours after eating, called late dumping. This is secondary to hypoglycemia from a postprandial insulin peak and can be managed with carbohydrate ingestion. Most patients with early dumping can be treated conservatively by initiating the dietary changes of frequent small meals that are high in protein and fat and low in carbohydrates. Administration of octreotide has been shown to help in some instances. The rare patient with intractable symptoms may be considered for operative therapy with the goal of delaying gastric emptying, which is best addressed by converting an antrectomy and Billroth reconstruction to a Roux-En Y reconstruction (❯ *Fig. 51-4*).

◘ Figure 51-4
Conversion of an antrectomy with Billroth X reconstruction to a Roux-en-Y reconstruction (Reprinted from Schwartz et al., 1989. With permission of the McGraw-Hill Companies)

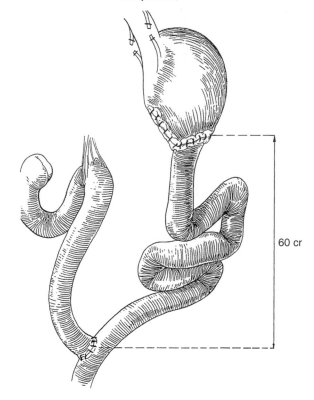

60 cr

Reflux of bile into the stomach is common after operations that eliminate the pyloric sphincter, but only about 2% of patients that undergo gastric ulcer surgery will experience alkaline reflux gastritis. Alkaline reflux gastritis typically presents with symptoms of postprandial, burning epigastric pain. Although a variety of medical treatments are available, none have been shown to be particularly effective in treating this problem. Surgical revision to a Roux-En Y reconstruction may be necessary to effectively treat this problem, if severe.

Afferent and efferent loop syndromes may develop after Billroth II reconstruction or gastroenterostomy. Patients will complain of postprandial epigastric pain and vomiting in both cases; however, only efferent loop syndrome will present with bilious vomiting. Both are related to mechanical obstruction of the limbs by kinking, anastomotic narrowing, or adhesions. In afferent loop syndrome, the detection of a distended afferent loop on CT is diagnostic. In this setting, operative intervention with a Roux-En Y reconstruction is appropriate.

Selected Readings

Ashley SW, Evoy D, Daly JM (1999) Stomach In: Schwartz SS (ed) Principles of surgery, 7th edn. McGraw-Hill, New York, p 1181

Csendes A, Lazo M, Braghetto I (1978) A surgical technic for high (cardial or juxtacardial) benign chronic gastric ulcer. Am J Surg 135:857–858

Doherty GM (2006) Gastric ulcer. In: Doherty GM, Way LW (eds) Current surgical diagnosis and treatment. 12th edn. McGraw-Hill, New York, p 517

Dooley CP, Larson AW, Stace NH, et al. (1984) Double-contrast barium meal and upper gastrointestinal endoscopy. A comparative study. Ann Intern Med 101:538–545

Eagon JC, Miedema BW, Kelly KA (1992) Postgastrectomy syndromes. Surg Clin North Am 72:445

Lickstein LH, Matthews JB (1997) Elective surgical management of peptic ulcer disease. Probl Gen Surg 14:37

McDonald MP, Broughan TA, Hermann RE, et al. (1996) Operations for gastric ulcer: a long term study. Am Surg 62:673

Ng EK, Lam YH, Sung JJ, et al. (2000) Eradication of Helicobacter pylori prevents recurrence of ulcer after simple closure of duodenal ulcer perforation: randomized controlled trial. Ann Surg 231:153–158

Schwartz SS, Rodney M, et al. (1989) Maingot's abdominal operations, 9th edn. McGraw-Hill/Appleton & Lange, New York, p 716

Siu WT, Leong H, Law BK, et al. (2002) Laparoscopic repair for perforated peptic ulcer: a randomized controlled trial. Ann Surg 235:313–319

52 Postgastrectomy and Postvagotomy Syndromes

Italo Braghetto

Pearls and Pitfalls

- Do not submit patients to gastric surgery without a comprehensive, careful evaluation.
- Any operation on the stomach alters normal digestive physiology and can cause symptoms and late sequelae.
- In the past, vagotomy and Billroth I or II gastric resections were used frequently for peptic ulcer disease or gastric cancer and were associated with some element of post gastrectomy/vagotomy syndrome in 25% of patients. These symptoms (diarrhea, early satiety, gastric stasis) were mild, self-limited, and only rarely needed operative treatment.
- Currently, the post-gastrectomy syndromes are rare, because peptic ulcer disease is treated medically.
- For severe, post-gastrectomy gastroparesis, near total gastrectomy with Roux-en-Y reconstruction can be used with successful results in highly selected patients.
- Post-vagotomy diarrhea must be treated with medical and dietary measures; no operative treatment has proven effective.
- Currently, minimally invasive operative procedures for gastric pathology obtain the best functional results.

Operations on the stomach that impair normal gastric and pyloric functions may alter gastrointestinal physiology markedly; collectively, this group of disorders is termed "postgastrectomy syndromes." Because the postgastrectomy disorders may be due to varying causes leading to either rapid or delayed gastric emptying and intestinal transit, it is important to differentiate these disorders by careful diagnostic studies, starting by taking a careful history from the patient.

Over the last 50 years, especially before recognizing the importance of *Helicobacter pylori* in the late 1980s/early 1990s, many acid-reducing operations were performed for peptic ulcer disease and gastric cancer. About 25% of these patients developed to some degree symptoms of one or more post-vagotomy/post-gastrectomy syndromes. We accumulated considerable experience with managing these disorders, but because only about 1% of patients were permanently disabled, few of these patients required remedial operations. In the last 2 decades, these complications have decreased in incidence and importance due in large part to the changes in the management and operative therapy for peptic ulcer disease; in fact, after 1995, very few elective operations for peptic ulcer have been performed as Stabile and Passaro predicted some years before. Similarly, gastric cancer appears also to be decreasing in many Western countries.

Interestingly, operations for emergencies due mainly to perforation of peptic ulcer disease have remained almost constant, and currently the operative treatment for this disorder can be performed in a conservative way by laparoscopy and omental patch; need for gastrectomy and/or vagotomy is deemed unusual. In similar fashion, elective operations for peptic ulcer disease have declined markedly and nearly disappeared over the last 30 years. This trend preceded the introduction of effective acid-suppressive medications such as H_2-receptor antagonists; these drugs, and the more recently developed proton pump inhibitors combined with antibiotic eradication of *Helicobacter pylori* have eliminated effectively the need for elective operative therapy of duodenal ulcer disease. What a remarkable change since the 1960s and 1970s!

Currently, most gastric surgery is performed for malignant diseases and morbid obesity. Advances in perioperative care as well as in operative techniques have decreased the mortality rate after total gastrectomy to less than 2%. Five-year survival after curative resection for gastric neoplasms is in the range of 30–40%, depending obviously on the type, stage, and extent of disease. With the current interest in performing minimally invasive and less aggressive procedures utilizing new technologies, better functional results have led to fewer "post-gastrectomy cripples." In addition, the classic Billroth I or II gastrectomies combined with truncal vagotomy often employed for operative treatment of peptic ulcer disease and for distal gastric cancer have been abandoned in favor of a Roux-en-Y reconstruction of gastrointestinal continuity due to the occurrence of related post-gastrectomy, bile reflux syndromes ("alkaline gastritis," "biliary gastritis," and reflux esophagitis).

Therefore, some of the post-gastrectomy/post-vagotomy syndromes are less common now than over the last 50 years. The physiologic consequences of loss of the stomach, as well as problems related to the method of restoration of gastrointestinal continuity, need to be understood, recognized, diagnosed, and treated if necessary according to the following alterations in gastrointestinal function: abnormal gastric emptying and intestinal transit, disturbed nutritional intake, and abnormal assimilation of ingested nutrients (digestion and absorption). Symptoms can vary considerably and may depend on individual susceptibility, co-morbidities present prior to operation, and the specific type of operative procedures performed. In addition to pathophysiologic changes in gastrointestinal function related to gastrectomy, vagotomy, and methods of reconstruction, it is necessary also to differentiate early or chronic complications due to technical mistakes from the expected physiologic changes of the gastric operation. Afferent loop syndrome, efferent loop syndromes due mesenteric hernias, and mechanical obstructions secondary to adhesive, fibrotic strictures or kinking of the jejunal loop occur not infrequently, can masquerade as post-gastrectomy syndromes, and will respond well to operative correction.

This chapter will review the different postgastrectomy/post-vagotomy syndromes based on the international literature.

Dumping Syndrome

Dumping has been classified into early and late forms based on the timing of the onset of symptoms after a meal. In patients with early dumping, symptoms start typically 10–30 min after ingestion of a meal. These patients generally have a mixture of gastrointestinal and vasomotor complaints. In contrast, the symptoms in patients with late dumping are primarily vasomotor and occur 2–3 h postprandial. Few patients have both early and late dumping symptoms. The incidence and severity of dumping varies greatly after the various types of gastric surgery. After proximal gastric vagotomy, dumping is quite unusual (<1%); in contrast, after truncal or selective vagotomy with destruction of the pylorus (pyloroplasty, gastroenterostomy, and antrectomy), about 20–30% of patients develop at least some bothersome symptoms, while about 5% have more severe symptoms that can be very severe in about 1%. Vagotomy of the proximal stomach plays a key role in dumping, because antrectomy alone (without vagotomy) and either a Billroth I or Billroth II reconstruction is complicated by dumping in only about 10% of patients. There is some evidence to suggest that clinically important dumping, even after vagotomy, is less common after Roux-en-Y drainage/reconstruction.

Diagnosis: Dumping is a clinical diagnosis that depends on the presence of typical symptoms. Abdominal pain is usually absent, but if present, an upper gastrointestinal contrast study and/or upper endoscopy should be performed to exclude stomal obstruction, afferent loop syndrome, or recurrent ulcer as a cause of postprandial pain. In most patients, any further evaluation is usually unnecessary, although a gastric-emptying study can be performed to document rapid gastric emptying. Currently, gastric emptying is assessed by radionuclide markers, including both liquid and solid components of a meal.

The Visick classification can be used to characterize the severity of symptoms after gastric operations and the success of treatment. Visick grade I is no symptoms, Visick II is mild to moderate symptoms not requiring treatment, Visick III is moderate to severe symptoms requiring medical treatment, while Visick IV involves very severe or persistent symptoms affecting quality of life markedly and requiring intense medical management and/or reoperation. Both motor and hormonal mechanisms are involved in the pathophysiology of dumping (❯ *Fig. 52-1*).

Treatment: The treatment of dumping syndrome is largely, in fact almost exclusively, dietary. Based on the known pathophysiologic changes, a diet low in carbohydrate content, "the dry diet routine," and eating small, frequent meals is the first line of treatment in these patients.

Recently, octreotide acetate, a long-acting somatostatin analogue, has been used in treating severe dumping symptoms. Successful resolution of symptoms is unusual, but can be dramatic in up to 20% of patients. Operative treatment is indicated only rarely, because symptomatic relief is usually obtained with medical therapy; moreover, symptoms rarely persist for more than 1 year after the gastric operations.

Many different remedial operations for dumping syndrome have been designed to slow gastric emptying. After vagotomy and pyloroplasty, attempts to reconstruct the pylorus may prove effective. For patients with previous Billroth I or II gastrectomy, Roux-en-Y conversion is the simplest and most effective operation. For patients who have undergone Roux-en-Y gastrojejunostomy, construction of a 10 cm, antiperistaltic jejunal segment within the Roux limb (Christeas' operation) has been suggested; however, although several groups have presented their experience with operative treatment of severe dumping syndrome, the success after these procedures has been disappointing and inconsistent.

Postvagotomy Diarrhea

Most all types of gastric surgery may result in diarrhea postoperatively, but the incidence of diarrhea is higher in patients who have undergone vagotomy. Truncal vagotomy has the highest incidence of around 20%, whereas the incidence after selective or highly selective vagotomy (which preserves vagal innervation to the small bowel) are 6% and 4%, respectively. Despite its presence, the diarrhea is truly

◘ Figure 52-1
Pathophysiology of dumping syndrome

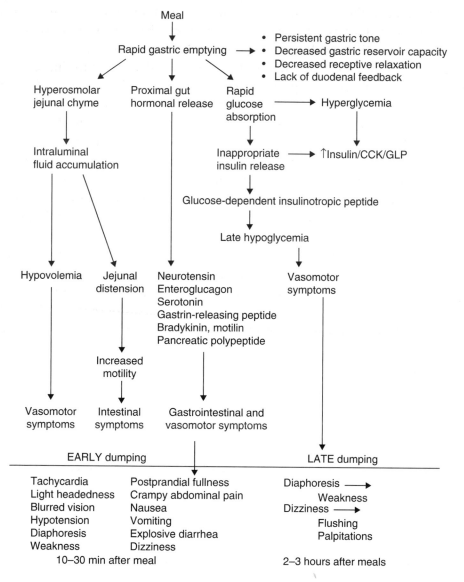

Meal

Rapid gastric emptying ⟶ • Persistent gastric tone
• Decreased gastric reservoir capacity
• Decreased receptive relaxation
• Lack of duodenal feedback

Hyperosmolar jejunal chyme   Proximal gut hormonal release   Rapid glucose absorption ⟶ Hyperglycemia

Intraluminal fluid accumulation   Inappropriate insulin release ⟶ ↑Insulin/CCK/GLP

Glucose-dependent insulinotropic peptide

Late hypoglycemia

Hypovolemia | Jejunal distension | Neurotensin Enteroglucagon Serotonin Gastrin-releasing peptide Bradykinin, motilin Pancreatic polypeptide | Vasomotor symptoms

Increased motility

Vasomotor symptoms | Intestinal symptoms | Gastrointestinal and vasomotor symptoms

EARLY dumping | LATE dumping

Tachycardia	Postprandial fullness	Diaphoresis ⟶
Light headedness	Crampy abdominal pain	Weakness
Blurred vision	Nausea	Dizziness ⟶
Hypotension	Vomiting	Flushing
Diaphoresis	Explosive diarrhea	Palpitations
Weakness	Dizziness	
10–30 min after meal		2–3 hours after meals

debilitating and only in a small fraction of these patients. Severe symptoms are characterized by frequent watery stools, occasionally explosive, often nocturnal, and not always associated with ingestion of a meal. Occasionally, the diarrhea can occur immediately after a meal concomitant with dumping symptoms. The initial diagnostic approach should include fecal white blood cell count, stool culture, and fecal titers for *Clostridium difficile*. For patients with persistent diarrhea, further studies should be performed to exclude steatorrhea, partial intestinal obstruction, and inflammatory bowel diseases, including fecal-fat studies, upper GI contrast series with small bowel follow-through, and either colonoscopy or barium enema.

Several etiologies for post-vagotomy diarrhea have been proposed, but the exact pathogenesis of this syndrome remains unclear. Gastric stasis leading to bacterial overgrowth, enteritis with malabsorption, changes in small bowel epithelial enzymatic content, decreases in mesenteric blood flow, and denervation of the extrahepatic biliary tree and small intestine leading to rapid transit of unconjugated bile salts into the colon where they inhibit water absorption have also been suggested, but solid experimental work has failed to support any of these theories. Most work suggests that the diarrhea is related to rapid intestinal transit without a true malabsorption.

Treatment: Dietary measures that can be effective include a decrease in the intake of both fluid and lactose-containing foods. Antidiarrheal agents, such as diphenoxylate with atropine or loperamide, the bile salt exchange resin cholestyramine, or a trial of octreotide may also be useful. Operative therapy is recommended rarely, because the vast majority of patients with diarrhea early after vagotomy improve with time or dietary changes alone. In our experience, 50% of patients with diarrhea after vagotomy present with mild diarrhea, 40% with more moderate diarrhea, and less than 5% present with daily or incapacitating severe diarrhea. Greater than 90% improve with only dietary modifications and/or medical treatment.

There is, however, the small sub group of patients with refractive postvagotomy diarrhea. Despite the observation that these patients are miserable, the concept of operative intervention should be approached with caution. Results with one or two, 10 cm anti-peristaltic jejunal interposition(s) are very controversial. In the 1980s, several authors presented successful outcomes claiming that their patients experienced relief from diarrhea; however, several required reoperation for pain or obstruction. Most experts avoid this operation currently. Another procedure reported for treatment of intractable postvagotomy diarrhea is the onlay-reversed-ileal graft designed to create a passive, nonpropulsive segment, thereby slowing small bowel transit; however, the experience in humans is quite limited. Others have attempted to slow transit (and gastric emptying) by conversion to Roux-en-Y gastric emptying but again with infrequent and inconsistent results. Unfortunately, no good treatment exists for these patients.

Alkaline reflux gastritis (biliary gastritis, biliary gastroesophageal reflux)

Enterogastric reflux is common after Billroth II gastrojejunostomy, but it also occurs after simple gastrojejunostomy, Billroth I anastomosis, or pyloroplasty. Nevertheless, true, symptomatic bile reflux gastritis is quite uncommon, in part, because many surgeons currently prefer Roux-en-Y gastrojejunostomy for reestablishment of gastrointestinal transit after gastrectomy and because gastrectomies are less common today. Which component of the refluxed enteric fluid is the injurious one is not clear, but bile salts are the likely candidate. Interestingly, the severity of the reflux or the severity of the histologic "gastritis" does not correlate with the presence or severity of symptoms. In addition, delayed clearance of bile is also thought to be important in the pathogenesis of this syndrome, and the clinician must be careful not to confuse post-vagotomy gastroparesis with bile reflux gastritis.

Clinical Presentation: The symptoms of bile reflux gastritis, although quite rare, are also characteristic. The primary symptom is a characteristic pain. Unlike peptic ulcer pain that is relieved by eating, or gastric ulcer pain that is exaggerated by eating, the pain of bile reflux gastritis is a constant epigastric pain. Bilious vomiting may occur, but the primary symptom is pain.

Diagnosis: Endoscopic examination with gastric mucosal biopsy and examination of the gastric anastomosis should be performed to help confirm the diagnosis but also to exclude other diagnoses such as afferent loop syndrome, one of the principal differential diagnoses in patients with bilious vomiting. The endoscopist will see bile pooling within the stomach and often an acutely inflamed, even ulcerated, mucosa. Mucosal biopsies will show intestinalization of the gastric glands, inflammation, and, on occasion, hemorrhage and ulceration, although the severity of the symptoms does not correlate with the histologic changes. Indeed, most all patients after a gastrectomy and with Billroth II reconstruction or after pyloroplasty or loop gastrojejunostomy will have some element of bile within the stomach and gastritis of varying severity. Many gastric surgeons recommend evaluation of gastric emptying, because the symptoms and endoscopic findings of post-vagotomy gastroparesis mimic many of those of bile reflux gastritis, and the treatment of such differs markedly. Scintigraphic assessment of the magnitude of reflux can also be obtained by tagging bile with a radioactive marker and determining the percentage of the secreted isotope refluxed into the stomach.

Treatment: Unfortunately, attempts at medical treatment are generally ineffective. The operative approach most often effective is diversion of bile away from the stomach. After a previous gastrectomy, this approach is best accomplished by converting gastric drainage to a Roux-en-Y limb of at least 70 cm (not just the classic 40 cm length). Some consideration may be given to a higher gastrectomy to decrease the possibility of future stomal ulceration. The Henley jejunal interposition limb between the gastric remnant and the duodenum has also been used to treat alkaline reflux gastritis, but we have no experience with this procedure. For patients with documented bile reflux gastritis after pyloroplasty alone (or the rare patient after cholecystectomy), the "duodenal switch" procedure can also be used; this procedure involves transaction of the junction of the first and second portion of the duodenum proximal to the entry of bile into the duodenum, oversewing the distal duodenum, and Roux-en-Y duodeno-jejunostomy (❯ *Fig. 52-2*).

Small Gastric-Remnant Syndrome

Early satiety with or without early postprandial vomiting is probably the most common postgastrectomy complaint and occurs often in the first 6 months after gastrectomy. Patients with this syndrome develop a characteristic pattern of early satiety, abdominal fullness, epigastric discomfort or pain, weight loss, nutritional deficiencies, and anemia. In addition, they will often have dumping symptoms. Conservative medical treatment is indicated in most patients and consists of symptomatic relief with

◼ Figure 52-2
Surgical options for treatment of alkaline gastritis

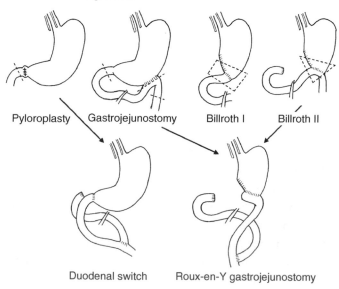

Pyloroplasty   Gastrojejunostomy   Billroth I   Billroth II

Duodenal switch   Roux-en-Y gastrojejunostomy

antispasmodic agents, dietary counseling, and reassurance, because as the GI tract adapts to this new anatomy, this symptom complex resolves gradually. A very small number of patients develop intractable pain and weight loss despite medical management. In these instances, the clinician should suspect gastroparesis, mechanical obstruction at the anastomosis, or the Roux stasis syndrome (see below). Although several types of surgically constructed complicated pouches have been designed to restore the reservoir function of gastric remnant, none has proven to be successful consistently.

Roux Stasis Syndrome/Post-Vagotomy Gastroparesis

Patients with the Roux-en-Y esophago- or gastrojejunostomy are at increased risk for delayed emptying secondary to the Roux stasis syndrome. Most investigators believe that this syndrome is secondary to abnormalities in motility of the jejunum distal to the site of transaction used to create the Roux limb which occurs primarily in patients who also have had a vagotomy; this syndrome is very unusual after, for instance, a Roux-en-Y gastric bypass which does not have a vagotomy. The symptoms include epigastric fullness, early satiety, abdominal pain, nausea, and vomiting not of bile but of ingested food. Indeed, these are the same symptoms and the same presentation as gastroparesis. Severe symptoms can lead to malnutrition and progressive weight loss. Gastric bezoars may develop. The spectrum of symptoms occurs to some extent in 10–50% in patients who have had a Roux drainage procedure combined with a vagotomy.

The medical management of this condition is disappointing and consists of dietary modification with smaller, more frequent meals and a more liquid-based diet; several drugs have been used but with highly variable results, including metoclopramide, domperidone (a dopamine antagonist), and cisapride (now no longer available). No completely satisfactory treatment for the Roux-en-Y stasis syndrome is available; attempts at intestinal electrical pacing, while successful in animals, have not worked in humans. When laboratory studies that incriminate the stomach (gastroparesis) as the cause of the stasis rather than the Roux-en-Y limb, near total gastrectomy has been advocated by some authors, and results have been encouraging. Therefore, the Roux-en-Y stasis syndrome should remain a diagnosis of exclusion, and remedial operations to resect the gastric remnant and re-establish the transit with a 40 cm long Roux limb have been proposed. About half the patients will have a reasonable result and be able to maintain their nutrition with oral intake; however, about half will require enteral feeding (distal to the Roux limb) or even total parenteral nutrition.

Prevention of Post-Vagotomy/Post-Gastrectomy Problems

❯ *Table 52-1* summarizes the most common symptoms after the various types of vagotomy and gastrectomy. Abnormalities discussed above in gastric emptying, intestinal transit, and enterogastric reflux resulting in abnormal digestion and nutrition account for the spectrum of post-vagotomy/post-gastrectomy symptoms and syndromes. Several modifications of the various classic operations have been evaluated in an attempt to prevent these symptoms. Various types of "neogastric pouches" have been constructed using the Roux limb in an attempt to provide a larger reservoir for ingested food; none has been demonstrated to impact consistently on postprandial eating habits, including J-shaped or S-shaped pouches, Omega loops, or interposition jejunal segments between the esophagus and the proximal duodenum. Similarly, the so-called uncut Roux limb has been evaluated in an attempt to

◘ Table 52-1

Late symptoms and complications after gastric surgery according to different techniques

	TV + A	SV + A	A alone	HSV
Malabsorption	+	++	+++	−
Loss of body weight	++	++	+++	−
Anemia	+	+	++	−
Dumping	++	++	+++	−
Diarrhea	+++	++	+	−
Cholelithiasis	+++	−	−	−
Alkaline reflux gastritis	++	++	+++	−
Gastric cancer	++	++	+++	−

TV = total vagotomy; A = antrectomy; SV = selective vagotomy; HSV = highly selective vagotomy.

prevent the Roux stasis syndrome. This procedure involves creating a loop gastro- or esophago-jejunostomy but stapling across the afferent limb to prevent pancreatobiliary secretions from refluxing into the stomach or esophagus, respectively. Then a side-to-side jejuno-jejunostomy is constructed between the afferent limb just proximal to the occluding staple line and the efferent limb at least 40 cm distal to the gastro- or esophago-jejunostomy. The concept behind this procedure is that by avoiding a complete transaction of the jejunum (to create a Roux limb), the motility of the jejunum downstream from the gastro- or esophago-jejunostomy will remain normal; the staple line prevents flow of enteric content but does not interrupt neuromuscular transmission in the wall of the jejunum across the staple line. Small series with this approach are encouraging.

Selected Readings

Braghetto I (1990) Late complications after surgery of duodenal ulcer. Cuad Chil Cir 34:82–95

Braghetto I, Bosch H, Csendes A (1986) Postoperative diarrhea after surgery for peptic ulcer. Rev Chil Cir 38:124–129

Braghetto I, Csendes A, Parada M, Lazo M (1983) Dumping syndrome. Rev Chil Cir 35:204–210

Carvajal S, Mulhivill SJ (1994) Postgastrectomy syndromes: dumping and diarrhea. Gastroenterol Clin NA 23:261–279

DeMeester TR, Fuchs KH, Ball CS, et al. (1987) Experimental and clinical results with proximal and-to-end duodenojejunostomy for pathologic duodenogastric reflux. Ann Surg 206:414–426

Eagon JC, Niedema BW, Kelly KA (1992) Postgastrectomy syndromes. Surg Clin NA 72:445–465

Liedman B, Hugosson I, Lundell L (2001) Treatment of devastating postgastrectomy symptoms. The potential role of jejunal pouch reconstruction. Dig Surg 18:218–221

Mackie CR, Jenkins SA, Hartley MN (1991) Treatment of severe postvagotomy/postgastrectomy symptoms with the somatostatin analogue octreotide. Br J Surg 78:1338

Schölmerich J (2004) Postgastrectomy syndromes-diagnosis and treatment. Best Proct Res Clin Gastroenterol 18:917–933

53 Bariatric Surgery

Silas M. Chikunguwo · Stacy A. Brethauer · Philip R. Schauer

Pearls and Pitfalls

- Obesity affects an estimated 1.7 billion people worldwide.
- Males and females in their twenties with a BMI >40 have 13 year and 8 year shorter life expectancies, respectively, than normal weight persons.
- Accepted criteria for bariatric surgery include a BMI ≥40 or a BMI 35–39 with active weight-related comorbidities and no active substance abuse or uncontrolled psychiatric issues.
- Currently bariatric surgery is the most effective, most durable treatment for weight loss.
- Bariatric surgery resolves the metabolic syndrome, decreases cardiovascular risk (~80%), and resolves or improves glucose intolerance, hypertension, dyslipidemia, sleep apnea, and gastro-esophageal reflux in over 80% of patients.
- Successful weight loss decreases markedly the risk of cardiovascular death and prolongs survival.
- The laparoscopic adjustable gastric band (LAGB) has the lowest morbidity and mortality rate of currently available bariatric procedures; weight loss at 5 years is ~45% of excess body weight.
- Laparoscopic sleeve gastrectomy, while effective as the first stage of a planned two-stage procedure for selected, high risk patients with super morbid obesity, has not yet been proven to be effective long-term as a primary bariatric procedure.
- Vertical banded gastroplasty is currently performed only rarely because of poor long-term weight loss and multiple complications/side effects.
- Malabsorptive procedures (biliopancreatic diversion and duodenal switch) have excellent and durable weight loss but a higher rate of complications; these procedures are best reserved for selected patients.
- Roux-en-Y gastric bypass is the most common procedure performed in the U.S. and the majority are now performed laparoscopically.
- All bariatric procedures have potential morbidity, both mechanical (operation-specific) and nutritional (malabsorption, micronutrient deficiency, vitamin deficiency: vitamin B_{12}, fat soluble vitamins) and thus, life-long medical follow up is mandatory.

Obesity is defined as the accumulation of excess body fat and is best quantified as body mass index (BMI, weight in kilograms divided by height in meters squared (kg/m^2)) (❷ *Table 53-1*). The obesity epidemic in developed countries throughout the world has spawned a tremendous interest in obesity research as well as a dramatic increase in the number of bariatric operations performed each year. Despite current efforts to prevent obesity, the percentage of overweight people in the world continues to rise and now rivals the number of underweight people. Severe obesity leads to multiple comorbid conditions (❷ *Table 53-2*) and decreased life expectancy, and currently, the only effective, durable treatment for this disease is bariatric surgery. Bariatric procedures performed today include

◘ Table 53-1
Classification of obesity

Severity	Body mass index (kg/m^2)	% Over ideal body weight
Overweight	25.0–29.9	
Obesity (Class 1)	30.0–34.9	>20%
Moderate obesity (Class 2)	35.0–39.9	>100%
Severe (Morbid) obesity (Class 3)	40.0–49.9	
Super morbid obesity	>50	>250%

◘ Table 53-2
Comorbidities associated with obesity

Cardiovascular	Coronary artery disease
	Hypertension
Peripheral vascular	Deep venous thrombosis
	Pulmonary embolism
	Thrombophlebitis
	Venous stasis disease
	Atherosclerosis
	Stroke
Pulmonary	Asthma
	Obstructive sleep apnea
	Obesity hypoventilation syndrome
Gastrointestinal	Gastroesophageal reflux
	Esophagitis
Hepatobiliary	Hepatic steatosis
	Non-alcoholic steatohepatitis (NASH)
	Cirrhosis
	Cholelithiasis
Neurologic	Migraines
	Pseudotumor cerebri
	Depression
Malignancy	Colon
	Breast
	Endometrium
	Prostate
Musculoskeletal	Degenerative joint disease
	Gout
	Carpal tunnel syndrome
Gynecologic/urologic	Irregular menstruation
	Polycystic ovarian syndrome
	Infertility
	Stress urinary incontinence
	Urinary tract infections
Metabolic/endocrine	Diabetes (insulin-resistant)
	Dyslipidemias

malabsorptive procedures (biliopancreatic diversion, duodenal switch), restrictive procedures (laparoscopic adjustable gastric banding, vertical banded gastroplasty, sleeve gastrectomy), or procedures that combine these two mechanisms (Roux-en-Y gastric bypass). Each procedure has its unique mechanism of action and associated risks and benefits. As more is learned about the pathophysiology of obesity and the biochemical changes that occur with weight loss after bariatric surgery, new less-invasive procedures will emerge undoubtedly. There is little doubt, though, that the problem of obesity will be present for years to come and that bariatric surgery will play an important role in managing this chronic disease entity.

Epidemiology

The epidemic of excess weight and obesity affects currently an estimated 1.7 billion people in developed countries throughout the world. As many as 60% of people in the United States are overweight, while the US has the highest prevalence of obesity worldwide (32%). This prevalence has increased dramatically over the last 2 decades, up from 15% in 1980. In the US, the prevalence of extreme obesity (BMI > 40) is 2.8% in men and 6.9% in women. Childhood and adolescent obesity has tripled since 1980 to a prevalence rate of 17%. Overall, the prevalence of obesity continues to increase at an alarming rate on a global scale, particularly in industrialized countries such as the United Kingdom, Australia, Germany, Russia, Columbia, Brazil, Italy, and Austria.

Costs of Obesity

The costs of obesity are enormous, both in terms of the economic impact of this disease and the medical consequences that result from comorbid conditions. The total cost attributable to obesity in the United States is over $100 billion annually. Worldwide, approximately 2.5 million annual deaths occur due directly to obesity-related comorbidities. The economic costs of obesity include direct medical costs of treating obesity illnesses and indirect costs due to lost workdays, productivity, and future income due to premature death. Epidemiologic studies suggest that, among African Americans, a higher BMI (32 for men, 37 for women) decreases life expectancy. The same study estimated that a Caucasian man in his twenties with a BMI over 45 will have a 22% reduction (13 years) in life expectancy, and a 20 year old Caucasian woman with a BMI of 45 will have 8 years of life lost to obesity. For each patient contemplating bariatric surgery, the risks of a bariatric procedure must be weighed against the long-term risks and costs of continued obesity and worsening comorbidities.

Surgical Management of Obesity

The dramatic increase in interest in bariatric surgery among surgeons and in the public occurred essentially between 1993 and 2003, when the number of bariatric procedures performed annually worldwide increased nearly four-fold to 145,000. Interestingly, membership in bariatric surgery societies has also increased by over 100%. Despite these increasing numbers of operations and the now well-documented successes of bariatric surgery to date, relatively few eligible patients are pursuing bariatric surgery. Currently, only about 1% of patients eligible for bariatric surgery in the United States have undergone a weight-loss procedure.

Indications for Bariatric Surgery

Patients with a BMI $\geq$40 kg/m^2 or a BMI $\geq$35 kg/m^2 with significant obesity-related comorbidities are candidates for bariatric surgery based on the 1991 NIH Consensus Guidelines. Typically, patients between the ages of 18–60 are considered for surgical weight loss. Carefully selected older patients and, increasingly, adolescents as well can benefit from bariatric surgery. Patients seeking bariatric surgery have, throughout their lives, failed multiple attempts at medical weight loss. In addition to meeting the basic criteria for surgery, these patients must also complete a thorough, multi-disciplinary, pre-operative evaluation designed to identify and optimally manage comorbid conditions and identify any contraindications to bariatric surgery.

Patients who cannot tolerate general anesthesia due to cardiac, pulmonary, or hepatic insufficiency are obviously not candidates for bariatric surgery. Patients must also demonstrate during their preoperative evaluation that they understand the associated changes in lifestyle required after surgery and are willing to comply with the post-operative diet, vitamin supplementation, and follow-up program. Most importantly, patients must understand that bariatric surgery is only a tool to help them lose weight in conjunction with good choices in food and adoption of an exercise program and not as a rapid solution to a lifelong problem.

Currently, no specific psychologic factors have been identified that predict success or failure reliably after bariatric surgery. Patient selection with regard to psychologic stability is based on the judgment of the psychologist/psychiatrist and the surgeon. Patients with active substance abuse or unstable psychiatric illness, though, are poor candidates for bariatric surgery.

Outcomes after Bariatric Surgery

Weight loss: Bariatric surgery is currently the most effective and durable method to treat severe obesity. Weight loss is most commonly measured as percent of excess weight loss (% EWL). Excess weight is defined as the amount of weight above the patient's ideal body weight (as determined by Metropolitan Life tables).

A meta-analysis by Buchwald and colleagues including over 10,000 patients found an average EWL of 61% for all patients undergoing bariatric surgery. Malabsorptive procedures had the greatest EWL (70%), while gastric banding (including open, non-adjustable gastric bands) had the least EWL (47.5%). The average EWL for Roux-en-Y gastric bypass in this analysis was 62%.

The Swedish Obesity Subjects (SOS) Study is an ongoing, prospective, controlled, matched-pair cohort study comparing surgery with nonsurgical treatment for obesity. The surgically treated patients underwent a variety of procedures, including vertical banded gastroplasty (70%), fixed or adjustable gastric banding (25%), and gastric bypass (5%). The treatment in the nonsurgical group varied widely as well, including intense behavioral therapy to no specific treatment according to the practices of their primary care physicians. Analysis at 10 years (641 surgical and 627 nonsurgical patients) showed that the control group had gained 2% of their original weight, while the surgical group lost 16% of their total body weight. Other studies have demonstrated durable weight loss beyond 15 years for gastric bypass and biliopancreatic diversion.

Comorbidity reduction: Bariatric surgery results in a decrease or resolution of many obesity-related comorbid conditions. The Metabolic Syndrome (abdominal obesity, atherogenic dyslipidemia, hypertension, insulin resistance or glucose intolerance, a proinflammatory state, and a prothrombotic state) comprises a constellation of serious cardiovascular risk factors; bariatric surgery improves or leads to resolution of all of these factors in over 80% of patients and decreases the risk for cardiovascular disease. Christou et al. conducted a matched cohort study comparing patients after bariatric surgery with a medically managed cohort and demonstrated an 82% decrease in cardiovascular risk 5 years after surgery. Similarly, diabetes also improves dramatically after bariatric surgery. Buchwald's meta-analysis showed that diabetes resolved in 99% of patients after biliopancreatic diversion, 84% after gastric bypass, 72% after gastroplasty, and 48% after gastric banding. About half of morbidly obese patients are hypertensive, and 80% of patients undergoing bariatric surgery will have resolution or improvement in their hypertension and their lipid profile after bariatric surgery.

Sleep apnea, obesity hypoventilation syndrome (Pickwickian Syndrome), and asthma improve or resolve in the majority of patients after massive weight loss. Gastroesophageal reflux is treated effectively by bariatric procedures. Gastric bypass is particularly effective in treating reflux (70–90% resolution of symptoms) and should be considered strongly instead of a fundoplication for morbidly obese patients with a primary complaint of severe gastroesophageal reflux.

Other comorbidities that improve or resolve after bariatric surgery include non-alcoholic steatohepatitis, venous stasis disease, lymphedema, pseudotumor cerebri, depression, polycystic ovarian syndrome, and stress urinary incontinence.

Life expectancy: Morbid obesity shortens the expected life span, but there is growing evidence that bariatric surgery alters the natural history of this disease. Retrospective, case control studies have demonstrated that 15 year survival is increased by one third for patients undergoing bariatric surgery compared with obese patients who do not have surgery. MacDonald et al. compared retrospectively obese diabetic patients who underwent gastric bypass (n − 154) to a similar group of obese diabetic patients who did not have bariatric surgery (n = 78); at 10 years of follow-up, there was a mortality rate of 9% in the surgical group (including perioperative deaths) but a 28% mortality rate in the non-surgical group, related to decreased cardiovascular deaths among patients who had gastric bypass. Similarly, in a matched cohort study of 1,035 gastric bypass patients and 6,746 age and sex-matched controls, Christou and colleagues reported a 5-year mortality in the surgical group of about 1% compared with 16% in the medically managed patients (89% relative risk reduction).

Perioperative mortality: Mortality rates after bariatric surgery depend on the patient's comorbidities and general risk, the procedure performed, and the surgeon and hospital volume of bariatric cases. The leading cause of death after bariatric surgery is pulmonary embolism (30–40% of deaths) followed by cardiac complications (25%) and anastomotic leaks (20%). The remaining perioperative deaths are due to respiratory, vascular, and hemorrhagic causes.

Restrictive procedures are associated with the lowest perioperative mortality rates (0.1%). A systematic review of the international literature revealed a 0.05% mortality rate after laparoscopic adjustable gastric banding; this procedure is considered the safest bariatric procedure performed today. The mortality rate for gastric bypass (open and laparoscopic) in Buchwald's meta-analysis was 0.5%. Malabsorptive procedures, such as biliopancreatic diversion and duodenal switch, are technically more demanding and are associated with a greater mortality rate than other bariatric procedures (1.1%), but these procedures tend to be performed on larger, higher risk patients.

Advanced age is also associated with higher mortality rates after bariatric surgery. In a review of Medicare patients undergoing bariatric surgery, one study found that patients older than 65 had 4.8% 30-day and 6.9% 90-day mortality rates, which were higher than after bariatric surgery in younger patients.

Restrictive Procedures

Laparoscopic Adjustable Gastric Banding

The Laparoscopic Adjustable Gastric Band (LAGB) utilizes a restrictive mechanism for weight loss by creating a small gastric pouch just below the gastroesophageal junction (❯ *Fig. 53-1A*). After opening the pars flacida along the lesser curvature of the stomach, a small window is created in the peritoneum at the base of the right diaphragmatic crus. Another small opening is created just above the angle of His and a blunt instrument is used to create a path for the band behind the cardia of the stomach. After the retrogastric tunnel is created, the band is pulled through and locked in place around the upper stomach just below the gastroesophageal junction. The fundus is then plicated over the band to the gastric wall

◘ Figure 53-1

Restrictive procedures: a. laparoscopic adjustable gastric band; b. sleeve gastrectomy; c. vertical banded gastroplasty. Malabsorptive procedures: d. biliopancreatic diversion; e. biliopancreatic diversion with duodenal switch. Combination procedure: f. Roux-en-Y gastric bypass (Reprinted with the permission of the Cleveland Clinic Foundation)

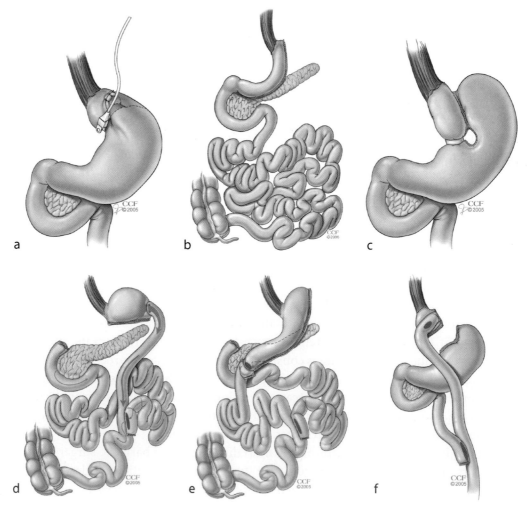

(not esophagus) above the band using three interrupted sutures, which helps prevent slippage or prolapse anteriorly. The plications should not cover the buckle of the band as this may increase the risk of band erosion. The tubing is attached to the port extracorporeally, and the port is sutured to the anterior rectus fascia. Typically, fluid is not added to the band until 1 month after surgery.

Advantages: A major putative advantage of the adjustable band is that the outlet of the gastric pouch can be titrated to weight loss and symptoms. This ability to vary the diameter of the pouch outlet avoids many of the chronic problems (severe reflux, dysphagia, vomiting, and maladaptive eating behaviors) seen with non-adjustable gastric banding. Regular follow-up is essential after the LAGB to achieve the optimal band tightness for each patient. The LAGB is the safest bariatric procedure with a mortality rate of 0.05% and a morbidity rate of 11%. This safety profile makes LAGB an attractive option for many patients and surgeons.

Weight loss after LAGB is more gradual than after gastric bypass, and maximal weight loss is achieved between 2 and 3 years (vs. 12–18 months after gastric bypass). Excess weight loss 3–5 years after LAGB ranges from 40% to 60% and is associated with improvements in most all weight-related comorbidities.

Complications: Major perioperative complications such as bleeding, gastric perforation, or thromboembolic events are rare after LAGB and occur in only 1–2% of patients. Late complications that occur after LAGB include device-related problems (port or tubing malfunctions in 5% of patients) or complications such as band slippage (5–15%) or band erosion (1%). Overall, complications require re-operation in 10–15% of patients undergoing LAGB.

Laparoscopic Sleeve Gastrectomy

Laparoscopic sleeve gastrectomy (LSG) is a relatively new procedure in bariatric surgery. It was introduced initially as a first stage procedure for very high-risk patients (BMI > 60) who ultimately underwent a RYGB. The intent of this first stage is to perform a relatively safe and simple procedure in a patient who cannot tolerate a prolonged anesthetic or who has anatomy that is unfavorable for performing a gastric bypass at that time because of cirrhosis, massive visceral fat, poor exposure due to hepatomegaly, or extensive intra-abdominal adhesions; this remains the primary, accepted indication for this restrictive procedure. But there is growing interest in using the LSG as a primary restrictive procedure. Sleeve gastrectomy has also been used in patients with inflammatory bowel disease, in whom the integrity of an anastomosis is a concern, and in patients with gastric or duodenal polyps in whom performance of a RYGB would make surveillance of this anatomy impossible.

In this procedure, a linear cutting stapler is used to tubularize the lesser curvature by creating a narrow gastric tube along the lesser curvature (❯ *Fig. 53-1B*). The remaining 75–80% of the gastric body and fundus are removed. Starting approximately 6 cm proximal to the pylorus, the lesser sac is entered through the gastrocolic ligament, and a linear cutting stapler is fired toward the angle of His. A Bougie dilator is used to size the sleeve. We currently use a 34 French Bougie and direct the tip into the pylorus after the initial vertical staple load is fired. Once the Bougie is in place, the stomach is divided adjacent to the dilator up to the Angle of His. The short gastric vessels are then divided and the now resected greater curvature of the stomach remnant is removed.

Advantages: This procedure provides a safe and relatively simple procedure for high risk patients or patients with massive hepatomegaly. The procedure has a relatively low complication rate and low mortality rate in the initial series published in very high-risk patients. In these series, patients had impressive initial decreases in weight (50–60% EWL), comorbidities, and anesthetic risk in the first year after LSG prior to the second stage procedure (RYGB). Although LSG has been studied as a primary procedure in lower BMI patients with reported EWL of 50–80% in the first year after surgery and improvement or resolution of many comorbidities, the durability of LSG beyond 1 year, has not been demonstrated. LSG as an effective, durable primary bariatric procedure is thus not yet established or accepted.

Complications: LSG appears to be safe and effective in the short term when used as a staged or a primary procedure. Overall, post-operative complications occur in 10–15% of patients and include strictures (most commonly at the gastric incisura), bleeding, and staple line leaks. Complication rates of LSG as a primary procedure are lower than those seen with the high-risk patients who undergo LSG as a staging procedure.

Vertical Banded Gastroplasty

This procedure (a form of "stomach stapling") involves the creation of a small, vertically oriented proximal gastric pouch, which empties into the main body of the stomach through a calibrated stoma (❯ *Fig. 53-1C*). The small pouch is created with a linear stapler and can be divided, although historically, the pouch has been created with an undivided staple line (or overlapping staple lines) using a combination of a circular stapler and a linear stapler fired upward from a window to the angle of His. A silastic or polypropylene band is placed around the outlet to provide fixed restriction of the outlet.

Although this procedure was popular in the 1980s and early 1990s, its demonstrated inferior weight loss compared with RYGB and long-term complications such as severe gastroesophageal reflux, nausea and vomiting, intolerance to solid foods, and weight regain in over half of patients who underwent this procedure have discouraged its current use. Many bariatric surgeons are seeing increasing numbers of patients who present for revision to RYGB after failing VBG (severe symptoms or weight regain).

Malabsorptive Procedures

Biliopancreatic Diversion and Duodenal Switch

These procedures work by limiting nutrient absorption (❯ *Fig. 53-1D*). In the biliopancreatic diversion (BPD), a 70% gastrectomy is completed and a long alimentary Roux limb from the proximal ileum is anastomosed to the remaining stomach. The biliopancreatic limb is connected to the alimentary limb about 100 cm from the ileocecal valve to create a short common channel. In the duodenal switch (DS) (❯ *Fig. 53-1E*), a sleeve gastrectomy is performed and a similar long alimentary Roux limb is anastomosed to the first portion of the duodenum. Again, a short common channel is created by connecting the biliopancreatic limb to the alimentary limb about 100 cm from the ileocecal valve.

Advantages: BPD and BPD with duodenal switch (BPD/DS) provide excellent long-term weight loss, with greater than 75% EWL maintained 15 years after the procedure. Though there is some adaptation of the common channel, the majority of patients are able to consume relatively normal quantities of food yet maintain their weight loss. In addition to weight loss, resolution of comorbid conditions exceed 80% and was superior to most other bariatric procedures in Buchwald's meta-analysis.

Complications: Although these procedures offer the best and most durable weight loss of any bariatric procedure performed today, higher complication rates, which include global protein/calorie malnutrition, anemia, micronutrient deficiency, diarrhea, stomal ulceration, metabolic bone disease, and a higher mortality rate, have limited their widespread use. Patients need to be followed closely, especially for fat-soluble vitamin deficiencies.

Gastric Bypass

The Roux-en-Y gastric bypass (RYGB) (● *Fig. 53-1F*) is the most commonly performed bariatric procedure in the United States (80%) and is performed open or, more commonly, laparoscopically. The primary mechanism of weight loss after gastric bypass is the restrictive component resulting from creating a small gastric pouch and small gastrojejunostomy and possibly initially by setting up a dumping physiology for ingestion of high caloric sweets. A global malabsorption is typically negligible with a standard 75–150 cm alimentary limb. The foregut bypass created with RYGB may have significant effects on appetite, long-term weight loss, and glucose metabolism, but these mechanisms are still being investigated.

The laparoscopic RYGB is performed using five or six trocars. The jejunum is divided 50 cm from the ligament of Treitz and a 150 cm Roux limb is measured. A side-to-side jejunojejunostomy is created and the mesenteric defect closed. A 15–30 ml gastric pouch is created using a linear cutting stapler, thereby completely separating the gastric pouch from the gastric remnant. After dividing the greater omentum, the Roux limb is delivered by most surgeons in an antecolic and antegastric orientation. The retrocolic position can be utilized if necessary to avoid tension on the gastrojejunostomy. The gastrojejunostomy can be created with a hand-sewn technique, a linear stapler, or a circular stapler.

Advantages: RYGB is generally a more effective weight loss operation than LAGB and results in 65–80% EWL at 2 years. Several studies have demonstrated 50% EWL 15 years after the operation. RYGB also results in improvement or resolution of obesity-related comorbidities in about 80% of patients, specifically, diabetes, hypertension, dyslipidemia, sleep apnea, asthma, metabolic syndrome, polycystic ovarian syndrome, gout, degenerative joint pain, pseudotumor cerebri, and stress urinary incontinence. Laparoscopic RYGB offers advantages over the open approach with fewer wound complications (incisional hernia, wound infection), fewer pulmonary complications, less postoperative pain, shorter hospital stay, and a faster return to normal activities.

Complications: Multiple large series of RYGB have reported perioperative mortality rates from zero to 2%, with the incidence of anastomotic leaks of ~2–5%, bleeding (0–4%), gastrojejunal stenosis (5–15%), marginal ulcers (1–5%), and bowel obstruction (1–10%). Complications requiring reoperation occur in 10–15% of patients after RYGB. Nutritional deficiencies, such as iron-deficiency anemia, vitamin B12 and D deficiencies, and calcium deficiency, can occur in one-third to one-half of patients after RYGB. Routine supplementation after surgery can prevent the majority of these deficiencies but patients require lifelong surveillance of their micronutrient status after gastric bypass.

Summary

Obesity is a complex disease with genetic, psychosocial, behavioral, and metabolic causes. Current medical therapy does not provide a satisfactory long-term solution for patients with severe obesity. Bariatric surgery is being performed in increasing numbers worldwide as the obesity epidemic grows. A variety of bariatric procedures are performed today and the mechanisms of action, risks, and benefits differ with each. The choice of procedure for a given patient is determined by their own preference, their willingness to accept slightly higher risks for more weight loss (or less weight loss after a lower risk procedure), and the surgeon's experience with specific operations.

Minimally invasive technologies are currently used for most bariatric procedures. Natural orifice transluminal and endoluminal bariatric procedures are being investigated currently. While most of these are in pre-clinical stages of development, the future of bariatric surgery may include endoluminal or transluminal procedures as either primary or adjunctive therapy.

Selected Readings

Brethauer SA, Chand B, Schauer PR (2006) Risks and benefits of bariatric surgery: Current evidence. Cleve Clin J Med 73:993–1007

Buchwald H, Avidor Y, Braunwald E, et al. (2004) Bariatric surgery: a systematic review and meta-analysis. JAMA 292:1724–1737

Chapman AE, Kiroff G, Game P, et al. (2004) Laparoscopic adjustable gastric banding in the treatment of obesity: a systematic literature review. Surgery 135:326–351

Christou NV, Sampalis JS, Liberman M, et al. (2004) Surgery decreases long-term mortality, morbidity, and health care use in morbidly obese patients. Ann Surg 240:416–423; discussion 423–424

NIH conference (1991) Gastrointestinal surgery for severe obesity. Consensus Development Conference Panel. Ann Intern Med 115:956–961

Ogden CL, Carroll MD, Curtin LR, et al. (2006) Prevalence of overweight and obesity in the United States, 1999–2004. JAMA 295:1549–1555

Schauer PR, Burguera B, Ikramuddin S, et al. (2003) Effect of laparoscopic Roux-en-Y gastric bypass on type 2 diabetes mellitus. Ann Surg 238:467–484; discussion 84–85

Sjostrom L, Lindroos AK, Peltonen M, et al. (2004) Lifestyle, diabetes, and cardiovascular risk factors 10 years after bariatric surgery. N Engl J Med 351:2683–2693

54 Gastric Adenocarcinoma

Yoshiro Saikawa · Masaki Kitajima

Pearls and Pitfalls

- Gastric cancer is one of the most common cancers worldwide.
- Protective factors against gastric carcinoma include dietary intake of fresh fruits and vegetables, vitamin C, and reduction of salt, pickling, and nitrates for food preservation.
- Factors that predispose to gastric cancer include *Helicobacter pylori* infection, natural carcinogens (e.g., nitrates), carcinogens from meat grilling or barbecuing, and dietary pro-carcinogens.
- Host-related factors associated with an increased risk of gastric adenocarcinoma include low serum ferritin levels and pernicious anemia, distal gastrectomy for benign ulcer, Barrett's esophagus, adenomatous polyps, and heritable and familial risks such as hereditary nonpolyposis colorectal cancer (HNPCC).
- Symptoms, if present, are non-specific for early gastric cancers, while more diagnostic symptoms occur in the advanced cancers.
- Imaging techniques, such as CT, US, EUS, and endoscopy, are helpful in determining appropriate treatment.
- Preoperative laparoscopy is beneficial for detection of peritoneal metastases, liver metatases, or locally advanced, unresectable diseases and may provide avoidance of a non-therapeutic laparotomy.
- Nutritional support through placement of a feeding jejunostomy may be beneficial.
- Staging systems for gastric cancer include: the American Joint Committee on Cancer/Union Internationale Contre le Cancer (AJCC/UICC), the Japanese Classification of Gastric Cancer, the World Health Organization Classification System, and the Lauren Classification System.
- Endoscopic mucosal or submucosal resection may be appropriate for selected patients with early gastric adenocarcinoma.
- Gastrectomy with lymph node dissection is the most widely used curative therapy.
- Surgical options must consider the extent of gastric resection, extent of lymph node dissection, and methods of reconstruction.
- Adjuvant chemotherapy and chemo-radiotherapy with several new drugs, such as CPT-11 and the taxanes, allow palliative control of gastric adenocarcinoma and may prove useful in the neoadjuvant setting.

Epidemiology and Carcinogenesis

At the beginning of 2000, gastric adenocarcinoma was the second most common cancer worldwide. Although the incidence varies dramatically from country to country, there is a general trend of declining incidence throughout the world, with decreases in gastric adenocarcinoma rates documented in many of the Western nations during the last century. The United States now has one of the lowest rates of gastric cancer in the world. Moreover, a remarkable shift in anatomic location has occurred from noncardia to cardial lesions. The incidences of proximal cardia and gastroesophageal (GE) junction adenocarcinomas have increased in the United States and Europe, suggesting a common pathogenesis distinct from the development of distal gastric carcinomas.

In contrast, the incidence of gastric adenocarcinoma in other countries is alarmingly high. In China, South America, Eastern Europe, Korea, and Japan, gastric carcinoma is the most common non-skin malignancy. Although most experts generally agree that diet and nutrition play a role in gastric carcinogenesis, the mechanisms that account for the observed patterns of geographic and temporal incidence have not yet been well established. Multiple studies designed to delineate the causes of gastric adenocarcinoma have identified a number of factors that appear to be involved (❯ *Table 54-1*). Factors that appear to provide a protective role include adequate nutrition, particularly intake of fruit and vegetables, vitamin C intake, and modern techniques of food processing and storage, thereby reducing spoilage and the need for salt-curing, pickling, and nitrates for preservation. In contrast, infection with *Helicobacter pylori* infection may be the most important factor worldwide that predisposes patients to gastric cancer. Other factors include natural carcinogens or precursors such as nitrates in food, the production of carcinogens during the grilling or barbecuing of meats, and the synthesis of carcinogens from dietary precursors in the stomach.

There are two general types of gastric adenocarcinoma: the intestinal type and the diffuse type. The intestinal type is more common and more often distal in the stomach, while the diffuse type carries a worse prognosis, tends to occur in younger patients, and can arise anywhere in the stomach, but especially in the cardia. Mucosal changes resulting from various kinds of environmental insults can lead eventually to atrophic gastritis, which, when present chronically, can induce intestinal metaplasia that appears to be a precursor state to the intestinal-type gastric adenocarcinoma. Within this setting, various host-related, environmental, and infectious factors have been implicated in the etiology of gastric adenocarcinoma. Host-related factors that may lead to an increased risk of gastric cancer include low serum ferritin levels and pernicious anemia. Although peptic ulcer disease does not appear to be related to increased risk, patients who undergo distal gastrectomy for benign ulcer disease are

◾ **Table 54-1**

Risk factors for gastric cancer

Definite-surveillance suggested	Possible
Familial adenomatous polyposis	Excess alcohol ingestion
Gastric adenomas	Gastric hamartomas
Gastric biopsy revealing high-grade dysplasia	High intake of salted, pickled, or smoked foods
Definite	Low intake of fruits and vegetables
Chronic atrophic gastritis	Ménétrier's disease
Gastric metaplasia on biopsy	Peutz-Jeghers syndrome
Helicobacter pylori infection	Tobacco smoking
Hereditary nonpolyposis colorectal cancer (Lynch II syndrome)	Questionable
	Benign gastric ulcers
Probable	Fundic gland polyps
History of subtotal gastrectomy (>20 years)	Hyperplastic polyps
Pernicious anemia	
Tobacco smoking (adenocarcinoma of cardia)	

reported to have a five-fold increased risk of gastric cancer in long-term follow-up. Barrett's esophagus is now accepted as a cause of gastric adenocarcinoma in the distal esophagus and gastric cardia, and adenomatous polyps have been associated with gastric adenocarcinoma. With regard to the risk of inheritable gastric adenocarcinoma, patients with hereditary nonpolyposis colorectal cancer (HNPCC) have an increased risk of gastric adenocarcinoma, while patients with familial adenomatous polyposis do not have a similar risk. In terms of environmental causes, food refrigeration has probably decreased the dietary exposure to various carcinogens, such as nitrates and nitrites, by reducing the bacterial and fungal contamination of food. Refrigeration has also led to a decrease in consumption of smoked, cured, and salted foods, thereby reducing the incidence of intestinal-type gastric adenocarcinoma. A higher intake of fruits and vegetables is known to be protective against gastric carcinogenesis, while a modest increase in risk has been reported for increased meat consumption, with a positive correlation with longer cooking times. Other environmental factors, such as smoking or industrial dust exposure, may also be associated with gastric adenocarcinoma. Chronic infections of the stomach, such as by *Helicobacter pylori* (HP) or Epstein-Barr virus, have been implicated repeatedly in epidemiologic studies, and a relationship between chronic infection and gastric carcinogenesis has been suggested by various studies.

Clinical Diagnosis and Pathologic Staging

Clinical Presentation

The symptoms of gastric cancer are often non-specific, usually without obvious symptoms during early stages, and often with only few or minimal symptoms that lead to diagnosis even at advanced stages. Due to the relatively large size of the stomach and abdominal cavity, mechanical symptoms such as obstruction or hemorrhage caused by a tumor mass are recognized only rarely until the tumor becomes large unless it is in the distal antrum. Non-specific symptoms, such as vague gastrointestinal distress, episodic nausea, vomiting, and anorexia, are common in patients without cancer and are often not taken seriously by the patient or physician, unless the symptoms are severe or progressive. Common symptoms at diagnosis are abdominal pain and weight loss. Although anemia is a frequent finding in gastric cancer patients, substantive upper gastrointestinal bleeding is uncommon. At advanced stages, proximally localized esophageal dysphasia is observed frequently, while nausea and/or vomiting may be due to circumferential involvement of either the stomach or the cardia that leads to mechanical obstruction.

Findings on physical examination, such as a palpable mass, jaundice (lymph node involvement in hepatoduodenal ligaments) or a Blumer's shelf (pelvic peritoneal metastasis), Krukenberg tumors (in ovaries), or periumbilical masses (peritoneal metastases) tend to occur in highly advanced, unresectable disease. Palpable lymphadenopathy of the left supraclavicular fossa (Virchow's node) can sometimes be observed without other complaints. Less common dermatologic findings include acanthosis nigricans and multiple seborrheic keratoses.

Clinical Staging with Imaging

To confirm the clinical staging of a gastric adenocarcinoma, patients should be evaluated in a stepwise fashion with physical examination, laboratory studies, computerized tomography (CT), endoscopic ultrasonography (EUS), and often, staging laparoscopy.

Physical examination should be directed toward evaluation of nutritional and performance states and detecting evidence of distant spread. Palpations for adenopathy in the supraclavicular fossa (Virchow node), the periumbilical area (Sister Mary Joseph node), and the left axilla (Irish node) are indicative of unresectable disease. The abdomen should be examined for the presence of palpable masses or ascites. A digital rectal exam may be performed to assess for masses or a Blumer's shelf in the pelvis. Laboratory studies should include complete blood count, electrolytes, blood urea nitrogen, and serum creatinine, as well as liver function tests. Tumor markers, such as carcinoembryonic antigen and CA 19-9, should be obtained to predict cancer state and malignant potential.

CT of the abdomen, pelvis, and chest (for proximal lesions) should be performed to evaluate the primary gastric neoplasm and to look for liver metastases, ascites, peritoneal nodules, and nodal metastases to allow assessment of clinical stage. EUS can be useful to assess both tumor T-stage and regional nodes. Endoscopy, CT, and EUS should be performed to confirm clinical staging. Accurate staging is imperative to guide the appropriate therapeutic strategy for gastric adenocarcinoma, ranging from endoscopic or laparoscopic intervention for early cancer to neoadjuvant or palliative chemotherapy for highly advanced malignancy.

Staging laparoscopy may be essential for complete staging and evaluation of peritoneal metastases, especially for patients with potentially resectable gastric cancer based on preoperative imaging and endoscopy. A feeding tube jejunostomy can also be placed during the staging laparoscopy; however, in the presence of ascites, the benefits of a jejunostomy tube should be considered carefully against the risks of abdominal and jejunostomy site complications.

Clinico-Pathologic Staging Systems

The AJCC/UICC System in Pathologic Staging (❯ *Tables 54-2* and ❯ *54-3*): The American Joint Committee on Cancer/Union Internationale Contre le Cancer (AJCC/UICC) system is the most widely used pathologic staging system for gastric cancer and evaluates the primary tumor (T), regional lymph nodes (N), and distant metastatic disease (M). T stage is divided into four levels based on the depth of penetration into the stomach wall. T1 tumors are the most superficial, with involvement only as deep as the submucosa. T2 tumors invade into the muscularis propria, and T3 tumors are into the serosa. T2 tumors are divided into T2a (invasion of the muscularis propria) and T2b (invasion of the subserosa). T4 tumors invade adjacent organs directly. N stage is divided into four levels based on the number of positive local lymph nodes: N0 = 0; N1 = 1–6; N2 = 7–15; N3 = >15, no longer on the site of nodal metastases. Patients with N3 nodal disease are classified as stage IV.

The classification of gastric carcinoma reported by the Japanese Research Society of Gastric Cancer defines nodal stage by anatomic location and proximity to the primary tumor, based on the division of six perigastric stations (right and left cardia, lesser and greater curvatures, and supra and infra pyloric), and five additional stations along the celiac vessels (celiac, hepatic, left gastric, splenic, hilum of the spleen). While the AJCC/UICC N staging was based on the Japanese system, proximity to the tumor may not necessarily reflect prognostic value in terms of nodal staging.

Lauren Classification System: The Lauren system is another major classification system for gastric adenocarcinoma that divides the disease into intestinal and diffuse types; however, cancers with a

◻ **Table 54-2**

TNM definition

Primary tumor (T)
• TX: Primary tumor cannot be assessed
• T0: No evidence of primary tumor
• Tis: Carcinoma in situ: intraepithelial tumor without invasion of the lamina propria
• T1: Tumor invades lamina propria or submucosa
• T2: Tumor invades the muscularis propria or the subserosa[a]
• T2a: Tumor invades muscularis propria
• T2b: Tumor invades subserosa
• T3: Tumor penetrates the serosa (visceral peritoneum) without invading adjacent structures[b,c]
• T4: Tumor invades adjacent structures[b,c]
• Regional lymph nodes (N)
• Regional lymph nodes include perigastric nodes found along lesser and greater curvatures and nodes located along left gastric, common hepatic, splenic, and celiac arteries. For pN, a regional lymphadenectomy specimen will ordinarily contain at least 15 lymph nodes. Involvement of other intra-abdominal lymph nodes, such as hepatoduodenal, retropancreatic, mesenteric, and para-aortic, is classified as distant metastasis.
• NX: Regional lymph node(s) cannot be assessed
• N0: No regional lymph node metastasis[d]
• N1: Metastasis in 1–6 regional lymph nodes
• N2: Metastasis in 7–15 regional lymph nodes
• N3: Metastasis in more than 15 regional lymph nodes
• Distant metastasis (M)
MX: Distant metastasis cannot be assessed
M0: No distant metastasis
M1: Distant metastasis

[a] Note: A tumor may penetrate muscularis propria with extension into gastrocolic or gastrohepatic ligaments, or into greater or lesser omentum, without extension through visceral peritoneum covering these structures. In this case, the tumor is classified T2. If there is extension through visceral peritoneum covering gastric ligaments or omentum, the tumor should be classified T3.

[b] Note: Adjacent structures of the stomach include spleen, transverse colon, liver, diaphragm, pancreas, abdominal wall, adrenal gland, kidney, small intestine, and retroperitoneum.

[c] Note: Intramural extension to the duodenum or esophagus is classified by the depth of greatest invasion in any of these sites, including stomach.

[d] Note: A designation of pN0 should be used if all examined lymph nodes are negative, regardless of total number removed and examined.

mixed histology containing components of both intestinal and diffuse disease have been described. Intestinal-type gastric cancer is also called the "epidemic" type, because it retains glandular structures and cellular polarity. Grossly, the intestinal type usually has a sharp margin, arises from the gastric mucosa, and is associated with chronic gastritis, gastric atrophy, and intestinal metaplasia. *Helicobacter pylori* and other environmental factors are thought to play major roles in its pathogenesis. The diffuse-type histology is associated with an invasive growth pattern with scattered clusters of uniformly-sized malignant cells that frequently infiltrate the submucosa. This diffuse type has little glandular formation, and mucin production is common. The infiltrative growth pattern observed in diffuse-type gastric cancers often leads to cancers without a mass and present as advanced linitis plastica. Endoscopically, such cancers may be difficult to identify without ulceration or mass formation. For example, linitis plastica is observed as a non-distensible, leather bottle-like appearance on the stomach.

World Health Organization Classification System: The World Health Organization (WHO) scheme divides Lauren intestinal-type gastric adenocarcinomas into papillary or tubular groups, and the

◘ Table 54-3

AJCC stage groupings

Stage 0
• Tis, N0, M0
Stage IA
• T1, N0, M0
Stage IB
• T1, N1, M0
• T2a, N0, M0
• T2b, N0, M0
Stage II
• T1, N2, M0
• T2a, N1, M0
• T2b, N1, M0
• T3, N0, M0
Stage IIIA
• T2a, N2, M0
• T2b, N2, M0
• T3, N1, M0
• T4, N0, M0
Stage IIIB
• T3, N2, M0
Stage IV
• T4, N1, M0
• T4, N2, M0
• T4, N3, M0
• T1, N3, M0
• T2, N3, M0
• T3, N3, M0
• Any T, any N, M1

Lauren diffuse-type into mucinous or signet ring cell groups. While this system is not frequently utilized worldwide, it offers more information than smaller classification schemes for gastric adenocarcinoma.

Treatment

Endoscopic Mucosal Resection and Endoscopic Submucosal Dissection

Techniques of endoscopic mucosal resection (EMR) for mucosal (M) cancer of the stomach are based on similar endoscopic techniques for resection of colonic polyps, while endoscopic techniques of submucosal dissection (ESD) have been developed recently for the treatment of T1 gastric adenocarcinoma and submucosal cancer (SM). Cure by endoscopic treatment of T1 tumors (M or SM tumors) may be achieved in patients without evidence of residual cancer or nodal disease. While the presence of nodal metastases is approximately 10% for T1 gastric adenocarcinomas, M cancers have a 1–3% incidence of positive nodes and SM cancers have an incidence of around 15%. Risk of nodal positivity is increased in patients with Borrmann tumor classification types 3–5, poorly differentiated or signet ring cell neoplasms, evidence of lymphatic invasion, or large tumor size (>2.0 cm).

In Japan, more than half of patients with gastric adenocarcinoma have early (T1) gastric cancer. This finding has been attributed to the use of sophisticated social education and mass screening programs. Endoscopic treatment has been performed successfully for T1 cancers, especially M gastric adenocarcinomas, while operative intervention is recommended for SM invasion, venous or lymphatic invasion, or positive margins after endoscopic resection. Worldwide, the use of minimally invasive procedures is dependent on economically appropriate costs and the health and welfare policies of each country.

Operative Indications and Curative Operations

Patient comorbidities should be reviewed when considering operative resection. Intervention is indicated when resection enables a beneficial outcome for the patient, aiming at either cure or palliation to improve quality of life (QOL). While recent developments in anticancer drugs and interventional endoscopic techniques have allowed control of tumor bleeding or mechanical obstruction in many patients with advanced gastric adenocarcinoma, palliative bypass or resection may be an option in selected patients.

When intervention is intended for cure, the extent of gastric resection, lymphadenectomy, role of splenectomy, and method of reconstruction should be determined according to location and histologic type of the neoplasm, as well as the disease stage. Gastrectomy remains the only treatment of invasive gastric cancer offering long-term survival.

Several prospective and randomized studies have failed to demonstrate a survival advantage of total gastrectomy compared with distal subtotal gastrectomy. Additionally, QOL after subtotal gastrectomy is superior to that after total gastrectomy. These findings have led to the preference for subtotal gastrectomy when an adequate margin can be obtained distant from the primary neoplasm.

The issue of lymph node dissection remains controversial in the surgical management of gastric adenocarcinoma. The extent of lymph node dissection is defined by the D (dissection) designation; D1 dissection includes only perigastric lymph nodes, while a D2 dissection also includes nodes along the named gastric arteries, including the hepatic, left gastric, celiac, and splenic arteries, and those in the splenic hilum. Dissections which include nodes along the porta hepatis, retropancreatic, and periaortic areas are classified as D3. Although retrospective studies from Japan suggest that extended lymphadenectomy can improve survival in patients with stage II or III disease with perioperative mortality rates of 1%, a Dutch prospective, randomized multi-center trial showed higher patient operative morbidity and mortality after D2 compared with D1 resections (43% and 10% vs. 25% and 4%, respectively, $p < 0.01$ each). Subset analysis (post hoc) of this latter study showed that survival of patients with stage II or IIIA disease was better after a D2 dissection, but the study was not powered to address this question adequately. The overall survival benefit of extended lymph node dissection may be around 5–8%, but obligates considerable operative morbidity and mortality rates, when splenectomy or distal pancreatectomy (to aid the lymphadenectomy) is performed. D3 lymph node dissections may be considered by experienced surgeons with excellent technique and low operative morbidity and mortality rates. Data from the American College of Surgeons indicate that the risk of mortality with a D3 resection is in the range of 8–9% across the United States, and thus D3 resections cannot be recommended routinely.

When necessary to achieve an R0 resection, resections of involved adjacent organs (colon, diaphragm, liver, pancreas) should be considered in centers with low operative mortality rates. The risk of mortality is increased to 15% when distal pancreatectomy and splenectomy are performed as concomitant procedures during gastrectomy in low volume hospitals.

Options for reconstruction after total gastrectomy include the standard Roux-en-Y esophago-jejunostomy, construction of a jejunal pouch, or jejunal interposition (with or without a pouch). While each of these approaches has its advocates, there are no large, controlled trials demonstrating superiority of one approach over the other. The most common reconstruction after total gastrectomy remains a simple esophago-jejunostomy to a Roux-en-Y limb, and in the absence of any conclusive data, it can be argued that the simpler procedure is probably the best. For subtotal gastrectomy, reconstruction options include a Billroth I-like gastroduodenostomy, a loop reconstruction (Billroth II), a jejunal inter-position, and a Roux-en-Y reconstruction. The choice depends on gastro-duodenal mobility as well as the size/volume of the gastric remnant; small gastric remnants are best drained by a Roux-en-Y limb to prevent bile reflux esophagitis after a B-II-type drainage. The anastomosis should be large enough to provide optimal emptying of the gastric remnant. The gastro-jejunostomy can be constructed utilizing a circular or linear stapler or by a hand-sewn technique. Debate continues with regard to anastomotic stricture and leak rates among the various techniques (stapler vs. hand-sewn).

Chemotherapy and Chemoradiotherapy for Gastric Cancer

Single agent treatments of 5-fluorouracil (5-FU), doxorubicin (DXR), mitomycin C (MMC), or cisplatin (CDDP) provide partial response rates of 10–30%. Response rates with 5-FU of up to 20% have been reported and with only mild toxicity. An oral "pro-drug" form of 5-FU composed of uracil and tegafur (UFT) has demonstrated a response rate of 28%, with a median survival of 6 months. When administered orally, UFT is tolerated better than 5-FU. Another oral 5-FU pro-drug currently under clinical trial is S-1, a combination of tegafur and 5-chloro-2,4-dihydropyrimidine (a dihydropyrimidine dehydrogenase inhibitor) and oteracil (anti-diarrhea). This drug has been evaluated in two Japanese Phase II trials for gastric cancer and showed response rates of 44–49% with a median survival of 7–8 months. While the results for S-1 are promising, further study in larger confirmatory trials is required.

Cisplatin (CDDP), a metal (platinum) with broad-spectrum, anti-tumor activity, offers response rates of 19–33%. Carboplatin, an analog of CDDP with less renal toxicity, has little activity as a single agent against gastric cancer, with only a 5% response rate, but a novel CDDP analog, oxaliplatin, is also now being studied. The topoisomerase I inhibitor irinotecan had a 23% response rate in a phase II trial. Microtubule agents known as taxanes (paclitaxel and docetaxel) have exhibited overall response rates of 17% for paclitaxel and 17–24% for docetaxel.

To improve overall survival and response rates, a number of combination chemotherapy programs have been investigated based on agents with known activity. Numerous patients have been treated with FAM (5-FU plus doxorubicin and mitomycin) since 1980, offering a 30% overall response rate and a 2% complete response rate. To increase the activity of 5-FU-based regimens, doxorubicin and methotrexate, along with 5-FU (FAMTX), have increased the response rate to 58%, with a complete remission rate of 12%; however, this regimen confers a relatively high mortality rate (3%). Nonetheless, the EORTC showed superiority of FAMTX to FAM in terms of response rate (45% vs. 9%, $p < 0.0001$), and median survival (10.5 months vs. 7 months).

Etoposide, doxorubicin, and cisplatin (EAP) were used in a Phase II trial for patients with advanced gastric cancer and gave a response rate of 64% (95% CI, 52% to 76%) and a complete remission rate of 21%; however, three subsequent Phase II trials of EAP showed excessive treatment-related mortality (6% to 14%) despite good efficacy (response rates: 43–72%). Subsequently, EAP and FAMTX were compared in a randomized Phase II trial that also observed excessive toxicities and treatment-related deaths (13%) for the EAP group.

Combined epirubicin, cisplatin, and 5-FU (ECF) have also been compared with FAMTX in a phase III trial. ECF had a greater response rate of 46% (95% CI, 37–55%), compared with 21% (95% CI, 13–28%) for the FAMTX group. In addition, ECF resulted in a superior median survival (9 vs. 6 for FAMTX, $p = 0.0005$). The combination of etoposide, leucovorin, and 5-FU (ELF) was assessed by the EORTC as part of a three-arm, randomized trial of FAMTX, ELF, and 5-FU plus CDDP, and showed response rates of 12%, 9%, and 20%, respectively, but with similar 7-month median survival times for all three groups.

To investigate combination chemotherapies based on the novel drugs irinotecan and cisplatin, several Phase I/II studies have been conducted using different regimens. The response rates of these trials were 42–58%, suggesting that such regimens may be effective in palliating gastric adenocarcinoma. Similarly, when the recently developed taxane drugs paclitaxel and docetaxel were added to a 5-FU and cisplatin regimen, a 51% objective response was achieved (95% CI, 37–66%).

Docetaxel-based chemotherapy regimens have also been studied extensively for gastric adenocarcinoma. Phase II trials using combined docetaxel and cisplatin had response rates of 33–56%, with median survival durations of 9–10 months. In addition, the combination of docetaxel, CDDP, and 5-FU (DCF) showed high response rates of 52–56% and is considered currently one of the best regimens. Japanese investigators recently tested the combination of S-1 and CDDP in a Phase I/II trial and demonstrated a response rate of 76%.

Radiation therapy is known to be effective against gastrointestinal cancers including gastric adenocarcinoma, but remains somewhat controversial in neoadjuvant and adjuvant settings. Because the sensitivity spectrum of chemotherapy may be different from that of radiotherapy, adjuvant radiotherapy may be effective against chemo-resistant cells that survive chemotherapy, as suggested by one American trial.

Selected Readings

Bonenkamp JJ, Hermans J, Sasako M, Velde van de CJ (1999) Extended lymph node dissection for gastric cancer. Dutch Gastric Cancer Group. NEJM 340:908–914

Bruckner HW, Morris JC, Mansfield P (2003) In: Kufe DW, Pollock RE, Weichselbaum RR, et al. (eds) Cancer medicine, 6 th edn. BC Decker, Ontario

Hans-Olov A, Hunter D, Trichopoulos D, et al. (2002) A textbook of cancer epidemiology, 1st edn. Oxford University Press, New York

Houghton J, Stoicov C, Nomura S, et al. (2004) Gastric cancer originating from bone marrow-derived cells. Science 306:1568–1571

Japanese Research Society for Gastric Cancer (1995) Japanese classification of gastric carcinoma, First English edition. Kanehara, Tokyo

Mullaney PJ, Wadley MS, Hyde C, et al. (2002) Appraisal of compliance with the UICC/AJCC staging system in the staging of gastric cancer. Union International Contra la Cancrum/American Joint Committee on Cancer. Br J Surg 89:1405–1408

Rustgi AK (2000) Neoplasms of the stomach. In: Cecil RL, Goldman L, Bennett JC (eds) Cecil textbook of medicine, 21st edn. W. B. Saunders, Philadelphia, pp. 738–741

55 Gastrointestinal Stromal Tumors

Francesco P. Prete · Ronald P. DeMatteo

Pearls and Pitfalls

- Gastrointestinal stromal tumor (GIST) is the most common mesenchymal neoplasm of the GI tract, while other intestinal sarcomas (lipoma, leiomyoma, and leiomyosarcoma) are infrequent.
- GIST is diagnosed by a combination of cellular morphology on hematoxylin-eosin staining and KIT immunohistochemistry. Rarely, GIST does not overexpress KIT and molecular evaluation may be necessary to render the diagnosis.
- Complete surgical resection is the standard treatment for primary, localized GIST and regional lymph nodes are involved rarely.
- The clinical behavior of GIST is variable, but nearly all lesions have the potential to behave in a malignant fashion (i.e., metastasize). The risk of GIST recurrence is increased with a mitotic rate > 5/50 high power fields, tumor size > 5 cm, and intestinal (vs. stomach) origin.
- The majority of GISTs have a mutation in the *KIT* proto-oncogene, or occasionally in *PDGFRα*, and effective tyrosine kinase inhibitors have been developed against both associated proteins.
- In metastatic GIST, imatinib mesylate (Gleevec) achieves stable disease or a partial response in over 75% of patients and is continued unless there is intolerance or resistance (progression). The median time of acquired resistance to imatinib is less than 2 years. Sunitinib (Sutent) is a second line agent.
- There may be benefit of resecting metastatic GIST that is stable on tyrosine kinase inhibitor (TKI) therapy.
- The value of imatinib as an adjuvant treatment is under investigation.

Presentation

Gastrointestinal stromal tumor (GIST) accounts for approximately 80% of all GI mesenchymal tumors. Originally considered to derive from smooth muscle, and variably classified as GI leiomyoma or leiomyosarcoma on the basis of light microscopy appearance, GIST was recognized widely as a distinct disease in the last decade, with the advent of immunohistochemical staining and ultrastructural evaluation. Currently, GIST is defined as a KIT-expressing or KIT-signaling driven primary spindle cell or epithelioid mesenchymal neoplasm of the GI tract, commonly harboring an activating mutation in either the *KIT* (italics denotes the gene as opposed to the protein) or platelet-derived growth factor receptor alpha (*PDGFRα*) gene, both of which encode for receptor tyrosine kinases.

Pathogenesis

KIT is a proto-oncogene that encodes for a transmembrane receptor glycoprotein with tyrosine kinase function. The KIT protein is expressed commonly by the intestinal interstitial pacemaker cells of Cajal (from which GISTs are believed to derive), hematopoietic cells, mast cells, and germ cells. KIT functions in differentiation, cell growth, and survival. In up to 90% of GISTs, a single gain-of function mutation is present in the *KIT* gene, leading to constitutive, ligand-independent activation of the receptor tyrosine kinase function. The most frequent sites of *KIT* mutation are in exon 11 of the gene (70%), which codes for the juxtamembrane domain of the KIT protein, or in exon 9 (10%). Exons 13 and 17 are rarely involved. KIT protein is expressed by the overwhelming majority (95%) of GISTs, and the antigenic determinant of the receptor (CD117 antigen) can be detected with simple immunohistochemical staining. A small subset of GISTs (5%) with otherwise typical clinicopathologic and cytogenetic features do not express detectable KIT protein and are CD117 negative. In a fraction of GISTs (approximately 3%), mutation occurs in *PDGFRα* but not *KIT*. *PDGFRα* mutation usually involves exon 12 (intracellular juxtamembrane region) or exon 18 (activation loop). These sites correspond to the *KIT* exons containing oncogenic mutations in many GISTs, and the downstream activation of intracellular intermediates and the cytogenetic changes occurring with tumor progression are similar to those from GISTs with *KIT* mutation. Overall, about 10% of all GISTs do not have a detectable mutation in either *KIT* or *PDGFRα* and are designated as wild-type with an unknown molecular pathogenesis. The presence of the constitutively activated mutant *KIT* isoforms (and some of the mutant *PDGFRα* isoforms) is clinically important, because the tumors are sensitive to the selective tyrosine kinase inhibiting agent imatinib mesylate, validating the molecularly targeted approach to cancer therapy.

Incidence and Anatomical Distribution

GIST is the most common mesenchymal neoplasm of the GI tract, but accounts for less than 1% of GI malignant neoplasms. The incidence is approximately 15 cases per million, with a prevalence of 129 cases per million. GIST represents about 20% of small-bowel malignant neoplasms (excluding lymphoma), 1–2% of gastric malignancies, and less than 1% of malignancies involving the esophagus, colon, and rectum. No racial predilection exists. Men are affected slightly more often than women. The majority of patients are between 40 and 80 years of age at the time of diagnosis (median 60 years), but the disease spans over a broad spectrum of age. GIST occurs rarely in adolescents or children. Approximately 60% of GIST occurs in the stomach, usually in the fundus. About 30% of tumors occur in the small intestine, and are most commonly found in the jejunum, followed by the ileum and the duodenum. Another 1–5% arise in the esophagus, and 5% are located in the colon and rectum. On rare occasions, GIST develops outside the gastrointestinal tract in the mesentery, omentum, or retro-peritoneum. GISTs are multicentric in fewer than 5% of cases. Rarely GISTs (mainly gastric, involving the body and the antrum) may occur in association with functioning extra-adrenal paraganglioma and pulmonary chondroma in the context of "Carney's triad", a rare syndrome of unknown etiology reported in young women. GISTs arising in this setting, even if metastatic, characteristically have a slower and more indolent clinical course than sporadic cases. These patients are wild-type for *KIT* and *PDGFRα*. GISTs related to the Neurofibromatosis type-1 syndrome seem to rely on the activation of alternative kinase pathways, and again the patients are wild-type for *KIT* and *PDGFRα*. *KIT* or *PDGFRα* germline mutations have been detected in at least a dozen kindreds with familial GIST in the world.

Clinical Features

There is a broad range of possible patient presentations in GIST. In the majority (about 70%) of cases, patients will seek medical attention because of nonspecific symptoms: nausea, early satiety, vomiting, abdominal discomfort, or vague abdominal pain. These symptoms reflect the typical growth pattern of GIST which, similar to other sarcomas, tends to displace but not invade adjacent structures. Consequently, a GIST is often clinically silent until it becomes large. Occasionally, an increase in abdominal girth or a palpable mass may be present. Overall, the mean duration of symptoms is 4–6 months. Small tumors (usually within 2–3 cm) are more likely to be incidentally detected in asymptomatic patients on radiologic imaging, abdominal exploration, or endoscopy. GIST may result in ulceration of the gut mucosa. After initial growth as a submucosal mass, GIST may then erode into the lumen of the intestinal tract and produce gastrointestinal bleeding. Blood loss is usually subclinical and may produce fatigue and microcytic anemia. However, up to 25% of patients present with acute GI hemorrhage. Large tumors that outgrow their blood supply may become necrotic and rupture into the peritoneal cavity, resulting in life-threatening hemorrhage. Other symptoms are particular to the site of tumor origin, so an esophageal GIST may cause dysphagia, or a rare periampullary GIST may result in biliary obstruction. Intestinal obstruction is uncommon; the tumor can act rarely as a lead point for intussusception. In the rectum, GISTs usually present as small, hard nodules less than 1 cm in diameter found incidentally during clinical examination. Large tumors can ulcerate and may mimic a rectal adenocarcinoma. The clinical behavior of any particular GIST is difficult to predict. With prolonged follow-up, it appears that almost any GIST presenting with clinical symptoms or signs leading to treatment has the potential to behave in a malignant fashion. On presentation, about 25% of GISTs have already metastasized. Metastases most commonly involve the liver, omentum, and the peritoneal cavity. Dissemination to the lungs and to extra-abdominal organs usually occurs late in the course of disease.

Diagnosis

Initial Assessment

The clinical diagnosis of GIST requires a high level of suspicion, as the patient's history and physical examination are usually nonspecific. Abdominal imaging (ultrasound, CT scan, or MRI) is usually performed because of a mass, abdominal pain, or other symptoms, and it is important to define the characteristics of a gastrointestinal mass, evaluate resectability, and determine distant spread of the disease. The possibility of a GIST should be considered when a circumscribed, vascular, exophytic mass is found in relation to the stomach or the intestine.

Cross-Sectional Imaging

Contrast-enhanced CT is useful to confirm and characterize an abdominal mass related to the gut. Oral and IV contrast should be administered to properly define the bowel margins. At CT scan, smaller GISTs present typically as hyperdense, well-defined solid masses with homogeneous attenuation, with uniform or rim-like bright enhancement after IV contrast. Occasionally, dense focal calcifications are present. Large tumors (>10 cm) present usually with enhancing borders of variable thickness and may contain irregular central areas of fluid as a result of necrosis or hemorrhage. In the majority of cases, the tumor margin appears smooth or lobular. The vessels surrounding large masses can appear stretched, but encasement is uncommon. CT can detect the presence or absence of metastatic disease in the liver, lungs, bone, and peritoneum. Liver metastases tend to appear hypodense in the portal phase but are hypervascular in the arterial phase.

MR imaging is useful for a low rectal mass or when the patient is intolerant to CT scan contrast. GIST appears isointense on T1-weighted and hyperintense on T2-weighted images, and again takes up contrast.

Upper Endoscopy

Endoscopy may be useful to characterize a gastric or duodenal lesion further. Small GISTs typically appear as a submucosal mass with smooth margins and a normal overlying mucosa. Sometimes they bulge into the gastric lumen and central ulceration is seen occasionally. Endoscopic ultrasound can be useful to define the local extension of a tumor incidentally discovered during endoscopy. However, sonographic characteristics alone provide insufficient information to assess the clinical behavior of the tumor.

Biopsy

If a suspected GIST appears resectable, preoperative biopsy is not required, because GISTs are soft and fragile and can easily bleed or rupture resulting in tumor dissemination. Most pathologists cannot reliably render a diagnosis of GIST from a percutaneous biopsy, especially when only a fine-needle aspirate is obtained or a necrotic portion of the tumor is sampled. The chance of bleeding or rupture is minimal in the case of endoscopic biopsy. A biopsy is preferred to confirm the diagnosis if metastatic disease is suspected, if there is a possibility that the diagnosis may be lymphoma, or if preoperative imatinib is considered prior to attempted resection in a patient who has a large locally advanced lesion thought to represent a GIST.

Pathologic Diagnosis

The diagnosis of GIST relies on the presence of characteristic morphologic findings on hematoxylin-eosin staining and the expression of the KIT receptor on immunohistochemistry, with central review by an expert in sarcoma pathology for equivocal cases. Three main morphologic types of GIST exist: spindle (70%), epithelioid (20%), and mixed spindle and epithelioid (10%). GIST tends to have bland morphologic features, which per se are not predictive of biologic behavior. CD117 immunohistochemistry is positive in up to 95% of cases, CD34 in 70% of cases, smooth muscle actin in 40%, S-100 in 5%, while desmin is mostly negative (2% of cases). KIT staining is generally intense and diffuse in GIST. Immunohistochemical examination is performed usually without antigen retrieval, as this can result in false positive staining for CD117. Molecular analysis for *KIT* or *PDGFRα* mutation is performed in cases of weak or absent CD117 staining, since this may occur in KIT-negative GISTs or other types of tumors. The optimal method for mutational analysis is still to be defined. Mutations in *KIT* exon 9 are

◘ Table 55-1

Estimation of malignant potential of GIST (Adapted from Miettinen et al., 2002, copyright 2002. With permission from Elsevier)

	Gastric		Intestinal	
	Size (cm)	Mitoses per 50 HPF	Size (cm)	Mitoses per 50 HPF
Likely benign	≤5	≤5	≤2	≤5
Intermediate	5–10	≤5	2–5	≤5
Probably malignant	>10	>5	>5	>5

HPF – high power fields.

typically of small intestine origin, while *PDGFRα* exon 18 mutations are typical of stomach and omental GISTs. The karyotype of GIST is characterized frequently by the deletions in chromosomes 14, 22 and 1p. The clinical behavior is variable. All GISTs are regarded as potentially malignant, with the possible exception of very small (<1 cm) tumors, and it seems appropriate to stratify GISTs according to their risk of progression rather than as benign or malignant. There is general consensus that mitotic rate, tumor size, and tumor site are the most important predictors (❯ *Table 55-1*). Gastric GIST tends to have a more favorable outcome than GIST of the small intestine. GIST with exon 9 mutation appears to be more aggressive than those with exon 11 mutation. No significant correlation has been shown between survival and sex, or intensity or distribution of the staining for CD117. The prognostic significance of grading in GISTs is not clear.

Treatment

Primary Localized Disease That is Resectable

The management of GIST depends upon the confidence in the preoperative diagnosis, tumor location, size, and clinical presentation (❯ *Fig. 55-1*). Since almost every GIST is considered to have malignant potential, nearly all of them should be resected. The management of small (<1 cm) tumors is unclear. The standard therapy for primary GIST is complete surgical resection. In the pre-imatinib era, the median survival was 66 months in patients who underwent complete gross resection of the primary disease and only 22 months in patients with incomplete or unresectable primary tumors. At laparotomy, the abdomen should be explored thoroughly, with particular attention to the peritoneal surfaces and the liver to exclude metastatic spread. Wedge resection of the stomach or segmental resection of the small intestine should be performed as opposed to wide resections. Although many primary GISTs may appear ominous on CT, they can often be lifted away from surrounding structures, since they tend to displace rather than invade adjacent organs. However, in case of dense adhesions, an en bloc resection should be considered. When a tumor arises in the esophagus, duodenum or rectum, where wedge resection may not be feasible, preference should be given to a wide resection. In extra-gastrointestinal GISTs (mesentery or omentum), en bloc complete resection of all the visible disease should be performed, encompassing any adherent organs. Intraoperative violation of the tumor pseudocapsule increases the risk of peritoneal recurrence and should be avoided. Thus, the tumor should be handled

■ Figure 55-1

Summary of present treatment and investigational pathway of gastrointestinal stromal tumor

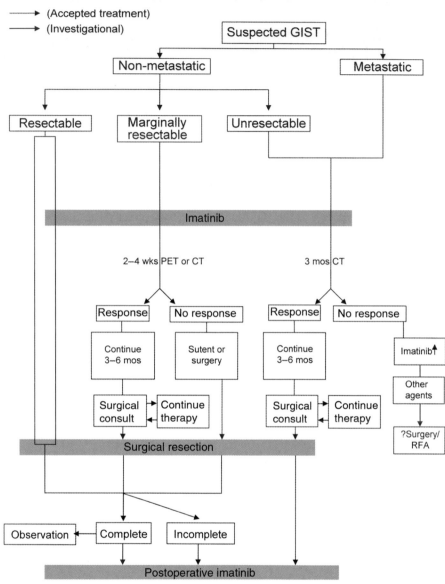

carefully, and meticulous surgical technique is necessary, because GISTs are soft and fragile. In general, every effort should be made to achieve negative resection margins, as positive margins may result in a higher risk of peritoneal relapse. It seems appropriate to consider re-excision after previous surgery with positive margins, but the risks and benefits of re-excision versus watchful waiting must be considered carefully. The management of a positive microscopic margin on the final pathology report depends also on whether the surgeon believes the finding reflects accurately the surgical procedure that was undertaken; for example, if a wedge resection was performed with a surgical stapler, the pathologist may not interpret the margin correctly once the staple line is cut away. Re-excision should also be considered following endoscopic removal of a GIST. The importance of negative surgical margins is uncertain for large GISTs, which may shed tumor cells into the peritoneum from anywhere along their surface. Since nodal metastases are rare, lymph node dissection is indicated only when nodal metastases are suspected. Often what is considered to be a lymph node is actually a satellite peritoneal metastasis. Laparoscopic resection of GIST is possible by experienced surgeons. Generally, laparoscopy should only be used for tumors < 5 cm to minimize intraoperative rupture.

Primary Localized Disease That Is not Resectable

The first-line treatment for patients with unresectable GIST (because of tumor proximity to important neurovascular structures, or risk of important functional consequences after resection of surrounding organs) is imatinib mesylate. If a GIST responds to imatinib and appears resectable, then surgery may be possible. CT scan is the preferred method to assess treatment response to imatinib. A scan is performed typically after 1 month of therapy to make sure that the patient is not in the 15% of patients who are resistant primarily to imatinib. In that case, sunitinib may be tried. Sufficient tumor shrinkage on either agent can require 6 or more months of therapy.

Primary Disease with Metastasis

In general, patients with a primary GIST and synchronous metastasis should be treated first with imatinib, even when all disease is technically removable. The exceptions include those with a low volume of metastatic disease or patients with symptoms.

Metastatic Disease

In patients presenting with metastatic disease, the first-line treatment is imatinib. Up to 80% of patients with metastatic GIST achieve a partial response or stable disease while receiving imatinib. Data from the pre-imatinib era demonstrate that surgical treatment alone of metastatic GIST almost never results in cure. Therefore, if resection becomes feasible, imatinib should be continued after surgery.

Imatinib Mesylate

Imatinib is a multi-kinase inhibitor, which acts on the tyrosine kinase BCR-ABL (involved in chronic myeloid leukemia) and on the protein kinases KIT and PDGFRα. The mechanism of inhibition is competitive. Competing with ATP for the binding to the catalytic site of the receptor, imatinib blocks the transfer of a phosphate group to the substrate, and therefore blocks the transduction of the signals generated by the activation of KIT or PDGFRα.

Imatinib should be started at the diagnosis of unresectable or metastatic GIST. The general starting dose of imatinib is 400 mg/day, although one study suggests a longer progression-free survival at a dose of 800 mg/day. In general, an increase of dose is not recommended in cases of stable disease. The dose can be increased if progression occurs after an initial response at 400 mg/day. Obtaining the maximum response to imatinib can require 3–12 months of therapy, with a median of 6 months.

At present, it is advised that imatinib therapy should be continued unless there is disease progression, drug intolerance, or patient non-compliance. In the event of surgery, the drug is stopped the day before surgery and resumed when oral medications are tolerated.

Side Effects

Overall, imatinib is well tolerated, and only 5% of patients undergo interruption of therapy because of toxicity. Toxicity is usually controllable and includes periorbital edema, rash, diarrhea, nausea, abdominal pain, and fatigue. Side effects are usually mild to moderate and transient, and can be managed without dose interruption. There is about a 5% risk of tumor hemorrhage. Neutropenia and liver toxicity are uncommon, but blood tests must be monitored routinely.

Evaluation of Response to Therapy

CT is the preferred method in evaluating the response to tyrosine kinase inhibitor (TKI) therapy, unless a very short-term follow-up of within 1–2 weeks is needed (e.g., to make a surgical decision for those with marginally resectable tumors). It is important to realize that response to molecular therapy in GIST is not always accompanied by a reduction in tumor diameter. The appearance of a new nodule in the context of a hypodense lesion, which represents early progression of disease (❷ Fig. 55-2), is also not interpreted properly if only external dimensions are considered. GIST treated with TKI can increase in volume as a consequence of myxoid degeneration of the tumoral content, intratumoral hemorrhage or edema of the lesion. A better marker of treatment response is tumor density; the tumoral mass often changes in appearance from hypervascular to hypoattenuating and homogeneous. In some cases,

◻ Figure 55-2

Acquired resistance to imatinib. The patient had multiple liver metastases and initially had a response to imatinib mesylate. Note the decrease in contrast enhancement at 6 months by CT scan. The presence of a small nodule (*solid arrow*) represents residual tumor. While still on imatinib, the patient progressed at 10 months (*solid arrow*) and the tumor extended down the right hepatic vein (*open arrow*) (Reprinted from Van der Zwan and DeMatteo, 2005. With kind permission of Lippincott Williams & Wilkins)

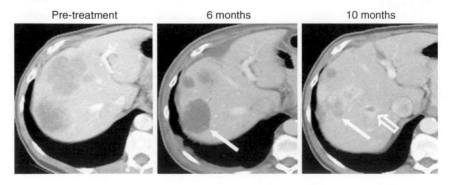

Pre-treatment   6 months   10 months

the initial density of the hepatic lesions can be similar to that of normal hepatic parenchyma, making them invisible on portal venous phases. Thus, noncontrast and arterial phase images are indicated. Responding liver lesions that decrease in density can become cystic and can be mistakenly interpreted as new lesions. Histologically, the cystic lesions contain hyaline degeneration and residual KIT-positive cells. The optimal criteria for the evaluation of the tumor response should include size, density and metabolic activity. When it is necessary to determine the early response to TKI, an 18-FDG PET scan can be performed. PET scan can demonstrate a response to TKI within a few days, while CT scan requires several weeks of treatment. Overall, however, nearly all patients can be managed by CT scan alone.

Prediction of Response Based on Mutation Status

The therapeutic response of GIST to imatinib appears to be related to the mutation status of *KIT* and *PDGFRα*. Typically, GISTs with exon 11 mutation have the highest chance of response to imatinib, while wild-type or exon 9 mutated GISTs have a lower chance. Little is known regarding the effect of imatinib on KIT-negative GIST, but there appears to be clinical benefit. Not all the *PDGFRα* activating mutations are biologically equivalent, as some are characterized by relative insensitivity to imatinib while others confer sensitivity. Because specific *PDGFRα* mutation analysis is typically not carried out in GIST, patients with advanced tumors that appear histologically compatible with GIST should not be denied a trial of imatinib if their tumor is KIT negative.

Clinical Applications

The efficacy of TKI therapy in advanced GIST has prompted interest in its use in the adjuvant setting for patients with primary disease at high risk of recurrence postoperatively, or as preoperative or induction therapy in patients with localized unresectable (or borderline resectable) tumors. Trials are ongoing to evaluate the role of molecular targeted therapy in these settings.

Neoadjuvant therapy is particularly attractive for patients with large or poorly placed tumors that are marginally resectable or tumors that would require extensive sacrifice of normal tissue. For instance, neoadjuvant imatinib may convert the resection of a rectal GIST from an abdominoperineal resection to a low anterior resection. While it is postulated that surgical resection might become a feasible option after imatinib therapy in some patients who present with initially unresectable disease, this concept has not been evaluated rigorously. Thus, neoadjuvant therapy should be tested in clinical trials. Neoadjuvant therapy used for patients with resectable disease with the goal of eradicating potential subclinical metastatic disease is another experimental approach.

Adjuvant Therapy

At present, adjuvant therapy with imatinib is investigational, and should not be employed in the routine postoperative treatment of patients after complete resection of high-risk tumors outside of clinical trials. Various studies are ongoing to evaluate the activity of imatinib as an adjuvant following the complete resection of a primary GIST. The American College of Surgeons Oncology Group (ACOSOG) is leading a Phase II intergroup trial testing the value of adjuvant imatinib at a dose of 400 mg/day for 12 months after complete macroscopic surgical resection in patients with high-risk primary GIST. High risk is defined as a tumor size ≥10 cm, intraperitoneal tumor rupture or hemorrhage, or multifocal tumors. Survival in this study will be compared with that of historical controls. The initial data from this trial have shown that imatinib is well tolerated in the adjuvant setting, and 83% of the patients completed the 12 months of imatinib therapy. In addition, a randomized, double-blinded Phase III ACOSOG intergroup trial is open for patients with tumors measuring at least 3 cm. Patients receive imatinib (400 mg/day) or placebo for 1 year after undergoing complete resection of their primary GIST. Patients assigned to the placebo arm will cross over to imatinib therapy in the event of tumor recurrence. The primary endpoint is recurrence-free survival between the two arms. EORTC is also conducting a trial to determine the benefit of adjuvant imatinib in moderate to high-risk patients.

Outcome

No prospective data exist regarding the outcome of patients with primary GIST and existing data are from the pre-imatinib era. Five-year survival rates range from 50% to 80%. In one report, median disease-specific survival was 60 months with primary disease, 19 months with metastatic disease, and 12 months with local recurrence. Complete resection is accomplished in approximately 85% of patients with primary disease. The availability of TKI therapy will undoubtedly improve these results.

Follow-Up

There is no standard postoperative follow-up in patients who undergo surgical resection of a primary GIST. In general, there is no proof that earlier detection of recurrent GIST improves survival. However, because there is now an effective treatment for patients with recurrent or metastatic disease, it appears reasonable to perform routine postoperative surveillance. The National Comprehensive Cancer Network (NCCN) consensus panel recommends CT scans of the abdomen and pelvis with intravenous contrast every 3–6 months during the first 3–5 years and possibly yearly thereafter. In metastatic disease, scans are undertaken typically every 3–4 months to assess response and monitor for resistance.

Recurrence

The majority of patients will experience tumor recurrence despite undergoing complete resection of their primary tumor. The median time to recurrence after surgery is reported to range from 18–24 months. The first site of recurrence of GIST is usually within the abdomen and involves the peritoneum and/or the liver. At the time of disease recurrence, approximately two-thirds of patients have liver involvement and half have peritoneal disease. Extraabdominal metastases (e.g., lung or bone) may develop later in the course of the disease. Typically, peritoneal disease is found to be more extensive than what is indicated on preoperative imaging. Removal of peritoneal metastases was usually followed by subsequent recurrence in the era before TKI therapy. Liver metastases from GIST are usually multifocal. Surgery alone has limited efficacy in recurrent GIST. Recurrent GISTs are now treated with TKI treatment and the median survival exceeds 5 years. Recurrence usually culminated in death within 18 months previously.

TKI Resistance

Resistance to imatinib or sunitinib occurs in patients who have had an initial therapeutic response. In patients with imatinib-resistant disease, KIT activation still plays a functional role in the majority of tumors. *KIT* exon 9 mutations, D824V substitutions in *PDGFRα* or the presence of a wild-type *KIT* gene are the most frequent causes of **primary resistance**, that can be observed in about 15% of cases and is defined as disease progression within the first 6 months of therapy with imatinib. This type of progression is usually multifocal. In the case of **secondary resistance**, disease progression occurs after the first 6 months of therapy with imatinib. Secondary resistance may be partial (the presence of a nodule of progressive disease in the context of one or a limited number of secondary lesions) or multifocal and diffuse. Selection of clones with secondary *KIT* or *PDGFRα* mutations appears to be the most common mechanism of imatinib resistance.

Management of Tumor Progression

Disease progression is determined with radiologic imaging. In the case of primary resistance, tumor pathology should be re-evaluated to confirm the diagnosis of GIST. Disease progression can be focal or multifocal. In patients who develop focal resistance to imatinib (i.e., one specific tumor begins to grow again), surgery should be considered, although the benefit of this approach is unknown. Alternatives to surgery for residual GIST liver metastases include radiofrequency ablation (RFA) and hepatic artery embolization. It is important to continue the therapy with imatinib, the dosage of which can be increased to 800 mg/day, if tolerated, with the purpose to prevent or delay the onset of further resistant clones. Dose escalation may also temporize multifocal disease progression in some patients. There is general agreement that multifocal resistance to imatinib should be treated with another targeted agent such as sunitinib. Sunitinib is a multi-kinase inhibitor acting on the KIT, PDGFR, VEGFR, RET and *fms*-related tyrosine kinase 3 (FLT3) receptors. In the initial clinical studies, sunitinib produced a partial response in 10% of patients and stable disease in about 60% with disease progression after imatinib. Sunitinib has more side effects than imatinib and include frequently fatigue (34%), diarrhea (29%), skin discoloration (25%), nausea (24%), anorexia (19%), stomatitis (16%), vomit (16%), cutaneous rash (13%) and anemia (12%). The efficacy of sunitinib raises the question of whether it may be more effective than imatinib as a first line agent. In particular, since sunitinib is more likely than imatinib to work in exon 9 mutation, consideration should be given to using it primarily in those patients.

Other Agents

A variety of other agents are being developed and tested for GIST. Everolimus (RAD001) is an inhibitor of mTOR. Other drugs include PKC412 (inhibits pKC, VEGFR, PDGFR, KIT isoenzymes), BMS 354825 (dasatinib – inhibits BCR-ABL, Src, KIT, PDGFR), AMG706 (inhibits KIT, PDGFR, VEGF, RET), and bevacizumab.

Selected Readings

Antonescu CR, Besmer P, Guo T, et al. (2005) Acquired resistance to imatinib in gastrointestinal stromal tumor occurs through secondary gene mutation. Clin Cancer Res 11:4182–4190

Antonescu CR, Viale A, Sarran L, et al. (2004) Gene expression in gastrointestinal stromal tumors is distinguished by KIT genotype and anatomic site. Clin Cancer Res 10:3282–3290

Debiec-Rychter M, Cools J, Dumez H, et al. (2005) Mechanisms of resistance to imatinib mesylate in gastrointestinal stromal tumors and activity of the PKC412 inhibitor against imatinib-resistant mutants. Gastroenterology 128:270–279

DeMatteo RP, Lewis JJ, Leung D, et al. (2000) Two hundred gastrointestinal stromal tumors: recurrence patterns and prognostic factors for survival. Ann Surg 231:51–58

Heinrich MC, Corless CL, Demetri GD, et al. (2003) Kinase mutations and imatinib response in patients with metastatic gastrointestinal stromal tumor. J Clin Oncol 21(23):4342–4349

Heinrich MC, Corless CL, Duensing A, et al. (2003) PDGFRA activating mutations in gastrointestinal stromal tumors. Science 299:708–710

Maki RG, Fletcher JA, Heinrich MC, et al. (2005) SU11248, a multi-targeted tyrosine kinase inhibitor, can overcome imatinib (IM) resistance caused by diverse genomic mechanisms in patients (pts) with metastatic gastrointestinal stromal tumor (GIST). Proc Am Soc Clin Oncol 23:9011 (abstract)

Miettinen M, El-Rifai W, Sobin LH, Lasota J (2002) Evaluation of malignancy and prognosis of gastrointestinal stromal tumors: a review. Human Pathol 33:478–483

Van der Zwan SM, DeMatteo RP (2005) Gastrointestinal stromal tumor: 5 years later. Cancer 104:1781–1788

Verweij J, Casali PG, Zalcberg J, et al. (2004) Progression-free survival in gastrointestinal stromal tumours with high-dose imatinib: randomised trial. Lancet 364:1127–1134

56 Gastric Lymphoma

John H. Donohue

Pearls and Pitfalls

- With rare exceptions, gastric lymphoma is no longer a surgical disease.
- Most low-grade MALT lymphomas respond completely to *H. pylori* eradication.
- MALT lymphomas require months to regress completely after successful *H. pylori* eradication. While monoclonal B lymphocytes may persist for years, clinical relapse is unusual without recurrent *H. pylori* infection.
- For gastric MALT lymphomas, resistance to *H. pylori* treatment can be predicted by genetic mutations, more extensive disease, and the presence of high-grade cytopathology.
- Unresponsive gastric MALT lymphomas can usually be salvaged with radiation therapy, cyclophosphamide, rituximab, or CVP ± rituximab chemotherapy.
- Regardless of treatment type, the 10-year survival of patients with gastric MALT lymphomas is ≥90% with 10-year event-free survivals of about 70%.
- High-grade gastric lymphomas (diffuse B-cell lymphomas comprise the majority) should be treated with combination chemotherapy (most often CHOP) ± radiation therapy.
- Operative therapy of gastric lymphoma is generally now restricted to patients with localized, residual, high-grade neoplasms after nonsurgical therapy or complications of the lymphoma (hemorrhage, obstruction, and perforation).
- Survival with high-grade gastric lymphomas is less than for MALT lymphomas and is stage-dependent (5-year overall survival: stage IE ∼ 90%, Stage IIE ∼70–80%, Stage IV ∼ 50%).

Basic Science

More than 90% of patients with gastric lymphoma have a *Helicobacter pylori* (*H. pylori*) infection. Despite the absence of lymphoid tissue in the stomach wall, a chronic *H. pylori* infection may cause a gastric mucosa-associated lymphoid tissue (MALT) lymphoma. Gastric MALTs contain a monoclonal population of B-cells, the proliferation of which is controlled by a small number of T-lymphocytes whose stimulation is dependent on the presence of the specific infecting strain of *H. pylori*.

In most gastric MALT lymphomas, *H. pylori* eradication results in cessation of the B-cell proliferation and eventual resolution of the lymphoma infiltrate. The presence of specific chromosomal translocation and other genetic changes (see ❷ *Fig. 56-1*) results in most failures of gastric MALT lymphomas to respond to *H. pylori* therapy and the progression of a MALT lymphoma to a high-grade gastric lymphoma. It is unknown how often pure high-grade lymphomas arise from a MALT lymphoma versus occurring *de novo*.

◘ Figure 56-1

Progression of gastric MALT lymphomas. Gastric MALT lymphomas occur with chronic H. pylori infection and the presence of H. pylori specific T-cells. B-cell proliferation becomes less dependent on H. pylori antigenic stimulation from the top to the bottom (late MALT and most t(1;14) and t(11;18) translocation MALTs are unresponsive to H. pylori therapy) (Adapted from Isaacson and Du 2004. Copyright 2004. With permission from Macmillan)

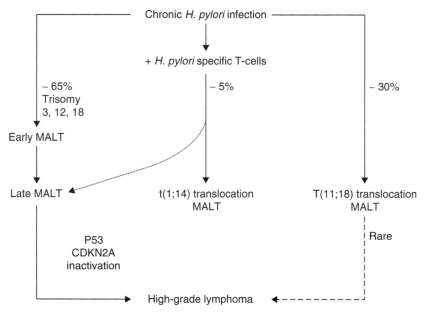

Clinical Presentation

Epigastric pain or dyspepsia is the most common symptom of gastric lymphoma. Clinically significant hemorrhage occurs in only a small number of patients. Advanced stage, high-grade gastric lymphoma may produce constitutional complaints of weight loss, fatigue, fevers, and nigh sweats (B symptoms) and/or an epigastric mass. Peripheral adenopathy is not present with primary lymphomas of the stomach. The absence of specific symptoms and signs make a clinical diagnosis of gastric lymphoma virtually impossible without a tissue biopsy.

Diagnosis

Upper gastrointestinal endoscopy (EGD) with biopsy is the diagnostic test of choice. Most gastric lymphomas infiltrate the stomach wall diffusely, similar to a diffuse gastric adenocarcinoma, but discrete masses, ulcerated tumors, and even polypoid lesions can all occur. The gastric biopsies should be evaluated for both the histologic type of lymphoma and the presence of *H. pylori*. Endoscopic ultrasonography (EUS) allows determination of both the depth of primary tumor invasion and the presence of nodal involvement (which can be documented with fine-needle aspiration). Findings of more extensive disease are especially helpful in MALT lymphomas, because they indicate the likely need for more treatment than just *H. pylori* eradication.

Once lymphoma of the stomach is diagnosed with a biopsy, computed tomography (CT) of the abdomen should be obtained for staging. A lymphangiogram is not indicated. Most experts

◙ Table 56-1

Musshoff staging system for gastric lymphomas

Stage	Disease extent
IE	Stomach only
IIEi	Perigastric nodes
IIEii	Para-aortic nodes
III	Spleen
IV	Distant site(s) (usually bone marrow)

E: extranodal lymphoma.

recommend a thorough head and neck evaluation to rule out involvement of the MALT tissues in Waldeyer's ring. A chest radiograph and bone marrow biopsy complete the staging process. The Musshoff modification of the Ann Arbor lymphoma staging system (see ❯ *Table 56-1*) is used for gastric lymphomas.

Treatment

Therapy for gastric lymphoma depends on the histology and is normally divided into treatment for low-grade gastric MALT lymphoma and high-grade lymphomas of the stomach. Because the vast majority of high-grade gastric lymphomas are diffuse B-cell types, only the treatment for this form of lymphoma will be discussed. T-cell lymphomas and other variants of B-cell lymphoma are quite uncommon, and their specific management will not be covered in this chapter.

MALT lymphomas: More than 90% of gastric MALT lymphoma patients are infected by *H. pylori*. *H. pylori* eradication is undertaken with a 2-week course of antibiotics, usually clarithromycin and amoxicillin (or metronidazole), plus a proton pump inhibitor to suppress acid secretion. Bismuth compounds are used less commonly than in the past. Confirmation of successful *H. pylori* elimination should be obtained with repeat gastric biopsies or a breath test. Repeat treatment with different antibiotics is indicated when the *H. pylori* infection is resistant to the first-line therapy.

The histologic resolution of MALT lymphomas requires an average of 3–6 months but on occasion may take up to 28 months. Repeat EGD with biopsies and EUS should be performed every three months until there is complete resolution (CR) of the neoplasm on imaging and microscopic evaluation. Endoscopic surveillance is continued after this every 6–12 months, because monoclonal B-cells are still present in ≥25% of MALT lymphoma patients after CR. After a histologic CR, less than 20% of patients will have a microscopic histologic relapse, and mostly when a monoclonal pattern of B-cells persists. Surprisingly, these microscopic recrudescences of disease normally resolve with a watch-and-wait approach. Macroscopic recurrent lymphoma in a MALT lymphoma patient with a CR is rare, unless there is recurrent *H. pylori* infection.

In the 10% of patients with gastric MALT lymphoma who are negative for *H. pylori* or those infected with *H. pylori* that does not respond to bacterial eradication therapy, other methods of treatment are indicated (see ❯ *Fig. 56-2*). Patients with a t(11;18) translocation (approximately 30% of all MALT tumors), including those with an *H. pylori* infection, are often resistant to treatment that eradicates *H. pylori*. Recent data suggest resistance of this genotype to therapy with oral cyclophosphamide agents. The MALT lymphomas that contain a component of high-grade lymphomas are also more likely not to respond to *H. pylori* eradication alone. Second-line therapies for resistant MALT lymphomas include radiation therapy (30 gray [Gy] in 150 cGy fractions over 4 weeks), oral cyclophosphamide (100 mg/day for 6–12 months), monoclonal anti-CD20 antibody (rituximab 375 mg/m^2 weekly x4) combination chemotherapy (cyclophosphamide, vincristine, and prednisone [CVP often with retuximab]) or combinations of these treatments. Some lymphomas with a component of high-grade lymphoma coexisting with a low-grade gastric MALT lymphoma will respond completely to *H. pylori* therapy, but there is greater probability that combination chemotherapy will be needed to produce a complete response. At least one recent report has noted a higher likelihood of eradicating residual microscopic, monoclonal B-cell proliferation after combined chemotherapy and radiation therapy for MALT, mixed MALT-high-grade, and pure high-grade gastric lymphomas.

High-grade gastric lymphomas: Patients with high-grade lymphomas require treatment with combination chemotherapy. Bulky disease, especially when residual disease persists, will benefit from the addition of radiation therapy. High-grade gastric lymphomas have diffuse, large-cell characteristics and respond best to R-CHOP chemotherapy (rituximab, cyclophosphamide, doxorubicin, vincristin, and prednisone). Rarer types of B-cell lymphomas and T-cell lymphomas should be treated in a fashion similar to the same histology at other primary sites. The management algorithm for high-grade, diffuse, large-cell gastric lymphoma is outlined in ❯ *Fig. 56-3*.

Outcome

Several randomized and nonrandomized prospective trials comparing operative treatment for clinical stage IE and IIE disease patients (some with and others without adjuvant therapy) versus nonsurgical

◘ Figure 56-2
Treatment of low-grade gastric MALT lymphomas

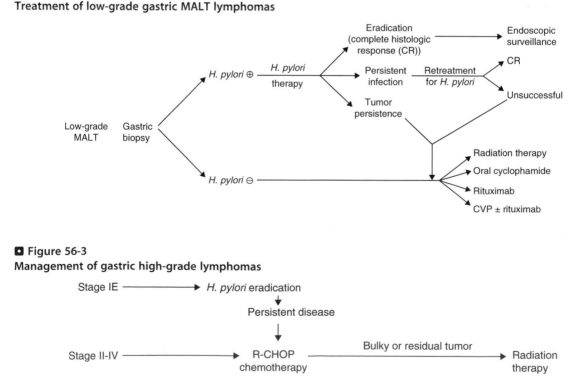

◘ Figure 56-3
Management of gastric high-grade lymphomas

therapy have shown patient survival to be the same or better for the nonsurgical treatment groups. In all studies, the frequency and severity of complications of the surgical group has been greater than for nonsurgical patients. These studies have hastened the move to defer operative intervention in patients with gastric lymphoma unless the patient has a rare complication from nonsurgical treatment or localized persistent lymphoma. Despite concerns about perforation and hemorrhage during the chemotherapy, these complications are rare in patients with gastric lymphoma. Operative therapy for gastric lymphoma is now the exception rather than the normal treatment for any stage of gastric lymphoma.

In clinical stage IE MALT lymphoma, 10-year survival is generally > 90% with *H. pylori* treatment or secondary therapies, when indicated. Treatment outcomes are similar for clinical stage IE high-grade gastric lymphomas. Mixed MALT high-grade and high-grade stage IIE gastric lymphomas have approximately a 70–80% chance of 5-year survival with nonsurgical therapy. Patients with stage IV gastric lymphoma have a 5-year survival of about 50%. Patients with T-cell or rarer types of high-grade B-cell lymphoma of the stomach generally have poorer outcomes than patients with diffuse large-cell lymphomas.

Selected Readings

Alpen B, Kuse R, Parwaresch R, et al. (2004) Ongoing monoclonal B-cell proliferation is not common in gastric B-cell lymphoma after combined radiochemotherapy. J Clin Oncol 22:3039 3045

Avilés A, Nambo J, Neri N, et al. (2004) The role of surgery in primary gastric lymphoma: results of a controlled clinical trial. Ann Surg 240:44–50

Alvilés A, Nambo MJ, Neri N, et al. (2005) Mucosa-associated lymphoid tissue (MALT) lymphoma of the stomach: results of a controlled clinical trial. Med Oncol 22:57–62

Chen LT, Lin JT, Tai JJ, et al. (2005) Long-term results of anti-*Helicobacter pylori* therapy in early-stage gastric high-grade transformed MALT lymphoma. J Natl Cancer Inst 97:1345–1353

Isaacson PG, Du M-Q (2004) MALT lymphoma: from morphology to molecules. Nat Rev 4:644–653

Koch P, Probst A, Berdel WE, et al. (2005) Treatment results in localized primary gastric lymphoma: data of patients registered within the German Multicenter Study (GIT NHL 02/96). J Clin Oncol 23:7050–7059

Lévy M, Copie- Bergman C, Gameiro C, et al. (2005) Prognostic value of translocation t(11;18) in tumoral response of low-grade gastric lymphoma of mucosa-associated lymphoid tissue type to oral chemotherapy. J Clin Oncol 23:5061–5066

Martinelli G, Laszlo D, Ferreri AJM, et al. (2005) Clinical activity of rituximab in gastric marginal zone non-Hodgkin's lymphoma resistant to or not eligible for anti-*Helicobacter pylori* therapy. J Clin Oncol 23:1979–1983

Nakamura S, Matsumoto T, Suekane H, et al. (2005) Long-term clinical outcome of *Helicobacter pylori* eradication for gastric mucosa-associated lymphoid tissue lymphoma with reference to second-line treatment. Cancer 104:532–540

Wündisch T, Thiede C, Morgner A, et al. (2005) Long-term follow-up of gastric MALT lymphoma after *Helicobacter pylori* eradication. J Clin Oncol 23:8018–8024

Yoon SS, Coit DG, Portlock CS, Karpeh MS (2004) The diminishing role of surgery in the treatment of gastric lymphoma. Ann Surg 240:28–37

Part 4

Small Bowel: Benign

57 Small Bowel Obstruction

Orlin N. Belyaev · Christophe Müller · Waldemar H. Uhl

Pearls and Pitfalls

- For patients with acute, crampy, abdominal pain and obstipation, always consider the possibility of small bowel obstruction (SBO).
- A detailed history, thorough physical examination, and characteristic findings on a plain abdominal film are usually sufficient to establish the diagnosis.
- Postoperative adhesions are the most common cause of SBO, followed by hernias and neoplasms.
- SBO should be differentiated from non-mechanical intestinal paralysis (ileus), especially in the postoperative period.
- The management of patients with SBO is based on intravenous resuscitation, nasogastric decompression, and expeditious surgery when necessary. "The sun should never rise and set on a SBO."
- All patients with complete bowel obstruction should immediately undergo operative intervention unless extraordinary circumstances such as terminal illness are present.
- A midline laparotomy is used as a standard. The surgical procedure should manage the intestinal segment at the site of the obstruction, the distended proximal bowel, and the underlying cause of SBO.
- A resection is the best and safest choice when doubt about bowel viability exists.
- Postoperative, immediate bowel stimulation with prokinetics, early mobilization, and removal of the nasogastric tube accelerate patient's recovery.
- The best prophylaxis of postoperative adhesions includes gentle handling of the distended intestine, avoiding introduction of foreign materials, careful repair of serosal defects, and copious lavage of the peritoneal cavity. Efficacy of all other methods, such as resorbable barrier membranes or chemical agents, has not yet been proven by randomized controlled trials.
- Decreasing the incidence of SBO requires an intentional search for and early elective repair of all abdominal wall hernias.

Introduction

Definition and Etiology

Small bowel obstruction is an interruption of the normal flow of luminal contents at the level of the small bowel caused by a mechanical blockage. SBO is a common medical problem and accounts for one of every five acute surgical admissions. The increasing number of patients undergoing laparotomy and their prolonged life expectancy have lead to peritoneal adhesions being the leading cause of SBO worldwide. Hernias and metastatic colorectal and ovarian cancer are the next most common causes. Adhesions, hernias, and metastatic cancer account for about 90% of all cases of SBO (● *Table 57-1*).

SBO can be incomplete (partial) or complete and simple or strangulated. A simple SBO is present when the bowel is occluded at a single point leading to proximal intestinal dilatation and distal intestinal decompression. Vascular compromise is unlikely with simple SBO. A closed-loop SBO is present when a bowel segment is occluded at two points, so that both the proximal and distal loops, as well as the bowel's mesentery are entrapped by a single constrictive lesion. A strangulated SBO is observed when the blood supply to a closed-loop segment becomes compromised, leading to ischemia and bowel necrosis. The small bowel, unlike the large bowel, perforates rarely when obstructed – and most often in cases of radiation enteritis or metastatic neoplasms.

Note: In parts of Europe, the term ileus is applied both to a mechanical obstruction and to atony of the bowel related to abdominal surgery or peritonitis; however, in most English-speaking countries, the term obstruction is reserved for the mechanical blockage arising from a structural abnormality that presents a physical barrier to the progression of gut contents. The term ileus probably should be reserved for the paralytic or functional obstruction.

Pathophysiology

Whatever the site and cause, SBO leads to rapid accumulation of luminal secretions, swallowed air, and gas from bacterial fermentation in the bowel segment proximal to the obstruction which becomes increasingly distended. Bacterial overgrowth, bowel edema, and loss of absorptive function follow,

◨ Table 57-1

Causes of mechanical small bowel obstruction

Extrinsic (most common)	Intrinsic	
	Intraluminal (rare)	Intramural (infrequent)
Adhesions	Milk curd obstruction	Neonatal atresia
Hernias	Inspissated meconium	Intussusception
• External	Foreign body	Small bowel neoplasms
• Internal	Worms (Ascaris lumbricoides)	• Primary – lipoma, leiomyoma, carcinoid, lymphoma, adenocarcinoma
• Incisional	Bezoar	
Metastatic cancer	Gallstone	
Volvulus	Small bowel tumors	• Metastatic – melanoma
Intraabdominal abscess		Hematoma
Intraabdominal hematoma		• Trauma
Intraabdominal drain		• Anticoagulant overdose
Tight fascial stoma opening		Stricture
		• Radiation enteritis
		• Crohn's disease
		• Tuberculosis
		• Complication of surgical anastomosis
		• Potassium tablets, NSAIDs

enhancing the third spacing of fluid, electrolytes, and proteins into the intestinal lumen. The overall effect is progressive dehydration, electrolyte imbalance, and systemic toxicity. Copious vomiting exacerbates fluid loss and electrolytic depletion. If the condition is not treated promptly, ischemia and necrosis of the small intestine may occur. Obstructed small bowel, unlike the large one, perforates rarely and this is usually due to compromised intestinal wall in cases of radiation enteritis or metastases.

Clinical Presentation

The most common symptoms of SBO are abdominal pain, vomiting, abdominal distension, and obstipation (❷ *Fig. 57-1*). Abdominal pain is the leading and most constant symptom. In simple SBO, the accompanying symptoms include periumbilical and intermittent pain and cramps, that waxes and wanes over 1 to 3 min intervals. It is believed that progression from a colicky to persistent, steady pain is a sign of impending strangulation. In general, pain increases in severity and depth as obstruction progresses. Distension, nausea, and vomiting usually develop after pain has already been existent for some time. In general, the more proximal the level of obstruction, the less the distension and the more rapid the onset of nausea and vomiting. Conversely, in patients with distal SBO, central abdominal distention may be marked, but vomiting is usually a late feature. Initially, the vomitus contains gastric juice, which is followed soon by bile, and finally, the vomitus contains feculent small bowel content. Absolute obstipation is a late feature, because the colon requires 12–24 h to empty after the onset of SBO. As a result, flatus and even passage of feces may continue after onset of symptoms. Hypotension, tachycardia, and oliguria correspond to fluid depletion, while tenderness, fever, and leukocytosis suggest strangulation. In the early stages, bowel sounds are usually high-pitched and occur in frequent runs as the bowel contracts to try to overcome the obstruction. A silent tender abdomen suggests perforation or peritonitis and is a late sign.

❏ Figure 57-1
Frequency of the leading symptoms of small bowel obstruction (Modified from Uhl W et al., 1998. With permission)

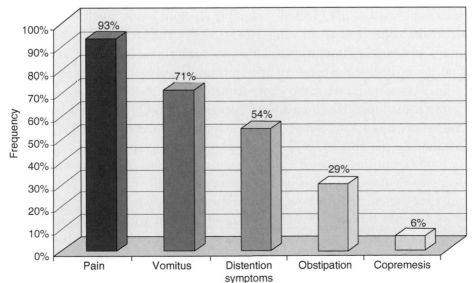

Diagnosis

A detailed history and a thorough physical examination will provide a correct diagnosis in more than three-quarters of affected patients. The patient should be queried of previous abdominal or pelvic surgery, prior radiation therapy, history of intraabdominal malignancy, inflammation, or trauma, as well as past episodes of bowel obstruction. All medications the patient is taking should be considered as causative, especially anticoagulants. The initial physical examination includes assessment of the patient's vital signs and severity of disease. A nasogastric tube, a urinary catheter, and an intravenous line are placed immediately. The volume and character of gastric aspirate and urine are noted. A full laboratory analysis is routine. The complete blood and chemistry profiles are not helpful in determining the presence or cause of SBO but are useful for the assessment of dehydration and the degree of metabolic derangement. Abdominal examination proceeds from observation to auscultation to palpation and percussion. Abdominal scars, asymmetry, and evidence of peristaltic waves on the abdominal wall should be noted. Auscultation is performed for several minutes – high-pitched bowel tones, tinkles, and rushes are suggestive of an obstruction. Their absence is typical of intestinal paralysis but may also indicate intestinal fatigue and atony from a long-standing obstruction or the development of peritonitis. A meticulous search is made for abdominal wall hernias, especially small inguinal and femoral ones, which are easy to overlook in obese patients. Proper genitourinary and rectal examinations are essential in the search for masses, fecal impaction, mucous, and blood. Patients with an ileostomy should have their stoma examined digitally to make sure there is no obstruction at the level of the fascia. Gentle percussion is performed to search for areas of dullness (suggestive of an underlying mass), tympany (distended bowel loops), and peritoneal irritation. No reliable way exists to differentiate simple from early strangulated obstruction on physical examination, but the more severe clinical course is usually suggestive of strangulation. Serial abdominal examinations are necessary to detect changes early.

An abdominal plain film series is used to confirm the diagnosis of SBO made by history and physical examination. Basic radiologic examination includes an upright chest X-ray to rule out the presence of free subdiaphragmatic air, as well as supine and upright abdominal films. If the patient cannot be placed into an upright position, a left lateral decubitus abdominal film should be obtained. The typical radiologic triad of SBO includes multiple air-fluid levels, small bowel distension, and a paucity of air in the colon and rectal vault (❯ *Fig. 57-2*). Thickened small bowel loops, mucosal "thumb-printing," pneumatosis intestinals and free peritoneal air are considered as evidence of strangulation. It is important to distinguish between small and large bowel gas. Valvulae conniventes are outlined in a distended small bowel and traverse the whole diameter of the bowel lumen. Gas in a distended colon outlines the haustral markings, which cross only part of the bowel lumen and typically interdigitate. Distended small bowel loops usually occupy the central abdomen, whereas distended large bowel loops are seen typically around the periphery. Valvulae conniventes are usually spaced closely and should be within 1–4 mm of each other, but this distance increases with small-bowel distention (the stretch sign). Even when distended, the valvulae conniventes in the jejunum are usually preserved; however, in a distended terminal ileum, they flatten, and the bowel often appears tube-like. Presence of air-fluid differential height in the same small-bowel loop and presence of a mean width greater than 25–30 mm are radiologic signs indicative of a high-grade or complete SBO. When both are absent, a partial SBO is likely or nonexistent. The more distal the obstruction, the more numerous the air-fluid levels. At different heights, the levels reveal a stepladder appearance. An increase in peristaltic activity can

▢ Figure 57-2
An upright abdominal x-ray of a patient with distal small bowel obstruction. The arrows indicate well-defined air-fluid levels and distended small bowel loops. Note the characteristic paucity of air in the colon

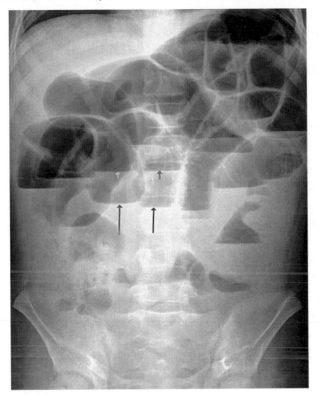

give rise to the string-of-beads sign in which the beads represent air trapped within the valvulae conniventes. The coffee-bean sign (a gas-filled loop) may be seen in closed-loop SBO.

A *small bowel follow-through series* and an *enteroclysis* (direct instillation of water-soluble contrast into the small intestine through a tube placed in the duodenum) can reliably and quickly detect SBO and remain the "gold standard" to differentiate partial from complete blockages but are not indicative of the etiology of obstruction. In cases of inconclusive plain films, a contrast-enhanced CT should be the next step in difficult-to-diagnose bowel obstructions. A CT is the study of choice if the patient has fever, tachycardia, localized abdominal pain, and/or leukocytosis. The CT is capable of revealing abscess, inflammatory processes, extraluminal pathology resulting in obstruction, and mesenteric ischemia. It can help to distinguish between ileus and mechanical SBO in postoperative patients and is the preferred method in patients with history of abdominal malignancy. CT rarely, however, shows the source of adhesive obstruction, because it cannot detect adhesions. The diagnosis of obstruction and determining its level is based on the identification of a dilated proximal loop and a collapsed distal loop of small bowel. Bowel wall thickening, portal venous gas, and pneumatosis are CT-signs of early strangulation. Magnetic resonance imaging (MRI) may be used as an alternative to CT in selected patients, e.g., with neoplasms or Crohn's disease; however, this method is complicated, time-consuming, expensive, and not available universally.

Ultrasonography is relatively inexpensive, easy, and quick to perform, but bowel gas and obesity pose problems, and the technique remains operator-dependent. It has no specific role in the diagnosis of an acute SBO but is used widely in the initial investigation of acute abdominal pain. Ultrasonography can often differentiate adynamic ileus of the postoperative state or peritonitis from a mechanical obstruction by depicting peristalsis. This method is preferred in young children, pregnant patients, and as a bedside test for the critically ill. With gallstone ileus, the classic triad of a calcified gallstone in an ectopic position, gas in the biliary tree (pneumobilia), and SBO may be demonstrated. Establishing the diagnosis and cause of SBO should always follow a simple but consistent algorithm in order to avoid mistakes and delay treatment (❷ *Fig. 57-3*).

Differential Diagnosis

Paralytic ileus, large bowel obstruction, acute pancreatitis, mesenterial infarction, and gastroenteritis should be excluded. Myocardial infarction, intracranial pathology, diabetic ketoacidosis, hyperthyroidism, uremia, and hypokalemia should also be kept in mind. Tricyclic antidepressants and atropine may cause similar symptoms as may peritonitis of any cause. Perhaps the greatest problem arises in the immediate postoperative period after any abdominal operation, in which it is difficult to determine whether the failure of gastrointestinal function to return to normal is due to a postoperative bowel atony or a mechanical obstruction. In paralytic ileus (a functional disorder seen most commonly after abdominal surgery but also associated with a myriad of acute medical conditions and metabolic derangement), the small bowel is distended throughout its length, and gas is present in the colon on plain films; pain is often not a prominent feature, and auscultation reveals absence of bowel sounds. If there is doubt as to whether a mechanical or functional obstruction exists, a water-soluble contrast study may be helpful. Postoperative ileus usually resolves spontaneously after 4 or 5 days. Intragastric

◘ Figure 57-3
Diagnostic-treatment algorithm for patients with suspected SBO

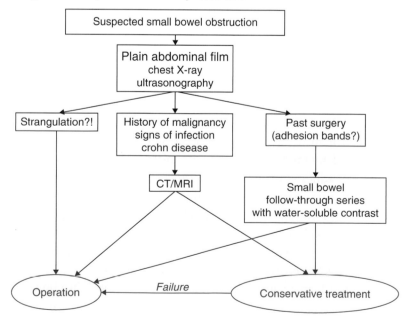

administration of water-soluble contrast may lead to the resolution of this condition in some patients. ❯ *Figure 57-4* offers a concise algorithm for cases of suspected early postoperative SBO.

Treatment

Initial treatment in the emergency department consists of aggressive fluid resuscitation using isotonic saline or lactated Ringer solution, bowel decompression, administration of analgesics, antiemetics, and antibiotic prophylaxis. Fluid resuscitation prior to operation is vital and may require more than 5 l of intravenous crystalloid; a central venous catheter may be preferable. Adequacy of resuscitation is judged by urine output and central venous pressure. Operative exploration in under-resuscitated patients is associated with increased mortality. Oxygen and appropriate monitoring of pulmonary and cardio-circulatory function is necessary. Continued nasogastric suction provides symptomatic relief, prevents aspiration, decreases the need for intraoperative decompression, and benefits all patients. Antibiotics should cover against gram-negative and anaerobic organisms.

A strangulated obstruction is a surgical emergency. A trial of conservatism should be considered carefully in cases of partial obstruction, terminal metastatic intraabdominal malignancy, recurrent adhesive obstruction, and diagnostic doubt about possible ileus in the early postoperative period. Obstructed patients should be observed for no more than 12–24 h and if frequent reassessments show no improvement, the patient should undergo operative exploration. The old rule "never let the sun rise and set on a small bowel obstruction" remains true today.

The nature of SBO determines the type and extent of operative therapy required. While incarcerated inguinal and femoral hernias often allow bowel resection through an inguinal incision, most other cases require exploratory midline laparotomy. A major critical step of the operation is the assessment of viability

◼ Figure 57-4
Diagnostic-treatment algorithm in postoperative patients with suspected SBO

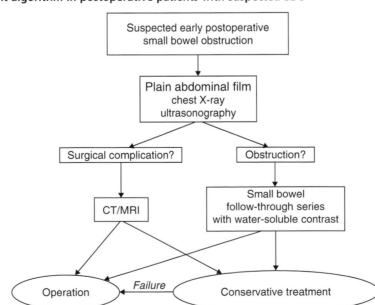

of the affected bowel segment after relief of the SBO. Any questionably viable bowel should be wrapped in warm, saline-soaked pads and a final assessment made 15–20 min later. Return of normal color, motility, and the presence of mesenteric pulses are signs indicating viability. Alternative but sophisticated and rarely used methods are the intravenous injection of fluorescein with subsequent illumination of the bowel and the standard Doppler ultrasonographic examination or the laser Doppler flowmetry. A resection is the best choice when doubt exists.

Recently, a laparoscopic approach has been used increasingly as a diagnostic and treatment tool for SBO. It is utilized predominantly in cases of adhesive obstruction and requires an experienced team to avoid iatrogenic complications. Experience is essential with laparoscopy, because this technique is not applicable as a standard procedure for SBO unless the surgeon is experienced.

Specific Problems

Intussusception in infants occurs usually in the first year of life and is usually a primary, idiopathic form. The treatment of choice is radiographic reduction with air or barium contrast, with operative treatment reserved for irreducible cases and those complicated with perforation. Adult intussusception is usually secondary and involves a pathologic leading point which is malignant in up to one-half of cases. Thus, most all adults with intussusception require operative exploration.

Patients with SBO secondary to end-stage malignancy present a special therapeutic problem and need highly individual assessment and treatment. When surgery is considered of little therapeutic benefit, continuous nasogastric tube drainage, rehydration, parenteral nutrition, octreotide, antiemetics, opiate analgesics, and comfort measures should be offered.

Early postoperative SBO is defined as that which occurs within 30 days of the initial operation. This condition is difficult to diagnose, because symptoms are often attributed to incisional pain and postoperative ileus. The most common etiology is adhesions; this variant of SBO usually resolves spontaneously within 1–2 weeks as the early formed adhesions undergo a process of spontaneous resolution during this period. This condition is managed safely by nasogastric decompression, and only patients with evidence of strangulation should be operated on expeditiously. Postoperative SBO should be distinguished from postoperative adynamic ileus.

In cases of inflammatory bowel disease, treatment is generally non-operative in combination with high-dose steroids. Parenteral treatment may be considered for prolonged periods of bowel rest. If non-operative treatment fails, resectional surgery of the strictured bowel segment will be necessary.

With radiation enteritis, non-operative treatment accompanied by steroids is usually sufficient in acute postradiation cases. If obstruction is a chronic sequel of radiation therapy, operative intervention is indicated.

Outcome

Complications related to the operative treatment of SBO include anastomotic leakage, sepsis, intraabdominal abscess, postoperative bleeding, wound dehiscence, aspiration, short-bowel syndrome (as a result of multiple resections or massive resection), and death (most often secondary to delayed treatment). Complete obstructions treated successfully non-operatively have a greater incidence of recurrence than those treated surgically.

Mortality and morbidity are dependent on the early recognition and correct diagnosis of obstruction, its etiology, the patient's age and comorbidities at presentation, and on delay in treatment. If untreated, a strangulated SBO causes death in 100% of patients. Thus, early operative intervention is essential. The mortality rate is 25% if the operation is postponed beyond 36 hours. If operation is performed within 36 h, the mortality decreases to 8%. With proper diagnosis and treatment of the obstruction, prognosis is good, and mortality under 3% can be achieved.

Selected Readings

Flasar MH, Goldberg E (2006) Acute abdominal pain. Med Clin N Am 90:481–503

Helton WS (1996) Intestinal obstruction. Chapter 6 in: Wilmore DW, Cheung LY, Harken AH, (eds) et al. SA Surgery CD. Scientific American, New York, pp. 1–22

Khan AN, Howart J (2004) Small-bowel obstruction. http://www.emedicine.com/radio/topic781.htm

Margenthaler JA, Longo WE, Virgo KS, et al. (2006) Risk factors for adverse outcomes following surgery for small bowel obstruction. Ann Surg 243:456–464

Nobie BA, Khalsa SS (2005) Obstruction, small bowel. http://www.emedicine.com/emerg/topic66.htm

Ottinger LW (1995) Small bowel obstruction. In: Morris PJ, Malt RA (eds) Oxford textbook of surgery CD. AND Electronic Publishing B.V/Oxford University Press, Rotterdam/Oxford pp. 961–965

Playforth RH, Holloway JB, Griffen WO (1970) Mechanical small bowel obstruction: a plea for earlier surgical intervention. Ann Surg 171:783–787

Quickel R, Hodin R (2006) Clinical manifestations and diagnosis of small bowel obstruction. Treatment of small bowel obstruction. In: Rose BD (ed) UpToDate 14.1. UpToDate, Watham

Uhl W, Herzog RI, Sadowski C, et al. (1998) The surgical treatment of small bowel obstruction. Zentralbl Chir 123:1340–1345

58 Motility Disorders of the Small Bowel

Reginald V. N. Lord · Lelan F. Sillin III

Pearls and Pitfalls

- A mechanical cause of intestinal obstruction should be excluded before the diagnosis of a functional intestinal obstruction is made.
- A thorough history and clinical suspicion are both important in recognizing and diagnosing small intestinal motility disorders.
- Whenever possible, enteral feeding is preferable to parenteral feeding.
- Postoperative ileus is normal, but prolonged ileus is not and needs to be investigated.
- The development of obstipation after apparent resolution of ileus, with passage of flatus or stool, is a sign of mechanical obstruction.
- Patients with intestinal "pseudo-obstruction" can have true, and even complete, non-mechanical bowel obstruction.
- Intestinal pseudo-obstruction may involve either part or all of the gastrointestinal tract.
- If the diagnosis of chronic intestinal pseudo-obstruction is not considered, unnecessary laparotomy is often performed.
- Patients with suspected primary intestinal pseudo-obstruction require very specialized evaluations to diagnose precisely the type of myopathy or neuropathy present.

Introduction

Classification of Small Bowel Motility Disorders

The two types of small bowel motility disorder included here are *paralytic* or *adynamic ileus* and the *chronic small intestinal hypomotility* or *pseudo-obstruction syndromes*. Intestinal pseudo-obstruction syndromes can be either primary or secondary motility disorders, whereas ileus occurs secondary to other pathology. Both pseudo-obstruction and ileus are characterized by abnormally delayed transport of gastrointestinal contents. Postoperative ileus is encountered very frequently by surgeons, unlike the rare chronic intestinal pseudo-obstruction syndromes. Despite promising recent research findings, the difficulty of conducting clinical studies of small intestinal motility means that the complex pathophysiology of both these conditions remains unclear.

Although it may be very difficult to distinguish paralytic ileus or intestinal pseudo-obstruction from mechanical small bowel obstruction due to adhesions, tumor, or other causes, there are important differences in the *typical* features of non-mechanical and mechanical bowel obstructions. These might alert a prudent surgeon and possibly avoid a non-therapeutic celiotomy in patients with pseudo-obstruction.

Paralytic Ileus

Ileus is defined as the temporary loss of gastrointestinal motor function. Ileus thus is an acute, reversible condition that results in a non-mechanical intestinal obstruction. Apart from its almost invariable development after intra-abdominal operations, paralytic ileus can occur after other major operations and after trauma, intra-abdominal or generalized sepsis, myocardial infarction, pneumonia, and electrolyte derangement. A list of causes is shown in ❷ *Table 58-1*. During resolution of ileus, contractile activity usually returns to the small bowel first, followed by the stomach, and only then the large bowel. The esophagus is not affected. Clinical features of ileus are usually less and may be absent after laparoscopic surgery compared with open abdominal operations.

The pathogenesis of ileus is not well understood. It is not simply a state of hypomotility, as evidenced by the fact that intestinal electrical and mechanical activity usually return rapidly after laparotomy, long before the clinical features of ileus disappear. Loss of both the contractile activity itself and the normal organization of contractile activity are important. Recent studies suggest that important etiologic factors are likely to include recruitment of inflammatory cells to the handled bowel, mast cell degranulation, and activation of inhibitory neural pathways. Also important may be the motilin-related peptide ghrelin, which has been identified as a strong promotility agent in postoperative ileus. Ileal resection and anastomosis results in the early loss, and later partial return, of electrical slow waves and phasic contractions in muscle near the resection area. This loss of electrical rhythmicity is associated with disruption to the network of interstitial cells of Cajal (ICCs), the "pacemaker" cells of the gut.

Clinical Presentation and Diagnosis

The diagnosis of ileus should be considered when signs of bowel obstruction develop in patients with known causes of ileus (see ❷ *Table 58-1*).

❏ Table 58-1

Causes of ileus

Abdominal surgery, especially laparotomy
Major non-abdominal operations
Intra-abdominal infection
Extra-abdominal infection, e.g. systemic sepsis, pneumonia
Peritonitis, e.g. anastomotic leak, bile peritonitis, perforated viscus
Retroperitoneal processes, e.g. pancreatitis, retroperitoneal hemorrhage, ureterolithiasis
Metabolic and electrolyte disturbances, e.g. hypokalemia, hyponatremia, hypomagnesemia, hypophosphatemia
Drugs, e.g. opiates, anticholinergic agents, autonomic blockers, psychotropic agents, general anesthesia
Renal failure
Spinal or orthopedic injury
Diabetic coma
Hypoparathyroidism

The clinical features of ileus are abdominal distension, obstipation, and either vomiting or a large quantity of nasogastric aspirate. Pain is usually absent, but, if present, it is non-colicky. In the postoperative setting, the pain is usually no more severe than would be expected with typical postoperative incisional pain and with the associated abdominal distension. Although the abdomen may be generally tender, it is usually not localized except at the wound. While the abdomen is typically silent on auscultation without the groans and rushes of a mechanical obstruction, tinkles are common, and a succussion splash may result from the large volume of fluid contained within the distended stomach or bowel. Plain erect and supine films of the abdomen show *both* small and large bowel dilatation with scattered air-fluid levels.

Distinguishing paralytic ileus from mechanical obstruction in the postoperative period may be difficult but is essential. Ileus should be managed nonoperatively, whereas mechanical obstruction may require operation, including urgent surgery in some patients. Careful examination and investigation of patients with continuing signs of obstruction after operation are important in order to detect complications responsible for an ongoing ileus (such as an anastomotic leak) and to detect mechanical obstruction. Mechanical obstruction in the early postoperative period may be caused by fibrinous adhesions or by an internal hernia. Patients with persistent clinical features of bowel obstruction must be evaluated to exclude a mechanical obstruction. Passing of flatus or stool, followed by a return to absolute constipation, may be a sign that mechanical obstruction has occurred. Similarly, severe or colicky pain, localized tenderness, radiographic findings of one or more loops of dilated small intestine with a deflated colon, or the absence of gas in the colon is each a sign of mechanical obstruction and not of ileus. Investigation by computed tomography (CT) with luminal contrast or a small bowel follow-through contrast examination may be needed to exclude mechanical obstruction.

Management

The management of ileus in the postoperative period is controversial. The standard treatment has been supportive, with nasogastric decompression, no oral intake, and intravenous fluids until the passage of flatus signifies resolution of ileus. In the absence of strong data showing that nasogastric aspiration reduces the duration of postoperative ileus, there is an increasing trend toward avoidance of nasogastric tubes postoperatively. Similarly, many surgeons now introduce a water or clear liquid diet before the passage of flatus. The management of patients with prolonged postoperative ileus or nonoperative ileus is not controversial. In these patients, the stomach should be decompressed with a nasogastric tube to relieve vomiting and reduce the risk of aspiration. Serum electrolytes should be checked regularly, medications that may induce ileus should be discontinued, and complications such as pneumonia or intra-abdominal sepsis should be excluded and treated aggressively when found. Ileus will resolve spontaneously if the underlying cause(s) is identified and treated successfully. Nutritional support, including TPN, is not usually needed but may be helpful in patients who have both a prolonged ileus and antecedent malnutrition.

There is no convincing evidence that any pharmacologic treatments are beneficial. Attempts to shorten the duration of ileus using prokinetic agents such as acetylcholine, cisapride, motilin, the motilin receptor agonist erythromycin, and other drugs have been disappointing. Cisapride has been reported to be beneficial occasionally, but the use of this drug is associated with a risk of life-threatening cardiac events and is no longer available. Recent studies suggest that effective pharmacologic therapies may be imminent. Promising agents include drugs that block peripheral opioid activity, leukocyte migration, or mast cell degranulation. As well as being a potent gastrokinetic agent, ghrelin also seems to accelerate postoperative small intestinal transit. The identification of the role of an inhibitory neural pathway involving sensory neurons of the lumbar dorsal horn of the spinal cord in the acute phase of postoperative ileus suggests other therapeutic targets. The initial suggestion that chewing gum might be a simple effective treatment for ileus has lost support after a randomized placebo-controlled trial found that chewing gum did not reduce the duration of postoperative ileus.

Intestinal Pseudo-Obstruction

Intestinal pseudo-obstruction is a term applied to a group of rare, incurable conditions that have in common permanent or recurrent hypomotility of either a part or the whole of the gastrointestinal tract. Although in sporadic cases the gut as a whole is abnormal, the most severely affected organ is usually the small intestine. Despite the name "pseudo-obstruction," patients with these conditions after previous abdominal surgery can also have true intestinal obstruction, sometimes requiring total parenteral nutrition (TPN). An increased awareness of these disorders by physicians has resulted in an increase in their recognized prevalence. With the exception of acute colonic pseudo-obstruction (Ogilvie's syndrome), intestinal pseudo-obstruction syndromes are chronic progressive diseases, with subacute and recurrent episodes in most patients that usually progress to chronic, non-resolving pseudo-obstruction.

Physiologically, both the fasted and fed motility patterns are abnormal. Migrating motor complexes (MMCs) are absent or abnormally infrequent during fasting, resulting in stasis, distension, and bacterial overgrowth. Similarly, postprandial motility is either markedly depressed, absent, or poorly coordinated.

The intestinal pseudo-obstruction syndromes are classified as either primary (idiopathic) or as secondary to a known disease. These syndromes are sometimes sub-classified according to whether they have primarily a neuropathic or a myopathic etiology. Familial visceral myopathies and, less frequently, familial neuropathies have both been described, with a clear autosomal inheritance in many myopathic cases. Sporadic idiopathic forms have been termed chronic idiopathic intestinal pseudo-obstruction (CIIP) for the neuropathic patients and nonfamilial hollow visceral myopathy for the myopathic patients. The natural history of CIIP was reported recently in a study of 59 patients followed for a mean 4.6 years. The diagnosis was made a median 8 years after symptom onset and only after most patients had undergone a therapeutic laparotomy for presumed mechanical obstruction. Long-term outcome was poor, and home TPN was needed for almost one third of patients.

A fibrotic myopathy is found in patients in whom the pseudo-obstruction is secondary to connective tissue diseases, with scleroderma being the most common of these disorders. Individuals with myotonic dystrophy, progressive muscular dystrophy, and other muscle diseases have gut involvement but may have few symptoms referable to the alimentary tract. The more common neuropathic causes are diabetes mellitus, hypothyroidism, amyloidosis, and medication use (antidepressants, antipsychotics, anti-Parkinsonian drugs, narcotics, and some antihypertensive and chemotherapeutic agents). Abuse of laxatives, especially those containing anthraquinone, can cause a chronic pseudo-obstruction that effects predominantly the colon. Pseudo-obstruction may also be secondary to a paraneoplastic syndrome.

Clinical Presentation and Diagnosis

Patients with intestinal pseudo-obstruction have a more gradual onset of progressively worsening intestinal obstruction or recurrent symptoms of subacute obstruction. Some patients come to attention only after complete cessation of bowel activity. Common symptoms include abdominal bloating, distension, and discomfort. Patients with colonic involvement may have severe constipation, although diarrhea may also occur as a result of bacterial overgrowth. Involvement of the foregut can cause nausea, vomiting, heartburn, dysphagia, and regurgitation. Children are seen frequently with failure to thrive and weight loss.

Except for those with a known causative disease such as scleroderma, the diagnosis of intestinal pseudo-obstruction is often not suspected or entertained early in its course. As a result, patients with these syndromes undergo exploratory laparotomy frequently to treat a presumed mechanical obstruction, and it is not uncommon for multiple laparotomies to have been performed without the correct diagnosis ever being reached. A careful history, including a detailed family and medication history, should prompt consideration of the diagnosis so that mechanical obstruction can be excluded by radiologic and endoscopic evaluation rather than by operation. The astute clinician may suspect intestinal pseudo-obstruction in the patient without a previous history of abdominal surgery, and thus no adhesions, in whom the clinical presentation is not characteristic of mechanical small bowel obstruction (i.e. slow onset, absence of crampy pain, history of less severe episodes). A slow-growing neoplasm causing a progressive mechanical obstruction may present with similar clinical features and needs to be excluded as does the diagnosis of sprue, which can mimic intestinal obstruction. Radiologic imaging will often show small bowel dilatation, although the diameter can be normal in early or mild cases. Foregut motility studies and gastrointestinal transit studies can be particularly helpful. If a full-thickness biopsy of the small bowel is needed to establish the diagnosis, a laparoscopic approach, in the appropriate setting, is preferred to reduce the risk of subsequent adhesions. The details of the tests used to establish the specific myopathic or neuropathic diagnosis in unclear cases are described in the review by Coulie and Camilleri.

Management

The treatment of known intestinal pseudo-obstruction syndromes is nonoperative. The goals of treatment are to provide nutritional support and improve intestinal motility. Attempts to provide nutritional needs with high caloric, high protein soft or liquid diets are indicated, along with vitamin and mineral supplementation. Antibiotic treatment is used for those with steatorrhea and diarrhea resulting from bacterial overgrowth. Promotility agents, including cisapride (if available), erythromycin, and metoclopramide, may be beneficial in some patients.

In those patients with the most severe myopathic disease and diffuse involvement of the gut, home TPN may be necessary. In patients with less severe disease, enteral feeding may be possible and is almost always preferable to parenteral feeding. Oral feeding can be supplemented or replaced by enteral feeding via a feeding jejunostomy. Surgical resection or bypass is much less effective for these syndromes than it is for isolated colonic hypomotility, but the rare patient with truly localized disease can benefit from resection. Studies of the regeneration of small intestinal motility in an animal model suggest that it may be preferable to construct an end-to-end rather than an end-to-side anastomosis.

Relief of distension and bloating by construction of a venting enterostomy has been reported to reduce the number of hospitalizations, nasogastric intubations, and laparotomies. This operation may even allow some patients to return to enteral feeding. In end-stage disease, small bowel transplantation may be lifesaving.

Selected Readings

Coulie B, Camilleri M (1999) Intestinal pseudo-obstruction. Annu Rev Med 50:37–55

de Jonge WJ, van den Wijngaard RM, The FO, et al. (2003) Postoperative ileus is maintained by intestinal immune infiltrates that activate inhibitory neural pathways in mice. Gastroenterology 125:1137–1147

Delaney CP, Weese JL, Hyman NH, et al. (2005) Phase III trial of alvimopan, a novel, peripherally acting, mu opioid antagonist, for postoperative ileus after major abdominal surgery. Dis Colon Rectum 48:1114–1125

Jones MP, Wessinger S (2006) Small intestinal motility. Curr Opin Gastroenterol 22:111–116

Matros E, Rocha F, Zinner M, et al. (2006) Does gum chewing ameliorate postoperative ileus? Results of a prospective, randomized, placebo-controlled trial. J Am Coll Surg 202:773–778

Murr MM, Sarr MG, Camilleri M (1995) The surgeon's role in the treatment of chronic intestinal pseudoobstruction. Am J Gastroenterol 90:2147–2151

Stanghellini V, Cogliandro RF, De Giorgio R, et al. (2005) Natural history of chronic idiopathic pseudo-obstruction in adults: a single center study. Clin Gastroenterol Hepatol 3:449–458

Trudel L, Tomasetto C, Rio MC, et al. (2002) Ghrelin/motilin-related peptide is a potent prokinetic to reverse gastric postoperative ileus in the rat. Am J Physiol Gastrointest Liver Physiol 282:G948–G952

59 Appendicitis

Matthew R. Dixon · Michael J. Stamos

Pearls and Pitfalls

- Although symptoms from appendicitis develop most commonly in the right lower quadrant, patients with long appendices or mobile cecums can develop pain throughout the abdomen.
- When treating suspected appendicitis in women, preoperative computed tomography or laparoscopic approach may be of great value given the broader possible differential diagnosis.
- Consider three diagnostic elements separately: history, physical examination, and laboratory/radiologic investigations. If two of the three support the diagnosis of appendicitis, the patient warrants operative evaluation.
- Computed tomography clearly demonstrating intraluminal contrast filling of the entire appendix *excludes* the diagnosis of appendicitis.
- Patients with a prolonged history of symptoms or a palpable mass suggestive of contained perforation may be best treated with non-operative management rather then urgent operation.
- The diagnosis of appendicitis can be challenging to establish in pregnant and immunocompromised patients; optimally, operative management should not be delayed in these patient groups.
- Care must be taken to identify with certainty the appendiceal-cecal junction to ensure complete appendectomy. Cecal mobilization may be required.
- Data establishing the role of interval appendectomy following successful nonoperative management of perforated appendicitis is evolving. Interval appendectomy may not be necessary for all patients.

Early Uncomplicated Appendicitis

Presentation

The typical patient with early appendicitis will present with vague periumbilical pain and anorexia during the first 24 h of symptoms. The pathophysiology of appendicitis is due to intraluminal appendiceal obstruction, most commonly from an appendiceal fecolith. Early in the course of the disease, the inflammation is limited to the visceral peritoneum, which does not localize the pain to the source in the right lower quadrant and results, instead, in vague discomfort. Patients may also give a history of nausea or vomiting, but patients with appendicitis usually describe the pain as preceding the nausea and vomiting. When nausea and vomiting occur first, gastroenteritis should be suspected. As the depth of inflammation progresses and begins to involve the parietal peritoneum, patients usually notice that the pain localizes to the right lower quadrant.

Diagnosis

When evaluating patients with appendicitis, it may be useful to consider three elements separately: history, physical examination, and laboratory/radiologic investigations. Many clinicians feel that if a patient has two of the three elements supporting the diagnosis of appendicitis, the patient warrants operative intervention. In addition to the classic history described above, patients with early appendicitis usually have a low-grade fever and mild tachycardia. Abdominal examination will usually demonstrate periumbilical or right lower quadrant tenderness with possible localized peritoneal signs. Pain may be most severe at the McBurney's point, a position two-thirds of the way from the umbilicus to the anterior superior iliac spine. In women, pelvic examination should be performed to exclude pronounced cervical tenderness and to evaluate for possible adnexal pathology.

Patients may have one of the following physical examination findings known to be associated with appendicitis:

- **Rovsing sign** – pain felt in the right lower quadrant on palpation of the left lower quadrant
- **Psoas sign** – pain at the waist with extension of the right hip and leg related to an inflamed pelvic appendix
- **Obturator sign** – pain with flexion and medial rotation of the right leg – related to an inflamed appendix in a pelvic location

Laboratory examination will generally show an increased white cell count with a "left shift". Urinalysis should be performed, although it should be remembered that some red cells in the urine may be found commonly with appendicitis secondary to ureteral inflammation and irritation. Urine B-HCG screen for pregnancy should be performed for all women. The overall differential diagnosis includes urinary tract infection and pyelonephritis, cecal diverticulitis, mesenteric adenitis in children, Crohn's disease involving the distal ileum, and gynecologic causes in women.

Additional work-up and treatment by gender: In several studies, the negative appendectomy rate for presumed appendicitis is substantially lower in men than in women due to the prevalence of gynecologic conditions mimicking appendicitis. Surgeons have accepted historically an overall negative exploration rate of 10% due to diagnostic uncertainty related to appendicitis. With the advent of computed tomography (CT), the ability to establish the diagnosis correctly has improved greatly, and the negative appendectomy rate has been decreased safely. Some authors have suggested that, with appropriate use of CT, the rate may be lowered to less than 2% (❷ *Figs. 59-1–59-3*). In the past, rectal contrast has been employed to facilitate intraluminal filling of the appendix; however, with the evolution of more sophisticated CT scanners, rectal contrast may not always be necessary. Moreover, the newest CT scanners may not require any contrast at all. While the authors do not advocate routine CT in all patients, selective liberal use of the CT is appropriate. Additional preoperative work-up suggestions will be discussed separately for men and women.

Male Patients

The differential diagnosis of right lower quadrant pain in otherwise healthy young men is quite limited. As long as the urinalysis does not suggest pyelonephritis, the literature suggests this is one patient

◘ Figure 59-1
Retrocecal appendicitis: non contrast-filled thickened appendix (arrow) adjacent to iliacus muscle

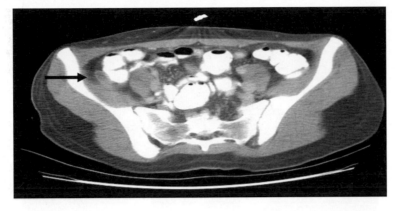

◘ Figure 59-2
"Arrowhead sign": note contrast "pointing" to appendiceal orifice, local cecal wall thickening, and thickened appendix medially (arrow)

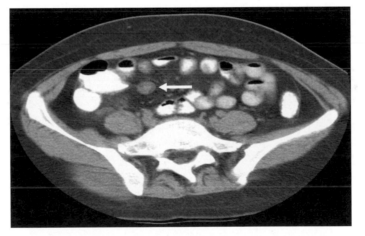

group that will not be helped generally by routine CT or other imaging studies when the clinical presentation is consistent with acute appendicitis. These patients may be taken to the operating room without additional work-up. A laparoscopic or open approach may be utilized depending on surgeon preference. For older male patients, for whom the differential diagnosis includes atypical diverticulitis and cancer, CT may be useful in avoiding an unnecessary emergency operation.

Female Patients

Women, particularly those of child-bearing age, presenting with symptoms consistent with appendicitis may actually have symptoms due to a gynecologic etiology such as ovarian torsion, ectopic pregnancy, ruptured luteal corpus cyst, or pelvic inflammatory disease. CT may be useful to confirm

◻ Figure 59-3
"Arrowhead sign": note contrast "pointing" to appendiceal orifice with non opacified thickened appendix extending retrocecally (arrow)

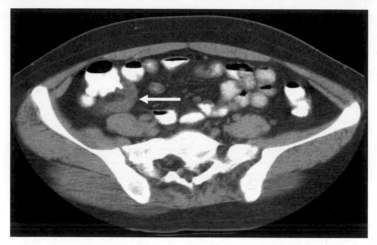

◻ Figure 59-4
Advanced perforated appendicitis with extraluminal gas and phlegmon

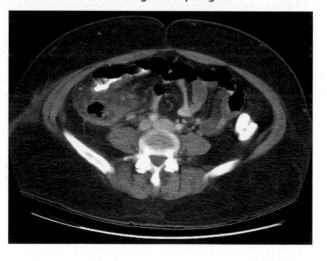

the diagnosis of appendicitis prior to operative intervention (❯ *Fig. 59-4*). Alternatively, a laparoscopic approach may be used, allowing for simultaneous evaluation of the uterus, tubes, and ovaries. In addition to bimanual pelvic examination, pelvic ultrasonography should be considered if the history suggests gynecologic cause, particularly if pelvic inflammatory disease is suspected.

Perforated Appendicitis

Several studies have demonstrated that perforated appendicitis may be suggested by clinical features such as long duration of symptoms (more than 48 h) and higher white cell counts and temperatures.

In the absence of diffuse peritonitis requiring urgent operative management, this patient group may be better investigated with CT to evaluate the degree of perforation and to guide a treatment strategy. CT findings of extraluminal gas, abscess, phlegmon, and wall thickening have been associated with perforation. A rationale underlying the nonoperative management of this group is that patients with long-standing perforation have contained the inflammation and may be treated safely with parenteral antibiotics. Immediate operation for a perforation with significant phlegmon and inflammation may require more extensive resection such as ileocectomy, thereby resulting in higher morbidity. Instead, patients with these findings can be treated with bowel rest, broad-spectrum parenteral antibiotics, and clinical monitoring without immediate operation during the peak of inflammatory response.

When CT demonstrates perforation with abscess, patients may be best treated initially with parenteral antibiotics (❯ Fig. 59-4). It is not necessary to drain all patients who present with an abscess because many periappendiceal abscesses will respond to antibiotic therapy alone, especially those that are multiloculated and/or <5–6 cm in size. Patients failing to improve after 48–72 h may then warrant percutaneous drainage under CT guidance instead of urgent operation.

The advantage gained by nonoperative management for those with the earliest signs of perforation on CT, such as specks of extraluminal gas without evidence of phlegmon, is likely to be more limited and unproven. Patients with an early perforation may be treated by nonoperative management or appendectomy. In contrast, patients with a large phlegmon or palpable mass should be offered conservative treatment initially.

Successful non-operative management of perforated appendicitis is assessed generally by three criteria: improvement in abdominal examination findings, resolution of elevated white cell count as well as body temperature, and ability to tolerate a diet. After successful management of perforated appendicitis, some authors have advocated interval appendectomy, which may be performed safely using either an open or laparoscopic approach with minimal morbidity. The data regarding the benefit obtained from routine interval appendectomy are mixed, because only a minority of patients will ever experience a recurrence. Some retrospective studies, including work performed by the authors, have suggested that recurrent appendicitis develops in a minority of patients and is likely to be clinically less severe when compared with the initial presentation. It is important to remember that underlying colonic malignancy is a possible cause of symptoms, and colonoscopy should be performed in older patients, as well as those with any clinical features suggestive of malignancy, including weight loss, change in bowel habits, and anemia.

Appendicitis in the Pregnant Patient

Appendicitis is not an uncommon event during pregnancy and occurs in approximately 1 in 1,500 pregnancies, making it the most common surgical condition encountered during pregnancy. Establishing the diagnosis during pregnancy can be more difficult and challenging for several reasons. First, the position of the appendix relative to the abdominal wall changes as the uterus expands. Therefore, the pain described during appendicitis in pregnancy assumes a position higher in the right upper quadrant, which may confuse the diagnosis. Despite the alleged changes in position, recent studies have indicated that, in the majority of patients with appendicitis at any stage of pregnancy, pain occurs within a few centimeters of McBurney's point. Second, physicians are often less likely to offer radiologic studies, such as CT, to pregnant patients. Finally, abdominal discomfort and alterations in appetite may be a normal feature of late pregnancy, hence, potentially delaying the diagnosis.

The principle which must be remembered when treating pregnant patients with possible appendicitis is to avoid perforation, if at all possible. Both maternal and fetal mortality, as well as the potential for preterm labor, increase substantially with perforated appendicitis.

A collaborative approach with an obstetrician may be useful in decision-making. Graded compression ultrasonography has been considered the first line imaging study. Patients in the second to third trimester may be evaluated safely with CT if the diagnosis is in question after ultrasonographic evaluation. A more difficult situation occurs when patients present in early pregnancy, prior to organogenesis, with possible appendicitis. CT is contraindicated in this group, and operative intervention should be offered liberally. Some have advocated accepting a higher rate of negative appendectomies in pregnant patients given the much higher rate of fetal loss in perforated appendicitis. Magnetic resonance imaging (MRI) has been mentioned in several recent studies as an alternative imaging modality after inconclusive ultrasonography, and may become used more widely for this group in the future when it is readily available.

Several retrospective studies with small numbers of patients have suggested that laparoscopy may be safely performed in pregnancy. In early pregnancy, a laparoscopic approach may be utilized, but this approach may become more difficult in patients late in pregnancy. In the latter, an open approach should be used.

Appendicitis in the Immunocompromised Patient

Diagnosing appendicitis in the immunocompromised patient is much more difficult, because the physical symptoms and clinical signs are usually muted and are more subtle when identified. Immunocompromised patients with right lower quadrant pain also have a much broader differential diagnosis, including viral and fungal colitides, as well as typhlitis in patients receiving chemotherapy. CT may be useful in this patient group to establish a more definitive diagnosis before embarking on an operation. Nonoperative therapy for perforated appendicitis is more dangerous in this population and should probably be reserved for those hemodynamically stable patients with palpable mass.

Operative Approach

Open Versus Laparoscopic Approach

Appendectomy has been performed traditionally with a right lower quadrant, muscle-splitting incision termed the McBurney incision. The muscles are split rather than divided to preserve the integrity of the abdominal wall after closure. A very small incision may be utilized, and the appendix may be found with palpation. On identification, a Babcock clamp is placed on the appendix, taking care to avoid iatrogenic perforation, and the appendix is then delivered through the incision. Cecal mobilization may be required, particularly when the appendix is located in a retrocecal position. Once the appendix is delivered through the incision, the mesoappendix and appendiceal base is divided and ligated between clamps. The appendiceal stump is usually inverted with a purse-string suture at the base. The abdominal wall may be closed in layers with absorbable suture; this closure includes the peritoneum, transversus abdominus, and internal oblique muscles, followed by the external oblique aponeurosis. A midline incision may also be chosen, allowing for extension in cases of widespread inflammation or more extensive surgery.

Laparoscopic approaches have become employed much more commonly. Laparoscopic appendectomy can be performed with three trocar sites after bladder and stomach decompression are achieved with urinary and nasogastric tube placement. One trocar is placed at the umbilicus, a second trocar at the suprapubic position, and a third trocar at the left lower quadrant. One of the trocars should be at least 10–12 mm to accommodate a laparoscopic stapling device (typically placed at the left lower quadrant) and to allow for specimen retrieval. If a 5 mm camera is available, the remaining trocars can be 5 mm. This approach allows the abdominal contents to be evaluated thoroughly before proceeding to appendectomy and provides an outstanding cosmetic result. The patient should be placed in Trendelenberg's position with right-side elevation to optimize appendiceal exposure. Colonic tenia or the distal ileum may be traced distally if the location of the appendix is unclear. Once the appendix is found, it may be grasped and laparoscopic scissors with cautery are then used to allow its full mobilization. Once the cecal-appendiceal junction is found clearly, a window may be created at the base with a laparoscopic dissecting instrument. The window should be large enough to accommodate a laparoscopic stapling device (endoscopic linear cutter). With the appendix retracted anteriorly and superiorly, two consecutive firings of the endoscopic linear cutter – one on the mesoappendix and another at the appendiceal base – complete the operation. A specimen retrieval bag is used to remove the specimen, and the area should be irrigated and checked for hemostasis. The 10–12 mm site can be closed with a laparoscopic fascial closer or closed in the standard fashion; the 5 mm sites require skin closure only.

Perforated Appendicitis

Appendectomy in the setting of perforation may be accomplished by either an open or laparoscopic approach with similar morbidity. Both approaches allow irrigation to be performed successfully and have been associated with similar postoperative complication rates. When operating acutely for perforated appendicitis in the patient with diffuse peritonitis or after failing nonoperative management, extensive inflammation extending to the cecum may be encountered. In these situations, partial or complete ileocectomy may be required. This procedure can be performed expeditiously with a stapling device. The right lower quadrant and pelvis should be irrigated thoroughly. Drains have been used by many surgeons, particularly when an abscess cavity is encountered. The data supporting the use of drains after appendectomy are limited. A recent meta-analysis concluded that drains are indeed harmful and should be omitted. Drain placement should be limited to cases with a large amount of residual inflammatory material after appendectomy and should not be used routinely. Skin incisions associated with conventional laparotomy are usually left open in the setting of perforation, or sutures may be placed to allow delayed primary closure. Skin incisions related to laparoscopic trocar sites may be closed primarily, even in cases of perforated appendicitis.

Selected Readings

Dixon MR, Haukoos JS, Park IU, et al. (2003) An assessment of the severity of recurrent appendicitis. Am J Surg 6:718–22

Jones K, Pena AA, Dunn EL, et al. (2004) Are negative appendectomies still acceptable? Am J Surg 188:748–754

McGory ML, Zingmond DS, Nanayakkara D, et al. (2005) Negative appendectomy rate: influence of CT scans. Am Surg 10:803–808

Oliak D, Sinow R, French S, et al. (1999) Computed tomography scanning for the diagnosis of perforated appendicitis. Am Surg 10:959–964

Oliak D, Yamini D, Udani VM, et al. (2000) Can perforated appendicitis be diagnosed preoperatively based on admission factors? J Gastrointest Surg 5:470–474

Pedrosa I, Levine D, Eyvazzadeh AD, et al. (2006) MR imaging evaluation of acute appendicitis in pregnancy. Radiology 3:891–899

Petrosky H, Demartines N, Rousson V, Clavien PA (2004) Evidence-based value of prophylactic drainage in gastrointestinal surgery. Ann Surg 240:1074–1085

60 Short Bowel Syndrome

Jon S. Thompson

Pearls and Pitfalls

- Short bowel syndrome (SBS) occurs after resection of sufficient small bowel to cause nutritional compromise (remnant <120 cm).
- The best treatment is prevention by minimizing the length of resection and preserving all viable small bowel.
- Postoperative management after extensive small bowel resection includes inhibition of hyperacidity, maintenance of fluid and electrolytes, and early enteral nutrition.
- Complication of SBS includes metabolic acidosis, cholelithiasis, nephrolithiasis, bacterial overgrowth, and parenteral nutrition-induced hepatic failure.
- Surgical treatment of SBS may involve restoring continuity and procedures for relieving obstruction or tapering and lengthening the intestine.
- Severe SBS, especially with associated hepatic failure, may best be treated with orthotopic small bowel transplantation.
- Avoid any unnecessary resections; reconstruct rather than resect shortened remnants.
- Avoid hasty decisions to resect reversibly ischemic bowel.
- Minimize extensive resection for inflammatory disease.
- Be certain to document not only the intestine that has been removed, but also the length and site of intestine that remains.
- Anticipating complications is important; consider prophylactic cholecystectomy, avoid blind loops, and prevent irreversible hepatic disease.

Pathophysiology

Short bowel syndrome (SBS) is a clinical condition resulting from extensive intestinal resection and characterized by malabsorption and malnutrition. In adult patients, SBS occurs generally when less than 120 cm of functional intestine remains. Several factors determine the severity and the spectrum of clinical features of the SBS, including the extent and site of the resection, presence of any underlying intestinal disease, the presence or absence of the ileocecal valve, the functional status of the remaining digestive organs, and potential for adaptation of the intestinal remnant. A number of pathophysiologic changes occur in SBS that may cause other specific metabolic problems of importance to the surgeon.

Clinical Presentation

A variety of conditions can lead to SBS. Postoperative complications have emerged as an increasing cause. Mesenteric vascular disease and the treatment of cancer, including radiation therapy, are other intestinal conditions that lead frequently to SBS (❷ *Table 60-1*). The initial clinical presentation of these patients depends heavily on the underlying diagnosis.

SBS results from a single massive small intestinal resection in approximately three fourths of patients. Patients undergoing massive resection are more likely to be elderly, present emergently, have mesenteric vascular disease, and have a worse nutritional and overall prognosis. One fourth of patients with SBS have multiple, lesser sequential resections. These patients usually have underlying intestinal disease which influences nutritional outcome.

Preventing the SBS should be the surgeon's first priority. The surgeon should be aware of the need for timely intervention in patients with mesenteric ischemia, early operation for intestinal obstruction to avoid resection, and minimizing resection in patients with underlying chronic, persistent conditions, such as Crohn's disease, that might eventually lead to SBS. Avoiding operation in patients with extensive adhesions or suspected frozen abdomen is also prudent.

Treatment

The appropriate management of patients with SBS, beginning even in the preoperative period, should minimize the predictable complications that might occur and improve prospects for future survival.

Preoperative management: Discussion with the patient and family about the potential consequences of the SBS, including the need for prolonged parenteral nutrition support, should be undertaken before operative decision making whenever possible. There are some patients, e.g., the elderly patient with extensive comorbidity or advanced malignancy, in whom it might be appropriate to consider not resecting diseased bowel that would result in SBS. Obviously, this can be a very difficult decision. For patients who have had previous resections and might predictably require further resection leading to the SBS, there should be greater discussion and consideration of management issues.

The surgeon should try to gain as much information as possible about preexisting anatomy and intestinal disease when considering further operative procedures in patients who have had previous intestinal resection. Contrast-enhanced studies of the intestinal tract are helpful in estimating the residual intestinal length and in assessing the presence of dilation, potential points of obstruction and mucosal disease. Preoperative ultrasonography of the gallbladder should be obtained when appropriate, because patients who have had previous resection are at increased risk for cholelithiasis.

▣ Table 60-1

Underlying disease in adult patients with short bowel syndrome

Postoperative resection	52	25%
Cancer/radiation	51	24%
Mesenteric vascular disease	46	22%
Crohn's disease	34	16%
Other benign conditions	27	13%
Total	210	

Nutritional status should be assessed so that appropriate nutritional support can be provided during the perioperative period.

In patients with acute intestinal conditions likely to require massive resection, management consists of stabilizing the patient hemodynamically and correcting fluid and electrolyte deficits. Preoperative antibiotics should cover colonic bacterial flora. Nasogastric decompression is usually appropriate. If an ostomy is anticipated and time permits, consultation with a stomal therapist and marking the optimal site for the ostomy should be done preoperatively. These stomas often become difficult-to-manage, high-output stomas, and proper construction and positioning are important. Bowel preparation should always be considered when a colon remnant is present, if this is feasible.

Intraoperative management: An important intraoperative strategy is to avoid extensive resection when it is not clearly necessary. Decisions about resection margins and management of intestinal lesions should not be carried out until the entire situation has been assessed fully. It may be appropriate to salvage even a few inches of small intestine in the setting of a severely shortened remnant, despite the potential morbidity of additional anastomoses. Strategies such as stricturoplasty, intestinal tapering, and serosal patching may be helpful in managing specific lesions that would otherwise require resection (❯ *Fig. 60-1*).

Management of the intestinal disease is an important intraoperative issue. When dealing with intestinal ischemia, any obstruction within or constriction of the mesentery should be relieved, and the bowel should be covered with warm, moist packs and observed for signs of viability. Palpation of pulses and the character of Doppler ultrasonic signals should be used to assess perfusion of the gut wall. Revascularization should be performed if necessary to preserve reversible ischemic bowel. Viability is assessed by improved color, visible mesenteric pulsations, and peristalsis. Intravenous injection of a fluorescent probe with visualization of fluorescent staining and with Wood's lamp to assess diffuse changes and the use of a Doppler ultrasonic flow probe to evaluate blood flow at the margins of

◼ **Figure 60-1**
Operative procedures for improvement of intestinal function in short bowel syndrome (Reprinted from Thompson et al., 1995. With permission)

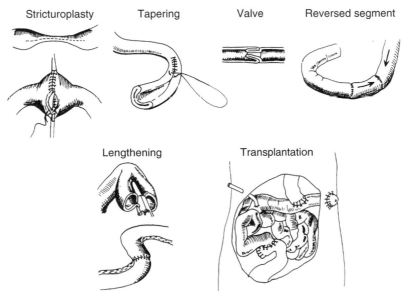

Stricturoplasty   Tapering   Valve   Reversed segment

Lengthening   Transplantation

the bowel continue to be the most useful modalities. Bowel which is obviously nonviable requires resection; however, when viability is uncertain and recovery of viability is a possibility, a second-look procedure should be considered in retaining questionable bowel.

Intestinal obstruction should be excluded intraoperatively if this possibility has not been adequately assessed preoperatively. This procedure may require passing a balloon-tipped catheter (e.g., Baker's tube or Foley catheter) through the intestinal tract to identify possible stenoses. In patients who already have a short bowel, there may be opportunities to reconstruct the bowel to eliminate blind loops, which can lead to stasis and bacterial overgrowth.

Formation of ostomies may be advisable when the patient is unstable, intestinal viability is questionable, and the patient will be left with a very shortened intestinal remnant, for example less than 90 cm. Duodenal or high jejunal ostomies create difficult management problems. Occasionally, tube decompression is required rather than a stoma. In general, restoring intestinal continuity should be considered strongly whenever distal viable bowel is present.

Because patients with SBS are at increased risk for development of cholelithiasis and acute biliary complications, a prophylactic cholecystectomy should be considered. This decision needs careful evaluation in the patient undergoing a massive resection in an emergent situation. Cholecystectomy would be performed more reasonably in patients who are undergoing elective procedures or who require subsequent reoperation.

Postoperative management: In the early postoperative period, the management of SBS involves primarily the management of the critically ill surgical patient who has undergone an extensive resection. The key issues are control of sepsis, maintenance of fluid and electrolyte balance, and initiation of nutritional support. As the patient recovers, important priorities become maintaining adequate nutritional status, maximizing the absorptive capacity of the remaining intestine, and anticipating and preventing the development of complications related to the SBS and its management.

Total parenteral nutrition (TPN) is usually required for nutritional support during the early postoperative period. Adjustments are necessary for fluid and electrolyte losses, which may be considerable. Most patients require approximately 35 kcal/kg/day and 1–1.5 g protein/kg/day with the appropriate electrolytes, minerals, trace elements, and vitamins. Beginning enteral nutritional support as early as possible once the ileus has resolved is very important, after which the proportion of enteral nutrients should be increased gradually over time. Luminal nutrition maintains intestinal function, maximizes intestinal adaptation, and minimizes complications related to TPN. In general, patients who have more than 180 cm of small intestine remaining will not require TPN or parenteral supplementation for an extensive period. The patients with approximately 90 cm of small intestine, and particularly those who have retained part or all of their colon, especially with an intact ileocecal valve, will require parenteral nutrition for less than 1 year; however, those who have less than 60 cm of small intestine are likely to require permanent TPN.

The transition from parenteral to enteral support requires careful monitoring. The goals are to maintain a stable body weight and prevent large fluctuations in fluid status. Careful monitoring should correct any metabolic abnormalities or nutrient deficiencies. Parenteral nutrition should be decreased gradually as enteral intake increases. A marked increase in gastrointestinal fluid losses in response to enteral feeding usually signifies that increasing the feeding further will not be tolerated. As parenteral requirements diminish, this therapy can be used intermittently until weaning is achieved.

The optimal diet for a patient with the SBS is determined by the length and location of the intestinal remnant, the underlying intestinal disease, and the status of remaining digestive organs. When the remnant is less than 90 cm, a program of more continuous enteral feedings may be necessary to achieve satisfactory nutrient intake. Initially, a high-carbohydrate, high-protein diet is appropriate to maximize absorption. Provision of simple nutrients will keep maldigestion from being a limiting factor during absorption. Fat requires more complex absorptive mechanisms, and stool fat will increase markedly when remnants are less than 60 cm. The initial diet should be hypo-osmolar to minimize gastrointestinal fluid losses, but it may eventually be increased later. Oral rehydration solution will improve absorption in patients with proximal jejunal remnants who are net secretors. If the colon is in continuity, less fat will be tolerated and dietary oxalate will need to be restricted, because the presence of fat malabsorption will lead to an increase in colonic absorption of oxalate with the possibility of renal complications (oxalate stones, oxalate nephropathy). The presence of a stoma may diminish markedly the ability to take in liquids orally due to diarrhea and perianal complications.

Luminal nutrients are important for maximizing the adaptive response of the intestine to resection. The intestinal remnant will increase its surface area and absorptive capacity in the 6–12 months after resection (❷ *Fig. 60-2*). Provision of fat and dietary fiber may be particularly important in this process. The role of other specific nutrients is currently under investigation. Glutamine is a conditionally essential amino acid that is trophic to the gut. While it is often employed in clinical protocols, its overall importance when given orally still remains unclear.

Growth factors may also stimulate the adaptive response and improve fluid absorption. These agents may accelerate adaptation or produce hyper adaptation (❷ *Fig. 60-2*). A growth hormone analog has been approved for this purpose. Glucagon-like peptide 2 (GLP-2) is being investigated in clinical trials.

Medical treatment should be directed at minimizing gastrointestinal secretion and controlling diarrhea. Dietary fiber is useful in many patients. Opiates such as codeine, Lomotil (diphenoxylate HCl and atropine sulfate), and loperamide may improve absorption via their antisecretory and antimotility effects. The somatostatin analogue, octreotide, should improve diarrhea, not only by reducing salt and water excretion but also by prolonging small bowel transit time and reducing gastric hypersecretion; however, because of potential side effects and cost, octreotide probably should not be continued indefinitely but rather should be maintained over the time of adaptation (6–12 months). H_2 receptor antagonists and proton pump inhibitors are useful to control the transient gastric hypersecretion and reduce fluid loss, primarily in the first few months after operation. Cholestyramine

◻ Figure 60-2

Schematic presentation of intestinal adaptation. SA: spontaneous adaptation; AA: accelerated adaptation, HA: hyperadaptation; AHA: accelerated hyperadaptation (Reprinted from Jeppesen, 2003. With permission)

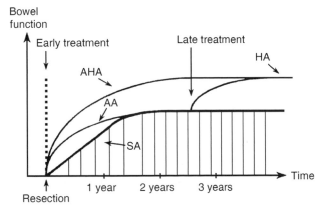

may be marginally beneficial for binding bile salts and ameliorating the bile salt-induced colonic diarrhea when the colon is in continuity. This approach is most effective when the patient has had an ileal resection of less than 100 cm.

Patients who have had a stoma formed at the time of their resection should be given consideration at a future time for establishing intestinal continuity. There are both advantages and disadvantages to restoring intestinal continuity. By restoring continuity, absorptive capacity may be increased and transit time prolonged. Energy from short-chain fatty acids reaching the colon may increase caloric intake. Having the colon in continuity is equivalent to having another 30 cm of intestine from a functional perspective. There are also psychologic advantages to eliminating the stoma. Furthermore, clinical evidence suggests that infective complications are reduced when the stoma is eliminated. In contrast, however, colonic bile acids may induce diarrhea with associated perianal complications and dietary restrictions. One must weigh the potential of a functional "perianal ileostomy" with intestinal restoration versus a permanent stoma. Patients with colon in continuity are at increased risk for nephrolithiasis. On balance, though, restoration of continuity is generally advisable when more than 90 cm of small intestine is present.

Approximately one half of patients who have SBS will eventually require repeat future intra abdominal operation, most commonly for intestinal complications. In these patients, careful planning should be carried out to avoid further resection. As mentioned previously, utilization of intestinal tapering to improve the function of dilated segments, employing stricturoplasty for strictures, and performing serosal patching for strictures and chronic perforations will help preserve the intestinal remnant. Other intestinal segments that might be recruited into continuity should be identified as well.

Surgical treatment for SBS has several specific goals. One objective is to improve the function of existing intestine by using the strategies mentioned previously. Obstruction should be sought and remedied, ideally by a nonresectional approach. Dilated dysfunctional segments, which may aggravate malabsorption and lead to bacterial overgrowth, should be eliminated (e.g., by tapering enteroplasty). Of note, intestine-lengthening procedures have been utilized in selected patients that permit using dilated segments of bowel to lengthen the intestinal remnant. Both transverse (STEP procedure) and longitudinal (Bianchi procedure) techniques of enteroplasty are often effective and appear to have durable long-term improvement.

Another goal of operative therapy has been to slow intestinal transit and thus improve absorption. This approach has been done with the use of a variety of techniques, including artificial valves and sphincters, reversing intestinal segments, interposing colonic segments in the small intestine, and other innovative approaches. The outcome of these procedures is less predictable, and they should be applied cautiously in carefully selected patients.

The ultimate operative treatment of SBS would be to lengthen the intestinal remnant. With recent improvements in immunosuppression, the outcome of intestinal transplantation is improving. Intestinal transplantation has now become an acceptable clinical approach to this problem in selected patients. Isolated intestinal transplantation is also indicated in patients with loss of vascular access and recurrent sepsis. Combined liver and intestinal transplantation is indicated in patients with irreversible liver failure and SBS.

The appropriate operation for the patient with SBS is determined by several factors, one of the most important of which is the type of nutritional support required. Patients who are able to sustain themselves with enteral nutrition alone should undergo operation only if they demonstrate worsening

■ Figure 60-3

Operative management of the short bowel syndrome (Reprinted from Thompson et al., 1995. With permission)

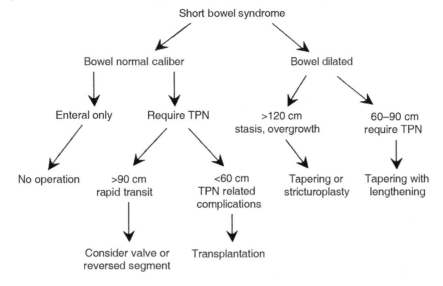

malabsorption, are at risk for requiring parenteral nutrition, or have overwhelming symptoms related to malabsorption. Patients who require parenteral nutrition but can tolerate a significant amount of enteral feeding may be candidates for operative therapy with the goal being to discontinue parenteral nutrition. Patients who develop significant complications while receiving parenteral nutrition should clearly be considered for operative therapy. Many of these patients, especially when children, will require either combined liver-small bowel transplantation or isolated small bowel transplantation. While liver disease is an obvious indication for transplantation, difficult vascular access and recurrent line sepsis are reasons for considering such therapy. Obviously, other patient-related factors, such as age and underlying disease, will also need to be considered carefully. Thus, the choice of operation for patients can best be tailored in relation to the length of the intestinal remnant, the degree of intestinal function, and the caliber of the intestinal remnant (❷ *Fig. 60-3*).

Complications

Metabolic complications of metabolic alkalosis and metabolic acidosis (including d-lactic acidosis) are common in patients with SBS related to their tremendous fluid and electrolyte fluxes and the need for specialized nutritional support. Hypocalcemia is commonly related to both impaired absorption and binding by intraluminal fat. Both hyperglycemia and hypoglycemia occur in patients requiring parenteral nutrition. Patients with SBS need to be monitored closely and regularly by a trained nutritionist to detect deficiencies of iron, other minerals, vitamins, and micronutrients.

Symptomatic cholelithiasis occurs in about one third of patients with SBS related to malabsorption of bile acids with the formation lithogenic bile, altered bilirubin metabolism, and biliary stasis. Thus, both pigment and cholesterol stones are found frequently. The natural history of cholelithiasis in this group of patients indicates that they tend to develop more biliary complications and require more complicated operative treatment. Cholelithiasis should always be suspected in patients with abdominal pain and abnormal liver function tests and evaluated with ultrasonography. In patients dependent on parenteral nutrition, intermittent injections of cholecystokinin may prevent stasis and reduce formation of sludge and gallstones. Early enteral nutrition should help reduce the risk of cholelithiasis. The risk of cholelithiasis increases when there is less than 120 cm and small intestine, when parenteral nutrition is required, and when the terminal ileum has been resected. Prophylactic cholecystectomy should be considered in these patients, either at the time of initial resection or at any subsequent laparotomy.

Patients with SBS develop a poorly understood form of gastric hypersecretion in the early postoperative period. This gastric hypersecretion is usually a transient phenomenon and should be treated with medical therapy directed at the increased acid secretion. The need for operative treatment is infrequent, but if required, a procedure such as a highly selective vagotomy may be desirable to avoid gastric resection.

Nephrolithiasis occurs in one third of patient with SBS, related in great part to reduced intraluminal free calcium and the resultant increased absorption of oxalate from the intestine. Because oxalate is absorbed from the colon, this complication occurs primarily in patients with a colon remnant in continuity. Management involves minimizing oxalate in the diet, minimizing intraluminal fat, providing oral calcium supplementation, and maintaining a high urinary volume.

Bacterial overgrowth may be a problem, but it is difficult to diagnose and requires a high degree of suspicion. Bacterial overgrowth decreases the luminal concentration of conjugated bile acids, impairs fat absorption, leads to secretory diarrhea from malabsorbed fatty acids, increases formation of short-chain fatty acids, and results in an increased osmotic load and gas production. It also impairs vitamin B_{12} absorption. The diarrhea of bacterial overgrowth is primarily a motor abnormality, which can be treated with intermittent antibiotic therapy; however, one should always consider a mechanical cause that may be relieved by operation.

Patient requiring long-term TPN or parenteral supplementation are at risk for catheter-related sepsis and catheter thrombosis, which can limit the clinician's ability to maintain nutritional support in the long term, when available access sites are exhausted. TPN-induced liver disease occurs in approximately 15% of adult patients on chronic TPN. This is a multifactorial problems related to the proportion of enteral calories, overfeeding, and recurrent sepsis. This form of liver disease can be minimized by increasing enteral calories, avoiding overfeeding, using mixed fuels (<30% fat), and eliminating nutrient deficiencies. Administration of ursodeoxycholic acid may also be beneficial. TPN-related liver disease in children with SBS is much more common than in adults and remains poorly understood. Treatment is not very effective and often requires strong consideration of liver-small bowel transplantation.

Outcomes

Permanent intestinal failure is likely in patients with small intestinal remnants less than 90 cm, or less than 30 cm with an intact colon. Permanent intestinal failure should lead to consideration of surgical treatment if severe symptoms or complication occur.

Survival in patients with SBS is approximately 85% at 2 years and 75% at 5 years. An end-jejunostomy, remnant length less than 50 cm, and mesenteric vascular disease have a negative impact on survival. Obviously, survival will also be influenced by patient age, other medical conditions, and underlying malignancy. TPN-induced liver disease has an average survival of only 1 year without transplantation.

Non transplantation procedures for improving intestinal function are successful in approximately 85% of patients. Intestinal lengthening improves intestinal function in 85% of patients early on, but success is less with long term follow up. Success is lowest (50%) in patients who undergo procedures for prolonging intestinal transit time.

One year patient survival after intestinal transplantation is approximately 85%, but decreases to 50% at 5 years. Isolated small intestine, combined liver-small intestine, and multi visceral transplantation (liver, small bowel, pancreas, stomach, colon) all have a role in selected patients. Isolated intestinal transplantation, in general, has a better prognosis than multiple-organ grafts.

Selected Readings

Byrne TA, Willmore DW, Iyer K, et al. (2005) Growth hormone, glutamine, and an optimal diet reduces parenteral nutrition in patients with short bowel syndrome. Ann Surg 242:655–661

Chan S, McCowen KC, Bistran BR, et al. (1999) Incidence, prognosis, and etiology of end-stage liver disease in patients receiving home total parenteral nutrition. Surgery 126:28

DiBaise JK, Young RJ, Vanderhoot JA, et al. (2004) Intestinal rehabilitation and the short bowel syndrome. Parts I and II. Am J Gastro 99:1386–1395, 1823–1832

Grant D, Abu-Elmagd K, Reyes J, et al. (2005) 2003 Report of the intestinal transplant registry: a new era has dawned. Ann Surg 241:607–613

Jeppesen PB (2003) Clinical significance of GLP-2 in the short bowel syndrome. J Nutr 133:3721

Messing B, Crenn P, Beau P, et al. (1999) Long-term survival and parenteral nutrition dependence in adult patients with the short bowel syndrome. Gastroenterology 117:1043

Thompson JS, Langnas AN, Pinch LW, et al. (1995) Surgical approach to the short bowel syndrome. Ann Surg 222:600–607

Thompson JS (2004) Surgical rehabilitations of intestine in short bowel syndrome. Surgery 135:465–470

Thompson JS, DiBaise JK, Iyer KR, et al. (2005) Postoperative short bowel syndrome J Am Coll Surg 201:85–89

61 Radiation and Surgery

Mary F. Otterson · Kathleen K. Christians

Pearls and Pitfalls

- Understanding the anatomy of radiation enteropathy is critical in elective cases. Preoperative imaging provides the road map.
- Maximize preoperative nutritional status with enteral (or parenteral) feeding. Micronutrient deficiencies, such as vitamin B 12, may infer the degree of intestinal damage.
- Bowel prep the patient prior to the procedure if possible, because strictures in the small intestine predispose to proximal intestinal bacterial overgrowth.
- Protect normal structures such as the ureter with ureteral stenting.
- Bypass the affected area if safe resection is not possible.
- Consider tissue transfer (plastic surgery) for difficult-to-heal wounds.

Introduction

Whether radiation exposure is therapeutic, accidental, or belligerent, the potentially profound effects produced by radiation alter the outcome of operative interventions. With an understanding of both normal tissue and oncologic radiobiology, the surgeon is both better able to make informed decisions regarding the patient who has been exposed and to apply the best procedures intraoperatively to avoid complications.

Gastrointestinal Radiobiology

Radiation effects may be divided into prodromal, acute, and late effects of radiation. Prodromal effects occur immediately after radiation exposure and prior to the development of acute histologic changes seen with radiation damage. The well-described effects of acute radiation are attributed to depletion of actively proliferating crypt cells and are associated with profound changes in absorption and secretion. Late effects of radiation are secondary to a combination of ischemic changes and fibrosis.

Within hours of a significant dose of radiation (approximately 400 Centigray [cGy]), prodromal effects of radiation can be detected. These acute symptoms include nausea, vomiting, abdominal cramping, and diarrhea. These effects are due, in part, to the release of serotonin from the enterochromaffin cells of the gut. In animal models (including primates), vomiting is associated with a series of contractions which begin in the mid small bowel and rapidly propel intestinal contents into the stomach immediately prior to emesis. The most striking contraction of this group is the retrograde giant contraction (RGC; ❯ *Fig. 61-1*). The RGC is a powerful contraction that originates in the mid small bowel and rapidly propels intestinal contents proximally into the stomach immediately prior to vomitus expulsion.

Abdominal cramping and diarrhea are associated with the giant migrating contraction (GMC; ❯ *Fig. 61-2*), another type of large amplitude contraction of the small intestine. GMCs are large amplitude contractions that push small intestinal contents into the colon and are associated with abdominal cramping. The GMC may propagate into the colon and, when the contraction reaches the distal colon, is associated with explosive diarrhea. Both Retrograde giant contractions RGCs and Giant migrating contractions GMCs are associated with radiation therapy but are seldom of concern to the surgeon.

◻ Figure 61-1
Both the RGC and GMC originate in the mid small bowel at strain gauge 6. The RGC propagates in a orad direction, propelling intestinal contents rapidly back into the stomach immediately prior to emesis. The numbers listed next to the strain gauge designation refer to the distance from the pylorus in centimeters (Reprinted from Otterson et al., 1988)

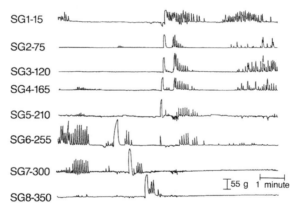

◻ Figure 61-2
Three GMCs originate in the duodenum and rapidly propel intestinal contents into the colon. The third GMCdoes not propagate beyond the mid small bowel at 130 cm distal to the pylorus (Reprinted from Otterson et al., 1988)

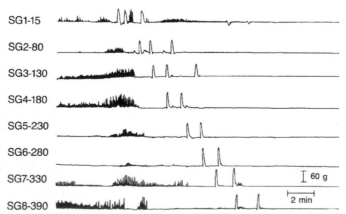

In the case of accidental radiation exposure, the total body dose needed to produce immediate effects of radiation approximates the lethal dose for bone marrow exposure. Thus, in the event of unplanned total body irradiation, vomiting is an indicator that fatal bone marrow suppression may have occurred. Any surgical intervention must proceed with this understanding. Profound bone marrow suppression after surgical intervention for trauma may necessitate exteriorization of intestinal injury as opposed to attempted anastomoses.

The acute effects of radiation are due to the rapid turnover of villous epithelium (5–6 days). Crypt cells are actively dividing cells which, if affected by radiation exposure, do not populate the villi as expected. After fractionated radiotherapy, crypt cell mitoses return to normal within 3 days and villi within 2 weeks of completion of radiotherapy and one can anticipate resolution of symptoms related to mucosal damage soon thereafter. The functional effects of acute phase radiation damage are the diminution of the absorptive capacity of the intestine. Malabsorption of fat, carbohydrates, protein, and bile salts correlate with the morphologic alterations produced by irradiation in small intestinal mucosa. This effect causes a period of reversible nutritional wasting and may produce dehydration. Bile salts are usually efficiently reabsorbed in the distal small intestine. Failure of the small intestinal mucosa results in dumping of primary bile salts into the colon where they are subjected to bacterial degradation. Secondary bile salts thus lead to bile salt-induced diarrhea by acting as cathartics and inhibiting water reabsorption. Expulsion of the watery feces decreases the enterohepatic bile salt pool and causes an increased synthesis of bile salts resulting in choleretic enteropathy. Binding bile salts with cholestyramine or similar agents may alleviate some of the profuse diarrhea that these patients experience. The drug must be within the gastrointestinal tract prior to the first concentrated release of bile.

Lactose intolerance may develop in patients receiving radiotherapy. Mature enterocytes are located at the tips of the villi and provide the enzyme lactase. These cells are missing during radiotherapy and continued ingestion of milk products may exacerbate diarrhea.

Late sequelae of radiation are influenced by the total radiation dose and the volume of bowel irradiated. Symptoms include crampy abdominal pain, bloody diarrhea, tenesmus, and malabsorption of fat and bile salts. Weight loss, obstruction, and occasionally perforation or fistula formation may occur. The area of bowel affected has more to do with bowel exposure than with intrinsic radio-sensitivity, i.e., the ileum and rectum are irradiated frequently because they are fixed in position in the pelvis where many disorders treated with radiation therapy occur. The sense of tenesmus may be treated with low doses of tricyclic antidepressants (amitriptyline, 10–25 mg administered at bedtime). Steroid suppositories may also relieve this irritating symptom. Some patients may improve with binding of bile salts using agents such as cholestyramine. Symptomatic relief is key in the management of patients with late sequelae from radiation.

Large vessels exposed to radiation display early vascular spasm which progresses to narrowing, thrombosis, and accelerated atherosclerosis. The microscopic features are obliterative endarteritis, fibrosis, and lymphatic and capillary ectasias. Occasionally, vascular surgical intervention is needed. The advent of minimally invasive stenting techniques may be appropriate, but long term studies in these irradiated patients is not likely to be forthcoming due to their limited numbers.

Patients who have survived cancer, radiation therapy, and chemotherapy often do not approach their next surgical procedure in optimum condition. In elective circumstances, anticipation of intra-operative issues, pre-operative preparation, and fully informed consent are essential. Surgical planning starts with a detailed history and physical examination. During physical assessment, the examiner should look for signs of malnutrition, weight loss, activity tolerance, numbness and tingling of the extremities, or radiation-induced skin changes. The tattoos marking the external focus points for the radiotherapy point to underlying tissue which is likely to be more severely affected. Co-morbid conditions such as diabetes and hypertension suggest accelerated disease processes.

Biochemical and hematologic assessments are helpful. Anemia may reflect subclinical bleeding or persistent bone marrow suppression. With the advent of safe and effective parenteral iron therapy, intravenous iron Dextran, combined with vitamin B_{12} and erythropoietin, may correct the patient's anemia. Although considered first line for treatment of anemia, oral iron irritates the gastrointestinal tract, and may affect appetite adversely and therefore may not be effective. Many patients find that oral iron therapy worsens their symptoms, resulting in poor compliance.

Along with avoidance of oral iron therapy, elimination of other drugs that produce mucosal damage should be considered. Nonsteroidal anti-inflammatory drugs, aspirin, and bisphosphonates may irritate intestinal mucosa or impede mucosal healing. Alternative therapies or routes of administration should be considered.

Decreased serum albumin is the greatest predictor of morbidity and mortality in the surgical patient. Causes of decreased serum albumin that should be investigated preoperatively include ongoing bleeding, serum loss from the damaged mucosa, malabsorption, and decreased oral intake due to partial small bowel obstruction (SBO). If operation is essential but elective, motivated patients may be able to enhance their nutritional status by sipping supplements to the point of adequate nutritional intake. If adequate nutrition cannot be achieved through oral supplementation, then preoperative total parenteral nutrition (TPN) may be necessary, which allows the patient to receive nourishment at the time of the admission and avoids further nutritional compromise during the postoperative period while awaiting return of bowel function.

Patients with bile salt malabsorption due to chronic radiation changes are at high risk for malabsorption of both fat soluble vitamins and Vitamin B_{12}. Cholestyramine, ½ to 1 scoop first thing in the morning with a possible repeat dose at evening, often decreases the diarrhea experienced by these patients. Either decreased serum vitamin B_{12} or an increased serum homocysteine level suggests a vitamin B_{12}/folic acid deficiency. Once vitamin B_{12} deficiency is diagnosed, the patient must understand that therapy will be life long. Vitamin B_{12} deficiency, through increased homocysteine levels, may predispose to premature cardiovascular disease, neuropathy, and gastrointestinal dysfunction.

Patients with sufficient terminal ileal dysfunction to have vitamin B_{12} deficiency may also have issues with absorption of fat soluble vitamin (vitamins A, D, E, K). Warfarin therapy must be monitored carefully due to its link to vitamin K. Malignancy and radiation damage to venous structures increases rates of deep venous thrombosis (DVT). Routine DVT prophylaxis is therefore recommended perioperatively or for prolonged hospitalization.

Prevention of Radiation Injury

As with many diseases, the best therapy is prevention (❯ *Fig. 61-3*). Preventing enteric exposure by: (1) performing radiation therapy prior to the operative resection; (2) optimizing positioning the patient during radiation therapy (i.e., prone, with a full bladder to push small intestine out of pelvis); (3) placement of omental flap in the area where radiation will be administered; or (4) placement of Vicryl mesh sling to suspend the intestines from the field of radiotherapy are all worthwhile endeavors.

■ Figure 61-3
This x-ray image shows the chronic radiation effects on exposed small bowel adjacent to the area of surgical excision. The patient received both internal and external irradiation for the treatment of uterine cancer

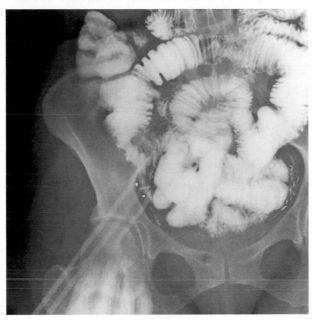

While described, the placement of tissue expanders is not commonly used to prevent exposure of the normal small and large intestine, probably because subsequent removal usually requires a second operation.

Early Surgery

If operation is planned after radiation, a window of 6–8 weeks post treatment is optimal. This period allows the hyperemic response of radiation to decrease and limits perioperative blood loss. The maximum tumor response to therapy is achieved during this interval. Surrounding tissues, although edematous, have not yet developed the fibrotic scarring and loss of normal tissue planes that characterize the late effects of radiation. Timing is key to optimal surgical results.

Late Surgery

Preoperative planning with the participation of subspecialties (urology, plastic surgery) is essential. Repeat pelvic surgery presents many challenges, especially after prior radiation therapy. Careful review of preoperative imaging to identify affected bowel and adjacent structures that may be displaced or adhesed is very important. Special attention should be given to the ureters which can be obscured by scar tissue. Preoperative ureteral stents can be a valuable addition for ease in identification during dissection and to both avoid and recognize ureteral injury. While the irradiated ureter may function well without injury, the transected irradiated ureter causes major technical difficulty and results in substantial disability for the patient. Involving the urologist during the planning process may help to avoid this unwanted complication.

Recurrent pelvic cancers in an irradiated field that necessitate operative intervention may leave the patient with a large potential space that will not heal. Preoperative consultation with a plastic surgeon can be useful. Gracilis muscle flaps are frequently used to fill in the space caused by an abdominal perineal resection. Use of a rectus muscle flap must be anticipated, because this flap can be thwarted by poorly positioned ostomies, laparoscopic port sites, or drains that interfere with blood supply of the planned flap. Vacuum-assisted wound closure devices may be employed to limit wound size once vascularized tissue is at the base of the wound. Careful multidisciplinary planning prevents the use of ill-thought-out procedures that would interfere with optimal treatment of these complicated patients.

Of the 5–15% of patients who develop chronic radiation enteropathy after abdominal or pelvic radiation, about one third of these patients require surgical intervention. Because of the high morbidity, operative intervention should be reserved for severe injury. These types of injury indications include high-grade obstruction, perforation, hemorrhage, intra-abdominal abscesses, and fistulas. While the timing and choice of operative techniques remain controversial, the goal of operation is limited resection of the entire diseased segment with primary anastomosis between the healthy bowel segments. Due to the diffuse nature of the intestinal injury and difficulty in distinguishing normal and irradiated intestine, limited resection is often difficult to achieve safely. If hemorrhage is not the indication for operation, the bypass may be performed more safely in such patients.

When undertaking operation for treatment of intestinal radiation damage, good surgical principles should be applied. Skin incisions in the field of prior radiation should be avoided. Adhesiolysis should also be avoided as it leads to further impairment of an already compromised blood supply and leads to increased risks of perforation and fistula. Whenever possible, anastomoses should be made between segments that are free of disease and with adequate blood supply, even should it require removal of a more generous length of involved bowel. This decision is often the most difficult. Anastomoses involving irradiated segments have leak rates as high as 50%. Distinguishing between normal and diseased segments of intestine is nearly impossible by gross intraoperative inspection, and while incompletely reliable, frozen section analysis of the margins may be helpful. The omentum may be incorporated at the anastomotic site to try to decrease the risk for leak. The surgeon should be prepared to perform an intestinal bypass rather than resection in an unfavorable abdomen.

Disabling symptoms associated with defecation or bleeding should be managed medically prior to any attempt at surgical correction. Formalin application to bleeding sites in chronic radiation proctitis is successful in greater than 80% of patients. A gauze pad soaked with 4% solution is applied to the affected rectum through a proctoscope for 2–3 min until the bleeding ceases. Care is taken to protect normal skin and tissue. Formalin installation (50 ml of Formalin for 30 s, total of 400–500 ml per session) with the placement of a balloon catheter cephalad to the treatment region to protect normal tissue with installation is also successful in 1 in 3 applications. Hyperbaric oxygen has 50–60% success rates in small retrospective studies. The disadvantage of hyperbaric oxygen remains its expense as well as limited access to this therapy.

Endoscopic management using both Nd:YAG laser or argon plasma coagulation for the control of hemorrhage has also been reported. The advantage of argon plasma coagulation is its availability, lesser expense, and limited tissue penetration (2–3 mm). The charred tissue produced by the argon coagulate interrupts current passing through the tissue, while the Nd:YAG laser energy continues to penetrate tissue until it is turned off. Complications of Nd:YAG laser include tenesmus, rectal stenosis, abdominal pain, prostatitis, and fistula formation.

Some patients elect or demand diversion of the fecal stream due to symptoms of severe radiation proctitis to provide some relief, especially if the perianal skin is affected. Endoscopy should be used to differentiate irradiated from normal bowel before the planning of the ostomy site. Use of endoscopic tattooing may help the surgeon locate the segment of colon to be utilized. Depending on distal strictures, a mucous fistula may be needed. If at all possible, a functioning, proximal ostomy should be constructed from normal tissue brought through a non-irradiated location of the abdominal wall. If diversion fails and resection of the rectum becomes necessary, the difficulty of this procedure cannot be over-emphasized. Sparing one rectus muscle (no stomas, no port sites, no drain placement) to fill the void left in the pelvis allows utilization of rectus as a vascularized flap into the pelvis. Consultation with a plastic surgeon, a urologist, and possibly a gynecologist should be considered. This type of surgery is best performed at a tertiary center.

Sometimes general surgeons become involved in procedures for urologic radiation damage, often involving fecal diversion for prostate-to-rectum fistulas and conduits for bladder and ureteral obstruction. Planning for this procedure requires imaging of the ureters, bladder, and colon-nearly simultaneously with three dimensional considerations to achieve optimal results for these unfortunate patients. This planning can be achieved with CT reconstruction or with creative fluoroscopic imaging.

Lymphoma can arise in segments of irradiated bowel. Rapidly increasing serum LDH levels suggest this diagnosis. While chemotherapy may treat this disorder, there is risk of transmural disease, and resection of perforated intestine in the setting of radiation enteropathy may be extremely difficult.

Management of Fistulae

Despite maximum preparation, optimum technique, and good perioperative care, some patients develop enteric fistulas. After recurrent malignancy is eliminated as a cause, control and treatment of the fistula is important. Re-operation, especially in the early postoperative time frame, may not be possible or advisable. Control of the fistula to prevent skin breakdown should be the first priority. Control may be accomplished with an ostomy appliance, wound manager, a catheter and drainage bag, or a vacuum-assisted wound closure device. Increasing the resistance of the fistula by increasing the length of the track to the skin in an enterocutaneous fistula may help. One technique to accomplish this involves re-approximating the skin edges around the fistula tract and controlling the fistula with a catheter. Decreasing the volume of effluent may help the fistula to heal; this can be accomplished by decreasing gastric and enteric secretions using proton pump inhibitors and somatostatin analogues. Keeping the patient NPO and initiating TPN may be necessary. A malnourished patient will not heal a fistula.

When the fistula tract has matured, evaluating the fistula with a fluoroscopic water soluble contrast study or a CT sinogram may identify the source of the fistula and determine whether there is a distal obstruction. If a partial distal obstruction exists in the early postoperative period, delay of any definitive procedure for 8–12 weeks is recommended. If there is no distal obstruction, the chances of healing the fistula are improved; hyperbaric oxygen therapy can be tried. Free flaps or omental flaps to provide a non-irradiated blood supply to the source of the fistula may be helpful. If operative intervention is needed, an ostomy may be necessary. Complex cases should probably be transferred to a tertiary referral center because of all the multidisciplinary services required.

Enterovesical fistulas in the setting of radiation damage are suspicious for recurrent malignancy. While relatively common in the case of inflammatory processes, fistulae from radiation damage take years to develop. Repair depends on the source of the fistula and the non-irradiated surrounding tissue.

Patients with enterovaginal fistulas seek surgical intervention less often than one would imagine. The degree of symptoms experienced by the woman is a function of the size of the fistula opening and the liquid content of the bowel movements. If the stool is liquid, bile salts binders (cholestyramine), the use of fiber, or oral opiates to constipate the patient may limit the symptoms. Surgical intervention for a radiation-induced rectovaginal fistula usually requires a diverting ostomy. Resection and repair in an irradiated field is not likely to be successful, particularly if the connection is between the low rectum and vagina because of the thickness of the tissue and the prior radiation. If the fistula is secondary to a loop of small or large intestine adherent to the vaginal cuff, surgical repair is more likely to be successful, because the offending loop of bowel may be resected.

Summary

No surgeon enjoys the prospect of procedures in the irradiated abdomen. Attention to perioperative preparation, medical optimization, and consideration of non-operative treatments and care for the entire patient is absolutely essential. These patients are generally more ill than other individuals but can be helped in many cases with appropriate surgical intervention.

Acknowledgment

Supported by a cooperative agreement with NIAID, AI067734.

Selected Readings

Cotti G, et al. (2003) Conservative therapies for hemorrhagic radiation proctitis: a review. Rev Hosp Clin Fac Med Sao Paulo 58:284–292

Galland RB, Spencer J (1986) Surgical management of radiation enteritis. Surgery 99:133–139

Kinsella TJ, Bloomer WD (1980) Tolerance of the intestine to radiation therapy. Surg Gynecol Obstet 151:273–284

Morgan V, et al. (2005) Amitriptyline reduces rectal pain related activation of the anterior cingulate cortex in patients with irritable bowel syndrome. Gut 54:601–607

Otterson MF, et al. (1992) Effects of fractionated doses of ionizing radiation on colonic motor activity. Am J Physiol 263:G518–526

Otterson MF, Sarna SK, Moulder JE (1988) Effects of fractionated doses of ionizing radiation on small intestinal motor activity. Gastroenterology 95:1249–1257

Plowman PN, Shand WS, Jackson DB (1984) Use of absorbable mesh to displace bowel and avoid radiation enteropathy, during therapy of pelvic Ewing's sarcoma. Hum Toxicol 3:229–237

Rowe GG (1967) Control of tenesmus and diarrhea by cholestyramine administration. Gastroenterology 53:1006

62 Splanchnic Venous Thrombosis

Götz M. Richter · Jens Werner

Pearls and Pitfalls

- Acute splanchnic or mesenteric venous thrombosis is a rare disease accounting for approximately 10% of all abdominal ischemic events.
- The splanchnic venous system represents all intestinal veins which drain ultimately into the portal circulation.
- In acute and subacute mesenteric occlusion, the presence or absence of clinical or laboratory signs of bowel necrosis mainly reflect the status and severity of the disease. Unfortunately, most of the symptoms are nonspecific and overlap with a variety of other abdominal emergencies.
- In chronic mesenteric occlusion, the extent of portal hypertension and its subsequent complications determine the clinical presentation; this holds true for both cirrhosis-related and non cirrhosis-related causes.
- The preoperative diagnosis of splanchnic thrombosis is made very rarely. Often the diagnosis is an unexpected result of imaging tests (mainly CT) for unclear abdominal pathologies.
- Treatment of acute splanchnic venous thrombosis requires immediate anticoagulation. Regional thrombolysis can be achieved via a catheter placed intraoperatively into the mesenteric vein or via a transjugular-intrahepatic porto-systemic stent (TIPS). In cases of local or diffuse peritonitis, patients need immediate laparotomy and bowel resection for irreversible ischemia.
- Chronic mesenteric venous thrombosis is a result of a hypercoagulable state, including protein C, protein S and antithrombin III deficiencies, and Factor V Leiden. Other conditions predisposing to thrombosis include portal hypertension, cirrhosis, pancreatitis, malignancies, and intra-abdominal infections. The underlying diseases should be identified and treated.
- Currently, portosystemic shunt operations are rarely indicated, because interventional radiologic alternatives exist. This approach is especially pertinent in those patients with good hepatic reserve who do not need liver transplantation in the near future. Alternatively, liver transplantation should be considered in those patients in whom cirrhosis is the underlying disease.

Historical Remarks

Acute splanchnic or mesenteric venous thrombosis is a rare but challenging clinical problem among abdominal emergencies. It was first recognized by Elliot in 1885 as a reason for intestinal gangrenous disease. In 1935, Warren and Eberhard were the first to establish the definite distinction between arterial and venous mesenteric thrombosis as causative factors for bowel gangrene. Grendell and Ockner demonstrated in a systematic analysis that mesenteric venous thrombosis accounts for approximately 10% of all abdominal ischemic events. Imaging techniques started to play an important diagnostic role before sonographic identification of splanchnic vascular pathology by B-mode and Doppler ultrasonography was introduced. As soon as helical computed tomography became available widely, the diagnosis of mesenteric, splenic, and portal venous thrombosis was obtained regularly with contrast-enhanced CT during the venous contrast phase. Ever since, several publications on surgical strategies in occlusive mesenteric disease have stressed the role of imaging in decision making and patient selection to improve therapy and outcome for abdominal emergencies and in elective situations. Furthermore, with the development of MRI and MRA, the visualization of normal and pathologic splanchnic vessels became available even in patients with contraindications against iodinated contrast material. The latest achievements to improve contrast and spatial resolution both in CT and MRI have helped to identify congested intestinal wall segments resulting from the lack of venous drainage, while describing correctly the arterial mesenteric vasculature. Using these imaging techniques, better algorithms for clinical management including the indication for conservative versus operative therapy particularly in patients in whom bowel ischemia is not suspected. Historically, symptomatic patients usually underwent laparotomy for suspected transmural necrosis and bowel perforation. With better imaging methods, these conditions are detected much easier or even ruled out without an operation. Furthermore, recent interventional radiologic advances in catheter technology and local pharmacomechanical thrombolysis have added treatment strategies which deal properly with the causative morphologic and hemodynamic problem by reestablishing free mesenteric venous flow.

Chronic splanchnic thrombosis presents with a distinctly different clinical pattern and is a diagnostic and management challenge as compared to acute or subacute forms. In 1988, Warren summarized for the first time the major differences between chronic, non-cirrhotic portal vein occlusion and cirrhosis-associated portal vein occlusion by characterizing the hemodynamic consequences and therapeutic options. In this clinical context, the complications from portal hypertension, such as esophageal or gastric variceal bleeding, play the predominant role. Hence, therapeutic options focus on endoscopic treatment of varices and surgical shunts. Because TIPS requires an patent portal circulation, it is usually not performed in chronic portomesenteric occlusion. Over the last 20 years, some case reports have emerged describing the use TIPS for treating highly focal portal or mesenteric venous occlusions or high grade stenosis in native or post liver transplantation vasculature.

Anatomic Background

The splanchnic venous system is best characterized as the venous tree of all intestinal veins which drain into the portal circulation. Hence, it shows distinct variations of its anatomic organization as compared to the arterial system. The superior and inferior mesenteric artery are completely independent vessels arising from the aorta at separate levels. The inferior mesenteric vein drains into the splenic vein very close to the confluens of the splenic and superior mesenteric vein. Thereby, both mesenteric veins draining the bowel are dependent on each other. In addition, segments of the ascending and descending large bowel have additional, retroperitoneal draining veins which are tributaries to the inferior vena caval circulation. All pancreatic venous vessels drain directly into the portal vein, and the veins of the pancreatic tail drain into the splenic vein. Similarly, almost all gastric veins are tributaries of the portal vein. The vessels from the lesser curvature drain via the coronary vein into the portal vein. Those of the greater curvature of the stomach reach the portal circulation via gastroepiploic veins which drain into the splenic vein. Typically, the veins of one anatomic bowel segment, e.g. ileal or gastric veins, form large, interconnecting loops in the mesentery ensuring a well-collateralized draining system. Furthermore, at the watershed region between the superior and inferior mesenteric venous drainage at the left colonic flexure, there are also venous collaterals that provide venous drainage between these two major intestinal veins. The symptoms of both, the acute and chronic occlusion of splanchnic veins, are dependent heavily on this anatomic background.

Pathogenesis

Besides its clinical presentation, acute and subacute splanchnic venous thrombosis have distinctly different causative factors compared to chronic occlusion. Various attempts have been made to classify and describe the etiology. Because of their similarities in clinical presentation and causative factors, acute and subacute forms of splanchnic venous thrombosis are discussed together and separated from chronic occlusion in this chapter.

In general, the acute and subacute forms represent the thrombotic venous effect of a procoagulant state. Primary and secondary thrombosis have to be discriminated. Primary thrombosis is generated by primary deficits in blood coagulation and imbalances of blood hemostasis, while secondary thrombosis is caused by local (mechanical) distortion of the venous drainage system regardless of the primary location within the portal tributaries. This classification tries to reflect the corresponding severity of the morphologic extent of venous thrombosis and the clinical symptoms. In spontaneous or primary mesenteric occlusion in young women, oral contraceptives play a major etiologic role and should be considered as a major co-factor for primary thrombosis as is smoking. The acute form of the Budd-Chiari syndrome can be considered in the same pathogenetic context, because it might result from the same coagulation disorders as primary splanchnic venous thrombosis alone. The Budd-Chiari syndrome represents an extremely difficult abdominal emergency associated with very high morbidity. A remarkable overlap between primary and secondary thrombosis might be found in patients who present with splanchnic venous occlusion days or weeks after splenectomy. This situation is particularly true in patients in whom splenectomy was performed for treatment of hemotologic disorders. The local venous trauma might add to the coagulation disorder. In addition, splenectomy alone can trigger delayed (total) mesenterico-portal thrombosis. In ❷ *Table 62-1*, the classification of primary and secondary splanchnic venous thrombosis is outlined in detail.

In chronic venous occlusion, the pathogenesis includes a vast variety of acquired and focal mesenteric venous pathologies. A reasonable classification approach is to discriminate between focal, cirrhosis-associated versus non cirrhosis-associated causative factors. This distinction reflects the different hemodynamic baseline of these two disease groups. In non-cirrhosis associated venous thrombosis, local venous infection (sterile and pyogenic), trauma, and tumor invasion play the predominant role for splanchnic venous obstruction. Liver parenchyma remains normal in cases with umbilical vein infection and subsequent portal vein thrombosis or in patients with pancreatic cancer and local invasion of the major mesenteric veins. Collaterals can develop gradually and maintain hepatopedal flow. By this phenomenon, multivessel thrombosis is prevented. In contrast, in cirrhosis-associated splanchnic thrombosis, both the causative factor and the hemodynamics are different. Thrombosis occurs secondary to long-lasting reversal of portal flow or on the basis of the development of a hepatocellular carcinoma and subsequent portal invasion.

◧ Table 62-1

Causative factors of splanchnic thrombosis

Primary thrombosis (inherited or acquired prothrombotic conditions)
Factor V Leiden
Protein C deficiency
Protein S deficiency
Prothrombin gene mutations
Antithrombin III deficiency
Antiphospholipid antibody development
Homocystenemia
Pregnancy
Post-pregnancy
Neuroendocrine neoplasms
Endocrine active neoplasm
Polycythemia vera
Essential thrombocythemia
Paroxysmal nocturnal hemoglobinuria
Secondary thrombosis
Inflammatory
Diverticulitis
Crohn's disease
Ulcerative colitis
Pancreatitis
Peritonitis
Postoperative
Splenectomy
Visceral resections
Variceal ligation, embolization
Trauma
Blunt abdominal trauma
Direct pancreatic trauma
Direct mesenteric root trauma
Direct duodenal trauma

Classification as acute or chronic splanchnic venous thrombosis might be difficult when previously established obstructive venous pathologies associated with portal or mesenteric venous hypertension promote or predispose to occlusion, or if a hypercoagulable state develops for any reason. Splanchnic venous thrombosis is observed frequently in recurrent chronic pancreatitis. In primary and acute splanchnic venous thrombosis, the origin of occlusion is in large mesenteric veins and tends to spread and propagate to smaller veins. It is of utmost importance to identify the functional status of the collateral pathways to provide a rationale for the clinical management by integrating the knowledge about the individual pathogenesis, the local extent of thrombosis, as well as ischemic or portal hypertensive consequences.

Hemodynamics

The simultaneous thrombotic occlusion of the three major splanchnic veins, the superior mesenteric, the splenic, and the portal vein, represents the most dramatic occlusive event in this vascular territory and is induced most frequently by coagulation deficits. Mortality can be as high as 70% due to intestinal congestive ischemia. Because acute onset of splanchnic venous thrombosis prevents the timely development of venous collaterals to relieve the increased intramural pressure within the bowel wall, hemorrhagic necrosis develops. As soon as the three major draining vessels are affected simultaneously, jejunal and ileal segments have no venous drainage and then depend on the mesenteric outflow via retroperitoneal venous connections of the ascending and descending colon and the periduodenal and pancreatic head collaterals. Therefore, bowel necrosis in splanchnic venous thrombosis most often affects distal jejunal and proximal ileal segments. The time course of the occlusion of the three major vessels determines the severity of the clinical course and its complications.

Splanchnic venous thrombosis associated with a coagulation disorder is often located in the small venous vessels and primarily interferes with the intramural drainage from the bowel. The thrombosis propagates downstream to involve the larger vessels. As long as the thrombosis does not involve all of the three vessels simultaneously, there might be time for collaterals to reach substantial size. In such cases of subacute thrombosis, relief of the venous hypertension via collaterals is just enough to prevent hemorrhagic bowel infarction despite the formation of symptoms from the pain of bowel wall conjestion and peritoneal irritation. Therefore, from the hemodynamic point of view, it is justified to discriminate a subacute form from an acute form of splanchnic thrombosis. Hence, splanchnic thrombosis secondary to local venous pathologies tends to have a more benign character. In most circumstances, the underlying disease has already allowed the development of collateral hepatopetal flow when unrelated to liver cirrhosis. This conditions holds true for most of the posttraumatic splanchnic venous pathologies, as well as mesenterico-portal occlusions secondary to pancreatitis or pancreatic cancer. Only the Budd-Chiari syndrome plays a different and much more life-threatening role. As long as the portal vein remains open, blood flow out of the liver might be maintained through hepatofugal flow via the coronary vein as the final outflow conduit. Portal occlusion in Budd-Chiari syndrome might occur when portal flow becomes stagnant as a result of the impaired hepatic vein outflow. Subsequently, when portal occlusion occurs in addition to the Budd-Chiari syndrome, no outflow out of the liver exists, and the liver can infarct within hours.

In chronic splanchnic venous occlusion, the hemodynamics are dominated by the sinusoidal liver pressure and the existence of a substantial portosystemic gradient. In liver cirrhosis, the collateral pathways, e.g. gastric or esophageal variceal systems, are essentially hepatofugal, but they require a patent portal vein as the primary conduit. Whenever a condition occurs which destabilizes this balance between intestinal hepatopetal flow toward the portal vein and hepatofugal flow along the (variceal) venous collaterals, the arterial inflow toward the liver determines its functional reserve.

Clinical Presentation

The etiologic factors causing splanchnic venous thrombosis determine its clinical presentation. In the acute and subacute forms, signs of bowel necrosis are the most important features. Unfortunately, most of the symptoms are nonspecific and overlap with a variety of other abdominal emergency conditions. Clinical signs of arterial and venous mesenteric thrombosis are different. Symptoms associated with arterial mesenteric occlusion are much more distinct and predictive of the underlying disease, while clinical symptoms of venous mesenteric occlusion are often nonspecific and non-diagnostic. If acute abdominal pain, local signs of peritonitis, and laboratory findings suspicious of infection are present, venous mesenteric occlusion should be considered in the differential diagnosis. Nevertheless, these symptoms overlap with other inflammatory diseases, including Crohn's disease, acute appendicitis, and others. In the subacute forms of splanchnic venous thrombosis, the leading clinical symptom is abdominal pain, but, pain is again nonspecific, and laboratory findings are mostly inconclusive as well. Therefore, the primary diagnosis is made very rarely. Often it is an unexpected result of imaging (mainly CT) for unclear abdominal complaints. In the acute form, the pain is colicky and located in the middle of the abdomen, because jejunal and ileal loops are involved most frequently. Fever and rebound tenderness are signs of transmural ischemia related to onset of infarction and subsequent complications. However, when subacute splanchnic venous thrombosis develops, the pain might last for a long time without progression to severe abdominal symptoms. In those cases, patients most often seek care several days after onset of symptoms. They report nausea, vomiting, diarrhea, and hematemesis. The most frequent sign in these patients is occult blood with hematochezia present in up to 20%. Sometimes and particularly in the subacute forms, there is postprandial worsening of the pain. In patients presenting with abdominal cramps and bloody diarrhea, the findings might be mistakenly associated with Crohn's disease. Endoscopy is often negative, and only CT and or MRI establish the diagnosis. In very rare cases, the onset of venous occlusion in small venous vessels does not progress to the major conduits and affects only the draining veins of one or only few loops. This small vessel venous thrombosis is often missed even on contrast-enhanced CT. Only the most recent generation of CT with multirow detector systems (16 detector rows and more) appear to provide enough spatial resolution in combination with contrast resolution to establish the diagnosis under such circumstances.

In chronic mesenteric venous occlusion, the extent of portal hypertension and its subsequent complications determine the clinical presentation. This finding holds true both for cirrhosis-related and non cirrhosis-related causes. Therefore, variceal bleeding, congestive gastritis, and ascites are found in both types of splanchnic venous thrombosis, while decreased liver function remains the hallmark of the cirrhosis-associated thrombotic event. In the latter, the functional reserve of the hepatic arterial system will determine worsening or stabilization of the already impaired liver function. In advanced cirrhosis, portal perfusion is reduced dramatically. Occlusion of the portal vein does not necessarily lead to catastrophic loss of liver function in contrast to the acute form of the Budd-Chiari syndrome.

Clinical Management

Acute mesenteric thrombosis: Treatment of acute splanchnic venous thrombosis requires immediate anticoagulation. In the absence of acute peritonitis and if no signs of bowel necrosis are detectable, long-term anticoagulation is the established treatment (❯ *Fig. 62-1*). In general, anticoagulation should be continued for the rest of the patient's life. In addition, antibiotic treatment as prophylaxis against bacterial translocation should be started as soon as the diagnosis has been confirmed.

Thrombolytic therapy has been advocated either systemically or via an indirect transarterial or direct porto-regional approach. Systemic thrombolysis is associated with the risk of generalized hemorrhagic complications, including intracerebral bleeding and severe intestinal bleeding. Thus, systemic therapy is restricted mainly to heparin treatment. Regional and direct thrombolysis can be achieved via a catheter placed intraoperatively into the mesenteric vein. An adjunctive or alternative technique is direct lysis through a transjugular-intrahepatic porto-systemic stent (TIPS) (❯ *Fig. 62-2*).

◘ Figure 62-1

CT demonstrating a chronic mesenteric vein thrombosis of the jejunum with unaltered flow within the venous branches of the ileum. Conservative treatment with anticoagulation was carried out successfully

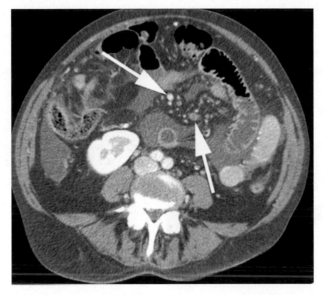

Both techniques allow placement of a catheter in the porto-mesenteric venous system to perform regional thrombolysis with high doses of urokinase or r-TPA and, even more important, over long time periods (up to 20 days). Over the past decade, the interventional catheter placement via TIPS has been often used as the first choice. Operative implantation of the catheter is reserved for those patients in whom the mesenteric veins are thrombosed over a long distance, making it difficult or even impossible to gain safe access transhepatically and for those patients who require immediate operative exploration for bowel infarction. Once an operative approach has been chosen, thrombectomy may be added before the regional thrombolysis via an intravascular catheter. This concept is a therapeutic option as long as the thrombus is not older than 3 days; endothelial cells lining of the mesenteric and portal veins are altered in the region of the thrombus and will be destroyed with subsequent re-thrombosis. Moreover, in most cases, the thrombus will already have extended far into the periphery even in case of timely diagnosis, so that thrombectomy is technically not feasible.

In cases of local or diffuse peritonitis, patients need immediate laparotomy. In those patients, resection of the small bowel and colon which are irreversibly ischemic must be performed with construcion of an ileostomy. An anastomosis should be avoided, because progression of the disease cannot be judged during the first operation but can be observed indirectly by the color of the ileostomy. Additionally, healing of an anastomosis is not guaranteed in ischemic and compromised tissue. If mesenteric venous thrombosis is identified as the underlying cause intraoperatively, a catheter for postoperative local thrombolysis should be inserted into the mesenteric venous system for local thrombolysis. Often, a second look operation is indicated to judge the viability of the remaining gut and by this, the effectiveness of the treatment.

Chronic mesenteric thrombosis: When mesenteric venous thrombosis is identified by imaging techniques, systemic anticoagulation with heparin should be instituted. The patient should undergo evaluation for a hypercoagulable state, including protein C, protein S and antithrombin III deficiencies, and Factor V Leiden. However, other well-known conditions predisposing to thrombosis include portal

◘ Figure 62-2

a. CT showing thrombosis of portal vein without portal vein flow. b. CT demonstrating thrombosis of superior mesenteric vein and splenic vein. c. A catheter was placed into the mesenteric vein for regional thrombolysis. d. The ischemic bowel was resected. e. Mesenteric venography showing the thrombosed superior mesenteric vein and portal vein with the catheter in place. f. TIPS performed for thrombolysis of the portal vein. g. Restored blood flow of the superior mesenteric vein and portal vein after successful thrombolysis. h. Follow-up CT 6 months after thrombolysis demonstrating long-term success of the regional thrombolysis with a patent portal vein

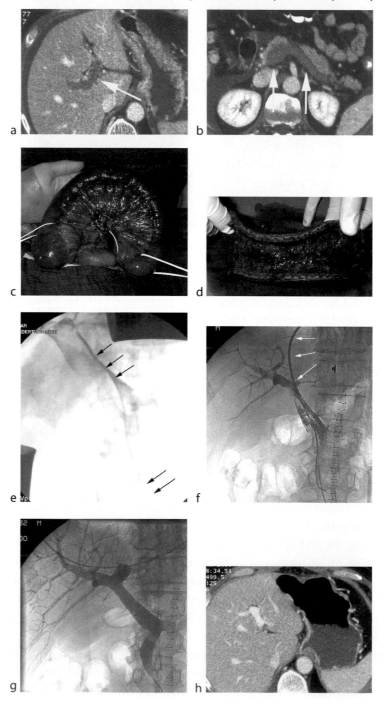

hypertension, cirrhosis, pancreatitis, malignancies, and intraabdominal infections. The underlying disease should be identified and treated. Emergency laparotomy should only be performed when bowel necrosis or infarction is suspected. In those cases, resection should be performed as described above.

Currently, portosystemic shunt operations are rarely indicated, because interventional radiologic alternatives exist for the treatment of Budd-Chiari syndrome and portal vein thrombosis. This approach is especially true in those patients with Budd-Chiari syndrome with good hepatic reserve who do not need imminent liver transplantation. Alternatively, liver transplantation should be considered in those patients in whom cirrhosis is the underlying disease. The choice between TIPS and a surgical shunt depends on the patient's hepatic reserve and possible timing to transplantation. If transplantation is expected within 1–2 years, TIPS is likely to successfully bridge the patient to liver transplantation without the need for surgical intervention. However, if transplantation is unlikely within 2 years, surgical shunting might be preferred, particularly in younger patients, because TIPS might require more shunt surveillance procedures and subsequent interventions.

Management of **bleeding esophageal varices** has also changed radically over the past decades. Primary treatment is endoscopic variceal sclerotherapy or endoscopic variceal ligation which have low complication rates. Similarly, the minimally invasive nature of TIPS and its successful implementation by interventional radiologists has further reduced the need of surgical shunt operations. TIPS is increasingly used routinely when endoscopic intervention has failed. Liver transplantation is recommended routinely for patients with advanced liver diseases. The time to transplantation is normally bridged with TIPS. Thus, surgical shunts are used more selectively. Surgical shunts are considered in the emergency setting when other modalities, including medical therapy, endoscopic control, or TIPS has failed, in the elective setting as a long-term bridge to liver transplantation, and as a definite treatment approach in patients with noncirrhotic portal hypertension as observed in the Budd-Chiari syndrome. Selective, distal splenorenal shunts are preferred in patients without ascites because of the lower risk of portosystemic encephalopathy. Side-to-side mesenterico or porto-caval shunts have the advantage of relieving ascites by decreasing the intrahepatic sinusoidal pressure and the portal venous pressure gradient.

Selected Readings

Abdu RA, Zakhour BJ, Dallis DJ (1987) Mesenteric venous thrombosis – 1911 to 1984. Surgery 101:383–388

Bilbao JI, Vivas I, Elduayen B, et al. (1999) Limitations of percutaneous techniques in the treatment of portal vein thrombosis. Cardiovasc Intervent Radiol 22:417–422

Demertzis S, Ringe B, Gulba D, et al. (1994) Treatment of portal vein thrombosis by thrombectomy and regional thrombolysis. Surgery 115:389–393

Elliot JW (1895) The operative relief of gangrene of intestine due to occlusion of the mesenteric vessels. Ann Surg 21:9–23

Grendell JH, Ockner RK (1982) Mesenteric venous thrombosis. Gastroenterology 82:358–372

Kumar S, Sarr MG, Kamath PS (2001) Mesenteric venous thrombosis. N Engl J Med 345:1683–1688

Orloff MJ, Orloff MS, Girard B, Orloff SL (2002) Bleeding esophagogastric varices from extrahepatic portal hypertension: 40 years' experience with portal-systemic shunt. J Am Coll Surg 194:717–28; discussion 728–730

Slakey DP, Klein AS, Venbrux AC, Cameron JL (2001) Budd-Chiari syndrome: current management options. Ann Surg 233:522–527

Warren S, Eberhard TP (1935) Mesenteric venous thrombosis. Surg Gynecol Obstet 61:102–121

Warren WD, Henderson JM, Millikan WJ, et al. (1988) Management of variceal bleeding in patients with noncirrhotic portal vein thrombosis. Ann Surg 207:623–634

63 Enterocutaneous Fistula

Feza H. Remzi · Victor W. Fazio

Pearls and Pitfalls

- Some 70–90% of enterocutaneous fistulas (ECF) are iatrogenic in origin.
- The management of ECF can be divided into three phases: acute, subacute, and repair with reconstruction.
- The likely presentation and recognition of a postoperative ECF usually occurs 5–10 days after an abdominal operation.
- With early postoperative ECF, fecal diversion with a proximal ileostomy or jejunostomy with or without repair is the procedure of choice, especially with an uncontrolled fistula.
- Note the "window period" before considering any surgical procedure (within 7–12 days from the most recent laparotomy). Within this "window period," severity of adhesions are usually milder, and repeat laparotomy is much easier (unless the first operation involved extensive adhesiolysis, then the window is 1–3 days).
- Initial management of the patient with a new fistula should be directed toward resuscitation and control of ECF drainage by pouching and skin protection; an enterostomal therapy nurse is indispensable.
- Computed tomographic or ultrasound-guided drainage for patients with localized sepsis and PEG tube insertion for small bowel obstruction are important strategies to avoid operation in patients past this window period.
- The subacute phase is the time from the control of sepsis until the time either the ECF heals spontaneously or the decision is made to proceed with repair.
- In the subacute phase, prompt initiation of either parenteral or enteral nutrition therapy is essential.
- Many ECF will close with conservative strategies; if fistula closure has not occurred after 4–6 weeks of nutrition, it is unlikely the fistula will close.
- Definitive repair should be delayed 4–6 months from the date of the initial procedure to allow for softening of adhesions.
- Prior to repair with reconstruction, patients require a complete work-up with nutritional and electrolyte deficiencies corrected, a radiologic road map, and marking by an enterostomal nurse.
- The operation may be a long procedure and may require senior assistance, as well as a multidisciplinary team (urologist, gynecologist, plastic surgeon).
- The goal of the initial phase of the operation is to free all adhesions, drain any remnant abscesses, and relieve any obstructed segment of bowel; leave the ECF management to the last portion of the procedure.
- Resection with anastomosis results in a greater rate of successful ECF closure.

- Consider a temporary high jejunostomy for a period of 3–6 months with parenteral alimentation in patients requiring multiple ECF repairs and residual sepsis.
- The primary aim in closing the abdomen is to provide a biologic cover (skin) over exposed small bowel loops; the expertise of a plastic reconstructive surgeon may be crucial.
- The recovery of these patients is difficult and involves active participation from multidisciplinary teams where the surgeon plays the primary role.
- The surgery of fistula is the surgery for adhesions and understanding the biology of this process – timing is everything.

Enterocutaneous fistula (ECF) involving the small bowel continues to be a challenging problem. Patients are often nutritionally depleted and require meticulous and skilled management to achieve fistula closure. An ECF is defined as an abnormal communication between intestinal lumen and skin. Enterocutaneous fistula may result from one of several conditions. Fully 75–90% of ECFs are iatrogenic in origin (❷ *Fig. 63-1*) and arise by postoperative leakage from an intestinal anastomosis or from an inadvertent enterotomy during a procedure for inflammatory bowel disease, small bowel obstruction, or operations complicated by severe adhesions or radiation injury requiring extensive adhesiolysis. In contrast, fistulas may be secondary to inflammatory or malignant abnormalities of the bowel wall or from extension from surrounding structures into the bowel wall. The more common intra-abdominal conditions include Crohn's disease, radiation enteritis, or extension of adjacent disease to normal bowel such as with malignant conditions. When these processes involve the abdominal wall,

■ Figure 63-1

Complex postoperative enterocutaneous fistula in patient with Crohn's disease

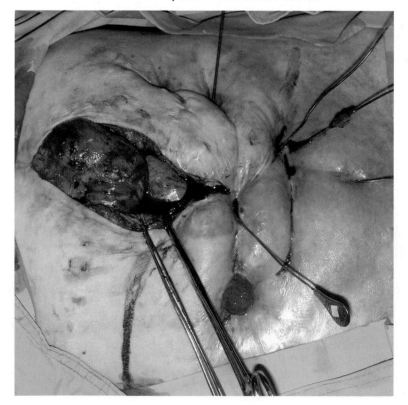

they can present as a spontaneous enterocutaneous fistula. This chapter focuses primarily on the management of postoperative ECFs; nevertheless, the majority of postoperative and spontaneous fistulas can be managed with the same basic principles of nutritional and surgical treatment despite their differing etiologies.

An ECF is often catastrophic to the health and quality of life of the patient. In the postoperative setting, patients are often septic and malnourished due to surgical stress and ongoing infectious processes. The goals of treatment in the patient with any ECF are closure of the defect and reconstitution of gastrointestinal continuity through an operative or nonoperative approach. Therefore, management of the ECF in the postoperative setting can be divided into three phases; acute, subacute, and repair with reconstruction.

Acute Phase

The presentation and recognition of a postoperative ECF usually occurs 5–10 days after an intra-abdominal operation. These patients usually have a prolonged initial recovery with persistent ileus and unknown source of fever; thereafter, the fistula presents with what usually looks like a wound infection, only later noted to be draining enteric content at the time of opening of the wound or after initial wound drainage and packing. With an early postoperative ECF, treatment will depend on the underlying cause, the volume of output (high output generally >500 ml vs. low output of <500 ml), time postoperatively, and presumed site of the fistula. Depending on the underlying cause, early reoperation with repair of an anastomotic leak, resection and reanastomosis, or fecal diversion in the form of an ileostomy or jejunostomy may be the procedure of choice. The time interval from the time of initial operation is also critical. It becomes important to note the favorable "window period" before considering any early reoperative procedure. We define this favorable window period as any time within 7–12 days from the most recent laparotomy. Within this favorable window period, the severity of adhesions is usually milder, and a repeat laparotomy with the intent of proximal intestinal diversion and/or repairing the fistula is justified; caring for a well-matured stoma is much easier than caring for an ECF. This approach will also increase the chance of enteral feeding rather than the need to manage the patient with parenteral nutrition and bowel rest with expectation of spontaneous closure of the ECF. After this window period, we usually defer any attempt of repeat laparotomy provided there is no associated peritonitis or ischemia of the intestine. If re-operation is chosen within or outside this window period, but the surgeon is confronted with a severe obliterative peritonitis precluding a safe adhesiolysis, it would be to the patient's benefit to accept defeat and end any further attempts at adhesiolysis with the intent of coming back at a minimum of 4–6 months later for re-exploration and definitive repair of the ECF, if spontaneous closure fails to occur. Aggressive attempts at complete adhesiolysis in patients with this type of obliterative peritonitis after the index surgery has the risk of further enterotomies, postoperative fistula formation, or worse, an extensive devascularization injury of the small bowel necessitating massive small bowel resection with the possible development of short bowel syndrome. An exception to the 10-day window period involves patients who develop an early ECF after an index operation that involved an extensive adhesiolysis; the favorable time window in these patients may be only 3 days.

The daily volume output of an ECF is also important. The greater the volume, the less chance of closure. An early, postoperative high output fistula suggests a more complete intestinal dehiscence or a distal intestinal obstruction and might precipitate an early re-operation. In contrast, a low output fistula suggests a less complete "diversion" of enteric content and might warrant a conservative, nonoperative approach to management.

Similarly, the presumed site of fistula may also be important. Proximal ECFs are more likely to have high output, less likely to close, will preclude oral feeding, and thus, may warrant a more aggressive operative approach. In contrast, a distal ECF is more likely low output, may allow oral nutrition, and would be more likely to close, depending, of course, on its etiology.

Whether the patient needs a relaparotomy versus a conservative approach, the initial management of the patient with a new ECF should be directed toward a timely and aggressive evaluation and resuscitation. Resuscitation is initiated with crystalloids to restore intravascular volume lost in the fistula drainage. Intravascular deficits may be exacerbated due to sepsis, intestinal obstruction, and edema in the bowel wall. Electrolyte imbalances should be replaced with frequent monitoring of serum electrolytes until stable levels are obtained. These imbalances usually involve potassium, sodium, magnesium, phosphate, calcium, and zinc. In addition to resuscitation, initial management of the ECF should include controlling the fistula drainage by pouching the opening (if possible) and protecting the surrounding skin. Control of the fistula output is often difficult, especially with multiple fistulas or with an open abdomen. An experienced enterostomal nurse therapist is indispensable in the care of the ECF patient during acute and subacute phases of these complex fistula and related wounds. The aim of the wound care is to obtain a pouchable effluent in order to minimize skin excoriation and the frequency of application of the stoma appliance.

Uncontrolled local or generalized sepsis, in association with malnutrition, are crucial determinants of mortality. Percutaneous drainage via computed tomography (CT) or ultrasound guidance is the initial management of choice in patients presenting with an ECF associated with a postoperative intra-abdominal abscess. This drainage may obviate the need for early operative intervention. A definitive procedure can be deferred with the drain left in to control further abscess formation. Aspirated material should be sent for microbiologic culture along with blood, urine, and sputum samples, if appropriate. In most instances, any change in the perioperative course clinically with features of systemic organ dysfunction is due to an undrained septic focus. Thus, prompt investigation and drainage should follow, by bedside ultrasonography or, if the patient is stable enough to be transported, by CT-guided drainage.

In select patients with complex multiple fistulas and an open abdomen who are usually beyond the "window period," pouching of the wound or the fistula alone and control of sepsis may not be possible. Also, re-laparotomy through the initial midline incision with adhesiolysis has the risk of further enterotomy, fistula formation, and devascularization of the small bowel with the possibility of causing a short bowel syndrome. In this group of patients, a left subcostal incision for creation of a high jejunostomy can be life-saving for the control of the chronic recurrent sepsis and may aid in the management of fistula-related drainage (❯ *Fig. 63-2*). We place this diverting stoma as far distally as possible and safe.

Subacute Phase

The subacute phase represents the time period from the control of sepsis until the time when the ECF heals spontaneously or the decision is made to proceed with definitive repair for re-establishment of gastrointestinal continuity. Once sepsis is controlled, initiation of full nutritional support is necessary. The availability of parenteral nutrition has reduced morbidity and mortality by permitting a period of conservative management during which many ECFs can be expected to close spontaneously.

◻ Figure 63-2
Creation of diverting high jejunostomy via left subcostal incision in patient with midline hostile abdomen with complex ECF and wound dehiscence

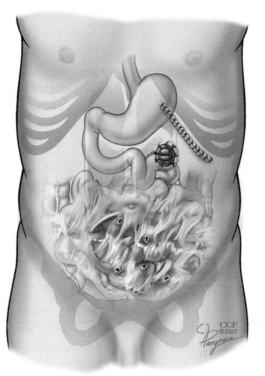

Closure is less likely if the fistula is complicated by inflammatory bowel disease, previous radiation therapy, malignancy, bowel discontinuity with large defects (greater >1 cm^2), distal obstruction, short fistula tracts with mucocutaneous continuity, persistent abscess, infection, foreign bodies such as nonabsorbable mesh, or granulomatous diseases/infections.

It is important to calculate accurately the patient's nutritional need to avoid underfeeding or overfeeding. Usually, 35–40 kcal/kg/day are required initially in men and 30–35 kcal/kg/day are required in women, but greater caloric requirements may be present if there is ongoing infection, underlying malnutrition, or if the patient has had multisystem trauma. Frequent use of metabolic cart analysis to measure resting energy expenditure can provide a more accurate estimate of caloric needs. The goal of nutritional support in this setting should be achieved with nitrogen equilibrium. The protein requirement of the patient with ECF is at least 1.5 g/kg/day. In complicated ECFs, consideration should be given to conducting a nitrogen balance study to measure protein needs more accurately.

Regular reassessments of the clinical progress of the patient and laboratory indicators of nutritional status are required to manage the nutritional progress of these patients. Weekly assessment of the transferin or prealbumin levels is helpful, because these protein concentrations serve as relatively acute phase indicators of the nutritional state of the patient. Parenteral nutrition formulas that will provide a calorie-to-nitrogen ratio of 100:1 to 150:1, while still supplying total caloric and protein needs should be utilized; ideally, 25–40% of total calories can be given as lipids. Fluid requirements for maintenance can be estimated from body surface area and adjusted for existing deficits and ongoing losses from the fistula. Weekly measurements of potassium, magnesium, sodium, and other common electrolytes are useful with supplementation if a deficiency is noted. Ideally, parenteral nutrition should be administered through a single-lumen central catheter.

For patients with a more proximal stoma, fistula output bypasses the majority of the distal small bowel, and this sets the stage for dehydration. The following advice is given to our patients on parenteral nutrition.

- Be aware of added risk factors for dehydration.
- Be aware of symptoms of dehydration – lassitude, fatigue, headache, nausea.
- Maintain intake of adequate oral liquids (if allowed), especially salty soups, electrolyte supplements, etc.
- Avoid high solid fiber/indigestible foods.
- Use liquid loperamide hydrochloride, diphenoxalate hydrochloride with atropine sulfate, liquid codeine, or tincture of opium dosed on a weight basis to thicken enteric output.

The use of somatostatin in the patient with an ECF has received much attention in recent years. Data provide mixed reports as to the overall effectiveness in promoting spontaneous fistula closure. There are data supporting the effectiveness of somatostatin in reducing fistula output, but fistula output does not always correlate with spontaneous closure rates; nevertheless, such decreases in volume and electrolyte losses can make the metabolic and electrolyte changes easier to manage. Therefore, we use somatostatin (100–600 μgm) and its analog octreotide only in patients with high output ECFs in whom the daily fluid requirements and electrolyte imbalance is difficult to regulate.

Early series of managing ECF reported the success of total parenteral nutrition in promoting fistula closure, and thus TPN remains the primary mode of nutritional support in the patient with an ECF to achieve either spontaneous closure or maintain nutritional neutrality until the definitive operative closure. Recent studies, however, have proven that enteral nutrition, when able to be given successfully, has a superior outcome, because it provides the advantages of preserving gastrointestinal mucosa, as well as supporting the immunologic and hormonal functions of the gut and the liver. Enteral feeding also avoids the problem of line sepsis with parenteral feeding. In our experience, we use enteral nutrition whenever possible, especially in patients with low output fistulas (<200 ml/day). For distal ECF, selected "elemental" enteral formulas that deliver pre-digested nutrients (glucose, amino acids, medium chain triglycerides) will minimize fistula output. In contrast, for very proximal ECF, enteral nutrition may be administered distal to the fistula using the residual gut; again, if all the pancreato-biliary secretions are diverted through the fistula, an elemental enteral formula is required unless the fistula output itself is re-administered distally. Although unpleasant and cumbersome, this approach will minimize volume, caloric, electrolyte, and bile salt/cholesterol losses. Nevertheless, while this approach may be the preferred mode of nutritional supplementation in the management of low output fistulas, enteral delivery that is manageable by the patient can be challenging technically, and cumbersome to find and adjust. There is some evidence to support the concept of delivering enteral nutrition at rates unable to supply total caloric needs alone, while still delivering the requisite caloric needs by parenteral nutrition. These lesser rates of enteral calories may maintain gut health and thereby aid recovery.

The fistula wound continues to require special care at this phase, because surgical procedures for permanent closure should not be performed through a septic, indurated, macerated, infected, or denuded abdominal wall. Once again, collaboration by a multidisciplinary approach with enterostomal nursing expertise is important in providing the continual support to these patients, their families, and healthcare workers.

As outlined during the acute and subacute phases of ECF management, strategies for successful resolution of ECF include control of sepsis with imaging-guided drainage and antibiotic therapy, skin protection with stoma care, maintenance of full nutritional supplementation, and fluid and electrolyte balance. In some patients, ECF closure can also be promoted with vacuum-assisted closure systems or fibrin glue, although these techniques have not been evaluated in large series and are not yet approved for this use. While many ECF will close with these conservative strategies, persistent fistulas require definitive surgical intervention. If fistula closure has not occurred after 4–6 weeks of adequate nutritional support and in the absence of sepsis, it is unlikely that fistula will close spontaneously. In most series, 80–90% of the fistulas that eventually close spontaneously will have done so by this time. Therefore, after 6–8 weeks, plans for operative repair should begin.

The timing of repair depends on the clinical situation, presence of multiple adhesions at the time of the original operation, and medical/nutritional state, as described above. This operative repair may involve a major laparotomy and should be delayed to allow resolution of intra-abdominal inflammatory adhesions for patients in the early postoperative phase. The postoperative peritoneal reaction is maximal from the second to tenth postoperative week and may be exacerbated and complicated by peritonitis or local reaction to the fistula formation. Retrospective studies have shown that mortality is doubled in patients who require re-operation during this subacute time frame of 2–10 weeks postoperatively. In many patients with a complicated ECF, it may be beneficial to delay operative repair of the ECF up to 6 months from the date of the initial procedure. This delay allows for adequate healing of any intrabdominal sepsis and for softening of adhesions, and a much easier operation which will result in a better outcome. An even longer delay may be prudent in patients with a long complicated postoperative course, intraperitoneal sepsis, and malnutrition. Clinical judgement is very important in such a setting.

During this subacute phase until the definitive repair is undertaken, the external drainage of a fistula can become demoralizing and humiliating for the patient. A multidisciplinary approach under the leadership of a surgeon with a trained, enterostomal therapy nurse, parenteral nutrition team, physical and occupational therapist, social worker, and even psychiatrist, are invaluable. Continued reassurance, availability, and affability from the physician will help in this situation. If necessary, psychotropic medications or treatment by psychiatric consulting services are beneficial.

Repair and Reconstructive Phase

Surgery for the definitive repair involves a major laparotomy. The patients and their family should be prepared emotionally and mentally for a prolonged recovery with the potential of recurrence and complications. Therefore, it is imperative that operations to correct an ECF be performed under optimal conditions. Optimal nutritional status and absence of associated sepsis are important parameters that must be obtained prior to definitive operative repair.

Avoiding the Unexpected

Patients need to have complete evaluation with deficiencies corrected whenever possible. The properly prepared patient should have adequate transferin, prealbumin, hemoglobin, and coagulation levels prior to operation. Diabetes should be controlled, and the patient should not be anemic. Blood should be available, because the majority of these patients have had prior transfusions, and it may be difficult to get proper cross-matched blood at the time of operation if it is needed. Parenteral nutrition should be continued until the date of operation; if a patient is on additional enteral nutrition, this should be stopped 48–72 h beforehand to decrease contamination or associated bowel distention that may complicate the laparotomy.

It is imperative to evaluate these patients fully and be prepared for unexpected findings at the time of definitive operative repair. It is our practice to study every orifice prior to operative repair; trying to dissect out all of the bowel may not be necessary. These tests usually include fistulograms, gastrograffin enemas, small bowel series, and stoma injection. It is imperative to rule out any distal obstruction or associated inflammatory bowel disease or other pathology such as radiation enteritis, malignancy, or granulomatous disease prior to operation. The use of CT is less helpful in delineating site or mucosal details in the evaluation of the fistula patient without sepsis at this stage of the management; in contrast, CT can be valuable in the search for abdominal abscess or associated pathology in the fistula patient prior to definitive surgery. These radiologic studies provide a road map to identify the anatomy and planes and may be crucial to avoid surprises in the operating room. Preoperative marking by an experienced enterostomal nurse is also prudent, even in patients in whom definitive repair is planned. On rare occasions, the repair may be tenuous, and a controlled, well-located proximal loop enterostomy may aid healing of the primary repair and allow an easier, early restoration of full intestinal continuity without the need for a full laparotomy. This loop enterostomy can be taken down by a more localized perisomal approach.

The Operative Repair

The operation may very well be a long procedure. Therefore, the first rule for the surgeon is not to overbook for that day. It would be important to schedule these complicated cases as the first case and not to schedule any other difficult case for that day. The surgical team should be prepared to obtain assistance from other disciplines such as gynecology, urology, plastics, and any other pertinent reconstructive teams. We usually position the patient in the Lloyd Davis stirrups with arms by the side and shoulder pads for extreme Trendelenburg position, especially for complex cases that involve the deep pelvis. We use ureteric stents liberally to avoid any unrecognized injury and to minimize the time required to identify the ureters during the operation. The availability of lighted retractors is also important. Access to the perineum is often necessary.

Technique of Adhesiolysis and Strategy of Relaparotomy, Repair, and Reconstruction

We begin the operation by entering the abdomen through the easiest place, usually the most cranial part of the abdomen from an area of new or prior midline incision. To accomplish this, we are not hesitant to make a big incision above the umbilicus up to the xyphoid level; the midline incision preserves as much of the abdominal wall as possible for any future stoma, and optimizes exposure and visibility. The goal of the initial phase of the operation is to free all adhesions, drain any remnant abscesses, and relieve all obstructed segments of bowel. Ideally, the entire of length of the small bowel from the ligament of Treitz to the cecum is freed of adhesions. The ECF are left in place until the bowel around them is freed. Our practice is to deliver the matted loops outside the abdomen, decompress the bowel, especially for interloop dissection, and use saline injection with hydro- and extrafascial dissection to avoid an inadvertent injury to the bowel. For hydro-dissection, we use sterile normal saline and a # 21 gauge long needle with a 10 ml syringe. The application of saline into the matted loops of small bowel or between the fascia creates a safer plane for sharp dissection and avoids inadvertent enterotomy. Sharp dissection from known to unknown, leaving the most difficult section untill last is our usual strategy. Immediate closure of all inadvertent enterotomies and repair of serosal tears will minimize the chance of missing or forgetting to repair these injuries after a long procedure, and avoids further leak with fistula formation in the postoperative period. Successful operation requires the resection of the ECF and associated diseased bowel, usually with a primary, handsewn anastomosis with absorbable sutures. The anastomosis should be distant from the site of any fistula or abscess cavity. In a recent study from our institution, resection with anastomosis resulted in a greater rate of successful ECF closure compared with fistula oversewing or wedge resection. In our past experience, a fistula was oversewn or wedge-resected when it was not thought possible to perform resection due to an inability to adequately mobilize the bowel itself; with this approach, the recurrence rate was unacceptable. If this is the case, or in patients with complex, multiple fistula sites, when the repair is close to any residual sepsis, or in patients with relatively suboptimal nutritional parameters (albumin is <3 g/dl), we strongly consider a temporary, diverting, proximal jejunostomy for a period of 3–6 months with parenteral alimentation.

Prior to abdominal closure, the entire bowel surface should be inspected again very carefully to be certain that no unrecognized injuries exist. It is sometimes useful to check the adequacy of repair by inflating air (via syringe) into the bowel after filling the abdomen with saline to look for air leaks. Irrigation with a copious amount of warm saline is important. This practice increases the body temperature and corrects the associated coagulopathy after prolonged dissection and recovery from the anesthesia. We use closed suction drains in patients with no associated sepsis, whereas silastic passive drains are preferred in patients in the presence of residual sepsis. In patients with a prolonged operation and extensive dissection due to severe adhesions, we prefer to place a gastrostomy tube to avoid discomfort and the complications associated with a long-term nasogastric tube in the management of postoperative ileus. If possible, the omentum should be placed between the anastomosis and the incision.

Abdominal wall closure in patients with complex ECF can be challenging due to prior abdominal wall loss secondary to sepsis, evisceration, or herniation. Bowel wall edema with distention can also complicate the primary closure in these patients, especially with marked fluid administration. A primary abdominal closure is the preferred technique where possible. We avoid using permanent prosthetic material for abdominal closure, as this can lead to further fistulization. The primary aim in closing the abdomen of these patients is to bring the fascia and, whenever possible, the skin back together. Ventral hernias can be repaired later with synthetic mesh. The lateral release of the external oblique aponeurosis (components separation) can be helpful to allow primary fascia closure. If primary fascia closure is not possible, we use a technique of mobilizing full thickness skin flaps as lateral as possible, and close the skin tension-free with polypropylene suture in vertical mattress fashion over dental roles and staples to avoid any skin tear or necrosis (❍ *Figs. 63-3* and ❍ *63-4*). When fascial approximation is not possible, it is important to lay the omentum or, or when no omentum is available, either a bioprosthesis like Alloderm or an absorbable polyglycolic acid mesh under this skin

◘ Figure 63-3
Abdominal wall closure at skin level with 1.0 polypropylene suture in vertical mattress over dental roles where primary fascia closure is not possible

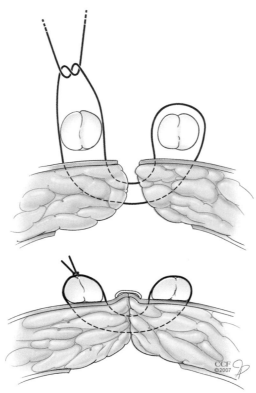

closure in case of wound breakdown; the omentum or the absorbable mesh can be covered with a skin graft or a vacuum-assisted dressing. We work with a plastic surgery team who has a special interest in and understanding of the pathophysiology of these complex cases; a musculocutaneous flap may be needed for primary closure or, in cases of direct exposure of the small bowel after the breakdown of the initial closure, a split-thickness skin graft. Skin grafting within less than 72 h is important to avoid any further breakdown and fistulization of the small bowel.

The recovery of these patients can be difficult and prolonged. Active participation from a multidisciplinary team is imperative. The surgeon plays the primary role with assurance and emotional and mental support. Parenteral nutrition support in the postoperative period is essential and should be given until ileus resolves.

Summary

The management of ECF is often a difficult problem. The principles of management involve control of sepsis and fistula output with adequate nutritional support. Early operative intervention in established ECF should be limited to abscess drainage and formation of a proximal defunctioning stoma for fistula effluent or sepsis control. The surgery of ECF is the surgery for adhesions, control of sepsis, and understanding the biology of this entire process – timing is everything. Definitive procedures for persistent ECF should be delayed to 4–6 months later with resection of the fistula and anastomosis of

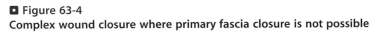

□ Figure 63-4
Complex wound closure where primary fascia closure is not possible

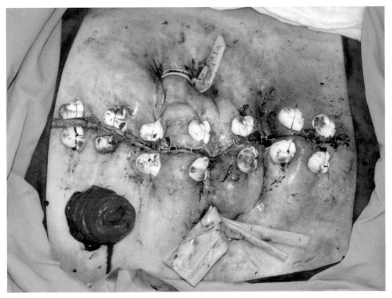

the healthy bowel. A low threshold is maintained for a defunctioning proximal stoma, particularly in the presence of residual sepsis, radiation enteritis, and Crohn's disease with multiple repair or resections. Operative and nonoperative management strategy, in the setting of a tertiary institution with access to multispecialty care, should result in a successful level of ECF closure with a low mortality and acceptable morbidity.

Selected Readings

Gibson SW, Fischer JE (2004) Enterocutaneous fistula. In: Fazio VW, Church JW, Delaney CP (eds) Current therapy in colon and rectal surgery. Mosby, St Louis, MO pp. 479–484

Gunn LA, Follmar KE, Wong MS, et al. (2006) Management of enterocutaneous fistulas using negative pressure dressings. Ann Plast Surg 57:621–625

Lynch CA, Delaney CP, Senagore AJ, et al. (2004) Clinical outcome and factors predictive of recurrence after enterocutaneous fistula surgery. Ann Surg 240:825–831

Makhdoom ZA, Komar MJ, Still CD (2003) Nutrition and enterocutaneous fistulas. J Clin Gastroenterol 31:195–204

Shetty V, Teubner A, Morrison K, Scott NA (2006) Proximal loop jejunostomy is a useful adjunct in the management of multiple intestinal suture lines in the septic abdomen. Brit J Surg 93:1247–1250

Worsey MJ, Fazio VW (2002) Reoperative pelvic surgery. In: Zuidema GD, Yeo CJ (eds) Shackelford's surgery of the alimentary tract, 5th edn, vol. 4. Elsevier, New York pp. 519–527

Part 5

Small Bowel: Malignant

64 Adenocarcinoma of the Small Bowel

Shailesh V. Shrikhande · Supreeta Arya

Pearls and Pitfalls

- Malignant neoplasms of the small intestine are uncommon and account for less than 1% of all gastrointestinal (GI) tract neoplasms.
- Thirty-five percent to 50% of small bowel neoplasms are adenocarcinomas.
- Small bowel adenocarcinoma (SBA) is found in decreasing order of frequency in the duodenum, jejunum, and ileum.
- Geographic correlation between large and small bowel cancer suggests shared etiologies.
- Hereditary cancer syndromes, such as familial adenomatous polyposis (FAP), hereditary non-polyposis colorectal cancer (HNPCC), and Peutz-Jeghers syndrome (PJS), are all linked to development of SBA.
- Crohn's disease is associated with an increased risk of SBA with a risk approximately 12-fold greater than the general population.
- Remember to consider a small bowel neoplasm when patients present with non-specific abdominal complaints or unexplained anemia.
- SBA is detected earlier than other small intestinal cancers. In particular, adenocarcinomas of the ampulla and the duodenum manifest earlier than SBA elsewhere in the jejunum and ileum. Thus, SBA in this region results in obstructive jaundice which aids in a somewhat earlier detection.
- Diagnostic tests to be used include upper gastrointestinal endoscopy, colonoscopy, computed tomography, and lastly a small bowel study to visualize the small bowel, especially if the upper and lower gastrointestinal studies are negative. Double contrast small bowel examination, or enteroclysis, is currently the best technique that can be employed for accurate information regarding the status of the small intestine.
- Operative resection is the treatment of choice and the only therapeutic modality with a curative potential.
- Pancreatoduodenectomy and local ampullary excision are the two available options for duodenal/ampullary disease.
- Local resection of periampullary neoplasms has a high rate of recurrence (5–30%) and requires an aggressive long-term postoperative endoscopic surveillance.
- Small bowel resection with wide surgical margins is the treatment for SBA located in the duodenum as well as in the jejunum and ileum.

- Distal ileal lesions may necessitate a right hemicolectomy.
- Five-year survival after resection is approximately 30% with a median survival of 20 months.
- Adjuvant treatment has no definite role in SBA except possibly in periampullary adenocarcinoma.

Introduction

The length of the small intestine is approximately 5 to 7 m and constitutes 60% of the gastrointestinal (GI) tract. Despite its length and an exposure to a wide spectrum of carcinogens, malignant neoplasms of the small intestine are uncommon and account for less than 1% of all GI tract neoplasms. The age-adjusted incidence of small bowel malignancies is 1/100,000 with a prevalence of 0.6%. Compared with other GI neoplasms, information about small intestinal malignant neoplasms is rather limited, and this is not surprising given that estimated malignant neoplasms of the small intestine are 40–70 times less common than colonic carcinoma. Despite the fact that the small intestine represents 90% of the absorptive surface of the GI tract, the average, annual, age-adjusted incidence of small bowel cancer is 50 times less common than colorectal cancer in the United States. While 35–50% of small bowel neoplasms are adenocarcinomas, 20–40% are carcinoids, 5–14% are lymphomas, and 15% are sarcomas (i.e. Gastrointestinal Stromal Tumors, or GIST). Small bowel adenocarcinoma accounts for 2% of GI neoplasms and 1% of GI cancer deaths.

The sites at highest risk of developing malignant neoplasms are the duodenum for adenocarcinoma and the ileum for carcinoids and lymphomas. Small bowel adenocarcinoma (SBA) is found in decreasing order of frequency in the duodenum, jejunum, and ileum. Recently, incidence data from the Surveillance, Epidemiology, and End Results (SEER) program (1973–2000) were used to analyze the four histologic types of small bowel cancer, viz., adenocarcinomas, carcinoid neoplasms, lymphomas, and sarcomas. This study observed that men had higher rates than women for all types of small bowel cancer. African-Americans had almost double the incidence of carcinomas and carcinoid neoplasms compared to Caucasians (10.6 vs. 5.6 per million people; 9.2 vs. 5.4 per million people, respectively). Furthermore, the geographic correlation between large and small bowel cancer suggested shared etiologies.

Risk Factors and Pathogenesis

In a study evaluating risk factors for SBA, the intake of bread, pasta, or rice appeared to increase directly the risk of small bowel cancer. In contrast, risk correlated inversely with coffee, fish, vegetables, and fruit. These results seem to suggest that dietary correlates of SBA are similar to those of colon cancer and at least of the same magnitude. While this particular study failed to confirm a definite association between smoking and alcohol consumption and development of small bowel cancer, other studies have shown that such a relationship exists. Epithelial cells of the GI tract are often exposed to toxic agents such as 7, 12-dimethylbenzanthracene (DMBA), the phenothiazines, and benzpyrene.

◘ Table 64-1

Clinical conditions predisposing to increased risk of small bowel cancer

Hereditary non-polyposis colorectal cancer syndrome (HNPCC)
Peutz-Jegher syndrome (PJS)
Familial adenomatous polyposis syndrome (FAP)
Crohn's disease
Celiac disease
Neurofibromatosis type I (NF-I)

Clinical Conditions Predisposing to Increased Risk of SBA

A number of clinical conditions are known to increase the risk of SBA. Hereditary cancer syndromes, such as familial adenomatous polyposis (FAP), hereditary non-polyposis colorectal cancer (HNPCC), and Peutz-Jeghers syndrome (PJS), are all linked to development of SBA. The lifetime risk of developing an HNPCC-related SBA is estimated to range 1–4%, which is 100 times greater than in the general population. Compared to the general population, SBA in the setting of HNPCC presents at an earlier age and carries a better prognosis compared to sporadic SBA. For PJS, a meta-analysis revealed a greater risk of gastrointestinal cancer and more specifically for SBA associated with PJS. There is evidence to suggest that PJS-related cancers have different underlying molecular genetic alterations compared with SBA that arise in the sporadic setting. Duodenal adenomas which are usually located around the ampulla of Vater for unknown reasons occur in 31–92% patients of FAP. Endoscopic examination at periodic intervals may be worthwhile to screen for early neoplasms in these FAP patients. Crohn's disease is also associated with an increased risk of SBA of 12-fold greater than the general population. In Crohn's disease, the small bowel neoplasms appear at a younger age compared to sporadic SBA and tend to be more common in the distal part of the small intestine where the Crohn's disease is usually active. Most SBAs associated with Crohn's disease are localized within an inflammatory stricture, where they are often responsible for obstructive disease. Risk factors for SBA in patients of Crohn's disease include male sex, previous surgical bypass loops, chronic fistulous disease, and long-standing disease of at least 10 years. Celiac disease has also been linked to development of SBA; however, its etiology remains uncertain. A distinctive feature of celiac disease-associated SBA is that the neoplasms tend to be localized in the jejunum and are often lymphomas. The various clinical conditions predisposing to SBA are listed in ❷ *Table 64-1*.

Molecular Genetics of SBA

The adenoma-carcinoma sequence in colorectal cancer represents a series of well-defined molecular changes consisting of activation of oncogenes and inactivation of tumor suppressor genes that accompany the histologic progression to invasive cancer. While similarities between small bowel and large bowel cancer suggest that they share many of the molecular changes of carcinogenesis, clear evidence is either lacking or limited. In a recent study evaluating the genetic pathway of SBA, Wheeler and colleagues investigated the expression of mismatch repair genes hMLH1 and hMSH2, the adenomatous polyposis coli (APC) gene, β–catenin, E-cadherin, and p53 in SBA. They did not observe any

◼ Table 64-2

Possible reasons for rarity of small bowel adenocarcinoma compared to colorectal cancers

Shorter bowel transit time with reduced exposure between mucosa and carcinogens
Large volume of secretions dilute insult of carcinogens on mucosa
Bacterial degradation of bile salts does not occur in small intestine
Lower level of anerobes in small intestine
Presence of abundant lymphoid tissue
Rapid proliferation of small bowel cells causes competitive inhibition of malignant cells at tumor site

mutations in the mutation cluster region (MCR) of the APC gene, which suggests that adenocarcinoma of the small intestine may follow a somewhat different genetic pathway to colorectal cancer. Furthermore, abnormal expression of β-catenin and E-cadherin suggested an early pathway in which mutations could be found in SBA. Overexpression of p53 is a frequent finding. Similar to colorectal cancer, this event reflects its important role in carcinogenesis in the small intestine. A number of studies have detected K-ras mutations in 14–83% of cases of SBA; however, this difference was reported over a wide range, because the number of duodenal adenocarcinomata within these studies were often of a small sample size. Some authors demonstrated complete concordance in K-ras mutations between tissues from adenocarcinomas and contiguous adenomas in their case series. This observation suggests a relationship between the conventional adenoma-carcinoma sequence and K-ras mutation in small bowel cancer. The oncogene c-neu is altered in approximately 50% of sporadic colorectal cancer cases; in SBA, 60% of these neoplasms were positive for this mutation. Furthermore, oncogene expression was noted to increase directly with tumor grade. Patients with c-neu positive neoplasms had a shorter survival compared to those with c-neu negative neoplasms. The potential reasons for the rarity of small bowel adenocarcinoma compared to colorectal cancer are provided in ❯ *Table 64-2*.

Clinical Presentation and Diagnosis

Unfortunately, small bowel tumors and cancers usually do not manifest with definite classic symptoms. Therefore, it is important to consider a small bowel tumor when patients present with non-specific abdominal complaints or unexplained anemia. The usual diagnostic tests used in the presence of such complaints are upper gastrointestinal endoscopy, colonoscopy, and lastly small bowel radiography to visualize the small bowel, especially if the upper and lower gastrointestinal studies are negative. Another symptom which an alert clinician could suspect and diagnose a small bowel tumor is that of insidious bowel obstruction – colicky abdominal pain and a sensation of abdominal distension. A plain x-ray of the abdomen during such episodes of "non-specific" abdominal complaints may reveal air fluid levels and point to a small bowel obstruction. Such a finding, however, indicates that the disease has progressed beyond the "early stage" of small bowel cancer. In early stage or asymptomatic small bowel cancers, plain x-rays of the abdomen have their limitations as does the barium meal follow-through which is widely available, simple, and inexpensive, but insensitive for detection of small or early SBA. Instead, double-contrast small bowel examination or enteroclysis is the best technique currently that can be employed for accurate information regarding the status of the small intestine. Barium and methylcellulose are infused in the small bowel under pressure which produces distension of the small bowel, thereby enabling the radiologist to follow the contrast material throughout its course in the small intestine. Furthermore, this examination offers the advantage of evaluating the mucosa for irregularities; hence this method is the best technique that is available widely and relatively inexpensive. Computerized tomography-aided enteroclysis, combining CT with enteroclysis, is considered an even better diagnostic test in small bowel cancers (❯ *Fig. 64-1*). The ability to image accurately a small intestinal neoplasm, independent of its size, anatomic localization, and growth characteristics, represents a major improvement in the diagnosis and management of small bowel cancer (❯ *Fig. 64-2*). The most recent investigational development has been the introduction of capsule endoscopy in addition to push enteroscopy, Sonde enteroscopy, and intraoperative or laparoscopically-assisted enteroscopy. Capsule endoscopy consists of a video capsule that is swallowed and transmits images from the small intestine. The major limitation with this technique is the lack of external control over the position and orientation of the capsule and the high cost of this technology. Push enteroscopy enables examination of the jejunum for 40–60 cm distal to the ligament of Treitz with the help of a longer endoscope. Intraoperative endoscopy is a variant of push enteroscopy in which the surgeon can

❏ Figure 64-1
Axial section of CT enteroclysis showing water distended normal small bowel loops with thin smooth walls

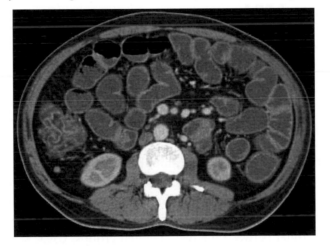

❏ Figure 64-2
Axial contrast enhanced CT showing concentric wall thickening in a short segment of small bowel (ileum) confirmed histologically to be adenocarcinoma (From the Archives of Department of Radiology, KEM Hospital, Mumbai, India. Courtesy of Professor Ravi Ramakantan)

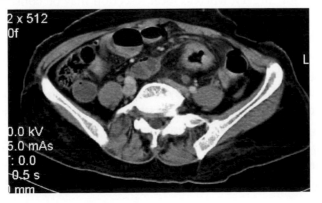

guide the endoscope inserted per orally or a colonoscope passed per rectum. Intraoperative endoscopy should, however, be the last resort for the clinician in suspected early stage small bowel cancer, because it is a major invasive procedure involving laparotomy.

In duodenal and ampullary adenocarcinoma, the presentation is somewhat different, and usually with signs and symptoms of upper abdominal pain, gastric outlet obstruction, and jaundice.

Treatment of SBA

SBA is detected earlier than other small intestinal cancers. In particular, adenocarcinomas of the ampulla and the duodenum manifest earlier than SBA elsewhere in the jejunum and ileum. Thus, SBA in this region results in obstructive jaundice which occasionally aids in a somewhat earlier detection. Despite this observation, the majority of SBA are metastatic at the time of diagnosis.

Surgical Treatment of SBA

Duodenal and Ampullary Adenocarcinoma

Operative resection is the treatment of choice and the only therapeutic modality with a curative potential. Pancreatoduodenectomy and local ampullary excision are the two available options. Local resection has a high rate of recurrence (5–30%) and requires postoperative endoscopic surveillance, which is the reason it is not considered as a first choice in the management of ampullary neoplasms. In a study evaluating 92 patients with cancer of the ampulla of Vater, 10 were treated with local resection, 49 with pancreatic resection, and 33 underwent only a laparotomy without resection. When the main outcome measures of postoperative morbidity and mortality, surgical radicality, and long-term survival were evaluated, the postoperative complication rate was significantly less after local resection, whereas mortality did not differ between the two operated groups. UICC stages were significantly less advanced in the local resection group; also, the frequency of positive resection margins and R0 resections was the same in both groups, as was long-term survival. The local recurrence rate, however, was 80% after local resection and 22% after pancreatic resection. The conclusion was that pancreatoduodenectomy should be the *preferred* operation for cancer of the ampulla of Vater in patients who are fit for major surgery, whereas local resection may be considered in carefully selected patients. A number of other earlier studies have also reached similar conclusions.

Because local resection is less invasive, it has been argued that it is potentially an equally effective alternative for cancers with favorable prognostic features. Thus, identification of these prognostic parameters may allow selection of some patients suitable for local resection. In a study evaluating 25 patients with primary adenocarcinoma of ampulla treated by pancreatoduodenectomy and local resection, it was observed that T-staging could predict the risk of tumor recurrence and could be determined accurately using endoscopic ultrasonography. Local resection was concluded to be a suitable alternative to pancreatoduodenal resection in patients with T1- and T2-adenocarcinomas with a maximum diameter of 3 cm or less. A word of caution about local ampullary resection is required. This procedure can be demanding and requires skill and understanding of the local anatomy;

it is inadvisable for an inexperienced general surgeon to proceed with this operation without advice from an experienced biliary-pancreatic surgeon.

In summary, with an operative mortality of 5% or less for pancreatoduodenectomy, it is currently the procedure of choice at most experienced centers for invasive carcinoma, foci of papillary adenocarcinoma in pre-excisional biopsies, or in ampullary adenomas with high-grade dysplasia. Ampullectomy is reserved for benign adenomas. It must be acknowledged that pancreatoduodenectomy is curative in 80% of patients with node-negative ampullary carcinomas; once 3-year survival is reached, long-term survival can be expected. The choice of treatment, however, depends on the level of surgical skill available, availability of endoscopic ultrasonography, and local expertise, patient compliance, and the presence or absence of co-existing familial adenomatous polyposis. Non-ampullary duodenal adenomas (FAP) can also be treated by a pancreas-preserving duodenectomy. An experienced biliopancreatic surgeon is crucial to ensure safe outcomes with use of this uncommon procedure.

❷ *Table 64-3* lists the outcomes of major series ampullary and duodenal adenocarcinoma treated by pancreatoduodenectomy. The various prognostic factors influencing survival in duodenal and ampullary adenocarcinoma are provided in ❷ *Table 64-4*. Patients with unresectable lesions should be treated symptomatically. Biliary obstruction and jaundice should be treated by endoscopic stenting (plastic/metallic stenting), while gastroduodenal obstruction is treated by palliative surgical gastric bypass.

◘ Table 64-3

Major series of outcomes after treatment of ampullary and duodenal adenocarcinoma with pancreatoduodenectomy

Tumor location	Author	5-year survival
Ampulla (overall)	De Castro SM et al., 2004	37%
Ampulla (overall)	Di Giorgio et al., 2005	64.4%
Ampulla (overall)	Roberts RH et al., 1999	46%
Ampulla (node negative)	Brown et al., 2005	78%
Ampulla (T1 and T2 lesions)	Brown et al., 2005	73%
Ampulla (well differentiated)	Brown et al., 2005	76%
Ampulla (node positive)	Brown et al., 2005	25%
Ampulla (T3 and T4 tumors)	Brown et al., 2005	8%
Ampulla (moderately/poorly differentiated)	Brown et al., 2005	36%
Duodenal	Schmidt et al., 2004	42% (3-year survival)
Ampulla		53% (3-year survival)
Duodenal	Sun et al., 2004	45.4%
Duodenal	Bakaeen et al., 2000	54%
Duodenal	Sohn et al., 1998	53%

◘ Table 64-4

Prognostic factors influencing survival in duodenal and ampullary adenocarcinoma

Lymph node positivity
Type of surgery (pancreatoduodenectomy vs. local resection)
Experience of the treating center in major resectional surgery
(<16 pancreatoduodenectomies/year)
Patient age (>75 years)
Patient reluctance for major definitive surgery (>75 years)

Jejunal and Ileal Adenocarcinoma

These lesions are treated by radical, segmental small bowel resection en bloc with the mesentery and its lymphatic drainage. Adequate proximal and distal pathologically negative margins must be ensured. Equally good results are achieved by both hand-sewn and stapler anastomoses. Terminal ileal lesions may have to treated by right hemicolectomy.

Management of Advanced Disease

Management of this state offers special challenges especially for those who are not eligible for palliative surgery. Treatment revolves around nasogastric aspiration, intravenous fluids, total parenteral nutrition, and in some cases antispasmodic agents.

Adjuvant Treatment for SBA

The leading cause of death from SBA is distant metastatic disease. This observation suggests that adjuvant chemotherapy should have a role in management of SBA. Unfortunately, no chemotherapy in use is of proven benefit, although many periampullary adenocarcinomas may be given adjuvant therapy with an occasional excellent result.

Conclusion

Early diagnosis is crucial for the definitive treatment of SBA. Oncologic surgery provides superior outcomes, thus, referral to specialist centers is to be preferred. According to a landmark study by the American College of Surgeons Commission on Cancer, the overall 5-year disease-specific survival of 5000 SBAs was 31% with a median survival of 20 months. Adjuvant chemotherapy is of unproven benefit in all SBA.

Selected Readings

Bakaeen FG, Murr MM, Sarr MG, Thompson GB, Farnell MB, Nagorney DM, Farley DR, van Heerden JA, Wiersema LM, Schleck CD, Donohue JH (2000). What prognostic factors are important in duodenal adenocarcinoma? Arch Surg. 135(6):635–641; discussion 641–2

Brown KM, Tompkins AJ, Yong S, et al. (2005) Pancreaticoduodenectomy is curative in the majority of patients with node-negative ampullary cancer. Arch Surg 140:529–532; discussion 532–533

de Castro SM, van Heek NT, Kuhlmann KF, et al. (2004) Surgical management of neoplasms of the ampulla of Vater: local resection or pancreatoduodenectomy and prognostic factors for survival. Surgery 136:994–1002

Delaunoit T, Neczyporenko F, Limburg PJ, Erlichman C (2005) Pathogenesis and risk factors of small bowel adenocarcinoma: a colorectal cancer sibling? Am J Gastroenterol 100:703–710

Di Giorgio A, Alfieri S, Rotondi F, et al. (2005) Pancreatoduodenectomy for tumors of Vater's ampulla: report on 94 consecutive patients. World J Surg 29:513–518

Frost DB, Mercado PD, Tyrell JS (1994) Small bowel cancer: a 30-year review. Ann Surg Oncol 1:290–295

Haselkorn T, Whittemore AS, Lilienfeld DE (2005) Incidence of small bowel cancer in the United States and worldwide: geographic, temporal, and racial differences. Cancer Causes Control 16:781–787

Howe JR, Karnell LH, Menck HR, Scott-Conner C (1999) The American College of Surgeons Commission on Cancer and the American Cancer Society. Adenocarcinoma of the small bowel: review of the National Cancer Data Base, 1985–1995. Cancer 86:2693–706

Jones DV, Skibber J, Levin B (1998) Adenocarcinoma and other small intestinal neoplasms, including benign tumors. In: Feldman M, Scharschmidt BF (eds) Sleisenger gastrointestinal and liver disease. W.B. Saunders, Philadelphia, pp. 1858–1865

Lewis JD, Deren JJ, Lichtenstein GR (1999) Cancer risk in patients with inflammatory bowel disease. Gastroenterol Clin North Am 28:459–77

Lynch HT, Smyrk TC, Lynch PM, et al. (1989) Adenocarcinoma of the small bowel in lynch syndrome II. Cancer 64:2178–2183

Roberts RH, Krige JE, Bornman PC, Terblanche J (1999). Pancreaticoduodenectomy of ampullary carcinoma. Am Surg. 65(11):1043–1048

Schmidt CM, Powell ES, Yiannoutsos CT, et al. (2004) Pancreaticoduodenectomy: a 20-year experience in 516 patients. Arch Surg 139:718–275; discussion 725–727

Sohn TA, Lillemoe KD, Cameron JL, Pitt HA, Kaufman HS, Hruban RH, Yeo CJ (1998). Adenocarcinoma of the duodenum: factors influencing long-term survival. J Gastrointest Surg. 2(1):79–87

Sun JJ, Wu ZY (2004). Treatment of 54 cases of primary malignant duodenal tumor. Zhonghua Wai Ke Za Zhi., 42 (5):276–278

Talamonti MS, Goetz LH, Rao S, Joehl RJ (2002) Primary cancers of the small bowel: analysis of prognostic factors and results of surgical management. Arch Surg 137:564–570; discussion 570–571

Vasen HF, Wijnen JT, Menko FH, et al. (1996) Cancer risk in families with hereditary nonpolyposis colorectal cancer diagnosed by mutation analysis. Gastroenterology 110:1020–1027

Wheeler JM, Warren BF, Mortensen NJ, et al. (2002) An insight into the genetic pathway of adenocarcinoma of the small intestine. Gut 50:218–223

Younes N, Fulton N, Tanaka R, et al. (1997) The presence of K-12 ras mutations in duodenal adenocarcinomas and the absence of ras mutations in other small bowel adenocarcinomas and carcinoid tumors. Cancer 79:1804–1808

65 Lymphoma of the Small Bowel

Wing-Yan Au · Raymond H. S. Liang

Pearls and Pitfalls

- Lymphoma of the small bowel present with local gastrointestinal or systemic symptoms, including malabsorption, mass lesions, bowel obstruction, bleeding, and/or systemic symptoms.
- The most common histology is diffuse large B-cell lymphoma, but mucosa-associated lymphoid tissue lymphoma (MALToma), mantle cell lymphoma, and mature T-cell lymphoma can occur.
- Surgical de-bulking is often required due to the size and complications caused by the lesions. An R0 resection may not be crucial, but lymphoma involvement of an anastomosis should be avoided for concern of leakage during chemotherapy.
- Lymphoma is a systemic disease, and systemic chemotherapy is needed, even for localized lesions with complete resection. For small or apparently unresectable lesions, biopsy followed by chemotherapy is preferred to extensive resection.
- An adequate wedge-type (not FNA) biopsy is necessary for histologic diagnosis, classification, and appropriate treatment. Specific treatment may be needed for different lineage and various histologic subtypes of lymphoma; thus, proper handling of the specimen is needed. Sending fresh tissue to the pathology laboratory is desirable for proper immuno-staining and molecular lineage clarification.
- Prognosis varies widely, depending on histology and stage.

Introduction

Lymphoma of the small bowel constitutes 2% of all extra-nodal lymphomas. Small bowel lymphoma, including ileocecal and multiple sites of involvement, accounts for about 20% of all small bowel malignancies and about 25% of all gastrointestinal lymphomas. Small bowel is the second most common site of lymphoma gut involvement, after the stomach. Primary intestinal lymphoma arises from lymphoid cells present in the Peyer's patches. The incidence of lymphoma decreases from the ileum to jejunum to duodenum. Lymphoma is a heterogeneous disease in terms of biology and clinical behavior due to the great variety of normal lymphocytes. The World Health Organization (WHO) classification divides lymphoma biologically into B- and T-/ natural killer (NK) cell lineages (◉ *Table 65-1*). The incidence of the various subtypes varies widely; some lesions appear to be peculiar to particular sites and ethnic groups. The common subtypes of lymphoma that occur in the gastrointestinal tract are highlighted below.

◘ Table 65-1

World Health Organization classification of lymphomas with the four main categories of B-cell, T-/NK- cell/Hodgkin/ and immunodeficiency-related lymphomas

Mature B cell neoplasms	Mature T/NK neoplasms	Immunodeficiency lymphoma
*Diffuse large cell lymphoma	Peripheral T cell NOS	HIV related
*Extranodal marginal zone (MALToma)	*T/ NK nasal/nasal type	Post transplant lymphoma
Follicular lymphoma	*Enteropathic T cell	Primary/secondary immune disorders
*Mantle cell lymphoma		
*Burkitt lymphoma		
Lymphoplasmacytoid/Waldenstrom	Anaplastic large cell	
Plasma cell neoplasms	Hepatosplenic T cell	Hodgkin's lymphoma
B-Prolymphocytic leukemia	Mycosis fungoides	Nodular lymphocyte predominant
Chronic lymphocytic leukemia/SLL	Primary cutaneous CD30 T cell	Lymphocyte rich classical
Hairy cell leukemia	Subcutaneous panniculitis	Classical
	T-large granular lymphocytosis	Nodular sclerosis classical
	T-prolymphocytic leukemia	Mixed cellularity

*Entities encountered in the small bowel.

Clinical Presentation

Most series report a peak presentation in the 7th decade with a 2:1 male predominance. Due to the inaccessibility of the small bowel to clinical examination, and endoscopic and radiologic imaging, the diagnosis of small bowel lymphoma may be difficult and is often delayed. Local symptoms are similar to those caused by other malignant or non-malignant intestinal lesions, including pain (85%), mass bowel obstruction due to intussusception (26%), bleeding (22%), and rupture (23%). For rapidly growing lesions, such as Burkitt's lymphoma and NK lymphoma, local symptoms can be dramatic. Lymphoma of the small bowel is a great mimicker of conditions, including tuberculosis and Crohn's disease, and may cause unexplained systemic features such as fever and weight loss (in one-third of patients), while defying extensive investigations. Late presentation is not unusual. An increased serum lactate dehydrogenase level (LDH) may be a clue. The use of PET (❯ Fig. 65-1) may be useful for localization of the disease. Certain subgroups of patients are at increased risk for specific small bowel lymphoma, including patients with celiac disease, those on immunosuppression due to transplantation, HIV infection, or congenital immunodeficiency, patients with nodular lymphoid hyperplasia of the intestine, and those of Middle Eastern descent. Due to the mucosa homing nature of small bowel lymphocytes, multiple sites of small bowel may be involved by lymphoma (10%) (❯ Fig. 65-2).

Pathology and Classification

According to Lee et al., two-thirds of the primary lymphomas of small intestine are of B-cell lineage, and 60–80% of both B- and T-cell small bowel lymphoma are classified as high-grade lesions (Lee et al., 2004). In most clinical and pathological series, gastrointestinal lymphomas are discussed as one single entity (Liang et al). However, in both etiological and clinical terms, the spectrum of origin and behavior of small bowel lymphoma are vastly different from that of gastric lymphoma. The prognosis and optimal treatment for each WHO category are also different and these clinical series are difficult to interpret without the pathological details.

■ Figure 65-1

CT and PET-CT images of the four different presentations of small bowel lymphoma. a. Multiple segments of bowel wall thickening in a patient with anemia. b. Acute perforation of the small bowel walled off by omentum resulting in an intra-abdominal abscess. c. Patient had a history of systemic lupus erythematosus on prolonged azathioprine. PET scan showed single focus of tumor in small bowel. Resection revealed Epstein Barr virus-positive immunosuppression-related lymphoma. d. Huge intra-abdominal mass in a patient with rapidly growing Burkitt's lymphoma

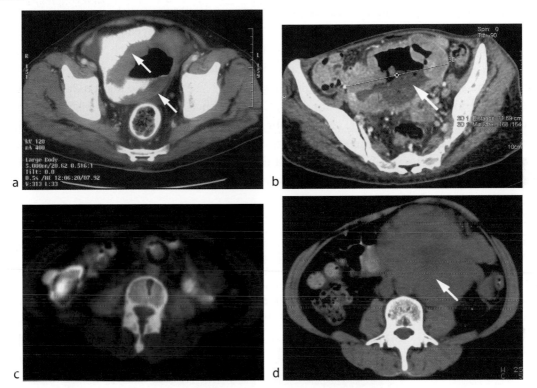

■ Figure 65-2

Endoscopic appearances. Two B-cell lymphomas involving parts of small bowel accessible by endoscopy (biopsies confirmed small bowel lymphoma). a. MALToma appearing as a duodenal polyp. b. Thickening of ileocecal fold by mantle cell lymphoma on multiple biopsies

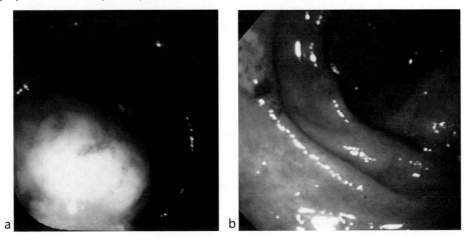

Diffuse large B-cell lymphoma: Similar to lymphomas of nodal origin, diffuse B-cell histology accounts for 50% of all small bowel lymphomas. Unlike those in the stomach, transformation from MALToma (Lymphoma of mucosa-associated lymphoid tissue) is uncommon. Regional lymph node involvement and systemic involvement occurs in 10–15% of patients. Histologically, sheets of large centroblasts or immunoblasts do not usually form follicular structure (❯ *Fig. 65-3A*). The cells are usually positive for CD20 and bcl-6, signifying a germinal center origin. The response to chemotherapy is good even though relapse, often extraintestinal, may occur in 30% of patients.

Low-grade lymphomas: MALTomas arise from the mucosa-associated lymphoid tissue in the submucosal region. Concomitant lymphoma may be present in the stomach, large bowel, and other mucosal areas, such as eye, lung, and salivary glands. Histologically, the malignant lymphoid cells are small in size and show distinct lympho-epithelial lesions (❯ *Fig. 65-3B*) and glandular destruction. The cells are positive for CD20 but negative for CD5, CD10 and bcl-6. Secondary transformation to large cells and diffuse histology may occur. The behavior is indolent, but eradication of gastric Helicobacter pylori may cause regression of the gastric forms. Both follicular lymphoma, as well as small cell lymphoma, may have primary and isolated small intestinal presentation. The prognosis is good, and their relation to the more common nodal and disseminated disease is undefined.

◼ Figure 65-3

a. Mucosal and submucosal infiltration by sheets of CD20-positive, diffuse large B cell lymphoma, stained brown by immunohistochemistry. There is no evidence of invasion of the mucosal villi (arrow). b. Hematoxylin and eosin staining showing diffuse large B cell lymphoma on high power. c. An NK cell lymphoma of small bowel presenting as perforation with sheets of lymphoma cells with necrosis. d. High power view showing angioinvasion by malignant NK cells (arrow) (Histologic appearances courtesy of Dr. Tony W. H. Shek, Queen Mary Hospital, Hong Kong)

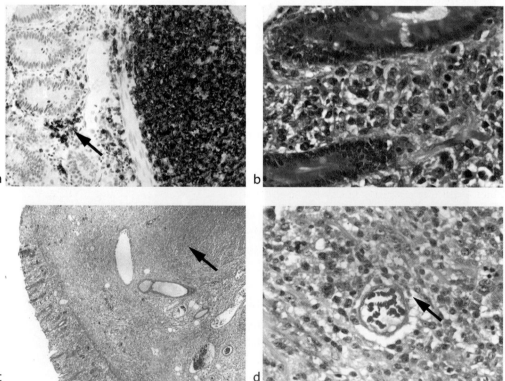

Mantle cell lymphoma: This is an aggressive lymphoma that arises from the mantle zone of the lymphoid follicle. Although a systemic disease, the malignant mantle cells home to the intestine and up to 70% of patients have small and large intestinal involvement at autopsy (lymphomatous polyposis). The growth is monotonous and cells are positive for CD5, CD20, and bcl-1. The disease usually runs a relentless, fatal, relapsing course.

Burkitt's lymphoma: This is a rare, but alarmingly rapid-growing progressive neoplasm. Classically occurring in a cervical, ovary, and neck node, it is also common in the small bowel. A classic "starry sky" appearance is evident on histology due to extensive cell apoptosis and mitoses. The cells express CD20 and Ki-67 and are also positive for Epstein Barr virus (EBV) in patients with HIV. Response to chemotherapy is rapid, and the whole lesion may disappear within hours. Despite such a rapid response, however, prognosis is poor with relapses occurring systemically and in the central nervous system. Aggressive treatment with hemopoietic stem cell transplantation may be required.

Lymphoplasmacytoid lymphoma: This is an indolent lymphoma that secretes monoclonal immunoglobulins (alpha chain disease). It is more commonly seen in certain ethnic groups, e.g., in patients of Middle Eastern descent (immunoproliferative small intestinal disease or IPSID) and is associated with bacterial overgrowth and malabsorption. Campylobacter jejuni has been implicated as the antigenic stimuli in some patients. The lymphoid cells show a classic plasmacytic differentiation. Chemotherapy and antibiotic treatment usually provide good disease control. Despite aggressive treatment, prognosis is poor for the transformed cases.

Mature T-cell lymphoma: This mixed group of disease constitutes 15–30% of all small bowel lymphomas, depending on the different ethnic groups and geographic areas. In Asian countries, peripheral T-cell lymphoma and NK-/T and EBV-positive nasal-type lymphoma predominate. The lymphoid cells are medium in size, positive for $CD3_E$, and negative for B-cell markers. EBV association is common for PTCL and invariable for NK lymphoma. The latter are also CD56 positive, accounting for its intestinal preference due to homotypic attraction. Due to its aggressive growth, bowel perforation is common, and the prognosis is poor. In Caucasians, enteropathic T-cell lymphoma may follow expansion of intraepithelial T-cells, resulting in celiac disease and refractory sprue. Gluten-free diet may reduce the risk. Prognosis is usually dismal due to its late diagnosis and malnutrition.

Imaging and Endoscopic Appearance

The small intestine is a difficult part of the body for imaging despite the use of intravenous, oral, and air contrast techniques of imaging. The diagnostic sensitivities of contrast radiography, computed tomography, and endoscopic biopsy are all reported to be over 75%, but up to 10–25% of small bowel lymphoma may only be detectable at operation, especially for the diffuse types. For lymphoma forming mass lesions (30%), mesenteric and retroperitoneal lymphadenopathy (50%), and bowel wall thickening (70%), CT is preferred over MRI. Most lymphomas are contrast-enhancing and homogeneous in attenuation, but large lesions may have areas of necrosis. In most cases, it is impossible to differentiate lymphoma from other neoplasms by imaging. The use of CT-guided core biopsy may obviate the need for open laparotomy for some bulky lesions. Although gallium scintigraphy may pick up lymphomatous lesions, its sensitivity in the small bowel is low. PET scanning is useful in high-risk patients and simplifies localization and staging. But PET scan may be negative for low-grade lymphomas, e.g., MALToma. The use of virtual endoscopy (MRI or CT) has not been evaluated. Because staging is an integral part of management, full staging by CT/MRI/PET screening of the thorax, abdomen, and pelvis is necessary.

The ability to perform endoscopic biopsy, coupled with imaging, may avoid the need for open laparotomy in treating some small bowel lymphomas, although concomitant involvement of the gastric and colonic regions, the regions most amenable to endoscopic access, is usually not be present. In addition, lymphoma usually does not extend to the parts of the duodenum and ileum assessable by endoscopy. The use of capsule endoscopy and small bowel enteroscopy for diagnosis of small bowel lymphoma is limited by their inability to obtain an adequate biopsy for histology. False negativity and inadvertent complications are common. The delay for definitive operative exploration may result in months of undiagnosed disease. Unlike malignant carcinomas, systemic chemotherapy is the standard treatment, and endoscopic ultrasonography for more precise TMN staging may not be necessary.

Staging, Treatment and Prognosis

The optimal treatment of small bowel lymphoma relies on both the histology and staging. For each histologic type, the prognosis is governed by clinical factors. The clinical Ann Arbor staging (I–IV) is used for nodal Hodgkin's lymphoma. Attempts have been made to modify it for the staging of other extra-nodal malignant lymphomas (❽ *Table 65-2*). Most small bowel lymphomas (80%) are confined to the intestinal area, although liver, pancreatic and peritoneal spread is not uncommon. The clinical prognosis is determined by the International Prognostic Index, which includes the clinical stage, age, LDH level, performance score, and number of extra-nodal sites (score: 0, best prognosis; 5, worst prognosis). The index is derived from patients with diffuse large cell lymphoma treated with curative intent, but has also been verified for other clinical groups, histology and sites. The overall 5-year survival of small bowel lymphoma is around 30–50%, but varies according to the pathology (worse for high-grade histology and much worse for T-cell lineage) and clinical prognostic factors (disease extent and treatment tolerance).

The optimal treatment of small bowel lymphoma has never been determined by prospective clinical trials. For both low- and high-grade lesions, prognosis is worse than that of gastric lymphoma. Operative resection is an important part of the initial management. Up to 80% of the patients would have a bowel resection, either electively or, more commonly, urgently for complications such as perforation, bleeding, and obstruction. But operative intervention may not be beneficial for patients

◨ Table 65-2

Staging of gastrointestinal lymphoma by Musshoff modifications of Ann Arbor criteria

Stage	Definition
Ia	One tumor area without perforation
Ib	Multiple tumors, no perforation
IIa	Gastric or mesenteric nodes involved
IIb	Perforation and adhesions
IIc	Frank peritonitis
III	Widespread thoracic/para-aortic/pelvic nodes
IV	Extra-lymphatic non-adjacent tissue involved

with bulky or disseminated disease. Palliative operative intervention or biopsy are required in 15% and 6% of patients, respectively. Nevertheless, in several multivariate analyses, the ability to perform a complete or de-bulking resection was a favorable prognostic factor. Chemotherapy, either alone or as part of multi-modality treatment, is used for over 90% of patients. Multi-agent chemotherapy (6–8 cycles) gives a synergistic effect and avoids overlapping toxicity. The agents used commonly are cyclophosphamide, anthracycline, vincristine, and steroids. Methotrexate, bleomycin, cytosine arabinoside, and *cis*-platinum are reserved for second-line treatment. All these regimes may cause gastrointestinal complications that require operative intervention, such as ileus (vincristine), mucositis (methotrexate), gastrointestinal bleeding and wound dehiscence (steroids), pancytopenia causing bleeding and infective typhlitis, acalculous cholecystitis, and peritonitis. Insertion of a central venous catheter is often required for delivery of chemotherapy, blood products, antimicrobials, and parenteral nutrition. For B-cell lymphomas expressing CD20, adding rituximab (anti-CD20) to the chemotherapy gives additional benefit. Radiotherapy can cause ileus and enteritis, but may be useful as adjuvant treatment (5–26%) for obstructive or residual diseases. With operative resection and chemotherapy, over 70% of patients achieve a remission. Relapses, usually extraintestinal, may occur. In patients with relapsing or disseminated disease, autologous or allogenic hematopoietic stem cell transplantation may be considered.

Selected Readings

Azab MB, Henry-Amar M, Rougier P, et al. (1989) Prognostic factors in primary gastrointestinal non-Hodgkin's lymphoma. A multivariate analysis, report of 106 cases, and review of the literature. Cancer 64:1208–1217

Koch P, del Valle F, Berdel WE, et al. (2001) Primary gastrointestinal non-Hodgkin's lymphoma: I. Anatomic and histologic distribution, clinical features, and survival data of 371 patients registered in the German Multicenter Study GIT NHL 01/92. J Clin Oncol 19:3861–3873

Koh PK, Horsman JM, Radstone CR, et al. (2001) Localised extranodal non-Hodgkin's lymphoma of the gastrointestinal tract: Sheffield Lymphoma Group experience (1989–1998). Int J Oncol 18:743–748

Lee J, Kim WS, Kim K, et al. (2004) Intestinal lymphoma: exploration of the prognostic factors and the optimal treatment. Leuk Lymphoma 45:339–344

Liang R, Todd D, Chan TK, et al. (1995) Prognostic factors for primary gastrointestinal lymphoma. Hematol Oncol 13:153–163

Lecuit M, Abachin E, Martin A, et al. (2004) Immunoproliferative small intestinal disease associated with Campylobacter jejuni. N Engl J Med 350:239–248

Nakamura S, Matsumoto T, Takeshita M, et al. (2000) A clinicopathologic study of primary small intestine lymphoma: prognostic significance of mucosa-associated lymphoid tissue-derived lymphoma. Cancer 88:286–294

Nomura K, Tomikashi K, Matsumoto Y, et al. (2005) Small bowel non-Hodgkin's lymphoma remaining in complete remission by surgical resection and adjuvant rituximab therapy. World J Gastroenterol 11:4443–4444

Stovroff MC, Coran AG, Hutchinson RJ (1991) The role of surgery in American Burkitt's lymphoma in children. J Pediatr Surg 26:1235–1238

66 Carcinoid of the Small Bowel

John R. Porterfield · David R. Farley

Pearls and Pitfalls

- The ileum harbors ~85% of small bowel carcinoid (SBC) neoplasms.
- Vague GI complaints are present typically for years prior to diagnosis.
- Less than 10% of SBCs present with "carcinoid syndrome."
- Laparotomy detects the majority of SBCs; a pre-op diagnosis is uncommon.
- Approximately 90% of patients with SBCs have evidence of metastases at exploration.
- Approximately 30% have multicentric disease.
- Most SBCs are <2 cm in diameter.
- Oncologic resection with primary anastomosis represents optimal therapy.
- Overall recurrence rate is 80%.

Background

It has been nearly 140 years since carcinoid neoplasms of the small bowel were first described. In 1867, Theodore Langhans described these lesions as *Drusenpolyp im Ileum* and Lubrarsch described "little carcinomata" in two patients in 1888. In 1907, the term Karzinoid was coined by Oberndorfer due to the morphologic similarities with adenocarcinomas; he was mistaken in his belief that these neoplasms were benign which we now know is not the case. Carcinoid neoplasms have been described throughout the entire gastrointestinal tract and foregut structures, which includes the thymus, bronchi, and lung. These neoplasms were classified in 1963 by Williams and Sandler according to their embryologic development and blood supply as foregut (celiac axis), midgut (superior mesenteric artery), and hindgut (inferior mesenteric artery) regions.

Carcinoid neoplasms arise from the neuroendocrine Kulchitsky cells found in the base of the crypts of Lieberkuhn and are a part of the APUD (amine precursor uptake and decarboxylation) system (❷ *Fig. 66-1*). These totipotent cells are capable of secreting multiple metabolically active hormones and biogenic amines, such as serotonin, histamine, tachykinins, dopamine, substance P, prostaglandins, and others. Serotonin, the most commonly secreted substance from small bowel carcinoids, is derived from its precursor 5-hydroxytryptophan and is metabolized to 5-hydroxyindole acetic acid (5-HIAA) excreted and quantifiable in urine.

Small bowel carcinoids are the second most common small intestinal neoplasm (#1 = adenocarcinomas). Thus, it is important to have a thorough understanding of the surgical and medical management of these unique neoplasms, because they are often discovered incidentally.

■ Figure 66-1

H&E low magnification views of submucosal small bowel carcinoid neoplasm (Courtesy of Dr. Gary L. Keeney, Mayo Clinic, Rochester, MN)

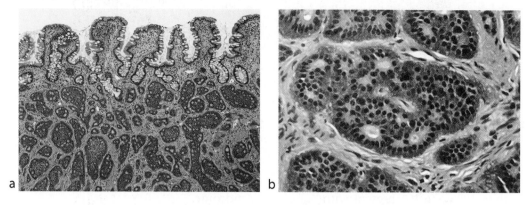

Clinical Presentation

Small bowel carcinoids (SBCs) present typically in the sixth or seventh decades of life with a slight male predominance. These neoplasms are nearly twice as common in black vs. white patients (incidence of 9.2 vs. 5.4 per million, respectively) according to a recent evaluation of the SEER (Surveillance, Epidemiology, and End Results) program. The most common anatomic part of small bowel is the ileum which harbors 85%. The typical presentation is 2–20 years of nonspecific gastrointestinal symptoms, abdominal pain, or intestinal obstruction. Patients have often been labeled with a variety of diagnoses, including irritable bowel syndrome, Crohn's disease, adhesive obstruction, lymphoma, and colitis. Less than 10% of patients present with true carcinoid syndrome characterized by cutaneous flushing, usually of the face, that cycles as quickly as every 10–30 min and begins resolution centrally. These episodes are associated often with tachycardia, diarrhea, sweating, and hypotension. SBCs may present with intestinal ischemia, an abdominal mass, or hepatomegaly, but this presentation is extremely rare. Because these submucosal neoplasms grow slowly, they do not cause symptoms typically until the disease has spread beyond the wall of the intestine, and, thus, greater than 90% are metastatic at initial presentation (❷ *Fig. 66-2*). Because SBCs are also multi-centric in 30% of patients, a meticulous exploration of the entire small bowel is necessary once the diagnosis is suspected.

These unique neoplasms can secrete a broad range of metabolically active substances that may be triggered by serotonin-rich foods such as coffee, cheese, alcohol, or exercise. Even patients with significant tumor burden may have minimal symptoms and evade detection through serologic testing because of their rapid "first pass" metabolism of these vasoactive substances in the liver. It is not until the secretory burden overwhelms the metabolic capabilities of the liver or the hormones are secreted directly into the systemic circulation via the hepatic veins from hepatic implants that the symptoms manifest. When carcinoid syndrome is present, the astute physician should also suspect the presence of nonendocrine malignancies found in 29% of patients with SBCs. Colorectal adenomas and carcinomas are associated most frequently with SBCs, but cancers of the breast, stomach, and lung are also seen. Therefore, chest radiography, mammography, and upper and lower gastrointestinal endoscopy are useful preoperatively.

◻ Figure 66-2
Computed tomography with extensive hepatic metastases from a primary small bowel carcinoid neoplasm

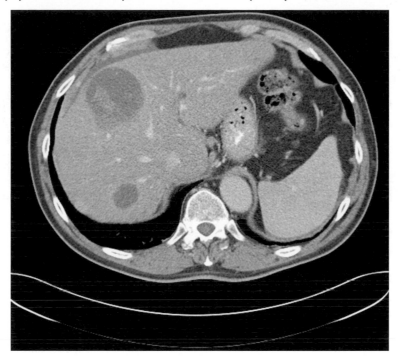

Diagnosis

While numerous preoperative studies aid in the diagnosis of SBCs, the vast majority of patients are diagnosed in the operating room. In order for the diagnosis to be made preoperatively there must be a high index of suspicion with application of multiple, semi-confirmatory tests. An increased 24 h urine 5-HIAA is the most reliable preoperative finding, yet nearly half of patients have normal levels preoperatively. Similarly, plasma serotonin, substance P, neurotensin, neurokin A, and neuropeptide K are all measurable with immunofluorescent neuropeptide assays, but their sensitivity is low because most such substances are not increased in the majority of patients. Unfortunately, the one marker that seems to be increased consistently, chromogranin A, is not specific to carcinoid neoplasms.

Because most carcinoid neoplasms are small (<2 cm), visualization with preoperative imaging is difficult. Contrast studies of the small bowel are usually unrewarding but may demonstrate one or more of the following findings: (1) solitary or multiple submucosal lesions; (2) mesenteric infiltration or retraction with or without lymphadenopathy; or (3) polypoid, mucosal-based masses. When these findings are present, the differential diagnosis includes SBCs, small bowel adenocarcinoma, lymphoma, Kaposi's sarcoma, and metastatic melanoma.

Even with the advent of high resolution computed tomography (CT) and magnetic resonance imaging (MRI), the primary neoplasms of SBCs are often undetectable; these cross-sectional imaging modalities with selective angiography, however, are beneficial in depicting the extent of metastatic disease and potential resectability. Lymph node metastases are often bulky and cause a swirling desmoplastic reaction in the base of the mesentery which accounts for the symptoms of ischemia due to the intense fibrosis and mass effect on the mesenteric vasculature (❯ *Fig. 66-3*). Hepatic

◘ Figure 66-3
Computed tomography of the abdomen with dense mesenteric fibrosis

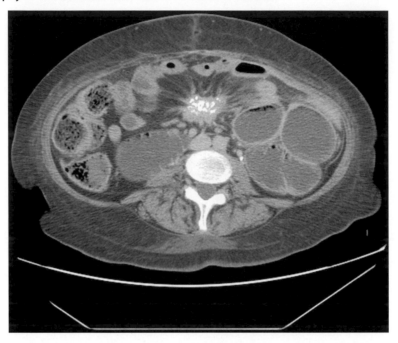

metastases are hypervascular, yet both contrast-enhanced CT and MRI tend to underestimate the burden of disease appreciable intraoperatively and pathologically (◉ *Fig. 66-4*).

Somatostatin receptor scintigraphy (OctreoScan) has been shown repeatedly to be the most sensitive imaging modality (~85%) for detecting carcinoid neoplasms. This noninvasive imaging modality relies on the density of somatostatin receptors and is able to detect tumors of ~1 cm diameter. The OctreoScan is not, however, able to determine the size of the neoplasms, because the image produced is a reflection of the density of the somatostatin receptors which may or may not correlate with the actual tumor size. Similarly, scintigraphy cannot detect those neoplasms that do not express the somatostatin receptors. Additionally, the first pass affect of the somatostatin analogue causes physiologic enhancement of the genitourinary system and spleen, which may produce sufficient background signal to hide lesions in the left upper quadrant and mid abdomen. Its use intraoperatively to guide or quantify the adequacy of resection is still under evaluation.

Preoperative Management

When the diagnosis is obtained preoperatively, it is crucial to recognize the characteristic symptoms of carcinoid syndrome to minimize morbidity and potential mortality. Asymptomatic patients may proceed to a curative resection with minimal preparation. In contrast, symptomatic patients are at risk for carcinoid crisis which is hallmarked by profound hypotension or bronchospasm during induction of general anesthesia or intraoperative manipulation of the neoplasm. The goal for preoperative management is to render the patients symptom-free with use of a somatostatin analogue. The majority (~75%) of symptomatic patients are able to be suppressed with octreotide at dosages ranging

◻ **Figure 66-4**

Magnetic resonance imaging of the liver with extensive hepatic metastases from a primary small bowel carcinoid neoplasm

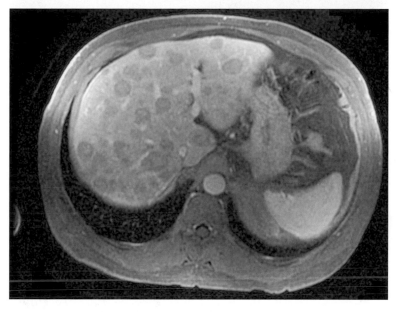

from 50 to 500 μg subcutaneously three times each day. The dosage should be titrated in accordance with symptom control. Longer acting somatostatin analogues are available (lanreotide and Sandostatin LAR) which allow dosing every 2 or 4 weeks, respectively. At the time of operation, previously suppressed patients should also receive a subcutaneous bolus of octreotide with induction of anesthesia and an additional 100 μg of octreotide should be immediately available to be administered intravenously in the setting of a carcinoid crisis. Additionally, the anesthesia team needs to be prepared to treat octreotide-induced bradycardia and heart block in the setting of a carcinoid resection.

The second facet regarding the preoperative evaluation is to exclude carcinoid heart disease. This rare but important complication occurs in approximately 5% of patients with SBCs and is characterized by heart murmurs and/or right-sided heart failure. Patients with hepatic metastases are at the highest risk for tricuspid insufficiency, because the secretions from the hepatic metastases are fed unaltered directly into the hepatic veins and thus directly to the heart. Transesophageal echocardiography should complete the preoperative evaluation, and carcinoid heart disease should be treated prior to abdominal exploration.

Operative Management

SBCs tend to be more aggressive and have a greater ultimate risk of death than carcinoids found in other locations. Given that these neoplasms are multicentric (30%) and usually (90%) metastatic, resection should proceed only after meticulous abdominal inspection with the goal of rendering the patient disease-free (❷ *Fig. 66-5*). The primary tumor should be resected with a wide tumor-free margin and excised en bloc with the maximal mesenteric resection to maintain an adequate vascular

◘ Figure 66-5
Intraoperative photograph of small bowel carcinoid neoplasm

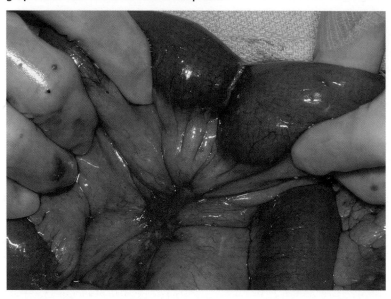

supply to the remaining bowel. Debulking of lymphadenopathy may be beneficial in delaying the mesenteric desmoplastic reaction and subsequent bowel obstruction or ischemia.

In the setting of hepatic metastases, palliative cytoreductive resection is beneficial for symptom control and is associated with increased survival when ≥90% of the tumor burden is removed. Sequential hepatic artery embolization may be considered when resection or in situ destruction (ablation techniques) is not a viable option to improve symptoms and slow the progression of the disease.

Postoperative Care

Care after a small bowel resection for a carcinoid neoplasm should be routine. The nasogastric tube is discontinued the evening of operation or the following morning. A liquid diet is initiated and advanced rapidly to a soft diet as tolerated. In patients who are asymptomatic preoperatively, there is no indication for postoperative somatostatin or other ongoing therapy. In contrast, patients who were symptomatic postoperatively should be continued on suppressive therapy. If there was significant debulking of the neoplasm, the dosage of somatostatin should be reduced to the lowest therapeutic dose.

In our practice, the timing of follow-up is driven by the clinical suspicion for recurrence at the time of resection. When the primary neoplasm and its associated nodal basin are resected without evidence of distant disease, patients are re-evaluated in 4–6 months. In the setting of distant disease where greater than 90% of the tumor burden was resected, we prefer a baseline set of imaging and laboratory studies within 2 months. Serial 24 h urine 5-HIAA concentrations and Chromogranin A levels are followed at each visit. We use CT for evaluation of the remaining small bowel and its associated mesentery. The best imaging for hepatic metastasis is MRI, while OctreoScans are used to survey for disease that may have spread beyond the abdomen.

In the setting of metastatic disease, many treatment options are available, but there is no magic bullet. Single agent chemotherapeutics (5-fluorouracil, doxorubicin, actinomycin D, dacarbazine, and streptozocin) have been little benefit. Combination chemotherapy, using streptozocin and 5-FU (±cyclophosphamide), produces biochemical and tumor response rates in only 8–25% of patients. No single or combination chemotherapy has demonstrated a response rate of greater than 15% when using the criteria of 50% reduction in bidimensionally measurable disease. This slow-growing neoplasm is essentially chemoresistant.

Carcinoid neoplasms are also usually radioresistant, but external beam therapy has been beneficial in symptom control in the brain, bone, and near the spinal cord, where local growth causes clinically significant pain or neurologic deficits. Recent advances in systemic receptor-targeted and metabolically directed radiotherapy have been utilized for unresectable patients. These agents consists of ^{131}I-MIBG or radiolabeled somatostatin analogues. Overall response rates range from 10% to 20%. The most likely use of these agents will be to slow the rate of progression to maintain a stable tumor burden.

While carcinoids from other regions have long-term survival, the overall 5-year survival for patients with SBC is 60%. When the disease presents with only regional disease, the 5-year survival is 90%; when inoperable liver metastases are present, the 5-year survival is approximately 50% and decreases further to 42% when there is accompanying mesenteric adenopathy. Therefore, when radical hepatic resection and metastasectomy is feasible technically, an aggressive resection should be pursued because the 5-year survival may extend to 70%.

Summary

Carcinoid neoplasms are the second most common small bowel neoplasm and are often discovered incidentally due to their myriad of clinical presentations. To establish the diagnosis preoperatively, physicians must be sensitized to the possibility of their presence when caring for patients with chronic, vague, and insidious abdominal symptoms. There are many investigative studies that may aid in the diagnosis, but none is pathognomonic or highly sensitive. An aggressive operative approach should be pursued; SBCs should be resected with wide margins to include the maximal mesenteric nodal basin. Patients with metastatic disease may be candidates for resection or image-guided destruction of the neoplasms, in light of the limited chemotherapeutic and radiotherapy options. Follow-up should be focused on detection of recurrent symptoms and imaging to detect treatable metastatic disease.

Selected Readings

Dilger JA, Rho EH, Que FG, et al. (2004) Octreotide-induced bradycardia and heart block during surgical resection of a carcinoid tumor. Anesth Analg 98:318–320

Hellman P, Lundstrom T, Ohrvall U, et al. (2002) Effect of surgery on the outcome of midgut carcinoid disease with lymph node and liver metastases. World J Surg 26:991–997

Kerstrom G, Hellman P, Hessman O (2005) Midgut carcinoid tumours: surgical treatment and prognosis. Baillieres Best Pract Res Clin Gastroenterol 19:717–728

Modlin IM, Kidd M, Latich I, et al. (2005) Current status of gastrointestinal carcinoids. Gastroenterology 128:1717–1751

Modlin IM, Lye KD, Kidd M (2003) A 5-decade analysis of 13,715 carcinoid tumors. Cancer 97:934–959

Oberndorfer S (1907) Karzenoide Tumoren des Dünndarms. Frankfurt Zeitschr Pathol 1:426–432

Que FG, Nagorney DM, Batts KP, et al. (1995) Hepatic resection for metastatic neuroendocrine carcinomas. Am J Surg 169:36–42

Williams ED, Sandler M (1963) The classification of carcinoid tumours. Lancet 1:238–239

Zar N, Garmo H, Holmberg L, et al. (2004) Long-term survival of patients with small intestinal carcinoid tumors. World J Surg 28:1163–1168

67 Stromal Tumors of the Small Bowel

Sherry J. Lim · Peter W. T. Pisters

Pearls and Pitfalls

- High index of suspicion of small bowel malignancy is necessary for early detection.
- Favorable prognostic factors: no tumor rupture, localized lesion, low-grade neoplasm, and tumor <5 cm.
- CT can often aid in differentiation between sarcoma, adenocarcinoma, carcinoid, and lymphoma.
- Primary therapy for patients with localized sarcomas and gastrointestinal stromal tumors (GISTs) is operative resection when feasible. At present, there is no defined role for adjuvant or neoadjuvant imatinib mesylate.
- Lymphadenectomy is not required for operative treatment of sarcomas.
- Care must be taken to avoid tumor rupture during resection.
- GISTs are almost always positive for CD117 (KIT), frequently for CD34, occasionally for SMA, and rarely for S-100 or desmin.
- Standard, first-line therapy for metastatic or unresectable GIST is imatinib mesylate.
- Second line therapy for imatinib resistant or intolerant GIST is sunitinib.

Introduction

Although the small intestine constitutes more than 75% of the intestinal tract, small bowel malignancies are rare. Indeed, small bowel neoplasms account for only 2–3% of digestive system cancers and less than 1% of all cancers diagnosed annually. According to the American Cancer Society, 6,000 cases of small bowel cancers are expected to be diagnosed in 2006. This number, however, may be a significant under-estimation of the true incidence of small bowel malignancies. The true incidence of gastrointestinal stromal tumors (GISTs) is unknown in the United States, but based on population studies completed in Europe, the true incidence of GISTs may be as high as 5,000–6,000 annually, of which 30% occur in the small bowel.

Adenocarcinomas are the most common small bowel malignancies (5.9 cases per million persons; 45% of all small bowel malignancies), followed by carcinoids (5.5 cases per million; 30% of all small bowel malignancies), lymphomas (3 cases per million; 15% of all small bowel malignancies), and sarcomas (1.7 cases per million; 10% of all small bowel malignancies). Unlike adenocarcinomas of the small intestine but similar to small bowel carcinoids and lymphomas, small bowel sarcomas are found most commonly in the jejunum and ileum; only 10% of small bowel sarcomas occur in the duodenum. This chapter will focus on the incidence, diagnosis, as well as current treatment recommendations for small bowel sarcomas. Particular attention to management of GISTs will be emphasized, because a treatment algorithm for this disease entity continue to evolve with new treatment paradigms.

Classification

Sarcomas develop from cells derived from the mesoderm. Mesenchymal cells can differentiate into fibroblasts, myoblasts, lipoblasts, chondroblasts, osteoblasts, etc., which then differentiate into the various mature cell lines. Unlike epidermal malignancies, where the extent of tumor invasion and the presence of metastasis predict the course of the disease and its treatment, the behavior of sarcomas can be predicted by the tumor grade based on morphologic criteria and classification based on cell of origin. Therefore, the histologic classification is important in defining the natural history, estimating prognosis, and selecting therapy.

Small bowel sarcomas, like other sarcomas, are classified on the basis of histology, cell of origin, and dominant cell pattern. Small bowel sarcomas include smooth muscle tumors (leiomyomas, leiomyosarcomas, leiomyoblastoma), neoplasms of the peripheral nerve sheath (schwannoma, paraganglioma), fibrous neoplasms (desmoid tumor, fibrosarcoma), and mixed neoplasms (❷ *Table 67-1*). Excluding GISTs (described below), the most common sarcomas of the small intestine are leiomyosarcomas (75%), followed by epithelioid leiomyosarcomas (7%), Kaposi's sarcomas (4%), sarcomas not otherwise specified (4%), and spindle cell sarcomas (3%). The diverse cellular morphology as well as the overlapping histology of sarcomas, makes classification based on morphology alone difficult. Therefore, immunohistochemistry has become an important adjunct to diagnosis (and eventual treatment).

Historically, GISTs were thought to be derived from smooth muscle cells, nerve cells, or other mesenchyme-derived cells; and as such, these neoplasms were classified previously as leiomyoblastomas, leiomyomas, or leiomyosarcomas. Since the 1990s, GISTs have been considered a distinct pathologic entity. These mesenchymal tumors result from neoplastic transformation of the interstitial cells of Cajal, which function as intestinal pacemaker cells. Mutation occurs in the *c-kit* proto-oncogene, which encodes for the type III receptor tyrosine kinase KIT. The most frequent mutation

❏ Table 67-1

Subtypes of gastrointestinal sarcomas

Leiomyoma
Leiomyosarcoma
Leiomyoblastoma
Schwann cell neoplasm
Paraganglioma
Desmoid tumor
Mesenchymal tumor
Mixed cell sarcoma
Stromal tumor of uncertain malignant potential
Gastrointestinal autonomic nerve tumor (GANT)
Gastrointestinal stromal tumor (GIST)
Fibrosarcoma

causing GISTs occurs in exon 11, which encodes the intracellular juxtamembranous region of the receptor. Other exon mutations have been observed, particularly in exon 9, with small bowel GISTs. These mutated KIT receptors are activated constitutively, leading to neoplastic development and progression. Advances in the understanding of GIST biology were instrumental in the development of imatinib as a targeted therapeutic tool.

Presentation

The mean age of patients with small bowel sarcomas is 53 years, while the mean age of patients with GISTs is 63 years; 80% of all GISTs are diagnosed after age 50. For all small bowel sarcomas, including GISTs, there is a slight male predominance (~55%). The majority of small bowel sarcomas are reported in white, non-Hispanic patients (85%). Among the ethnic groups, African-Americans have a higher prevalence in both small bowel sarcomas and GISTs.

The symptoms of GISTs and other small bowel sarcomas at presentation depend on the size and location of the tumor and include vague abdominal pain, bleeding, increased abdominal girth, or, rarely, obstruction. Because most of the clinical symptoms that occur are nonspecific in nature, diagnosis is often delayed. Furthermore, many patients with small bowel sarcomas are asymptomatic, and the neoplasms are diagnosed incidentally as a result of imaging studies performed for another condition or at the time of unrelated laparotomy.

Diagnosis

The differential diagnosis of a small bowel mass includes adenocarcinoma, carcinoid, lymphoma, malignant melanoma, GIST, or sarcomas such as leiomyoma, leiomyosarcoma, malignant peripheral nerve sheath tumor, and schwannoma, as well as benign conditions such as fibromatosis and inflammatory myofibroblastic tumor. Once a small bowel mass is found or suspected, contrast-enhanced computed tomography (CT) is recommended and may facilitate differentiation between adenocarcinoma, carcinoid, and lymphoma. Importantly, radiographic findings of malignancy, such as invasion to adjacent structures or distant metastasis, may be identified. On CT, most small bowel sarcomas, including GISTs, appear as well-defined extraluminal or intramural masses with varying attenuation depending on the size. Small tumors are typically enhancing homogeneous masses, while larger tumors (>6 cm) may have central areas of necrosis or hemorrhage. In the small intestine, sarcomas often appear as intraluminal masses or intraluminal polyps and may show extension into the adjacent mesentery. Sarcomas can often be distinguished from adenocarcinomas and lymphomas, because adenocarcinomas are usually annular lesions, while lymphomas are accompanied typically by lymphadenopathy. Radiographically, additional tests, such as upper gastrointestinal series with small bowel follow-through and enteroclysis, may be necessary to distinguish carcinoid from other small bowel malignancies.

If a pretreatment diagnosis is required, a biopsy can often be performed endoscopically or percutaneously. In addition to histopathologic evaluation, immunohistochemical characterization of the tumor can assist with classification of small bowel sarcomas. This is particularly true for diagnosis of GISTs. Immunohistochemical evaluation has become essential in the diagnosis of GISTs and should include staining for CD117 (KIT), CD34, smooth muscle actin (SMA), desmin, and S-100 to distinguish between GISTs, smooth muscle neoplasms (leiomyoma and leiomyosarcoma), schwannoma, and fibromatosis (❯ *Table 67-2*). In addition to CD117 positivity (95%), GISTs may demonstrate immunopositivity for CD34 (65%), SMA (35%), and S-100 (5%). True KIT-positive GISTs, however, are rarely positive for desmin.

Histologically, there are three categories of GISTs: spindle cell type (70%), epithelioid type (20%), and mixed type. These neoplasms are classified as very low-, low-, intermediate-, or high-risk based on anatomic site (gastric versus small bowel), size, and mitotic rate. A commonly used classification system is outlined in ❯ *Table 67-3*.

Prognosis

The 5-year, disease-specific survival rate in patients with small bowel sarcomas is about 35%, with a median, disease-specific survival duration of 32 months. Factors associated with a better prognosis are complete (R0) operative resection without tumor rupture, localized lesion, low tumor grade, and size <5 cm. Despite aggressive surgical resection, patients with tumor rupture, contiguous organ invasion, and high tumor grade are at increased risk for recurrence.

Treatment for Non-GISTs Sarcomas

Complete operative resection is the mainstay of therapy for localized disease. Extensive lymphadenectomy is not indicated, because lymph node metastases are seen only rarely in sarcomas; however, en-bloc resection of the lesions to achieve tumor-free margins should be attempted for potentially

◘ Table 67-2

Immunophenotypes of GIST and other spindle cell neoplasms of the GI tract (Adapted from Fletcher et al., 2002)

Tumor	KIT (CD117)	CD34	Smooth muscle actin	S-100 protein	Desmin
GIST	+++	++	+	+	Very rare
Leiomyosarcoma	–	+	+	Rare	+
Schwannoma	–	+	–	+	–
Fibromatosis	–	Rare	+	–	Rare

GIST, gastrointestinal stromal tumor; GI, gastrointestinal.

◘ Table 67-3

Potential malignant behavior of small bowel GISTs (Adapted from Miettinen et al., 2002)

	Size (cm)	Mitoses per 50 HPF
Benign	≤2	≤5
Intermediate	>2–5	≤5
Malignant	>5	>5

HPF, high-power fields; GIST, gastrointestinal stromal tumor.

curative resections. Localized disease and complete surgical resection are independent variables in overall survival (50 months vs. 15 months). Even when contiguous organ involvement or peritoneal implants were encountered at the time of operation, the ability to achieve complete resection conferred an overall survival advantage (36 months vs. 21 months). For high-grade sarcomas, unresectable lesions, and recurrent disease, a protocol-based treatment should be offered to patients in attempt to downstage the disease or convert an unresectable neoplasm to a resectable one.

Treatment for GISTs

Though the treatment algorithm continues to evolve, current treatment of primary and metastatic GISTs involves a combination of operative resection, imatinib mesylate, and close monitoring (❏ *Fig. 67 1*).

Operative Therapy

Like other sarcomas, complete resection is the primary treatment for patients with localized GISTs. GISTs can be friable and fragile, so care must be taken to avoid rupture or tumor shedding during resection, because this has been linked to an increased risk of peritoneal recurrence. Although some GISTs appear large on CT, they may have a small stalk or base, because these neoplasms tend to grow in an extraluminal fashion without invasion of adjacent structures (❏ *Fig. 67-2*).

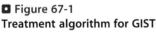

❏ Figure 67-1
Treatment algorithm for GIST

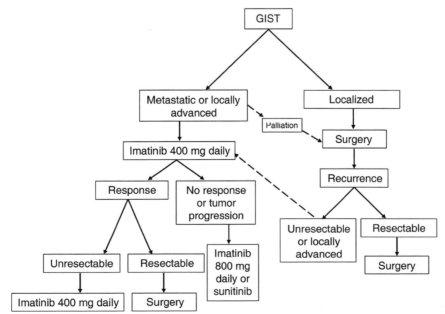

⬛ Figure 67-2
Large mid-jejunal GIST with a small base and no evidence of local invasion to adjacent organs at the time of exploration

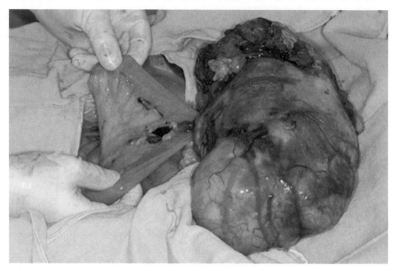

The goal of operative resection is to achieve macroscopically and microscopically negative surgical margins (R0). Therefore, if the neoplasm is locally advanced at the time of surgery, en bloc resection of adjacent involved organs may be required. In contrast to adenocarcinomas, lymph node metastases are rare in GISTs, and thus, lymphadenectomy is not warranted.

In a study by Dematteo et al., 200 patients with GISTs were evaluated for operative resection. A complete R0 resection was achieved in 80 of the 93 patients with localized primary GISTs and in 34 of the 94 patients with metastatic or locally recurrent disease. Patients with localized GISTs who underwent complete R0 resection had a 5-year, disease-specific survival of 54%, with a median survival of 66 months. In contrast, patients with incomplete resection or unresectable neoplasms had a median survival of only 22 months. A subset of patients with metastatic disease who underwent complete resection had a median survival of 16 months versus only 5 months for patients who had an incomplete resection or unresectable disease.

Disease recurrence is usually intraabdominal and is seen first in the liver or on the peritoneal surface. Extraabdominal metastases may occur later in the course of the disease. The treatment of recurrent disease usually involves primary therapy with imatinib mesylate in conjunction with selective use of operative resection.

Imatinib

Primary Therapy for Metastases

Imatinib mesylate (Gleevec), which was used first in patients with chronic myeloid leukemia, is a small molecule inhibitor of ABL-kinase, KIT, and platelet-derived growth factor A and B. Imatinib binds to the intracellular portion of KIT and inhibits cell signaling. When imatinib is used to treat metastatic

GISTs, partial responses are achieved in 50% of patients, and stable disease is achieved in an additional 30%. The 2-year, overall-survival rate is reported to be 75% in patients with metastatic GISTs treated with imatinib. The current standard dose of imatinib is 400 mg daily. Patients whose neoplasm progresses while receiving the standard dose are considered for a dose escalation or are offered second-line therapy with sunitinib (Sutent). Even though imatinib is well tolerated by patients, most patients experience some adverse effects, including edema (74%), nausea (52%), diarrhea (45%), myalgia (40%), and abdominal pain (26%).

Adjuvant Therapy

Currently, there is no defined role for adjuvant imatinib therapy after complete resection of localized GIST. Phase II and III clinical trials are under way to better define the possible role of adjuvant imatinib. The American College of Surgeons Oncology Group (ACOSOG) is conducting a single-arm, phase II clinical trial (Z9000) of adjuvant imatinib for patients with completely resected high-risk GISTs. Accrual began in June 2001 and was completed in September 2003 with enrollment of 110 patients. Primary and secondary end points being evaluated are overall survival and recurrence, respectively. A report of the primary end-point analysis is expected in late 2006.

Also under way is ACOSOG Z9001, a phase III, randomized, double-blind trial of adjuvant imatinib versus placebo after resection of localized GISTs. Inclusion criteria for this study include

■ Figure 67-3
Clinical trials of adjuvant therapy for GIST conducted by the American College of Surgeons Oncology Group (ACOSOG). (a) Z9000 is a phase II trial for patients with completely resected high-risk GISTs. (b) Z9001 is a phase III randomized, double-blind study of adjuvant imatinib versus placebo for patients with completely resected primary GISTs ≥3 cm

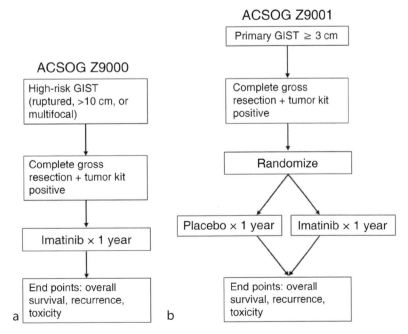

■ Figure 67-4

A phase III randomized study of adjuvant imatinib versus placebo following complete surgical resection of GIST by the European Organization for Research and Treatment of Cancer (EORTC 62024)

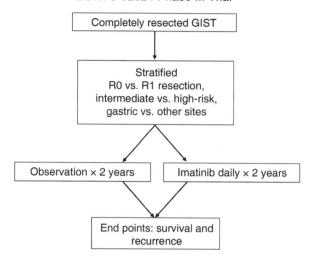

tumor size ≥3 cm, CD117-positivity, and complete (R0) operative resection. Patients are assigned randomly to receive either imatinib (400 mg daily) or placebo for 1 year. The primary end point is disease-free survival (❷ *Fig. 67-3*). In addition, a European, phase III trial (EORTC 62024) is evaluating 2 years of adjuvant imatinib (400 mg daily) compared with observation (❷ *Fig. 67-4*).

The results of these trials will provide important information on the toxicities of imatinib in a setting of the adjuvant therapy and will define whether there is any clinical benefit to 1 or 2 years of adjuvant imatinib. In the absence of prospective, randomized trials supporting use of imatinib after complete operative resection, there is no present role for adjuvant imatinib treatment outside of clinical trials.

Neoadjuvant Therapy

There is also currently no defined role for preoperative (neoadjuvant) therapy with imatinib. Preoperative imatinib, however, may warrant consideration in specific patient subgroups, including patients with large rectal GISTs and patients with large, locally advanced primary neoplasms. In these unique situations, imatinib-related responses may improve the R0 resection rate or facilitate organ preservation.

At the moment, there are no randomized trials evaluating preoperative imatinib treatment. The Radiation Therapy Oncology Group has an ongoing, phase II trial (S0132) evaluating pre- and postoperative imatinib for patients with localized or recurrent GISTs. The protocol involves 8 weeks of preoperative imatinib followed by resection and postoperative imatinib for 2 years. The end points are tumor response to imatinib therapy and disease-free survival. This trial will provide insight into the feasibility and toxicities of preoperative therapy with imatinib.

Selected Readings

DeMatteo RP, Lewis JJ, Leung D, et al. (2000) Two hundred gastrointestinal stromal tumors: recurrence patterns and prognostic factors for survival. Ann Surg 231:51–58

Fletcher CD, Berman JJ, Corless C, et al. (2002) Diagnosis of gastrointestinal stromal tumors: a consensus approach. Hum Pathol 33:459–465

Gold JS, DeMatteo RP (2006) Combined surgical and molecular therapy: the gastrointestinal stromal tumor model. Ann Surg 244:176–184

Hirota S, Isozaki K, Moriyama Y, et al. (1998) Gain-of-function mutations of c-kit in human gastrointestinal stromal tumors. Science 279:577–580

Howe JR, Karnell LH, Scott-Conner C (2001) Small bowel sarcoma: analysis of survival from the National Cancer Data Base. Ann Surg Oncol 8:496–508

Kosmadakis N, Visvardis EE, Kartsaklis P, et al. (2005) The role of surgery in the management of gastrointestinal stromal tumors (GISTs) in the era of imatinib mesylate effectiveness. Surg Oncol 14:75–84

Miettinen M, El-Rifai WE, Sorbin LH, et al. (2002) Evaluation of malignancy and prognosis of gastrointestinal stromal tumors: a review. Hum Pathol 33:478–483

Ng EH, Pollock RE, Munsell MF, et al. (1992) Prognostic factors influencing survival in gastrointestinal leiomyosarcomas. Implications for surgical management and staging. Ann Surg 215:68–77

Van Glabbeke M, Verweij J, Casali PG, et al. (2005) Initial and late resistance to imatinib in advanced gastrointestinal stromal tumors are predicted by different prognostic factors: a European Organization for Research and Treatment of Cancer-Italian Sarcoma Group-Australasian Gastrointestinal Trials Group study. J Clin Oncol 23:5795–5804

Part 6

Colon and Rectum: Benign

68 Large Bowel Obstruction

Angelita Habr-Gama · Fábio Guilherme Campos

Pearls and Pitfalls

- Differentiation of mechanical large bowel obstruction (LBO) from colonic pseudo-obstruction is crucial.
- Colonoscopic examination is a beneficial diagnostic and potentially therapeutic modality.
- The most frequent cause of LBO is colorectal cancer, and the most frequent site is the sigmoid colon followed by splenic flexure.
- Volvulus of the sigmoid colon is the second most frequent cause of LBO and occurs most commonly in elderly, chronically constipated patients.
- Timing, grading, site of obstruction, competency of the ileocecal valve, presence of ischemia or perforation, presence of locally advanced or metastatic disease, and operating skill influence the prognosis of patients and choice of the procedure.
- Obstructing right colon cancer can be treated usually with primary resection and anastomosis; however, a protective ileostomy should be considered in selected patients.
- Obstructing left colon cancer is more likely to necessitate resection with end colostomy; in selected patients, a primary resection and anastomosis may be considered.
- Subtotal colectomy with ileorectostomy may be an acceptable operation in selected elderly patients with an obstructing left colon cancer.
- On-the-table colonic lavage can be used to facilitate resection and primary anastomosis for an obstructing left colon when the proximal colon looks reasonable; the presence of feces in the colon does not appear to increase the rate of complications.
- Sigmoid volvulus may be treated successfully by endoscopic decompression unless there is associated ischemia; however, elective resection should be considered in the future.
- LBO secondary to diverticular disease is rare and may be managed by a one-stage procedure when conservative management fails.

Large Bowel Obstruction

Large bowel obstruction (LBO) is a common condition that may be caused by mechanical conditions such as colorectal cancer, volvulus, diverticular disease, fecal impaction, inflammatory or vascular diseases, hernias, adhesions, carcinomatosis, or by functional disturbances (pseudo-obstruction). This chapter focuses on the clinical features, diagnosis, and management of LBO.

Clinical Features

The classic symptoms of LBO include obstipation, abdominal pain, and marked abdominal distension. Vomiting occurs generally late in the evolution of the condition. These symptoms and clinical findings depend on several factors, such as rapidity of the onset of the obstruction, cause and degree of obstruction, presence of co-morbid conditions, and the competency of the ileocecal valve. When a closed loop LBO is present, either by a colonic volvulus or a competent ileocecal valve, colonic distension is greater and is associated with a markedly increased risk of ischemia and perforation. Perforation may occur in the region of the neoplasm or proximally in areas of distended ischemic colon, most frequently in the thin-walled cecum. Many surgeons consider a closed loop LBO to be a surgical emergency. If the ileocecal valve is incompetent, patients are more likely to present with findings similar to small bowel obstruction and are less likely to present with ischemic colonic complications.

On physical examination, usually there is marked abdominal distension, often without much discomfort or tenderness to palpation. Auscultation may demonstrate obstructive bowel sounds, but with chronic obstruction, the bowel sounds may be diminished. On palpation, usually no mass is evident with a colonic volvulus or with an obstructing colon cancer (the colon cancer may be relatively small, <10 cm), but with diverticulitis, the suggestion of a mass and local tenderness may be present. On digital rectal or proctoscopic examination, a rectal or a low sigmoid tumor, presence of impacted feces, or evidence of extrinsic compression may be identified.

In addition to the clinical examination and routine laboratory evaluations, plain abdominal radiographs are helpful in determining the next diagnostic and therapeutic approach. The presence and location of gaseous distension of the colon, the diameter of cecum, fluid levels, association with small bowel dilation, and the presence or absence of gas in the rectum are essential for evaluation of LBO (❯ Fig. 68-1). If this study is inconclusive or if more information is sought, a multi-slice CT with intravenous and rectal contrast is a useful method for diagnosing the cause and site of obstruction. If CT is not available, water-soluble contrast enema can be used. Oral gastrointestinal contrast examination provides no useful information and should not be used.

General Principles of Management

The majority of patients with mechanical LBO require an urgent or emergent operation; indeed complete LBO should be considered a surgical emergency. The timing of operative intervention is dependent on the diagnosis, the general condition of the patient, the presence of a competent ileocecal valve, and signs of ischemia and perforation.

The first step in the treatment is fluid and electrolyte ressuscitation. A nasogastric tube is advised to prevent further entry of orally ingested gas into the colon. When operative intervention is required, it is important to assume that adequate ressuscitation efforts have been initiated and that appropriate prophylactic measures are taken. Perioperative broad-spectrum antibiotics, prophylaxis for deep vein thrombosis, and an indwelling urinary catheter are important. The patient is placed preferably in a litothomy position, and a midline incision performed. After opening the peritoneum, the abdominal cavity should be inspected carefully and the cause of obstruction and as well the viability of the involved bowel segments must be confirmed. In patients with massive luminal distension, decompression with a

□ **Figure 68-1**
a. Complete closed loop obstruction with gross distension of the cecum and right colon. b. An incomplete LBO with distension of small bowel

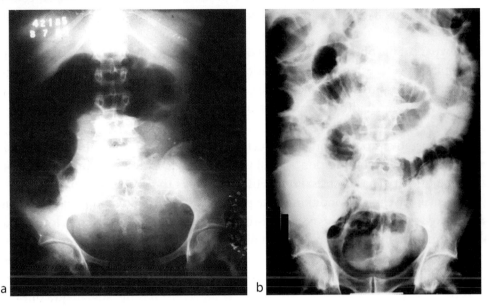

a   b

suction tube helps the manipulation of the bowel. If the small bowel is also distended, its contents should be decompressed back into the stomach and aspirated through the nasogastric tube.

Specific Causes of LBO and Treatment

Colorectal Cancer

Colorectal cancer (CRC) is the most common cause of LBO. In about 10% of patients with CRC, acute intestinal obstruction may be the presenting diagnosis. Obstruction is more common in the left colon due to its more solid contents, smaller luminal diameter, and less distensible bowel wall. The splenic flexure and sigmoid colon are the most common sites for obstruction. Patients presenting with an obstructing CRC have an increased risk of perioperative morbidity and mortality. Perforation occurs in 15% of patients and is associated with decreased long-term disease-free and overall survival, often because of both the perforation and locally advanced disease.

Treatment: For many years, a three-stage procedure was considered to be the best approach for an obstructing CRC. In the first stage, the colon was decompressed proximally by an external stoma. Colonic resection is then performed at a second stage, and the bowel continuity re-established in the third stage of this approach. With this approach, however, about 30% of patients were never able to undergo the third stage due to patient refusal, prohibitive medical comorbidities, or development of an advanced malignancy. Currently, the majority of surgeons agree that primary resection, with or without immediate restoration of colonic continuity, can be performed safely under favorable conditions.

There is now consensus that primary right colectomy and immediate anastomosis is a safe alternative in the majority of patients with an obstructing or near-obstructing right colon cancer.

Contraindications of primary resection with anastomosis are an unstable patient, presence of intraperitoneal sepsis, or concern about the viability of the bowel. Under these circumstances, the tumor should be resected, an end ileostomy performed, and the proximal end of the transverse colon closed or brought out as a mucous fistula near or at the same site as the ileostomy to facilitate restoration of intestinal continuity.

Intestinal bypass of the obstructing segment or loop ileostomy should be reserved for patients with fixed, large neoplasms with extensive local invasion or for patients with a prohibitively high risk for a prolonged anesthetic. Despite the acceptance that radical operations for obstructing right colon cancer are safe, mortality and morbidity in emergent operations is greater than that observed for elective operations.

The optimal operative strategy for an obstructing left colon cancer remains controversial. Opinions are divided between initial decompression by a colostomy followed by resection or an immediate resection with or without a primary anastomosis. Factors that may affect the operative approach may include the surgeon's experience, the clinical condition of the patient, and availability in the hospital resources.

The *three-stage procedure* (❷ *Fig. 68-2*) is associated with higher overall cost, longer hospital stay, considerable cumulative morbidity, and a mortality rate of 31%. Currently, the tendency is to reserve this approach for high-risk patients or for situations where surgical expertise in emergent colorectal procedures is lacking. In contrast, resection without primary anastomosis (the classic *two-stage procedure*) as described by Hartmann or Mickulicz (❷ *Fig. 68-3*) has the advantages of early resection of the cancer, relief of obstruction without the risk of anastomotic complications, a shorter overall hospital stay, and faster recovery. Disadvantages of the two-stage approach include the cost and morbidity of the second operation, and the necessity of another hospitalization and recovery period. Nevertheless, this two-stage approach is probably the most commonly performed approach for left-sided obstructing CRCs and appears especially suited for patients with a perforated left colon cancer and those patients with a compromised nutritional or medical state. This Hartmann's operation is generally reserved for neoplasms located in the high rectum or low sigmoid colon when the remaining rectal stump can be closed. For neoplasms in the upper sigmoid or descending colon, resection with exteriorization of both ends brought out through separate wounds is generally advocated to facilitate later restoration of intestinal continuity.

▢ Figure 68-2
Three-stage procedure for obstructed left colon cancer. a. Colostum; b. resection; c. colostomy closure

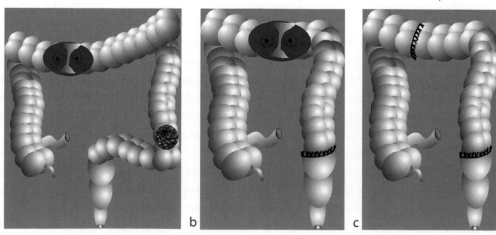

a   b   c

■ Figure 68-3
Two-stage procedure for obstructed left colon cancer. Hartmann's operation

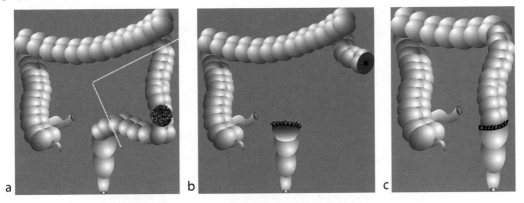

■ Figure 68-4
Segmentar resection and primary anastomosis

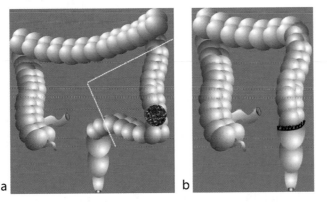

A *one-stage procedure* of segmental resection with primary anastomosis has been advocated increasingly over the past few years despite alleged concerns of anastomotic complications in an unprepped bowel or the presence of bacterial contamination (❏ *Fig. 68-4*).

The use of *intraoperative colonic lavage* has engendered acceptance of resection with primary anastomosis. This procedure is time-consuming, requires take down of one or both colonic flexures, and can be messy; however, operative mortality with this approach is low (4%), which compares favorably with the overall morbidity of the two-stage colostomy decompression procedures. Comparisons of this approach to the two-stage approaches are limited by selection bias, because patients undergoing two-stage are generally sicker with more medical comorbidity. Although several controlled trials have demonstrated that mechanical bowel preparation may not be necessary prior to an *elective* primary colonic anastomosis, the need for fecal evacuation in an obstructed colon is believed necessary but not proven.

Subtotal colectomy with ileosigmoidostomy or ileorectostomy is another form of one-stage procedure (❏ *Fig. 68-5*). This approach is the most appropriate operation for patients with synchronous right and left colon cancers, or when the cecum has serosal tears or ischemia related to the LBO. This approach is more difficult technically and should be reserved for selected patients with previous excellent bowel function and anorectal control, low surgical risk, absence of peritonitis, and operations to be performed

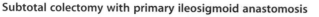

■ Figure 68-5
Subtotal colectomy with primary ileosigmoid anastomosis

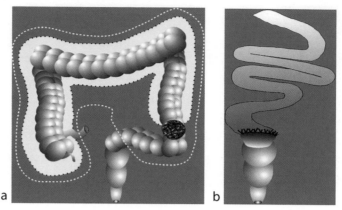

a   b

by experienced surgeons. Bowel frequency and anal function must be assessed by history prior to the operation, because diarrhea and fecal incontinence may occur and may be difficult to control, particularly in the elderly.

The Scotia Study Group conducted a prospective trial to compare subtotal colectomy with segmental resection and primary anastomosis after intraoperative lavage for left colon cancer. The perioperative mortality and morbidity did not differ between these groups; however, 4 months postoperatively, the number of bowel movements was much greater in the subtotal colectomy group. Thus, at our institution, favorable short- and long-term results with subtotal colectomy have encouraged our use of this approach but only in selected patients with obstructing colon cancer.

Other Treatment Options

Temporary methods of colonic decompression may convert an otherwise urgent operation to an elective one. Use of a transanal rectal tube and placement of an expandable luminal stent have been described. Endoscopic metallic endoluminal stent may also be used as a definitive palliative treatment in the setting of unresectable disease or in patients with prohibitive operative risk. Several series have reported a low morbidity and a high rate of clinical success in avoiding emergent operations in up to 94% of patients and allowing colonic decompression, bowel preparation, and elective resection; however, complications such as stent migration, pain, bleeding, intestinal perforation, and recurrence of obstruction have been reported.

Volvulus

Volvulus is defined as the abnormal rotation of a segment of bowel around its mesentery resulting in a complete or partial obstruction. The incidence of colonic volvulus varies depending on the region of the world, the socioeconomic status, age, and the presence of mental handicaps. In Western Europe and

North America, volvulus accounts for only 2–5% of all LBOs with 80% of those occurring in the sigmoid colon. Among certain populations in Africa, Iran, and Eastern Europe, however, volvulus is the most common cause of intestinal obstruction.

Sigmoid Volvulus

Predisposing factors for sigmoid volvulus include both congenital and acquired conditions. In all cases, redundancy of the bowel, an elongated mesocolon, and approximated points of fixation are present. In developed countries, sigmoid volvulus is seen most frequently in elderly, institutionalized, or chronically constipated patients treated with excessive use of laxative, psychotropic, or sedative drugs. Dietary factors such as ingestion of an excessively large bulk diet may also explain the differences in geographic distribution of the disease. In countries as in South America where Chagas' disease is frequent, sigmoid volvulus represents the most frequent complication of megacolon.

Complete volvulus requires torsion of the intestine of more than 180°. When the rotation is less than 90°, there is a simple twisting of the sigmoid colon over the rectum. A rotation of more than 180° around its mesenteric axis is followed by axial torsion of the bowel above the posterior fixation point. The magnitude of this axial torsion is twice that observed in the mesentery, as demonstrated by Groth, who suggested this to be the most important factor in producing intestinal obstruction.

Once obstruction occurs, the proximal colon distends with air and fluid, the extent of which depends on the competency of the ileocecal valve. As distension of the proximal colon and/or the volvulated colon increases, occlusion of intramural vessels can result in ischemia. As transmural ischemia develops, peritonitis with perforation may follow, either in the proximal colon (if the ileocecal valve is competent) or in the volvulated segment. Plain roentgenograms generally demonstrate a large, air and fluid-filled loop of bowel projecting into the right upper quadrant with loss of haustrations and the presence of other air-fluid levels in the abdomen (❂ *Fig. 68-6*). Depending on the competence of

◘ Figure 68-6
a. Sigmoid volvulus; b. sigmoid volvulus with radiologic signs of peritonitis

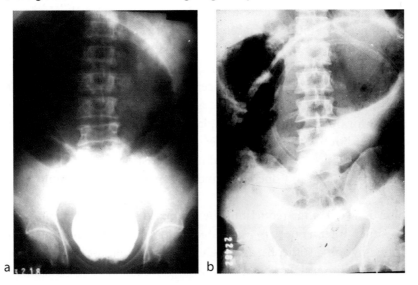

the ileocecal valve, there may be multiple distended loops of small bowel. Contrast enema studies demonstrate the typical bird-beak deformity.

Treatment: When there is no clinical or radiologic signs of peritonitis, conservative management is usually indicated initially. Endoscopic reduction of the sigmoid volvulus is based on the knowledge that the obstruction due to axial torsion causing distention can be decompressed effectively and de-torsed via an intraluminal approach. This technique requires passage of a nasogastric or rectal tube into the volvulated loop using the sigmoidoscope. The decompression tube should be left in place for several days to prevent recurrence of the volvulus; frequent irrigation ensures tube patency. Endoscopic decompression allows the opportunity for bowel preparation and elective operation. The overall success of endoscopic tube decompression initially is around 75–90%.

Emergent laparotomy is indicated in patients with evidence of ischemia, perforation, or failed endoscopic reduction. The choice of surgical procedure depends on the viability of the colon. When the sigmoid colon is viable and the colon proximal to the volvulus is viable and not too dilated, good results with resection and primary end-to-end anastomosis as an emergency procedure have been obtained in good risk, selected patients. In the presence of ischemia of the sigmoid colon, a Hartmann's procedure is the procedure of choice without primary anastomosis. Exteriorization of the colon distal to the volvulated segment is usually not possible, and therefore closure of the rectal stump is preferable.

Cecal Volvulus

Cecal and right colon volvulus represent only 1–10% of all acute causes of LBO and is less common than sigmoid volvulus. A cecal volvulus arises from an axial twist of the cecum on its mesentery, resulting in obstruction with the potential for vascular compromise and gangrene. Typically, cecal volvulus involves the terminal ileum, cecum, and the ascending colon, and on abdominal radiography, the dilated obstructed loop projects into the left upper quadrant. This type of cecal volvulus must be differentiated from a cecal bascule in which the cecum folds anteriorly and superiorly onto the ascending colon. Excessive mobility of right colon, typically due to congenital anomalies of fixation (the so-called floppy cecum), is prerequisite for the development of cecal volvulus.

Treatment: Spontaneous resolution of a cecal volvulus occurs in less than 2% of patients, and thus some form of intervention is necessary. When there is no sign of peritonitis, treatment options include colonoscopic decompression, cecopexy, cecostomy, and ileocolonic resection.

Although colonoscopic decompression has been reported with success, favorable results have not been obtained uniformly. While this conservative approach may be appropriate for selected patients with contraindications for operative intervention, laparotomy is required for the majority of patients. If the dilated segment of bowel is non-viable after reduction, resection is the appropriate treatment. Primary anastomosis or end ileostomy with distal mucous fistula may be performed according to the clinical condition of the patient and operative findings (peritonitis, contamination, and the quality of proximal bowel).

When the colon is viable after reduction, the optimal treatment remains controversial. Simple reduction without other intervention is associated with an inordinately high rate of recurrence. Cecopexy is advocated by some surgeons, although recurrence rates of up to 30% have been reported unless a very wide, long, peritoneal flap-based fixation is performed. Tube cecostomy has the advantage of fixation of the bowel to the abdominal wall while also allowing maintenance of cecal decompression. Whereas recurrence rates are low, morbidity is increased compared with other procedures. Overall, we favor colectomy with primary anastomosis in young or relatively healthy patients, and reserve cecopexy and cecostomy for elderly, poor risk patients.

Acute Colonic Pseudo Obstruction

Acute colonic pseudo obstruction or Ogilvie's syndrome is a condition characterized by symptoms and signs of LBO but without any mechanical obstruction. It is characterized by acute, massive dilation usually limited to the cecum and right colon. Without prompt colonic decompression, the dilated colon may result in perforation, peritonitis, and death. The syndrome may be a primary condition caused by an underlying motility disorder such as familial visceral myopathy or a disorder affecting the innervation of smooth muscle. Secondary pseudo-obstruction is much more frequent and may be the result of metabolic disturbances, cardiovascular disease (especially complicating myocardial infarctions), the postoperative state after orthopedic, urologic, or renal transplantation surgery, or conditions that are inflammatory, neurologic, or endocrine-related. Additional contributing factors include opiates, psychotropics, anticholinergics, and chemotherapic agents.

Patients with acute colonic pseudo-obstruction present with abdominal distension and progressive discomfort which may develop acutely or gradually. Clinical features may be similar to those observed in mechanical obstruction.

Plain abdominal radiographs demonstrate diffuse gaseous distension of the colon. Often there are few or absent fluid levels. The diameter of the cecum correlates with the risk of perforation and determines timing and aggressiveness of intervention. When the diameter is less than 10 cm, management may be conservative, with placement of a nasogastric tube, fluid and electrolyte resuscitation, identification of contributing factors, and serial abdominal x-rays. Rectal tube decompression and pharmacologic stimulation of the motility of the bowel with neostigmine have demonstrated effectiveness.

Colonoscopy is useful as an aid to diagnosis, allows decompression, and facilitates luminal tube placement for continued decompression. Colonoscopic decompression or aggressive neostigmine therapy is indicated for patients with a cecal diameter of ≥ 10 cm. Colonoscopy is our preferred initial approach and may be performed without mechanical bowel preparation and with minimal insufflation of air. Colonic decompression with placement of a colonic tube provides initial success in up to 80% of patients; however, repeated colonoscopy may be necessary for recurrences.

Laparotomy is required for patients who do not response to conservative methods and for those with signs of perforation or ischemia. If at laparotomy a small cecal perforation with little spillage is encountered, a tube cecostomy may be used. The success rate of tube cecostomy has been reported as 100% and has the lowest mortality rate among the operative procedures. These cecostomy tubes need to be of a large diameter and require frequent irrigation to clear the lumen of stool to allow ongoing decompression. For patients with free perforation or ischemic colon, resection of the segment and exteriorization are usually necessary. These procedures have high rates of complications and mortality due to both the presence of the complication itself and to the presence of other medical conditions, and thus a primary ileocolostomy should be undertaken only in selected patients. Percutaneous cecostomy has been proposed, although it is associated with as yet undefined risk of complications.

Diverticular Disease of the Colon

Intestinal LBO is quite rare in diverticular disease of the colon, occurring in less than 10% of all cases. It may occur in patients with acute diverticulitis with a peridiverticular abscess, pericolic annular fibrosis in chronic disease, or by angulation and consequent adhesive fixation of the inflamed bowel to the lateral wall of the pelvis. Small bowel obstruction may also occur if a segment of bowel adheres to the inflamed sigmoid colon.

Patients with obstruction caused by an acute episode of diverticulitis and an associated abscess may be treated with intravenous antibiotics, bowel rest, and image-guided percutaneous drainage. For those patients with a complete LBO, emergent laparotomy is usually required. The most frequently used operative intervention is resection of the diseased segment with immediate anastomosis with or without a diverting loop ostomy depending on operative findings, patient condition, and preference of the surgeon.

Other Causes of Large Bowel Obstruction

Fecal Impaction

Fecal impaction is more common in elderly patients, those who have been bedridden for an extended time, or institutionalized patients. This type of fecal impaction is a common complication of Chagasic megacolon and in younger patients with megarectum (❯ Fig. 68-7). Symptoms include chronic constipation with frequent small liquid feces and occasional incontinence. Abdominal palpation may detect an abdominal mass, usually in the left iliac fossa. A hard bolus of feces usually can be also felt by digital examination of the rectum.

◗ Figure 68-7
Megacolon with fecaloma

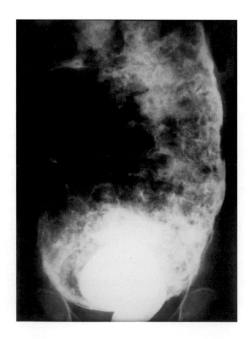

Treatment usually consists of digital manipulation, enema with oil or paraffin, magnesium sulfate, or phosphate enema. These methods generally are successful, although in some patients, disimpaction under general anesthesia may be necessary. Rarely, laparotomy is required to prevent or treat the complications of fecal impaction, such as complete intestinal obstruction or stercoral perforation.

Ischemic Stricture

Ischemia of the colon may be caused by occlusion of the inferior mesenteric artery by thrombosis, embolus, low output states, iatrogenic causes such as aortic surgery or therapeutic embolization, or after an episode of ischemic colitis. Despite these causes, vascular occlusion rarely is a cause of complete LBO. Treatment consists of wide resection of the ischemic segment back to healthy vascularized bowl; primary restoration of continuity depends on local conditions and overall patient health. After aortic surgery in which the inferior mesenteric artery has been occluded, cognizance of an adequate vascular supply of the remaining colon should be confirmed before restoring intestinal continuity after resection of the strictured area.

Crohn's Disease

LBO caused by Crohn's disease is also extremely rare, although strictures of the large colon are common. When LBO occurs, differentiation from CRC may be difficult or impossible even after colonoscopic examination. Sometimes the diagnosis of Crohn's disease is made only at laparotomy or after resection. Treatment consists of segmental resection if the stricture is localized or total colectomy in the presence of extensive disease. A primary anastomosis is for LBO complicating Crohn's disease is not recommended often due to the high incidence of anastomotic dehiscense.

Radiation Damage

In contrast to small bowel obstruction, LBO is extremely rare after radiation therapy. The distal colon may, however, become obstructed by a fibrous stricture, usually in the proximal rectum after pelvic irradiation. Operation must be carried out with caution because of adhesions, fibrosis, and difficult manipulation of the rectum in the pelvis. Inadvertent enterotomy is not a rare event. Resection may be technically impossible and a diverting stoma may be the procedure of choice.

Selected Readings

Bokey EL, Chapius PH, Fung C, et al. (1995) Postoperative morbidity and mortality following resection of the colon and rectum for cancer. Dis Colon Rectum 38:480–487

Habr-Gama A, Haddad J, Simonsen O, et al. (1976) Volvulus of the sigmoid colon in Brazil: a report of 230 cases. Dis Colon Rectum 19:314–320

Lopez-Kostner F, Hool GR, Lavery I (1997) Management and causes of acute large-bowel obstruction. Surg Clin N Amer 77:1265–1286

Martinez-Santos C, Lobato RF, Fradejas JM, et al. (2002) Self-expandable stent before elective surgery vs. emergency surgery for the treatment of malignant colorectal obstructions: comparison of primary anastomosis and morbidity rates. Dis Colon Rectum 45:401–406

Rabinovici R, Simansky DA, Kaplan O, et al. (1990) Cecal volvulus. Dis Colon Rectum 33:765–769

The SCOTIA Study Group (1995) Single-stage treatment for malignant left-sided colonic obstruction: a prospective randomized clinical trial comparing subtotal colectomy with segmental resection following intraoperative irrigation. Br J Surg 82:1622–1627

Smothers L, Hynan L, Fleming J, et al. (2003) Emergency surgery for colon carcinoma. Dis Colon Rectum 46:24–30

Tuech JJ, Becouarn G, Cattan F, Arnaud JP (1996) Volvulus du côlon droit. Plaidoyer pour l'hémicolectomie droite. J Chir 133:267–269

69 Chronic Ulcerative Colitis

Simon P. Bach · Neil J. Mortensen

Pearls and Pitfalls

- Ulcerative colitis (UC) patients admitted in relapse should be managed jointly by an "aggressive" physician and a "conservative" surgeon.
- If emergency surgery is required, a subtotal colectomy and end ileostomy should be performed. Leave a long closed sigmoid stump within the subcutaneous tissues at the lower pole of the wound. Decompress the rectum with a Foley catheter.
- Thromboprophylaxis should be strongly considered in all patients admitted with UC due to the increased risk of deep venous thromboses and thromboembolic events.
- Surveillance colonoscopy is performed optimally with the patient in remission to avoid sampling regenerative areas with histological features that might be misconstrued as dysplasia. Also, report recent cyclosporin treatment to the pathologist in order to facilitate the diagnosis of "pseudodysplasia".
- Incomplete endoscopic excision of any dysplastic colonic lesion within an area of colitis or the discovery of flat dysplasia in association with or remote from a dysplastic mass (regardless of resectability) is an indication for proctocolectomy. High grade flat dysplasia is a relatively rare indication for colectomy and patients with low grade flat dysplasia should be observed.
- The ileal pouch-anal anastomosis should ideally be positioned 2–3 cm above the anal margin. In practice this distance is roughly equivalent to the length of the distal two phalanges of the index finger.

Basic Science

Ulcerative colitis (UC) is characterized by chronic mucosal and submucosal inflammation of the colon and rectum. While the etiology of UC is yet to be elucidated, several associations are observed. There is a family history of either UC or Crohn's in 15% of patients. It is hypothesized that a hierarchy of inflammatory bowel disease (IBD) genes exist. One level may confer susceptibility to IBD in general, separate genes specify for UC or Crohn's while others modulate clinical features, such as disease distribution and the presence of extra-intestinal manifestations. Genetic influences are likely to interact with environmental factors. For instance UC occurs more commonly in non- or ex-smokers. Presentation is more frequent in the winter months, possibly as a result of an infectious agent. Appendicectomy is associated with a reduced risk of developing UC. Whether surgery is protective or patients destined to develop UC experience appendicectomy less frequently remains unclear. A unifying hypothesis is that UC follows an inappropriate, genetically determined response by the mucosal immune system to unspecified luminal antigens.

Clinical Presentation

UC is a relapsing and remitting disease confined to the colon and rectum. Disease activity is highly variable, ranging from chronically active colitis to a "burnt out" disease with protracted remission. Sex distribution is equal. Most patients present between 15 and 30 years of age although in a small proportion it occurs for the first time in their 60s and 70s, usually with localized proctitis. Onset of loose bloody stools with mucus and pus is usually gradual and reflects underlying inflammation of the colorectal mucsa. Abdominal cramping, bloating and increased stool frequency indicate more widespread enteric involvement. Patients may experience urgency or urge incontinence. Stool frequency is a particularly good indicator of disease severity. Systemic symptoms of anorexia, malaise and weight loss are similarly useful when assessing severity as are signs of tachycardia, fever, abdominal distension and tenderness. It should be remembered that steroid treatment may mask many of these findings.

Diagnosis of Ulcerative Colitis

Blood Tests: Anemia, leukocytosis and thrombocytosis indicate severe disease. Hypokalemia and dehydration may complicate prolonged diarrhea. Poor nutritional intake results in hypoalbuminemia. C reactive protein (CRP) > 45 mg/l or erythrocyte sedimentation rate (ESR) > 30 mm/h are additional markers of disease severity.

Stool Microscopy and Culture: Stools should be examined for *E. coli*, *Campylobacter*, *Salmonella* or *Entamoeba histolytica* in addition to *Clostridium difficile* toxin. Cytomegalovirus (CMV) is detected following intestinal biopsy and immunohistochemical staining (seronegativity negates the need for this test).

Radiological Diagnosis: Plain films are largely used to evaluate colonic calibre and to rule out perforation. A diameter of > 6 cm is considered abnormal.

Endoscopic Diagnosis: Although there is a risk of perforation in acute disease, initial endoscopic assessment provides an accurate tissue diagnosis and helps determine the extent and severity of inflammation. In the acute setting, flexible sigmoidoscopy is usually the investigation of choice, being relatively easy and safe to perform. Ultimately the colon should be surveyed until macroscopically normal tissue is reached. In UC, circumferential inflammation extends proximally from the anal verge. This is in contrast to Crohn's colitis where 40% of patients demonstrate rectal sparing. The pattern of involvement in UC is rectum alone in approximately 40%, left colon in 40% and total colitis in 20%. The distribution of disease is not static and may increase or decrease after initial assessment. Biopsies taken from normal and abnormal areas avoid underestimating the extent of colonic involvement, although the significance of microscopic inflammation proximal to macroscopic disease remains uncertain. Mucosa affected by UC initially exhibits a granular appearance with loss of vascular markings secondary to intramural edema. Bleeding often occurs spontaneously or following contact with the endoscope. Numerous shallow erosions or microulcers may be apparent, and their size and extent mirror disease severity. Repeated cycles of relapse and remission lead to clumps of hyperplastic, regenerating mucosa interspersed between areas of ulceration that give rise to "pseudo-polyps" otherwise termed "inflammatory polyps". Clinicians should be aware that *bone fide* UC may present initially with features suggestive of Crohn's disease. Prominent inflammation of the transverse colon in severe UC gives an impression of rectal sparing, and partial treatment with steroid enemas may compound this effect. Fissuring or transmural ulceration is another feature of fulminant UC. Lastly, one quarter of patients with active subtotal UC exhibit discontinuous inflammation at the appendiceal orifice. This appendiceal "skip lesion" is considered to be a normal variant of UC.

Histological Diagnosis: UC is characterized by isolated mucosal inflammation; the muscularis propria and serosa remain unaffected except in fulminant disease. Inflammatory cells congregate within crypts and alongside dilated vessels of the lamina propria. Secondary infection of inflammatory debris within the crypt lumen is thought to drive the formation of crypt abscesses. While these lesions are characteristic of UC they are a non-specific feature of large intestinal inflammation. Crypt abscesses can point directly into the intestinal lumen or alternatively rupture in a submucosal plane causing ulceration. Crypt architecture is distorted and goblet cells are lost giving rise to mucin depletion. These histological features may become unevenly distributed as the patient improves giving a false impression of segmental disease. A degree of crypt distortion will usually persist once remission is achieved. This is a histopathological hallmark of UC.

Differential Diagnoses: Infectious colitides usually arises as a result of an isolated infection that is self limiting within a period of 14 days and of insufficient duration to cause crypt distortion. Immunocompromised hosts, such as AIDS and UC patients, treated with immunosuppressive agents are prone to develop longer lasting infection, often of viral origin. Protozoal infections also have a tendency to persist if untreated. It is estimated that in 10–20% of patients with relapsing UC, pathogens are seen on stool testing. It remains unclear whether these pathogens trigger or mimic relapse but some will respond to appropriate antibiotic therapy. Fulminant colitis complicated by CMV infection may respond to antiviral treatment using gancyclovir. Major differential diagnoses are outlined in ❯ *Table 69-1*.

Assessing the Severity of Ulcerative Colitis: Complete assessment of disease activity involves evaluation of symptoms, physical examination, measurement of laboratory indices and endoscopy. Scoring systems draw together key elements of this assessment to stratify patients according to their disease severity. They provide a basis for the consistent delivery of treatment protocols, especially

◻ **Table 69-1**
Differential diagnoses of ulcerative colitis

Infectious	Bacterial	*Campylobacter, Escherichia coli, Clostridium difficile, Salmonella, Shigella, Yersinia, Chlamydia* or *Gonococcus*
	Viral	Rotavirus, CMV, Herpes simplex
	Protozoal	*Entamoeba histolytica, Cryptosporidium* or *Giardia*
Non-infectious	Drug induced	NSAIDs eosinophilic infiltrate – eosinophilic infiltrate
	Diverticular	Characteristic distribution, rectal biopsies are normal
	Ischemic	Rectal biopsies should be normal
	Radiation	History of radiation and telangiectasia
	Microscopic colitis	Triad of watery diarrhea, endoscopically normal mucosa and collagenous or lymphocytic infiltrate (most pronounced in the proximal colon). Minority of cases associated with drug ingestion or coeliac disease

within randomized controlled trials. Truelove and Witts first classified relapses of UC according to criteria listed in ❯ *Table 69-2*. This system is easy to remember and may aid identification of the sick patient.

◘ Table 69-2

Classification of disease severity in ulcerative colitis (Modified from Truelove and Witts, 1955)

	Mild	Moderate	Severe	Fulminant
Stools per day	<4	4–6	>6	>10
Rectal bleeding	Infrequent	Intermediate	Frequent	Continuous
Temperature	<37.5°C	Intermediate	>37.5°C	>37.5°C
Heart rate	<90 bpm	Intermediate	>90 bpm	>90 bpm
Hemoglobin	>10 g/dl	Intermediate	<10 g/dl	Transfusion
ESR	<30 mm/h	Intermediate	>30 mm/h	>30 mm/h

Special Features of Ulcerative Colitis

Extra-intestinal Manifestations: 20% of patients with UC manifest associated conditions of the joints, liver, eyes or skin. IBD-associated peripheral arthritis is the commonest extra-intestinal manifestation of UC. It produces a transient and asymmetrical inflammation of the large joints (knees, ankles, elbows, wrists). Synovitis mirrors the course of colitis and is cured by colectomy. The axial skeleton may be affected by ankylosing spondylitis (AS) or isolated sacroiliitis. AS is a seronegative arthropathy of the sacroiliac and vertebral facet joints. Its prevalence in UC is 1–5% and two thirds of affected individuals are HLA-B27 positive. Axial arthritis does not resolve following successful treatment of colitis.

Primary sclerosing cholangitis (PSC) is a serious condition that causes fibrous stricturing of the entire biliary tree in 5% of patients with UC. Asymptomatic elevation of alkaline phosphatase may be the first indication of liver disease. Abdominal pain, intermittent episodes of jaundice and pruritis develop later. The diagnosis is confirmed by a characteristic magnetic resonance cholangiopancreatography (MRCP) or endoscopic retrograde cholangiopancreatography (ERCP) and compatible liver biopsy. Hepatic failure gradually ensues over a 5–10 year period and it is independent of the course of colitis. Biliary stenting and rarely, surgery may be required to relieve obstruction, and orthotopic liver transplantation can be performed in end-stage disease. Unfortunately, a significant proportion of patients develop cholangiocarcinoma which has a very poor prognosis. The risk of colorectal cancer is also increased 10-fold compared to those with UC alone.

Iritis, episcleritis and anterior uveitis complicate UC relatively rarely. Prompt access to specialist services and appropriate treatment with topical and/or oral corticosteroids leads to resolution of symptoms in the majority of cases without any permanent damage.

Pyoderma gangrenosum is a skin condition occasionally associated with UC. Painful violaceous plaques merge to form solitary ulcers with an undermined purple border. Any area can be affected but the lower limbs are especially vulnerable as are any previously injured areas of the skin. Systemic steroid therapy or intralesional steroid injection have been used to treat this for many years although the condition will slowly improve following colectomy. More recently, tacrolimus ointment (an immune modulator that inhibits calcineurin) has been used with some success. Cyclosporin and infliximab also show activity in this disorder. Erythema nodosum produces tender red nodules on the shin that are also prone to ulceration. Treatment includes bed-rest and anti-inflammatory medication.

UC and Neoplasia: Large bowel malignancy ultimately complicates UC in 5% of patients. Risk becomes clinically significant once the disease has been present for 8–10 years. Subsequent risk accumulates at a rate of 0.5–1.0% per year. It is estimated that 2% will develop cancer at 10 years, 8% at 20 years and 18% after 30 years. The magnitude of risk may be decreasing due to the effects of screening, prophylactic surgery and anti-inflammatory maintenance therapy. Nonetheless, a family history of colorectal cancer combined with pancolitis mark subjects at high risk. Frequency and severity of relapse are also considered significant factors. Those with PSC are at highest risk of colorectal cancer.

The best surrogate for development of colorectal cancer in UC is the discovery of dysplasia in large intestinal mucosal biopsies. This provides the rationale for colonoscopic surveillance. Dysplasia associated with UC is classified microscopically as either low, (LGD) or high, (HGD) grade depending upon the degree of cytological and architectural disturbance. Endoscopic classification depends upon whether the lesion is raised or flat with further subdivision of raised lesions according to their macroscopic appearance. Raised areas resembling conventional adenomas are designated as adenoma-like lesions or masses (ALMs). These pedunculated or sessile polyps are usually amenable to endoscopic resection. Areas that demonstrate pronounced irregularity are termed dysplasia-associated lesions or masses (DALMs). These include plaques, velvety patches, areas of nodular thickening and broad based masses. Such lesions are typically not endoscopically resectable in their entirety. Sporadic adenomas may be encountered within non-inflamed portions of the colon. These are managed in a conventional way.

The majority of UC related lesions (~80%) are ALMs and in such cases COMPLETE local excision and surveillance yields a good prognosis, irrespective of the degree of dysplasia. Continued surveillance will identify further ALMs in 50–60% of patients and flat dysplasia may occur in a small proportion (< 5%). DALMs are usually more challenging to remove endoscopically due to their irregular morphology. Ultimately, completeness of endoscopic resection will govern prognosis, and categorizing lesions as ALMs or DALMs is perhaps of secondary importance. This management strategy must be underpinned by careful endoscopic assessment of the whole colon by an experienced practitioner with facility to use dye-spray techniques. Adherence to these principles uncovers otherwise "occult" colonic lesions. Indications for proctocolectomy following the discovery of a dysplastic mass are (1) incomplete excision of that mass or (2) discovery of multifocal flat dysplasia of any grade at sites either near to or remote from the index lesion. Biopsy samples must be taken beyond the perimeter of a sessile mass to uncover patients who possess a wider field change. The incidence of underlying malignancy in those who undergo proctocolectomy for DALM is in the order of 30–40%.

The finding of HGD in otherwise flat mucosa is an indication for proctocolectomy as the risk of underlying malignancy is in the order of 40%. This is a relatively unusual finding as isolated HGD is more often associated with some form of discernable lesion. Management of LGD in the absence of a macroscopic lesion is more controversial as its natural history is still hotly debated. It should be appreciated that there is significant inter-observer variability in the reporting of LGD even amongst experienced gastroenterological histopathologists. One problem is that biopsies taken from regenerative mucosa following an exacerbation of UC may be mistaken for LGD. Some institutions favor immediate proctocolectomy for LGD based upon studies demonstrating a 20% risk of occult malignancy at presentation with 50% disease progression in 5 years. A more conservative approach consists of intensified surveillance with colonoscopy at 6-monthly intervals even in cases of multifocal flat LGD.

Thorough endoscopic examination by an experienced clinician obviates the need for routine colectomy for LGD. Dye-spray techniques help to identify malignant lesions that are otherwise invisible. This strategy has been safely adopted in specialist centers with rates of disease progression between 3 to 10% at 10 years. The patient's attitude towards surgery, risk of occult cancer and increased endoscopic surveillance should also be taken into account and used to guide treatment in these circumstances.

Screening for Malignancy: Colonoscopy is advocated for patients with long-standing colitis. Surveillance programs have been derived empirically and much heterogeneity exists in the application and delivery of this service. Evidence based guidelines produced in the UK recommend that patients with pancolitis start surveillance 8–10 years following the onset of symptoms. Examinations are recommended every 3 years during the second decade of UC, 2-yearly in the third and annually in the fourth. Smaller intervals reflect the notion of an exponential rise in cancer incidence over time although this view has recently been challenged. Patients with isolated left sided disease may begin surveillance later at 15–20 years. Due to the higher risk of malignancy in patients with PSC, annual surveillance is recommended from the outset. Guidelines in the UK state that random biopsy samples (2–4 in number) should be taken at 10 cm intervals throughout the colon and rectum. Another favorable strategy is to perform careful inspection of the whole colon with dye-spray, targeting macroscopically abnormal areas for biopsy. Colonoscopy should optimally be performed with the patient in remission as regenerating mucosa may display atypical features that mimic dysplasia, although in practice this is often difficult to achieve. Cyclosporin treatment may also cause pseudo-dysplasia and the pathologist should be informed where this drug has been used.

Thromboembolism: Patients with UC have a threefold increased risk of developing pulmonary embolism compared to normal controls. This risk is manifest at a young age. Thrombocytosis, dehydration, nutritional deficiencies, presence of inflammatory cytokines, immobility and surgery have all been implicated. Antithrombotic stockings and prophylactic heparin should be prescribed routinely for inpatients with UC, especially those undergoing surgery. Pneumatic calf compression devices are used intra-operatively.

Treatment for Ulcerative Colitis

Treatment of patients with UC is dependent upon disease location (proctitis vs. left sided disease vs. pancolitis), severity (mild, moderate, or severe) and the presence of complications. Medical treatment is aimed at inducing and then maintaining remission. Surgery is usually considered appropriate for those with refractory disease or where neoplastic lesions are found within the colon. In children, growth retardation can prompt colectomy in order to correct malnutrition.

Medical Treatment

Aminosalicylates constitute first line therapy for both the induction and maintenance of remission in mild to moderate UC. They are thought to exert topical anti-inflammatory and immunomodulatory effects. Mesalazine induces remission in 70% of patients with mild to moderate UC at a dose of 4 g/day, although at 6 weeks this figure drops to 30%. In predominantly left sided disease, steroid (prednisolone

5 mg) or mesalazine (1 g daily) are also administered topically per rectum. Suppositories reach the upper rectum and foams to the distal sigmoid (these preparations may be combined) while enemas extend up to the splenic flexure. Patients who fail to respond after 2 weeks are given oral prednisolone 20 mg daily which is then reduced over the course of a month as symptoms improve. Mesalazine is continued to maintain remission. Two-year therapy may be appropriate for those with left sided disease whereas indefinite therapy is considered for patients with pancolitis. 5-ASA compounds reduce relapse rates from 80% to 30–50% and in addition the incidence of neoplastic transformation may also be reduced.

Moderate flares of UC are treated using oral prednisolone (40 mg daily). A reducing dose is continued for 4–6 weeks. Hospitalization with administration of parenteral hydrocortisone (200–400 mg/day) or prednisolone (60 mg daily) should be considered in those who do not improve or have severe disease from the outset. Aminosalicylates are generally poorly tolerated in this type of patient. Antidiarrheal agents may precipitate megacolon and should also be avoided. With steroid therapy clinical improvement typically occurs over 7–14 days. Those who promptly relapse are treated with azathioprine or 6-mercaptopurine. There is evidence to suggest that these drugs are effective in reducing corticosteroid dose and may also help maintain remission in patients with UC. They may take 3 months to reach full activity. Non-responders have their diagnosis reconfirmed by stool culture and sigmoidoscopy with biopsy. Intravenous cyclosporin may help avoid surgery in those with refractory UC. More than 50% of patients respond over 2–5 days. Oral cyclosporin must then be used to maintain remission and allow tapering of steroids and establishment of azathioprine. Infliximab may similarly be used to treat severe steroid resistant flares. Three infusions at 0, 2 and 6 weeks are recommended for induction. Responders receive maintenance therapy with infliximab infusions every 8 weeks.

Surgical Treatment

About 25% of patients with UC ultimately require colectomy. Patients usually submit to surgery during a particularly severe exacerbation of the disease or following a protracted period of ill-health and steroid dependence. In the acute setting, colectomy most often follows failure of medical treatment for severe and extensive colitis. Toxic dilatation (colon > 6 cm), perforation and hemorrhage are less common indications for colectomy. The decision to operate is taken jointly and involves daily communication between the gastroenterology and surgical teams. Patients receiving high-dose intra-venous steroids, and who have a stool frequency of > 8 per day on the third treatment day are likely to require colectomy. Similarly, those with a stool frequency of 3–8 stools per day who have a CRP > 45 mg/l are unlikely to settle. Failure to respond after 5–7 days or any significant deterioration during this period is an indication for colectomy. Patients who initially respond but promptly relapse with the reintroduction of diet are also likely to require colectomy.

In the acute setting, ile-pouch anal anastomosis (IPAA) surgery should be avoided. It is customary to instead perform subtotal colectomy with an end ileostomy. The diseased rectum is left in situ, for resection at a later date once the patient has regained health and steroids have been withdrawn. Emergency colectomy may be performed using an open or laparoscopic approach. The colon is mobilised and vessels taken relatively close to the bowel wall. The sigmoid stump is stapled and left long allowing it to be secured with sutures in the subcutaneous space at the lower pole of the wound. Any stump dehiscence will then result in an easily manageable fistula rather than a pelvic abscess. Occasionally the stump must be left short in cases of sigmoid hemorrhage. In all cases, a Foley catheter is used to decompress the rectum for a period of 3 or 4 days.

Three operative strategies are in common use for the definitive surgical treatment of UC patients. (1) Proctocolectomy plus end ileostomy removes all diseased tissue at the expense of a permanent stoma. This option is undertaken in patients with poor sphincter function. It is also used in those patients who are happy with their ileostomy following subtotal colectomy and do not wish to consider a pouch. (2) Subtotal colectomy plus ileorectal anastomosis (IRA) is a compromise procedure in which a minimally diseased rectum is retained. The rectum must be distensible and retain its capacity to act as a reservoir. This can be confirmed using flexible sigmoidoscopy or a contrast enema. There should be no evidence of colonic dysplasia or malignancy. These criteria are seldom met and this option is rarely used. Function is difficult to predict following IRA and one quarter of patients suffer from unacceptable stool frequency as a consequence of persistent rectal inflammation. Long-term endoscopic follow up of the retained rectum is essential due to the risk of malignant change. (3) Finally, IPAA has become the standard of care for patients with ulcerative colitis who ultimately require colectomy. This approach is popular with patients as it avoids the necessity for a long-term stoma. Pouch surgery aims to deliver 5 or 6 semi-formed bowel motions per day, with no night time evacuation and no incontinence. Successful outcomes are built upon sensible patient selection, clear pre-operative counseling, an operative strategy appropriate to the patient and expedient management of any complications.

Patient Selection for Ileal Pouch Surgery

Age: Large case series have shown that surgical complications and pouch preservation rates appear to be independent of age at operation, whilst continence and quality of life are generally a little worse with advancing years. IPAA surgery is performed routinely in well motivated elderly individuals without symptomatic disturbance of the anal sphincters.

Indeterminate Colitis: A definitive histopathological diagnosis of UC or Crohn's is not always possible following colectomy for colitis. In 10–15% of all surgical specimens a diagnosis of indeterminate colitis (IndC) is made. A diagnosis of Crohn's disease will be made subsequently in 4–15% of patients initially labeled as IndC. Clinicians make every effort to define this population prior to embarking upon ileal pouch surgery. While the majority of patients with IndC obtain good results from IPAA surgery, pelvic sepsis and pouch failure may occur more frequently. This is largely due to the emergence of patients with Crohn's disease. At 10 years, 85% of those with IndC retain their pouch. The consensus amongst most surgeons is that patients with *bona fide* IndC are suitable candidates for pouch surgery if fully informed of the risks involved. Special attention should be paid to any suspicious history of pelvic sepsis or perineal fistula as these patients are more likely to manifest Crohn's and in our opinion should not be considered for IPAA surgery.

Crohn's Colitis: Crohn's disease remains an absolute contraindication to IPAA as the overall failure rates approach 50%. There may be a role for pouch surgery in a highly selective group of patients with Crohn's colitis who possess a normal anus, have no small bowel disease and are prepared to accept the increased risks of failure and reoperation.

Dysplasia or Cancer in the Proctocolectomy Specimen: The presence of dysplasia or potentially curable cancer either within the colon or high in the rectum does not preclude IPAA. Mucosectomy and a hand-sewn pouch-anal anastomosis rather than stapling are considered for patients with multiple tumors or multifocal dysplasia especially when these lesions encroach upon the rectum. Following mucosectomy dysplastic cells may survive deep within the muscular rectal cuff and these may re-present as "pouch tumors". For this reason, reconstructive pouch surgery is probably inadvisable when dealing with low rectal tumors.

Technique of Ileal Pouch Surgery

Pouch Design: Parks and Nicholls originally devised a triple limb "S"-shaped pouch. This was relatively complicated to construct and suffered from kinking of the efferent limb if left too long. Alternative designs have included the high capacity "W" pouch, the "H" pouch and the "J" pouch. The majority of surgeons now favor the J pouch due to ease of construction, economical use of terminal ileum and reliable emptying. Functional results are equal to those of other reservoir designs. The pouch is formed from the terminal 40 cm of ileum using several applications of a linear, cutting stapler to join the antimesenteric borders of two 20 cm ileal limbs.

Mucosectomy vs. Double Stapling: Stripping of the columnar mucosa above the dentate line has been advocated in order to prevent recurrence of UC. Mucosectomy, combined with a per-anal hand-sewn anastomosis allows precise placement of the pouch-anal anastomosis at the dentate line. This technique is more complex to perform and may be associated with higher rates of sphincter damage and incontinence. Mucosectomy also entails excision of the anal transition zone (ATZ), an area of cuboidal epithelium richly innervated by sensory nerve endings that mediate anal sampling reflexes. The "double stapled" IPAA technique preserves this theoretically important area with no requirement for prolonged anal dilation. A transverse stapler fired from above, separates the rectum from the top of the anal canal. The stapling instrument should be positioned 2–3 cm above the anal margin, a distance roughly equivalent to the length of the distal two phalanges of the index finger. This helps to avoid an error of judgement that places the anastomosis too high resulting in a pouch-rectal anastomosis. A circular EEA stapler inserted via the anus joins the ileal reservoir to the upper anal canal. Many surgeons favor the double staple technique as this is a simpler operation and may have a lower risk of failure.

One, Two or Three Stage IPAA: To date, most surgeons have favored the creation of a temporary defunctioning loop ileostomy following IPAA surgery as this avoids catastrophic pelvic contamination in the event of anastomotic dehiscence. Pouch failure rates from St Marks were higher in patients without a covering stoma; 15% versus 8%, although Toronto have published contrasting figures with less than 1% of one-stage pouches failing. To omit a defunctioning ileostomy is an exercise in risk management. Large series indicate that anastomotic separation occurs in approximately 5–15% of patients while complication rates for ileostomy closure range from 10% to 30%. Small bowel obstruction, wound infection and anastomotic leakage are most prevalent. In practice, stomas are omitted in approximately 15% of cases based upon the perceived risks (steroids, nutrition, age, anemia etc.), uneventful surgery and discharge arrangements.

Laparoscopic IPAA: Conventional open surgery utilizes a long midline incision for access to the splenic flexure and pelvis. The laparoscopic approach is more elegant as trauma to the abdominal wall is minimized. In the short term, wound related complications, such as pain and infection, may be reduced. Over a more protracted period the risk of symptomatic adhesions and incisional herniation may be diminished. There is little doubt that cosmetic appearance is enhanced. To date, rigorous assessment of these endpoints using large clinical trials has been hindered by the relative complexity of these techniques. Accelerated recovery programs have delivered reduced hospital stays for elective IPAA patients somewhat negating the benefits of laparoscopic over open surgery in this regard.

Acute Complications of IPAA

Acute Sepsis: Fever in a patient recovering from IPAA surgery should arouse suspicion of pelvic sepsis. This remains a relatively common acute complication and failure to react in a timely fashion is likely to compromise pouch function and may lead to its eventual failure. Septic complications usually result from anastomotic dehiscence or the presence of an infected pelvic hematoma. Digital examination may reveal the anastomotic defect or localized tenderness overlying an indurated or fluctuant mass. CT or MRI can be used to gauge the extent of sepsis. A trial of broad spectrum antibiotics is appropriate for relatively small abscesses. More sizeable collections are considered for radiological drainage. Failure to settle would prompt examination under anesthesia. The anus is inspected using an Eisenhammer anal speculum (Seward, London, UK). Anastomotic breakdown is usually detected without difficulty. The underlying area is then probed to determine the extent of any associated abscess cavity and suction applied to clear its contents. Larger defects may be amenable to digital examination followed by placement of a catheter for irrigation and drainage. Regular re-examination under anesthesia may be required to be confident that the cavity remains clean. The vagina must also be inspected for evidence of fistulation, especially if the IPAA was stapled.

Re-laparotomy is reserved for cases where CT-guided drainage and minor surgery have failed to control sepsis and also for those who deteriorate quickly with signs of generalized peritonitis. Major leaks require a proximal diverting loop ileostomy to be formed if one is not already in place. Consideration should be given to exteriorizing of the pouch if complete anastomotic disruption has occurred. If gross ischemia occurs, it is best to resect and exteriorize the ileum.

Rates of pelvic sepsis are much higher for patients with UC undergoing IPAA than for those with familial adenomatous polyposis (FAP) who are subject to the same operation. High dose corticosteroids (systemic equivalent of > 40 mg prednisolone per day) have been implicated in the causation of anastomotic failure. Steroids may impair healing at the anastomosis, promote infection or merely label patients in poor clinical condition. It is customary to avoid IPAA formation and instead perform subtotal colectomy in those patients who are acutely unwell and receiving high dose corticosteroids.

Hemorrhage: Primary intraluminal hemorrhage may follow formation of a sutured or stapled pouch and it is therefore important to carefully inspect the mucosal surface before the pouch-anal anastomosis is constructed. Reactionary intraluminal hemorrhage, within 24 h of surgery is likely to originate from the suture or staple lines. Irrigation of the pouch with a 1:200,000 adrenaline solution controls the majority of clinically significant hemorrhages. Continued bleeding necessitates a return to the operating room. The pouch is inspected using an Eisenhammer speculum, proctoscope or sigmoidoscope. Suction and irrigation are used to accurately locate the bleeding point which is then sutured or injected with 1:100,00 adrenaline solution. Secondary hemorrhage is less common and usually heralds pelvic sepsis. The pouch should be inspected in theater with special attention to the ileoanal anastomosis for evidence of localized anastomotic breakdown. Bleeding points are under-run and collections drained, preferably via the original defect. A small mushroom or Foley catheter may then be placed trans-anally into the cavity.

Intra-abdominal hemorrhage may arise from mesenteric vessels or the pelvic side wall. The rectal stump may bleed following hand-sewn pouch-anal anastomosis. In exceptional circumstances inspection of the lower pelvis is facilitated by detachment of the pouch. The stump is approached endo-anally using a Lone Star retractor (Lone Star Medical Products Inc, Houston, TX). The pouch may then be exteriorized as a left iliac fossa mucous fistula if re-anastomosis is considered unsafe. Uncontrollable pelvic hemorrhage requires packing of the cavity with a follow-up 48 h later.

Chronic Complications and Outcome Following IPAA

Mucosal Adaptation and Pouchitis: Pouchitis is a relapsing, acute-on-chronic inflammatory condition presenting with diarrhea (may be bloody), urgency, abdominal bloating, pain or fever. The etiology is unknown although recurrent UC in areas of colonic metaplasia and bacterial overgrowth are possible mechanisms. Interestingly, this condition does not seem to affect pouches in patients with FAP. Patients with new symptoms suggestive of pouchitis should be investigated by endoscopy and biopsy. Endoscopic appearances are similar to those of UC. Histologically signs of acute inflammation (polymorphonuclear leucocyte infiltration) with superficial ulceration, superimposed onto a background of chronic inflammatory changes are typical. Once the diagnosis is established then it would be reasonable to instigate empirical therapy for relapses.

The cumulative probability of pouchitis, determined on the basis of symptomatology, endoscopy and histopathology is in the order of 20% at 1 year, 30% at 5 years and 40% at 10 years. Differential diagnoses include undiagnosed Crohn's disease, especially in the presence of prominent ulceration, with pre-pouch ileitis or fistula formation. Alternatively, bacterial/ viral infections, cuffitis, pelvic sepsis, a low volume reservoir, pouch outlet obstruction and incomplete emptying, can produce similar symptoms. Stool examination, MRI and isotope or contrast pouchogram may help to elucidate the nature of malfunction.

Most cases respond to oral metronidazole or ciprofloxacin. Two thirds of patients develop further attacks and 5% become chronic sufferers. Maintenance therapy may be effective for those who promptly relapse although prolonged treatment with metronidazole is inadvisable due to the risk of peripheral neuropathy. The probiotic VSL-3 may be taken orally with some evidence that relapse rates are decreased. Those who fail to respond may be offered oral or rectal corticosteroids. Oral or topical mesalazine may also be used. Consideration should be given to removing the pouch where function is very poor as a consequence of chronic pouchitis. Chronic pouchitis accounts for 10% of all pouch failures.

Cuffitis: The ATZ forms a relatively small proportion of the anal canal. Conventional double-stapled restorative proctocolectomy therefore leaves 1.5–2.0 cm of columnar epithelium above the ATZ (❯ *Fig. 69-1*). Recurrent UC within the columnar cuff is termed "cuffitis" and it arises in 9–22% of patients. Cuffitis may lead to increased stool frequency, bloody discharge, urgency and discomfort. Mesalazine suppositories may be helpful in improving these symptoms. Dysplasia or carcinoma may theoretically arise within unresected columnar mucosa. Reports do exist of adenocarcinomas situated below the level of the IPAA but these lesions are generally associated with the presence of severe dysplasia or malignancy within the original proctocolectomy specimen. Routine surveillance of the

◘ Figure 69-1

Distribution of epithelial subtypes in a typical double-stapled pouch-anal anastomosis (Reprinted from Thompson-Fawcett et al., 1998. Copyright 1998. With permission from Wiley)

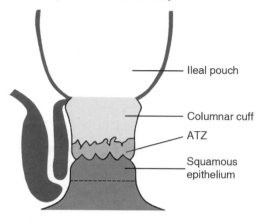

anal canal is not advocated for the first 10 years following IPAA unless the patient has a previous history of dysplasia or malignancy.

Small Bowel Obstruction: In a large series from Toronto, the risk of small bowel obstruction (SBO) outside of the perioperative period was reported as 6% at 1 year, 14% at 5 years and 19% at 10 years. Laparotomy was required in one third of patients, and in the majority of cases small bowel was adherent to the pelvis or a previous stoma site. About 20% of patients who underwent laparotomy and adhesiolysis developed further episodes of SBO. One quarter of these had a further laparotomy. A water soluble contrast enema may help to determine the site, nature and degree of obstruction. This investigation may also be of therapeutic benefit. Alternatively, CT scan with oral contrast provides similar information.

Chronic Pelvic Sepsis: Pelvic sepsis is estimated to complicate 10–20% of IPAA procedures. Long term manifestations of pouch sepsis include a variety of fistulae (pouch-anal anastomotic, pouch vaginal, pouch perineal or proximal pouch) and anastomotic stenosis. Functional outcome is likely to be worse and long term ileostomy may be required.

Fistulae arising between the IPAA and vagina occur relatively rarely. Operative trauma, postoperative pelvic sepsis and undiagnosed Crohn's disease are all implicated. Unsuspected Crohn's should be actively sought as rates of healing are worse (25% vs. 48%) and pouch failure more common (33% vs. 14%) amongst this subgroup. Principals of management include local drainage of the tract using a seton with fecal diversion in selected cases based upon the degree of uncontrolled sepsis. Several options are available to the surgeon for definitive treatment. Transanal ileal advancement flap is appropriate for a pouch that remains mobile with success rates reported in the order of 50%. Transabdominal advancement of the ileoanal anastomosis with closure of the defect is necessary when the pouch cannot be mobilized from below. Per-anal access to fistulae arising within the anal canal may be difficult, especially where an anastomosis has been placed at the anorectal junction. For this reason the transvaginal route is favored by some as access is easier and damage to the anal sphincters may be avoided. Fistulae that arise as a consequence of previously unrecognized Crohn's disease may be treated with infliximab, although recurrence remains a problem.

Anastomotic stricture may complicate leakage, tension or ischemia at the IPAA. It is important to perform an adequate examination under anesthesia prior to ileostomy closure in addition to the pouchogram. For those using the pouch, symptoms of straining, diarrhea and anal or abdominal pain suggest stricturing of the anastomosis. It may be possible to attempt dilatation at the time of pouchoscopy. Alternatively, application of Hegar's dilators under anesthesia treats most cases successfully. Particularly long or tight strictures may not respond to these measures and further biopsies should be taken to exclude Crohn's disease. Per-anal pouch advancement is considered once all sepsis has been eradicated if the pouch is not tethered. This technique is also used to close fistula tracks situated at the level of the stricture. Otherwise re-laparotomy and mobilization of the pouch with re-anastomosis is the sole option.

Sexual Dysfunction: Erectile function is a parasympathetic response mediated by the erigent nerves, while ejaculation is a sympathetic event mediated by the hypogastric nerves. These structures may be damaged during pelvic dissection as they lie behind the parietal facial envelope, close to the mesorectal plane. One may avoid contact with the pelvic nerves using a close rectal dissection. This approach is highly vascularized and for this reason many surgeons prefer to dissect in the more anatomical mesorectal plane. Sexual dysfunction affects 3% of men following pouch surgery and for this reason sperm banking should be recommended. Sildenafil (Viagra) has been shown to help erectile dysfunction but will not impact upon retrograde ejaculation.

Fecundity and Pregnancy: UC commonly affects young females of reproductive age. Neither the disease itself nor the medical treatments currently available (apart from salazopyrin in men) are thought to compromise fertility. Fertility rates are lower in women who have had pouch surgery when compared those who undergo medical management. About 40% of women will have difficulty becoming pregnant following IPAA. It may be possible to delay proctectomy until a family has been established or alternatively anti-adhesion products may combat tubal obstruction.

Vaginal delivery has been associated with occult sphincter injury in 30% of patients. Females with an ileal pouch might risk incontinence following vaginal delivery. The Cleveland Clinic have reported that sphincter injury occurs more frequently in those who choose vaginal delivery rather than cesarean section with rates of 50% and 13% respectively but no difference in pouch function was apparent at 5 years. For the duration of the pregnancy, stool frequency, incontinence and pad usage gradually increase with pouch function returning quickly to normal in most cases. It seems reasonable to conclude that while vaginal delivery confers no functional disadvantage in the medium term there is concern that sphincter integrity is indeed compromised. Long-term implications remain unmeasured and therefore uncertain.

Pouch Failure: Complication rates for IPAA of about 30–40% are relatively high. Fortunately, most of these problems can usually be resolved. Pouch excision or indefinite retention of a defunctioning stoma defines failure. Institutional pouch failure rates have notably fallen over the past 20 years presumably following improvements in patient selection and surgical technique. Long term failure occurs with a frequency of 5–10%. A consistent theme that emerges from the large institutional series is that early pouch failure is associated closely with the occurrence of perioperative pelvic sepsis while that occurring later is often secondary to poor function or following an unexpected diagnosis of Crohn's disease. The success of redo pouch surgery for UC has improved with approximately half to three quarters of patients now retaining a functional pouch in the long term. When considering revision, it is necessary to evaluate the sphincters, assess pelvic soft tissue compliance, make a judgement regarding the likely diagnosis (Crohn's or UC) and determine the patient's general health and wishes. It is clear that redo-IPAA surgery may benefit patients with an excessively long efferent ileal spout or those with a tortuous stricture. It is perhaps less clear whether revision is as beneficial to those with ongoing septic complications. Even in the best hands, redo-IPAA surgery carries an appreciable morbidity rate. Not surprisingly outcomes are worse both in terms of overall failure and function when compared to first time surgery; nonetheless this procedure remains a valid alternative to a defunctioning stoma or pouch excision.

When faced with the proposition of removing an ileoanal pouch should be considered that 62% of 68 cases treated at St Marks suffered significant morbidity and one patient died. The single most common complication following pouch excision was non-healing of the perineal wound. Readmission within 5 years was the norm with 20% of patients requiring reoperation for small bowel obstruction, stoma complications or hemorrhage.

Selected Readings

Bernstein CN (2006) Natural history and management of flat and polypoid dysplasia in inflammatory bowel disease. Gastroenterol Clin North Am 35:573–579

Lim CH, Dixon MF, Vail A, et al. (2003) Ten year follow up of ulcerative colitis patients with and without low grade dysplasia. Gut 52:1127–1132

Parks AG, Nicholls RJ (1978) Proctocolectomy without ileostomy for ulcerative colitis. Br Med J 2:85–88

Rubio CA, Befrits R (2004) Low-grade dysplasia in flat mucosa in ulcerative colitis. Gastroenterology 126:1494; author reply 1494–1495

Rutter MD, Saunders BP, Schofield G, et al. (2004) Pancolonic indigo carmine dye spraying for the detection of dysplasia in ulcerative colitis. Gut 53:256–260

Rutter MD, Saunders BP, Wilkinson KH, et al. (2006) Thirty-year analysis of a colonoscopic surveillance program for neoplasia in ulcerative colitis. Gastroenterology 130:1030–1038

Thompson-Fawcett MW, Warren BF, Mortensen NJ (1998) A new look at the anal transitional zone with reference to restorative proctocolectomy and the columnar cuff. Br J Surg 85:1517–1521

Travis SP, Farrant JM, Ricketts C, et al. (1996) Predicting outcome in severe ulcerative colitis. Gut 38:905–910

Truelove SC, Witts LJ (1955) Cortisone in ulcerative colitis: final report on a therapeutic trial. Br Med J 2:1041–1048

Yu CS, Pemberton JH, Larson D (2000) Ileal pouch-anal anastomosis in patients with indeterminate colitis: long-term results. Dis Colon Rectum 43:1487–1496

70 Crohn's Disease of the Small Bowel and Colon

Jenny Speranza · Steven D. Wexner

Pearls and Pitfalls

- Crohn's disease is a transmural inflammatory condition of the GI tract.
- The disease can affect the entire GI tract from the mouth to the anus and present a myriad of extraintestinal manifestations.
- Medical therapy is the principal treatment for exacerbations and active disease.
- Surgery is indicated when the patient is refractory to medical therapy, has intractable adverse sequelae of medical management, or desires to discontinue medical therapy.
- Bowel conservation is a fundamental tenet of surgery.
- Presenting features include: abdominal pain, fever, diarrhea, weight loss, anorexia, vomiting, chronic malnutrition, and fatigue.
- Affects the young in 2nd and 3rd decades of life but also has a bimodal distribution and equal gender predominance.
- Distal ileal involvement is most common at 41%, small bowel disease in 27%, colonic involvement in 27%, and isolated perianal involvement in 3.4% of patients.
- Diagnosis is most often made with a combination of physical exam, contrast radiographic studies, endoscopy, and histopathology.
- Histopathology of the small bowel will exhibit "fat wrapping"; mesenteric thickening and granulomas are pathognomonic.
- Colonoscopic exam may grossly reveal skip areas, linear deep ulcerations, and stricture formation. Histologically granulomas will be definitive of Crohn's disease.
- Surgical intervention is used to treat the complications of the disease such as perforation, abscess, and fistula.
- Intraoperative ureteric catheters are advised in surgical patients with severe inflammation presenting with a large phlegmon.
- Bowel margins should be resected to grossly normal tissue.
- The mesentery should be carefully thinned and suture ligated to avoid hematoma formation.
- The quality and length of both resected and retained bowel should be accurately documented during surgery.
- Whenever possible intra-abdominal abscesses should be percutaneously drained prior to surgery to assist in control of inflammation.
- Strictureplasty should always be considered in patients with recurrent or extensive disease and in patients who have or are in imminent danger of having short bowel syndrome.

- Isolated colonic disease with rectal sparing may be best treated by subtotal colectomy with ileorectal anastomosis.
- Segmental colectomy should only be done in selected cases since recurrence has shown to be increased as compared to proctocolectomy.
- Severe perianal disease will ultimately necessitate proctectomy in 25% of patients with perianal involvement.

Introduction

Crohn's disease was originally described in 1932. Crohn's disease is a transmural inflammatory condition that can affect the entire gastrointestinal tract from the mouth to the anus with a myriad of extraintestinal manifestations. Although there have been suggestions of immunologic, genetic, and environment effects, the etiology is still unknown. Medical therapy is the mainstay of treatment at the current time. Although efficacy is variable, side effects of such therapy may be extreme. Surgery is reserved to treat complications of the disease, complications of medical therapy or the intractability of disease despite medical therapy. Since there are many components of care required in treating Crohn's patients, it is best that such patients be treated in a tertiary center with a multi-specialty approach to the disease.

Presentation

Crohn's disease typically presents with abdominal pain, distension, nausea, vomiting, chronic diarrhea, weight loss, fever, and general malaise. On physical examination, a tender mass in the right lower quadrant often signifies the presence of terminal ileal/small bowel disease. Although quite rare (1–3%), duodenal involvement will present with duodenal or gastric outlet obstruction. When Crohn's disease is isolated to the colon, patients can have pain, diarrhea, bloody bowel movements, and anemia, along with extraintestinal manifestations. Enterocolonic fistula is usually a result of small bowel disease and the colon is otherwise normal. If there is perianal involvement, there can be multiple fistulous tracts, linear ulcerations and abscesses, enlarged skin tags, and stricture of the anal canal. Perianal disease often precedes the onset of small bowel disease by several years. Perianal involvement is more common in patients with colonic manifestations than with small bowel disease.

Epidemiology

Crohn's disease usually presents in the 2nd and 3rd decades of life, although a bimodal distribution has been described with the second onset in the 5th and 6th decade of life. The incidence is 1–6 per 100,000 population. The prevalence is higher among Ashkenazi Jews (10 cases per 100,000 persons per year) and in cooler climates areas, such as Scandinavia, the United Kingdom, Germany, and the northern United States. Genetics have also been implicated since the disease has been shown to affect first-degree relatives. Women and men seem to be equally affected. The distribution of Crohn's disease is varied 41% of patients will have distal ileal involvement, 27% have small intestine involvement only, 27% have colonic involvment, and 3.4% have anorectal involvement.

Diagnosis

A patient often presents to the colorectal surgeon with an established diagnosis. At that time it is important to determine the extent and activity of the disease. This analysis can often be accomplished by radiographic and endoscopic studies. A small bowel series can determine extent of small bowel disease, giving location and assessing stricture and fistulous disease. CT scan with oral and intravenous contrast can help define enterocutaneous fistulas, as well reveal and possibly drain localized abscesses. A contrast enema can identify colonic strictures, fistulae, cobblestoning, and ulceration. Colonoscopic examination is vital when assessing the colon, as well as to intubate the terminal ileum and obtain biopsies throughout the colon. Findings on colonoscopy often reveal rectal sparing, stricture formation, skip areas, deep linear ulceration, and fissures. Although granulomas identified by endoscopic biopsies will confirm the diagnosis, they are rarely found. Upper endoscopy is also important in evaluating the esophagus, stomach, and duodenum. Endoanal ultrasound can evaluate fistulous disease using hydrogen peroxide to further delineate complex fistulae. MRI is useful in further identifying complex perianal disease.

Histopathology

On macroscopic exam the bowel appears thick-walled, granular, and friable. "Fat wrapping" is often seen encroaching from the mesentery toward the antimesenteric border of the bowel. The mesentery may be thickened and foreshortened with adenopathy adjacent to diseased small bowel. Strictures frequently reveal deep linear ulcerations on the mucosal surface. Microscopic granulomas are pathognomonic for Crohn's disease, although they are present in only two-thirds of all patients. Transmural inflammation is also pathognomonic of the entity.

Medical Management

The goals of medical treatment of Crohn's disease are to treat manifestations of the disease, while minimizing the morbidity of the therapeutic agents. Therapy is aimed at minimizing inflammation with medication and providing nutritional support. Sulfasalazine and 5-ASA compounds can help induce and maintain remission of disease. Antibiotics, such as metronidazole and ciprofloxacin, are beneficial in treating perianal disease. Corticosteroids are used for acute exacerbation of disease, but have detrimental side effects and are not intended for long-term use for suppression. Immunosuppressant agents, 6-MP, azathioprine, methotrexate, and cyclosporine are used when first-line agents are not effective. These agents have been shown to induce remission, but also have multiple side effects. Infliximab has been shown to promote healing of Crohn's fistulas, but administration of this medication requires careful surveillance due to serious adverse effects. Total parenteral nutrition can be beneficial in strengthening the malnourished patient.

Surgical Indications

Indications for surgery include patients, abscesses, obstruction, perforation fistulization, resistance to or intolerable complications of medical treatment, and growth retardation. Approximately 80% of patients with Crohn's disease require surgery within 20 years of onset. The cumulative rate of intestinal resection was shown to be 44%, 61%, and 71% at 1, 5, and 10 years after diagnosis, respectively. Because short gut syndrome can become a potential danger with repeated bowel resections, bowel-preserving surgery and avoiding surgery until it is an absolute necessity are major tenets for treating Crohn's disease.

Pre-Operative Planning

CT scan of the abdomen can allow for preoperative percutaneous drainage of abscess collection. This step can help decrease inflammation and sepsis, in addition to providing total parenteral nutrition, to improve the patient's nutritional status and wound healing ability prior to surgical intervention. Patients should undergo stoma marking by a stoma therapist prior to the procedure. Mechanical bowel prep is given if the patient is not obstructed. In the presence of severe inflammation and phlegmon, we employ the use of ureteric catheters to help identify and avoid the ureters.

Surgical Management

Small Bowel

Surgery for small bowel disease is the primary modality for treatment of complications of Crohn's disease, such as strictures, fistulae, abscess, and phlegmon. Bowel preservation is the principle goal of management. The bowel should be evaluated from the ligament of Treitz to the ileocecal valve; measurement should be documented for disease extent and normal bowel. Bowel resection limits are evaluated by gross examination. Histologic margins have not been proven to affect recurrence. Fazio et al. prospectively examined two groups of patients having margins of small bowel that were not diseased grossly with either a 2 cm or 12 cm margin. No significant difference in recurrence rates between the two group was noted. When dividing thickened Crohn's mesentery, it is important to score the peritoneum and carefully palpate vessels. Suture ligating can help ensure hemostasis, as the vessels in this thickened tissue have a tendency to retract, with subsequent hematoma formation and further loss of small bowel.

When treating strictured small bowel, Heineke-Mikulicz type strictureplasty is preferred in short segment disease (❷ *Figs. 70-1–70-3*). If there are multiple short strictures in a small segment of bowel, it may be advantageous to resect a continuous piece of bowel rather than having numerous strictureplasties in one area. For long-segment strictures, resection or long strictureplasty are two options. Long strictureplasty is as safe and effective as short strictureplasty. Shartari et al. followed 62 patients

◘ Figure 70-1

A longitudinal incision over the stricture, on the antimesenteric border of the small bowel, extends 3–5 cm beyond the edges of the stricture on each side (Reprinted from Wexner et al., 2001. With permission)

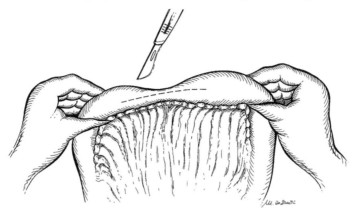

◘ Figure 70-2

The lumen is spread apart and inspected (Reprinted from Wexner et al., 2001. With permission)

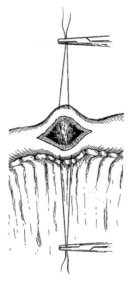

undergoing strictureplasty for jejunoileal disease over a 20-year period. Twenty-one patients underwent long strictureplasty, while 41 patients received strictureplasty. No significant differences were found in the 3, 5 and 10 year disease free rates for the long and short strictureplasty. For disease involving fistulous communications to adjacent organs, skin, or bowel, the basic premise is to resect the diseased bowel and to repair the involved organ, if possible. The "bystanding" organ need not be resected if there is no gross disease; in such circumstances, a wedge resection or suture closure may suffice.

When gastroduodenal disease is present, the complication is usually a stricture of the duodenum causing an outlet obstruction. Although this is a rare event, a gastrojejunostomy can be created with or without vagotomy.

⬛ Figure 70-3

A Heineke-Mikulicz-type stricturoplasty. The longitudinal incision is closed transversely using a single layer of interrupted polydioxan 3–0 sutures (Reprinted from Wexner et al., 2001. With permission)

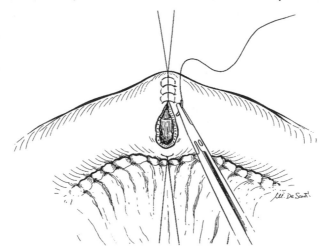

Surgical Management

Colonic Crohn's

With colonic involvement, surgical intervention is dependent on the severity and location of the disease. In the emergent setting of toxic colitis, total abdominal colectomy with end ileostomy is warranted. Colectomy with ileorectal anastomosis may be warranted if there is rectal sparing and otherwise normal small bowel. Segmental colectomy can be performed in select cases, such as terminal ileal disease, with limited involvement of the right colon. Segmental colectomy can also be used in cases of ileosigmoid fistulas, when the ileum is diseased and the colon is normal. Although the above options of segmental colectomy are occasionally feasible, segmental colectomy has been shown to have a significantly shorter time to recurrence and increased risk of recurrence, compared with proctocolectomy. Fichera et al followed 55 patients who underwent segmental colectomy, 49 total abdominal colectomy, and 75 proctocolectomy. Total proctocolectomy patients had significantly lower morbidity, lower risk of recurrence, and longer time to recurrence.

Surgical Management

Perianal Crohn's

Perianal Crohn's should be treated based on the presenting signs and symptoms. Patients with chronic fistulae and perianal disease may need temporary diversion of the fecal stream. Treatment of mild disease such as an abscess will require incision and drainage, which can be accomplished with a small incision and use of a drain or Mallenkot catheter. Fistula tracts should be identified either by examination under anesthesia, endoanal ultrasound, or MRI. Once the tract is known, a seton of 0 ethibond can be placed within the tract while the sepsis and inflammation abate. These setons can be left in place for long periods of time to provide effective drainage and limit possible incontinence from fistulotomy. Fistulotomy should only be used for patients with a documented minor amount of sphincter involvement. For definitive treatment of transsphincteric fistulas in patients with Crohn's disease, the endorectal advancement flap has been applied with good results (Shatari et al., 2004). Joo et al. evaluated outcomes of 31 endorectal advancement flaps between January 1991 and December 1995. The results were found to be more favorable if there was no small bowel Crohn's disease (25% versus 87% of patients with no small bowel involvement). Asymptomatic skin tags and hemorrhoids should not be removed secondary to poor wound healing in these patients. Severe ulceration and complex fistulous disease may ultimately require proctectomy. Galandiuk et al. demonstrated that the presence of colonic disease and anal strictures were predictors of eventual permanent diversion.

Surgical Management

Laparoscopic Surgery for Crohn's Disease

With an elective surgical procedure, laparoscopic surgery is gaining popularity as the procedure of choice for treating Crohn's disease. The benefits of minimally invasive surgery for Crohn's disease have been shown in multiple studies to decrease postoperative pain, reduce length of hospital stay, and hasten recovery. Conversion rates remain low, between 10% and 28%. In one study, laparoscopic ileocolic resections were shown to have significantly decreased rates of small bowel obstruction over 5 years compared with open ileocolic resections. At our institution, ileocolic resection is the procedure of choice for treating ileocolic Crohn's disease in select cases.

Surgical Management

Crohn's Disease Recurrence

Despite advances in medical and surgical care, Crohn's disease continues to be a complex and vexing condition to treat. Medical management can help maintain remission for some patients, but with a myriad of serious side effects. Surgical intervention, even when used sparingly to treat complications of the disease, results in recurrence of disease. Bernell et al. (2000) retrospectively assessed 1936 patients and found that three of four Crohn's patients will need intestinal resection at some time. In addition, the extent of disease at diagnosis and presence of perianal fistula increase the risk of recurrence after surgery. Yamamoto examined factors affecting Crohn's disease recurrence. Smoking was associated with a significant decrease in postoperative recurrence of disease. In addition, 5-ASA was shown to slightly lower the recurrence rate.

Selected Readings

Bergamaschi R, Pessaux P, Arnaud JP (2003) Comparison of conventional and laparoscopic ileocolic resection for Crohn's disease. Dis Colon Rectum 46:1129–1133

Bernell O, Lapidus A, Hellers G (2000) Risk factors for surgery and postoperative recurrence in Crohn's disease. Ann Surg 231:38–45

Delaney CP, Fazio VW (2001) Crohn's disease of the small bowel. Surg Clin North Am 81:137–158

Fazio VW, Marchetti F, Church JM, et al. (1996) Effect of resection margins on the recurrence of Crohn's disease in the small bowel. A randomized controlled trial. Ann Surg 224:563–573

Fichera A, McCormack R, Rubin MA, et al. (2005) Long term outcome of surgically treated Crohn's disease: a prospective study. Dis Colon Rectum 48:963–969

Galandiuk S, Kimberling J, Al-Mishlab T, et al. (2005) Perianal Crohn's disease predictors of need for permanent diversion. Ann Surg 241:796–802

Joo JS, Weiss EG, Nogueras JJ, et al. (1998) Endorectal advancement flap in perianal Crohn's disease. Am Surg 64:147–150

Wexner SD, Reissman P, Bernstein MA (2001) Surgery of Crohn's disease including strictureplasty. In: Baker RJ, Fischer JE (eds) Mastery of surgery 4th edn. Lippincott, Williams & Wilkins, Philadelphia, pp. 1442–1457

Yamamoto T (2005) Factors affecting recurrence after surgery for Crohn's disease. World J Gastroenterol 11:3971–3979

71 Acute Colonic Pseudo-Obstruction

Raul Martin Bosio · Anthony J. Senagore

Pearls and Pitfalls

- Colonic pseudo-obstruction refers to a clinical syndrome of colonic dilation in the absence of a mechanical obstruction; the presentation may mimic an acute large bowel obstruction.
- Pseudo-obstruction occurs primarily in hospitalized patients, with an incidence as high often >20% after selected surgical procedures or trauma.
- The pathogenesis of this syndrome is not fully elucidated; however, an imbalance in the autonomic regulation of the colon has been suggested.
- Physical findings include a distended, tympanitic abdomen with present but diminished bowel sounds.
- When combined with clinical examination, abdominal x-rays are usually diagnostic or highly suspicious.
- Colon ischemia and subsequent perforation, which occurs in 3–15% of patients, is the most important complication and has a mortality of about 50%.
- The radiographic findings are of marked distention of the proximal colon with the descending and sigmoid colon of normal caliber.
- A water-soluble contrast enema or colonoscopy should be performed to exclude mechanical causes.
- Initial management includes nasogastric tube decompression, replacement of fluid and electrolyte imbalances, and serial abdominal films; more than 85% of patients recover with conservative management.
- Persistence of symptoms for more than 48 h or a cecal diameter > 12 cm requires intervention, which may include use of neostigmine, colonoscopic decompression, or, rarely, operative intervention. A cecal diameter exceeding 12 cm is associated with an increased risk of ischemia/perforation.
- The use of neostigmine has been associated with a success rate of 90%, leading several groups to advocate its use early in the treatment plan; however, a sustained response is maintained in only 70% of responders.
- Colonoscopic decompression is another effective option, with a primary success rate of about 73–83%; a 4% morbidity has been reported after colonoscopic decompression.
- Colonic resection as opposed to tube cecostomy is indicated after failure of conservative treatment or when clinical findings raise concern of ischemia.

Introduction

First described in 1948 by Sir H. Ogilvie, colonic pseudo-obstruction refers to a clinical situation that resembles an acute large bowel obstruction, with a dilated proximal colon on abdominal films, but in the absence of a mechanical obstruction. Approximately 60% of patients diagnosed with colonic pseudo-obstruction are critically ill in the setting of major trauma or after major surgical procedures. Colonic pseudo-obstruction can also occur in bedridden patients or those on high dose narcotics. The patients are predominantly males in their sixth or seventh decade of life. Both intraperitoneal and extraperitoneal operative procedures have been associated with the development of this syndrome, with urologic, orthopedic (hip, knee, and spinal surgery) and gynecologic procedures (Caesarean section) among the most frequent. As a common feature, in about half of the patients in a postoperative setting, the spine or the retroperitoneum has been traumatized or manipulated. Among 400 nonsurgical patients, a retrospective review identified non-operative trauma (11%), systemic infections (10%), and cardiac failure (myocardial infarction, congestive heart failure) (10%) as the most common medical conditions associated with this syndrome. Among a variety of signs and symptoms, the most prominent clinical feature is marked abdominal distention due to massive colonic dilation. Although the pathogenesis of acute colonic pseudo-obstruction is not fully elucidated, autonomic dysregulation of the colon has been implicated (see below). Spontaneous resolution occurs in about 85% of the patients managed by supportive measures; however, patients need to be monitored closely because spontaneous cecal perforation occurs in 15%, with associated mortality of 50%.

Pathophysiology

An imbalance in autonomic regulation of the colon, resulting in dysmotility, has been suggested in the pathogenesis of this syndrome. The parasympathetic nervous system stimulates colonic motility, whereas sympathetic nerves targeting either the myenteric plexus or the smooth muscle inhibit contraction. Vagal innervation of the colon extends up to the splenic flexure, with the distal segments of the colon receiving parasympathetic supply via lumbar nerves from spinal segments S2–S4 (sacral parasympathetic nerves). A transient decrease in the parasympathetic drive, combined with an increased sympathetic input to the colon, has been proposed as the mechanism of this syndrome. Abdominal films usually demonstrate a markedly dilated ascending and transverse colon with the distal colon being of normal caliber. Based on colonic innervation and these radiographic findings, a disruption of parasympathetic input, possibly combined with increased sympathetic inhibitory input to the colon, may be responsible for this functional obstruction. While most investigators believe this disorder to be a dysmotility of the proximal colon, some groups believe that this syndrome represents a disorder of the distal colon with an inhibitory reflex to the proximal colon. In either case, the drugs (i.e., neostigmine, pyridostigmine) that increase parasympathetic activity may produce prompt colonic decompression in patients with acute colonic pseudo-obstruction.

Diagnosis

Prominent abdominal distension is the most characteristic clinical feature of this syndrome. Nausea, vomiting, low-grade fever, and abdominal discomfort or pain may be present. Increasing abdominal pain should be evaluated carefully, because it may imply bowel ischemia or perforation. Physical examination reveals a markedly distended, tympanitic abdomen with mild diffuse tenderness. The presence of bowel sounds and the passage of small amounts of flatus and stool do not exclude the diagnosis. The presence of peritoneal signs usually correlates with ischemia or bowel perforation, requires urgent operative intervention, and is associated with a high mortality.

Abdominal x-rays demonstrate a distended large bowel affecting the ascending colon and, to a variable degree, transverse colon up to the splenic flexure (❷ *Fig. 71-1A*). A water-soluble contrast enema is usually essential in confirming the diagnosis and excluding a mechanical obstruction. This study may induce colonic decompression and contribute to the treatment of the syndrome. If there is concern for ischemia or perforation, the study is contraindicated. Once the diagnosis has been established, plain abdominal films should be obtained every 12 h to monitor colonic diameter closely. A cecal diameter of ≥12 cm or a transverse colon diameter of ≥9 cm are associated with an increased risk of ischemia and may indicate the necessity of more active treatment.

Treatment

As with many medical conditions, early diagnosis and treatment is of great importance in acute colonic pseudo-obstruction. A fivefold increase in the risk of mortality has been reported with prolonged colonic distention (more than 6 days), secondary to ischemia and subsequent bowel perforation. Treatment includes supportive measures, pharmacologic treatment, endoscopic or percutaneous procedures, and operative exploration (❷ *Fig. 71-2*). Recently, a prospective, randomized, placebo-controlled trial demonstrated that administration of polyethylene glycol upon resolution of symptoms after either neostigmine or endoscopic decompression may decrease the risk of recurrence of this syndrome.

◘ Figure 71-1
a. Abdominal radiograph showing a distended ascending and transverse colon in a patient with acute colonic pseudo-obstruction. b. Abdominal films post treatment with neostigmine

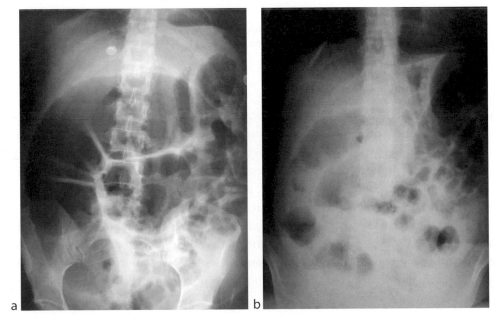

a   b

■ Figure 71-2

Suggested treatment algorithm for acute colonic pseudo-obstruction

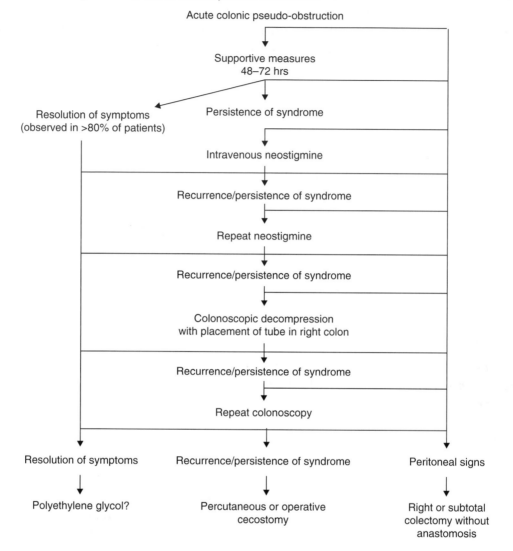

Initial management: Supportive measures refer to placement of a nasogastric tube, suspension of oral intake, discontinuation of medications that may adversely affect gastrointestinal motility, such as opiates and anticholinergics when possible, correction of fluid and electrolyte disorders, and patient mobilization. The efficacy of a rectal tube is questionable, because a rectal tube does not reach the distended segments of the colon. Resolution of acute colonic pseudo-obstruction with the above conservative measures would be expected in about 85% of patients.

Pharmacologic treatment: Persistent or progressive colonic distention after 48–72 h of treatment or a cecal diameter >12 cm usually necessitates a more active approach. Pharmacologic and endoscopic procedures constitute valid treatment options. Similar success rates with reduced morbidity makes pharmacologic treatment superior to colonoscopic decompression as a second step after failure of conservative management.

Many drugs for the treatment of this syndrome (i.e., erythromycin, cisapride, and metoclopramide, among others), targeting motilin or 5-HT4 receptors among others, have been studied in clinical trials. Most of these reports, however, included only small numbers of patients and failed to show consistent results. More than 30 years ago, Catchpole proposed the combination of a sympathetic blocker (guanethidine) and a parasympathomimetic agent (neostigmine) as a treatment for gastrointestinal motility disorders secondary to autonomic dysfunction. This concept was later applied to acute colonic pseudo-obstruction. Although no clinical improvement was observed after guanethidine, colonic decompression was reported after administration of neostigmine. The first randomized, double-blind, placebo-controlled trial for patients who had not responded to conservative measures with a cecal diameter > 11 cm was published in 1994. Clinical and radiologic response occurred in 91% of patients who received neostigmine, compared with no objective improvement in the placebo group. Cross-over of seven patients from the placebo group to treatment with neostigmine demonstrated success in all but one of these patients.

The rationale behind the use of neostigmine is that it inhibits acetylcholinesterase, an enzyme that hydrolyzes acetylcholine at the neuromuscular junctions. Neostigmine, a reversible competitive inhibitor of acetylcholinesterase, binds to the active site of the enzyme, blocking access to the neurotransmitter and causing a relative increase in acetylcholine, thereby enhancing cholinergic transmission and smooth muscle contraction. Various reversible acetylcholinesterase inhibitors with a short half-life are available, including neostigmine, pyridostigmine, and physostigmine, which can be administered intravenous, orally, and subcutaneously. Most published data, however, support the use of intravenous neostigmine. Oral pyridostigmine has been used in chronic syndromes such us myasthenia gravis. However, erratic absorption and variable bioavailability may occur with oral administration in patients with acute colonic pseudo-obstruction where prolonged fasting and superimposed partial small bowel ileus may negatively affect absorption. Physostigmine crosses the blood-brain barrier and affects the central nervous system, and therefore, is usually not considered in the treatment of this syndrome.

Neostigmine is usually administered in a 2.5 mg dose intravenously over a period of 1–3 min or as an infusion over a period of 30–60 min; the latter is associated with a lower risk of bradycardia. Patients should be under cardiac monitoring for a period of 30–60 min after injection with atropine available for brachycardia. Mechanical obstruction of the colon must be ruled out before initiation of treatment. Side-effects associated with the use of this drug include bradycardia, salivation, sweating, restlessness, nausea, abdominal pain, hypotension, and bronchoconstriction. Relative contraindications to its use involve heart rate < 60 beats/min, systolic blood pressure < 90 mmHg, use of beta-blockers, severe bronchospasm, or known hypersensitivity to this drug, recent myocardial infarction, acidosis, or a serum creatinine > 3 mg/dl due to the renal excretion of the drug.

Colonic decompression is observed usually within minutes after neostigmine administration; evacuation of flatus and stool occurs in about 90% of patients within 30 min (❯ Fig. 71-1B). A sustained response, however, generally drops to 61–80%. In one study, six patients who recurred and the three non-responders received a second dose of neostigmine. Five out of the six patients that recurred had a sustained response, with no clinical improvement among the other three patients.

Endoscopic treatment: Colonoscopic decompression is usually the next step after failure of neostigmine or when the use of neostigmine is contraindicated or associated with severe side-effects. The presence of peritoneal signs or pneumoperitoneum is obviously a contraindication to its use. Colonoscopy is usually challenging and should be performed with extreme caution by experienced colonoscopists.

Sedation and analgesia is generally administered, although use of opiates should be minimized. Dual channel colonoscopes or colonoscopes with accessory channels of large diameter may contribute to suctioning of gas and stool; air insufflation should be kept to a minimum. The mucosal appearance and viability should be evaluated to determine the presence of ischemia or indirect signs of necrosis, such as a dusky mucosa. These findings generally indicate the need to terminate the procedure and proceed to operative intervention.

Complete colonoscopy, though preferable because it allows assessment of cecal mucosa, is not always necessary, provided right colon decompression is successful at the end of the procedure. Strong consideration should be given to leaving a large bore transanal decompression tube in the proximal colon. Geller et al. reported an overall success rate of 88% after colonic decompression, but found that sustained decompression was maintained in only 25% of patients in whom a decompression tube was not placed. Using a guide wire and, if possible, under fluoroscopy control minimizes loop formation and confirms that the tube has reached the right colon. The tube is usually left in place for 72 h, and should drain by gravity, but needs to be flushed every 6–8 h to prevent clogging.

In a review analyzing outcomes of endoscopic decompression in 292 patients, a 69% rate of initial decompression, including patients with and without decompression tube insertion, was observed. Recurrence was about 25%, but was greater when a decompression tube was not left in the right colon. Overall success rate, including patients who required more than one colonoscopy, varied between 73% and 88%. Morbidity after endoscopic treatment, primarily colonic perforation, has been observed in about 5% of patients.

Operative treatment: Operative intervention is indicated after failure of the above-mentioned treatments or in patients with peritoneal signs or free air. Intraoperative options include creation of a cecostomy in the absence of perforation or a right or a subtotal colectomy when there are findings of ischemia or colonic perforation. Cecostomy can be accomplished percutaneously under fluoroscopic control, as a combined endoscopic-radiologic procedure, by laparotomy (even under local anesthesia), or by laparoscopy. Percutaneous cecostomy may avoid the risk associated with a laparotomy or laparoscopic procedure. Mortality secondary to leakage and abdominal wall cellulitis has been reported after this procedure and needs to be considered; therefore, most surgeons have abandoned cecostomy as definitive therapy in most patients and especially those with ischemia. Diverting ileostomies or transverse colostomies do not always resolve colonic distention and should not be considered as viable options. Colonic resection with end ileostomy and either closure of the distal colon or mucous fistula formation should be considered the gold standard. No matter what operative procedure is used, the operative mortality is about 50%.

In summary, colonic pseudo-obstruction can masquerade as an acute large bowel obstruction, but occurs in the absence of a mechanical obstruction. The etiology appears to be a dysmotility related to an imbalance in the autonomic regulation of colonic motility. A markedly distended abdomen, secondary to massive colonic distension, constitutes the most prominent clinical feature. Abdominal x-rays contribute to the diagnosis and will show a markedly distended proximal colon. Initial supportive therapy leads to resolution in about 85% of patients. Neostigmine and colonoscopic decompression constitute treatment options after failure of supportive measures. Operative treatment is indicated after failure of pharmacologic and endoscopic procedures or when clinical findings raise concern of ischemia or colonic perforation, but has an associated mortality of 50%. The operative procedure usually involves a proximal colectomy, but a tube cecostomy may be utilized in select patients.

Selected Readings

Chevallier P, Marcy PY, Francois E, et al. (2002) Controlled transperitoneal percutaneous cecostomy as a therapeutic alternative to the endoscopic decompression for Ogilvie's syndrome. Am J Gastroenterol 97:471–474

De Giorgio R, Barbara G, Stanghellini V, et al. (2001) Review article: the pharmacological treatment of acute colonic pseudo-obstruction. Aliment Pharmacol Ther 15:1717–1727

Eisen GM, Baron TH, Dominitz JA, et al. (2002) Acute colonic pseudo-obstruction. Gastrointest Endosc 56:789–792

Mehta R, John A, Nair P, et al. (2006) Factors predicting successful outcome following neostigmine therapy in acute colonic pseudo-obstruction: a prospective study. J Gastroenterol Hepatol 21:459–461

Ponec RJ, Saunders MD, Kimmey MB (1999) Neostigmine for the treatment of acute colonic pseudo-obstruction. N Engl J Med 341:137–141

Saunders MD, Cappell MS (2005) Endoscopic management of acute colonic pseudo-obstruction. Endoscopy 37:760–763

Saunders MD, Kimmey MB (2005) Systematic review: acute colonic pseudo-obstruction. Aliment Pharmacol Ther 22:917–925

Sgouros SN, Vlachogiannakos J, Vassiliadis K, et al. (2006) Effect of polyethylene glycol electrolyte balanced solution on patients with acute colonic pseudo obstruction after resolution of colonic dilation: a prospective, randomised, placebo controlled trial. Gut 55:638–642

Tenofsky PL, Beamer L, Smith RS (2000) Ogilvie syndrome as a postoperative complication. Arch Surg 135:682–686; discussion 686–687

72 Surgical Therapy of Constipation

Joe J. Tjandra · Henry Yeh

Pearls and Pitfalls

- The definition of constipation includes fewer than three bowel movements per week, straining at defecation, and/or hard pellet-like stools.
- Constipation includes a constellation of symptoms influenced by local culture, geography, socio-economic background, and the patient's personality.
- Coexistence of weight loss and rectal bleeding suggests colorectal cancer.
- Diagnosis should attempt to differentiate an extra-colonic or systemic cause from a mechanical or functional colonic cause.
- The key to treatment is appropriate diagnosis.
- Mechanical causes include diverticular stricture, colonic neoplasm, occult rectal prolapse, and rectocele.
- Functional causes include slow transit constipation, irritable bowel disease, psychologic disorders, and pelvic floor dysfunction.
- Diagnosis may involve combinations of colonoscopy, scintigraphic transit studies, anorectal physiologic testing, and defecating proctography.
- Medical therapy for simple constipation involves a high liquid intake and increased dietary fiber.
- Pelvic floor dysfunction is best managed by biofeedback therapy with a regular, structured program that includes a planned process of re-learning.
- Operative therapy can be effective in patients with slow transit constipation (total abdominal colectomy/ileorectostomy) and rectocele (transvaginal or transanal).

Constipation

Constipation is a symptom or a constellation of symptoms influenced by a myriad of factors. These etiologies are as varied as culture, geographic, and socio-economic background, as well as the personality of the individual. A full dietary history and appraisal of the symptoms is important. If the symptoms are of new onset and in the presence of other associated abdominal symptoms, especially weight loss and rectal bleeding, then appropriate investigations should be instituted to exclude a colorectal cancer, diverticular disease and other less common conditions (❷ *Table 72-1*).

Due to the wide variation in the interpretation of constipation, it is defined commonly as passing fewer than three bowel movements per week, inordinate straining during defecation, incomplete evacuation more than 25% of the time, or hard pellet-like stools more than 25% of the time, with the symptoms lasting more than 12 months. Constipation is common, with a prevalence of 10% in

◻ Table 72-1

Causes of constipation (Adapted from Seow-Choen and Tjandra, 2001)

Mechanical colonic causes

- Neoplastic
- Benign stricture (ischemic or anastomotic)
- Colonic volvulus
- Diverticular disease (stricture)

Dietary

- Poor fiber intake
- Inadequate fluid intake

Medications

- Neuropsychiatric medications, e.g. anticonvulsants, anti-Parkinsonian drugs, antidepressants, antipsychotics
- Narcotics and opiates
- Calcium channel blockers
- Antacids
- Barium sulfate
- Iron tablets

Functional

- Irritable bowel syndrome
- Psychologic disorders
- Slow transit constipation
- Ogilvie's syndrome

Anorectal/pelvic disorders

- Mucosal prolapse syndrome
- Paradoxic puborectalis contraction (anismus)
- Rectocele

Metabolic and endocrine

- Diabetes mellitus
- Hypercalcemia
- Hyperparathyroidism
- Hypokalemia
- Hypopituitarism
- Hypothyroidism
- Scleroderma

Neurogenic

- Peripheral
  Hirschsprung's disease
  Autonomic neuropathy
  Chagas' disease
- Spinal
  Cauda equina tumor
  Multiple sclerosis
  Paraplegia
- Central
  Cerebrovascular accidents
  Parkinson's disease
  Cerebral neoplasms

Western societies. Most patients seek help from pharmacists, general practitioners, and naturopaths, while only about 5% are ever referred to gastrointestinal specialists.

The key in management is to identify the underlying etiology of constipation, which can be quite complex. It is important to exclude mechanical bowel obstruction due to a neoplasm or stricture (❂ *Table 72-1*), which would mandate operative intervention. The focus of this chapter is on functional disorders of the bowel and pelvic floor, which can affect the lifestyle of the affected individuals severely. A systematic workup is extremely important. The first order of evaluation is to differentiate between an extracolonic or systemic cause from a colonic or intestinal cause, and then to differentiate between a mechanical colonic cause and a functional bowel disorder, and finally, to assess the relative role of slow gastrointestinal transit, pelvic floor dysfunction and irritable bowel syndrome. A full anorectal examination is mandatory in most patients. A colonoscopy is generally indicated in patients over the age of 40–45 with clinically significant symptoms.

Diagnosis

The diagnosis of constipation should be established. The severity of the symptoms would dictate the extent of investigations. Past treatment(s) should be documented, and may provide insight into the severity of the disorder. Documenting the nature of constipation might also help determine the underlying pathogenesis (❂ *Table 72-1*). Difficult evacuation requiring digital evacuation of stool would suggest pelvic floor disorder, while a chronic history of abdominal bloating and/or infrequent bowel movement would suggest a delayed intestinal transit. In contrast, a short history of changes in bowel pattern, especially if accompanied by rectal bleeding, a family history of colorectal neoplasm, and/or weight loss, would suggest a more sinister cause, such as a colorectal neoplasm. A mechanical cause such as a neoplasm usually produces a change in bowel habit rather than chronic constipation. With severe symptoms, special investigations are required (see below).

A full physical examination may determine whether a more systemic cause of constipation exists (❂ *Table 72-1*). Abdominal examination might identify abnormal masses. Anorectal examination would determine whether there is a rectocele present, mucosal rectal prolapse, megarectum, or inappropriate pelvic floor contraction or excessive perineal descent on straining. Proctoscopy will help identify a rectal neoplasm, occult rectal prolapse on straining, or presence of solitary rectal ulcer syndrome.

Pelvic floor disorders such as a rectocele may be corrected by biofeedback therapy, and occasionally, by operative intervention. Abdominal surgery such as a colectomy for slow colonic transit is rarely indicated. Most patients will respond to dietary changes that include an increased intake of liquid and fiber. Simple bulk-forming laxatives might suffice (❂ *Table 72-2*). For patients persistently troubled by constipation, further investigations are indicated as below.

Intestinal Versus Extra-Intestinal or Systemic Cause

Most extra-intestinal or systemic causes (❂ *Table 72-1*) can be excluded by a careful medical history, review of medications used or tried in the past, and physical examination. Systemic causes such as hypothyroidism or Parkinson's disease should be entertained and can be identified readily. In some patients, despite the presence of or correction of extra-intestinal causes, the constipation may be so severe that its presence mandates further gastrointestinal investigations.

◼ Table 72-2

Common laxatives

Bulking agents
Bran
Methylcellulose
Lubricants
Liquid paraffin
Osmotics
Lactulose
Magnesium citrate
Epsom salts
Sodium phosphate
Picosulfate
Stimulants
Herbal laxatives
Senna
Biscodyl
Castor oil
Rectal preparations
Enemas
Suppositories

Intestinal Causes: Mechanical Versus Functional

The diagnosis of a functional cause of constipation is made only after exclusion of mechanical causes (❷ *Table 72-1*). It is most important to exclude a colorectal neoplasm by a detailed history and physical examination, anorectal examination, proctoscopy, and, if indicated, colonoscopy. Recurrent diverticulitis might suggest a diverticular stricture. Double contrast barium enema (❷ *Fig. 72-2*), combined with a sigmoidoscopy, might be an alternative to a colonoscopy and provides a good image of the topography of the colon and its redundancy. In addition, this contrast radiograph technique provides better definition of diverticular disease than a colonoscopy. A pelvic floor dysfunction can be recognized by digital rectal and perineal examination. Occult rectal prolapse, solitary rectal ulcer syndrome, and rectocele all suggest pelvic floor dysfunction, which might occur in isolation or in conjunction with gastrointestinal dysmotility. Symptomatic rectocele presents as a bulge into the vagina during defecation, and the patient often needs to digitate to help with fecal evacuation.

Treatments of various mechanical colonic disorders are covered in other chapters.

Functional Bowel Disorder

When a mechanical cause of constipation has been excluded, a functional bowel disorder is likely responsible for the chronic constipation.

A gastrointestinal transit study will help delineate the "motility" and emptying of the stomach, small bowel, and colon. The transit studies can be performed by radio-opaque markers or by scintigraphy. Marker studies evaluate primarily colonic transit and involve ingestion of 20 markers followed by serial plain radiographs of the abdomen. The test takes 7 days to complete or less if the markers are fully eliminated before 7 days. A transit time of greater than 72 h is considered to be "delayed transit," compared with a mean transit time of 36 h in normal subjects.

Scintigraphic transit studies require the ingestion of a meal mixed with technetium-99m and indium-111 in a delayed-release capsule. The capsules containing technetium-99m are used to assess gastric and small bowel transit, while the capsules containing indium-111, which dissolve in the ileocolic region, help to assess colonic transit.

Pelvic floor function is best evaluated using anorectal physiologic testing. Resting and squeeze anal canal pressures are measured, as well as the rectal compliance and the balloon expulsion test. Surface electromyography will help determine if there is anismus or paradoxic function of pelvic floor. These tests together, rather than individually, provide a global assessment of whether there is any pelvic floor disorder. If identified, pelvic floor biofeedback therapy can be helpful. Absence of a recto-anal inhibitory reflex could suggest the rare adult presentation of Hirschsprung's disease. A definitive diagnosis requires a full-thickness rectal biopsy from the posterior anorectal junction.

Defecating proctography may allow the identification of pelvic floor disorders, such as occult rectal intussusception, rectoceles, and enteroceles. These disorders may respond well to operative intervention in appropriately selected situations.

If gastrointestinal dysmotility and pelvic floor disorders are excluded, and there has been no mechanical cause or systemic cause to the constipation, some patients have constipation related to irritable bowel syndrome or other psychosomatic syndromes. Multi-disciplinary management should then involve a gastroenterologist, psychologist, dietician, physiotherapist, and social worker (❯ *Fig. 72-1*).

Medical Therapy for Constipation

The vast majority of patients with constipation have "simple" constipation, which can be identified with a careful history and physical examination. Dietary manipulation, a high liquid intake, and physical activity are the backbone of management of chronic constipation. Increased dietary fiber, up to 20 g/day, is helpful. Prudent use of laxatives (❯ *Table 72-2*) such as oral sodium phosphate might improve the quality of life, but the use of oral or transanal laxatives should be monitored closely.

Slow Transit Constipation

About 10% of patients with severe constipation who present to our specialized center have slow transit constipation; it should be acknowledged, however, that this is a referral practice of highly screened patients. In such patients, excess dietary fiber actually accentuates the bloating and abdominal discomfort. A multi-disciplinary approach, as indicated earlier, is adopted. These patients have often used most laxatives by the time they present to a specialized center. A coordinated prescription of osmotic laxative (lactulose, magnesium citrate) and sodium phosphate enema may be helpful. Due to the chronicity of the problem, stimulant laxatives, such as senna or bisacodyl, are less favored. Newer 5-HT uptake inhibitors have shown some success. These patients often have severe constipation that

■ Figure 72-1
Overall approach to the patient with constipation

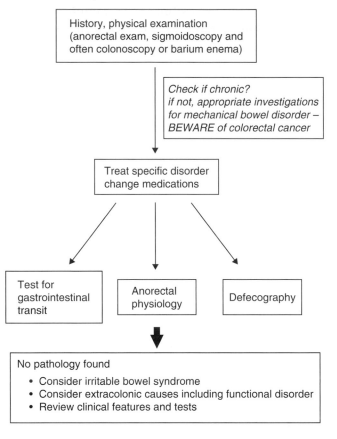

History, physical examination
(anorectal exam, sigmoidoscopy and
often colonoscopy or barium enema)

Check if chronic?
if not, appropriate investigations
for mechanical bowel disorder –
BEWARE of colorectal cancer

Treat specific disorder
change medications

Test for
gastrointestinal
transit

Anorectal
physiology

Defecography

No pathology found
• Consider irritable bowel syndrome
• Consider extracolonic causes including functional disorder
• Review clinical features and tests

■ Figure 72-2
Barium enema showing a stenosing cancer in rectosigmoid junction of the colon

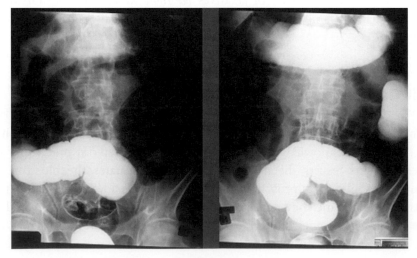

substantially affects their lifestyle. Ultimately, many patients need a more vigorous laxative such as polyethylene glycol, oral sodium phosphate, or picosulphate preparation. Even these vigorous laxative tend to become less effective with time, and many patients require repeated hospital admissions for relief of pain and fecal impaction. Finally, operative intervention is considered as an alternative.

Pelvic Floor Disorders

Pelvic floor retraining involves biofeedback but requires a strong commitment of the patient. A multidisciplinary approach, involving physiotherapist, dietician, surgeon, gastroenterologist, and psychologist, is likely to be the most effective therapy. Pelvic floor biofeedback therapy enhances the appropriate pelvic floor function with pushing and fecal evacuation. The duration of pelvic floor training varies, but a regular structured program with a process of planned, repeated relearning is best.

Surgical Therapy for Functional Bowel Disorder

Slow Colonic Transit Constipation

A highly selected group of patients with slow colonic transit will benefit from abdominal colectomy and ileorectal anastomosis. In one series, patients were evaluated extensively with a firm diagnosis of slow transit constipation and good results were obtained. Of 74 patients who underwent operation, 97% were satisfied with the results of colectomy, and all patients were able to pass a stool spontaneously. The morbidity includes the future possibility of small bowel obstruction (9%) and a prolonged ileus (12%). In patients with combined slow colonic transit and pelvic floor dysfunction, pelvic floor retraining should precede operative intervention. Preoperative bowel preparation is often more complex, requiring a protracted bowel cleansing, often with a 48 h liquid.

The operation of choice is a total abdominal colectomy, removing the colon from the terminal ileum to the rectosigmoid junction and constructing an ileorectal anastomosis. This procedure can now be performed laparoscopically. A less extensive procedure, such as a segmental colectomy or less extensive colectomy with an ileosigmoid anastomosis, produces much inferior functional results and should be avoided. It is essential that the anastomosis is to the rectum itself. Prior to definitive colectomy, it is sometimes helpful, as a bridge, to provide a diverting ileostomy for 6 months or so, to ensure that there is a good response when the colon is bypassed. Presence of a concomitant disorder of slow small bowel transit or gastroparesis is an absolute contraindication to abdominal colectomy with ileorectostomy.

In the early postoperative period, the stools are loose and may be frequent, though incontinence is rare. More than 90% of patients have semisolid stools by 4 months, and approximately 30% of patients use some form of antidiarrheal medications to control stool frequency in the first 6 months after operation. With time, the stool tends to become more solid and the frequency of bowel movements decreases.

Rectocele

Rectocele, defined as herniation of the anterior rectal and posterior vaginal wall into the vaginal lumen, can be treated by operative repair. While a rectocele can be asymptomatic, it may also contribute substantially to obstructed defecation and is often associated with mucosal rectal prolapse. Various operative techniques using transvaginal, transanal, transperineal, or transabdominal approaches with or without prosthetic mesh have been described to repair the rectocele. The operative results are variable between studies due to variability in patient selection and operative techniques. Repair of rectocele is performed commonly by the gynecologist via the vaginal route, especially if there is a significant enterocele.

Transanal repair of rectocele is equally effective for smaller rectocele, and especially when there is associated mucosal-rectal prolapse. Transanal resection of the rectal wall, the STARR procedure (stapled trans-anal rectal resection), is currently under study as the operative procedure to treat obstructed defecation syndrome, which is commonly associated with mucosal rectal prolapse and rectocele. With meticulous protection of the posterior wall of the vagina, an approximately 5×7 cm rectal mucosal flap is resected using the circular stapler. In principle, the rectovaginal septum is strengthened, and the redundant rectal mucosal tissue is resected.

Hirschsprung's Disease

Adult presentation of Hirschsprung's disease is quite rare and usually involves short-segment disease. Ultrashort segment disease in an adult will respond to anorectal strip myectomy where a posterior strip of anal sphincter is resected, which also allows for a histologic diagnosis.

Sacral Nerve Stimulation

Sacral nerve stimulation has been used to treat fecal incontinence since 1995. The same technique suggests that it might help to modulate the sensory responses in the rectum and pelvic floor, and thereby, help with fecal evacuation. There are two active trials, in Melbourne and in Europe, to evaluate this approach. Results are encouraging, but investigators await Level 1 evidence of efficacy.

Selected Readings

Fazio VW, Tjandra JJ, Church JM, et al. (1992) Clinical conundrum of solitary rectal ulcer. Dis Colon Rectum 35:227–234

Nyam D, Pemberton J, Ilstrup D, Rath D (1997) Long-term results of surgery for chronic constipation. Dis Colon Rectum 40:273–279

Ommer A, Albrecht K, Wenger F, Walz MK (2006) Stapled transanal rectal resection: a new option in the treatment of obstructive defecation syndrome. Langenbecks Arch Surg 391:32–37

Seow-Choen F, Tjandra JJ (2001) Chronic constipation. In: Tjandra JJ, Clunie GA, Thomas RJS (eds) Textbook of surgery, 2nd edn. Blackwell, Oxford, pp 628–632

Tjandra JJ, Fazio VW, Petras RE (1993) Clinical and pathological factors associated with delayed diagnosis in solitary rectal ulcer syndrome. Dis Colon Rectum 36:146–153

Tjandra JJ, Ooi BS, Tang CL, et al. (1999) Transanal repair of rectocele corrects obstructed defecation if it is not associated with anismus. Dis Colon Rectum 42:1544–1550

73 Diverticulitis

Daniel L. Feingold · Richard L. Whelan

Pearls and Pitfalls

- The proximal margin of resection is determined by visualizing and palpating healthy descending colon.
- The distal margin of resection is the most proximal healthy rectum such that a true colorectal anastomosis is performed.
- During sigmoid resection, the left ureter is in jeopardy and must be identified accurately and preserved.
- Minimal access surgery offers substantial benefits over traditional open surgery in the setting of diverticulitis.
- In cases where a mucosal-based neoplasm has not been ruled out, a cancer-type operation should be performed.
- Three-stage operations (drainage, resection, reconstruction) are of historic interest only and should be avoided.
- Laparoscopic-assisted operations for complicated "benign" diverticular disease can be more challenging than resections for malignant disease.
- In the vast majority of cases, full mobilization of the splenic flexure is necessary if a full sigmoid resection is to be carried out.
- When presented with an acutely inflamed sigmoid colon or in the presence of a phlegmon or severe fibrotic reaction, initiate the mobilization in an uninvolved area, identify the critical structures and then work towards the disease.
- Consider ureteral stenting when operating on a patient with a phlegmon, severe fibrotic reaction, or colovesical fistula.
- When performing laparoscopic-assisted resection, if the inflammatory phlegmon is large or if the pelvic dissection proves very difficult, use of a hand-assist technique is advised.

Diverticulitis is an inflammatory process that will eventually affect 10–25% of patients with diverticulosis of the colon. Most likely due to the distribution of acquired diverticula in patients in the Western world, the vast majority of episodes of diverticulitis occur in the sigmoid colon. In contrast, in Africa and Asia where the incidence of diverticula in the left colon is much less common, the distribution of diverticular disease favors the right colon. Not only has the incidence of sigmoid diverticulitis increased over the past century, due to the age-related nature of the disease, the prevalence has increased with the aging population as well.

Pathophysiology, Clinical Presentation, and Evaluation

The pathophysiology of diverticulitis has been described through anatomic and histologic studies demonstrating the formation of false, pulsion diverticula within the colon wall where vasa rectae penetrate the inner, circular muscle layer, resulting in points of structural weakness through which mucosa can herniate. Lack of dietary fiber and the relatively high intraluminal pressure associated with the narrow sigmoid colon are thought to predispose to the formation of diverticula at these points of compromised, structural integrity.

The inflammatory process of diverticulitis is the consequence of microperforation caused by "impacted," inspissated stool within a diverticulum; the range of clinical manifestations and presentations varies considerably. Acute, uncomplicated diverticulitis is characterized by localized inflammation, while complicated diverticulitis includes abscess or phlegmons, gross perforation, and generalized peritonitis. Sub-acute and chronic sequelae of complicated diverticular inflammation include fistula formation and large bowel obstruction due to fibrosis of the diseased sigmoid colon resulting in a stricture.

The clinical presentation of diverticulitis depends on the acuity and severity of the inflammation. The triad of left lower quadrant pain, fever, and leukocytosis is the most common manifestation of acute, uncomplicated disease. The redundancy and course of the sigmoid colon may result in right-sided symptoms, making the diagnosis potentially more difficult. Patients with complicated disease may also have a palpable phlegmon, evidence of large bowel obstruction, symptoms of fistulization, or manifestations of sepsis caused by perforation and peritonitis. The differential diagnosis includes inflammatory bowel disease, ischemic or infectious colitis, colon neoplasia, and a variety of genitourinary and gynecologic processes. Successful initial non-operative treatment allows for a thorough diagnostic workup that, in the majority of patients, can exclude other potential diagnoses.

At presentation, patients are evaluated typically with abdominopelvic computed tomography (CT) utilizing oral and intravenous contrast (❯ *Fig. 73-1*). Whereas this imaging modality can demonstrate reliably the inflammatory changes of the colon and surrounding tissues suggestive of diverticulitis, the clinician should consider other diagnoses as well that can present with similar findings, because the medical and operative treatment for these alternative diagnoses can be substantially different. CT is most helpful in identifying localized intra-abdominal abscesses and other complicated disease; this finding will enable percutaneous drainage of these collections, thus preventing the need for emergent or urgent operation in the acute setting (which usually requires a colostomy) and allows a more elective, one-stage resection and primary anastomosis in the near future after further evaluation. Once the acute inflammatory process has resolved, colonoscopy can be performed to evaluate the colon to rule out malignancy and confirm the diagnosis. Sigmoidoscopy and colonoscopy are usually contraindicated in the acute setting, owing to concerns that air insufflation or endoscope insertion may exacerbate the infection. Another complimentary study that may be useful in certain situations is a water-soluble contrast enema. Clearly, care must be taken in the acute setting when instilling the contrast during an enema study.

Treatment

The majority of patients with uncomplicated diverticulitis may be treated on an outpatient basis with oral antibiotics; recurrences can be anticipated in approximately one third of patients. Medical therapy (often referred to by the misnomer "conservative" treatment) utilizes any of a number of single or

◘ Figure 73-1
CT with contrast demonstrating uncomplicated diverticulitis with fat stranding of the mesentery and thickening of the sigmoid colon

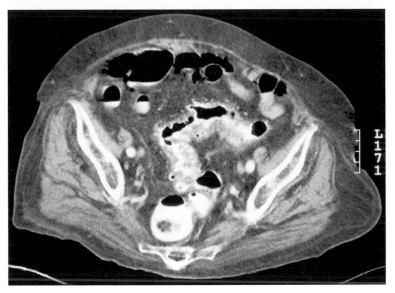

multi-drug regimens covering gram-negative rods and anaerobic bacteria. Typically, patients with recurrent episodes of uncomplicated inflammation and many patients with exacerbations of chronic complicated disease can be managed medically in anticipation of a planned, elective operation. Of course, acute septic complications (such as free perforation with generalized peritonitis) mandate emergent operation.

According to the most recent consensus statement on the management of diverticulitis by the American Society of Colon and Rectal Surgeons, operative intervention is indicated after two documented episodes of uncomplicated disease or after a single bout of complicated disease. These recommendations are based on thorough review of the data addressing the recurrence, morbidity, and mortality from published series with long-term follow up and take into consideration the purported increasing risks incurred with successive episodes of inflammation and the coincident decreased response rates to non-operative management. Review of the literature, however, demonstrates continuing controversy over operative indications in the setting of diverticulitis and hinges on the considerations of risk of recurrence and failure rates of non-operative, medical management.

The recommendations regarding operative therapy for young patients with diverticulitis are based, for the most part, on anecdotal or limited retrospective reviews and remain controversial. Early reports described a more virulent form of the disease in young patients with substantially increased rates of recurrence and complications; thus, sigmoid resection was advised after resolution of the first episode of uncomplicated diverticulitis. Taking into consideration the more effective, non-operative therapies available currently and the marginal quality of the literature in support of early operate therapy, the treatment algorithm utilized by the authors and most surgical societies no longer discriminates therapeutic decisions based on age at presentation.

Otherwise healthy patients with a clear diagnosis of uncomplicated diverticulitis may be evaluated and treated on an outpatient basis with oral antibiotics and a liquid diet. Those who fail to improve with outpatient therapy, who have a questionable diagnosis, or who have medical co-morbidities precluding outpatient treatment require admission. Excluding the minority of patients who present with feculent peritonitis or complete bowel obstruction who require emergent intervention, the management of patients with acute diverticulitis who require hospitalization consists of bowel rest, broad-spectrum intravenous antibiotics, fluid resuscitation, and pain control. The majority of these patients will respond to non-operative care and should undergo further evaluation and treatment in the near future in an elective situation as outlined above. In general, once the decision is made to proceed with elective resection, it may be helpful to consider delaying operation for approximately 6 weeks. Although this practice has not been assessed objectively, proponents believe this waiting period may permit improvement, or even resolution, of the acute inflammatory response and, in addition, allow for nutritional recovery and an easier operation.

Although there has been intense debate about which surgical approach is preferred for diverticulitis, the surgical literature is now replete with studies documenting the feasibility, safety, improved short term outcome, and comparable long-term outcomes of elective, laparoscopic-assisted colectomy when compared with traditional open resection provided the surgeon has mastered techniques requiring advances laparoscopic skills. Thus, presently, minimal-access sigmoid resection with colorectal anastomosis appears to be the operative method of choice in the elective setting. When feasible and practical, it is the preference of the authors to utilize the laparoscopic-assisted method, whereby patients undergo a mobilization, devascularization, and distal bowel transection laparoscopically, followed by specimen extraction and anastomosis via as small an incision as possible.

For obese patients, patients with a bulky specimen, or those in whom the pelvic dissection proves very difficult, a hand-assisted approach is preferred. The rationale for this choice is that in these situations, using standard laparoscopic methods to their fullest, the majority of these patients, in the end, will require an incision 8 cm or larger. The hand-assisted approach facilitates dissection, is easier to teach and learn, and, in the authors' opinion, shortens the operation. Thus, it seems logical to employ a hand-assisted technique once it is clear that an incision as large as your glove size will be needed in the end or if it is evident that completion of the operation via purely laparoscopic means is unlikely.

Operative Techniques

The technical challenges, added degree of difficulty, a need for advanced laparoscopic skills and training associated with minimal-access approaches have limited their use in the general surgical community, thus far, such that the majority of sigmoid colectomies are still accomplished via open technique. Of note, certain fundamental principles regarding colectomy for diverticulitis apply regardless of the operative approach utilized. Pre-operatively, it is advised that patients undergo bowel preparation, per routine, and that an appropriate intravenous antibiotic be administered peri-operatively. Once the abdomen is accessed, the sigmoid colon is mobilized from its lateral and retroperitoneal attachments, and the left ureter is identified and preserved. Confidently visualizing the course of the ureter prior to transecting the mesenteric vascular pedicle is critical to avoid technical misadventure. Intense retroperitoneal inflammation can obscure the ureter and make dissection quite difficult. In this situation, we recommend identifying the ureter in a more cephalad location, away from the inflammation, to establish the plane between the uretogonadal bundle and the mesentery and then to follow the plane into the pelvis. In this fashion, the ureter may be dissected away safely from the disease. In selected patients when a hostile retroperitoneum is anticipated based on review of the clinical history or the preoperative CT, the surgeon should consider strongly the placement of bilateral ureteral stents.

Traditionally, for sigmoid resection, proximal vascular transection is carried out at the level of the main sigmoidal artery after the take-off of the left colic artery from the inferior mesenteric artery (❯ *Fig. 73-2*). An alternative method calls for mid-mesenteric dissection and transection of the individual sigmoidal branches, thereby preserving the main sigmoidal and superior hemorrhoidal arteries. This latter method differs from the conventional approach only with regard to the level of the vascular transection. The colon must still be fully mobilized with the left uretogonadal bundle well visualized and dissected away from the mesentery. This approach is not feasible when the colonic inflammatory process involves the entire mesentery or when the pelvic anatomy is unclear. The purported advantages of a mid-mesenteric transection are that the blood supply to the rectum is preserved, and the hypogastric nerves are protected, because the plane dorsal to the superior hemorrhoidal vessels is not violated. This dissection has not been well studied in an objective manner, but, theoretically, it may decrease colorectal anastomotic leak rates (due to the preserved rectal blood supply), and it may decrease the risk of sexual or bladder dysfunction as compared with conventional dissection.

Mid-mesenteric division can be tedious and is facilitated by using several ancillary devices such as a bipolar diathermy and tissue division device, an ultrasonic scissors, hemostatic clips, and/or a linear stapler. One of the shortcomings of the mid-mesentery transection method is that the rectum is not mobilized posteriorly, because the presacral plane is not dissected. Therefore, there may be a tendency to perform the distal transection of the bowel more proximally than would be the case if the rectum were mobilized partially. Care must be taken to ensure that the entire sigmoid colon is resected and that a true colorectal anastomosis is constructed to avoid leaving any diverticula-bearing sigmoid colon.

◻ Figure 73-2
The anatomy of the inferior mesenteric artery (IMA)

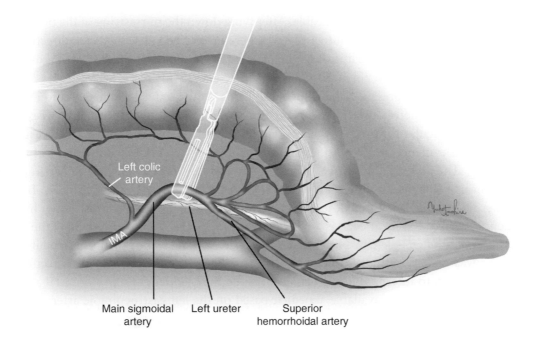

Another ramification of avoiding the posterior rectal mobilization is that it can, on occasion, be quite difficult to pass the circular stapler trans-anally up to the proximal limit of the Hartmann pouch because of the curve of the rectum. It is advised that the feasibility of insertion of the circular stapler be assessed by passing trans-anally the metal stapler sizing instruments. There are two options if full insertion of the stapler proves problematic: resect more rectum or carry out a limited posterior mobilization, beginning well caudal to the sacral promontory (so as to avoid the hypogastric nerves).

It is important to recognize that diverticular resection can be very difficult if the inflammatory process or the resulting fibrotic reaction obliterates the usual anatomic planes. Therefore, if minimally invasive methods are being used, conversion may be necessary if the pelvic dissection proves too difficult. In this situation, we recommend strongly that the splenic flexure be mobilized fully and the mesentery divided proximally using laparoscopic methods, if feasible, prior to conversion. If these steps of the operation are performed using minimally invasive methods, then, in almost all situations, the operation can be completed using open methods via a limited, infra-umbilical incision.

Depending on the redundancy of the bowel and the length of colon to be resected, splenic flexure mobilization is performed to allow an adequate tension-free reach of the remaining descending colon to the level of the anastomosis. Adequate resection requires flexure takedown in the vast majority of patients. Once the bowel is mobilized completely and the relevant vasculature addressed, the next step is to determine the appropriate margins of resection. Failing to resect distally to the level of the rectum increases the recurrence rate of diverticulitis considerably, whereas retaining diseased proximal colon jeopardizes anastomotic integrity and may also lead to recurrence. The rectosigmoid junction, described as the confluence of the taenia, usually occurs below the level of the sacral promontory. It is important to appreciate that although the rectum is devoid of diverticula, it may be inflamed secondarily, and the distal margin of resection must be made through healthy rectum as determined by intra-operative inspection and palpation.

Using the laparoscopic-assisted approach, the specimen is delivered via an enlarged port incision, an additional low Pfannenstiel incision, or, in the case of hand-assisted cases, via the hand-port incision. Next, a functional end-to-end circular stapled colorectal anastomosis is carried out using the largest diameter stapler that proves feasible. After tying down the pursestring of the proximal bowel around the stapler anvil, it is important to assess whether any retained diverticula fall directly across the projected path of the circular staple line. If so, the diverticula should be displaced in towards the central rod or outwards, away from the position of the anticipated staple line.

Colovesical fistula: The presence of a colovesical fistula requires specific consideration with regard to the operative plan. Whereas ureteral stents are not required for the vast majority of resections for uncomplicated diverticular disease, these stents are used often for patients with a colovesical fistula, especially if there is evidence on CT of inflammatory changes in the retroperitoneum or at the level of the pelvic inlet. The fistula most often can be taken down bluntly using a finger-fracture type technique, although sharp dissection may be required sometimes to separate the tissues. In the event that a bladder wall defect is identified, it is repaired with absorbable suture; most often, however, no defect is demonstrated. Rarely, if ever, is a partial bladder resection required. To allow the bladder to heal, the urinary catheter is left in place for approximately 5 days and, in those patients in whom bladder repair was carried out, a cystogram is obtained. To reduce the risk of fistula recurrence, it is helpful, when feasible, to interpose healthy tissue between the bladder and the colorectal anastomosis. If a robust greater omentum is available, a pedicle based on the left gastroepiploic artery is mobilized.

In the absence of an adequate omentum, if deemed necessary, a rectus sheath flap can be mobilized, preserving the caudal blood supply.

Perforated acute diverticulitis with diffuse peritonitis: While there is general consensus regarding the management of recurrent uncomplicated diverticulitis, associated localized collections, and colovesical fistulas, the optimal management of perforated diverticulitis with diffuse peritonitis still remains somewhat controversial. This controversy is due, in part, to the rarity of the entity (it accounts for 1–2% of patients with acute diverticulitis) and, therefore, a paucity of data. In addition, the morbidity and mortality associated with emergent operative intervention in this setting make it difficult to reach a uniform consensus regarding the most appropriate operation. Hinchey developed a classification of diverticulitis to aid the description of intraoperative findings (❷ *Table 73-1*).

Through the mid-1970s, the standard operation for Hinchey class 3 or 4 diverticulitis, corresponding to purulent and feculent peritonitis, respectively, was a three-stage approach, with the initial washout of the abdomen and diversion of the fecal stream with a transverse loop colostomy. Subsequently, a second operation for sigmoid resection, performed after the patient recovered, was followed by a third operation for colostomy reversal. The justification for this three-stage approach was to perform as minimal of an operation as possible during the acute phase of the illness when patients were often clinically unstable and in critical condition. This three-stage approach has been abandoned due to the unreasonably high complication rates associated with leaving the septic source in place.

Currently, recommended treatment of choice for Hinchey class 3 or 4 diverticulitis is open sigmoid resection with end-colostomy and formation of a Hartmann pouch. In this setting, it is beneficial to resect the sigmoid down to the most proximal healthy rectum in anticipation of future colostomy reversal. Given the potential operative difficulties and morbidity associated with end-colostomy reversal in this setting, a reasonable alternative to the Hartmann procedure is on-table lavage and primary anastomosis with or without diverting loop ileostomy. Clearly, this approach is contingent on the patient's status and ability to tolerate a more extensive operation. The purpose of the lavage is to evacuate as much of the stool column from the colon as possible so as to decrease the contamination from the fecal load in the event of a leak at this high-risk colorectal anastomosis.

Colonic obstruction secondary to diverticulitis: Patients with a critical diverticular stricture of the sigmoid colon often present with a large bowel obstruction indistinguishable from an obstructing sigmoid colon cancer. Often, despite attempts to carry out colonoscopy or contrast enema, a definitive diagnosis cannot be made, and an urgent intervention is required. Prior to operation, an attempt at endoluminal stenting should be considered. In situations where stenting is not available or an attempt at decompression is not successful, operation is required. Laparotomy in this situation is facilitated by decompressing the large bowel early in the operation through a colotomy in the proximal sigmoid or

◻ Table 73-1

Hinchey classification of complicated acute diverticulitis

Stage	Characteristics
I	Pericolic or mesenteric abscess
II	Walled-off pelvic abscess
III	Generalized purulent peritonitis
IV	Generalized fecal peritonitis

transverse colon. Alternatively, early transection of the sigmoid colon with on-table lavage may be performed. Whereas sparing of the superior hemorrhoidal artery may be advocated in the setting of known diverticular disease, if malignancy has not been excluded, a formal oncologic resection must be performed, with mobilization of the rectum via the presacral plane and division of the main sigmoidal vessel.

Summary

Sigmoid diverticulitis encompasses a spectrum of disease that can be challenging to manage both medically and operatively. The laparoscopic-assisted approach to sigmoid colectomy has marked clinical benefits over the traditional open operation and should be considered in patients with uncomplicated disease as well as in selected patients with complicated disease provided the surgeon has the advanced laparoscopic skills necessary for this approach. Successful operation requires an advanced understanding of the anatomy, as post-inflammatory changes can obliterate tissue planes and make for difficult dissection.

Selected Readings

Benn PL, Wolff BG, Ilstrup DM (1986) Level of anastomosis and recurrent colonic diverticulitis. Am J Surg 151:269–271

Chapman JR, Dozois EJ, Wolff BG, et al. (2006) Diverticulitis: a progressive disease? Do multiple recurrences predict less favorable outcomes? Ann Surg 243:876–883

Milsom JW, Bohm B, Nakajima K (eds) (2006) Laparoscopic colorectal surgery. 2nd edn. Springer, New York

Welch JP, Cohen JL, Sardella WV, Vignati PV (eds) (1998) Diverticular disease: management of the difficult surgical case. Williams & Wilkins, Baltimore, MD

74 Pilonidal Disease

David E. Beck

Pearls and Pitfalls

- Pilonidal disease is an acquired condition associated with an inflammatory or foreign body reaction to entrapped hairs or a disrupted hair follicle in subcutaneous tissue of intertriginous areas within the gluteal or natal cleft.
- The condition usually presents in young hirsute adults.
- The differential diagnosis includes skin infections such as hidradenitis, anorectal abscess or fistulas, and Crohn's disease.
- The goal of treatment is removal of the foreign body (i.e. hairs) and infection (associated abscess) while providing optimal conditions for wound healing.
- Acute abscesses are managed with incision and drainage.
- Chronic disease is initially managed with unroofing with attempts to keep incisions off the midline, while keeping the wound as small as possible to diminish healing time.
- In selected patients with limited disease, excision and primary closure is an option.
- Recurrent disease may require excision and flap closure.
- Antibiotics have little role except to treat associated cellulites.
- Wound care and removal of hair (by shaving or depilatories) assists healing and reduces recurrence.

Basic Science

Pilonidal disease is an acquired condition of the subcutaneous tissue of intertriginous areas, such as the gluteal or natal cleft (midline sacrococcygeal area). Several etiologic factors have been associated with pilonidal disease. The inflammatory or foreign body reaction is produced by hairs or disrupted hair follicles that are forced or pulled into the subcutaneous tissue. Keratin plugs and other follicle debris may contribute to the inflammation of the hair in the midline internatal cleft pits. The inflammation around the hair follows the path of least resistance and often tracks in a cephalad and lateral direction, thus forming secondary tracks and openings. Vagrant hairs from the region gather in the gluteal cleft and into the sinus. If the sinus cavity fails to heal promptly, epithelium migrates into the sinus from the edges of the follicle and forms an epithelial lined tube. The sinus is susceptible to recurrent infection.

Clinical Presentation

Pilonidal disease is more common in men and tends to occur between puberty and 40 years of age. Physical examination typically reveals one or more small (1–2 mm) dermal pits at the base of the intergluteal cleft (❯ *Fig. 74-1*). Tracking from the pits (usually in a cranial and lateral direction) will appear as areas of induration. Pilonidal disease has three common presentations. Nearly all patients have an episode of acute abscess formation (polymicrobial infection). With an associated abscess, the diseased area may be tender and erythematous, and draining pus may be evident. The more extensive the disease, the more prominent the findings. When this abscess resolves, either spontaneously or with medical assistance, many patients will develop a pilonidal sinus. Although most sinus tracts resolve, a small minority of patients will develop chronic or recurrent disease after treatment. Treatment methods vary for each stage in pilonidal disease.

Treatment

Abscess

Abscesses must be drained. In one study, simple incision and drainage of first-episode acute pilonidal abscesses resulted in an improvement in symptoms in all patients and complete eradication in 58% of patients within 10 weeks of the procedure. Between 20% and 40% of patients develop recurrent disease after this form of treatment. Bascom has reported a recurrence rate of only 15% by excising the epithelial pits with small 7 mm incisions 5 days after initial incision and drainage.

Incision and drainage of acute abscesses is readily performed in an office setting using local anesthesia. A 10–30 ml solution of 1% lidocaine (Xylocaine HCl) with 1:100,000 epinephrine is injected

◘ **Figure 74-1**
Pilonidal cyst disease. Dermal pits associated sinus and abscess (From Beck et al., 2003. With permission)

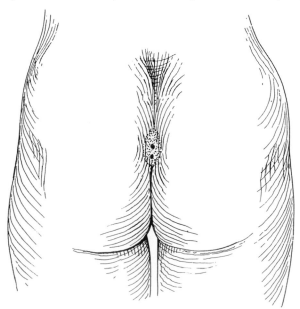

as a field block around the area of inflammation with a 25-gauge needle. In cases of simple abscess with minimal cellulitis, incision, drainage, and curettage of the wall of the cavity will provide definitive treatment. Cultures of the abscess contents may be taken, but the use of antibiotics is rarely required. The wound is initially packed open with plain gauze to prevent premature closure of the skin over the cavity. The wound is kept clean by irrigating the area twice daily with warm water using a shower attachment, sitz bath, or even a Water-Pik. It is important to painstakingly dry the area by blotting the skin dry or using a hair dryer to avoid maceration. The skin in the gluteal cleft is shaved before drainage and then during weekly office visits. Also during office visits, granulation tissue is cauterized and removed. Success in treatment results from diligent wound care by both the patient and the physician.

Sinus

Up to 40% of acute pilonidal abscesses treated by incision and drainage form a chronic sinus that requires additional treatment. The predominant organisms cultured from pilonidal sinuses are anaerobic and seldom require antibiotic therapy. A prospective randomized trial comparing a single preoperative dose of cefoxitin with no antibiotic prophylaxis in excision and primary closure of chronic pilonidal sinuses failed to show a benefit with antibiotic prophylaxis. The majority of pilonidal sinuses resolve, regardless of treatment option, by age 40. It is theorized that changes in body habitus (altered and increased fat deposition alters the gluteal cleft) and softening of body hair account for this change with age.

There is debate about the best method of treatment for a nonhealing pilonidal sinus. A review of articles published in the last 30 years on the treatment of pilonidal disease divided the procedures and analyzed them by broad category (❷ *Table 74-1*). Closed techniques (injection with phenol or coring-out follicles and brushing the tracts) required shaving of the area but could be performed on an outpatient basis. Mean healing time was about 40 days and recurrence rates were slightly higher than other forms of treatment. **Laying open** (unroofing) the tracts with healing by granulation resulted in average healing times of 48 days and required frequent outpatient dressing changes. The incidence of

◨ Table 74-1

Comparison of techniques by time to healing and recurrence rate based on minimal follow-up in several review articles (Reprinted from Beck et al., 2003. With permission)

Procedure	Number of series	Number of patients	Mean time to healing (days)	Mean recurrence rate	
				<1 Year follow-up (%)	>1 Year follow-up (%)
Debridement of epithelial pit	13	955	44	14	18
Laying open sinus	14	716	48	4	13
Laying open sinus and cauterizing base of sinus	4	630	36	3	13
Excision to fascia	12	572	72	14	13
Excision to fascia and marsupialization of edges	8	538	26	6	4
Primary midline closure	22	872	19	8	15
Primary oblique closure	8	1,983	9	1	3
Flap closure	16	536	15	2	8

recurrent sinus formation was less than 13% with this technique (❯ *Fig. 74-2*). Addition of cauterization of the cavity decreased the average healing time to 36 days and slightly reduced the reported recurrence rates. **Wide and deep excision** of the sinus alone resulted in an average healing time of 72 days and similar recurrence rates as for simple laying open of the sinus with wound granulation (❯ *Fig. 74-3*). When partial closure of the wound (marsupialization) is added to wide and deep excision of the sinus, healing time decreases to an average of 26 days. Excision and primary closure resulted in wound healing within 2 weeks in successful cases (19 days overall). However, up to 30% of patients failed primary wound healing and the average recurrence rate for these experienced authors was 15%. With **excision and primary closure** using oblique or asymmetric incisions, the mean healing time dropped to 9 days and the recurrence rate was less than 3%.

Bascom reported less than 10% recurrence with excision of enlarged follicles, with corroborating results by other authors using the same technique. This procedure involved an incision lateral to the

⬛ Figure 74-2
Unroofing of sinus. Removes skin and subcutaneous tissue overlying the cavity. a, sagittal section, b, cross-sectional view (From Beck et al., 2003. With permission)

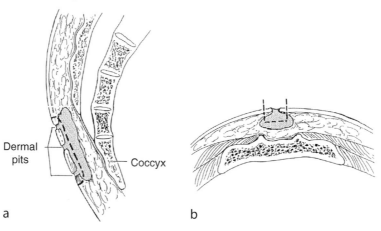

⬛ Figure 74-3
Wide and deep excision of sinus to the fascia. a, sagittal section, b, cross-sectional view (From Beck et al., 2003. With permission)

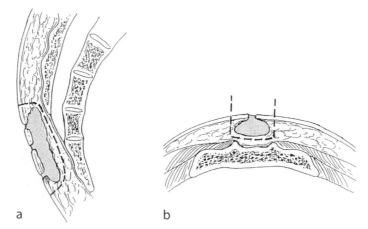

midline to scrub the chronic cavity free of hair and granulation tissue (❂ *Fig. 74-4A*). Removal of the small midline pits was carried out with small 7 mm incisions (❂ *Fig. 74-4B*). When epithelial tubes were present, they were removed through the lateral incision. The lateral wound was then left open but the midline incisions were closed with a removable 4-0 polypropylene subcuticular suture (❂ *Fig. 74-4C*).

A nonoperative or conservative approach has been suggested as an alternative to conventional excision. In this approach, meticulous hair control by natal cleft shaving, improved perineal hygiene, and limited lateral incision and drainage for treatment of abscess has resulted in a significant reduction in the number of excisional procedures and occupied-bed days. As an added benefit, there is improved patient tolerance and near normal work status during treatment. This concept merits further investigation.

Complex or Recurrent Disease

Even with proper treatment, a small subgroup of patients are left with persistent, nonhealing wounds. Repeated treatment of complex or recurrent disease with conventional measures rarely results in satisfactory healing. A number of more aggressive treatments have been described to treat complex or recurrent disease, including wide excision and split-thickness skin grafting, excision and Z – plasty, and myocutaneous or fasciocutaneous flaps. As a group, these **flap techniques** have resulted in primary healing in less than 15 days in 90% of cases. There are, however, disadvantages to these aggressive approaches. Nearly all of these techniques require hospitalization and general anesthesia. In addition, up to 50% of those procedures requiring skin flaps for wound coverage or closure develop loss of skin sensation or flap tip necrosis.

An extremely rare complication of nonhealing pilonidal disease is squamous cell carcinoma arising from the sinus tract. Most of these tumors are slow-growing but with a tendency to aggressive local invasion. Cases typically present after years of long-standing, untreated pilonidal disease. Patients with advanced disease, including inguinal metastasis, had a poor prognosis and most died within 16 months. Long-term survival has been reported in patients treated with aggressive surgical resection, and adjuvant radiation therapy, and chemotherapy to help reduce local recurrence.

Conclusion

Pilonidal disease has three basic presentations: acute abscess, simple sinus, and complex or recurrent disease. Simple incision and drainage of an acute abscess will result in relief of symptoms in nearly all patients. Additional steps at this point may help reduce recurrence rates. Treatment of a simple pilonidal sinus is eventually effective, regardless of surgical techniques. Of the many options, wide excision of the sinus tract to the fascia, without flap coverage or marsupialization, should be avoided. This procedure is associated with prolonged healing and comparable recurrence rates when compared with less-morbid procedures. Satisfactory treatment of complex or recurrent disease is possible but often requires an aggressive approach. The use of asymmetric incisions or skin flaps results in reliable primary healing and a low recurrence rate, but has a high rate of flap complications.

■ Figure 74-4
Bascom procedure. a, Lateral incision and debridement of cavity. b, Removal of a midline pit with a small incision after lateral debridement. c, Closure of midline wounds without closure of the lateral incision (From Beck et al., 2003. With permission)

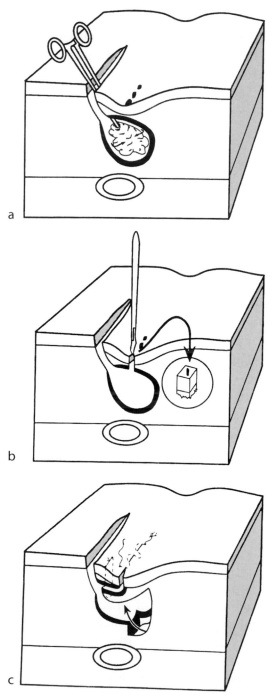

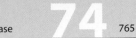

Selected Readings

Allen-Mersh TG (1990) Pilonidal sinus: finding the right track for treatment. Br J Surg 77:123–132

Armstrong JH, Barcia PJ (1994) Pilonidal sinus disease: the conservative approach. Arch Surg 129:914–919

Bascom J (1980) Pilonidal disease: origin from follicles of hairs and results of follicle removal as treatment. Surgery 87:567–572

Beck DE, Karulf RE (2003) Pilonidal disease. In: Beck DE (ed) Handbook of colorectal surgery, 2nd edn. Marcel Dekker, New York, pp 391–404

Hanley PH (1980) Acute pilonidal abscess. Surg Gynecol Obstet 150:9–11

Jensen SL, Harling H (1988) Prognosis after simple incision and drainage for a first episode acute pilonidal abscess. Br J Surg 75:60–61

Mosquera DA, Quayle JB (1995) Bascom's operation for pilonidal sinus. J R Soc Med 88:45–46

Patey DH, Scarff RW (1946) Pathology of postanal pilonidal sinus: its bearing on treatment. Lancet 2:484–486

Sondenaa K, Andersen E, Nesvik I, Soreide JA (1995) Patient characteristics and symptoms in chronic pilonidal sinus disease. Int J Colorectal Dis 0:39–42

Sondenaa K, Nesvik I, Gullaksen FP, et al. (1995) The role of cefoxitin prophylaxis in chronic pilonidal sinus treated with excision and primary suture. J Am Coll Surg 180:157–160

75 Anal Fissure and Fistula

Herand Abcarian

Pearls and Pitfalls

Anal fissure

- Most often mistakenly diagnosed as hemorrhoids.
- Almost always located in the midline (90% post, 5% ant, 5% both).
- If a fissure is located in non midline position, suspect Crohn's disease, TB, AIDS, syphilis, or blood dyscrasias.
- Internal sphincter spasm or hypertrophy is the etiologic factor (increased anal resting pressure at manometry).
- Overshoot phenomenon in response to defecation results in typical post cibal pain lasting from minutes to hours (diagnostic of fissure).
- Surgical treatment of choice is lateral internal sphincterotomy (LIS) which is less likely to cause keyhole deformity seen after midline sphincterotomy.
- Pharmacologic sphincterotomy may be effective temporarily but with high recurrence/persistence rates and eventual need for LIS.

Anal fistula

- Overwhelming majority are of cryptoglandular origin after development of an anorectal abscess.
- 1% caused by Crohn's disease, TB, fungal infections, trauma, or foreign bodies.
- Park's classification (1976) is the most useful guide in planning therapy and predicting prognosis.
- Horseshoe fistulas with multiple openings should be differentiated from hidradenitis suppurativa which normally does not communicate with the anal canal.
- Goodsall's rule (1901) locates the primary opening unless the anatomy is distorted by prior operation.
- Prolonged antibiotic therapy is ineffective and may result in c. diff. colitis.
- The aim of surgery is cure. Too conservative an approach leads to persistence/recurrence of fistulas, while too aggressive an operative approach may lead to incontinence or false passage.
- Intersphincteric fistulas are readily amenable to fistulotomy (sphincterotomy), while extrasphincteric fistulas are not amenable to fistulotomy.
- Fistulotomy in transsphincteric and suprasphincteric fistulas may result in fecal incontinence. These fistulas require alternative surgical approaches, avoiding sphincterotomy.

Anal Fissures

Anal fissure was originally described by Recamier in 1829, who noted its relationship to anal contracture and recommended anal dilatation as treatment. Anal fissure can be diagnosed easily by its symptoms, i.e. pain lasting from minutes to hours after bowel movements and slight bleeding of a bright red nature. Patients and many physicians mistake the sentinel tag (pile) of an anal fissure for hemorrhoids and resort to topical anesthetic creams and suppositories which are totally ineffective.

Anal fissures can be seen easily as a longitudinal midline anal split or ulcer by gentle spreading of the buttocks laterally. Digital rectal examination is unnecessary because it will cause severe pain often lasting for many hours. If a fissure or ulcer is seen in non midline location, one should suspect more complex etiologies such as Crohn's disease, AIDS, TB, syphilis, or blood dyscrasias. An appropriate work-up, including examination under anesthesia, biopsy, dark field examination, or culture, is necessary in such patients. In acute anal fissure, the base of the fissure consists of the corrugator ani muscle which is pink, but in chronic anal fissure, the exposed white fibers of the internal sphincter line the base of the fissure. While the acute anal fissure might respond to sitz baths and stool softeners, chronic anal fissure is almost always associated with a tight, hypertrophied internal anal sphincter and much less likely to heal permanently without operative intervention.

Evolution of the Surgical Treatment of Anal Fissure

Since the original description of anal stenosis in conjunction with anal fissure, dilation or enlargement of the anal canal by fissurectomy and/or sphincterotomy were recommended routinely. In the 1930s Miles described the pectin band, which he thought was part of the external sphincter constricting the anal canal and advocated its division or excision. At the same time Nesselrod in the US advocated excision of the anal fissure and anoplasty for treatment of fissures, but added a small midline sphincterotomy to correct the anal stenosis which he ascribed to scarring due to repeated breakdowns and healing of the anoderm.

Eisenhammer in 1959 described the importance of the internal sphincter in the etiology of anal fissure. Midline internal sphincterectomy with or without fissurectomy were popularized by Parks, Goligher, and Lane. Stewart and Samson in the US and Hughes in Australia advocated "coverage" of the fissurectomy wound with skin flaps and V-Y plasty. The main complication of midline sphincterotomy is a keyhole deformity of the anus which results in varying degrees of fecal incontinence.

With the advent of anorectal manometry, Schuster and Whitehead demonstrated that patients with anal fissure had an abnormally high anal resting pressure. Also, after initial relaxation in response to defecation, the internal sphincter undergoes an "overshoot phenomenon" contracting strongly for a prolonged period of time and return to the baseline pressure after many hours. This overshoot is responsible for the prolonged post cibal pain experienced by patients with anal fissure.

In 1971, Notaras in London popularized the subcutaneous lateral internal sphincterectomy (LIS). Healing of the fissure which was not excised occurred in 2–3 weeks, and the keyhole deformity was avoided. A comparison of large numbers of patients undergoing fissurectomy and midline sphincterotomy verses LIS confirmed the superiority of the latter technique. Currently, LIS performed either with the closed technique or through an open incision in the anoderm is the procedure of choice for chronic anal fissure. With either technique, the fibers of internal sphincter distal to the dentate line

◘ Figure 75-1

Technique of open lateral internal sphincterotomy. a. Typical posterior midline fissure. b. Incision in lateral anal wall. c. Division of distal IS (from dentate line caudad). d. Completed sphincterotomy with intact external sphincter

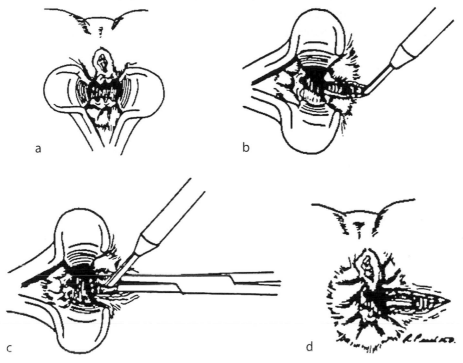

a   b   c   d

are divided down to the anal verge leaving the external sphincter undisturbed. This procedure has been associated with >95% healing rate and less than 2% complication rate consisting of infection or fistula (❷ *Fig. 75-1*).

Surgical versus "Pharmacologic Sphincterotomy"

In mid-1980s, two reports of patients who had had LIS were published, warning about an alarmingly high (30%) rate of flatus incontinence and a 5% incidence of involuntary fecal soilage. Because of medicolegal implications of fecal incontinence after anorectal surgery, chemical and pharmacologic alternatives have been sought to replace surgical sphincterotomy. Nitroglycerin (glyceryl trinitrate GTN) was the first such agent used in the treatment of anal fissure. Application of GTN in varying concentrations results in transient relaxation of the internal anal sphincter and lowering of anal resting pressure. To be effective, the GTN application must be repeated 2–3 times daily. The major drawback of GTN is its incidence of severe headaches in 10–30% of the patients leading to discontinuation of the treatment. Ideally, the concentration of GTN should not exceed 0.2%, and a small fingertip-sized amount of ointment should be "swiped" on the anal canal (not inserted) in recumbent position. The patient may experience a transient feeling of warmth or rush in the head (secondary to generalized vasodilatation) and should remain recumbent for 2–3 min before resuming activity. The low concentration and application in the recumbent position help reduce the incidence of headache to below 5%. In a prospective, randomized trail in Canada, LIS was far superior to GTN and resulted in a 95%

healing rate with LIS vs. 29% in GTN-treated patents. Most patients failing GTN healed after LIS; moreover, in a quality of life questionnaire, the patients rated LIS far superior to GTN. There was no difference in anal continence at 6 weeks or 6 months between the two groups. Recent preliminary reports in a small number of patients demonstrated similar vasodilation and smooth muscle relaxation after using a low concentration of Sidenafil (Viagra®) ointment in patients with anal fissure. Sidenafil is potentially more effective than GTN, but also costlier.

In an attempt to alleviate the side effect of GTN, calcium channel blockers have been used to induce relaxation of the internal sphincter. Application of 2% Diltiazem or Nifedipine gel induces a 25–30% decrease in internal sphincter pressure, but the transient nature of this effect requires application of the gel on the anal area three or four times daily. Studies have shown superiority of this product over the lidocaine/steroid mixture with no significant side effects from the use of calcium channel blockers.

Maria and Brisinda reported excellent results from injection of small amounts of botulinum toxin into the internal sphincter. Botulinum toxin blocks the production of acetylcholine in the muscle resulting in muscle paralysis. The onset of relaxation (pain relief) is usually early, within a few hours, and lasts for 3–4 months. The injection has to be repeated due to tachyphylaxis (similar to its use in achalasia), and accidental injection into the external sphincter carries a risk of major anal incontinence (albeit transient).

An international consensus conference held during Digestive Disease Week in 2001 concluded that LIS is the treatment of choice for anal fissure. GTN was associated with too high an incidence of headaches, botulinum toxin was potentially dangerous especially in inexperienced hands, and calcium channel blockers and bethanechol needed further studies to confirm their routine use in "chemical sphincterotomy."

Finally in an elegant meta-analysis of all randomized, controlled trials to assess the efficacy and morbidity of medical therapies for fissure, Nelson reported on 21 different comparisons in 35 trials including 9 agents: GTN, isosorbide dinitrate, botulinum toxin, diltiazem, nifedipine, hydrocortisone, lidocaine, bran, and placebo, as well as anal dilatation and surgical sphincterotomy. The advantage of GTN over placebo was not statistically significant. Nifedipine and diltiazem were not better than GTN in curing fissures. Botulinum toxin, compared with placebo and GTN, was no better than either. LIS was more effective then medical therapy, stimulating the conclusion that "medical therapy for chronic anal fissure, acute fissures, and fissures in children may be applied with a chance of cure that is only marginally better than placebo and for chronic fissure, far less effective than surgery."

Anal Fistulas

Anal fistulas originate from infection in anal glands and therefore are cryptoglandular in origin. Anal glands, described by Hermann and Defosses in 1880, open into anal crypts, branch out laterally and inferiorly, and terminate in the intersphincteric space. Obstruction of drainage combined with the rich bacterial environment result in an abscess which begins in the intersphincteric space and follows a path of least resistance for spread. Extension of an abscess caudad results in perianal abscess. If the abscess extends through the external sphincter it will present as an ischiorectal abscess. Cephalad extension is uncommon as are high intermuscular and supralevator abscesses. Fewer than 1% of abscesses are not of cryptoglandular origin and are caused by Crohn's disease, TB, fungal infection, trauma, and foreign bodies (❯ Fig. 75-2).

◘ **Figure 75-2**
Anorectal abscess fistulas based on cryptoglandular origin. 1. Submucosal; 2. high intermuscular; 3. supralevator; 4. ischiorectal; 5. perianal

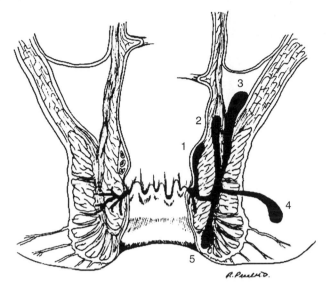

Spontaneous rupture or surgical drainage of abscess may result in healing, healing and recurrence, or nonhealing and persistence as a fistula. This is the reason why some proctologists call an anorectal abscess a fistulous abscess or an abscess-fistula. Anorectal fistulas have been classified in many different ways (low vs. high, simple vs. complex, etc.) in various texts, however the classification by Parks' et al. in 1976 is the most useful guide in planning therapy and predicting success and prognosis after surgery (❯ *Fig. 75-3*).

Diagnosis of anal fistula is not difficult. Persistent leakage of blood and pus after spontaneous or surgical drainage of abscess is pathognomonic. The primary opening of a fistula is often seen at a posterior midline crypt at the dentate line; these fistulas can be seen easily with an anoscope but just as easily missed during sigmoidoscopy or colonoscopy. Goodsall's rule (1901) is helpful in locating the primary opening unless the normal anatomy is distorted or altered by prior surgery. According to the rule, all fistulas located anterior to a line drawn transversely through the anal canal terminate radially in the anus. In contrast, secondary openings posterior to this line or if they are located more than 3 cm from the anal canal would take a curved path and end in the posterior midline. If the surgeon is unsure of the path of the fistula tract in the operating room, injection of dilute solution of hydrogen peroxide with or without a few drops of methylene blue will produce bubbles exiting from the priory opening. Computed tomography, magnetic resonance imaging, and endorectal ultrasonography with or without injection of peroxide is rarely needed in primary fistulas but are occasionally helpful in patients with persistent fistulas despite multiple surgical interventions. Similarly, fistulography is reserved for complex or recurrent fistulas. There is no medical treatment for anorectal fistulas. Repeated cauterization of the tract and use of various antibiotics are ineffective and only delay the inevitable.

Surgical Treatment

If a fistulous tract can be identified easily during drainage of an abscess, the surgeon may choose to perform primary fistulotomy. Primary fistulotomy has a low (5%) complication rate, a low (2–3%)

☐ **Figure 75-3**
Classification of anal fistulas. a. Intersphincteric; b. transsphincteric; c. suprasphincteric; d. extrasphincteric

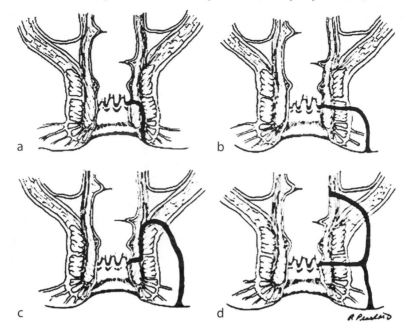

recurrence rate, and reduces the number of sick days and need for additional surgery. In the hands of less experienced surgeons, simple drainage of an abscess will relieve the symptoms and postpone the treatment of the fistula to a later date. Alternately, if a fistula is identified, the surgeon may choose to leave a thick, braided, non-absorbable suture tying it loosely as a marking Seton. Although a cutting Seton, i.e. a Seton tied tightly around the sphincter mechanism to allow a slow cutting through the sphincter like a cheese cutter is preferred by some, many surgeons choose a staged fistulotomy using a Seton. In this procedure, a portion of the sphincter muscle is divided and the remainder circled with a loose Seton. Six to 8 weeks later, the patient is returned to the operating room and examined under anesthesia. If the divided muscle has healed adequately, the remaining portion is divided and the Seton is removed. In a large series of anal fistulas treated with staged fistulotomy, the recurrence rate was 2%, and the incontinence rate was minimal.

The aim of operative intervention for anal fistulas is cure. Too conservative an approach leads to persistence and/or recurrence, while overzealous surgery may result in incontinence or false passage, which have led to the following questions in the treatment of anal fistulas. Is fistulotomy (sphincterotomy) always necessary? When should it be avoided? Should it be a second line versus first line therapy?

Utilizing the Park's classification as a treatment guide, one could conclude that:

(a) Intersphincteric fistulas should be treated with simple internal sphincterotomy because this is no different from the procedure recommended for anal fissure.

(b) Transsphincteric and suprasphincteric fistulas, if treated with primary or staged fistulotomy, will end up with varying degrees of fecal incontinence, ranging from minimal to significant. These fistulas are suitable for alternative surgical approaches avoiding sphincterotomy.

(c)   Extrasphincteric fistulas are not amenable to fistulotomy and need to be addressed through a parasacrococcygeal or York Mason approach most probably with a diverting colostomy. Extrasphincteric fistulas secondary to Crohn's disease may respond to Infliximab infusion:

Alternatives to Fistulotomy (Sphincterotomy)

1.   The endorectal advancement flap operation was designed originally for low recto-vaginal or anoperineal fistulas secondary to obstetric injuries. This procedure can be expanded to include fistulas in Crohn's disease which open at the dentate line, provided the rectum is normal in gross appearance and by biopsy. The procedure is impractical in the posterior quadrant especially in men where adequate mobilization of the rectal wall is quite difficult. In this operation, a rectal flap based superiorly is raised. This should include some fibers of the smooth muscles; mucosal flaps without some muscle have poor blood supply and will necrose or retract easily. The internal sphincter is closed over the primary opening, and the external opening is drained with a small caliber mushroom catheter. The rectal flap is then advanced caudad and sutured to the dentate line with polyglycolic or polyglactin sutures. The advantage of this procedure is its almost 80% success rate and preservation of continence. The disadvantage is a recurrence rate averaging 20% and an occasional anterior ectropion or horseshoe abscess involving the perineum.

2.   Dermal Island Flap Anoplasty. In this procedure, an island flap based on subcutaneous blood supply is raised connecting the internal to the external fistulas openings. After adequate mobilization, the primary opening of the fistula is debrided and closed with absorbable fine sutures. The dermal flap is then advanced into the anal canal and sutured to the rectal mucosa, covering the primary opening. This technique can be utilized in all four quadrants of the anal canal, in pouch-anal fistulas after ileal pouch anal anastomosis for ulcerative colitis, and in patients with Crohn's disease with normal rectum. The success rate of dermal island flap anoplasty is 80%, and recurrence can be treated with a second attempt. If the internal opening is situated higher than usual, a dermal flap can be combined with an endorectal advancement flap (❷ *Fig. 75-4*).

3.   Fibrin Sealant. The use of autologous fibrin sealant in the treatment of anal fistulas was first reported in 1993. Commercially produced fibrin sealant products became available worldwide in the mid-1990s, and initial trials on 79 patients showed 82% success rate in intersphincteric, 62% in transsphincteric and extrasphincteric fistulas, but only 33% in Crohn's related or recto-vaginal fistulas. No complications or incontinence was reported. Recurrences occurred as late as 8–11 months after operation.

    The technique of use of fibrin sealant for closure of fistulas is simple. The entire fistula tract is debrided using a small curette or cytology brush. A silk suture is passed through the tract and the dual chambered catheter is tied to the silk and passed from outside inward until the tip extends just beyond the internal opening. Fibrinogen and thrombin are injected simultaneously until a "pearl" is formed at the internal opening. The catheter is then withdrawn gradually while the injection continues until a pearl forms at the external opening. The sealant is allowed to set for 5 min. Then a dressing of Vaseline gauze is applied, and the patient is sent home (❷ *Fig. 75-5*). No excessive activity and sitz baths are allowed for 72 h. Fibrin sealant can be used to treat all

◘ **Figure 75-4**
Dermal island flap anoplasty. a. Outline of dermal flap; b. mobilized flap, closure of internal opening; c. flap advanced and sutured to rectal mucosa

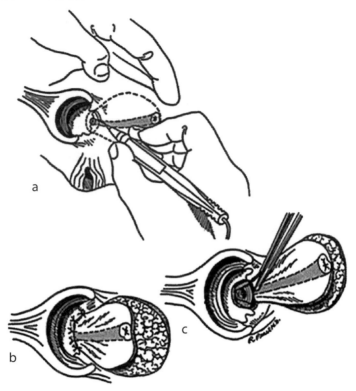

fistulas, but it is most effective in long tracts and least successful in short wide tracts such as rectovaginal fistulas. The results of fibrin sealant use in treatment of anal fistulas is listed in ❯ *Table 75-1.*

Early expulsion of fibrin plug and infection in the fistula tract have been blamed for the failure of this modality. In a prospective, randomized trail of 75 patients, fibrin sealant plus antibiotic, fibrin sealant plus closure of the internal opening, and fibrin sealant plus antibiotics and closure of the internal opening were evaluated. Mean follow-up was 27 months. The success rate of fibrin sealant and closure of internal opening was superior to the other two groups but not better than historical results of fibrin sealant alone. Closure of the internal opening is therefore recommended when it is either large or distally placed. At this time, fibrin sealant can be recommended for most transsphincteric fistulas and may be repeated once if it fails. If the fistula persists or recurs after the second treatment, a flap procedure, Seton drainage, or an anal fistula plug may be recommended.

4. Prolonged Seton Drainage is suitable for fistulas where sphincterotomy is inadvisable or contra-indicated. Ideal indications include extrasphincteric fistulas, Crohn's fistulas with grossly diseased rectum, complex fistulas in patients with AIDS, or other poor risk and debilitated patients. Placement of a silastic Seton (e.g. vessel loop) in the fistula tract which is kept in for 12–18 months allows for the tract to epithelialize and prevents recurrent abscesses. Currently Crohn's fistulas are

◻ Figure 75-5
Closure of fistula-in-ano with fibrin sealant. Dual chemical catheter inserted into secondary opening existing from primary opening prior to injection of sealant

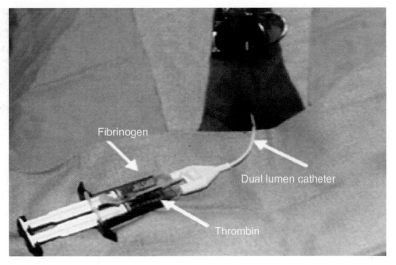

◻ Table 75-1
Success rate of fibrin sealant in treatment of anal fistulas

Author (year)	#pts	Success (%)
Hjorturp (91)	23	74
Abel (93)	10	60
Venkatesh (99)	30	60
Aitola (99)	10	0
Pately (00)	69	74
Cintron (00)	79	61
Zamora (01)	24	33
Lindley (02)	42	69
Sentovich (02)	48	69
Buchanan (03)	22	14
Singer (05)	76	21–40

best treated with infusion of infliximab. If so, the Seton is removed after the second infusion to allow closure of the fistula if it is going to respond to medical management.

5. Anal Fistula Plug. Several studies have reported early favorable experience using a porcine small intestinal submucosal collagen plug. After irrigating the fistula tract with hydrogen peroxide, a Seton is passed through the tract and tied to the plug, which is then pulled from inside out. The plug is trimmed and the internal opening is closed with a Z stitch incorporating the internal sphincter and passing through the fistula plug so that the plug is fully covered and not left exposed. The external end of the plug is also trimmed flush with the secondary opening and left unsutured. Success rates of 60–80% have been reported. These results need further confirmation in large number of patients with longer follow-up period (❯ *Fig. 75-6*).

◘ Figure 75-6

Closure of fistula in ano-with anal fistula plug. Anal fistula plug placed in anterior midline transsphincteric fistula prior to suturing it in place

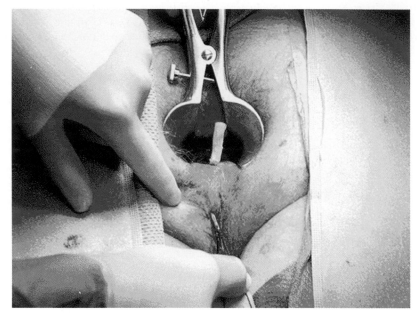

6.   Parasacrococcygeal (York Mason) approach is suitable for extrasphincteric fistulas secondary to trauma, recurrent pouch-anal fistulas, and infected retrorectal cysts. In very complex cases, prior or concomitant fecal diversion should be considered. The advantage of this approach is it provides a virgin operating field but the disadvantage is its technically challenging nature, risk of infection, and the unfamiliarity of most surgeons with the anatomy and technique.

In conclusion, the principal of surgical treatment of anal fistulas is to "DO NO HARM". The surgeon must use a procedure which preserves continence, considering that not every fistula needs a fistulotomy and that recurrence is preferable to incontinence. The surgeons treating fistulas must become familiar with many alternatives or be prepared to refer difficult and complex cases to more experienced specialists.

Selected Readings

Aguilar PS, Placencia G, Hardy TG, et al. (1983) Mucosal advancement flap in the treatment of anal fistula. Dis Colon Rectum 28:496

Brisinda G, Maria G, Bentivoglio AR (1999) A Comparison of injection of botulinum toxin and topical nitroglycerine ointment for the treatment of chronic anal fissure. N Engl J Med 341:65

Del Pino A, Nelson RL, Abcarian H, et al. (1996) Island flap anoplasty for treatment of transsphincteric fistula-in-ano. Dis Colon Rectum 39:224

Gorfine S (1995) Treatment of benign anal disease with topical nitroglycerine. Dis Colon Rectum 48:453

Johnson EK, Gaw JU, Armstrong DN (2006) Efficacy of anal fistula plug vs. fibrin glue in closure of anorectal fistulas. Dis Colon Rectum 49:371

MacElwain JW, MacLean MD, Alexander RM (1975) Experience with primary fistulotomy for anorectal abscess: a report of 1000 cases. Dis Colon Rectum 18:646

Nelson R (2004) A systemic review of medical therapy for anal fissure. Dis Colon Rectum 47:422

Ramanujam PS, Prasad ML, Abcarian H, et al. (1984) Perianal abscesses and fistulas: a study of 1023 patients. Dis Colon Rectum 27:593

Richard CS, Gregoire R, Plewes EA, et al. (2000) Internal sphincterotomy is superior to topical nitroglycerin in the treatment of chronic anal fissure: results of randomized controlled trial by the Canadian colorectal surgery trials group. Dis Colon Rectum 43:1048

Singer M, Cintron JR, Abcarian H, et al. (2005) Treatment of fistulae in ano with fibrin sealant in combination with intra-adhesive antibiotics and surgical closure of the internal fistula opening. Dis Colon Rectum 48:799

76 Polyposis Syndromes of the Colon

Andrew Latchford · Sue Clark · Robin K. S. Phillips

Pearls and Pitfalls

- Management of individuals with polyposis syndromes and at-risk family members within organized registries reduces mortality.
- Meticulous colonoscopy technique, with dye spray, polyp count and biopsy is important in clinical diagnosis.
- Failure to identify a mutation in a causative gene does not exclude the diagnosis of a polyposis syndrome.
- It is important to distinguish familial adenomatous polyposis (FAP) arising as a new mutation (with no background family history) from mutY human homolog (MYH) associated polyposis as the different modes of inheritance (autosomal dominant vs. recessive) fundamentally affect management of the family.
- In FAP there are several options for prophylactic surgery, but the aim is to prevent rather than treat cancer, and surgery should be performed usually during teenage years.
- With advances in the management of the large bowel, duodenal and periampullary cancers and desmoid tumors have become the commonest causes of death in FAP.
- 90% of patients with FAP develop duodenal and ampullary adenomas, but just 5–10% develop cancer at these sites.
- Surgery for intra-abdominal desmoid tumor is hazardous and associated with high recurrence rates; it should be avoided if possible, and if necessary be performed in specialist centers.
- In Peutz-Jeghers syndrome (PJS) failure to perform enteroscopy and polyp clearance at laparotomy results in a high re-laparotomy rate.
- PJS is associated with a high risk of gastrointestinal and a number of extra-intestinal malignancies; clinical suspicion should be high.
- Most cases of juvenile polyposis can be managed endoscopically.

Colonic polyposis syndromes have been recognized for many years and have been characterized clinically and pathologically to varying degrees (❯ *Table 76-1*). These syndromes are associated with increased risk of colorectal and other cancers and are inherited. Their study has not only improved the understanding and management of these conditions, but has also been influential in elucidating the underlying mechanisms of colorectal cancer, in general.

◻ Table 76-1

Summary of polyposis syndromes of the colon

Syndrome	Polyp type	Inheritance	Extracolonic cancer	Management of colon
FAP	Adenoma	AD	Yes	Surgery
MAP	Adenoma	AR	Yes	Surgery/colonoscopy
JP	Hamartoma	AD	Yes	Colonoscopy/surgery
PJS	Hamartoma	AD	Yes	Colonoscopy
CS	Hamartoma	AD	Yes	Colonoscopy
BRRS	Hamartoma	AD	No	Colonoscopy
HP	Hyperplastic	Not known	No	Colonoscopy

Adenomatous Polyposis Syndromes

Familial Adenomatous Polyposis

Familial adenomatous polyposis (FAP) was one of the first recognized polyposis syndromes and is the best characterized.

It is also the most common, with an estimated incidence of approximately 1:10,000.

Genetics

FAP is a highly penetrant, autosomal dominant disorder caused by a germline mutation in the adenomatous polyposis coli (APC) gene. This tumor suppressor gene is located on chromosome 5q21, and encodes a 312-kDa protein, the function of which remains to be fully characterized. It has a role in cell adhesion and is involved in regulating the Wnt pathway. When APC is mutated, this pathway is activated causing altered expression of genes that affect proliferation, migration and apoptosis. APC has a role in controlling the cell cycle, thus suppressing tumorigenesis. Finally, by stabilizing microtubules, APC maintains chromosomal stability; when mutated defects in mitotic spindles and chromosomal missegregation lead to aneuploidy.

Clinical Features

The development of adenomatous colorectal polyps is the hallmark of FAP. Polyps usually develop in late childhood and adolescence. Attenuated FAP refers to those cases where less than 100 polyps are present and classical FAP where greater than 100 polyps are observed. In the absence of an identified APC/mutY human homolog mutation, FAP is diagnosed on clinical grounds if > 100 adenomatous polyps are found in the large bowel. Polyps are more numerous on the left side of the colon. Although colorectal polyps may present with diarrhea, gastrointestinal (GI) bleeding or pain, the majority of cases remain asymptomatic until cancer develops.

Although FAP is typified by the development of large bowel polyps, a generalized disorganization of tissue regulation is present, resulting in adenomas elsewhere in the GI tract and the extra-colonic manifestations associated with the syndrome. Some have little clinical significance (such as gastric fundic gland polyps, osteomas, sebaceous cysts, congenital hypertrophy of the retinal pigment epithelium

(CHRPE), supernumerary teeth), whereas other extra-colonic manifestations represent a significant cause of morbidity and mortality. Desmoid tumors affect around 15% of patients with FAP and are benign tumors of myofibroblastic origin. Desmoid disease and duodenal cancer are the most important causes of mortality in patients with FAP who have undergone colectomy.

Several genotype–phenotype correlations have been observed consistently (❯ *Fig. 76-1*). Mutations at codon 1309 are associated with a more severe colonic phenotype and increased risk of colorectal cancer, which develops at an earlier age. Far 5′ and 3′ mutations are associated with a more attenuated colonic phenotype, and 3′ mutations have been shown consistently to be associated with an increased risk of desmoid disease.

◼ Figure 76-1
Genotype–phenotype correlation in FAP

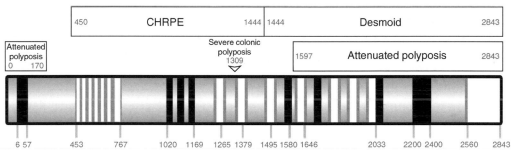

Cancer Risk

Unless prophylactic surgery is performed, there is a nearly 100% progression to colorectal cancer by 35–40 years of age. Isolated reports exist in the literature of cancer developing in childhood.

About 90% of patients will develop duodenal adenomas by 70 years of age and of these, duodenal cancer develops in 5–10%. The risk of duodenal cancer varies according to the stage of duodenal disease, as might be expected (❯ *Table 76-2*). For those with stage 4 disease there is a 36% risk of developing duodenal cancer by 10 years.

A number of extra-gastrointestinal neoplasms are associated with FAP, including adrenal adenomas, a variant of papillary thyroid cancer, hepatoblastomas and medulloblastoma. Although patients with

◼ Table 76-2
Spigelman staging of duodenal adenomas in FAP

No of polyps	Size of polyps (mm)	Histology	Dysplasia	Points
1–4	1–4	Tubular	Mild	1
5–20	5–10	Tubulovillous	Moderate	2
>20	>10	Villous	Severe	3
Total points	**Spigelman stage**	**Interval to next duodenoscopy**		
0	0	5 years		
1–4	I	5 years		
5–6	II	3 years		
7–8	III	1 year		
9–12	IV	6 months		

FAP have often markedly increased risks of developing these cancers, they remain a relatively minor cause of morbidity and mortality since the absolute lifetime risk is low.

Diagnosis

Management of families with FAP in a specialized registry allows gathering of pedigree data to identify at-risk individuals. Current techniques allow identification of the causative APC mutation in 70% of clinically affected individuals. Once the mutation has been identified predictive testing in at-risk relatives is straightforward and reliable.

In the UK, the standard practice is to offer predictive testing around the age of 12–14 years. There is rarely a need to perform testing sooner, as polyps do not usually start to develop before this age, and an earlier diagnosis does not alter management. An exception to this is an at-risk child who develops bowel-related symptoms or anemia; genetic testing and colonoscopy should be performed promptly.

After a positive predictive test, colonoscopy is performed to assess polyp burden—an important factor in deciding the timing and type of prophylactic surgery. Surgery can usually be delayed until a socially and educationally convenient time in the teens.

In a family in which no mutation has been identified, clinical screening by annual flexible sigmoidoscopy is started at 14 years. Additional colonoscopy at 5-yearly intervals is added from 20 years.

About 20% of cases of FAP have no family history and are due to a new mutation. The diagnosis is initially made clinically if over 100 large bowel adenomas are present.

Management

There is no doubt that prophylactic colectomy before the age of 20 should be recommended in virtually all patients with FAP and extends life expectancy by 30 years. The main issue is what operation should be performed (Clark and Phillips, 1996).

The choice is between colectomy and ileorectal anastomosis (IRA) and proctocolectomy with ileoanal pouch anastomosis (IPAA). Colectomy and IRA is an operation with low morbidity and good functional outcome. The main drawback is the risk of developing rectal cancer in the future. Surveillance of the rectal remnant by flexible sigmoidoscopy should be performed every 6 months and larger lesions removed. If rectal polyps become too numerous then therapy with an non-steroidal anti-inflammatory drug (NSAID; sulindac or celecoxib) may be used or consideration should be given to completion proctectomy and ileoanal pouch. Cancer risk in the rectal remnant is related to age and polyp density.

IPAA surgery seems an attractive alternative in that it theoretically obviates future colorectal cancer risk. However a cuff or small islands of at-risk rectal mucosa may be retained; it is also becoming increasingly clear that there is a risk of developing pouch adenomas and cancer. Thus annual surveillance of the pouch and rectal cuff with flexible sigmoidoscopy is recommended. In addition, pouch surgery is associated with a higher surgical complication rate and less satisfactory function than an IRA, risk of male sexual dysfunction, reduced female fertility and the need for a temporary ileostomy. These risks are sometimes difficult to accept in the context of an essentially healthy adolescent facing prophylactic surgery.

For those over 25 years, high density of rectal polyposis or the presence of a codon 1309 mutation predict high risk of rectal cancer, and IPAA is recommended. For most others IRA is a reasonable option. Both procedures are increasingly being performed laparoscopically, which make them more acceptable. In very exceptional cases with high risk of desmoid development and a low polyp burden, endoscopic surveillance with NSAID therapy may be considered to delay or avoid surgery.

Patients with a rectal cancer sufficiently low to preclude a sphincter preserving procedure will require abdominoperineal excision combined with total colectomy and ileostomy. IPAA may be an option in a higher rectal cancer, but the stage of disease and need for radiotherapy may preclude this. Colectomy should be performed if a colonic cancer is present, but a proctectomy is not always necessary. The factors guiding decision making in this scenario are the same as in prophylactic surgery.

The management of the duodenum remains a challenge. Patients should undergo regular upper GI tract surveillance from the age of 25, with frequency determined by the Spigelman stage (❯ *Table 76-2*). Surveillance should be performed with a side-viewing endoscope (due to the distribution of polyps and the need to assess the ampulla) and by an endoscopist experienced at assessing the duodenum in FAP. Endoscopic therapy may be considered for lesions greater than 1 cm or those with worrying histological features. For those with stage 3 disease, celecoxib may reduce polyp burden (Phillips et al. 2002) but patients need to be counseled adequately regarding the potential cardiovascular and cerebrovascular risks. For those with disease that is not manageable endoscopically or who have stage 4 disease, prophylactic duodenectomy should be considered. After surgical or endoscopic intervention in the duodenum/ampulla there is a risk of recurrent disease and continued endoscopic surveillance is required.

MYH Associated Polyposis

MYH associated polyposis (MAP) was first described in 2002 and its genetic and clinical features are yet to be fully characterized. The true incidence of MAP is not known but it is thought to account for 10–30% of patients who appear to have FAP clinically but in whom no germline APC mutation can be identified.

Genetics

MAP is inherited in an autosomal recessive manner, with high penetrance, and is caused by biallelic mutations in the MYH gene, which codes for a protein involved in the repair of DNA that has been damaged by reactive oxygen species generated during aerobic metabolism.

Homozygous or compound heterozygous germline mutations are required to develop the MAP phenotype. Patients who are heterozygotes for germline MYH mutations do not display polyposis but may have an elevated cancer risk. The heterozygous carrier frequency in the UK population is estimated to be around 1%.

Clinical Features

As with FAP, the hallmark of MAP is the development of colorectal adenomas. Although initially it was thought to be similar to an attenuated FAP phenotype, it is now clear that there may be wide variation, with up to thousands of colonic adenomas being present in some cases. Both duodenal adenomas and cancers have been reported but seem to occur less frequently than in FAP. Osteomas and CHRPE have both been observed but there are no reports of desmoid tumors in MAP.

Cancer Risk

A number of series have confirmed an increased risk of colorectal cancer associated with biallelic MYH mutations, with a risk up to 50-fold that of those with no MYH mutations. In the largest reported cohort of MAP, 65% of patients developed colorectal cancer at a median age of 45 years.

There is much debate regarding the cancer risk in heterozygotes. Initially it was felt that they did not carry an increased cancer risk and did not develop polyposis, as one would expect with a classical autosomal recessive pattern of inheritance. However, it has now been reported that heterozygotes may have an increased colorectal cancer risk (odds ratio 1.5–3).

Management

Currently there are no standard guidelines on how these patients should be managed. There is a wide variation in colonic phenotype and management should be tailored to the individual patient. For those who have been confirmed by genetic testing to have biallelic mutations, annual colonoscopy is recommended. Many of these patients will undergo surgery, the type of operation performed depending on tumor burden and site of disease, as for FAP. Some patients with a sparse colonic phenotype may prefer to opt for colonoscopic surveillance, but need to be counseled appropriately on long-term cancer risk. In view of the reports of increased cancer risk in heterozygotes current recommendation is a baseline colonoscopy at the time of diagnosis, and then 5-yearly until 80 years of age.

There are no data to confirm whether duodenal surveillance is effective in patients with MAP, however, it is recommended that bi-allelic carriers undergo duodenal surveillance identical to that of patients with FAP.

Other Polyposis Syndromes

A number of other polyposis syndromes have been described. Peutz-Jeghers syndrome (PJS) and juvenile polyposis (JP) are the commonest, while Cowden syndrome (CS) and Bannayan-Riley-Ruvalcaba Syndrome (BRRS) are very rare. Hyperplastic polyposis (HP) is increasingly recognized, but remains poorly understood.

Peutz-Jeghers Syndrome

Genetics

PJS is genetically heterogeneous. Germline mutation in the LKB1 gene (also called STK11), has been identified as the cause of PJS but is detected in only 50% of patients. LKB1 is involved in regulation of cell polarity and proliferation and also has a role in inhibiting the Wnt signaling pathway.

Clinical Features

The reported incidence of PJS varies widely but is likely to be around 1:100,000. The association of mucocutaneous pigmentation with intestinal polyposis typifies PJS. Traditional diagnostic criteria are histological confirmation of characteristic gastrointestinal polyps and two out of three of the following:

— Small bowel polyps
— Family history of PJS
— Pigmented macules on the buccal mucosa, lips or digits

The polyps of PJS have a typical histopathological appearance and may occur throughout the GI tract but are most commonly found in the jejunum, where they cause bleeding and anemia or obstruction, either directly or by intussusception. They may be found at extra-intestinal sites, such as the kidney, ureter, gallbladder, nasal passages and bronchus. Pigmented lesions occur in over 90% of patients and vary in size, number and color. These lesions generally develop in infancy and may fade after puberty. Although most frequently observed on the buccal mucosa, lips and digits, these lesions may also be seen in the rectum, vulva and conjunctiva.

Cancer Risk

It is now firmly established that there is an increased cancer risk in PJS. In the largest analysis of 419 individuals there was an 85% risk of developing a cancer by the age of 70. The most common cancers were gastrointestinal in origin and the risk of colorectal cancer was 3%, 5%, 15%, and 39% at ages 40, 50, 60, and 70, respectively. An increased risk of all GI tract, pancreatic, breast and gynecological cancers has been observed with reported risks at 70 years of 57%, 11%, 45%, and 18%, respectively. Adenomatous foci may be seen within PJS which may progress to cancer along the adenoma-dysplasia-carcinoma pathway. However it is not clear whether in fact most GI cancers arise in polyps or in the "normal" mucosa, which may be unstable due to mutated LKB1.

Management

The two main problems facing the clinician caring for individuals with PJS are the lifetime risk of cancer and the management of small bowel polyps, particularly the need to prevent repeated emergency laparotomies and subsequent loss of small bowel.

Panenteric examination is recommended every 3 years (more frequently for those with a particularly dense phenotype), with removal of any significant lesions at the time of upper GI and lower GI examinations. Video capsule endoscopy is used for small bowel imaging and removal of small bowel polyps when they reach 1–2 cm in size (earlier if associated with symptoms), is recommended (❍ *Fig. 76-2*). Removing significant polyps reduces the future rate of intussusception/obstruction and the need for emergency surgery (Edwards, 2003); it may reduce occult GI blood loss and may alter the

Figure 76-2
PJS on table enteroscopy

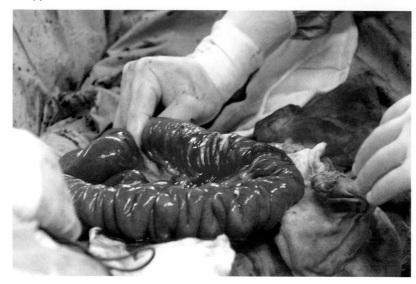

risk of developing cancer. In most patients, prophylactic colonic surgery is not required and endoscopic surveillance and treatment will suffice.

Cervical and breast screening is recommended as per national guidelines, unless there is a family history of breast cancer when screening by MRI at a younger age should be considered. Self-examination of the breasts/testes is to be encouraged.

Juvenile Polyposis

This is a clinically and genetically heterogeneous condition that affects 1 in 100,000–160,000 people. It is distinct from solitary juvenile polyps, which develop in 1–2% of children and adolescents. Although cases of carcinomatous change have been described in a solitary juvenile polyp, it is accepted that patients with such solitary lesions are at no increased relative risk of colorectal carcinoma or death compared with the general population.

Genetics

JP is an autosomal dominant condition with incomplete penetrance. Two genes have been implicated, with some families having mutation identified in SMAD4 and others in BMPR1A.

The remaining 60% of cases of JP are termed mutation negative. Both SMAD4 and BMPR1A mutations cause disruption of the transforming growth factor β (TGF β) signal transduction pathway, which regulates apoptosis and growth inhibition responses.

Clinical Features

JP can be diagnosed, in the absence of extra-intestinal features consistent with CS or BRRS, when the following criteria are met:

(a)   > 5 juvenile polyps of the colon or rectum
(b)   Juvenile polyps in other parts of the GI tract
(c)   Any number of juvenile polyps and a positive family history

Furthermore three distinct phenotypes exist each with a different disease course. In its most severe form, patients present in infancy with GI bleeding, intussusception or protein losing enteropathy. The entire GI tract is involved and characteristically no family history is found, probably because the condition is fatal. The other phenotypes may present at a later age (5–15 years) and affect either the colon and rectum alone or the entire GI tract. Both these phenotypes may present as acute or chronic GI bleeding, anemia or abdominal pain. In a review of 272 patients with JP, the colorectum was involved in 98%, the stomach in 14%, duodenum in 2% and jejunum/ileum in 7%.

Cancer Risk

JP is associated with a significant malignant potential, predominantly affecting the GI tract. St Mark's Polyposis Registry data have shown that the cumulative risk of cancer was 68% by 60 years of age. The largest review assessed reports on 271 patients with JP and found that the overall incidence of carcinomas was 17% (47 patients). The large bowel was the site at which most of these developed, but gastric, duodenal and pancreatic cancers were also reported. The risk of malignancy appears to start when patients are in their 20s.

Management

The mainstay of management for those with JP is regular GI tract surveillance. Patients and at-risk family members should undergo colonoscopy and esophagogastroduodenoscopy at 1–3-yearly intervals depending on polyp number and symptoms. Colonic polyps can usually be managed by endoscopic polypectomy. If severe dysplasia or invasive cancer is found, or if polyps are too numerous or causing symptoms (especially anemia or protein losing enteropathy), then colectomy is recommended. In the majority of cases IRA is sufficient, but if there is carpeting of the rectum or rectal cancer then IPAA will be necessary. Long term endoscopic surveillance of the rectal stump or pouch is required for those who have undergone surgery.

Similarly, the management of the upper GI tract is dependent on disease severity and symptoms. In most cases endoscopic polypectomy suffices, however with diffuse gastric disease subtotal or total gastrectomy may be required. Small bowel polyps may require removal by enteroscopy or surgery.

In addition to GI tract surveillance, patients should annually undergo review and check hemoglobin concentration, as long-term studies suggest that symptoms or anemia usually precede the development of malignancy.

Cowden Syndrome and Bannayan–Riley-Ruvalcaba Syndrome

These very rare syndromes have considerable clinical and genetic overlap, and may represent different ends of the spectrum of a single disorder. Up to 60% of patients with CS will develop gastrointestinal polyps, which are indistinguishable from the JPS polyp. However, it is the extraintestinal manifestations that are most striking, especially the mucocutaneous lesions which affect 80–90% of patients. Of these, facial trichilemmomas, acral keratosis, palmarplantar keratoses and oral papillomas are the most common. In addition, breast and thyroid cancers are particularly common, but the risk of gastrointestinal malignancy is unclear.

Intestinal polyposis affects 45% of patients with BRRS. Other features include multiple hemangiomas, macrocephaly, developmental delay, pseudopapilloedma, lipomas and pigmented papules on the penis. There are no reports of increased risk of malignancy in patients with BRRS.

Both CS and BRRS are inherited in an autosomal dominant manner but with incomplete penetrance. Germline PTEN mutations are found in up to 80% of patients with CS and also in BRRS. PTEN acts as a tumor suppressor gene and is associated with a number of malignant tumors.

We would suggest an initial upper GI endoscopy and colonoscopy at 25 years of age, and thereafter as guided by polyp burden or if symptoms develop. Regular breast and thyroid screening is recommended in CS.

Hyperplastic Polyposis

Hyperplastic polyps are the most frequently observed colorectal polyps. The incidence of such polyps increases with age, occurring in 70–80% of individuals over 60 years of age. These lesions have been considered to be an inconsequential finding, with no malignant potential. However, recent literature supports the concept that there is a morphologically and genetically distinct type of hyperplastic polyp, which may be pre-malignant.

Clinical Features

HP, sometimes called metaplastic polyposis, has no extracolonic features. Various definitions have been used but the WHO definition is widely accepted:

1. At least 5 histologically proven hyperplastic polyps proximal to the sigmoid colon, of which 2 are greater than 10 mm
2. Any number of hyperplastic polyps occurring proximal to the sigmoid colon in an individual with a first degree relative with HP
3. More than 30 hyperplastic polyps distributed throughout the colon

HP is a heterogeneous condition, most commonly diagnosed in the 6th and 7th decades of life.

Genetics

The WHO definition of HP includes familial aggregation, thus intimating that this may be an inherited disorder. However, only few cases with familial clustering have been reported and it is still not clear whether this truly is an inherited disorder.

Cancer Risk

An increased risk of colorectal cancer in patients with HP is supported by a number of published series. The reported risk has been between 50–70%. Cancers may arise through a serrated neoplasia pathway, leading to microsatellite-unstable and typically right-sided colon cancer.

Management

Given the rarity of this condition and the conflicting literature, it remains unclear how best to manage these patients. Colonoscopic surveillance is advocated 1–3-yearly depending on the number and size of hyperplastic polyps identified. Given the WHO definition it is reasonable to offer screening colonoscopy to first degree relatives of affected patients.

Selected Readings

Agnifili A, Verzaro R, Gola P, et al. (1999) Juvenile polyposis: case report and assessment of the neoplastic risk in 271 patients reported in the literature. Dig Surg 16:161–166

Al Tassan N, Chmiel NH, Maynard J, et al. (2002) Inherited variants of MYH associated with somatic G:C to T:A mutations in colorectal tumours. Nat Genet 30:227–232

Clark SK, Phillips RKS (1996) Desmoids in familial adenomatous polyposis. Brit J Surg 83:1494–1504

Edwards DP, Khosraviani K, Stafferton R, et al. (2003) Long-term results of polyp clearance by intraoperative enteroscopy in the Peutz-Jeghers syndrome. Dis Colon Rectum 46:48–50

Groves CJ, Saunders BP, Spigelman AD, Phillips RKS (2002) Duodenal cancer in patients with familial adenomatous polyposis (FAP): results of a 10 year prospective study. Gut 50:636–641

Hearle N, Schumacher V, Menko FH, et al. (2006) Frequency and spectrum of cancers in the Peutz-Jeghers syndrome. Clin Cancer Res 12:3209–3215

Nielsen M, Franken PF, Reinards THCM, et al. (2005) Multiplicity in polyp count and extracolonic manifestations in 40 Dutch patients with MYH associated polyposis coli (MAP). J Med Genet 42:e54

Phillips RKS (1995) Familial adenomatous polyposis: the surgical treatment of the colorectum. Semin Colon Rectal Surg 6:33–37

Phillips RKS, Wallace MH, Lynch PM (2002) A randomised, double blind, placebo controlled study of celecoxib, a selective cyclooxygenase 2 inhibitor, on duodenal polyposis in familial adenomatous polyposis. Gut 50:857–60

77 Clinical Management of Patients with Fecal Incontinence

Ian G. Finlay

Pearls and Pitfalls

- Fecal incontinence usually has a multifactorial etiology; consequently, all patients having surgery should be fully investigated.
- Irritable bowel syndrome is a common cause of incontinence.
- Obstetric anal sphincter injuries during child birth should be repaired under good light sources with anesthetic facilities by an experienced surgeon soon after the delivery.
- Sacral nerve stimulation is an exciting new development but the mechanism is an yet unclear are unknown.
- Many patients respond to treatment with amitriptyline or biofeedback.
- Less than 10% of patients referred for surgery require an operation.
- Do not offer surgery to patients in whom the principal symptom is incontinence for liquid stool.
- Patients who undergo surgery should be warned that all recognized operations have the potential to make the symptoms worse.
- Patients with irritable bowel syndrome have a poor outcome after surgery.
- Beware of performing a hemorrhoidectomy in patients with perineal descent.
- Avoid anal stretch operations, since they risk producing diffuse disruption of the internal anal sphincter.

Introduction

Fecal incontinence is a disabling and distressing condition that affects all age groups. It is more common in women than men with the highest prevalence in the elderly. It has been estimated to affect 1–2% of the population over 40 years of age.

Mechanism of Continence

Fecal control is maintained by an extraordinary and complex sphincter mechanism that is not fully understood. It is, however, recognized as comprising of the following components—an internal anal sphincter, an external anal sphincter, pelvic floor muscles and a sensory and motor nerve supply.

The internal anal sphincter (IAS) is an involuntary smooth muscle under autonomic control (sympathetic innervation is excitatory, whereas parasympathetic supply is inhibitory). The function of the IAS is to keep the anal canal closed. Injury to the IAS leads to leakage of mucous and fecal staining rather than incontinence.

The external anal sphincter (EAS) encircles the IAS and is continuous with the puborectalis muscle and other muscles of the pelvic floor. It is of note that during surgical dissection, there is no visible separation between the EAS and the puborectalis. The EAS is under voluntary control as a consequence of innervation from the pudendal nerve with connections to the ventral horn of S2 (Onuf's nucleus) and the corticospinal pathways. The motor neurons of Onuf's nucleus are unusual since they are tonically active during sleep. The integrity of the nerve supply to the EAS may be determined on clinical examination by either stroking the perianal skin or asking the patient to cough; both should cause spontaneous contraction of the EAS. The EAS (in conjunction with the pelvic floor) may be contracted voluntarily by the patient to avert the call to stool but this can only be maintained for less than a minute. Consequently, the principal symptom in patients with an EAS defect is the inability to avert the call to stool leading to urgency.

The muscles of the pelvic floor provide a "sling support" for the rectum and pelvic organs and are composed of a sheet of striated muscle. Four component parts of the muscle have been identified; the puborectalis, pubococcygeus, iliococcygeus and ischiococcygeus. The nerve supply is uncertain but includes ventral fibers from S2 and S3, which enter the muscle posteriorly where they may be vulnerable to stretch-injury during childbirth. When contracted, the puborectalis causes an angle of approximately 90° to develop between the anal canal and the rectum. This is probably the most important single factor contributing to the continence of solid stool, but has no beneficial effect in controlling liquids, since in contrast to solids they flow easily around bends.

It would appear therefore, that the control of loose stool or diarrhea is provided by voluntary contraction of the striated muscles (EAS and pelvic floor muscles) explaining the observation that the control of liquid stool is precarious even in normal subjects. This is important in clinical practice since many patients who seek advice regarding symptoms of incontinence are only symptomatic when they have loose stool. Such patients are unlikely to respond to surgical intervention and treatment should be directed towards alleviating the cause of the diarrhea.

It is an extraordinary fact that the anorectum in conjunction with the sphincter muscles can function such that it is possible for humans to expel gas in a downward direction while maintaining control of solids. The probable explanation for this phenomenon is that the puborectalis contracts vigorously producing an acute angle of less than 90° between the anal canal and rectum. The external anal sphincter also contracts resulting in "a retort shape". Air is then pushed from the rectal chamber by transiently raising intra-abdominal pressure above sphincter pressure. This process is aided by the abundance of sensory fibers at the mucocutaneous junction in the anal canal that have been considered to contribute to the mechanism of continence.

The exact mechanism, whereby rectal filling is detected and results in the call to stool is poorly understood but can be sensed by both the stretch receptors of the pelvic floor and "sampling" in the anal canal. This would explain why patients who have undergone a restorative proctectomy with anal canal mucosectomy have a near normal perception of pouch filling.

Etiology of Fecal Incontinence

There are numerous causes of fecal incontinence; the most important are given in ❯ *Table 77-1*. Patients rarely have a single abnormality and the cause of symptoms is invariably multifactorial necessitating careful clinical examination and investigation. In addition, it has been the author's experience that patients who have had episodes of incontinence suffer from anxiety and apprehension that it may occur again, thereby complicating both clinical assessment and the efficacy of treatment.

IAS defects or weakness leading to symptoms of fecal staining may be associated with autonomic neuropathy secondary to conditions such as diabetes or excessive alcohol consumption. The internal anal sphincter may also be deliberately divided at surgery in the operation of internal sphincterotomy or inadvertently during hemorrhoidectomy producing a "gutter deformity". Diffuse disruption of the IAS may occur after an anal stretch operation but fortunately this procedure is now used rarely.

The EAS may be subject to trauma but the most frequent and important cause of injury occurs during childbirth. Post partum perineal injuries that involve the EAS are defined as third degree tears while those that also involve the rectal mucosa are classified as fourth degree tears. The risk of sustaining a tear is increased if the birth is complicated or prolonged; risk factors include multiparity, prolonged second stage of labor (more common with the routine use of epidural anesthesia), large babies and the use of forceps. Severe perineal tears have been reported to occur in 0.6–0.9% of deliveries.

The attendant at the delivery has a duty of care to identify the presence of a sphincter tear. When a tear is found it should be repaired in good light under appropriate anesthesia by trained personnel. Evidence suggests that if patients have an immediate repair of a third or fourth degree tear then subsequent incontinence to solid stool is infrequent (<5%) but leakage of liquid stool or gas has been reported in up to one third of patients. This contrasts with the poor results reported for delayed repairs by Hajivassiliou and others. Missing a sphincter injury at the time of delivery, therefore, has serious consequences probably because the divided muscle ends retract and are difficult to identify in scar tissue during a later operation.

Despite guidelines highlighting the need for careful post partum examination, it is now recognized that minor sphincter tears are missed frequently. Several studies using ultrasound have reported occult internal and external sphincter injuries in over a third of all women who have had a vaginal delivery. Most of these patients, however, are asymptomatic.

◘ Table 77–1

Causes of fecal incontinence

Congenital
Congenital anomalies including agenesis of the anorectum
Acquired
Fecal impaction and spurious diarrhea
Anorectal cancer and villous adenoma
Conditions causing autonomic neuropathy, e.g. diabetes
Irritable bowel syndrome
Inflammatory bowel disease
Rectal prolapse
Fistula in ano
Sphincter injury to internal or external anal sphincters (childbirth, anorectal surgery or trauma)
Sphincter and pelvic floor neuropathy (childbirth, demyelinating spinal injury cerebral vascular injury)

Childbirth also causes a neuropathic injury to the pelvic floor. Electromyographic studies have shown that all vaginal deliveries cause a degree of injury to the pelvic floor muscles but this is more extensive in complicated deliveries and is cumulative with multiple births. Patients who suffer severe neuropathy have features of perineal descent leading to an obtuse anorectal angle. This condition is often named idiopathic fecal incontinence (IFI) but there is now sufficient evidence to attribute it to childbirth. IFI is associated with prolonged pudendal nerve conduction time leading to weakness of the EAS and reduced squeeze pressures in the anal canal. Paradoxically, as a consequence of the pelvic floor weakness, patients with IFI may also have difficulty emptying the rectum necessitating straining; this in turn causes further damage to the pudendal nerve. It is not uncommon, therefore, for these patients to complain of both "incontinence and difficulty in emptying". Since the neuropathy affects the entire pelvic floor, the patient may also have incontinence of urine with a vaginal/ uterine prolapse.

Loss of rectal support may cause a rectal intussusception or even an overt rectal prolapse. The exact cause of rectal prolapse is unknown but many of the features observed in IFI are also found in patients with rectal prolapse. Rectal prolapse is a common cause of incontinence that merits surgical treatment. In contrast, there is debate regarding the significance of the presence of a midrectal intussusception if diagnosed by proctography, since it is unlikely to be the cause of incontinence.

Congenital abnormalities are an unusual but important cause of incontinence since they affect young adults who often seek a surgical solution. The severity of the abnormality varies but pelvic MRI may help to define whether there is any evidence of either the IAS or EAS (usually absent) or evidence of the pelvic floor musculature (usually present). It is extraordinary and important for our understanding of the physiology of continence that these patients, who have no IAS or EAS may have relatively few symptoms thereby confirming the importance of the pelvic floor in the mechanism of continence.

It is the "way of nature" that human organs have considerable reserve function and are able to sustain a considerable degree of deterioration before symptoms develop. So it is in the anorectum; substantial loss of a component of continence may occur before the patient becomes symptomatic (see ❯ Fig. 77-1). For example, the anal sphincter (IAS and EAS) may be divided partially at a fistula operation in the majority of cases with few consequences. The exception is the female patient who already has a pelvic floor neuropathy from previous childbirth and in whom even a minor sphincter division may cause symptoms. It is for this reason that all patients with anorectal pathology require experienced and careful assessment.

It has been shown recently that up to 50% of patients with incontinence presenting for assessment have an abnormality of both rectal sensation and colonic motility. These patients have a hypersensitive rectum with low maximum tolerated volumes on balloon distension. This gives rise to symptoms of severe urgency. These patients also have evidence of colonic hypermotility in response to standard stimuli such as ingestion of food or the injection of neostigmine. In brief, they have irritable bowel syndrome fulfilling the Rome criteria. It has been shown that IBS was either the principal cause or a major contributing factor in 50% of patients who had been referred to a colorectal clinic for the investigation of incontinence. It is important to identify the presence of IBS since it has a deleterious effect on the efficacy of surgical treatment. It is the author's experience that surgical treatment of incontinence should, if possible, be avoided in patients with IBS.

◘ Figure 77-1

Continence of solids is dependent on the interaction of various components, including the internal/external anal sphincter, pelvic floor and an intact neurological supply. Since their functions overlap, some loss of a component may occur without the development of clinical incontinence

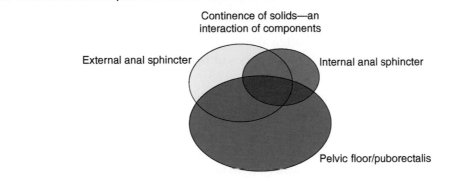

Continence of solids—an
interaction of components

External anal sphincter   Internal anal sphincter

Pelvic floor/puborectalis

Investigation of Patients with Incontinence

All patients with fecal incontinence for whom surgery is being considered should be investigated. Patients who have had a change of bowel habit require a colonoscopy to exclude neoplastic conditions such as villous adenoma, carcinoma and inflammatory bowel disease.

Ano-rectal physiology studies may identify pudendal nerve neuropathy and abnormalities of rectal sensation. Hyper and hyposensitivity of the rectum are both recognized to lead to incontinence. Anal canal pressures are recorded frequently, but their value in clinical decision making has been questioned. Complex studies of rectal compliance are principally research tools but can be helpful in cases of megarectum.

Evacuating proctography is less useful in investigating patients with incontinence than in those with outlet obstruction disorders but may show an unexpected rectal intussusception or prolapse. It also provides objective evidence for perineal descent. It is the author's practice to proceed to an examination under anesthesia in patients in whom occult prolapse is suspected. Only those patients in whom the rectum may be easily drawn through the anus are then considered for surgical correction.

Anorectal ultrasound examination is an indispensable investigation in patients with incontinence. In experienced hands, a clear image of the integrity of the IAS and EAS may be obtained. This may include a spectrum of abnormality from minor atrophy to complete disruption.

MRI can be useful in selected patients including those with congenital abnormalities when it aids in defining the anatomy. It also has an important role in assessing patients with complex fistula in ano who may have residual sepsis contributing to their symptoms of leakage.

Treatment

Treatment is based upon careful clinical assessment. It is important to identify the cause or in most cases, causes, for the incontinence.

Medial Management of Incontinence

Many patients with minor incontinence only require reassurance and will respond to the judicious use of anti-diarrheal agents. Patients with spurious diarrhea secondary to fecal impaction should be treated with enemas or bowel washouts. This is an important group to diagnose since patients with incontinence secondary to impaction are often reluctant to accept that the cause is "constipation". Clinicians should be aware that although most common in the elderly, this condition can occur at any age.

It is especially important to identify those patients with IBS since they are numerous and often respond to a small dose of amitriptyline. It is unknown whether the efficacy of this treatment is due to a central or peripheral effect. It is the author's practice, however, to prescribe treatment even in cases of doubt because of the beneficial effects observed. Indeed, amitriptyline has been shown to be efficacious in the treatment of incontinence in the absence of irritable bowel symptoms. This observation merits further investigation.

Symptom improvement has also been reported by post menopausal women when they commence hormonal replacement therapy. Female patients who have evidence of a pelvic floor neuropathy may attribute the onset or exacerbation of their symptoms to the menopause. It has been postulated that symptoms develop as muscle tone diminishes due to fall in estrogen levels.

In addition to oral medicines, there are a variety of commercial products available including anal plugs that may be used to treat patients with minor leakage.

The technique of biofeedback has been reported to improve symptoms but the mechanism of action is unknown. It is of note in this respect that physiotherapy has been shown to be ineffective in treating fecal incontinence but is of benefit in patients with urinary incontinence. Since biofeedback is relatively simple and non invasive, it should be used before more invasive techniques.

Surgical Management

Surgery is indicated in less than 10% of patients who undergo investigation for fecal incontinence. It is important that patients are carefully apprised before surgery with regard to the risks as well as the potential benefits of the operation. In particular, all patients should be warned that there is a risk that surgical intervention could make the symptoms worse.

Internal Anal Sphincter Repair and Correction of an Anal Canal Deformity

Internal anal sphincter disruption in isolation most commonly results from surgical intervention such as internal sphincterotomy or hemorrhoidectomy (gutter defect).

Repair of the IAS after sphincterotomy has been reported to be effective. This, however, has not been the experience of the author who has found the results of surgery disappointing. Furthermore, there is a high risk that surgery to the IAS may make the symptoms worse. In contrast, surgical correction of a gutter or key-hole deformity after hemorrhoidectomy is often highly successful. Although defects may be directly repaired, a cutaneous advancement flap is usually required.

Generalized disintegration of the IAS after manual dilatation of the anus does not have a surgical solution and it for this reason that anal stretch should be avoided.

External Anal Sphincter Repair

The availability of endoanal ultra-sonography has led to the identification of increasing numbers of patients with an external anal sphincter defect. Although these can occur as a consequence of anal trauma, the majority are secondary to perineal tears during childbirth. The resulting defect may be partial or complete. Since the sphincter is under tension, a complete division allows retraction of the muscle ends and may lead to a defect that is half the circumference of the anal canal in size. In such circumstances, the ends become embedded in scar tissue making mobilization to facilitate an adequate repair difficult.

EAS defects often occur in association with IAS defects, pelvic floor weakness, pudendal nerve neuropathy and symptoms of irritable bowel syndrome. Although these associated abnormalities are not necessarily a contraindication to attempting a sphincter repair, they may contribute to a poor outcome. It is the author's preference to repair an IAS defect en-bloc with the EAS. The literature has produced conflicting reports regarding the effect of pudendal nerve neuropathy on outcome. Some studies have suggested no detrimental effect; others have suggested a profound effect. Consequently, the presence of a pudendal nerve neuropathy should not prevent the surgeon from attempting a repair. However, in the author's experience, the presence of diarrhea-predominant IBS will limit the results of a repair and should be treated before attempting surgery.

Several techniques have been reported for EAS repair. In the first instance, it is necessary to identify the scar tissue within the defect and dissect laterally until pliable and mobile muscle is identified. Care must be taken in large defects to avoid injury to the pudendal nerves that enter in the 3 and 9 o'clock positions. The presence of nerves limits the extent of the dissection. Indeed it has been shown that injudicious dissection may cause pudendal nerve neuropathy leading to a poor long-term outcome. For this reason, some surgeons use a nerve stimulator to identify the exact site of the pudendal nerves.

Having identified the muscle ends (see ❷ *Fig. 77-2*), it is necessary to reconstitute the anal sphincter. The author usually uses an overlap repair but on occasion, a "keel" type repair may be employed. The type of suture material used varies between surgeons; the author now uses PDS since non-absorbable sutures such as prolene often need to be removed at a later stage. Fast-absorbing sutures are also avoided because early disruption of the repair has been observed. The author recommends the frequent use of a defunctioning colostomy if a major repair is undertaken. This prevents fecal impaction with disruption of the repair and is more comfortable for patients. It should be noted that the only randomized trial, albeit including only small numbers of patients, showed no benefit with the use of a stoma. However, that study included patients who had undergone only limited repairs.

Early reports suggested that the efficacy of surgery for EAS repair was excellent with continence restored in approximately 70% of patients. Unfortunately, these results are not maintained and after 10 years of follow up, only 10–30% of patients remain continent. Sometimes, it is evident that the failure is due to disruption of the repair. Although repeat repairs may be attempted, the surgery is technically difficult and the outcome likely to be poorer than those obtained after primary repairs.

◼ Figure 77-2

An example of an anterior anal sphincter repair for trauma after childbirth (showing the ends of muscle after mobilization that will be brought together)

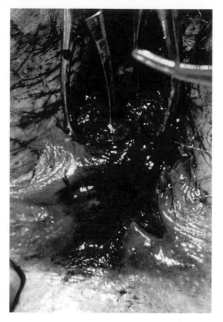

Post Anal Repair

Patients with pelvic floor neuropathy present evidence of perineal descent and an obtuse ano-rectal angle. The operation of posterior anal repair, devised by Parks, aims to recreate an acute anorectal angle by plication of the pelvic floor muscles behind the anus after an intersphincteric dissection. Early reports suggested that the procedure was highly efficacious in restoring continence with success rates of over 70% but later reports were less favorable and the procedure is now rarely used.

Rectal Prolapse Surgery

Rectal prolapse is a relatively common cause of fecal incontinence although it produces other distressing and compelling symptoms. Consequently, surgical repair is usually recommended for patients who are otherwise fit. The condition is characterized by a neuropathy of the pelvic floor muscles, diastases of the levator ani muscles and a patulous anal sphincter.

Although over 100 different operations for rectal prolapse have been described they share common principals. Surgery may be undertaken by either the abdominal or perineal route. The former involves dissection of the rectum followed by fixation and in some cases excision of the redundant bowel. These operations are highly effective in correcting the prolapse but often produce a poor functional outcome with approximately 50% of patients suffering from severe constipation. Indeed this may be the mechanism whereby incontinence is corrected. In an attempt to avoid constipation, sigmoid colectomy has been advocated but this can increase the risk of postoperative incontinence. It is the author's practice to avoid colectomy in patients undergoing surgery for rectal prolapse when incontinence is the predominant symptom. Despite this selective approach, approximately one-third of patients who have undergone abdominal rectal prolapse surgery will suffer from incontinence.

Perineal operations are usually reserved for patients who are unfit for abdominal surgery since they are less effective at correcting the prolapse. There is however, evidence that the functional results are superior with less constipation and incontinence.

Stoma

Since fecal incontinence is such a socially devastating symptom, the option of creating a stoma should not be overlooked. Used in conjunction with techniques such as colonic irrigation a stoma may greatly improve the quality of life for these patients.

Artificial Bowel Sphincters

At present, there are two artificial bowel sphincters available for use in patients with fecal incontinence. The first is the artificial bowel sphincter or ABS; an ingenious design first used in urinary incontinence. The device has three component parts: a cuff that encircles the anus, a constant pressure balloon and a hydraulic control pump. For evacuation, the patient depresses the pump thereby transferring fluid from the cuff to the balloon. This fluid then "bleeds" back slowly closing the device.

The ABS has been shown to be highly effective in restoring continence; indeed such is the efficacy that patients often report difficulty with emptying. Unfortunately, the reported complication rate including infection and erosion has been high. Despite this, some surgeons have reported success. It has been suggested that serious complications of infection and erosion may occur because the device is implanted in the perineum. Further, the cuff can create localized areas of high pressure when wrapped around the bowel.

A new artificial sphincter known as the PAS (prosthetic anal sphincter) has been designed by the author and colleagues that aims to overcome the difficulties encountered with the ABS. The device utilizes a constant pressure balloon like the ABS, but the cuff component is implanted in the pelvis where it reproduces the action of the puborectalis (see ❷ *Fig. 77-3*). The cuff of the PAS differs from the ABS having been designed specifically to avoid localized areas of high pressure. Early clinical studies have been encouraging and the product has only recently come on the market.

Dynamic Gracilis Muscle Transposition

Attempts have been made to improve continence in patients with deficient anal sphincters by using the gracilis muscle to wrap around the anal canal. One or both muscles may be used (see ❷ *Fig. 77-4*). Although initial reports were promising the technique proved to be disappointing with longer follow up. In particular, patients either lacked control or were unable to empty the rectum because the muscle produced adynamic constriction.

In an attempt to improve the outcome, the gracilis muscle was electrically stimulated, to change the characteristics of the muscle from "fast to slow twitch" fibers that were less likely to fatigue. The operation performed in expert hands can be highly effective in restoring continence. Unfortunately the

◨ Figure 77-3
The PAS device in the open (left) and closed (right) positions

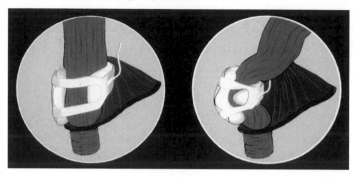

◨ Figure 77-4
The gracilis muscle is first mobilized from the thigh, carefully preserving the neuro-vascular bundle

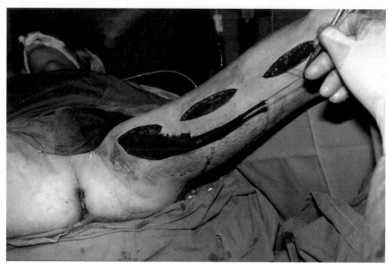

operation has high complication rates limiting the value of the procedure. Since the advent of sacral nerve stimulation, it is rarely used.

Sacral Nerve Stimulation

Of all the treatments for fecal incontinence to emerge over the past 25 years, sacral nerve stimulation (SNS) is perhaps the most promising.

Sacral nerve stimulators were first used in the early 1980s to treat urge incontinence of urine. It was noted that there was also an improvement in bowel function in these patients. SNS was first reported to have been used in patients with fecal incontinence in 1995. Since then it has been used and reported to be successful in patients who have suffered incontinence from a variety of causes including spinal cord injury, idiopathic degeneration, post rectal prolapse repair, after low anterior resection and even in patients with a sphincter defect. Although the numbers of patients in these studies was small, improved continence for liquid and solid stool was reported in 50–75% of patients.

SNS has the advantage that patients may have a trial of treatment using a temporary electrode before being subjected to the surgical procedure of placing a permanent electrode. It is usual to attempt to place the electrode through the third sacral foramen, although both the second and fourth have also been used successfully. Open implantation has recently been superseded by percutaneous techniques but it remains necessary to make a subcutaneous pocket for the stimulator. Currently, work is being undertaken to compare unilateral with bilateral stimulation and to define the optimal settings for the stimulator.

It is important to note that at present the mode of action of SNS is unknown. In particular it is unknown whether it has a peripheral or central action. There is some evidence, however, that it may modify rectal motility and sensation. This would be especially interesting given the high number of patients with fecal incontinence who have IBS. Studies have suggested that SNS does not work as a placebo although it would be interesting to compare SNS with traditional treatment such as amitriptyline in a randomized crossover trial.

SNS is arguably the most promising treatment available at present for the treatment of fecal incontinence but it should be remembered that many treatment options have previously been reported as demonstrating potential only to disappoint with long term follow up. Given current knowledge, SNS should be tried first after failed medical management with implantation of artificial sphincters reserved for SNS failures.

Selected Readings

Chapman AE, Geerdes P, Hewett P, et al. (2002) Systematic review of dynamic gracioplasty in the treatment of faecal incontinence. Br J Surg 89:138–153

Donnelly V, Fynes M, Campbell D, et al. (1998) Obstetric events leading to anal sphincter damage. Obstet Gynaecol 92:955–961

Finlay IG, Richardson W, Hajivassiliou CA (2004) Outcome after implantation of a novel prosthetic anal sphincter in humans. Br J Surg 91:1485–1492

Fitzpatrick M, Behan M, O'Connell PR, O'Herlihy C (2000) A randomised clinical trial comparing primary overlap with approximation repair of third degree tears. Am J Obstet Gynecol 183:1220–1224

Ganio E, Masin A, Ratto C, et al. (2001) Short term sacral nerve stimulation for functional anorectal and urinary disturbances: results in 40 patients: evaluation of a new option for anorectal functional disorders. Dis Colon Rectum 44:1261–1267

Hajivassiliou CA, Carter KB, Finlay IG (1996) Anorectal angle enhances faecal incontinence. Br J Surg 83:53–56

Jarrett MED, Varma J, Duthie G, et al. (2004) Sacral nerve stimulation for faecal incontinence in the United Kingdom. Br J Surg 91:755–761

Lehur PA, Zerbib F, Neunlist M, et al. (2002) Comparison of quality of life and anorectal function after artificial sphincter implantation. Dis Colon Rectum 45:508–513

Malouf AJ, Norton CS, Engel AF, et al. (2000) Long term results of overlapping anterior anal sphincter repair for obstetric trauma. Lancet 355:260–265

Perry S, Shaw C, McGrother C, et al. (2002) Prevalence of faecal incontinence in adults aged 40 years or more living in the community. Gut 50:480–484

Poen AC, Felt-Bersma RJ, Strijers RL, et al. (1998) Third degree obstetric perineal tear: long term clinical and functional results after primary repair. Br J Surg 85:1433–1438

Sultan AH, Monga AK, Kumar D, Stanton SL (1999) Primary repair of obstetric anal sphincter rupture using the overlap technique. Br J Obstet Gynaecol 106:318–323

Swash M (1993) Faecal incontinence; childbirth is responsible for most cases. BMJ 307:636–637

78 Pruritus Ani

Santhat Nivatvongs

Pearls and Pitfalls

- Idiopathic pruritus ani can be intractable.
- Hand washing with mild soap (best with glycerine soap) is the optimal way to clean the perianal area (unless the patient is allergic to soap which is rare).
- Applying Capsaicin cream is a novel treatment, start with 0.025%.
- Proper use of methylene blue injection should be considered as a last resort.
- Soaking in water is not cleaning.
- All anal wipes contain chemicals and do not help.
- Traditional washing with a soapy wash cloth without washing it off with water is a bad practice which gives soap a bad name.
- There is no evidence that eating or drinking certain kinds of food or liquid is the cause of pruritus ani.

Pruritus ani is not a disease but a symptom of itching of the perianal skin. It is estimated to occur in approximately 1–5% of the population, with a male-to-female ratio of about 4:1. The onset of the condition is most commonly in the fifth and sixth decades of life. Most patients have only a mild form of the condition and respond quickly to proper treatment. To treat pruritus ani rationally, one must have a clear-cut concept of the etiologic factors involved in its production.

Clinical Manifestation

Itching, usually combined with burning, is the prominent complaint. The itching may occur any time of the day or during sleep. Anything that keeps the anal skin moist causes itching. The itch-scratch cycle usually creates abrasions of the perianal skin, resulting in seepage of serum which further irritates the perianal skin.

Careful history taking usually uncovers clues of the problem. Often, the patient has more problems at night or in hot, humid weather, although this is not always the case. The itching may also be exacerbated by friction from clothing, wool, and nylon. With time, the condition may progress to an unrelenting itching and burning with an insurmountable urge to scratch. Poor anal hygiene is often a major contributing factor. Questions about the patient's cleaning habits and how the perianal skin is cleansed are important to ask. Wiping with toilet paper only spreads and smears feces to the perianal skin. All cleaning wipes contain chemicals that also damage the sensitive perianal skin. Specific dietary ingredients and neurogenic, psychogenic, and idiosyncratic reactions with pruritus should be suspected whenever another factor is not identified readily. Because the diagnosis is made by exclusion, inquiries about diabetes, antibiotic use, and vaginal and anal discharge may establish the factors responsible for the symptoms. Stress and anxiety often exacerbate pruritus ani. Common complaints revolve around family, work, and finances.

Physical Findings

In the early stage, examination of the perianal skin reveals minimal erythema and excoriation. As the symptoms progress, the perianal skin becomes friable, inflamed, and weeps from excoriation. Poor anal hygiene may be apparent with staining of stool or mucus and a wet anal area. In the later stages, the typical findings of long-standing idiopathic pruritus ani include thickened, whitish, ulcerated, or abraded perianal skin from scratching, with deep furrows with radial ridges of perianal skin.

Flexible sigmoidoscopy or colonoscopy should be performed to rule out associated diseases, particularly in patients with chronic pruritus ani who are older than 50 years of age. Daniel and co-workers found associated colorectal disease in 35% of patients with chronic pruritus ani, including rectal cancer in 11%, proctitis in 5%, squamous cell carcinoma of anus in 5%, inflammatory bowel disease in 5%, adenomatous polyp in 4%, anal diseases in 2%, and colon cancer in 2%.

Etiologic Factors

Pruritus ani can be divided into secondary type and idiopathic type. With proper history, examination, and patch tests, the causes of the itching will be discovered eventually. The idiopathic type is diagnosed by means of exclusion.

Secondary Pruritus Ani

From Within Anorectum

Prolapsing hemorrhoids (grade 3 or 4) cause a mucous discharge which, if not washed off, irritates the perianal skin. Treatment with rubber band ligation or hemorrhoidectomy is indicated. Anal fissures cause seepage of serum from the ulcer and thus should be treated conservatively with bulk agents and warm sitz baths, nitroglycerin or nifedipine paste, or if unresponsive to these measures, lateral internal sphincterotomy. Discharge from an anal fistula is also caustic to the anal skin. Fistulotomy usually cures the problem. Other surgically correctable conditions include anal skin tags and prolapsed hypertrophied anal papillae.

Fecal incontinence, especially of liquid stool, can be a major problem. Radiation proctitis may cause leakage of mucus and liquid stool. Patients with pruritus ani have an abnormal rectal inhibitory reflex and abnormal, transient, internal sphincter relaxation. Whether these abnormalities are the cause or the effect remains unknown. Heavy coffee drinking causes relaxation of the internal sphincter, which may cause seepage of mucus and liquid stool. The main management of these problems is to eliminate the cause.

Anal hygiene is important in these situations. Patients should be discouraged from sitting in water to relieve itching, because it causes maceration of the skin. Instead, washing with water by hand with or without glycerine soap is the best way to clean and relieve the irritation. In patients who have incomplete evacuation of the stool, irrigation of the anal canal with bulb syringe to wash away stool from the anorectum after each bowel movement is helpful to prevent seepage of stool. Dietary measures to firm the stool should be initiated. For radiation proctitis, cortisone retention enemas may be helpful.

From Outside the Anorectum

Sweating, particularly in overweight patients and in patients with a deep natal cleft, causes maceration of skin with potentially bacterial or fungal invasion. Wearing tight or non-porous underwear also traps the moisture. An irritating vaginal discharge should also be excluded. Proper washing with mild soap and water by hand will improve the condition.

From Perianal Skin Disease

In a study of patients with pruritus ani, Dasan and co-workers found 34 of 40 patients to have an underlying dermatosis which accounted for their symptoms, the most common form being psoriasis. Many of these patients also have a high incidence of sensitization to previously used topical preparations on patch testing. These patients should be referred to a dermatologist for proper tests and management.

Anal condyloma acuminata can be diagnosed easily and should be treated with excision and/or electrocautery. Perianal Paget's disease and Bowen's disease can cause intense itching and mimic a dermatitis; a biopsy should often be performed to confirm or exclude the diagnosis. Treatment consists of a wide local excision; in the case of Bowen's disease, electrocoagulation has become the treatment of choice.

Radiation to perianal area, such as for carcinoma of the prostate and cervix, damages the skin causing erythema, ulceration, and seepage. The problem is usually temporary and improves with time. The area should be kept clean by hand washing. Cortisone cream often helps as well.

Idiopathic Pruritus Ani

This category includes all patients with no known cause of the condition. Typically, the patients have long-standing disease. The appearance of the perianal area varies from pale but otherwise normal looking, to ulcerated and seepy, to thickened with deep furrows. Many of these patients are excessively clean and have tried all kinds of topical preparations including over-the-counter cream and steroid preparations. All these agents should be stopped.

Oztas and co-workers showed that washing with a liquid cleanser (Protex liquid cleanser; Colgate-Palmolive) was as effective as topical steroids. Using a liquid cleanser, however, is unnecessary; proper hand-washing with soap (preferably glycerine soap) and water is excellent treatment. The patients should be instructed *not* to use a wash cloth. This regime should be done after each bowel movement and whenever there is discharge or sweat in the perianal area. Also any psychologic aspect should not be overlooked. In some patients, the anal itching may be the primary behavior, and this eventually perpetuates to the itch-scratch cycle. Dietary measures are helpful for many patients with pruritus ani with the goal to achieve a bulky, formed stool. Fungus infection of the perianal skin is usually a secondary involvement from the moist and poor hygiene and is aggravated by antibiotic usage for this and other conditions.

Topical Capsaicin

This approach is a novel treatment for idiopathic intractable pruritus ani. Capsaicin is a natural alkaloid extracted from red chili peppers. There is an over-the-counter topical analgesic cream (0.075% and 0.025%) commonly used for arthritis pain relief. Topical application of Capsaicin in therapeutic dose (0.075%) to pruritus ani produces profound loss of intraepidermal fibers within 24 h. Nerve terminals regenerate and reinnervate if Capsaicin application is discontinued; repeated application is often required.

The perianal area should be washed clean. Initially, the lower concentration of the cream should be tried first, applying a thin film to the itching area three to four times a day.

The Last Resort

When all etiologic factors have been excluded and other treatments have failed, one should consider injection of the perianal skin with methylene blue as the last resort. The solution for injection is prepared as follows:

10 ml of 1% methylene blue
5 ml normal saline
15 ml 0.25% bupivacaine with 1:200,000 epinephrine

The mixture is injected subdermally and subcutaneously in the anoderm and perianal skin. In their preliminary experience with 23 patients, Eusebio and colleagues found that cellulitis developed in three patients, and full thickness skin necrosis developed in three others when a 0.5% methylene blue solution alone was used; nevertheless, 21 of 23 patients had relief of their itching.

Methylene blue causes necrosis of nerve endings, and the injected area becomes numb for about 1 month. This temporary denervation breaks the itch-scratch cycle and allows the skin to heal and return to normal. Because the methylene blue solution alone can cause tissue necrosis, it should be mixed and diluted as described above. The patient should be warned that his or her urine will turn blue for a few days. The skin in pruritus ani appears to have a low resistance to infection. The injected area should be cleansed with antiseptic before the injection. In some patients, prophylactic antibiotics should be considered as well.

Selected Readings

Anand P (2003) Capsaicin and menthol in the treatment of itch and pain: Recently cloned receptors provide the key. GUT 52:1233–1235

Daniel GL, Longo WE, Vernava AM (1994) Pruritus ani. Causes and concerns. Dis Colon Rectum 37:670–674

Dasan S, Neill SM, Donaldson DR, Scott HJ (1999) Treatment of persistent pruritus ani in a combined colorectal and dermatological clinic. Br J Surg 86:1337–1340

Eusebio EB (1991) New treatment of intractable pruritus ani (Letter). Dis Colon Rectum 34:289

Eusebio EB, Graham J, Mody N (1990) Treatment of intractable pruritus ani. Dis Colon Rectum 33:770–772

Lysy L, Sistiery-Ittah M, Israelit Y, et al. (2003) Topical capsaicin – a novel and effective treatment for idiopathic intractable pruritus ani: a randomized, placebo controlled, crossover study. GUT 52:1323–1326

Oztas MO, Oztas P, Onder M (2004) Idiopathic perianal pruritus: washing compared with topical corticosteroids. Postgrad Med J 80:295–297

79 Rectovaginal Fistulas

Richard Cohen · Alastair Windsor · Kumaran Thiruppathy

Pearls and Pitfalls

- Rectovaginal fistulas cause an underappreciated morbidity to affected women.
- The incidence of these fistulas in underdeveloped countries is underappreciated.
- The most common causes are traumatic obstetrical injuries during childbirth, postoperative causes, radiation therapy, invasive malignancies, and diverticulitis.
- Rectovaginal fistulas are classified as simple or complex and involve either the upper, middle, or lower third of the rectovaginal septum.
- Etiology and techniques of repair depend on location of the fistula.
- Lower third rectovaginal fistulas are usually repaired by a perineal approach, either transanal or transvaginal.
- Upper third rectovaginal fistulas are approached trans-abdominally.
- Approach to middle third rectovaginal fistulas depends on etiology; some can be repaired via a perineal approach, others require a trans-abdominal approach.
- Complex rectovaginal fistulas often require temporary or permanent proximal colonic diversion.
- Techniques of repair may involve resection, flap advancement, or primary repair.
- The function of the anal sphincter should be evaluated preoperatively in all patients.

Introduction and Etiology

There are few afflictions, unattended with danger to life, which give rise to greater anxiety or produce more disagreeable results than cases of rectovaginal fistula. Tanner 1855.

A rectovaginal (RV) fistula is an abnormal communication between the epithelial surfaces of the vagina and the anal canal or rectum. These fistulas cause considerable morbidity to afflicted individuals and a severe headache to the treating surgeons, because recurrence with the need for perseverance and multiple procedures is often required. Although these fistulas are believed to be a rare condition, they are hugely underestimated worldwide.

The management of RV fistulas depends on the etiology as well as the anatomic configuration. RV fistula due to underlying pathology (Crohn's disease, tuberculosis, postradiotherapy) are much more difficult to manage, because there is an inherent resistance to healing within the tissue. This chapter will not, however, address pouch-vaginal fistulas after ileopouch anal procedures.

Most rectovaginal fistulas are acquired, although congenital RV fistulas do occur (❷ *Table 79-1*). Obstetric trauma is the leading cause of RV fistulas worldwide. The incidence increases dramatically across developing countries where obstetric care is sparse. Risk factors include the use of forceps or

◘ Table 79-1

Etiology of RV fistula

- Congenital causes
- Acquired causes
  - Inflammatory bowel disease
    - Ulcerative colitis
    - Crohn's disease
  - Postoperative causes
    - Colorectal procedures (anastomoses near vaginal vault)
    - Gynecologic surgery
  - Traumatic
    - Obstetric trauma
    - Foreign bodies
    - Penetrating injuries
  - Infection and inflammation
    - Diverticular disease
    - TB
    - Cryptoglandular sepsis
  - Pelvic irradiation
  - Neoplasms
  - Idiopathic
  - Miscellaneous
    - Coital injury
    - Fecal impaction

other assisted methods of delivery, perineal tears, or an episiotomy that extends into the rectum. Long and difficult labor can cause weakness, necrosis, or tearing, which result in fistulas with the adjacent structures, such as the bladder, urethra, rectum, or perineum. These complex/difficult labors are most frequent in primiparous and young women and can result in low RV fistulas.

Other traumatic causes include blunt or penetrating perineal trauma. Traumatic fistulas respond well to treatment. If the RV fistula is secondary to a foreign body, removal of the foreign body usually results in spontaneous healing.

Diverticular disease is a disease of an aging population; 30% of people ≥60 years old suffer with the condition, of whom some will develop fistulas. As 40–60% of diverticula are found in the sigmoid, which is also the most mobile part of the colon, it is this site which is most associated with colovaginal fistulas. In contrast to colovaginal fistulas which occur in women who have undergone a previous hysterectomy or some other form of pelvic surgery, RV fistulas secondary to diverticulitis are much less common, but when they occur, they cause high vaginal lesions.

Inflammatory bowel disease (ulcerative colitis and Crohn's disease) is associated with formation of external and internal fistulas. The incidence is far greater in Crohn's disease where the disease is transmural and abscess formation is more common. It is estimated that 80% of patients with Crohn's disease will develop some form of internal fistula, but less than 10% will develop RV fistulas. This discrepancy is due to the low incidence of Crohn's disease involving the rectum. The incidence of RV fistula in ulcerative colitis is about 4%. These fistulas arise primarily or, more often, in relation to a peri-rectal abscess and/or fistula and manifest most commonly as complicated peri-anal sepsis.

Malignancies are a rare cause of RV fistulas and may be due to primary, recurrent, or metastatic disease. The most common offending cancers are rectal, cervical, vaginal, and uterine. A history of any of these or other perineal cancers in the presence of a RV fistula requires a biopsy of the fistula.

With more liberal use of pelvic radiation therapy for adjuvant and neoadjuvant treatment of advanced rectal and gynecologic malignancies, there is an increasing incidence of radiation injury in the rectum with a high incidence of progression to fistula formation. The incidence of radiation-induced RV fistulas had varied between 1% and 6%. These RV fistulas are usually in the mid or upper vagina and occur within 2 years of the radiation treatment. Radiotherapy causes irreversible tissue and vascular damage resulting in poor tissue quality, poor healing, and inflammation. Radio-necrotic ulceration occurs, inducing fistula formation. The degree of radiation damage is dependent on patient and treatment factor. The incidence of RV fistulas increases with radiation-related parameters such as total dose and overlapping radiation portals, patient factors (radiation effects are worse in thin patients and children), patient co-morbidities, especially diabetes and malnutrition, and iatrogenic factors, including chemotherapy and previous pelvic or abdominal surgery.

A variety of infectious conditions can lead to RV fistulas. Commonly implicated are peri-rectal abscess or fistula and peri-anal abscesses. Less common conditions are tuberculosis, lymphogranuloma venereum, and Bartholin gland abscess.

Classification

Anatomy

The rectovaginal septum is the thin septum separating the anterior rectal wall and the posterior vaginal wall (❷ *Fig. 79-1*). The caudal portion of the septum comprises the perineal body, an important supporting structure linking muscles that extend across the pelvic outlet and providing support to the pelvic floor and pelvic diaphragm. Disruption or attenuation of this structure can lead to prolapse of pelvic viscera and formation of cystocele and rectocele. The anal sphincters are located in the posterior portion of the perineal body and can be compromised by an initial insult or during treatment.

Proximal to the perineal body, the septum is of variable thickness, often with a cephalic extension. The septum consists of three separate layers, including the posterior vaginal wall, the anterior rectal wall and mesorectum, and, in between, a thin, dense fascial layer consisting of collagen, smooth muscle, and coarse elastin. This inner layer helps provide the RV septum with durability and strength.

■ **Figure 79-1**
Rectovaginal fascia

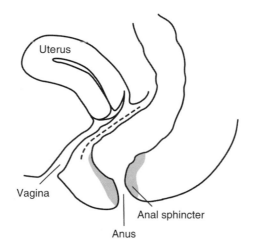

RV fistulas can also be complicated by involvement of neighboring structures, such as the bladder, sigmoid colon, or small bowel in the pouch of Douglas.

Classification

RV fistulas have been classified in many different ways, according to their etiology, size, anatomic location, or indeed, the various surgical approaches. Alternatively, they can be classified into simple or complex fistulas, depending on the ease with which treatment can be given (see ❯ *Table 79-2*).

The rectovaginal septum can be divided conveniently into thirds. The lower third anterior to anal sphincter complex and perineal body, the middle third involving the thin fascial layer, and the upper third covered posteriorly with peritoneum. Simple RV fistulas include small (<2.5 cm in diameter), lower third (❯ *Fig. 79-2*), or middle third (❯ *Fig. 79-3*) fistulas resulting from infection or trauma. Large (>2.5 cm), high fistulas involving the upper third of the septum (❯ *Fig. 79-4*) are considered complex, as well as those caused by inflammatory bowel disease, cancer, or radiation, congenital fistulas, or those involving other organs. RV fistulas that have failed multiple prior repairs are also classified as complex.

Presentation

The symptoms of RV fistula range between minimal egress of flatus and vaginal discharge to the passage of feces per vagina. The volume and character of the discharge varies and depends on the size, site, and etiology of the fistula. Patients may present with nonspecific signs. Acute exacerbation of inflammatory conditions (diverticulitis or inflammatory bowel disease) or abscesses may present with abdominal pain, low grade fever, nausea and vomiting, or diarrhea. On examination, a pelvic mass may be palpable and can be inflammatory or caused by a neoplasm.

Management

For successful management of these patients, it is essential to address several important principles. First is to confirm the presence of the fistula. Second is to define the anatomy, size, site, and complexity of

◼ **Table 79-2**

Classification of rectovaginal fistulas

Simple fistula
• <2.5 cm
• Lower or middle third
• Infective or traumatic origin
Complex fistula
• >2.5cm
• Upper third lesion
• Neoplastic, inflammatory, radiation
• Congenital fistulas
• Other organ involvement
• Multiply recurrent fistulas

■ Figure 79-2
Low rectovaginal fistula

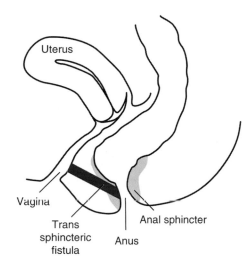

■ Figure 79-3
Mid rectovaginal fistula

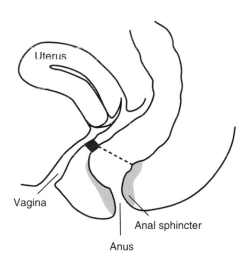

the fistula, especially addressing the presence of multiple fistulas and other organ involvement. Third, it is crucial to determine etiology and other underlying pathology. And finally, involvement and functional capacity of the anal sphincter is of vital importance.

Diagnosis

The diagnosis is made invariably on the history taken from the patient. Examination and investigations may be used to confirm the diagnosis and delineate the anatomy of the problem. The most useful

◼ Figure 79-4
High rectovaginal fistula (in a patient who has had a hysterectomy)

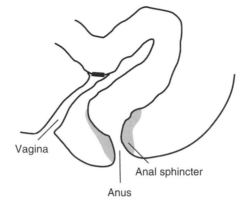

Vagina

Anal sphincter

Anus

investigation may be a careful examination under anesthesia. Imaging with retrograde contrast radiographs, computed tomography (CT), and magnetic resonance imaging (MRI) helps to further define local anatomy.

Clinical Examination

Careful examination in the clinic can be helpful, bearing in mind that the area can be very excoriated and sore. Digital rectal examination complemented with bimanual pelvic examination may reveal scars, defects, or masses on the anterior rectal wall and posterior vaginal wall. Proctosigmoidoscopy may demonstrate the fistula itself or underlying inflammatory bowel disease or malignancy. Insufflation of air into the rectum at proctosigmoidoscopy can produce audible air escaping from the vagina through a fistula. When indicated, colonoscopy is a useful tool in evaluating the proximal colon looking for related colonic pathology (e.g., Crohn's disease).

Examination under anesthetic (EUA) may be the most useful examination available to the surgeon faced with a RV fistula. Careful, comprehensive, and painless assessment of the lower anorectum and entire vagina can be carried out without embarrassment or discomfort to the patient. Fistula probes and hydrogen peroxide may help to delineate tracks and locate internal openings. Rectocele can be assessed, and a catheter can be left in high tracks to allow targeted fistulography.

Retrograde barium enema radiographs can be useful in the study of rectovaginal fistulas. Although the usual barium contrast can be too thick for many fistulas to fill, the other findings add valuable information in the diagnosis of other GI pathologies such as inflammatory bowel disease, diverticular disease, or malignancies. Vaginograms may prove successful in identifying small and multiple RV fistulas. The technique is performed by placing a Foley catheter into the vagina, inflating the catheter to form a seal, and instilling contrast into the vagina. As contrast flows into the vagina, the fistula and involved bowel can then be imaged.

High-resolution CT and MRI have come to play an invaluable role in the delineation of complex fistulas. Cross-sectional imaging is employed routinely when underlying pathology or other organ involvement is suspected. These non-invasive imaging techniques allow a quick and effective way of assessing GI and extra-gastrointestinal structures. MRI of the pelvis is particularly useful for evaluating the elusive mid and upper third fistula, because the inflammatory reaction shows up as a bright white signal on a black background.

Anal Sphincter

Before planning operative correction of an RV fistula, it is crucial to know the state and function of the anal sphincter complex. The sphincter can be assessed on digital examination in the awake patient, but a more formal evaluation by endorectal ultrasonography and/or anorectal physiology is usually indicated.

Treatment

Medical therapy: While operative therapy is usually required to treat an RV fistula, it is important to ensure maximal medical therapy of any underlying inflammatory bowel disease or unusual infection such as tuberculosis. It is best to adopt a multidisciplinary approach in these patients involving gastroenterologist and, if necessary, other colleagues in gynecology, infectious diseases, etc., depending on the etiology of the RV fistula.

Surgical therapy: Operative treatment of RV fistula is approached differently according to the etiology. For infections, the treatment involves drainage of the site with appropriate antibiotic coverage. For certain non-reconstructible RV fistulas, proximal colonic diversion is most appropriate. For lower third RV fistulas that are repairable, the fistula can be closed by a perineal approach using a transvaginal repair, a transperineal repair with sphincter reconstruction, transanal repair, or an interposition graft (Martius graft). For upper third RV fistulas, an abdominal approach is best using either resection, mucosectomy, and coloanal sleeve anastomosis or an anterior resection and omental interposition. On rare occasions, an ablative excision (abdominoperineal excision) is required. Mid third RV fistulas can be approached from the perineum, but when they involve a previous anastomosis or radiotherapy sites, they are often managed via an abdominal approach.

Lower third RV fistula: Most of these fistulas are either post-obstetric or cryptoglandular in origin and can be managed from a perineal approach. The operative plan depends on the competence of the anal sphincter. If the anal sphincter requires a concomitant repair, a perineal operation is advocated, with excision of the fistula and laying open the sphincter muscles anteriorly. The anorectal mucosa is then repaired, and an overlapping anterior sphincter repair is carried out before closing the vagina. This approach has the added advantage of providing the bulky sphincter repair to sit between the anorectal and vaginal repairs. It is also a useful procedure when simple transanal or transvaginal flaps have failed.

If the anal sphincter complex is intact, a transvaginal or transanal flap repair can be performed. The authors prefer the transvaginal route, because the access is far greater than struggling through the anal canal. An incision is made in the posterior fourchette of the vagina, and the rectovaginal septum is carefully dissected out well above the level of the fistula. Care is taken to avoid the vaginal veins, which need to be oversewn if injured. The fistula-bearing vaginal mucosa is then excised and the fistula into the anorectum cored out. The rectal defect is repaired as per any bowel anastomosis; the authors prefer interrupted 3/0 polyglactin suture material. The rectovaginal septum can be plicated with

2-0 polydiaxone and the vaginal flap brought down to the vaginal skin with polyglactin sutures. The vagina can be packed for 24 h if dissection is difficult, in which case bladder catheterization is required.

In patients who have had previous attempts at repair, a useful modification is the use of a labial fat pad graft (Martius graft). The dissection is as above, but the left hand labia is also incised allowing dissection of the labial fat pad. This fat pad has both proximal and distal blood supply but will survive on its distal vessels, thereby allowing full mobilization. The fat pad can then be swung to interpose in the rectovaginal septum between the anorectal and vaginal repairs.

It is possible and occasionally necessary to perform repeat attempts at closure until success is achieved. The authors have seen successful closure of RV fistula after multiple transanal and transvaginal failures. In a recent series of 17 patients with RV fistula, of which 13 were a postsurgical complication, 16 (94%) were treated successfully by these approaches.

The role of a defunctioning stoma in the management of RV fistula is debated and unproven. The authors believe that it is not necessary to suggest a defunctioning stoma in a first time attempt at closure if there is no underlying bowel pathology. In contrast, after previous attempts at repair and in the presence of diseases such as Crohn's disease or post radiation, we advocate the use of a defunctioning stoma. Our approach is based on the empiric assumption that the chance of success would be greater if fecal flow were taken out of the equation. The luminal pressures of a patient straining at stool after a complex fistula closure can only put strain on a delicate situation.

In very symptomatic patients where all else has failed, ablative excision via abdominoperineal excision of the anorectum using an intersphincteric technique can be employed. In the presence of Crohn's disease, the perineal wound can cause continuing trouble, and the authors advocate the use of myocutaneous flaps in difficult cases.

Upper third and middle third RV fistula: These types of RV fistulas require an abdominal approach. The abdomen is opened via a midline laparotomy, and a full assessment of the peritoneal cavity is made, looking for evidence of an otherwise unappreciated inciting cause. The required operation usually falls into one of two categories, either a colovaginal fistulation from diverticular disease or invasive malignancies into the vault of the vagina after a previous hysterectomy, or fistulation from the rectum into vagina, either from an anastomosis or after prior therapy. In the former circumstances, traditional resection of the diseased segment of colon with a sigmoid colectomy or high anterior resection is advocated. Care must be taken to separate the newly formed anastomosis from the repaired vaginal vault to minimize risk of re-fistulation. Interposition of omentum is a useful trick. In the latter situation, the key is to ensure maximum separation of the vaginal repair from any anastomosis using the technique of a coloanal pull-through. The rectum is transected below the level of the fistula, and the remaining rectal remnant mucosa is excised either from above or below as appropriate. The proximal, undiseased colon "pulled through" the rectal muscle cuff is anastomosed by hand from below to the dentate line. A defunctioning ileostomy is often prudent.

Selected Readings

Bahadursingh AM, Longo WE (2003) Colovaginal fistulas. Aetiology and management. J Reprod Med 48:489–495. Review

Bangser M (2006) Obstetric fistula and stigma. Lancet 367:535–536

Casadesus D, Villasana L, Sanchez IM, Diaz H, Chavez M, Diaz A (2006) Treatment of rectovaginal fistula: a 5-year review. Aust N Z J Obstet Gynaecol 46:49–51

Grissom R, Snyder TE (1991) Colovaginal fistula secondary to diverticular disease. Dis Colon Rectum 34:1043–1049

Hudson CN (1970) Acquired fistulae between the intestine and the vagina. Ann R Coll Surg Engl 46:20–40

Lindsey I, Guy RJ, Warren BF, et al. (2000) Anatomy of Denonvilliers' fascia and pelvic nerves, impotence, and implications for the colorectal surgeon. Br J Surg 87:1288–1299. Review

Rahman MS, Al-Suleiman SA, El-Yahia AR, et al. (2003) Treatment of rectovaginal fistula of obstetric origin: a review of 15 years' experience in a teaching hospital. J Obstet Gynaecol 23:607–610

Tahzib F (1983) Epidemiological determinants of vesicovaginal fistulas. Br J Obstet Gynaecol 90:387–391

80 Pseudomembranous Colitis

Lisa M. Colletti

Pearls and Pitfalls

- Antibiotic-associated diarrhea is common; in the outpatient setting, this is most commonly due to the antibiotic. In the inpatient setting, it is most commonly due to *Clostridium difficile.*
- *Clostridium difficile* colitis should be considered in all hospitalized patients with new onset diarrhea; failure to treat this disease can have substantial morbidity and mortality.
- *Clostridium difficile* colitis produces a range of symptoms from minor self-limited diarrhea to colonic perforation and sepsis.
- All antibiotics and many antineoplastic agents can predispose to the development of *Clostridium difficile* colitis.
- Development of *Clostridium difficile* colitis is not associated with duration or dose of antibiotic treatment.
- Diarrhea is the presenting sign in *Clostridium difficile* colitis.
- Risk factors for *Clostridium difficile* colitis include: advanced age, antibiotic therapy, immunocompromised state, ICU stay, burns, uremia, and enteral feeding.
- Diarrhea may be absent in patients with severe *Clostridium difficile* colitis causing ileus or toxic megacolon.
- Toxic megacolon due to *Clostridium difficile* colitis causing hypovolemic shock, cecal perforation, and/or toxic dilation of the colon with secondary sepsis is a surgical emergency with a 10–20% mortality rate.
- Diagnosis of *Clostridium difficile* colitis is made by testing a stool sample for toxin A and B or visualization of pseudomembranes on sigmoidoscopy.
- *Clostridium difficile* can rarely affect the ileum or jejunum in the post-colectomy patient.
- Treatment for *Clostridium difficile* colitis includes fluid resuscitation, discontinuing the offending antibiotic, and administration of metronidazole.
- Antidiarrheal agents should NOT be used in the treatment of *Clostridium difficile* colitis, as they may inhibit clearance of the toxins.
- Oral vancomycin is an alternative treatment for *Clostridium difficile* colitis; the drug of choice is currently metronidazole in an effort to prevent the development of bacteria drug resistance to vancomycin in other enteric bacteria (i.e. enterococcus).
- Operative intervention is necessary for the patient with toxic megacolon due to *Clostridium difficile* colitis; the procedure of choice is total abdominal colectomy with ileostomy.

Introduction

The incidence of antibiotic-associated diarrhea varies from 5% to 39%, depending on the antibiotic used, and most cases in outpatients are due to the antibiotic and not to a specific bacteria. In contrast, most hospital or nursing home outbreaks of antibiotic-associated diarrhea are secondary to *Clostridium difficile*. *Clostridium difficile* causes 300,000–3,000,000 cases of diarrhea and colitis in the United States every year, and its incidence appears to be increasing. In addition, it is the fourth most common nosocomial infection reported to the Centers for Disease Control and Prevention. This disease is associated commonly with the use of antibiotics. Although clindamycin, ampicillin, and cephalosporins are associated most commonly with development of *Clostridium difficile* colitis, any antibiotic can predispose a patient to this infection. Antibiotics alter the balance of normal gut flora and allow overgrowth of *Clostridium difficile*. The clinical presentation can vary from asymptomatic colonization to a mild diarrhea to fulminant disease, with high fever, severe abdominal pain, and toxic megacolon, sometimes with perforation. The most sensitive and specific test for *Clostridium difficile* infection is a tissue culture assay for the cytotoxicity of toxin B, however, detection of the toxin by ELISA (enzyme-linked immunoassay) is more rapid and inexpensive. Oral metronidazole or oral vancomycin are the drugs of choice for treatment, and most affected patients respond well to medical therapy. Approximately 15–25% of patients will relapse and require repeat treatment. Recurrent disease can be difficult to treat.

Epidemiologic Features

Clostridium difficile is a gram-positive, spore-forming anaerobic bacillus; interestingly, it was not implicated with antibiotic-related diarrhea until the late 1970s. *Clostridium difficile* is the cause of approximately 25% of cases of antibiotic-associated diarrhea and virtually all cases of pseudomem-branous colitis. Most cases of *Clostridium difficile*-associated diarrhea occur in hospitals or nursing homes; the incidence of this infection in the outpatient setting is much lower, however, it does occur. Clindamycin is the most common antibiotic associated with this infection, however, it is also associated commonly with use of ampicillin, amoxicillin, and cephalosporins. While these antibiotics are the most common etiologies for *Clostridium difficile*-colitis, this disease can develop with the use of virtually any antibiotic. Other predisposing factors include advanced age, bowel ischemia, recent bowel or abdominal surgery, Cesarean section, burns, uremia, malnutrition, chemotherapy, malignancy in general, shock, and possibly enteral feeding. After controlling for antibiotic use, patients receiving enteral feeding have a 20% chance of testing positive for *Clostridium difficile*, while a control group tested positive only 8% of the time. Patients fed distal to the stomach were at increased risk compared to patients who were fed intragastrically.

The spectrum of disease ranges from an asymptomatic carrier state to diarrhea without colitis, to colitis with or without the presence of pseudomembranes, to toxic megacolon, colonic perforation, and death.

Pathogenesis

In general, *Clostridium difficile* is a non-invasive pathogen, although rare cases of actual tissue invasion have been reported in children with malignancy or a compromised immune system. The first step in development of *Clostridium difficile* colitis is disruption of the normal colonic flora, most commonly by use of antibiotics, although this disrupted intraluminal milieu can be related to use of antineoplastic or immunosuppressive drugs. Colonization occurs via the fecal-oral route. The spores are ingested, are able to survive the acid environment of the stomach, and germinate in the colon; overgrowth of *Clostridium difficile* then occurs with toxin production and development of diarrhea and colitis. Symptoms of colitis may occur as early as the first day of antibiotic use or 6 weeks or longer after the antibiotics are stopped.

Some strains of *Clostridium difficile* do not produce toxins and are therefore do not cause colitis. The strains that cause clinical disease produce both Toxin A and Toxin B; indeed, it is these toxins that are largely responsible for symptomatic disease. Toxin A binds to mucosal receptors and disrupts cytoplasmic microfilaments. Toxin B then enters the damaged mucosa and causes hemorrhage, inflammation, and necrosis. Full tissue damage requires the presence of both toxins. In patients with severe or fulminant disease, inflammation involves the deeper layers of the colonic wall, resulting in toxic megacolon and possible perforation. Severity of associated illness and decreased levels of serum IgG antibody to toxin A increase the severity of colitis. In animal models, antibodies against Toxin A prevent toxin binding, neutralize the secretory and inflammatory effects, and limit or prevent clinical disease. The immune response to Toxin B is less well-understood, but anti-Toxin B antibodies also protect against *Clostridium difficile* colitis. Cellular immunity appears to be less important in this process, however, it has not yet been studied in detail.

Infants and young children commonly have *Clostridium difficile* in their fecal flora but have no symptoms related to *Clostridium difficile* toxin. As an individual ages, the prevalence of *Clostridium difficile* in the fecal flora decreases for unknown reasons. While asymptomatic carriers of *Clostridium difficile* are an important reservoir of the bacteria, clinical symptoms only develop in about one third of colonized patients, and asymptomatic colonization may be associated with a decreased overall risk of developing symptomatic colitis. *Clostridium difficile* spores persist in the environment for years, which explains why contamination by these spores is common in hospitals and long-term care facilities, especially in rooms occupied previously by infected/colonized individuals.

Early histologic changes due to *Clostridium difficile* toxins include patchy epithelial necrosis and exudates of fibrin and neutrophils. Epithelial necrosis with ulceration develops, with associated overlying pseudomembrane containing cellular debris, leukocytes, fibrin, and mucin (gross appearance: ❯ *Figs. 80-1A* and *B*; microscopic appearance: ❯ *Figs. 80-2A* and *B*).

❑ **Figure 80-1**
a, b. Gross pathology of florid pseudomembranous colitis due to *Clostridium difficile*

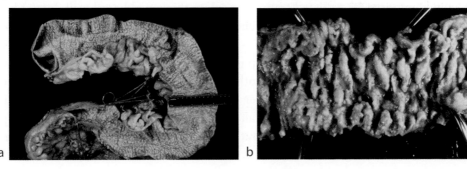

a　　　　　　　　　　　　　　　b

◘ Figure 80-2
a, b. Microscopic section of severe pseudomembranous colitis due to *Clostridium difficile.* **The pseudomembrane of dead leukocytes, mucosal epithelial cells, mucus, and adherent fibrin is obvious in the upper portion of photograph**

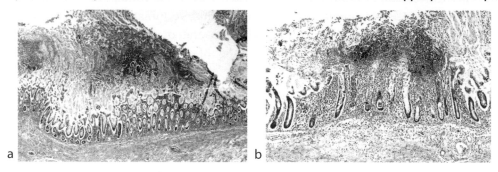

Clinical Presentation

Clostridium difficile diarrhea or colitis usually presents within 1–2 weeks of antibiotic treatment, although the presentation can vary from 1 day to 6 weeks. The symptoms can be quite variable and may include abdominal pain, low grade fevers, and diarrhea, which may be watery, mucoid and may contain blood. The spectrum of the colitis varies from colitis without pseudomembranes, pseudomembranous colitis, to fulminant colitis. Some individuals harbor both the bacteria and the two toxins yet never become symptomatic. Mild to moderate disease is usually associated with abdominal cramping, without other systemic manifestations. Moderate to severe colitis presents with profuse diarrhea, abdominal distention, abdominal pain, and occasionally, occult GI bleeding. Dehydration, electrolyte depletion, and hypoproteinemia due to a protein-losing colonopathy may occur with prolonged or severe disease. Systemic symptoms such as fever, malaise, nausea, and anorexia are usually observed. Fulminant colitis occurs in 1–3% of patients and presents with ileus, toxic megacolon, and perforation; death can occur in this form of disease. In addition, because of ileus and loss of colonic muscular tone, there may be a decrease in diarrhea in this form of disease. Other complications can include GI hemorrhage, sepsis, and pneumatosis coli. Overall, mortality is low (2–5%) but is considerably higher in elderly or debilitated patients (10–12%). For patients with fulminant colitis or toxic megacolon, mortality approaches 30–80%.

In about 10% of patients, the disease is localized to the proximal colon and therefore is more difficult to diagnose. Patients with toxic megacolon typically present with an acute abdomen, localized rebound tenderness or guarding, no diarrhea, and no abnormalities on sigmoidoscopy. Abdominal films should be obtained to exclude free intraperitoneal air. The supine film in patients with toxic megacolon usually demonstrates a dilated transverse colon, thickened bowel wall, loss of haustra, and occasionally pseudopolyps. Contrast enema or endoscopy should not be pursued in patients when perforation or toxic megacolon is suspected.

Occasionally, this clinical picture can develop in neutropenic patients secondary to antineoplastic agents and can occur in the absence of antibiotic use; this presentation is typically ileocecitis or typhilitis caused by *Clostridium difficile*. Another severe form of *Clostridium difficile* colitis can be seen in women undergoing Cesarean section; altered colonic motility associated with pregnancy, in addition to the opiates given for post-operative pain management, well as the pre-operative prophylactic antibiotics contribute to development of *Clostridium difficile* colitis. This form of *Clostridium difficile* colitis is often associated with toxic megacolon in the absence of diarrhea. Another situation in which *Clostridium difficile* is a common etiologic agent is in the setting of enterocolitis associated with Hirschsprung's disease in infants and children.

Although the vast majority *Clostridium difficile* disease manifests as a colitis, *Clostridium difficile* enteritis is an established entity, albeit rare, that should not be overlooked in the post-colectomy patient. Several reports have documented fatal cases involving enteritis of both ileum and jejunum.

Diagnosis

Staphylococcal enterocolitis is a more uncommon cause of antibiotic-associated diarrhea but should be suspected when tests for *Clostridium difficile* are negative, and gram-positive cocci are seen on a stool smear. Neutropenic enterocolitis or typhilitis is the most common etiology of diarrhea and abdominal pain in patients receiving chemotherapy, particularly in the setting of neutropenia. Crohn's disease and ulcerative colitis can also mimic antibiotic-associated colitis, and an active *Clostridium difficile* infection in these patients can also cause what appears to be a flare of the primary disease. Other disease in the differential diagnosis of antibiotic-associated colitis include chemical colitis, ischemic colitis, and other infections, such as Campylobacter, Salmonella, Shigella, Escherichia coli, Listeria, and cytomegalovirus.

The diagnosis of *Clostridium difficile* colitis is based on a combination of clinical findings, laboratory tests, and occasionally, endoscopy. Fecal leukocytes may be seen on a stool smear, but their absence does not exclude *Clostridium difficile* colitis. Culture of *Clostridium difficile* is difficult and a poor choice for diagnosis, as may people are asymptomatic carriers.

The most sensitive and specific test for diagnosis of *Clostridium difficile* is a tissue culture assay for cytotoxicity of toxin B, using preincubation with neutralizing antibodies to show the specificity of the cytotoxicity. This test is 94–100% sensitive and 99% specific. This test is expensive, requires tissue culture facilities, and takes 1–3 days to run. Enzyme-linked immunosorbent assays (ELISA) are much easier, faster, and cheaper to conduct. These assays detect either toxin and have a sensitivity of 71–94% and a specificity of 92–98%. In 5–20% of patients, more than one stool sample may be required to detect the toxins. If *Clostridium difficile* is suspected and the first ELISA is negative, 1–2 additional stool samples should be sent. If ELISA remains negative, but the clinical index of suspicion is high, then the cytotoxicity test should be performed; this test will detect an additional 5–10% of cases missed by ELISA.

Radiologic imaging may be helpful in suspected cases of fulminant colitis. Plain abdominal x-rays may reveal ileus and/or a dilated colon and should also be obtained to rule out free air (❯ *Figs. 80-3A* and *B*). Diffusely thickened or edematous colonic mucosa can sometimes be detected on abdominal computed tomography (CT) or as "thumbprinting" on plain abdominal x-rays. CT may also demonstrate colonic distention, thickening, or pericolonic inflammation and may be most helpful in cases where *Clostridium difficile* is localized to the proximal colon. A barium enema should not be performed because there is a high risk of perforation, especially with megacolon.

Sigmoidoscopy or colonoscopy is reserved for special situations such as the need to exclude another disease, need for rapid diagnosis, or in situations where a stool sample cannot be obtained

◘ Figure 80-3
a, b. Plain abdominal radiograph of a patient with toxic megacolon due to severe *Clostridium difficile* enterocolitis; dilation involves primarily transverse colon

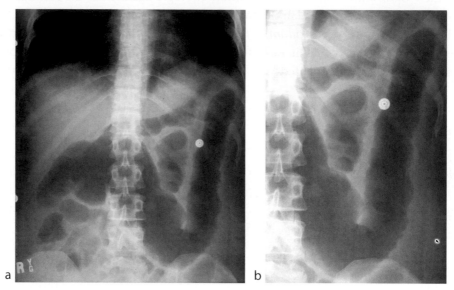

due to ileus. One should remember, however, that sigmoidoscopy may be normal in patients with mild disease. In more severe colitis, pseudomembranes should be visible, although in 10% of cases, only the right colon may be involved. Most patients have some abnormality of colonic mucosa, ranging from minimal erythema or edema, to ulcerated mucosa, often with nodular exudates, which will eventually coalesce to form yellowish "pseudomembranes". Due to the increased risk of perforation, endoscopy should not be the first diagnostic intervention.

Treatment

Antibiotic treatment should be discontinued if possible and supportive therapy with fluids and electrolyte replacement instituted. Precautions of enteric isolation are recommended. Antiperistaltic and opiate drugs should be avoided, as they may mask symptoms or may worsen the course of the disease. Diarrhea resolves spontaneously, without specific antimicrobial therapy, in 25% of patients.

Antimicrobial treatment is indicated in any patient with other associated illness and in all cases of moderate to severe disease. In the appropriate clinical setting, antimicrobial treatment should be instituted before lab results confirm *Clostridium difficile*. Oral metronidazole or oral vancomycin are the drugs of choice; *Clostridium difficile* is sensitive uniformly to vancomycin. Rare cases of resistance to metronidazole have been reported. Because of the risk of selecting vancomycin-resistant enteric organisms, such as enterococcus, initial therapy with metronidazole is preferred at doses of 250–500 mg three times per day for 10–14 days. Therapy with metronidazole or vancomycin is effective in 95% of patients, although 10–20% of patients relapsed subsequently.

With severe ileus or toxic megacolon, intravenous metronidazole should be used, at doses of 500 mg given every 8 h. Although intravenous therapy with vancomycin is not effective, this drug may be given rectally.

Despite successful treatment of the initial episode of *Clostridium difficile* diarrhea, 15–25% of patients will relapse after completing antibiotic therapy. Treatment of recurrent diarrhea includes conservative therapy without antibiotics, re-treatment with specific antibiotics against *Clostridium difficile*, use of anion binding resins, probiotics (therapy with "friendly" microorganisms), or immunoglobulin therapy. Conservative treatment of recurrent diarrhea is preferable to resumption of metronidazole or vancomycin, because these agents perpetuate the disturbance of the normal colonic flora; however, most patients are not able to tolerate ongoing diarrhea and will demand treatment. Persistent or worsening diarrhea, with confirmed *Clostridium difficile* infection, is an indication for more active treatment.

The most common therapy for recurrent *Clostridium difficile* diarrhea is a second course of the same antibiotic used to treat the first episode. Ninety-two percent of patients respond to a single course of repeat therapy. For patients with multiple recurrences, a prolonged course of vancomycin or metronidazole should be successful. Other treatment for persistent or recurrent disease include anion exchange resins such as cholestyramine to bind *Clostridium difficile* toxins, and biotherapy with probiotics aimed at restoring the "normal" colonic flora; these agents may include brewer's or baker's yeast taken by mouth, lactobacillus GG given as a concentrate in skim milk, a mixture of colonic bacteria in saline administered rectally in enema form, oral administration of non-toxigenic *Clostridium difficile*, and Saccharomyces boulardii, given as a capsule. No good, controlled studies have evaluated the efficacy of probiotic therapy.

Evidence now suggests that the immune response to *Clostridium difficile* toxin plays a major role in host susceptibility to this disease. Serum antibodies to *Clostridium difficile* toxin are low in patients with recurrent *Clostridium difficile* diarrhea. For these patients, treatment with normal, pooled, intravenous gamma globulin containing IgG anti-Toxin A was associated with a marked increase in serum antitoxin antibody and resolution of diarrhea. This therapy remains experimental.

Operative intervention is only required for *Clostridium difficile* colitis in about 3% of patients and only in those with more severe disease. More severe colitis is associated with advanced age, malignancy, renal failure, chronic pulmonary disease, immunosuppression, use of anti-peristaltic drugs, hypoalbuminemia, hemoconcentration, and significant increases or decreases in the patient's white blood cell count. Indications for operative intervention include acute abdomen, sepsis, multiorgan failure, hemorrhage, toxic megacolon, perforation, or deterioration despite aggressive medical treatment. Pneumatosis coli does not necessarily mandate operative treatment if it responds to aggressive medical treatment.

At laparotomy, the colon is edematous and distended. The serosa can appear normal despite severe mucosal disease. Segmental resections and diverting ileostomy without colonic resection have been described; however, these operations often fail, and n additional operative intervention is required, and mortality increases. Therefore, the operation of choice is a total abdominal colectomy with end ileostomy and Hartmann's pouch. Mortality for these patients is high, partly due to delay in diagnosis and need for total colectomy. In addition, the risk of local complications, such as perforation, increases substantially in patients with fulminant colitis which does not respond to medical therapy. Therefore, all patients with severe *Clostridium difficile* colitis whose condition does not respond to medical treatment within 48–72 h should be considered for operative intervention.

Selected Readings

Barbut R, Petit JC (2001) Epidemiology of *Clostridium difficile*-associated infections. Clin Microbiol Infect 7:405–410

Fekety R (1997) Guidelines for the diagnosis and management of *Clostridium difficile*-associated diarrhea and colitis. American College of Gastroenterology, Practice Parameters Committee. Am J Gastroenterol 92:739–750

Kelly CP, Pothoulakis C, LaMont JT (1994) *Clostridium difficile* colitis. N Engl J Med 330:257–262

Kyne L, Kelly CP (2001) Recurrent *Clostridium difficile* diarrhea. Gut 49:152–153

Lipsett PA, Samantaray DK, Tam MT, et al. (1994) Pseudomembranous colitis: a surgical disease? Surgery 116:491–496

McFarland LV (1998) Epidemiology, risk factors and treatments for antibiotic-associated diarrhea. Dig Dis 16:292–307

Morris LL, Villalba MR, Glover JL (1994) Management of pseudomembranous colitis. Am Surg 60:548–551

Yassin SF, Young-Fadok TM, Zein NN, Pardi DS (2001) *Clostridium difficile*-associated diarrhea and colitis. Mayo Clinic Proceed 76:725–730

81 Toxic Megacolon

Bruce G. Wolff · Anne Marie Boller

Pearls and Pitfalls

- Initial medical management, in the absence of peritonitis or perforation, is appropriate and consists of supportive care, intravenous fluids, antibiotics, and steroid therapy.
- All narcotic medications (antidiarrheal, anticholinergic, and some antidepressant agents) should be discontinued upon suspicion of toxic megacolon.
- Associated underlying conditions and diseases include:
  - Ulcerative colitis
  - Crohn's disease
  - Bacterial infections such as Clostridium difficile colitis
  - Viral (CMV) and parasitic infections (Entamoeba histolytica, Cryptosporidium)
- CT scan may prove useful in demonstrating subclinical abscesses or perforations.
- Colonoscopic decompression is not recommended.
- Emergent surgical intervention is required for progressive dilatation or increasing systemic toxicity, perforation, peritonitis, hemorrhage, or failure of medical therapy.
- Surgical intervention is recommended with persistent colonic dilatation after 48–72 h of medical therapy.
- Subtotal colectomy with an end-ileostomy is the procedure of choice in the emergent or urgent setting.
- Toxic megacolon which progresses to peritonitis and perforation is associated with an increased mortality rate.
- Delay in surgical intervention is associated with an increased mortality rate.
- Although controversial, toxic megacolon as the initial presentation of inflammatory bowel disease has been associated with a grave prognosis.
- Even "successful" medical management has been associated with recurrent bouts of toxic megacolon and the necessity for subsequent emergent surgical intervention.

Introduction

Toxic megacolon is a potentially fatal complication of inflammatory, ischemic, and infectious colitis. Early recognition, appropriate therapy, and surgical intervention are paramount when this diagnosis is suspected. Classically, toxic megacolon is defined as segmental or total colonic dilation greater than 6 cm, accompanied by signs of systemic toxicity and acute colitis. In 1950, Marshak et al. first described toxic megacolon in the literature as a complication with specific clinical features in relation to ulcerative colitis. Since this time, the diagnosis of toxic megacolon has been recognized in association with multiple different underlying diseases, including ulcerative colitis, Crohn's disease, pseudomembranous colitis, and additional infectious causes of colitis. Toxic megacolon requires immediate surgical consultation, as a delay in its diagnosis and the implementation of appropriate surgical interventions increases the risk of complications and associated mortality. In a study from the Mayo clinic which followed 38 patients with toxic megacolon managed nonoperatively, Grant and Dozois found a 29% incidence of recurrent bouts of toxic megacolon or colitis, which most often required emergent, subsequent surgery. Their results led them to the conclusion that medical management of toxic megacolon should be "regarded almost exclusively as preparation for imminent surgery."

Incidence

Exact estimations of the incidence of toxic megacolon are difficult to determine given the various underlying diseases responsible for the disorder, the lack of prospectively collected data, and the referral bias manifested by centers publishing reports regarding their experience with toxic megacolon. Although traditionally toxic megacolon was associated exclusively with ulcerative colitis, it is now recognized in association with Crohn's disease and most inflammatory causes of colitis. Grieco et al. cited the lifetime incidence of toxic megacolon in patients with ulcerative colitis between 1% to 2.5%, and in Crohn's disease between 1% to 6%. Current incidence rates associated with antibiotic-induced pseudomembranous colitis and subsequent toxic megacolon are estimated in up to 3%, although this number increases accordingly with the rising prevalence of this diagnosis.

Etiology

Although the majority of recognized cases are associated with ulcerative colitis, it is now recognized that a wide array of underlying diseases and causes of colitis may progress to toxic megacolon (❯ *Table 81-1*). In addition to the diagnoses of inflammatory bowel disease, specifically ulcerative colitis and Crohn's disease, this includes the bacterial and viral causes of colitis such as *Clostridium difficile*, Salmonella, Shigella, Campylobacter, Cryptosporidium, Entameba histolytica, Yersinia and Cytomegalovirus. In contrast to *Clostridium difficile*, the remaining etiologies of bacterial colitis are rarely associated with the development of toxic megacolon. In HIV compromised patients, the diagnosis of CMV colitis is most frequently associated with the development of toxic megacolon, although Kaposi's sarcoma has also been implicated in this setting. Cytomegalovirus also has been documented in the development of toxic megacolon in the setting of immunocompromised patients and ulcerative colitis. Ischemic colitis, especially associated with cancer chemotherapy, has been associated with the development of toxic megacolon.

Several risk factors have been noted in the development of toxic megacolon. In inflammatory bowel disease patients, the major risk factor is the severity of the underlying colitis. While ulcerative colitis typically involves the colonic mucosa, the underlying colitis and inflammation associated with toxic megacolon progresses transmurally in affected patients. Medications associated with toxic megacolon and inflammatory bowel disease include sulfasalazine, 5-aminosalicylic acid (5-ASA) and corticosteroids. Premature discontinuation of these medications, or a decrease in the dosage, may also be associated

◻ **Table 81-1**
Causes of toxic megacolon

Inflammatory bowel disease	
	Ulcerative Colitis
	Crohn's disease
Bacterial infection	*Clostridium difficile*
	Shigella
	Salmonella
	Yersinia
	Campylobacter
Viral infection	Cytomegalovirus
Other	Ischemic colitis
	Immunodeficiency
	Kaposi's sarcoma

with toxic megacolon. Additional risk factors include barium enemas, antimotility medications, anticholinergics, and some antidepressants. Colonoscopy in the setting of suspected toxic megacolon is not recommended due to historic reports of its association with the development of the disorder.

Pathogenesis

While the exact mechanism responsible for the development of toxic megacolon is unclear at this time, there are likely several contributory factors. Severe inflammation associated with toxic megacolon progresses transmurally into the smooth muscle. The inflammation causes dysfunction of the associated smooth muscle and subsequent dilatation. It has been postulated that the severity of the dysmotility and dilatation are directly correlated with the degree of transmural inflammation. Metabolic disturbances and hypokalemia, which occur with toxic megacolon, are more commonly thought of as markers of disease progression, rather than inherent to the pathogenesis of the disease.

Nitric oxide (NO), a vasodilator, may contribute to the pathogenesis of toxic megacolon. Mourelle and colleagues studied the activity of nitric oxide synthase in a rat model and in humans affected by ulcerative colitis and toxic megacolon. The rat model revealed a correlation between inducible nitric oxide generation and impaired smooth muscle contractility. The human cohort studied colonic tissue from three different sets of patients: those with active pancolitis, toxic megacolon, and nonocclusive colon neoplasms. Toxic megacolon specimens were associated with inducible nitric oxide synthase in the muscularis propria of the affected colon. Excessive nitric oxide produced by NO synthase may be responsible for the colonic atony and dilatation associated with toxic megacolon.

Clinical History

The clinical picture of toxic megacolon may present as pancolitis or segmental disease. The diagnosis is equally prevalent in both genders and may occur at any stage of inflammatory bowel disease, with a notable portion of patients manifesting toxic megacolon as the initial presentation of their disease.

Toxic megacolon is defined as *dilatation of the colon ≥6 cm in the setting of acute colitis*, with the concomitant onset of systemic toxicity. Patients will present with clinic findings consistent with acute colitis, including diarrhea which is often bloody, abdominal pain, and cramping. These symptoms may precede colonic dilatation by a week or more. Progression to toxic megacolon may be accompanied by increasing distention, fever, tachycardia, an increased white blood cell count, or anemia. Jalan and colleagues established criteria for the diagnosis of toxic megacolon (❷ *Table 81-2*). These criteria include the aforementioned clinical criteria with at least one of the following additional criteria: dehydration, mental changes, electrolyte disturbances, or hypotension. In this setting, patients may or may not manifest signs of peritonitis.

Immunocompromised patients, including HIV patients, may have minimal signs or symptoms on clinical examination. Medications should be reviewed for steroid usage and specifically, as possible risk factors, including antidiarrheal medications, narcotics, anticholinergics, and some antidepressants. All such medications, including narcotics, should be discontinued in a setting of suspicion for toxic megacolon.

Electrolyte disturbances are frequently present. Laboratory studies will reveal an elevated white cell count and anemia. Hypokalemia and hypoalbuminemia reflect ongoing diarrhea losses and dehydration. Stool cultures should be sent for *Clostridium difficile* toxin and blood cultures should be drawn. Endoscopy is indicated in the work up only when pseudomembranous or CMV colitis is suspected, and only on a limited basis. The high risk of perforation precludes the use of colonoscopy.

The clinical picture is supported by radiographic findings. Abdominal radiographs will demonstrate colonic dilatation ≥ 6 cm. Normal haustra may be absent on evaluation of the plain radiograph. The transverse colon is most frequently affected by the dilatation due to its superior and anterior anatomical position; however, the bowel gas may redistribute with patient position. Small bowel dilatation has been implemented in patients at high-risk for developing toxic megacolon. CT scans are useful in the evaluation of toxic megacolon. The presence of abscess and microperforations are discernible on CT scan but may be indiscernible on plain radiograph. Submucosal edema, wall thickening, ascites, and assessment of colonic and small bowel dilatation may also be accurately assessed with this modality. Toxic megacolon associated with pseudomembranous colitis may be more effectively evaluated with a CT scan, as many of the more subtle abscesses and small perforations have not been shown on plain film.

◼ Table 81-2

Criteria for toxic megacolon (Modified from Sheth and LaMont (1998). Copyright 1998. With permission from Elsevier)

Jalan's criteria	
Fever	>101.5°F (38.6°C)
Heart rate	>120 beat/min
WBC	>10.5 (10^9/l)
Anemia	
Plus one of the following:	
	Dehydration
	Mental status changes
	Electrolyte disturbances
	Hypotension

Management

A high index of suspicion and early intervention are crucial to the successful management of toxic megacolon. Medical management, surgical consultation, and appropriate surgical intervention are all required.

Medical management should be initiated immediately on suspicion of toxic megacolon. Bowel rest, nasogastric and bladder decompression, and intravenous fluid resuscitation are begun simultaneously with a surgical consultation. A long intestinal tube may be placed under fluoroscopic guidance. All narcotic medications, antimotility agents, and anticholinergics are discontinued. Appropriate broad-spectrum antibiotics are initiated and all previously administered antibiotics are halted, especially in bacterial colitis cases such as *Clostridium difficile.* Stress ulcer therapy and deep venous thrombosis prophylaxis are started at admission. Daily electrolyte values and abdominal films should be ordered and reviewed for signs of improvement or clinical degeneration. Patient repositioning to the prone or knee-elbow position multiple times throughout the day has been advocated to assist in decompressing the bowel. Total parental nutrition has not been shown to affect outcomes in patients with toxic megacolon, but is associated with septic and line-associated complications.

Intravenous corticosteroids should be started in the inflammatory bowel disease patient with toxic megacolon. Jalan and colleagues reviewed and compared ulcerative colitis patients treated with supportive care and those treated with steroids. Their retrospective analysis revealed a higher remission rate and better overall mortality within the group of patients who received steroids.

Patients whose condition does not improve in 48–72 h should proceed to surgery. Signs of perforation, persistent fever, signs of systemic toxicity, or ongoing transfusion requirements would indicate an earlier necessity for surgical intervention. Conversely, some patients who show an improvement in their colonic dilatation, without the onset of systemic complications, may be treated conservatively for as long as 7 days without surgical intervention.

Those requiring surgery due to ongoing dilatation or lack of clinical improvement should receive an elective subtotal colectomy and end ileostomy. Mortality rates decrease significantly when perforation is avoided (2–8% vs. 40%) and surgical intervention is elective (5%) and not emergent (30%). Dozois and Grant recognized that nearly one-third of their patients suffered a second episode of toxic megacolon, strengthening their assertion that "medical management of toxic megacolon should be regarded almost exclusively as a preparation for imminent surgery." Furthermore, their findings highlighted two additional groups who should be considered for surgery after the initial assessment: inflammatory bowel disease patients whose initial presentation occurs in the setting of toxic megacolon, and pregnant patients who present with toxic megacolon.

Conclusion

Toxic megacolon is a devastating manifestation of ischemic, infectious, and inflammatory colitis. Continuous monitoring and surgical surveillance is warranted in order to manage these patients appropriately. Timely surgical intervention decreases the mortality associated with toxic megacolon and improves patient outcomes.

Selected Readings

Caprilli R, Vernia P, Latella G, Torsoli A (1987) Early recognition of toxic megacolon. J Clin Gastroenterol 9:160–164

Dallal RM, Harbrecht BG, Boujoukas AJ, et al. (2002) Fulminant Clostridium difficile: an underappreciated and increasing cause of death and complications. Ann Surg 235:363–372

Gan SI, Beck PL (2003) A new look at toxic megacolon: an update and review of incidence, etiology, pathogenesis, and management. Am J Gastroenterol 98:2363–2371

Grant CS, Dozois RR (1984) Toxic megacolon: ultimate fate of patients after successful medical management. Am J Surg 147:106–110

Greenstein AJ, Sachar DB, Gibas A, et al. (1985) Outcome of toxic dilatation in ulcerative and Crohn's colitis. J Clin Gastroenterol 7:137–143

Grieco MB, Bordan DL, Geiss AC, Beil AR, Jr (1980) Toxic megacolon complicating Crohn's colitis. Ann Surg 191:75–80

Imbriaco M, Balthazar EJ (2001) Toxic megacolon: role of CT in evaluation and detection of complications. Clin Imaging 25:349–354

Jalan KN, Sircus W, Card WI, et al. (1969) An experience of ulcerative colitis. I. Toxic dilation in 55 cases. Gastroenterology 57:68–82

Latella G, Vernia P, Viscido A, et al. (2002) GI distension in severe ulcerative colitis. Am J Gastroenterol 97:1169–1175

Marshak RH, Lester LJ (1950) Megacolon a complication of ulcerative colitis. Gastroenterology 16:768–772

Mourelle M, Casellas F, Guarner F, et al. (1995) Induction of nitric oxide synthase in colonic smooth muscle from patients with toxic megacolon. Gastroenterology 109:1497–1502

Mourelle M, Vilaseca J, Guarner F, et al. (1996) Toxic dilatation of colon in a rat model of colitis is linked to an inducible form of nitric oxide synthase. Am J Physiol 270:G425–430

Sheth SG, LaMont JT (1998) Toxic megacolon. Lancet 351:509–513

82 Colonic Volvulus

Chrispen D. Mushaya · Yik-Hong Ho

Pearls and Pitfalls

Sigmoid Volvulus

- More common than, appreciated, it represents the third most common cause of large bowel obstruction in the West; however, elsewhere, it may be the most common cause.
- Usually presents in elderly *males*; however, there is a young male predominance in areas with high incidence.
- Presenting signs and symptoms include: gross abdominal distension (may cause cardiac and respiratory embarrassment), colicky abdominal pain, and constipation.
- Plain abdominal x-rays show "omega"/inverted "coffee bean" sign or "Northern exposure" sign.
- Early recognition of imminent gangrene is crucial; non-gangrenous volvulus can be decompressed endoscopically with staged elective sigmoid colectomy.
- Gangrenous colon requires resuscitation and emergent sigmoid colectomy. Primary anastomosis is not recommended; a Hartmann's procedure is the preferred treatment.
- A subtotal colectomy should be considered as the primary procedure if there is concomitant megacolon or megarectum, because this will reduce the risk of recurrence after sigmoid colectomy alone.

Cecal Volvulus

- Much less common! Usually in elderly *female* patients.
- Vomiting is prominent (because of involvement of terminal ileum); colicky abdominal pain and abdominal distension are other features.
- X-ray signs of volvulus on right side may be subtle and require a high index of suspicion.
- The diagnosis is often made only at laparotomy.
- Right hemicolectomy (primary anastomosis or stoma as appropriate) is indicated; reduction alone results in high risk of recurrence.

Sigmoid volvulus was first described as far back as the Ebers Papyrus in 1500. Colonic volvulus usually occurs in the sigmoid colon and less commonly in the cecum, however, volvulus occurs, rarely in the transverse colon and splenic flexure.

Pathogenesis

Anatomic variation involving a freely mobile colonic mesentery and a narrow base allows volvulus to occur. Other risk factors include chronic constipation, megacolon, neurologic diseases, adhesions, Hirschsprung's disease, Chagas' disease, ischemic colitis, ileus, and pregnancy. In areas with a high incidence of sigmoid volvulus, such as Africa, a diet high in fiber and carbohydrates results in large fecal bulk and gas content, which predisposes the sigmoid mesentery to twist, leading to chronic sigmoiditis. This cicatricial reaction further narrows the base of the mesentery, increasing the risk for volvulus. The degree of torsion varies with more than 360 degrees in over 50% of the patients, most commonly in a counterclockwise manner (❯ *Fig. 82-1*). Cecal volvulus is predisposed by an incomplete embryologic bowel rotation and retroperitoneal fixation, the so called floppy cecum, which occurs in about 10% of adults.

Closed-loop obstruction causes early gangrene with an attendant high morbidity and mortality. Anaerobic bacteria produce massive amount of endotoxins which easily traverse the compromised bowel and highly permeable peritoneum to enter the circulation. Progression to perforation and generalized peritonitis in the elderly, frail patient is almost universally fatal.

Sigmoid Volvulus

Clinical presentation: In most Western countries, sigmoid volvulus is the third most common cause of colonic obstruction after cancer and diverticulitis, and accounts for about 5% of all colonic obstructions. In many areas of the developing world, including Africa, Asia, Eastern Europe, South America, and the Middle East, sigmoid volvulus is the most common cause (~50%) of large bowel obstruction. The most common presentation in the West of a frail, elderly, 70- to 80-year-old male (63%) contrasts

◗ Figure 82-1
Sigmoid volvulus with 360° counterclockwise torsion, forming a knot

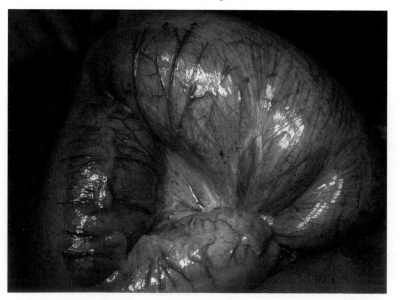

with the younger 40-year-old male in countries where sigmoid volvulus is more common. This condition is rare in children, occurring predominantly in males (90%) with a mean age of 10 years; in this age group, sigmoid volvulus is often associated with ileosigmoidal knotting in which the small bowel mesentery becomes chronically inflamed from recurrent twisting of the sigmoid mesentery. These children often suffer from worm infestation. Acute, marked, abdominal distension is an important feature, so much so as to cause cardio-respiratory compromise in some patients. Constipation tends to be absolute, but vomiting is unusual unless there is ileosigmoidal knotting. Abdominal pain is initially colicky and centered in the left lower quadrant, but becomes more diffuse as the condition progresses. Emptiness can be seen or felt in the left iliac fossa in as many as 28% of patients. The differential diagnosis involves other causes of large bowel obstruction, including colorectal cancer, diverticulitis, pseudo-obstruction, and constipation with megacolon.

Patients tend to have multiple medical co-morbidities and are often institutionalized for psychiatric conditions, making their clinical condition more desperate. Over 50% of patients have at least one clinically important operative risk factor. It must be emphasized that gangrene occurs in the twisted sigmoid loop in up to 20% of patients and is an ominous factor predisposing to morbidity and mortality. Fever, hemodynamic compromise, or peritonitis should raise suspicion for colonic gangrene. In severe cases, the abdominal distension may cause respiratory compromise (❷ *Fig. 82-2*).

Diagnosis: A confident diagnosis of sigmoid volvulus can be made on abdominal x-rays in 60–75% of patients. The characteristic "omega" or inverted "coffee bean" sign or shape is formed by grossly dilated and closely opposed sigmoid loops, and the "Northern exposure" sign, formed by dilated sigmoid colon that ascends cephalad to the transverse colon, is virtually pathognomonic (❷ *Fig. 82-3*). If the diagnosis is in doubt, a water-soluble contrast enema will show a "bird beak" sign from the characteristic obstruction at the rectosigmoid junction. CT of the abdomen is employed rarely and shows a "whirl pattern" of the dilated sigmoid loop around the mesocolon and a "bird beak" shape

❑ Figure 82-2
Sigmoid volvulus with marked abdominal distension causing acute respiratory compromise

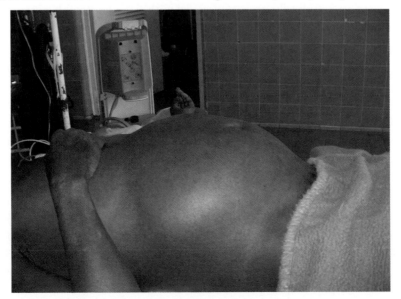

◼ Figure 82-3
"Coffee bean" sign of sigmoid volvulus on plain x-ray

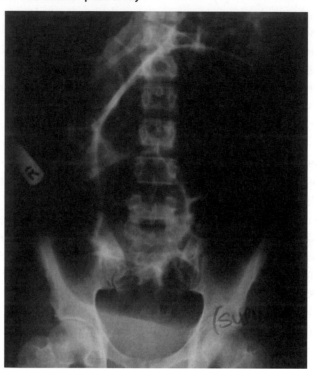

formed from the affected segments. In lieu of contrast or complex radiologic investigations, a flexible sigmoidoscopy can be both diagnostic and therapeutic.

Treatment: When the bowel is *not* gangrenous, management involves non-operative relief of obstruction by endoscopic decompression. This approach allows for optimizing the frail, elderly patient with significant co-morbidities so that an elective operation can be performed to prevent recurrence. Decompression is typically more successful with use of a flexible sigmoidoscope, although the colonic twist usually occurs about 15–25 cm from the anal verge and should be accessible with a rigid sigmoidoscope. A well-lubricated rectal tube can be advanced carefully and gently beyond the torsion to deflate the volvulus. If a flexible instrument is used, the endoscope is passed carefully beyond the twist, and the distended bowel is deflated by suction. The deflated bowel will untwist spontaneously, but it is prudent to leave a tube for decompression until the patient is prepared for elective surgery to reduce the risks of early recurrences. In one report, 86% of patients who did not undergo operative intervention developed recurrent volvulus within a median of only 2.8 months.

Elective sigmoid colectomy is advised within the same hospital admission, but only after optimization of co-morbidities. Pre-operative workup should include a complete colonoscopy, as appropriate; a repeated bowel preparation is not necessary if the operation is timed in close proximity, and the patient kept on clear fluid oral intake. Pre-operative antibiotics against Gram negative bacteria and anaerobes are usually given on induction of general anesthesia; regional anesthesia can be employed safely in selected patients if indicated by co-morbidities. A mini-laparotomy with a 4–5 cm, muscle-slitting incision in the left iliac fossa enables the procedure to be performed easily and expediently with similar invasiveness as the laparoscopic approach. Provided that the diagnosis is correct, the redundant sigmoid colon is identified easily and exteriorized fully through the incision. There is no need to ligate the sigmoidal vessels at the base of the sigmoid mesentery. Instead, the latter can be divided effectively at the level of the skin incision; the resultant adhesions should then prevent recurrence of volvulus. The sigmoid mesentery is always thickened, and special care must be taken to avoid bleeding from slipped ligatures (❯ *Fig. 82-4*). A functional, end-to-end anastomosis can then be performed expediently. When performed properly, the entire operation can be completed safely. When there is concomitant megacolon or megarectum, a subtotal colectomy is recommended as the primary procedure to reduce the risk of recurrence after a sigmoid colectomy alone. In such circumstances and when the expertise is available, a laparoscopic approach may be suitable. Other methods to prevent recurrences of sigmoid volvulus after decompression include colopexy, laparoscopic or open sacral fixation, and mesosigmoidoplasty. These procedures have not stood the test of time and are not accepted widely.

Emergent operative intervention is indicated if endoscopic decompression fails or is contraindicated. The latter applies when the obstruction has been present for more than 72 h or when gangrenous bowel is suspected by clinical features described above (often accompanied by an increasing leukocytosis); under these conditions, the risk of perforation from endoscopic manipulation will be high. Delay in treatment is equally detrimental, however, and the patient must be resuscitated aggressively for an urgent laparotomy. Preoperative preparation includes intravenous fluid resuscitation, bladder catheterization, nasogastric tube insertion, correction of electrolyte imbalances, and administration of broad spectrum antibiotics. A lower midline incision is recommended for rapid access with minimal blood loss. The bowel may or may not be viable, but the sigmoid volvulus can be detorsed and a sigmoid resection performed. The fecal load in the colon can be evacuated manually, and a primary anastomosis can still be undertaken in select patients with very good results, even on rare occasions when the bowel is gangrenous. Elaborate measures such as on-table lavage are seldom necessary and prolong the operative time in these sick patients. In most patients, when the patient's

☐ Figure 82-4
Thickened sigmoid mesentery in volvulus

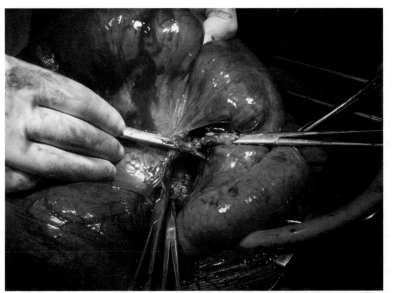

general condition remains unstable or when there is gross peritoneal soiling, a Hartmann's procedure is the procedure of choice. A double-barrel or loop colostomy diversion proximal to a primary anastomosis can be an alternate consideration.

Outcomes: The patient should show objective improvement by postoperative day 4, otherwise an anastomotic leak should be suspected. The overall hospital mortality is about 6–14%; the greatest mortality occurs in patients undergoing emergent resection and primary anastomosis in the presence of gangrenous sigmoid colon.

Cecal Volvulus

Clinical presentation: Cecal volvulus is a much more uncommon cause of bowel obstruction, being responsible for less than 2% of intestinal obstructions. The patient is usually an elderly lady, although in endemic areas, patients present at a younger age. Clinical features depend on the degree and duration of the twist. The "floppy" or "mobile" cecum syndrome occurs when patients present with acute right lower abdominal pain, which resolves after passing a large gush of flatus. These patients usually have a history of similar attacks in the past. In contrast, if the volvulus is complete, the patient will present with clinical features of small intestinal obstruction with colicky abdominal pain, constipation, abdominal distension, and especially vomiting. When the cecum becomes gangrenous, the clinical presentation is more ominous; findings of peritonitis may be florid and perforation becomes an imminent risk. The cecal bascule is a different anatomic entity which includes an upward and anterior twist of the cecum. Cecal bascule shares many similarities with cecal volvulus, including a tendency to give rise to intestinal obstruction.

Diagnosis: Because cecal volvulus is uncommon, a high index of suspicion is needed to make the diagnosis. The abdominal x-ray findings include right-sided colonic distension and obstruction or a "coffee bean" sign pointing to the left upper quadrant. Small bowel dilation may be prominent as well. If gangrenous bowel is not suspected, a contrast enema may demonstrate the volvulus with a sharp cut off "beak" sign; this test has a diagnostic sensitivity approaching 90%. The contrast enema may also reduce the volvulus in some patients. An abdominal CT is rapidly becoming the preferred imaging modality, because it shows the characteristic dilated cecum with air fluid levels ("coffee bean" sign) and progressive tapering of bowel loops at the site of the volvulus ("bird beak"). In addition, signs of mural ischemia suggestive of gangrene may be evident as well, although the sensitivity for ischemia is not high.

Treatment: If the diagnosis is suspected preoperatively, which is not always the case, an initial effort at non-operative treatment can be attempted. This approach is suitable only when the patient presents early, and ischemic bowel is not suspected. Reduction by barium enema reportedly been successful, although this approach is not advised as a treatment option in most patients. Endoscopic decompression can be employed, but again, this approach is known to have a limited success rate of less than 30% and requires experienced endoscopists. The risk of perforation is high.

The surgical options in these patients are variable and depend on the patient's condition at presentation, the intra-operative findings, and the surgeon's experience. Because cecal volvulus is not a common condition, no randomized trials are available to guide management. If the bowel is viable, manual detorsion of the volvulus can be performed, but simple detorsion of the volvulus has a recurrence rate of over 70%. Cecopexy is another well-described technique, where the cecum and ascending colon are anchored or pexed broadly to the lateral parietal peritoneum with suture fixation. The recurrence rate after this technique is as great as 40%. Surgeons who favor this approach claim that this is an easy and quick procedure, hence, the patient spends less time under anesthesia. Moreover, preservation of the terminal ileum and ileocecal valve results in less physiologic disturbance. The seromuscular sutures are difficult to place, however, and are poorly retained in edematous tissue. Cecostomy is an option, but carries a high risk of postoperative mortality. Leakage around sutures and cecal necrosis leading to loss of fixation around the cecostomy tube is not uncommon.

When bowel ischemia occurs, resection is necessary, and in most patients a primary anastomosis with well-vascularized bowel is possible. In some patients, however, it may be safer to fashion a stoma because an anastomotic leak will confer disastrous consequences. Where the patient is treated in an elective setting, laparoscopic colectomy can be considered if a skilled laparoscopist is available.

Outcomes: An excessively mobile cecum, together with other factors which include chronic constipation and a high fiber diet, suggest the occurrence of a cecal volvulus. Colonic distension with cecal displacement during pregnancy may also cause this condition in susceptible individuals.

Ideal patient care is largely determined by the particular case merits, and hence, the judgment of the treating physician. Most patients with cecal volvulus are difficult to diagnose preoperatively, and many patients are operated on with the presumptive diagnosis of peritonitis or small bowel obstruction. Adequate preoperative fluid and electrolyte resuscitation is important, especially if there is gangrenous bowel, which adversely affects the outcome of the patient.

Operative options depend largely on the experience of the surgeon, although it is generally agreed that colectomy will avoid recurrence. The ideal operative option remains controversial, but most surgeons favor ascending colectomy. In a series in which a right hemicolectomy was performed, the postoperative mortality was 7% and the morbidity was 20%, mainly attributed to sepsis.

Selected Readings

Atamanalp SS, Yildirgan MI, Basoglu M, et al. (2004) Sigmoid colon volvulus in children: review of 19 cases. Pediatr Surg Int 20:492–495

Ballantyne GH (1982) Review of sigmoid volvulus: history and results of treatment. Dis Colon Rectum 25:494–501

Catalano O (1996) Computed tomographic appearance of sigmoid volvulus. Abdom Imaging 21:314–317

Chung YFA, Eu K-W, Nyam DCNK, et al. (1999) Minimizing recurrence after sigmoid volvulus. Br J Surg 86:231–233

Tuech JJ, Pessaux P, Regenet N, et al. (2002) Results of resection for volvulus of the right colon. Tech Colopoctol 6:97–99

Utpal D, Ghosh S (2003) Single stage primary anastomosis without colonic lavage for left-side colonic obstruction due to acute sigmoidal volvulus: a prospective study of one hundred and ninety-seven cases. ANZ J Surg 73:390–392

83 Rectal Prolapse and Solitary Rectal Ulcer

Susan Galandiuk

Pearls and Pitfalls

- Always examine patients in the upright straining position; prolapse may not be apparent in other positions.
- Full thickness prolapse can be differentiated from hemorrhoidal disease by the concentric rings of mucosa, unlike the "clusters" associated with hemorrhoids.
- In the absence of overt prolapse, but with symptoms suggestive of constipation and straining, a defecating proctogram may be helpful in identifying the source of the problem.
- In the presence of non-relaxing puborectalis syndrome, operative intervention will be doomed to failure if paradox muscle function is not first corrected through biofeedback.
- Failure to reduce and treat overt rectal prolapse may lead to permanent sphincter damage.
- In the majority of patients, one can only assess the restoration of sphincter function to its baseline 6 months following correction of rectal prolapse.

Clinical Presentation

Straining is the common denominator among rectal prolapse, procidentia and solitary rectal ulcer syndrome. Rectal prolapse, while very common in the nursing home population, is approximately six times more common in women than in men. The highest incidence in women starting in the 5th and subsequent decades. Women who are particularly at high risk are those who have had multiple vaginal deliveries and especially those who have had a hysterectomy. In some studies, more than half of the patients with prolapse have a history of constipation and a history of straining. If not corrected and not reduced, rectal prolapse can lead to permanent injury of the anal sphincter due to stretching. Prolapse should therefore, always be reduced and should be repaired soon after diagnosis. Most patients with prolapse have several common anatomic abnormalities including: (1) relative separation or diastasis of the levator ani muscles; (2) a deep cul-de-sac; (3) redundant sigmoid colon; (4) a narrow small caliber rectum with loosening of the normal posterior and lateral attachments, that allows the rectum to "telescope" out as a prolapse; and (5) a weakened anal sphincter. Prolapse in children is different from that in adults and will be addressed separately at the end of this chapter.

Diagnosis

Symptoms: Other than the obviously prolapsing rectum, loose discharge or incontinence for mucus is a typical symptom in cases of rectal prolapse. Due to trauma to the prolapsing rectal mucosa, rectal bleeding is common. With the close proximity of the bladder, in women, due to pelvic floor laxity, there is often an associated cystocele. In assessing the patient's symptoms, one should therefore inquire regarding difficulty urinating, urinary incontinence and urinary tract infections. In most patients with rectal prolapse, the prolapse acts almost like a "plug" and causes significant constipation. The degree of impairment of fecal continence may therefore be more difficult to ascertain.

Physical examination: Rectal prolapse is an embarrassing situation, and unless the patient is very frail and old and doesn't care, demonstration of rectal prolapse to a physician is typically associated with anxiety and embarrassment on the part of the patient! It is best demonstrated in the upright position while straining and this is best done on a toilet. Unless the prolapse is huge, it may not be apparent in other positions. Almost all patients with rectal prolapse will have a lax anal sphincter. Rectal prolapse can be differentiated from hemorrhoids by the concentric rings characteristic of full thickness prolapse in contrast to hemorrhoids (❯ *Fig. 83-1*).

Patient evaluation: Evaluation of the patient should assess the colon in order to exclude pathology such as cancer and polyps. Because of the significant constipation and difficulty cleansing the colon, subsequent difficulty clearing barium, and frequently impaired sphincter function, barium enemas are frequently nearly impossible to perform in these patients. The pre-operative evaluation can be performed on 2 different days with two different sets of tests performed: (1) defecating proctography and then at another time; (2) pudendal nerve terminal motor latency testing, anorectal manometry, endoanal ultrasound and colonoscopy. With a defecating proctogram, thick barium paste is inserted into the rectum. Barium is used to mark the vagina, and contrast is instilled into the bladder. Dynamic views during straining and defecation demonstrate whether there is appropriate puborectalis muscle relaxation. The defecating proctogram allows for assessment of associated vaginal vault prolapse and determination of whether a cystocele is present. With the close proximity of the pelvic organs, failure to correct an associated vaginal prolapse could, for example, act as a lead point for a prompt recurrence of

◘ Figure 83-1

Full thickness rectal prolapse. Note the concentric folds characteristic of full thickness prolapse, which contrast to the clusters of "bundles" characteristic of prolapsing grade III or IV hemorrhoids

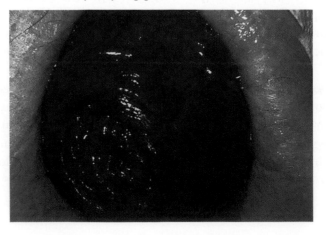

rectal prolapse. Performing a sacrocolpopexy, cystocele repair or bladder suspension in conjunction with a urogynecologist or gynecologist may therefore be important in lessening the risk for postoperative recurrence.

If anorectal physiology testing is not available, only colonoscopy is performed in addition to defecating proctography. This excludes proximal pathology as the cause of constipation. If available, pudendal nerve terminal motor latency testing can demonstrate whether or not there has been injury to the pudendal nerve from chronic stretch injury and prolapse of the rectum. This is very simply assessed by an electrode that is strapped to the index finger of the examiner that allows one to deliver an electrical signal to the pudendal nerve and measure the time delay for an electrode to measure contraction of the anal sphincter. Prolongation of this time indicates nerve injury. Anorectal manometry allows for objective assessment of internal and external anal sphincter function and endoanal ultrasound allows the examiner to document the degree of sphincter atrophy and also any unsuspected anterior obstetrical injury, which is often present. This information is helpful in predicting what anal sphincter function the patient will have after correction of the rectal prolapse. Pudendal nerve terminal motor latency testing, anorectal manometry and endoanal ultrasound, each take about 5 min to perform and are typically done prior to the colonoscopy.

Treatment

Non-operative Therapy

Unless the prolapse is small and the patient can reduce it after every bowel movement, non-operative therapy in my experience is uniformly unsuccessful and is doomed to failure. Non-operative therapy is generally directed at treating the constipation, minimizing straining and reducing the prolapse whenever it occurs.

Deciding on the Type of Surgery for Rectal Prolapse

Few conditions have generated so many operations for their correction as has rectal prolapse. Important with respect to the treatment of this condition is the fact that no matter how it is corrected surgically, there is over a 10% recurrence rate. The younger the patient, the higher the recurrence, due to the longevity of the subject. An important factor with respect to recurrence is the fact that many of these patients are chronic strainers. This and the already weakened pelvic floor are both high risk factors for recurrence.

Operative repair of rectal prolapse is divided into two broad categories of procedures: (1) perineal procedures with or without correction of the levator diastasis, and (2) abdominal procedures with fixation of the rectum with or without resection. Generally speaking, perineal procedures are reserved for older patients since they are associated with (1) loss of the rectal reservoir capacity, (2) more sphincter trauma, and (3) a higher recurrence rate. Perineal procedures can, however, be done under local anesthesia with IV sedation and are therefore suitable for even the most ill and moribund patients. Trans-abdominal procedures with or without resection are reserved for younger patients and are associated with a lower risk of recurrence.

Perineal Proctectomy

In the older debilitated patient, perineal proctectomy is the procedure of choice. Although it has a slightly higher recurrence rate, it has a low complication rate and can be performed under local anesthesia with intravenous sedation. If there is an extremely lax pelvic floor or extreme diastasis of the levator muscle, a levator plication can be performed during the same approach by plicating the levator muscle using non-absorbable suture prior to performing the colo-anal anastomosis. The entire rectum and lower sigmoid colon can be removed transanally using this approach. The downside of this procedure is that in many cases much or even the entire reservoir capacity of the rectum is removed. The symptom of fragmentation with frequent small bowel movements is common following this procedure. Although the use of the circular stapler has been reported by some, the handsewn approach is simple, safe and cost effective. With this approach, the rectal prolapse is pulled out as far as it will come using Babcock clamps, and the rectal wall transected full thickness approximately 1 cm above the dentate line using the electrocautery (❷ *Fig. 83-2A*). While the distal rectal wall is tagged using stay sutures of 2-0 polyglycolic acid, the proximal rectum is retracted distally (❷ *Fig. 83-2B*). The rectal mesentery is then systematically clamped, divided, and ligated. The proximal bowel is slowly divided, as quadrant tacking sutures are placed and a one layer interrupted hand-sewn coloanal anastomosis is performed using 2-0 absorbable suture (❷ *Fig. 83-2C*). Although patients have a lax anal sphincter during and at the conclusion of surgery, in approximately 50% of patients there will be a restoration of normal anal sphincter tone within 6 months of surgery. In the interim, fiber products and antidiarrheals are frequently necessary to adjust bowel function to maintain continence by providing for fewer, bulkier bowel movements. ❷ *Table 83-1* shows a summary of recurrence, morbidity and mortality data for perineal proctectomy.

Abdominal Procedures

As with low anterior resection, and ultra low anterior resection in which the majority of the reservoir capacity of the rectum is removed, patients with perineal proctectomy have fragmentation and frequent small volume bowel movements. High recurrence rates are also reported. For these reasons, in younger patients who have an expected greater longevity, transabdominal populations are more suitable. These maintain the reservoir capacity of the rectum and involve both fixation of the rectum to the sacral promontory to minimize the chance of recurrent prolapse, as well as resection of the redundant bowel to reduce the incidence of postoperative constipation. Abdominal procedures can either be done via open or laparoscopic approaches. An extensive rectal mobilization to induce fixation or scarring of the rectum to the sacral hollow is common to all of these procedures. Some fixation procedures such as the Ripstein procedure that have involved sling-type fixation of the rectum to the sacral promontory have been associated with a higher degree of postoperative constipation either due to the sling being too snug or due to sling fibrosis. In addition, in the existence of pre-existing constipation, the persistence of constipation is more common following rectopexy alone than following resection and rectopexy. Other methods of fixation, such as the polyvinyl alcohol sponge that has been popular in Britain have not been used extensively in the United States. The most common abdominal procedure in the United States is abdominal rectopexy with sigmoid resection as originally described by Frickman in 1955. A summary of the recurrence rates, morbidity and mortality for Ripstein rectopexy and resection rectopexy are shown in ❷ *Tables 83-2* and ❷ *83-3*, respectively.

◘ Figure 83-2

a. Perineal proctectomy is begun by inducing prolapse and grasping the prolapsed rectum with Babcock or Allis clamps. A full thickness incision is made through the rectal wall approximately 1 cm proximal to the dentate line using the electrocautery. As the bowel is divided, the distal rectum is tagged with stay sutures of absorbable suture material. I prefer 2-0 polyglycolic acid. **b.** Once the rectal wall is transected, traction is applied and the proximal rectum is pulled downward. The mesentery of the bowel is then systematically clamped, divided and ligated using absorbable suture. **c.** Once the prolapsed rectum has been resected, a single layer anastomosis is created between the proximal rectum or colon and the distal rectum using interrupted absorbable 2-0 polyglycolic acid suture. Four quadrant stay sutures are applied to the proximal colon to facilitate suturing

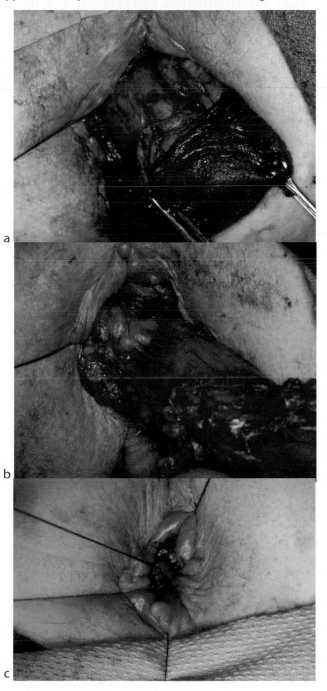

a

b

c

The Delorme procedure in which a mucosectomy is performed on the prolapsed rectum and the muscle wall plicated is not widely performed. It has been associated with a recurrence rate much higher than that reported for other procedures. The Thiersch procedure is used in children by placing absorbable suture around the distal rectum as a mechanical "vise" to keep the rectum from prolapsing, but this is not effective in adults and is essentially of historic interest.

Management of Fecal Incontinence Persisting > 6 Months Post-operatively

Nothing surgical should be done for 6 months postoperatively with respect to fecal incontinence following correction of rectal prolapse. During this time, normal restoration of sphincter tone can occur. If, however, the patient remains incontinent after this time, there are several treatment options;

◘ Table 83-1

Summary of results for perineal proctectomy for rectal prolapse (Data from Goligher, 1980)

	No. (%)
Patients reported	402
Calculated recurrence	30 (7)
Post-operative mortality	3 (1)
Complications	50 (12)
Follow-up (range in years)	1–17

◘ Table 83-2

Summary of results for Ripstein procedure for rectal prolapse (Data from Goligher, 1980)

	No. (%)
Patients reported	2,058
Calculated recurrence	60 (3)
Post-operative mortality[a]	8 (1)
Complications[b]	327 (19)
Follow-up (mean years)	5

[a]Only reported for 947 patients.
[b]Only reported for 1,748 patients.

◘ Table 83-3

Summary of results for sigmoid resection and rectopexy for rectal prolapse (Data from Goligher, 1980)

	No. (%)
Patients reported	243
Calculated recurrence	6 (2.5)
Post-operative mortality	2 (1)
Complications[a]	13 (6)
Follow-up (mean years)[b]	3.5

[a]Only reported for 226 patients.
[b]Only reported for 215 patients.

the first being an anterior sphincteroplasty if the patient has an obvious sphincter defect from a previous obstetrical injury that is demonstrated on endoanal ultrasound. Depending on patient age and pudendal nerve terminal motor latency, this may or may not be a viable option. In other words, if the patient is elderly, has a significant sphincter defect and significant nerve damage, functional results are likely to be poor. In this case, a better choice might be fecal diversion or implantation of an artificial anal sphincter (Acticon, American Medical Systems, Minnetonka, MN). This is an FDA-approved prosthetic device that yields functional results superior to sphincteroplasty in the presence of nerve injury, multiple sphincter defects or significant sphincter atrophy. In these cases, significant improvement from a sphincteroplasty would be unlikely. Postoperative infection is, however, a significant complication of this procedure. Other prosthetic products are available in Europe. Stimulated graciloplasty that was evaluated in clinical trials in the United States is not FDA-approved in the United States but is available in Europe.

Complications of Uncorrected Rectal Prolapse

If rectal prolapse is not corrected, incarceration of the hernia sack contents such as small bowel or even necrosis of the rectum can ensue, and in this case urgent surgery, rectal resection and colostomy are necessary (❯ *Fig. 83-3*). If rectal prolapse is not corrected, it can lead to significant stretch injury to the anal sphincter and to trauma to the pudendal nerve. When the rectal prolapse is eventually corrected, severe disabling incontinence may result that does not improve over time and requires further surgical intervention.

Solitary Rectal Ulcer Syndrome

The occurrence of chronic straining can lead to the presence of solitary rectal ulcer syndrome or levator ani syndrome. The solitary rectal ulcer syndrome is an increasingly recognized nomenclature for a variety of rectal problems in which chronic constipation is common. This is also known as

◻ Figure 83-3
Incarcerated rectal prolapse containing small bowel in the cul de sac. Initially, an attempt was not made to reduce this in a timely fashion

non-relaxing puborectalis muscle syndrome. Upon defecation, rather than relaxing in the normal fashion, the puborectalis muscle either does not relax or contracts, leading to straining and prolapse of the anterior rectal wall on the non-relaxed puborectalis muscle and chronic trauma. Rectal bleeding, mucus per rectum and tenesmus are common. The anterior rectal ulcer when seen is typically chronic and may appear polypoid rather than ulcerative. Dysfunctional defecation is a hallmark of the disease and used by many to explain the ulceration. This abnormal muscle behavior can be modified by biofeedback, it is not treated surgically. Attempts to treat this surgically without correction of the underlying abnormal muscle behavior result in prompt recurrence of the problem postoperatively. This problem may occur as early as adolescence. It is frequently characterized by bleeding and by the severe pain and tenesmus associated with the ulcer. Surgery may be necessary in cases in significant bleeding. Defecating proctography will often reveal obstructed defecation. A trial of anti-inflammatory 5-amino salicylic acid suppositories may be helpful. If there is internal prolapse, correction of this is occasionally warranted.

Prolapse in Children

Prolapse in children is a different situation than in adults. The incidence is highest in the first 2 years of life and declines thereafter in contrast to the frequency in adults. A variety of predisposing causes have been proposed, including a failure of the rectosigmoid to follow the sacral curve; constipation, diarrhea, and excess laxative use. Boys are affected slightly more frequently than girls, and this is most frequently mucosal prolapse rather than full thickness prolapse. The mucosa may project as much as 4 cm beyond the anus, but is easily reduced. Unlike adults, rectal prolapse in children is a self limited disease and disappears with time. Treatment in the pediatric age group typically is directed at correcting constipation. Proper defecating habits and avoidance of laxatives and suppositories seem to work best. Various surgical procedures are used, including the Thiersch procedure in which an absorbable suture is placed to act like a "vise" and prevent prolapse. Resection is rarely needed.

Summary

Problems related to anatomic pelvic relaxation and functional issues with constipation and laxative use occur commonly worldwide. Rectal prolapse and its surgical treatment should take into consideration both patient age and associated pelvic floor defects. The operation must be matched to the individual patient. Irrespective of the procedure, recurrence is common.

Selected Readings

Altemeier WA, Culbertson WR, Schowengerdt CJ, Hunt J, (1971) Nineteen years' experience with the one-stage perineal repair of rectal prolapse. Ann Surg 173:993–1006

Beahrs OH, Theuerkauf FJ, Hill JR (1972) Procidentia: surgical treatment. Dis Colon Rectum 15:337–346

Frykman HM (1955) Abdominal proctopexy and primary sigmoid resection for rectal procidentia. Am J Surg 90:780–789

Goldberg SM, Gordon PH, Nivatvongs S (1985) Complications of surgery after complete rectal procidentia. In:

Ferrari BT, Ray JB, Gathright JB (eds) Complications of colon and rectal surgery, prevention and management. W.B. Saunders, Philadelphia pp 251–266

Goligher JC (1980) Surgery of the anus, rectum and colon, 4th edn. Balliere Tindall, London, pp 224–258

Gordon PH (1999) Rectal procidentia In: Gordon PH, Nivatvongs S (eds) Principles and practice of surgery for the colon, rectum, and anus, 2nd edn. Quality Medical Publishing, St. Louis, MO, pp 503–540

McMahan JD, Ripstein CB (1987) Rectal prolapse. An update on the rectal sling procedure. Am Surg 53:37–40

Neill NE, Parks AG, Swash M (1981) Physiological studies of the anal sphincter musculature in faecal incontinence and rectal prolapse. Br J Surg 68:531–536

84 Ischemic Colitis

Mario A. Abedrapo Moreira · Gonzalo Soto Debeuf

Pearls and Pitfalls

- The etiology of ischemic colitis is usually related to a low flow state.
- The symptoms of ischemic colitis are usually non-specific.
- One of the key points in diagnosis is a high index of suspicion by the clinician, especially in patients with risk factors.
- Currently, there are no sensitive or specific laboratory tests for detection of early ischemic colitis.
- Colonoscopy within the first 3 days of symptoms is the best diagnostic method for ischemic colitis.
- For patients without evidence of transmural ischemia, an initial trial of conservative management may be employed; conservative non-operative treatment is successful in the majority of patients with ischemic colitis (non-transmural ischemia).
- Careful observation with repeated evaluation is necessary in patients managed conservatively to assure absence of progressive disease.
- Only 15–20% of the patients require emergency operation, with mortality rates of 50–60% (transmural ischemia).
- Segmental resection of the ischemic colon with proximal diverting colostomy is recommended when emergency operation is required.
- A late sequela of ischemic colitis successfully managed conservatively is a colonic stricture.

Introduction

The colon is the most common segment of the gastrointestinal tract where compromised blood flow produces clinically apparent ischemia. Ischemic colitis (IC), first described in 1963 by Boley, consists of a wide spectrum of clinical, endoscopic, and histopathologic alterations that range from a transient intramural ischemia of the colon to transmural necrosis; the latter is associated with a high mortality. This disease occurs typically in elderly patients when, as a result of inadequate tissue blood flow, the metabolic demands of the tissue supersede the delivery of oxygen, resulting in colonic ischemia. Most frequently, a non-occlusive diminution of the colonic blood flow is present, although occlusive factors can also be involved. The diagnosis of IC requires a high degree of clinical suspicion and confirmed by colonoscopy, the diagnostic method of choice. Most patients have intramural ischemia and a good prognosis, requiring only conservative management, whereas when transmural ischemia is evident, aggressive operative resection is indicated.

Epidemiology and Etiology

Approximately 1 in 2,000 acute hospital admissions are attributed to IC. The incidence of IC has been reported between 4.5 and 44 cases per 100,000 person-years. This incidence, however, may be under-estimated due to the difficult diagnosis, especially in mild cases. In fact, after aortic surgery, in only 50% of patients with endoscopic and histologic confirmation of IC was the diagnosis suspected initially. IC is the most frequent form of ischemic changes of the gastrointestinal tract, representing approximately 50–60% of such cases. Generally, IC affects elderly people in the seventh and eight decades, with 90% of patients being older than 60 years of age. Irrespective of age, risk factors include cocaine use, hypercoagulable states, vasculitis, trauma, and marathon runners. There is a slight predilection for women (55–64%) in most reported series. In many cases, the exact etiology of IC is difficult to find. The most common etiology of IC is a hypoperfusion state secondary to shock or cardiac failure. Additional etiologies include mesenteric arterial thrombosis or embolism producing an occlusive type of ischemia. IC may also develop after procedures where technical factors may contribute, such as vascular surgery (especially those after repair of an abdominal aortic aneurism) and left colectomy (◉ *Table 84-1*).

◘ Table 84-1

Etiology of ischemic colitis

I.	Non-occlusive factors	
	1.	Idiopathic
	2.	Shock
		(a) Septic
		(b) Hemorragia
		(c) Cardiogenic
		(d) Hypovolemic
	3.	Drugs
		(a) Catecholamines
		(b) Diuretics
		(c) Digitalis
		(d) Estrogens, oral contraceptives
		(e) NSAIDs
		(f) Cocaine
	4.	Colon obstruction
		(a) Colon cancer
		(b) Fecal impaction
II.	Occlusive factors	
	1.	Arterial
		(a) Embolus
		(b) Thrombosis
		(c) Post aortic reconstructive surgery
		(d) Trauma
		(e) Vasculitis
	2.	Venous
		(a) Hypercoagulable status
		(b) Pancreatitis

Pathophysiology

Perfusion of the colon and rectum depends on inflow from the mesenteric arteries (superior and inferior) and on the internal iliac vessels. In the region of the splenic flexure, the arc of Riolan and the marginal artery of Drummond join the superior and inferior mesenteric systems, producing a zone potentially vulnerable to ischemia (also called the watershed area) where the blood supply between both arterial territories is suboptimal. Up to 30% of the patients do not have a sufficient communication between both systems, predisposing this area of the splenic flexure to ischemia. Despite this, IC is usually not confined to the splenic flexure, and any segment of the colon can be affected, leading some to question whether IC is really an ischemic phenomenon at all. IC occurs most commonly in the descending and sigmoid colon (40%), followed by the transverse colon and splenic flexure (17%), the splenic flexure alone (11%), the right colon (12%), and the rectum (6%). The ischemia is secondary to alterations of the systemic circulation or of the mesenteric circulation itself. The colon is particularly sensitive to decreased mesenteric blood flow, because the colonic circulation does not have an adequate self-regulation and because there is poor microcirculation in the muscular walls. The histologic alterations consist initially of edema and hemorrhage of the mucosa and submucosa, with the potential for progression to ulceration, transmural ischemia, necrosis, and eventual perforation. In cases of non-transmural colonic ischemia, parietal fibrosis with secondary colonic stricture may develop in the long term.

Clinical Presentation

The central point in the clinical presentation and diagnostic evaluation of the patient with IC is clinical suspicion. The clinician must consider the diagnosis of IC in elderly patients with abdominal symptoms and risk factors such as recent aortic surgery (ligated inferior mesenteric artery), patients in shock and under the effect of vasoconstrictor drugs (diminution of the mesenteric and specially colonic blood flow), and patients with predisposing factors to mesenteric insufficiency (atherosclerotic vascular disease, ischemic heart disease, congestive heart failure). Although this is the classic history of a patient with IC, this diagnosis must also be considered in young patients (especially women) using cocaine or oral contraceptives, patients with known vasculitis or hypercoagulable states, and in long distance runners. The clinical presentation is dependent frequently on the degree of colonic ischemia. IC should be suspected in patients with risk factors who present with slight to moderate abdominal pain (2/3 of the patients), bloody diarrhea (2/3 of the patients), nausea/vomiting (1/3 of the patients), or abdominal distention. The pain is generally sudden in onset, crampy, located in the left side of the abdomen, and associated with urge to defecate. Rectal bleeding, red or darker, according to the location of the ischemia, is generally self-limiting, and transfusion is required only rarely. Initially, the patient with IC is generally stable, without hemodynamic compromise and without signs of peritonitis, reflecting the fact that most of the patients do not have transmural ischemia; however, when transmural ischemia is present, the patients will develop peritoneal signs, and the risk of perforation is imminent.

Diagnosis

Patients with suspected IC must undergo appropriate evaluation to confirm the diagnosis. The biochemical markers are generally non-specific; however, leukocytosis may be present. Serum lactate determination deserves special mention due to its frequent use when intestinal ischemia is suspected. Although it is true that serum lactate increases in some patients with advanced IC, the serum lactate level is non-specific and lacks adequate sensitivity. Second, in intestinal ischemia, lactate is removed from the portal circulation by the liver; therefore, its utility is extremely low, especially in the initial phase of IC.

In the evaluation of patients with abdominal pain, abdominal and chest radiographs may be useful to exclude other diagnoses, such as visceral perforation or intestinal obstruction. The radiographic findings in IC are also generally non-specific. Air/barium contrast enemas have the risk of further decreasing the effective colonic blood flow by increasing the parietal pressure, may interfere with subsequent study by computed tomography (CT), and are not recommended when IC is suspected. CT of the abdomen and pelvis allows for screening of other abdominal pathologies and, in the case of IC, can demonstrate a non-specific segmental thickening of the colonic wall, air within the colon wall, or free air. Angiography is generally not useful because of its low sensitivity. Colonoscopy is the preferred diagnostic modality in patients with suspicion of IC.

In emergency cases, in which the colon cannot be prepared (e.g., patients in the intensive care unit), careful endoscopic examination requires gentle water flush to clean the colonic mucosa for inspection. Minimal insufflation of the colon during colonoscopy is necessary to avoid perforation when transmural ischemia is present. In more clinically stable patients where time allows, it may be possible to give an oral bowel preparation prior to endoscopy. The endoscopic study must be made as early as possible to determine presence of ischemia and allow appropriate intervention to avoid progressive ischemia or perforation. The endoscopic view is fundamental for the diagnosis, evaluation of the magnitude of the ischemia, management, and follow-up of the patient. In mild cases, the mucosa and submucosa appears edematous and erythematous with hemorrhagic nodules or with disrupted zones of mucosa, submucosa, and abundant fibrin. In advanced cases, the colonic mucosa is edematous with a greenish, grayish, or even black appearance corresponding to transmural ischemia or frank necrosis. Patients treated conservatively must be followed endoscopically based on the initial degree of ischemia and the patient's clinical evolution.

Patient Management

Most patients have a slight, reversible ischemia that never progresses to transmural disease. When the definitive diagnosis is made, all potentially contributing factors contributing to the ischemia must be corrected. Treatment includes intestinal rest, rehydration, optimization of cardiac function, and discontinuation of vasoconstrictor drugs. Although there is no evidence-based proof of the benefit of antibiotic use in IC, their use is recommended typically because of the theoretic protection against bacterial translocation and because of the possible progression toward gangrene. The patient requires regular and frequent (every 6–8 h) clinical, endoscopic, and laboratory reevaluation in order to detect signs of ischemic progression. In the case of ischemic progression despite aggressive conservative management, operative intervention is recommended. Other indications for urgent operative intervention are patients who present with peritoneal signs, patients diagnosed with transmural necrosis during colonoscopy, fulminate colitis, and, rarely, massive lower GI bleeding. Typically, a segmental colectomy is adequate, resecting the ischemic colon with a margin of normal, non-ischemic bowel and performing a proximal diverting colostomy. The distal end may be matured as a mucous fistula or can be left in the abdomen as a Hartmann's pouch. Only in cases of ischemia of the right colon and in hemodynamically stable patients should a ileocolic primary anastomosis be considered. Indications for semi-elective operative intervention are for those patients with persistent symptoms and signs of colitis for more than 2 weeks, patients who develop a protein-losing colopathy, or patients with recurrent septic episodes attributable to the IC. In these patients, a segmental colectomy with a primary anastomosis may be performed according to the clinical condition of the patient. Finally, there are also indications for elective colectomy, such as chronic IC with development of colonic stricture or the unusual patient with chronic segmental colitis. When symptomatic, segmental resection with primary anastomosis is warranted (❯ *Table 84-2*).

Prognosis and Results

Of all patients with IC, approximately 80–85% have a non-transmural ischemia. Of them, 70% recover completely with conservative therapy and are asymptomatic after 1–2 weeks. Nearly 10% eventually will go on to develop a symptomatic ischemic stricture that requires operative resolution, and up to 20% will develop a chronic ischemic colitis that also will need a partial colectomy (❯ *Fig. 84-1*). Patients

◘ Table 84-2
Operative indications in ischemic colitis

1. Acute
   (a) Peritonitis
   (b) Massive lower GI bleeding
   (c) Fulminant colitis
2. Subacute
   (a) Segmental colitis with persistent symptoms
   (b) Protein-losing colopathy
   (c) Recurrent sepsis attributable to IC
3. Chronic
   (a) Symptomatic stricture
   (b) Symptomatic segmental IC

◘ Figure 84-1
Classification of ischemic colitis

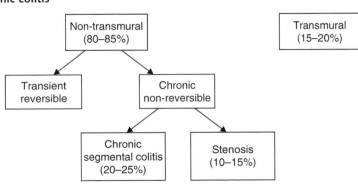

who require emergency operation because of transmural disease (15– 20%) have a mortality rate near to 50–60% because of sepsis or related complications. The factors associated with a poor prognosis after operative treatment of IC are early hemodynamic instability, IC secondary to aortic surgery (mortality approaching 80%), IC after operations employing extracorporeal circulation (mortality of 75%), and total colonic ischemia (mortality of 70%).

Conclusion

A high clinical suspicion and early endoscopic diagnosis are the most important determining factors in evaluation and management of the patients with IC. Most patients with IC will require only conservative management. Nevertheless, those patients who have a rapid progression of transmural disease require prompt and aggressive surgical treatment. This group of patients has a high mortality associated generally with their frequent and complex co-morbidities, sepsis, and multiple organ failure.

Selected Readings

Brandt LJ (2000) AGA technical review on intestinal ischemia. Gastroenterology 118:954–968

Church J (1995) Ischemic colitis. In: Church J (ed) Endoscopy of the colon, rectum and anus. Igaku-Shoin, New York/Tokyo, 328–331

Higgins PDR, Davis KJ, Laine L (2004) Systematic review: the epidemiology of ischemic colitis. Aliment Pharmacol Ther 19:729–738

MacDonald PH (2002) Ischemic colitis. Best Pract Res Clin Gastroenterol 16:51–61

Medina C, Vilaseca J, Videla S, et al. (2004) Outcome of patients with ischemic colitis: review of fifty-three cases. Dis Colon Rectum 47:180–184

Sreenarasimhaiah J (2005) Diagnosis and management of ischemic colitis. Current Gastroenterology Reports 7:421–426

85 Hemorrhoids

Francis Seow-Choen · Kok-Yang Tan

Pearls and Pitfalls

- Hemorrhoidal tissue is a normal anatomical structure that is only of concern when symptomatic.
- Factors predisposing to hemorrhoids include: hereditary factors, straining during defecation, squatting during defecation, and pregnancy.
- Use of a high fiber diet is controversial and may aggravate symptoms.
- Other sinister colorectal conditions may mimic hemorrhoid symptoms.
- Only symptomatic hemorrhoids require treatment.
- Hemorrhoids are traditionally divided into 4 degrees. Each degree should, however, be subdivided into large and small piles.
- Some small fourth-degree hemorrhoids may be treated conservatively, however, large first-degree piles may require operative intervention.
- Single pedicle rubber band ligation is efficacious and superior to injection sclerotherapy.
- Stapled hemorrhoidopexy is efficacious in most patients that require operative intervention.
- Patients with filiform skin tags or singular hemorrhoid prolapse should be treated with conventional operative excision.

Pathophysiology

Hemorrhoidal tissues are derived from the anal vascular cushions. Hemorrhoids are present as normal structures in every individual beginning in fetal life. These vascular cushions consist of mucosa, submucosal fibro-elastic connective tissues, smooth muscle, and arterio-venous channels. These arterio-venous channels, which control the size of the anal cushions, are involved in the fine control of continence to liquids and gases, and function normally when they are in their proper position in the anal canal. Fixation is by submucosal smooth muscle and elastic fibers, which act as suspensory ligaments anchoring the anal cushions to the anal sphincters.

Even totally asymptomatic people can engorge their anal cushions massively by bearing down. Performing a Valsalva maneuver during proctoscopy will confirm this fact. Vascular engorgement of anal cushions is also made more obvious by straining in the squatting position. We believe that the propensity of the Asian population to have larger hemorrhoids (piles) is in part related to many Asian toilets being of the squatting type. Prolonged and repeated straining on a sitting toilet also results in engorgement of these cushions. As such, reading in the toilet and prolonged and repeated straining with chronic constipation or frequent diarrhea also predispose to symptomatic hemorrhoids. Pregnancy and delivery exert tremendous pressure or bearing down and are also common causes of large, congested, and prolapsed piles.

Once prolapse occurs, further engorgement of these arteriovenous channels occurs. This leads to pain and inflammation. Anal spasm then prevents reduction of the prolapsed tissue and edema, and inflammation and thrombosis ensue. As long as thrombosis has not occurred, these engorged cushions will shrink rapidly once they are reduced into the anal canal.

Chronic prolapse occurs when there is repeated prolapse and congestion of the hemorrhoids and the hemorrhoidal suspensory ligaments are sheared and fragmented. (❯ *Fig. 85-1*) The vascular cushions can then prolapse easily, and when anal sphincters contract, there is further aggravation of edema and congestion. In genetically predisposed individuals, symptomatic prolapse may occur at a much younger age without conscious straining of stool.

Clinical Presentation

Many patients remain asymptomatic despite having prolapsed hemorrhoids. Hemorrhoids should not be treated unless they are symptomatic.

The most common symptoms of hemorrhoids are bleeding, prolapse, pain, and perianal pruritis.

While most patients suffering from piles are aware of bleeding symptoms, it is often remarkable that many are unaware as to whether their hemorrhoids are prolapsed or not. This may not be entirely surprising, considering that not everyone is aware of the normal anatomy of the anal region. Many patients with large prolapsed hemorrhoids will answer in the negative when asked if they had any prolapsed hemorrhoids. Prolapse may be reducible spontaneously after defecation, may require digital reduction, or may be irreducible. Pain may be caused by acute thrombosis of the prolapsed tissue, edema, or strangulation. Pain may also be secondary to concomitant anal fissures. Bleeding occurs when the vascular channels within the hemorrhoidal tissues rupture. This may occur at any stage of prolapse. Patients often complain of fresh blood dripping after defecation; others experience staining only on wiping. Perianal pruritis is commonly due to mild fecal or mucus discharge around the perianal area, which leads to perianal inflammation or dermatitis.

◼ Figure 85-1

Prolapse of hemorrhoids results from partial or complete rupture of suspensory ligaments which anchors the hemorrhoidal tissues above the anorectal junction

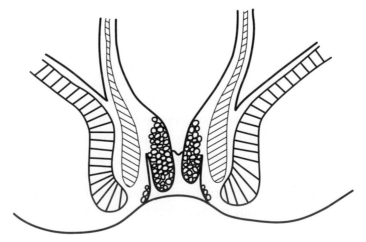

It is important to note that hemorrhoids are very common and may coexist with other more sinister colorectal conditions. Rectal cancer may present with symptoms similar to those of hemorrhoids. Indeed, there have been patients who were treated for bleeding hemorrhoids and were later found on colonoscopy to harbor rectal cancers.

Any patient who has blood or mucus mixed with stools, change in bowel habits, abdominal symptoms, or a family history of colorectal cancer should undergo endoscopic evaluation. We recommend colonoscopy in patients above 40 years of age. Younger patients should at least have a sigmoidoscopy, as one encounters young patients, even those without a family history, with silent colorectal cancer or inflammatory bowel disease.

Diagnosis and Staging of Hemorrhoids

The diagnosis of hemorrhoids is clinical. A proper anorectal examination is essential to assess fully the severity of the hemorrhoids and exclude concomitant anorectal pathology. We examine our patients in the left lateral position with good lighting. Careful inspection of the perianal region and anus is performed to exclude anal fissures, fistulae, and tumors. This examination is followed by proctoscopy with a wide and beveled Graeme-Anderson proctoscope.

Prolapsed piles are conveniently graded into the various degrees of prolapse for purposes of treatment (❯ *Table 85-1*). First-degree hemorrhoids are due to circulatory disturbances within the anal cushions leading to engorgement and swelling of the hemorrhoidal tissues. These hemorrhoidal tissues are located anatomically at the anorectal junction in the submucosal plane and are fixed in place by perihemorrhoidal condensed fibers of the longitudinal layer of the internal anal sphincter. These fibers are especially thick at the dentate line, where they are known as the suspensory ligaments of Parks. Partial rupture of these ligaments allows the hemorrhoidal tissues to slide downward during defecation; however, because there is sufficient residual contractile activity in intact fibers, hemorrhoids are withdrawn spontaneously after defecation. These are considered to be second-degree hemorrhoids.

In third-degree hemorrhoids, these ligaments are ruptured almost completely. Once prolapsed, spontaneous reduction is not possible, and manual reduction is required. The perianal skin is stretched in fourth-degree hemorrhoids, and thus, complete reduction is not possible or prolapse recurs immediately after reduction.

Patients often have mixed degrees of prolapse, with one portion at a different severity from the others. Surgeons normally assign the degree of prolapse as that of the most severely affected hemorrhoid.

◘ Table 85-1

Classification of internal hemorrhoids

Degree	Description
1	Hemorrhoids protrude into anal canal and often bleed, but do not prolapse
2	Hemorrhoids may protrude beyond anal verge with straining or defecation, but reduce spontaneously when straining ceases
3	Hemorrhoids protrude spontaneously or with straining, and require manual reduction
4	Hemorrhoids chronically prolapse and cannot be reduced. They usually contain both internal and external component and may present with acute thrombosis or strangulation

Physicians should be aware that at every level of prolapse, the hemorrhoidal tissues can be large or small. Hence, there are large first-degree hemorrhoids which may demand therapy because of incessant bleeding and small fourth-degree hemorrhoids that are asymptomatic and do not require treatment.

Treatment

Two important issues are worthy of re-emphasis. First, in the assessment of hemorrhoidal symptoms, it is very important to ensure that symptoms are not attributed to hemorrhoids prior to screening the rectum. Second, hemorrhoids are treated on the basis of symptoms and not just on the degree of prolapse. The degree of prolapse and the size of the hemorrhoids help to determine the appropriate therapy.

Nonoperative Treatment

Because hemorrhoids have an important function in fine-tuning continence, one should first use non-operative methods of treatment if hemorrhoids are prolapsing minimally. The first thing to do is to correct toilet habits. Sitting toilets are preferred to squatting toilets. Reading and other habits that emphasize straining or prolong the time required for defecation should be discouraged.

Although many health authorities recommend a high fiber diet as a treatment for constipation, our experience has been that in up to 60% of patients, high fiber diet often aggravates constipation by producing bigger, harder, and more compact stools. Many constipated patients actually require a decrease or stoppage of dietary fiber to ease the act of defecation. Adequate fluid intake is essential and must be encouraged. Many patients with prolapsed hemorrhoids drink inadequate fluids secondary to various lifestyle reasons.

Micronized diosmin and hesperidin (Daflon 500) have pharmacologic properties that include venous contraction, reduction in blood extravasation from capillaries, and inhibition of the inflammatory response. These properties have proven to reduce hemorrhoidal symptoms. Thus, these agents can be useful as primary treatment and also as an adjunct to other forms of treatment.

Rubber band ligation is useful for first-and second-degree hemorrhoids that are not too large but sufficiently symptomatic for patients to seek treatment. One or two small rubber bands are applied to the pedicle of the hemorrhoid tissue *above* the dentate line. This results in a pulling inwards of the bulk of the hemorrhoid tissue (❷ *Fig. 85-2*). Four to 5 days later, the ligated tissue necroses and sloughs off. The wound then undergoes fibrosis with resultant fixation of the mucosa and prevention of engorgement and prolapse. Banding is 60–80% effective, but there is a 2–5% risk of secondary hemorrhage occurring 4–7 days postoperatively.

Sclerosant agents used include phenol (5%) in almond oil or sodium tetradecate. These solutions are injected into the submucosa of the pedicle. We do not favor this method, because we find that the results are inferior to those of rubber band ligation. The injection needle causes bleeding, which on occasion may be dramatically brisk. There is also the risk of intra-vaginal or prostatic injection. We do not recommend infrared photocoagulation unless patients are in coagulopathy. Similarly, cryotherapy is not recommended by us, as it is associated with an unpleasant and odorous discharge. Hemorrhoidal artery ligation using a Doppler-guided anoscope shows promise with regard to technical ease and effectiveness. Further studies are needed on these novel surgical approaches.

☐ **Figure 85-2**
Rubber band ligation of hemorrhoids. A small rubber band is applied to the pedical of the hemorrhoidal tissue above the dentate line

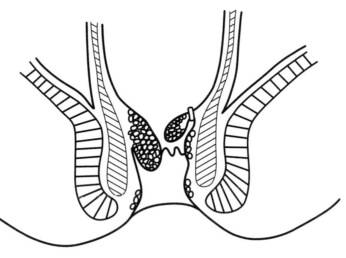

Operative Treatment

When the hemorrhoids are large and are at the third- or fourth-degree stage, operative management gives the most durable results. Traditionally, conventional operative excision of these hemorrhoids is recommended. There are numerous techniques that have been described pertaining to whether the wound after excision should be left open to granulate or closed primarily with sutures. There are also different techniques described with regard to the equipment used to perform the excision. The aim, however, is to excise the prolapsing hemorrhoidal tissue by dissecting it off the internal sphincter, while preserving adequate mucocutaneous bridges between the excision margins.

We believe that this form of treatment is not ideal for the following reasons. First, conventional operative excision focuses only on the symptoms without addressing the pathophysiology of hemorrhoids. The primary aim of restoring normal physiology is to restore the fixation of congested anal cushions rather than to excise them completely. Second, conventional excision is associated with substantial pain and discomfort from the time of operation and up to 3 months postoperatively. There are also frequent cases of anal incontinence, especially in the first few months after operative resection. Finally, operative excision in patients with massive circumferential hemorrhoids often results in residual or recurrent symptoms even after the performance of a Whitehead hemorrhoidectomy.

Nonetheless, excision is still performed widely. In this regard, we have found open hemorrhoidectomy using diathermy to give the best results. A trial using lateral sphincterotomy with hemorrhoidectomy to reduce sphincter spasm after excision demonstrated increased rates of incontinence and this is no longer performed. Another recent randomized, controlled, double-blind trial from Singapore using glyceryl trinitrate ointment on the postoperative wound showed that the wound healing rate was faster in the glyceryl trinitrate ointment group compared with placebo, although there was no significant difference in the pain and analgesic use. Excision using the Harmonic Scalpel and the Ligasure has been shown in recent trials to have marginal benefits in terms of operative blood loss, but larger studies and cost analysis are not available to justify their widespread use.

◘ Figure 85-3
Stapled hemorrhoidopexy excises redundant lower rectal mucosa, reduces the prolapsed hemorrhoidal tissues, and fixes them back into their proper place

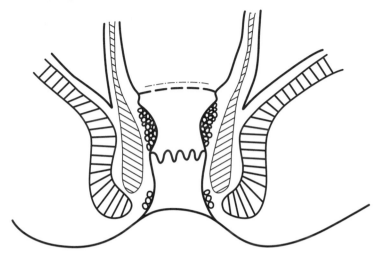

Compared with operative excision, however, stapled hemorrhoidopexy corrects the primary pathology, resulting in resolution of hemorrhoidal symptoms; this approach is now our preferred technique for patients with advanced piles. This technique excises redundant lower rectal mucosa, impressively reduces the prolapsed hemorrhoidal tissue, and fixes the prolapse back into its proper place on the wall of the anal canal (❷ *Fig. 85-3*). Fixation onto the muscle wall of the anal canal may be important to prevent subsequent dislodgement and recurrence. Once reduced, the engorged hemorrhoidal tissues decongest and shrink rapidly. We have found a modification of this technique suitable for acute thrombosed hemorrhoids as well. The preservation of the anal cushions within the anal canal may contribute to the low rate of incontinence after this operation.

Even stapled hemorrhoidopexy on its own may not deal with massive circumferential hemorrhoidal prolapse. Prolapse more that 3–4 cm beyond the anal verge may not be housed adequately in the staple gun, and much residual hemorrhoidal tissue will remain prolapsed. Residual skin tags or external components may also result in less than ideal outcome. Various novel techniques to deal with these difficult issues have been described, ranging from elliptical mucosal excision after stapling to mucosal excision before insertion of the purse-string. Minor complications of acute urinary retention and bleeding occur in about 5% of patients undergoing operative excision or stapling. Postoperative pain requiring readmission and anorectal stricture occurs in 1–2% of patients. The recurrence rate after a median follow-up of 16 months was 0.3%. These results confirm the safety and efficacy of stapled hemorrhoidopexy.

Conclusion

In the treatment of hemorrhoids, an understanding of the pathophysiology is essential and efforts should be directed at restoring the weakened support for anal cushions in order to produce the best results.

Treatment should be instituted only if symptomatic, and efforts to exclude concomitant sinister colorectal disease should not be spared. Rubber band ligation remains the best non-operative option, while stapled hemorrhoidopexy is efficacious for most patients who require operative intervention.

Selected Readings

Ho YH, Tan M, Seow-Choen F, Goh HS (2000) Micronized purified flavonidic fraction compared favorably with rubber band ligation and fiber alone in the management of bleeding hemorrhoids. Randomized controlled trial. Dis Colon Rectum 43:66–68

Lloyd D, Ho KS, Seow-Choen F (2002) Modified Longo's hemorrhoidectomy. Dis Colon Rectum 45:416–417

Ng KH, Ho KS, Ooi BS, et al. (2006) Experience of 3711 stapled hemorrhoidectomy operations. Br J Surg 93:226–230

Seow-Choen F (2002) Surgery for hemorrhoids: ablation or correction. Asian J Surg 25:265–266

Tan KY, Sng KK, Tay KH, et al. (2006) Randomized double blind clinical trial 0.2 percent glyceryl trinitrate ointment on wound healing and pain reduction after open diathermy hemorrhoidectomy. Br J Surg 93:1464–1468

Thomson WHG (1975) The nature of hemorrhoids. Br J Surg 62:542–552

Part 7

Colon and Rectum: Malignant

86 Premalignant Polyps of the Colon and Rectum

David J. Maron · Robert D. Fry

Pearls and Pitfalls

- Most colorectal cancers arise from benign polyps that transform histologically into neoplasms.
- The "adenoma-carcinoma sequence" describes the process by which a benign polyp develops into an invasive cancer.
- The removal of benign polyps detected during colonoscopy has been shown to decrease the incidence of colorectal cancer.
- The possibility of a polyp containing carcinoma increases with size and with villous architecture.
  - A tubular adenoma smaller than 1 cm has a less than 5% chance of containing cancer.
  - A villous adenoma larger than 2 cm has a greater than 50% chance of containing cancer.
- Familial adenomatous polyposis (FAP) is a hereditary syndrome caused by a mutation in the APC gene and characterized by over 100 polyps arising in the colon and rectum; the incidence of colorectal cancer approaches 100%.
- Attenuated familial adenomatous polyposis is characterized by a significant risk for cancer, but with colorectal polyps (average of 30).
- Patients suspected of having attenuated familial polyposis, but in whom genetic testing fails to reveal an APC mutation, should be investigated for an MYH genetic mutation.
- Hereditary nonpolyposis colorectal cancer syndrome (HNPCC) is caused by a mutation in DNA repair genes and is associated with an increased cancer risk of not only colorectal cancer, but other organ sites including: endometrium, stomach, gall bladder, kidney and small intestine.
- Cancer incidence in patients with HNPCC can be decreased by surveillance colonoscopy, performed every 2 years after age 20 and annually after age 35.
- Colon cancer in the patient with HNPCC should be treated by abdominal colectomy and ileorectal anastomosis.
- The risk of metastases from cancer arising in a colorectal polyp can be assessed by determining the depth of invasion into the polyp (Haggit's level).

Introduction

A colorectal polyp may be defined as a mass that arises from the surface of the intestinal epithelium and projects into the intestinal lumen. These lesions may be characterized by their gross appearance as sessile (relatively flat) or pedunculated (with a stalk). The histological pattern of the epithelium of a polyp may also be used to further describe the lesion. The epithelium of a colorectal polyp is generally characterized by pathologists as being of one of three common varieties: tubular (with branched, tubular appearing glands), villous (with long frond-like projections of surface epithelium), or tubulovillous (containing both tubular and frond-like epithelium). Tubular adenomas are the most common polyps of the large bowel (comprising about three fourths of all polyps), and are typically pedunculated. About 15% of polyps are tubulovillous, and a slightly lesser number are villous adenomas, which are most often sessile.

The basic definition of a polyp given above is usually used to initiate a discussion of benign, or at least minimally invasive, early neoplasms. However, a "mass of surface epithelium that projects into the lumen of the intestine" also describes the majority of cancers of the large bowel. Although polyps may bleed and can (rarely) cause obstructive symptoms by serving as a lead point for an intussusception, their importance lies in the close relationship between benign growths and invasive cancer of the large bowel. The purpose of this chapter is to examine that relationship in the light of evidence that has been gathered by surgeons, gastroenterologists, pathologists, epidemiologists, and molecular geneticists, with emphasis on relatively recent observations and discoveries that have enhanced our understanding of that relationship.

The Adenoma-Carcinoma Sequence

Although a quarter of a century ago there was considerable controversy over the concept that a benign polyp is a precursor to cancer, the evidence from many fronts provides such strong support for the adenoma-carcinoma sequence that this concept is generally unquestioned today. It is naïve to assume that all colorectal polyps are predestined to become cancerous, and there have been documented cases (especially in the Japanese literature) that occasionally large bowel cancers can arise directly from the mucosa without being associated with a benign precursor. Nevertheless, our understanding of the process of colorectal carcinogenesis assumes the fact that most cancers arise from benign polypoid precursors.

Evidence that supports the notion that benign polyps may be premalignant include the observation that microscopic examination of a colonic cancer will often reveal elements of a benign tubular or villous adenoma adjacent to, and often inseparable from, the cancer. In fact, the pathologist may often describe the cancer as "arising from a villous adenoma."

The incidence of both benign polyps and colon cancers increases with patients' age, with the polyps' rising incidence preceding that of the cancers' by about 7–10 years. This suggests a 7–10-year "dwell time" for a benign polyp to acquire malignant characteristics.

Colonic polyps occur more frequently in patients who have colorectal cancer. At least one third of patients with a colorectal cancer will have a polyp elsewhere in the large bowel. Removal of benign polyps by screening colonoscopy reduces the expected incidence of colorectal cancer in the population undergoing screening.

Large polyps are found to contain cancer much more often than small polyps, and the larger the polyp, the higher the chance that it is cancerous. The histological pattern of the polyp is also important; a tubular adenoma smaller than 1 cm in size has less than a 5% chance of containing invasive cancer, while the risk of cancer in a tubular adenoma larger than 2 cm is at least 35%. A villous adenoma larger than 2 cm has an approximately 50% chance of containing cancer.

Patients with familial polyposis, in which there are literally hundreds of adenomatous polyps throughout the colon, will invariably develop colorectal cancer if not treated. The adenomatous polyps in these patients are indistinguishable from the colorectal polyps that occur in the general population, both histologically and by genetic markers.

Perhaps most convincing of all these observations in the support of the adenoma-carcinoma sequence is the discovery of the molecular model of carcinogenesis by Fearon and Vogelstein, which describes the step-by-step progression from normal epithelium through benign adenoma to invasive cancer at the molecular level (❷ *Fig. 86-1*).

◘ Figure 86-1
Model of colorectal carcinogenesis (Modified from Corman, 1998. With permission; after Fearon and Vogelstein, 1990. Copyright 1990. With permission from Elsevier)

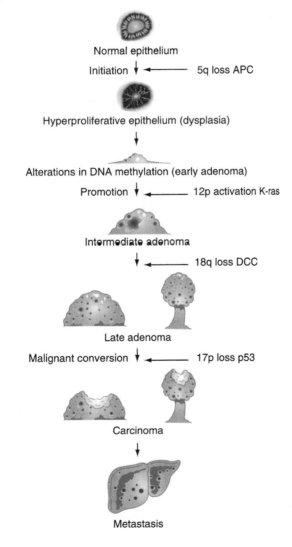

Normal epithelium

Initiation ↓ ⟵——— 5q loss APC

Hyperproliferative epithelium (dysplasia)
↓

Alterations in DNA methylation (early adenoma)

Promotion ↓ ⟵——— 12p activation K-ras

Intermediate adenoma

↓ ⟵——— 18q loss DCC

Late adenoma

Malignant conversion ↓ ⟵——— 17p loss p53

Carcinoma
↓

Metastasis

Polyps and Hereditary Colorectal Cancer Syndromes

APC-Associated Polyposis Syndromes

There are several recognized inherited syndromes which predispose a carrier to colorectal cancer. APC-associated polyposis syndromes include *familial adenomatous polyposis (FAP), attenuated FAP, Gardner's syndrome, and Turcot's syndrome.* These syndromes are all caused by mutations in the APC gene, located on chromosome 5q. FAP is characterized by hundreds to thousands of adenomatous polyps arising in the large bowel, usually appearing after puberty and increasing in number with age. Patients with this syndrome will invariably develop colorectal cancer if not treated, with a mean age of cancer in untreated patients of 39 years. The appropriate surgical treatment depends somewhat upon the number of polyps involving the rectum, but there is no controversy involving the importance of removing the colon that is harboring the numerous benign appearing adenomatous polyps, one or more of which will certainly progress to cancer. The rectum may be preserved in some instances (by abdominal colectomy with anastomosis between the ileum and rectum) with the understanding that surveillance (proctoscopy) is required every 6 months to detect and eradicate any polyps that subsequently arise. If the rectum should harbor too many polyps to consider this approach (which is usually the case), the appropriate treatment is restorative proctocolectomy with ileal pouch anal anastomosis.

Attenuated FAP is characterized by a significant risk for colorectal cancer, but with fewer polyps (average of 30) than classic FAP. The polyps tend to be located more proximally in the colon than in classic FAP, and the average age of cancer diagnoses in individuals with attenuated FAP is 50–55 years (10–15 years later than in patients with classic FAP, but earlier than in patients with sporadic colorectal cancer). Management is significantly different than that of FAP, but the importance of recognizing the syndrome and the risk associated with numerous premalignant polyps is obvious. Abdominal colectomy with ileorectal anastomosis is the preferred treatment for individuals with this syndrome, but segmental colectomy with annual colonoscopy to remove any new polyps is an acceptable approach for some patients.

Gardner's syndrome is FAP associated with osteomas and soft tissue tumors (epidermoid cysts, fibromas, desmoid tumors). Usually these tumors are innocuous, but retroperitoneal or mesenteric desmoid tumors arising after colectomy may be very problematic. The treatment of desmoids arising in patients with FAP includes surgical excision, radiation, nonsteroidal anti-inflammatory drugs (NSAIDS), anti-estrogens, and cytotoxic chemotherapy.

Gardner's syndrome was once thought to be a distinct clinical entity, but it is now recognized that mutations in the APC gene are responsible for both classic FAP and Gardner's syndrome. Some correlation exists between extraintestinal growths and the mutation location in APC.

Turcot's syndrome is the association of CNS tumors, usually medulloblastomas, with colorectal polyposis. The numbers of polyps that occur, as well as the phenotypic features of Gardner's syndrome and Turcot's syndrome, relate to the location of the APC mutation. (Two thirds of Turcot's syndromes are associated with APC mutations, but one third are associated with HNPCC mutations, described below. The CNS tumors in individuals with HNPCC are usually glioblastoma multiforme.)

APC-associated polyposis syndromes are inherited in an autosomal dominant fashion. Approximately 75–80% of patients with APC-associated polyposis will have an affected parent, with the remaining individuals representing a new mutation. Molecular genetic testing of APC detects disease-causing mutations in up to 95% of probands with typical FAP.

Chemoprevention with FAP

Several studies have demonstrated temporary regression of adenomas in patients with FAP treated with nonsteroidal anti-inflammatory drugs (NSAIDs). Celecoxib received accelerated Food and Drug Administration approval based on data showing a reduction of polyp burden in individuals with FAP, although the clinical benefit of this COX-2 inhibitor was not proven. Unfortunately, these somewhat optimistic results were tempered with data showing that refecoxib, a COX-2 inhibitor, increases the risk of cardiovascular events.

COX-2 inhibitors are unlikely to play a role in colorectal cancer prevention in the general population, but they currently are recommended by some for FAP patients with a low polyp burden in the rectum who have been treated with abdominal colectomy and ileorectal anastomosis in the hopes of delaying or preventing the need for proctectomy.

MYH-Associated Polyposis

MYH is a DNA repair gene that corrects DNA base pair mismatch errors in the genetic code prior to replication. Mutations in the MYH gene are associated with a high risk of colorectal cancer and a syndrome of premalignant polyposis similar to that seen with attenuated FAP. However, the disorder is inherited in an autosomal recessive manner, so two copies of the gene must carry a mutation. If an APC mutation is not identified in a patient suspected of having FAP or attenuated FAP, molecular genetic testing of MYH should be considered.

Hereditary Non-polyposis Colorectal Cancer

HNPCC is an autosomal dominant colorectal cancer syndrome with polyps that appear grossly similar to APC-associated polyps that arise with somewhat greater frequency in the proximal colon. The "dwell time" during which cancer arises in these polyps appears to be relatively short, and apparently benign polyps have progressed to cancer within the time span of a year ("accelerated carcinogenesis"). There are far fewer colorectal polyps appearing in this syndrome than in patients with FAP, but there is an increased incidence of other malignancies, including cancer of the endometrium, ovary, stomach, small intestine, pancreas, ureter and renal pelvis. HNPCC is caused by mutations in DNA mismatch repair genes, primarily MLH1, MSH2, and to a lesser frequency MSH6 and PMS2. Microscopically the tumors appear aggressive (poorly differentiated, Signet cells), and the tumors are characterized by microsatellite instability (MSI) that can be demonstrated on testing a tumor block from the cancer.

A family history is critical to detect patients with HNPCC. Before the genetic mutations responsible for the syndrome were recognized, the diagnosis was made based upon three elements known as the Amsterdam criteria: (1) colorectal cancer in three family members (first-degree relatives),

(2) involvement of at least two generations, and (3) at least one affected individual being younger than the age of 50 at the time of diagnosis. The initial Amsterdam criteria has since been modified, recognizing the risk of other cancers found in the syndrome. The modified Amsterdam criteria considers not only colorectal cancer, but also endometrial, ovarian, gastric small intestinal, pancreatic and upper urinary tract cancers.

Patients with known or suspected HNPCC should have surveillance colonoscopy every 2 years beginning at age 20, and annually after age 35. In women, periodic vacuum curettage is begun at age 25, as well as pelvic ultrasound and determination of *CA-125 levels*. Annual tests for occult hematuria should also be obtained, because of the risk of upper urinary tract cancer.

Annual colonoscopy with removal of benign polyps has been shown to decrease the cancer incidence in patients with HNPCC. If colon cancer is detected, abdominal colectomy with ileorectal anastomosis should be considered. Women with known HNPCC who develop colon cancer should consider hysterectomy and bilateral oophorectomy at the time of colectomy.

The hereditary colorectal cancer syndromes account for only a small portion of all colorectal cancer. However, the identification of the genetic causes of these particular cancers, and the observations of the progression from normal mucosa to benign polyp to invasive cancer that occurs has provided insight into the development of nonhereditary colorectal carcinogenesis. The genetic abnormalities that cause APC, MYH and HNPCC syndromes are known to arise spontaneously and play a major role in the pathogenesis of noninherited colorectal cancer.

Genomic Instability

Colorectal cancer arises as a multistep progression sequence at both the molecular and morphologic levels. This observation is not incompatible with the view that many (even most) benign polyps remain forever benign and do not progress to cancer. It does not exclude the fact that cancer can arise directly from the epithelium, without a benign polypoid precursor, although this form of pathogenesis is relatively uncommon. However, most colorectal cancers arise from a polyp that acquires certain alterations transforming it from a benign growth to a lesion capable of invasion and metastasis.

It is also generally accepted that genetic and epigenetic alterations promote colorectal cancer formation because they provide a clonal growth advantage to the cells that acquire these alterations. A key molecular step that occurs early in the pathogenesis of colorectal cancer is the loss of genomic stability. Three significant forms of *genomic instability* have been identified in colon cancer: (1) microsatellite instability (MSI), (2) chromosome instability (CIN), and (3) chromosomal translocations. In addition to genomic instability, a form of epigenomic instability has been identified that results in the aberrant methylation of tumor suppressor genes. Much research is ongoing regarding the exact role of genomic and epigenomic instability in the process of tumorigenesis. It is not clear whether genomic instability commonly initiates the adenoma-carcinoma sequence or whether it arises during this process and facilitates the development of cancer. However, both CIN and MSI can be observed in adenomas, so it would appear that at least in some cases chromosomal instability appears during adenoma initiation but before progression to frank cancer.

CIN is the most common type of genomic instability observed in colorectal cancer, occurring in approximately 85% of tumors. However, despite the high incidence of CIN in colorectal cancer and the fact that aneuploidy is a well-known characteristic of cancer, our understanding of the significance of chromosomal disarray is still incomplete. It is not clear if aneuploidy is a nonspecific occurrence arising during carcinogenesis which is tolerated by the tumor, or if the chromosomal disarray reflects an active process of CIN that is an important factor in tumorigenesis.

Colorectal Polyps: Assessment of Virulence

The treatment of an adenomatous or villous colorectal polyp is removal, usually by colonoscopy; distal polyps may be removed through a transanal approach. Pedunculated polyps are usually removed by severing the stalk with a snare passed through the colonoscope. Sessile polyps may not be amenable to excision using endoscopic techniques, although in some circumstances it is possible to elevate the polyp from the underlying muscularis with saline injection, thus permitting transluminal excision without perforation of the bowel wall. However, large sessile polyps often require segmental colectomy for complete removal, even if the presence of cancer is not confirmed prior to resection.

In view of the preceding discussion, polyps should be considered premalignant, and consideration given to assessment of the presence of cancer, and to its virulence, or metastatic potential of a cancer found in the polyp. Careful histological assessment of the polyp may reveal the presence of malignant cells. If these cells are confined to the muscularis mucosae (whether the polyp is pedunculated or sessile), the potential for metastases is negligible, such a finding is usually termed "atypia", and polypectomy is sufficient treatment. However, malignant cells penetrating the muscularis mucosae possess the ability to metastasize, and such polyps contain "invasive cancer". Appropriate treatment of such polyps requires consideration of the risk of lymph node metastasis and local recurrence. Haggitt proposed a classification for polyps containing cancer based upon the depth of invasion. Haggitt's criteria is as follows (❯ *Fig. 86-2*):

▫ Figure 86-2
Anatomic landmarks of pedunculated and sessile polyps (Reprinted from Haggitt et al., 1985. Copyright 1985. With permission from the American Gastroenterological Association)

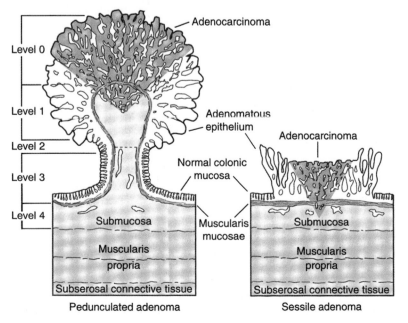

Level 0:   Cancer cells do not invade the muscularis mucosae (carcinoma-in-situ or intramucosal carcinoma)

Level 1:   Cancer penetrates the muscularis mucosae (into submucosa), but is confined to the head of the polyp

Level 2:   Cancer invades the level of the neck of the polyp (junction between the head and stalk)

Level 3:   Cancer invades the stalk

Level 4:   Cancer invades the submucosa below the stalk but above the muscularis propria

By this classification, all sessile polyps with invasive carcinoma are classified as Haggitt's Level 4.

Other factors to be considered when assessing the risk of metastases from a polyp containing cancer include the cellular differentiation of the tumor (poorly differentiated cancer is more virulent than well differentiated, with moderately differentiated cancer assuming carrying an intermediate risk). Invasion of the lymphovascular spaces by cancer cells is also a poor prognostic factor, with at least a 10% chance of metastases to lymph nodes even if the cancer appears confined to the submucosa.

A pedunculated polyp with invasion to Haggitt's Levels 1, 2, and 3 has a low risk of lymph node metastasis or local recurrence, and complete excision of the polyp is adequate if the cancer is not poorly differentiated and there is no invasion of the lymphovascular channels in the specimen. Sessile cancers containing invasive cancer have at least a 10% chance of lymphatic metastasis, and generally require resection of the involved segment of intestine.

Selected Readings

Burt RW, Leppert MF, Slattery ML, et al. (2004) Genetic testing and phenotype in a large kindred with attenuated familial adenomatous polyposis. Gastroenterology 127:444–451

Corman ML (ed) (1998) Colon and rectal surgery, 4th edn. Lippincott-Raven, Philadelphia, p 593

Fearon ER, Vogelstein BL (1990) A genetic model of colorectal cancer tumorigenesis. Cell 61:759–767

Grady WM (2006) Genomic instability and colorectal cancer. Current Colorectal Cancer Reports 2:66–71

Haggitt RC, Glotzbach RE, Soffer EE, et al. (1985) Prognostic factors in colorectal carcinomas arising in adenomas: Implications for lesions removed by endoscopic polypectomy. Gastroenterology 89:328–336

Haggitt RC, et al. (1985) Prognostic factors in colorectal carcinomas arising in adenomas: implications for lesions removed by endoscopic polypectomy. Gastroenterology 89:328–336

Vogelstein B, Fearon ER, Hamilton SR, et al. (1988) Genetic alterations during colorectal tumor development. N Engl J Med 319:525–532

Wang L, Baudhuin LM, Boardman LA, et al. (2004) MYH mutations in patients with attenuated and classic polyposis and with young-onset colorectal cancer without polyps. Gastroenterology 127:9–16

87 Management of Colon Cancer

Robin S. McLeod · Robert Gryfe

Pearls and Pitfalls

- There is strong evidence that colorectal cancer screening with fecal occult blood testing reduces cancer related mortality and decreases the incidence of colon cancer in average risk individuals.
- Taking a family history is essential in individuals with colorectal cancer since 15–20% will have a family history of colon cancer. This information may change the management of the individual with cancer and change screening recommendations in family members.
- Familial adenomatous polyposis accounts for approximately 1% of colorectal cancers while HNPCC accounts for between 3% and 5% of colorectal cancers.
- Deaths due to colorectal cancer have decreased in the past 20 years in western countries.
- Laparoscopic colon resections can be performed safely with less pain and a modest decrease in time to the return of gastrointestinal function and length of stay and similar long-term outcomes.
- There is Level I evidence that mechanical bowel preparation is unnecessary in patients having colon resections.
- Patients with cancers that have microsatellite instability (MSI) have a better prognosis although these same individuals do not appear to derive benefit from 5-fluorouracil-based adjuvant chemotherapy.
- Colectomy and ileorectal anastomosis may be the procedure of choice in individuals who have obstructing or perforating cancers and those who have synchronous cancers, HNPCC or attenuated familial adenomatous polyposis.
- Outcome is similar irrespective of the anastomotic configuration and whether it is stapled or handsewn.

Epidemiology, Incidence, Genetics

Colon cancer is among the most common cancers in the Western World. In the USA, it is estimated that more than 145,000 individuals were diagnosed with colorectal cancer in 2005 and more than 55,000 deaths were attributed to the disease; thus, making colorectal cancer the third most common cancer among males and females. Cancer is fundamentally a genetic disease in which a number of genetic alterations present in a cancer cell allow for its uncontrolled growth, evasion of cell death, local invasiveness and metastatic potential. Approximately 20% of individuals with colorectal neoplasia will have an affected first degree family member but only 5% of all patients with colorectal cancer will have an identifiable inherited genetic disorder. Inherited syndromes that predispose to colorectal cancer are generally categorized based on the presence of large numbers of adenomatous polyps, few (if any) adenomatous polyps or the presence of hamartomatous polyps (❯ *Table 87-1*). Rational treatment recommendations for patients with inherited colorectal cancer syndromes are tailored to these variable disease phenotypes.

Although genetic abnormalities are fundamental to cancer development, various behavioral risk factors have been identified which are associated with colorectal cancer. Physical activity has been shown to be protective against the development of polyps. Smoking, alcohol consumption and dietary factors have all been causally linked with colon cancer. Controversy exists as to whether fiber or animal fat content is the important factor in diet since diets high in fiber tend to be low in animal fat and vice versa. It is therefore difficult to disassociate these two factors.

Staging of Colon Cancer

Several staging systems have been described but the most widely used system is the TNM Staging System developed by the American Joint Commission on Cancer (AJCC). To be considered invasive, cancers must extend into the muscularis mucosae. Malignant cells superficial to this layer lack malignant potential and such lesions are considered to be carcinoma in situ or to be dysplastic. Four stages are recognized (❯ *Table 87-2*) and the prognosis worsens as the stage increases. Although a number of variables have been shown to have prognostic significance, the depth of invasion and

❑ Table 87-1

Inherited colorectal cancer syndromes and their associated genes

Syndrome	Associated gene
Adenomatous polyposis syndromes	
Familial adenomatous polyposis (FAP)	APC
MYH-associated polyposis (MAP)	MYH
Nonpolyposis syndrome	
Hereditary nonpolyposis colorectal cancer (HNPCC)	MSH2, MLH1, MSH6, PMS2
Hamartomatours polyp syndromes	
Peutz-Jeghers syndrome (PJS)	LKB1
Juvenile polyposis syndrome (JPS)	SMAD4, BMPR1A
Cowden disease, including Bannayan-Ruvalcaba-Riley syndrome	PTEN

❑ Table 87-2

AJCC staging classification

	Depth	Nodal status	Distant metastasis
Stage 1	T1, 2	N0	M0
Stage 2	T3, 4	N0	M0
Stage 3	Any T	Any N (except N0)	M0
Stage 4	Any T	Any N	M1

TX, primary tumor cannot be assessed; T0, no evidence of primary tumor; Tis, carcinoma in situ; T1, tumor invades into submucosa; T2, tumor invades into muscularis propria; T3, tumor invades through muscularis propria; T4a tumor perforates visceral peritoneum; T4b tumor directly invades other structures; NX, regional lymph nodes cannot be assessed; N0, no regional lymph nodes; N1, 1–3 regional lymph nodes; N2, more than 4 regional lymph nodes; N3, regional lymph nodes along a named vascular trunk; MX, presence of distant metastasis cannot be assessed; M0, no distant metastases; M1, distant metastases.

the status of the nodes are the greatest independent predictors of outcome in colon cancer. The degree of differentiation (moderate or poorly differentiated) and the presence or absence of lymphovascular invasion are also considered to be predictors of outcome. While no genetic marker has yet to gain widespread acceptance in terms of prognosis, high frequency-microsatellite instability (MSI-H), observed in approximately 15% of sporadic colorectal cancers and most cases of HNPCC, has been consistently observed to be prognostic of improved survival independent of clinical factors such as tumor stage and grade. Additionally, while it appears that patients with microsatellite stable (MSS) cancers derive a survival benefit from adjuvant 5-fluorouracil-based chemotherapy, patients with MSI-H cancers do not appear to benefit similarly.

Prevention of Colorectal Cancer

Primary Prevention

Despite strong epidemiological evidence that populations consuming diets high in animal fat and low in fiber have an increased risk of colorectal cancer, to date, modifications to diet and administration of supplements with fiber, vitamins and minerals have not been shown to decrease the risk of polyps or cancer. This apparent discrepancy may be because there is a complex association between dietary factors, and trials have tended to include only adults; modify or supplement only one or a few factors; and tend to be relatively short in duration such that a therapeutic effect may be missed.

There are several non experimental studies and randomized controlled trials assessing the effective ness of aspirin and other non steroidal anti-inflammatory agents. NSAIDS are potent inhibitors of cyclooxygenase (COX) enzymes and animal studies suggest that they produce their antineoplastic effect through both COX dependent and independent pathways. Most studies have included individuals who had a previous cancer or polyp. There appears to be some benefit in this group, although there is no evidence to date that the frequency of colonoscopic surveillance can be decreased. Furthermore, the side effects of these drugs, including gastrointestinal bleeding and cardiovascular complications, mean that further studies are required to ensure that the benefits outweigh the risks. There is also evidence from one trial that calcium may decrease the risk of adenomas (but not cancer) but this trial has inadequate power to determine whether the risk of cancer is reduced and furthermore, does not address the issue of whether colonoscopic surveillance recommendations can be modified.

Secondary Prevention

There are several screening options available including fecal occult blood testing (FOBT), flexible sigmoidoscopy, barium enema and colonoscopy. Other tests such as fecal DNA studies and virtual colonoscopy are promising but have not been adopted for general use. Screening recommendations vary depending on the personal and family history of the individual.

In average risk individuals (i.e., those without a personal or family history of colon cancer), it is usually recommended that screening be started at age 50 years. Fecal occult blood testing lacks sensitivity and specificity but it is the easiest test to perform. There is Level I evidence that annual or biennial screening with FOBT decreases cancer specific mortality as well as the incidence of colon cancer. However, approximately 1,000 individuals must be screened for 10 years to prevent one death. The evidence is less strong for the other modalities but they have been recommended as follows: (1) flexible sigmoidoscopy every 5 years, (2) combined FOBT and flexible sigmoidoscopy every 5 years, (3) colonoscopy every 10 years, and (4) double contrast barium enema every 5 years.

For individuals with a first degree relative with colon cancer, it is generally recommended that screening colonoscopy be performed starting at age 40 years or 10 years younger than the earliest age of diagnosis in the family. Individuals at risk for HNPCC should have colonoscopy every 1–2 years beginning at age 20–25 years. However, the evidence supporting this recommendation is weak. Finally, individuals who are at risk for familial adenomatous polyposis should have genetic testing if the mutation has been identified in the proband. If so, then genetic testing in the at-risk relative can be performed with 100% accuracy. Those individuals who are known to carry the APC gene or are at-risk but cannot have genetic testing require annual flexible sigmoidoscopy beginning in puberty.

Preoperative Evaluation

Patients presenting with a colon cancer require evaluation of their entire colon since polyps and synchronous cancers may be present in up to 30% of individuals and might alter management decision making. Endoscopic examination is preferred since it may also be therapeutic if another lesion is found. In some instances, it may not be possible to evaluate the proximal colon because the cancer has narrowed the lumen. If so, a careful inspection should be performed intraoperatively and colonoscopy performed post operatively. Since many colon cancer procedures are now performed laparoscopically, the tumor should also be tattooed with India ink so that it is readily identifiable at the time of surgery.

To assess the patient for metastatic disease, a CT scan should be performed. This may provide valuable information regarding the presence of metastatic disease as well as the extent of local lesion invasion. If CT scanning is not available, an ultrasound may be performed. A chest x-ray or CT scan of the chest should be performed to assess the lungs for metastatic disease.

Perioperative Care

There is Level I evidence supporting many of the perioperative measures prescribed in patients undergoing colorectal cancer surgery. Recent evidence suggests that a mechanical bowel preparation may not only be unnecessary but harmful to patients. Guenga and colleagues performed a Cochrane review that included nine trials and 1,592 patients. Following colonic surgery, both leak (2.9% vs. 1.6%; OR 1.80, 95% CI 0.68–3.26) and wound infection rates (7.4% vs. 0.4%, OR 1.46, 95% CI 0.97–2.18) were insignificantly higher in the cohort having bowel preparation.

The need for prophylactic antibiotics is well accepted. Various routines have been studied including different combinations and different routes of administration (oral or intra-venous). What is well established is that antibiotics should be administered prior to the skin incision being made so there are adequate tissue levels. Secondly, post-operative antibiotics do not appear to be required. Intraoperative doses may be required only when the case is greatly extended. There is also level I evidence that intra-operative warming reduces the risk of wound infections by approximately 50% as well as decreasing the risk of cardiac complications. Supplemental oxygenation given both pre and intraoperatively also appears to be effective in reducing the risk of surgical site infections by 50%. In addition, clipping rather than shaving may be preferable. Similarly, prophylaxis against the development of thromboembolic complications is required. Kehlet and colleagues have been proponents of "fast track" surgery (❷ *Table 87-3*). They have been able to show that functional capabilities return earlier and length of hospital stay can be reduced with a fast track approach.

Surgical Therapy

Surgical resection remains the mainstay of treatment of cancers of the colon. Since cancers spread locally, through the lymphatics and hematogenously, the oncological principles of colon cancer surgery include resection of the tumor with adequate resection margins plus removal of all lymph node bearing tissue. Depending on the site of the cancer, the segment of colon resected may vary. For most cancers, a segmental resection and primary anastomosis can be performed. However, if the patient has more than one cancer, has a family history of HNPCC or attenuated FAP, or has no family history of colon cancer but is young (i.e., less than 40 years), a colectomy and ileorectal anastomosis is often recommended depending on the site of the cancer. This is based on the rationale that the risk of a second primary cancer is high and also, surveillance of the rectum can be performed more easily. If colectomy and ileorectal anastomosis are performed the anastomosis should be carried out at the sacral promontory. Removing more of the rectum might result in a poor functional result. For patients with familial adenomatous polyposis, colectomy with ileal pouch anal anastomosis is the preferred option by most experts. However, colectomy and ileorectal anastomosis may be an acceptable option in patients who have few or no polyps in their rectum and whose family history is negative for more numerous polyposis or desmoid tumors.

For cancers of the right colon, a right hemicolectomy is performed with ligation of the ileocolic vessels. In most instances, it is necessary to mobilize the hepatic flexure in order to complete the anastomosis. Cancers of the hepatic flexure and proximal transverse colon are treated usually with an extended right hemicolectomy with ligation of both the ileocolic and middle colic vessels. For technical

◻ Table 87-3

Care program in patients undergoing resection with fast-track care

Preoperatively	Information of surgical procedure, expected length of stay and daily milestones for recovery
Day of surgery	Mobilized at 2 h
	Drink at 1 l h
	Two protein-enriched drinks
	Solid food
Postoperative day 1	Mobilized > 8 h
	Drink > 2 l
	Four protein enriched drinks
	Solid food
	Remove bladder catheter
	Plan discharge
Post operative day 2	Normal activity
	Remove epidural catheter
	Discharge after lunch

reasons, it is easier to perform an anastomosis between the terminal ileum and distal transverse or descending colon for transverse colon cancers rather than attempting to mobilize the hepatic flexure and perform a colo-colonic anastomosis. Left sided lesions require ligation of the inferior mesenteric vessels or their branches. There is no strong evidence to suggest that a high ligation of the inferior mesenteric vessels improves outcome but in many situations it is technically easier to divide the vessels at the origin of the inferior mesenteric artery rather than more distally. Splenic flexure cancers and cancers high in the left colon are often difficult to mobilize, particularly if they are large. The left branch of the inferior mesenteric artery must be divided to remove the lymph nodes. While theoretically, an anastomosis can be performed between the proximal transverse colon and proximal sigmoid colon, in reality this may be difficult and an ileosigmoid anastomosis may be necessary.

The type of anastomosis can be done at the discretion of the surgeon. There is level I evidence that sutured and stapled anastomoses can be performed with similar complication rates with the exception of stricture which is somewhat more common in stapled anastomoses. However, strictures usually are not significant and do not cause symptoms. Similarly, the configuration of the anastomosis may be based on the surgeon's preference: side to side, end to end or end to side. For sigmoid cancers, the patient should be placed in stirrups in the lithotomy position so one has the option of performing an end to end anastomosis by passing a circular stapler per anum. Otherwise the patient can be placed in the supine position unless one expects invasion of other organs.

The complication rate following elective surgery for colon cancer tends to be low. The leak rate in most series is less than 5%. Thus, it is unusual in the elective situation that a defunctioning ileostomy is required except in situations where there is a perforation, an abscess or contamination of the abdomen, if a multivisceral resection is performed or other unusual findings are encountered.

Laparoscopic Versus open Resection

Laparoscopic colon resection was first described in 1991. It has been adopted much slower than other laparoscopic abdominal procedures such as cholecystectomy and anti reflux procedures likely because it can be a technically challenging procedure. Early reports, however, suggested that laparoscopic assisted colectomy is associated with less pain, lower analgesic requirements, and a more rapid recovery. However, there was hesitancy in adopting the approach because of early reports of recurrences occurring at the site of port sites. In 1995, Ortega and colleagues reported a port site recurrence rate of 1.2% in 504 patients registered in The American Society of Colon and Rectal Surgeons database. Further concerns were raised about whether an adequate oncological resection could be performed laparoscopically since the oncological outcomes far outweigh the early functional outcomes in importance.

Multiple randomized controlled trials have been performed in Europe, South America, Asia, Australia and North America over the past decade. At present, mainly short term results are available. These results suggest that laparoscopic resection takes longer to perform, but time to pass flatus, time until solid diet is tolerated, and time to hospital discharge are decreased by approximately 30%. In absolute terms these differences are approximately 30–60 min longer for surgery but approximately 1 day shorter in the other outcomes in the laparoscopic group. Pain and narcotic requirements are similarly reduced. Interestingly though, both the CLASICC and the COST studies were not able to demonstrate differences in quality of life using several validated instruments between the two groups of patients.

Early data suggest that laparoscopic procedures can be performed equally as well and safely as open procedures with several studies showing similar numbers of nodes harvested as well as post-operative complication rates being similar or even lower. To date, four trials have reported long term data with follow-up of 1,528 patients for between 3.5 and 5 years. Reza and colleagues combined the data from these trials and reported no difference in overall mortality (OR 0.81, 95% CI 0.58–1.11); cancer related mortality (OR 0.70, 0.28–1.72) or recurrence (OR 0.88, 0.61–1.27).

The COST trial is the largest trial to report long-term outcome data. Overall, survival was 86% in the laparoscopic group and 85% in the open-colectomy group with no significant differences between groups in the time to recurrence or survival for patients with any stage of cancer. On the other hand, Lacy and colleagues reported a significantly higher cancer-related survival in patients in the laparoscopic group with the improvement being mainly due to improved outcome in the Stage III group of patients.

The evidence to date suggests that laparoscopic colectomy is an acceptable alternative to open surgery for colon cancer. Short term outcomes are modestly better, patient satisfaction appears to be high with a laparoscopic approach and oncological results appear to be similar. Laparoscopic colectomy is being quickly adopted by surgeons yet it is a difficult procedure to master and there is a definite learning curve. Some guidelines suggest that a surgeon should perform at least 20 laparoscopic colectomies in patients with benign disease before undertaking a laparoscopic colectomy for malignant disease. Even that number may be inadequate and certainly patients should be chosen carefully during the early phase of adoption.

Most procedures are actually laparoscopic assisted procedures. For malignant disease, the colon should be mobilized and vessels taken intracorporally before exteriorizing the bowel to do the anastomosis. Most authors recommend making an adequate incision and using a wound protector to exteriorize the bowel to minimize the chance of a local recurrence.

Special Situations

Obstructing Cancers

Cancers are the most common cause of large bowel obstruction. Left sided cancers are more likely to cause obstruction, but obstruction may be caused by cancers at virtually any location. Obstructing cancers tend to be large and are usually associated with a poorer prognosis with many already having distant metastases.

Treatment will depend to some extent on whether the patient is partially obstructed or completely obstructed. If possible, it is always worthwhile to delay surgery to allow the obstruction to resolve. However, if the patient is completely obstructed, emergency surgery may be necessary. For patients with right sided obstructing lesions, a right hemicolectomy with a primary anastomosis can usually be performed unless there are extenuating circumstances. A defunctioning stoma is not necessary. Treatment options for obstructing lesions of the left colon include the following: Hartmann procedure, subtotal colectomy and ileorectal or ileosigmoid anastomosis or a washout procedure followed by resection and anastomosis. In rare circumstances, a defunctioning colostomy alone may be the preferred option but it should probably be reserved for patients with significant comorbidities or who are systemically unstable or as a palliative procedure. Each of the other procedures has both advantages and disadvantages. The Hartmann procedure is the standard operation and is probably the most straight forward procedure. Mobilization of the splenic flexure, which might be difficult if the bowel is greatly distended, is not required. It is the preferred option for unstable patients or those in whom it might not be safe to perform an anastomosis. The disadvantage of a Hartmann procedure is that a second operation is required. In fact, reconstruction is never performed in a large proportion of patients who are elderly or have comorbidities. Colectomy and ileorectal or ileosigmoid anastomosis eliminates the need for a second operation. Furthermore, it eliminates stoma problems and deals with a synchronous cancer if present and unsuspected. It, however, should not be performed if the resection line is below the sacral promontory or in elderly patients as functional results might be suboptimal. In younger patients, it is probably the procedure of choice. It may also be required if there are ischemic changes or tearing of the caecal serosa due to the obstruction.

Theoretically, colonic washout followed by segmental resection and anastomosis is the best option. However, surgery for obstructing cancers is usually performed in the middle of the night and the washout tends to be tedious and fraught with mishaps so this technique has not gained popularity with many surgeons. If undertaken, the resection is performed in the usual way. Intravenous tubing is then threaded into the appendix and anesthetic tubing is inserted into the bowel at the proximal resection margin. An umbilical tape is used to fasten securely the tubing. The distal end of the anesthetic tubing is placed in a bucket. The splenic flexure needs to be mobilized so one can assist with the passage of the fluid and stool. Several liters of saline are required to wash out the colon but once completed, an anastomosis is performed.

The operative morbidity and mortality following emergency or urgent surgery for obstructing cancers is higher than following elective surgery and vary widely depending on the site of the tumor and the type of procedure performed as well as the status of the patient. Furthermore, obstructing cancers tend to be more advanced than non obstructing cancers and therefore a curative operation may be possible in only half of them. Long term survival is also significantly lower, even when adjusted for stage. Some authors have reported the survival is approximately half of that of non obstructing cancers.

Perforation

Perforation is an uncommon complication but portends a poor prognosis. The perforation may be at the site of the tumor or may occur secondarily at a proximal site, usually the caecum, in obstructing cancers. There may be invasion of other structures and organs. Primary resection is the preferred treatment and if there is a contained perforation, it may be possible to undertake a primary anastomosis. Otherwise, a colostomy or an anastomosis with a defunctioning stoma may be necessary. If the perforation is in the right colon due to an obstructing left sided lesion, a subtotal colectomy is required.

Resection in the Setting of Metastatic Disease

Approximately 25% of patients with colon cancer present with Stage IV disease. Of those, it is estimated that approximately 20% have potentially resectable primary lesions. In the vast majority of these patients, their metastatic disease is not resectable and therefore surgery, if it were performed, would be for palliative purposes only. If the patient is symptomatic (bleeding, anemia or obstruction) from the primary lesion, surgery is indicated. In the asymptomatic patient, there is controversy as to whether surgery is worthwhile. With modern chemotherapeutic regimens, median survival in this group is approximately 20 months and during this time the patient may become symptomatic from the lesion. Theoretically, surgical removal of the primary might improve survival, improve quality of life, obviate the need for surgery and likely a stoma in the future when patients may have more advanced disease and are less well systemically. On the other hand, only 10% of patients who are not resected seem to require surgery in the future. Operative mortality tends to be low but not insignificant. Results of treatment (surgery and chemotherapy vs. chemotherapy alone) are available from only a few retrospective studies which may be biased by patient selection. These results suggest that there may be a small improvement in survival in the surgery group but there are no data pertaining to quality of life. Thus, at the present time, decision making must be individualized based on the burden of metastatic disease present, the site and symptomatology of the primary tumor, the ease with which it could be resected and the age and comorbidities of the patient.

Follow-Up

Patients having curative resections for colon cancer are at risk of recurrence. There is some evidence from a small number of trials that more intensive post-operative follow-up leads to a small survival benefit. The benefit is likely due to the early diagnosis and resection of recurrent, limited disease, particularly in the lungs, liver and locally. However, it is not clear what tests or group of tests are optimal nor what the optimal timing of tests is due to the heterogeneity of the trials. There is further uncertainty since the risk of recurrence varies depending on the stage of the disease, and therefore, the follow-up regimen should perhaps be altered depending on the stage of the disease.

The rationale for surveillance is first, to detect recurrence of the cancer, and secondly, to detect polyps or other cancers at an early stage since metachronous cancers may occur in up to 5% of patients. The evidence supporting surveillance of the colon is stronger than for other sites. Based on the National Polyp Study, it is recommended that a colonoscopy be performed 1 year following surgery (unless the colon was not fully evaluated preoperatively and then colonoscopy should be performed earlier) and if that is normal, then at 3 and 5 year intervals.

Otherwise, recommendations for surveillance are somewhat arbitrary. Cancer Care Ontario, in Canada, recommends follow-up in patients with Stage IIb or III cancers when they are symptomatic and at 6 monthly intervals provided they can tolerate the diagnostic tests and surgery if recurrent disease is detected. Patients with earlier disease likely require less intense follow-up. Furthermore, if patients are deemed too old or unfit for surgery, then follow-up examinations are unnecessary.

Prognosis

Based on SEER data from the USA, the overall survival of colon cancer is approximately 65%. However, survival varies according to the stage of the disease. Thus, the mean 5-year survival of patients with Stage I disease is over 90%, with Stage II disease is approximately 75–80%, Stage III disease is 50–60% and Stage IV disease is less than 5%.

References

Figueredo A, Rumble RB, Maroun J, et al., and members of the Gastrointestinal Cancer Disease Site Group (2004) Follow-up of patients with curatively resected colorectal cancer. Practice Guideline Report #2–9, www:Cancer care Ontario/program in evidence-based care

Geerts WH, Pineo GF, Heit JA, et al. (2004) Prevention of venous thromboembolism: the Seventh ACCP Conference on Antithrombotic and Thrombolytic Therapy, http://www.chestjournal.org/cgi/content/full/126/3_suppl/338S

Selected Readings

The Clinical Outcomes of Surgical Therapy Study Group (2004) A comparison of laparoscopically assisted and open colectomy for colon cancer. N Engl J Med 350:2051–2059

Gryfe R (2006) Clinical implications of our advancing knowledge of colorectal cancer genetics: inherited syndromes, prognosis, prevention, screening and therapeutics. Surg Clin N Am 86:787–817

Guenaga K, Atallah AN, Castro AA, et al. (2006) Mechanical bowel preparation for elective colorectal surgery. The Cochrane Database of Systematic Reviews, vol 3

Jacobsen DH, Soone E, Andreasen J, Kehlet H (2006) Convalescence after colonic surgery with Fast-Track vs. Convention Care. Colorectal Dis 8:683–589

Reza MM, Blaxco JA, Andradas E, et al. (2006) Systematic review of laparoscopic versus open surgery for colorectal cancer. Br J Surg 93:921–928

Sanga S, Yao M, Wolfe MM (2005) Non-steroidal anti-inflammatory drugs and colorectal cancer prevention. Postgrad Med J 81:223–227

Schwent W, Haase O, Neudecker J, Muller JM (2006) Short term benefits for laparoscopic colorectal resection. The Cochrane Database of Systematic Reviews, vol 3

Song F, Glenny AM (2006) Antimicrobial prophylaxis for colorectal surgery. The Cochrane Database of Systematic Reviews, vol 3

Winawer S, Fletcher R, Rex D, et al. (2003) for the US Multisociety Task Force on Colorectal Cancer. Colorectal cancer screening and surveillance: clinical guidelines and rationale-update based on new evidence. Gastroenterology 124:544–560

88 Appendiceal Epithelial Neoplasms and Pseudomyxoma Peritonei, a Distinct Clinical Entity with Distinct Treatments

Paul H. Sugarbaker

Pearls and Pitfalls

- Appendiceal epithelial malignancies present as either a malignant mucocele of the appendix or as a perforated appendiceal malignancy.
- If the disease presents as a contained process, then surgical removal of the mucocele with negative margins and negative appendiceal lymph nodes offers a curative approach to the disease process.
- In a majority of patients, the mucocele has perforated and epithelial cells in mucoid ascites have distributed themselves throughout the abdomen and pelvis (pseudomyxoma peritonei syndrome). Patients with pseudomyxoma peritonei syndrome should be treated with cytoreductive surgery which includes peritonectomy procedures and intraperitoneal chemotherapy washing usually with hyperthermic mitomycin C.
- The pseudomyxoma peritonei syndrome may present with large volume disease requiring knowledgeable selection of patients for this combined approach.
- Use of systemic chemotherapy in patients with mucinous appendiceal carcinomatosis remains controversial in the absence of a definitive clinical trial.
- In the absence of further evidence, these patients with aggressive carcinomatosis from appendix cancer are treated with systemic chemotherapy after cytoreduction and perioperative intraperitoneal chemotherapy.

Background Clinical Science

In the 9th International Classification of Disease (ICD-9) revised in 2004, primary epithelial neoplasms of the appendix are grouped together with colorectal malignancy. In future revisions, appendiceal neoplasms may be reclassified as a distinct clinical entity, because of profound differences in natural history and pathology of colorectal cancer compared with appendiceal neoplasms. Consequently, there are profound differences in the treatment of these two disease processes. ❷ *Table 88-1* contrasts the clinical and pathologic features of colorectal cancer and appendiceal neoplasms. The clinical presentation, histology, extent of tumor invasion, and difference in tumor differentiation separate colorectal cancer and appendiceal neoplasms as distinct pathologic and clinical diseases.

◘ Table 88-1

Contrast of the clinical and pathologic features of colorectal cancer and appendiceal neoplasms

Feature	Colon	Appendix
Mean age of onset (years)	68	48
Peritoneal dissemination at onset	10%	85%
Adenocarcinoma histology	85%	10%
Mucinous histologic type	10–15%	90%
Minimally invasive	1%	75%
Signet ring adenocarcinoma	1/1000	1/10
Adenocarcinoid	0%	2.5%
Differentiation of adenocarcinoma		
Well-differentiated	10%	80%
Moderately differentiated	80%	10%
Poorly differentiated	10%	10%

The age of onset of appendiceal epithelial neoplasms is lower than colorectal cancer with a mean age for initial presentation of 48 years. Although the proportion of patients with an unruptured mucocele is not known, many of these patients have peritoneal dissemination at the time of their initial presentation. The great majority of the tumors are of a mucinous histopathologic type. Also, about 75% of appendiceal neoplasms are minimally invasive, such that they layer out on the peritoneal surfaces rather than invade into parietal peritoneum or visceral structures. There is, however, a wide spectrum of aggressiveness, and some patients show signet ring morphology or poorly differentiated cancer with dissecting mucus penetrating deeply through the peritoneal layer of structures in the abdomen and pelvis. Because they usually present with peritoneal dissemination, even the most minimally aggressive of these malignancies should be regarded as a uniformly fatal condition, sometimes over several decades, unless unique, specialized treatments are initiated.

Management of a Mucocele

The clinical presentation of a mucocele is usually nonspecific. Up to 50% are found incidentally at the time of operation, and about half of patients will be asymptomatic. In those with symptoms, 30% will have abdominal pain, 15% an abdominal mass, 15% weight loss, 10% nausea, vomiting, or both, and the remainder acute appendicitis. Presence of symptoms suggests a higher incidence of cystadenocarcinoma.

Diagnostic Studies

Diagnosis of a mucocele, often made by computed tomography of the abdomen, is characterized by a well-encapsulated cystic mass 2–20 cm in diameter that occurs usually in the right lower quadrant. Curvilinear mural calcification is present about 50% of the time. Enhancing nodules in the mucocele wall suggest cystadenocarcinoma. In women, these findings are accompanied by enlargement of the ovaries from mucinous, tumor cell entrapment within the ovarian tissues (pseudomyxoma ovarii). Mucoceles of benign origin are rarely larger than 2 cm. A mucocele caused by cystadenoma or cystadenocarcinoma is usually larger and associated with a 20% incidence of perforation. Mucinous ascites in the pelvis and in right upper quadrant between liver and right hemidiaphragm indicates rupture of the mucocele and pseudomyxoma peritonei syndrome.

Diagnosis of a mucocele is sometimes made by an ultrasonography based on a sausage-shaped cystic structure in the appendiceal region but may include images suggesting mucous ascites. The target lesion imaged by ultrasonography is secondary to a thickened appendiceal wall. In some patients, multiple echogenic layers along the dilated appendix may be pathognomonic for mucocele.

An Intact Mucocele is a Benign Process

One of the cardinal principles of surgical management of an appendiceal mucocele is that an intact mucocele presents no future risk for the patient. In contrast, just the opposite is true if the mucocele has ruptured and epithelial cells escape into the peritoneal cavity. In the review by Misdraji and colleagues, none of 39 patients with intact mucoceles had progression of disease; however, patients with epithelial cells in the mucus within the peritoneal cavity developed mucinous neoplasms on peritoneal surfaces. Thus, it is crucial to maintain the mucocele intact during operations. When a mucocele is visualized at the time of laparoscopic examination, although it may be possible to remove it intact without rupture, the safer approach is to convert the laparoscopic examination to an open laparotomy for safe mucocele excision to prevent rupture of the mucocele and seeding of trocar sites.

Conversion of a laparoscopy to a laparotomy for excision of a mucocele aids in managing this disease process in two ways. First, this approach ensures that a benign process will not be changed to a malignant one by rupture of the mucocele. Second, it allows the surgeon to explore more thoroughly the remainder of the abdomen to exclude the presence of mucoid fluid accumulations. These accumulations are most commonly found in the right retrohepatic space or deep in the pelvis. Also, mucinous tumor nodules within the omentum are very common. Another site where mucoid neoplasms can accumulate is the in cul-de-sac created in the left paracolic space just above the junction of the sigmoid and descending colon. Thorough exploration of all these anatomic sites may be difficult by laparoscopic examination. An open laparotomy enables palpation and direct inspection of all sites that are of high risk for progression of the mucinous carcinomatosis.

At the time of laparoscopy or laparotomy for mucocele, all mucinous fluid within the abdomen should be harvested carefully for a cytospin of the fluid collected. If epithelial cells are found outside the appendix within the mucoid fluid, the diagnosis of pseudomyxoma peritonei syndrome or mucinous peritoneal carcinomatosis of appendiceal origin is established.

Right Colectomy is not Required in the Management of Mucinous Appendiceal Malignancies

In the past, all patients with epithelial malignancy of the appendix have been recommended for right colectomy. This practice was suggested on the basis of retrospective data; right colectomy appeared to produce a survival advantage. But recent prospective data by Gonzalez-Moreno and associates[3] showed that in treating appendiceal mucinous carcinomatosis and the pseudomyxoma peritonei syndrome, there is no survival benefit with a right colectomy. The standard of practice of right colectomy with appendiceal mucinous neoplasms has changed such that open operation for removal of mucoceles associated with mucinous carcinomatosis should not be extended for a right colectomy.

Although appendiceal epithelial malignancies can metastasize to regional lymph nodes, this pattern for mucinous appendiceal neoplasms is unusual. Nevertheless, a second important part of the open laparotomy for an appendiceal mucocele is the generous resection of the appendiceal lymph nodes. The entire mesoappendix should be resected with the appendiceal mucocele to provide additional information about the natural history of the disease. The indications for a right colectomy in these patients would be the gross appearance or frozen sections showing malignancy in the appendiceal or the ileocolic lymph nodes.

Similarly, the base of the appendix should be evaluated carefully when removing the mucocele. If there is any doubt about extension of the tumor mass longitudinally through the appendix, frozen sections of the surgical margin is indicated. Another indication for a right colectomy or, preferably, a cecectomy, is a positive margin at the appendectomy site.

Mucocele Progression and the Pseudomyxoma Peritonei Syndrome

Perforated mucoceles may be associated with mucoid material in the peritoneal cavity. This mucoid material may be acellular or can contain cells with either low- or high-grade dysplasia. Patients with appendiceal mucinous neoplasms with peritoneal dissemination have a lethal condition without treatment. Gough and colleagues established that there is no disease-free survival in the absence of either intraperitoneal 5-fluorouracil or intraperitoneal 32-phosphorus. More recently, Misradji and associates[1] showed a median survival of 5–8 years; at 10 years, only a few patients were available for study.

Combined Treatment for the Pseudomyxoma Peritonei Syndrome

About half of patients with mucinous neoplasms of the appendix have perforation at the time of exploration with mucinous peritoneal carcinomatosis or pseudomyxoma peritonei found at the time of appendectomy. In the past, this was a lethal condition without exception. More recently, peritonectomy combined with hyperthermic intraperitoneal chemotherapy has been employed to treat pseudomyxoma peritonei and peritoneal carcinomatosis. The essential features of this approach are diagrammed in ❷ *Fig. 88-1*. The surgeon is responsible for removing as much neoplasm on peritoneal surfaces as possible. This approach of cytoreductive therapy involves a greater and lesser omentectomy and splenectomy combined with peritonectomy procedures to strip neoplasm from the abdominal gutters, pelvis, right subhepatic space, and right and left subphrenic spaces.

Perioperative Intraperitoneal Chemotherapy

After the operative cytoreduction and with the abdomen open, the peritoneal space is washed extensively by the surgeon's hand using gauze debridement of all surfaces. This is done in the presence of a warm mitomycin C chemotherapy solution (❷ *Fig. 88-2*). Also, a window of time exists in which all

□ Figure 88-1
Approach to the treatment of peritoneal carcinomatosis from appendix cancer

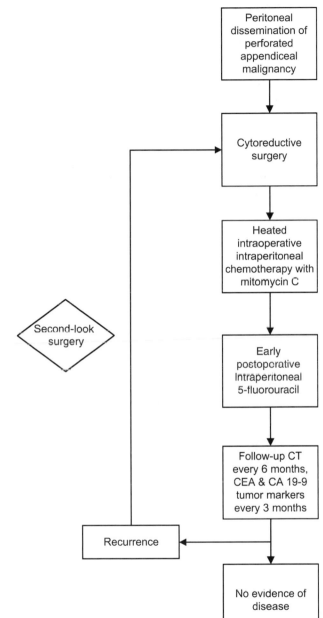

intraperitoneal surfaces are available for intraperitoneal chemotherapy utilizing 5-fluorouracil in the early postoperative period. Uniformity of treatment with intraperitoneal chemotherapy to all peritoneal surfaces, including those surfaces dissected by the surgeon, can be achieved if the intraperitoneal chemotherapy is used during the first postoperative week. As the 5-fluorouracil chemotherapy solution is indwelling in the early postoperative period, intraperitoneal distribution is maximized by turning the patient alternately onto his or her right and left side as well as into the prone position.

◘ Figure 88-2
Intraoperative hyperthermic intraperitoneal chemotherapy. The skin edges are suspended on a self-retaining retractor. Warm (41–42°C) chemotherapy solution is circulated while distributed manually throughout abdomen and pelvis

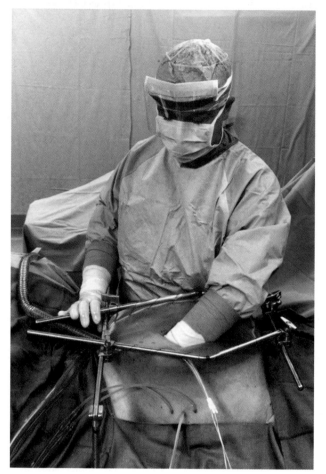

    This perioperative intraperitoneal chemotherapy (combination of heated, intraoperative mitomycin C and early postoperative 5-fluorouracil) has been utilized in over 850 patients and has not been associated with an increased incidence of anastomotic disruptions. In patients with prior operative procedures who require many hours of lysis of adhesions, there is an increased incidence of postoperative bowel perforation, presumably a result of the combined effects of damage to small bowel from electrosurgical dissection of adhesions (seromuscular damage) and effects of intraperitoneal chemotherapy on the intestine (mucosa and submucosa damage). In patients with high-grade, appendiceal mucinous peritoneal carcinomatosis, intravenous chemotherapy is also recommended after combined treatment is completed. Usually capecitabine and oxaliplatin for 6 months are appropriate. In selected patients, usually those who require ostomy closure, a second-look operation is recommended at 6 months after the cytoreduction with perioperative chemotherapy. If at staging celiotomy small tumor foci are found on peritoneal surfaces of the abdomen or pelvis, the nodules are resected, and a final intraperitoneal chemotherapy treatment is performed.

Peritoneum as the First Line of Defense in Carcinomatosis

It is important that definitive treatment of peritoneal carcinomatosis or pseudomyxoma peritonei be instituted in a timely fashion. Each non-definitive (debulking) operative intervention makes potentially curative cytoreductive surgery more difficult. Respect for the peritoneum as the first line of defense of the host against carcinomatosis is a requirement of optimal results using the peritonectomy procedures. Also, the relative sparing of the small bowel seen early in the natural history of peritoneal carcinomatosis and pseudomyxoma peritonei disappears after several surgical procedures have been performed. The fibrous adhesions that result inevitably will become infiltrated by neoplastic cells, leading to extensive involvement of the small bowel. Eventually, effective cytoreductive therapy is impossible, and the effects of intraperitoneal chemotherapy are not adequate to keep the patient disease-free.

Results of Treatment with Cytoreductive Surgery and Intraperitoneal Chemotherapy

The results of this aggressive combined treatment for peritoneal surface dissemination of appendiceal malignancies are unexpectedly good. The mean follow-up of our 385 patients with appendiceal malignancy was 38 months; all appendiceal malignancy patients including adenomucinosis and mucinous adenocarcinoma subtypes were included. All had documented peritoneal surface disease, and a majority had large volume disease. After completion of cytoreductive surgery, the abdomen was inspected for the presence of residual disease. A completeness of cytoreduction score (CC) was obtained based on the size of individual tumor nodules remaining. A CC-0 score indicated no visible tumor remaining; CC-1 indicated tumor nodules less than 2.5 mm; CC-2 indicated tumor nodules between 2.5 mm and 2.5 cm; and CC-3 indicated tumor nodules larger than 2.5 cm or a confluence of implants at any site. In ❷ *Fig. 88-3*, the survival of patients with CC-0 and CC-1 is compared with those with an incomplete cytoreduction (CC-2 and CC-3). Survival differences were statistically significant; patients with tumor nodules smaller than 2.5 mm in diameter were more likely to survive in the long term than were those with an incomplete cytoreduction. There were no differences in survival between patients with CC-2 and CC-3.

■ Figure 88-3
Survival by cytoreduction of appendiceal malignancy with peritoneal dissemination (Reprinted from Sugarbaker and Chang (1999). With kind permission of Springer Science and Business Media)

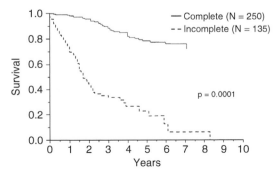

Survival by Histology

From specimens removed at the time of cytoreductive surgery and whenever possible from review of the primary appendiceal malignancy, a histologic assessment was made. Histologic subtypes of adenomucinosis, hybrid, and mucinous adenocarcinoma have been described. Adenomucinosis includes minimally aggressive peritoneal neoplasms that produce large volumes of mucous ascites usually with a primary appendiceal neoplasm described as a cystadenoma. Hybrid malignancies showed adenomucinosis combined with isolated foci of mucinous adenocarcinomas (less than 5%). Mucinous adenocarcinoma involves a truly invasive process, often of the signet ring morphology with poor differentiation.

❯ *Figure 88-4* shows the survival distribution of these appendix malignancy patients by histology. Survival differences were evident between patients with adenomucinosis and those with hybrid or mucinous adenocarcinoma. No differences were noted between patients with hybrid and mucinous adenocarcinoma histology. A noninvasive histopathology is extremely important in selecting patients most likely to benefit from the treatment strategy of aggressive combined therapy.

Survival by Prior Surgical Score

When the previous operative notes on these patients were reviewed, a judgment was made regarding the anatomic sites of previous surgical dissections. The summation of these dissections from all prior surgical interventions was recorded on a diagram of the abdominopelvic regions which allowed an assessment of the anatomic locations in which previous surgery had been performed. In patients with a prior surgical score (PSS) of 0, diagnosis of peritoneal carcinomatosis was obtained through biopsy only or by laparoscopy plus biopsy. PSS 1 indicated only a previous exploratory laparotomy, while PSS 2 indicated exploratory laparotomy with some resections, usually greater omentectomy with or without right colectomy. With a PSS of 3, patients had an attempt at a complete cytoreduction, usually involving a greater omentectomy, right colectomy, hysterectomy, and bilateral salpingo-oophorectomy with the possibility of other resections from both abdominal organs or parietal peritoneal regions. Patients with PSS scores of 0 through 2 had an improved survival compared with those with a PSS of 3. When analyzed by a multivariate type analysis, complete versus incomplete cytoreduction proved the most important variable with a relative risk of 9.98.

■ Figure 88-4
Survival by histology of appendiceal malignancy with peritoneal dissemination. (Reprinted from Sugarbaker and Chang (1999). With kind permission of Springer Science and Business Media)

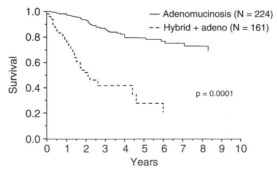

Morbidity and Mortality

Extensive cytoreductive surgery combined with early postoperative intraperitoneal chemotherapy presents a major physiologic insult. Nevertheless, operative mortality remains at 2% in this group of patients. Pancreatitis and fistula formation represent the major complications. Anastomotic leaks were no more common in this group of patients than in a routine general surgical setting (2.4%). Substantial morbidity was 20%. There was no morbidity or mortality associated directly with the intraperitoneal chemotherapy. Rather, the incidence of complications depended on the extent of the operation, number of peritonectomy procedures, and time required to complete the cytoreduction.

Selected Readings

Gonzalez-Moreno S, Sugarbaker PH (2004) Right hemicolectomy does not confer a survival advantage in patients with mucinous carcinoma of the appendix and peritoneal seeding. Br J Surg 91:304–311

Gough DB, Donohue JH, Schutt AJ, et al. (1994) Pseudomyxoma peritonei: long-term patient survival with an aggressive regional approach. Ann Surg 219:112–119

Misdraji J, Yantiss RK, Graeme-Cook FM, et al. (2003) Appendiceal mucinous neoplasms: a clinicopathologic analysis of 107 cases. Am J Surg Pathol 27:1089–1103

Sugarbaker PH (2003) Peritonectomy procedures. Surg Oncol Clin N Am 12:605–621

Sugarbaker PH, Chang D (1999) Results of treatment of 385 patients with peritoneal surface spread of appendiceal malignancy. Ann Surg Oncol 6:727–731

Sugarbaker PH, Alderman R, Edwards G, et al. (2006) Prospective morbidity and mortality assessment of cytoreductive surgery plus perioperative intraperitoneal chemotherapy to treat peritoneal dissemination of appendiceal mucinous malignancy. Ann Surg Oncol 13:635–644

Sugarbaker PH, Ronnett BM, Archer A, et al. (1997) Pseudomyxoma peritonei syndrome. Adv Surg 30:233–280

89 Anal Cancer

Graham Branagan · Brendan Moran

Pearls and Pitfalls

- Eighty-five percent of anal cancers arise in the anal canal with 15% in the anal margin.
- Eight-five percent of anal canal cancers are squamous cell carcinomas (SCC).
- Anal intraepithelial neoplasia (AIN), thought to be a precursor of SCC, is associated with human papillomavirus infection of the perianal skin and anal canal, and iatrogenic immunosuppression in patients who receive an organ allograft.
- Delay and misdiagnosis are common as the signs and symptoms of SCC of the anal canal are similar to those of common, benign perianal conditions, such as hemorrhoids or fissures.
- Histological diagnosis often requires examination and biopsy under anesthesia.
- A record should be made of: (1) position and size of the tumor, including the extent of the tumor within the rectum, perineum, and ischiorectal fossa; and (2) fixity of the tumor to surrounding structures.
- Optimal staging of patients with anal cancer includes a pelvic magnetic resonance imaging (local invasion and pelvic/inguinal lymphadenopathy) and abdominal/thoracic computed tomography for distant spread. This could be complemented by sentinel node biopsy where local expertise exists.
- Compared with surgery, primary chemoradiotherapy offers superior local control and survival with the added benefit of avoiding a permanent stoma in many patients.
- Patients with severe anal symptoms may require fecal diversion, best performed laparoscopically.
- Studies have confirmed the benefits of both combined chemoradiotherapy over radiotherapy alone and that of mitomycin.
- Debate continues regarding the most appropriate radiotherapy dose and overall treatment time.
- Radical salvage surgery by abdominoperineal resection (APR) is the only option offering the possibility of long-term survival for patients with persistent or recurrent disease.
- The major morbidity after salvage APR is perineal wound problems.
- A vertical rectus abdominis flap to primarily close the defect has excellent primary healing rates and acceptable morbidity.

Introduction

The anus is composed of the anal margin and the anal canal. The anal margin extends from the anal verge outwards to include 5 cm of perianal skin. The anal canal extends from the anorectal ring to the anal verge and is usually 3.5–4 cm in length. At the proximal end of the anal canal is a transition zone known as the dentate line, where the squamous lining of the anus meets the glandular mucosa of the rectum. The fundamental distinction between the anal canal and anal margin is important as early squamous tumors of the anal margin can be treated by a similar approach to that of skin lesions by wide local excision with an 80% 5-year survival.

Anal cancer is a rare disease accounting for less than 4% of all anorectal neoplasms, with an annual incidence of 1 per 100,000 population. Historically, anal cancer is more common in women and the elderly. However, the incidence is rising dramatically in the young, especially among the male homosexual population. Incidence rates among this population are 25–30 times that of the general population. Infection with the human immunodeficiency virus (HIV) significantly increases the risk of developing anal cancer, whilst HIV-positive homosexual males have a relative risk 84 times that of the general population.

The etiology of anal cancer seems to be more closely related to genital malignancies than other malignancies of the gastrointestinal tract. Data suggest associations between incidence of anal cancer and infection with human papillomavirus (HPV), lifetime number of sexual partners, cigarette smoking, genital warts, receptive anal intercourse, and infection with HIV.

Anal intraepithelial neoplasia (AIN) is thought to be a precursor of squamous cell carcinoma (SCC) of the anus, similar in many respects to cervical intraepithelial neoplasia. AIN is associated with HPV infection of the perianal skin and anal canal, including the anal transition zone. As infection with these oncogenic viruses persists, the anal tissues may progress through low-grade to high-grade dysplasia and eventually cancer. Long-term follow up suggests that approximately 5% of advanced AIN undergoes malignant change. AIN is also associated with iatrogenic immunosuppression in patients who receive an organ allograft with an estimated increased risk for developing anal cancer of between 10 and 100 times that of the general population. Treatment aims to eradicate AIN and prevent development of anal cancer. Available treatment options include HPV-based vaccines, immunomodulation, local ablation and surgery. However, reported success rates are variable and larger randomized trials are needed. Surgery is associated with significant recurrence rates, especially in HIV positive patients.

Eighty-five percent of anal cancers arise in the anal canal with the remainder arising in the anal margin. Eight-five percent of anal canal cancers are SCC. Approximately, 10% are adenocarcinomas of the anal ducts or glands, behave similarly to low rectal adenocarcinomas and are treated in the same fashion. Other rare anal tumors include melanomas, sarcomas and neuroendocrine tumors.

Anal melanoma is a particularly aggressive tumor that does not respond to chemotherapy or radiotherapy and prognosis is poor. There appears to be no advantage in abdomino-perineal resection (APR) over simple wide local excision of these tumors with median survival rates of 17 and 21 months, respectively.

Clinical Presentation and Diagnosis

Misdiagnosis and delays in diagnosis are common as the signs and symptoms of SCC of the anal canal are similar to those of common, perianal conditions, such as hemorrhoids or fissures. Physicians should be alerted by persistent symptoms that do not respond to treatment.

The majority of patients present with either bright red rectal bleeding (60%) and/or perianal pain (60%). Other common presenting symptoms are the presence of a mass (25–30%) and pruritus or anal discharge (25%). Anal cancers are often locally aggressive with spread to adjacent organs. At first presentation 30–50% of patients will have locally advanced disease. Symptoms of tenesmus or fecal incontinence suggest involvement of the anal sphincter. The passage of feces or offensive discharge per vagina in females is suggestive of a recto-vaginal fistula. Other organs at risk of invasion are the urethra and the prostate gland in men.

A careful inspection of the perianal region, digital rectal examination and proctosigmoidoscopy are of paramount importance. A record should be made of the position and size of the tumor either at the anal margin or within the anal canal, including the extent of the tumor within the rectum, perineum and ischiorectal fossa. Other important details are the fixity of the tumor to surrounding structures, such as the vagina, prostate and pelvis. In some patients it may be possible to palpate enlarged mesorectal lymph nodes. Both groins should be carefully palpated to check for inguinal lymphadenopathy. Recording these details is important as they act as a reference for further examination after chemoradiotherapy.

A histological diagnosis is mandatory and may be best performed during an examination under anesthesia (EUA), which may also facilitate the careful examination described above. Evaluation of the remaining colon has been demonstrated as not to be necessary.

Systemic spread of anal cancer is usually via the lymphatics and less commonly via the bloodstream. Distal anal canal cancers (below the dentate line) spread to the inguinal and femoral node basins whereas proximal cancers drain to mesorectal, internal iliac and para-aortic nodes. About one third of patients with anal cancer will have palpable inguinal nodes but only half of these will have metastases.

Clinically palpable nodes should be evaluated histologically which has been done historically by fine-needle aspiration cytology. Recently some clinicians have advocated the use of sentinel node biopsy techniques to stage these patients more accurately.

Staging and Imaging

Staging of anal cancer patients is based on information gained from pre-treatment clinical, endoscopic and radiological assessments. It is performed using the Union Internationale Contre le Cancer/American Joint Committee on Cancer (UICC/AJCC) TNM classification (2002) (❷ *Table 89-1*).

Tumor stages T1–T3 are defined on the basis of size, and imaging has little role to play in the staging of these lesions. However, imaging is of paramount importance in determining the presence and extent of invasion into surrounding structures (T4). Magnetic resonance imaging (MRI) and endoanal ultrasound (EUS) are useful in this respect as they are both able to distinguish the different layers of the bowel wall and identify the interface between the outer layer of the bowel and surrounding structures.

EUS is a relatively inexpensive investigation but the availability of the necessary expertise is limited and the procedure is operator dependent. There is a learning curve with experience of over 50 patients recommended to achieve good results.

MRI is now used extensively in the staging of rectal cancer, particularly in Europe. However, the experience of MRI staging of anal cancer is limited. Although more expensive than EUS, MRI has two distinct advantages. Firstly, MRI has multiplanar capability allowing sagittal and coronal imaging (❷ *Fig. 89-1*). Secondly, tumor visualization can be enhanced by intravenous/intraluminal contrast and fat suppression imaging techniques. There are no published data comparing EUS with MRI in staging anal cancer but data from studies in rectal cancer have shown benefits in local staging of advanced disease by MRI.

Local response to therapy is based usually on clinical assessment but can be augmented by EUS. Magnetic resonance imaging (MRI) has been shown to be accurate in assessing the extent of recurrent

◘ Table 89-1

Union Internationale Contre le Cancer/American Joint Committee on Cancer (UICC/AJCC) TNM classification (2002)

Primary tumor (T)
TX: Primary tumor cannot be assessed
T0: No evidence of primary tumor
Tis: Carcinoma in situ
T1: Tumor < 2 cm in greatest dimension
T2: Tumor between 2 and 5 cm in greatest dimension
T3: Tumor > 5 cm in greatest dimension
T4: Tumor of any size that invades adjacent organs, e.g., vagina, urethra, bladder (involvement of the sphincter muscle alone is not classified as T4)

Regional lymph nodes (N)
NX: Regional nodes cannot be assessed
N0: No regional lymph node metastases
N1: Metastasis in mesorectal lymph node or nodes
N2: Metastasis in unilateral internal iliac and/or inguinal node or nodes
N3: Metastasis in mesorectal and inguinal nodes and/or bilateral internal iliac and/or inguinal nodes

Distant metastases
MX: Distant metastases cannot be assessed
M0: No distant metastases
M1: Distant metastasis

Stage grouping
Stage 0: Tis N0 M0
Stage 1: T1 N0 M0
Stage 2: T2/3 N0 M0
Stage 3: T4 N0 M0, any T N1 M0
Stage 4: T4 N1 M0, any T N2 M0, any T N3 M0

local disease. Abdominal and pelvic computed tomography (CT) or MRI scanning have high sensitivity for identifying pelvic, inguinal and retroperitoneal lymphadenopathy. However, neither modality is accurate at characterizing lymphadenopathy as benign or malignant.

Current treatment of primary anal cancer does not involve surgical resection and thus the histological status of the lymph nodes is not known. The status of the pelvic nodes is clinically less important than the status of inguinal nodes as the former are included routinely as part of the primary pelvic radiotherapy fields. The approach to management of inguinal nodes remains open to debate. Prophylactic groin irradiation has been shown to decrease the incidence of metachronous inguinal metastases but the majority of patients will probably be overtreated with this regime, receiving larger doses of radiation and an increased risk of toxicity, especially when combined with chemotherapy.

Several authors advocate the use of lymphatic mapping by sentinel node biopsy (SNB) to identify the status of inguinal nodes. This technique is based on the premise that the sentinel node is the first to receive drainage from a primary tumor and is the node most likely to contain metastatic disease. Hence the presence of a negative sentinel node suggests that the remainder of the draining nodal basin is at minimal risk of containing metastases.

Published data for the use of SNB in anal cancer are limited but 5 small series have been reported including a total of 84 patients. In the largest series the sentinel node was identified in all 33 patients and was histologically positive in 7 (21%). None of the patients with histologically negative sentinel nodes received groin irradiation and at 18 months follow up none had developed inguinal metastases.

◘ Figure 89-1
Coronal and sagittal MRI images of a patient with a T4 cancer invading vagina

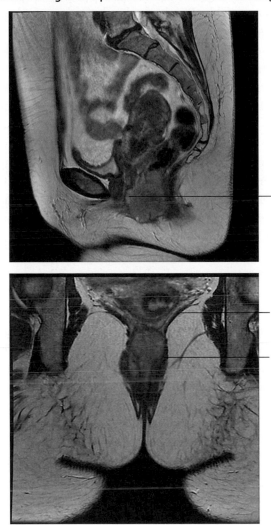

Anterior edge of
T4 tumour
invading posterior
vaginal wall

Levator ani

Tumour arising in anal
canal, destroying internal
sphincter

Advocates of SNB suggest that the technique allows a more selective approach to treatment of the inguinal nodes in anal cancer.

Distant metastases are present in 10% of patients at diagnosis with the most common sites being liver and lung. The liver can be assessed by either CT or MRI and the chest by CT.

An optimal approach to staging of patients with anal cancer is to undertake a pelvic MRI to assess local invasion and both pelvic and inguinal lymphadenopathy with an abdominal and thoracic CT to assess for distant spread. This could be complemented by sentinel node biopsy where local expertise exists.

Treatment and Outcomes

Historically, treatment of most patients with anal cancer was by abdominoperineal resection (APR) of the rectum and anal canal, with local excision reserved for patients with well-differentiated tumors smaller than 2 cm or tumors confined to the mucosa and submucosa. APR was a radical surgical option with significant morbidity and formation of a permanent end colostomy. It resulted in local treatment failure in 30–50% of patients and 5-year survival of 50–70%. Local excision was suitable for less than 10% of patients with anal cancer and reported results were variable. Results for local excision of advanced lesions were extremely poor with local recurrence rates greater than 60% and few 5-year survivors.

Pioneering work by Nigro et al. in the 1980s has led to the adoption of combined chemoradiotherapy as the recommended first-line treatment for SCC of the anal canal. In this study patients with locally advanced anal cancers were treated with neoadjuvant external beam radiotherapy and concurrent chemotherapy with fluorouracil (5-FU) and mitomycin C. Complete pathological responses were observed in 81% patients.

Subsequent studies have confirmed the benefits of combined chemoradiotherapy over radiotherapy alone (❯ Table 89-2). Both the European Organisation for Research and Treatment of Cancer (EORTC) trial and the UK Coordinating Committee on Cancer Research (UKCCCR) Anal Cancer Trial (ACT)1 demonstrated that chemoradiotherapy is more effective than radiotherapy alone in terms of local control, with a clear improvement in colostomy free survival. However, neither trial demonstrated any difference in overall survival between the two groups.

Currently, debate continues regarding the most appropriate radiotherapy dose and overall treatment time. Recent data suggest that the shortening of radiotherapy treatment times by eliminating the gap between the initial phase of radiotherapy and subsequent boost dose results in improved local control.

The use of mitomycin C is associated with significant toxicity including prolonged thrombocytopenia. However, the Radiation Therapy Oncology Group (RTOG 87-04) trial reported a higher complete response rate (92% vs. 85%), better local control (72% vs. 51%), improved disease-free survival (73% vs. 51%) and a lower colostomy rate (9% vs. 22%) in the group that received mitomycin C and 5-FU in combination with radiotherapy compared with the group that received radiotherapy and 5-FU alone (❯ Table 89-2). Overall 4-year survival was similar (75% vs. 70%) but toxicity (Grade 4 + 23% vs. 7%) was significantly greater in the mitomycin arm.

Cisplatin is superior to mitomycin C as a radiosensitizer with greater activity against squamous cell solid tumors. It also has a more favorable side-effect profile with less myelosuppression. There are some data to suggest that cisplatin based regimes may be superior to those containing mitomycin C with similar local control and survival rates, but reduced toxicity. However, the numbers are small and

◼ Table 89-2

Results of randomized clinical trials of chemoradiation in anal cancer

Trial	N	DXT (phase 1)	Boost	Chemotherapy	Outcome
UKCCCR ACT I	585	45 Gy in 20–25 fractions	15 Gy after 6 weeks	5-FU days 1–4 and 29–32; mitomycin day 1	Significant improvement in local control in chemoradiotherapy group ($p < 0.0001$)
EORTC	110	45 Gy in 25 fractions	15–20 Gy after 6 weeks	5-FU days 1–5 and 29–33; mitomycin day 1	Significant improvement in local control in chemoradiotherapy group ($p < 0.02$)
RTOG	291	45–50.4 Gy in 25–28 fractions	None	5-FU days 1–4 and 29–32 (both groups); mitomycin days 1 and 29 (1 group only)	Significant improvement in local control with mitomycin ($p < 0.001$)

UKCCCR ACT I: UK Coordinating Committee on Cancer Research Anal Cancer Trial; EORTC: European Organisation for Research and Treatment of Cancer; RTOG: Radiation Therapy Oncology Group; 5-FU: fluorouracil.

most of the trials involving cisplatin use higher radiation doses than mitomycin based trials. Several trials investigating the role of cisplatin in the treatment of anal cancer are currently under way. In particular, two large phase III randomized trials, RTOG 98-11 and the UKCCCR-ACT II trials are comparing mitomycin C-based with cisplatin-based chemoradiotherapy.

The maximum clinical and pathological response to chemoradiotherapy may not be reached until 6–9 months after completion of treatment. Hence, patients that have residual tumor clinically on completion of treatment require intense follow-up examination every 6 weeks. Tumors that persist or progress require biopsy. For patients with a complete clinical response, any new growth requires a biopsy to exclude recurrence.

Persistent disease is defined as tumor that remains after maximum treatment response or tumor that recurs within 6 months of a complete response. Recurrent disease is defined as tumor that reappears more than 6 months after a complete response.

Although surgery is no longer the primary treatment for anal cancer it still has an important role in the management of these patients. As already described, EUA and biopsy of the primary tumor is required for most primary tumors, and SNB is increasingly accepted as optimal staging of the inguinal lymph nodes. Formation of a temporary colostomy may be necessary in patients who have incontinence of feces due to invasion of the sphincter by advanced tumor or those who are at risk of continence problems secondary to the acute side, effects of pelvic radiotherapy. Currently, laparoscopy with laparoscopic stoma formation is the best method for peritoneal and liver surface imaging, with rapid recovery compared to open surgery.

Finally, for patients with persistent or recurrent disease that cannot have or do not respond to further chemotherapy and/or radiotherapy, radical salvage surgery in the form of APR with wide skin margins is the only option offering the possibility of long term survival. Patients being considered for salvage surgery require careful assessment. Where clear resection margins cannot be achieved, radical excisional surgery should not be considered as there is no survival benefit and significant risk of morbidity. In these cases, diversion of the faecal stream by a defunctioning stoma may be necessary for palliation.

Overall survival after salvage surgery ranges from 24% to 53% with most of the reported series having small numbers. The largest reported series of 57 patients demonstrated a 5-year survival of 33% with median survival of nearly 3 years. Patients with curative resection (negative margins and no new intraoperative metastases) had a 5-year survival of 40% with a median survival of over 4 years.

Factors which predicted poor outcome after salvage surgery included positive resection margins (0% 5-year survival, median survival 10 months), nodal disease at surgery (11% 5-year survival, 8 months median survival) and tumors which were large (> 5 cm) or invaded adjacent organs (0% 5 year survival, median survival 19 months). Most reported series demonstrate worse outcomes for patients with persistent disease (5-year survival 56–82%) compared with patients with recurrent disease (5-year survival 23–33%).

The major morbidity after salvage APR is perineal wound complications almost certainly related to the radiotherapy component of the initial treatment. Perineal breakdown occurs in 30–60% of patients resulting in persistent non-healing wounds for 6–9 months or longer. The large perineal wounds resulting from radical salvage APR present problems due to a combination of the difficult anatomical position, the propensity for infection and the potential need for further management of the underlying pathology. This has led to the introduction of plastic surgical techniques which aim to reduce this considerable complication rate. Local flaps, such as the posterior thigh flap, tensor fascia lata flap and vastus lateralis flap have been used. However, there is a complication rate of 20–50% for these flaps and they do not always have sufficient bulk to close the defect.

Currently, the most commonly used technique is the use of a trans-pelvic vertical rectus abdominis myocutaneous (VRAM) flap based on the inferior epigastric vessels, providing a long pedicled flap with a large bulk of muscle. There are a number of small series reporting excellent primary healing with acceptable morbidity with VRAM flaps.

The treatment of the inguinal node basins may differ with the advent of SNB. Currently, some centers irradiate the groins as part of the pelvic radiotherapy regime. Others pursue a "watch and wait" policy after careful clinical assessment of the groins and fine needle aspiration cytology of any suspicious nodes. SNB allows more accurate staging of these nodes and a selective policy for groin irradiation.

For patients with synchronous groin node disease, chemoradiotherapy results in disease control in 65–90% patients. For persistent inguinal disease, block dissection of the groin can be offered, although in an irradiated field this procedure has high morbidity. In patients who have not received groin irradiation, metachronous or recurrent groin disease can be treated with radiotherapy and additional chemotherapy or with inguinal node dissection.

Currently, treatment of distant metastatic disease is palliative with a uniformly poor prognosis. Complete response to treatment is rare and duration of response usually short. Palliative radiotherapy and chemotherapy have a role to play in the management of symptomatic metastases.

Conclusion

Whilst no longer the primary modality of treating patients, surgery still has an important role to play in the management of patients with anal cancer and the surgeon remains a key member of the multidisciplinary team. The majority of patients present to surgeons with local anal symptoms and confirmatory histological diagnosis may require biopsy under anesthesia. Chemoradiotherapy offers good disease control and 5-year survival and avoids a permanent stoma in the majority of patients. Individual patients with severe anal symptoms may require fecal diversion prior to chemo-radiotherapy. In selected patients with persistent or recurrent disease, radical salvage surgery may be necessary and in specialized units is associated with reasonable 5-year survival and good palliation in incurable cases.

Selected Readings

Abbasakoor F, Boulos PB (2005) Anal intraepithelial neoplasia. Br J Surg 92:277–290

Bell SW, Dehni N, Chaouat M, Lifante JC, et al. (2005) Primary rectus abdominis myocutaneous flap for repair of perineal and vaginal defects after extended abdomino-perineal resection. Br J Surg 92:482–486

Damin DC, Rosito MA, Schwartsmann G (2006) Sentinel lymph node in carcinoma of the anal canal: a review. Eur J Surg Oncol 32:247–252

Mackay SG, Pager CK, Joseph D, et al. (2003) Assessment of the accuracy of transrectal ultrasonography in anorectal neoplasia. Br J Surg 90:346–350

Nilsson PJ, Svensson C, Goldman S, Glimelius B (2002) Salvage abdominoperineal resection in anal epidermoid cancer. Br J Surg 89:1425–1429

Roach SC, Hulse PA, Moulding FJ, et al. (2005) Magnetic resonance imaging of anal cancer. Clin Radiol 60:1111–1119

Welton ML, Sharkey FE, Kahlenberg MS (2004) The etiology and epidemiology of anal cancer. Surg Oncol Clin N Am 13:263–275

Yue-Kui B, Wen-Lan C, Ji-Dong G, et al. (2004) Surgical salvage therapy of anal canal cancer. World J Gastroenterol 10:424–426

90 Rectal Cancer: Issues for the 21st Century, a Practical Update for the Surgeon

Richard J. Heald

Pearls and Pitfalls

- Mobility of the tumor (on pubo-rectal sidewall) remains the key physical sign.
- Think embryology: What is removed is an intact envelope of the midline hindgut with its surrounding lymphovascular "mesentery."
- Circumferential surgery is the key – move from one quadrant to another.
- As Goethe said, "Man recognizes only what he knows." Learn the "holy plane" by careful visualization and three-directional traction to open its avascular areolar "cobweb."
- Learn the hypogastric plexuses and preserve them.
- The plane leads to the visceral muscle tube of the internal sphincter. Triple stapling is expensive but safe and a washout below to seal the specimen wise.
- Never forget to do both rectal and vaginal examinations before neo-adjuvant treatment and always on the table at the start of surgery. Mobility is the key.
- If you lose the "holy plane" or make something bleed go across the pelvis 180° and develop the plane elsewhere, whilst maintaining pressure on the bleed.
- Avoid tearing from excessive traction.
- During the circular stapling never catch any external sphincters. Be sure you can see the edge of the anvil through the single layer of anorectal smooth muscle.
- It is usually wiser to defunction the very low anastomosis.

Introduction

There can be few areas of surgical practice around which change seems so frenetic but yet in which cynics might feel that hard evidence of survival benefit so slow to appear. Rectal cancer offers more opportunity for improvement in outcome, both in terms of cure and in the reduction of "collateral damage," than any of the other common malignancies. Nevertheless, competing pressures from the various disciplines that are now involved have created more unanswered questions and less truly convincing hard evidence of real benefit than we need for the many decisions we must help our patients to make. Examples of outstanding and pressing areas of confusion include:

- Radiotherapy (RT)
- Should it be short course or long?
- Conformal anal preserving or conventional?
- Should it be combined with chemotherapy?
- Which combinations of drugs and how should the two modalities be scheduled?
- The criteria for selection and the use of modern imaging modalities
- Should a rectal cancer operation in 2006 ever be undertaken without a fine slice magnetic resonance imaging (MRI)?
- The emergence of the "complete response" phenomenon (cCR)
- Should we be following Habr-Gama's lead and observing selected cases with the now widespread use of chemoradiotherapy (CRT) combinations?

All of these add to the already rich tapestry of surgical challenges and potential improvements to which this chapter seeks to provide an update. In the background is the understanding in the minds of many experienced surgeons that details of their operative technique probably matter more to most patients than the decisions that may be made at a distance on their behalf by distinguished members of the multidisciplinary team (MDT). Perhaps the most worrying aspect of advances into the 21st century is the staggering escalations in cost that the involvement of other disciplines has brought with it. Many European cancer centers now regard preoperative chemo-radiotherapy as the "new European standard" so that the first 5 years of the new century have seen the cost of these therapies surpass the total cost of hospitalization, surgery and all other aspects of the patient's management added together. The second 5 years of the new century are likely to see this situation become even more out of proportion with even more potentially devastating financial implications for the funding of cancer care especially in poorer countries. A further serious consequence of multiple therapies with changes and modifications that appear almost monthly is that the practice of "evidence-based medicine" becomes impossible because so many aspects of care are changing simultaneously. Fortunately there is much that can be achieved by the affordable application of MRI staging, refinements in surgical technique, and the introduction of histopathological audit.

Preoperative Assessment and Work Up

It is self-evident that each patient must be assessed clinically with particular regard to comorbidity that may influence operative decisions. By government edict most patients are now discussed by a MDT covering the whole range of relevant specialists although specialist advice on comorbidity is often not available at such meetings. Key elements of this presurgery conference about each patient are a full computed tomography (CT) scan of the chest and abdomen with particular reference to the detection of metastatic disease. In the UK the Pelican Centre has been working for a number of years on the MERCURY project which has demonstrated close correlation between specialist preoperative fine slice phased array coil MRI examinations and the subsequent histology. For tidy comparison the whole specimen is not cut right open by the surgeon but preserved intact, fixed, and subsequently sliced axially to conform with the preoperative axial images. Where the necessary radiological and histological skills have been developed in the same hospital the focal point of most MDT discussions is now these special MRI scans, which show very accurately the relationship of the cancer and its extramural extensions to the enveloping mesorectal fascia which will subsequently guide the surgeon's "holy plane" dissection around the total mesorectal excision (TME) specimen. The operator's grasp of the anatomy and the levels in the pelvis is much enhanced by reference to these scans if they are skillfully presented. It should not be forgotten, however, that these fine slice examinations do not generally extend up to the root of the inferior mesenteric artery, so that some lymph nodes, which might be removed in a good TME may not be assessed by this method. Similar limitations apply to all the routine RT pelvic fields, so that high nodes escape irradiation and the dissection around the aortic root of the inferior artery becomes more important. The MERCURY study reports the practice of a network of hospitals in three countries (England, Germany, and Wales) and centered on the Pelican Centre in Basingstoke in using a minimum of 1 mm mesorectal clearance within the mesorectal fascia on MRI as the principal indication for avoiding preoperative RT (predicted clear margins). Exception is made when there is extensive intra-mesorectal disease, either N2 lymphatic spread or extensive extramural venous invasion, all factors known to increase the risk of local failure. Somewhat arbitrarily also the involvement of internal iliac nodes visualized on MRI is taken as an indication for preoperative chemo-radiotherapy, since the management of such nodes surgically is generally avoided except in Japan.

Choice of Operation – Clinical and Radiological Assessment

Local excision. This is probably most safely restricted to T1 cancers in the anorectal area or possibly more advanced tumors in people in whom the risk of a major operation or of major adjuvant therapy tips the balance towards a relatively minor procedure. We consider that the combination of local excision with chemo-radiotherapy is currently suspect in relation to the hazard of converting an entirely curable early lesion into a preventable late disaster.

Transanal endoscopic microsurgery (TEM) has been extensively practiced in some centers and claims for its suitability for some T2 tumors have been made by certain specialists. The excision of a disk of rectal wall in the upper anal canal and distal rectum is considered by our unit to be intrinsically dangerous in that it may compromise the peri-mesorectal "holy" plane if a subsequent anterior resection and TME were to become necessary.

Anterior resection (AR) and abdominoperineal excision (APE). Advances in imaging have in no way diminished the need for the surgeon to establish the following by digital examination:

1. The size and the mobility of the primary tumor in relation to the pubo-rectal sling in the conscious patient and therefore tone in the pubo-rectal sling (i.e., not simply examination under anesthetic when the pelvic floor may be relaxed).
2. The position and the size of the cancer and its relationship to left or right pelvic sidewalls, prostate, vesicles or vagina in front, and the coccyx and sacrum behind. Mobility on the vaginal wall is particularly important to establish since we do not consider its excision necessary unless it is threatened or invaded by the cancer.
3. The discrete nature and palpability of the precise distal margin of the cancer together with an assessment of the amount of healthy normal mucosa below the tumor and above where the surgeon judges the dentate line to be.

The palpable lower edge of a rectal cancer is almost invariably its microscopic lower edge.

Selection for sphincter preservation. It is the author's opinion that most cancers with (a) a discrete distal margin, which is mobile on the pubo-rectal sling with the patient awake and (b) in whom there is 1–2 cm of clear smooth anorectal mucosa between an anorectal discrete edge and the dentate line, will be best treated, in expert hands, by the TME operation. After the full mesorectal mobilization achieved by this operation, provided the patient has a healthy functioning anal sphincter, an ultralow stapled reconstruction with a colon pouch or side to end anastomosis will provide good or acceptable anorectal function. This, however, may not be true in the new century if the patient has undergone, or later undergoes, radiation therapy – as is now very common in European practice. Data from Sweden suggest that incontinence and frequency of bowel function is rather common after anterior resection procedures in patients who have undergone RT. Frank discussion of these risks with the patient is now essential.

Technical Advances in Total Mesorectal Excision

The basic steps of TME have been fully described elsewhere. The surgeon who is likely to achieve the best results is the one who is prepared to take infinite pains to perfect the creation of a perfect cancer specimen according to the embryological principles which underlie the concept of TME. The "holy plane" around the mesorectum was created in utero when the midline hindgut, distinct from the essentially paired embryonic parities, returned into the abdominal cavity during intrauterine life. All the surgical planes around gut derivatives – pancreas, duodenum, retromesocolic on right or left, the holy plane itself within the pelvis, etc. – are recognizable as dissection planes and provide the key to optimal curative colorectal cancer surgery. This is most particularly true in rectal carcinoma where the main field of spread is usually locoregional, metastases are so often late, and intra-peritoneal spread somewhat uncommon.

If the concept is so simple, how can there be continuing "advances" in the 21st century? Quintessentially these are those improvements that surgeons are making in every field of surgery but applied here to *das koncept der TME totalen mesorectalen excisionen.* Firstly there can be few procedures where it is so true that two really experienced specialist surgeons achieve better results and more perfect specimens than one senior with an inexperienced assistant. This was one of the secondary observations on the data collected for the MERCURY project. Most of the relevant technical advances relate to newer methods of visualizing accurately what we are actually doing. Thus in open surgery improvements in the shaping and illumination of retractors, based on the St. Mark's pattern and the reversed mesorectal retractor with built-in fiber-optic illumination designed by Bolton Surgical, are significant. The use of a pair of retractors, both illuminated but one concave and the other convex, combines the provision of excellent illumination with traction and counter-traction in the difficult depths of the human pelvis. The addition of a third direction of retraction further helps to put areolar tissue continuously on stretch so that it may be divided in an avascular manner by modern diathermy dissection. All these methods combined with the effective aspiration of smoke and the creation of a dry operation field facilitate better and more anatomically correct surgery for this technically challenging malignancy. In addition to this there have been major advances in the use of electro-coagulation and ultrasonic hemostatic devices such as Ligasure. The application of these same principles in laparoscopic surgery is little short of revolutionary in its impact on the potential of the laparoscope in the whole of colorectal surgery. It is interesting in this regard that open surgery and laparoscopic surgery are both making progress but it is the retraction which remains the greatest problem in laparoscopy and the hemostasis which still represents the greatest problem in open surgery. Probably each discipline can learn from the other so that the next few years will see better and better mesorectal specimens with more consistently clear surgical margins. At the present time, however, it is probably sensible to warn laparoscopic surgeons against attempting to excise large cancers in the true pelvis, most particularly in large male patients or patients with a narrow small pelvis. It is literally true that the planar anatomy of the lower pelvis is only now being fully understood because the planes are difficult to demonstrate in the cadaver and difficult to develop during live surgery due to access and bleeding. It is interesting that in laparoscopic surgery the lessons of open surgery are being applied by many of the leading exponents, i.e., sharp monopolar diathermy dissection and more sophisticated methods of opening up tissue planes by ingenious traction and counter-traction devices.

Abdominoperineal Excision

Whilst this has been frequently described elsewhere there are developing ideas which are appropriate for this "update." It has been observed by Quirke and others that the frequently published poor results that are often achieved in APE correlate with a much higher incidence of margin involvement by cancer on the histological specimens than is observed in anterior resection TME specimens. Interestingly these apply both to the perineal and the TME component of the APE – an operation which should encompass the whole mesorectum and the enveloping levators and sphincters. This has led to widespread calls for a more cylindrical operation specimen and the careful avoidance of the development of a "waist" on the APE specimen. This waist comes about because the peri-mesorectal holy plane tapers into the top of the two-layered sphincter mechanism and it is around this area between the dentate line and about 5 cms above it that perforation of the bowel or involvement of the specimen margin most commonly occurs. The author's view is that modern MRI can demonstrate reasonably clearly whether the outside of the sphincter complex is threatened at any point by the carcinoma and it is in these cases that preoperative CRT should be considered – rather than after all ultralow cancers undergoing APE as is practiced in many centers. The specific disadvantage of giving RT to patients undergoing APE is that delayed perineal wound healing becomes extremely common.

It is the author's personal opinion that the widespread advocacy of "cylindrical APE" has perhaps pushed us towards removing more ischio-rectal fat than is really necessary. It appears logical, provided the outside of the sphincter complex is not penetrated by cancer, as visualized on MRI, to preserve most of the ischio-rectal fat and dissect in the recognizable plane just outside the anal sphincters and to follow the levator ani muscles up to their point of origin on the inner aspect of the obturator internus muscles. Many surgeons believe that this can be best done and the best "waist-free" specimens achieved with the patient in the prone jackknife position for the perineal dissection. Removal of the coccyx may also be a wise precaution, particularly in the more advanced cancers, as the larger "hole" thus created makes it safe to deliver the upper part of the specimen first without risking rupture of the cancer which is an operative error to be avoided at all costs. Laparoscopy for the abdominal dissection has obvious advantages in APE, which are not so clear when the method is used for anterior resection, because this perineal delivery of the specimen makes an abdominal incision completely unnecessary. Furthermore, it is desirable to discontinue dissection from the abdominal aspect in APE at the point of origin of the levator muscles around to the coccyx at the back, i.e., the most difficult and challenging part of peri-mesorectal dissection. As in anterior resection, however, the anterior plane remains a major dissection challenge, and anterior tumors have a higher incidence of local failure than posterior or posterolateral tumors.

High Anterior Resection and Mesorectal Transection (Partial Mesorectal Excision)

Partial mesorectal excision (PME) applies to rectal cancers with their lower margin above between 10 and 14 cm from the anal verge according to the size and build of the patient. The degree of extra mobilization that can be achieved by avascular dissection is the final determinant. The decision as to whether a TME or a PME is to be undertaken is made after every avascular component of the dissection has been completed down to the point which used to be described as the "lateral ligament." At this point, where the inferior hypogastric plexus is on the pelvic sidewall, surgeons in the past have used big clamps to divide what are often called the "lateral stalks." Provided peri-mesorectal dissection is pursued in a TME operation very precisely only small vessels are generally found here and no middle rectal artery of any significant size actually exists except in a small minority of patients (Sato & Sato). After dissection has proceeded to this level, if there is a 5 cm mesorectum available distal to the lower edge of the tumor, the mesorectum may be divided at this point using ligasure or ligation. This is only a worthwhile exercise if it enables a significantly higher anastomosis to be effected, as this will obviate the need for a temporary loop stoma. Indeed the whole procedure becomes a less "major" operation with clear advantages for the patient.

The Colon Pouch and the Coloplasty

Each of these methods has been widely described elsewhere and each provides satisfactory improvement in the functional outcome of the very low anastomosis. If a pouch is to be used, however, we would counsel against it being larger than around 2×6 cm for fear of obstructed defecation developing over time. This is the only risk of pouch surgery which may get worse rather than better over time.

Anastomotic Leakage and the Temporary Stoma

The author's extensive traveling and performance of TME in different countries has given him an insight into the variations that exist in attitudes to this problem. It has been made very clear throughout the world that the principal risk factor for anastomotic leakage is the lowness of the anastomosis, i.e., its proximity to the anal sphincters themselves. Rullier put the difference at eight times increase in risk for anastomoses below 6 cm. This places most true TME operations, as opposed to PMEs for higher tumors, in the high-risk category. Multiple discussions in China reveal the fact that there and probably in many parts of the world the defunctioning stoma is not routine but the use of a wide bore soft tube drain for 7 days or more is standard practice against the risk of fecal fistula. In Europe, however, the defunctioning stoma for the ultralow anastomosis has become very widespread indeed whilst drainage is generally restricted to low tension suction drainage for only 2 days to evacuate potential hematoma in the pelvic space. Many factors are relevant to these differences. RT is rarely used in China where anal stretch is considered a convenient and cost-effective method of protecting the anastomosis. The latter is, however, considered inappropriate in Europe by most colorectal authorities who consider that it may lead to long-term anal incontinence. Reconstitution of the pelvic peritoneum in some parts of the world has been common and may be relevant in helping to confine the leakage within the pelvis but this does become virtually impossible if a full TME is undertaken along the lines that have been described by us. Our own view is that significant leakage should be avoided if possible and its consequences minimized since clinically detectable leakage in our own series not only increases mortality but also diminishes the chance of good ano-rectal function. We therefore advocate either ileostomy or colostomy with closure at 6 weeks – before adjuvants if these are planned.

As in so many aspects a multitude of factors contributing to anastomotic leakage make reliable hard data unobtainable. One long-standing misconception has, however, been recently corrected by workers from Orebro in Sweden. They have confirmed that defunctioning does not only minimize or abolish the consequences of a low leak, but it also reduces the risk of this actually occurring. Risk factors which should be borne in mind and which probably make defunctioning in Western practice imperative include smoking, widespread vascular disease, and diabetes. Operative factors that are certainly relevant include pulsatile blood supply on the colonic side of the anastomosis, lack of tension and adequate length to fill the pelvis with redundant colon, optimal hemostasis within the pelvic cavity, and possibly the use of effective suction drainage to remove any blood, which does so readily collect. Good stapling technique and the use of either a colon pouch or a side to end anastomosis are probably important.

The Complete Pathological Response

A "new dilemma" is posed by the apparent complete disappearance of the cancer. This is compounded by the progressive but variable timescale of the down-staging process which continues over many months after the CRT has finished. Somewhat arbitrarily only 6–10 weeks delay is usual before operating – a time perceived as a "window of opportunity." Radical surgery is considered mandatory because regrowth within the irradiated area is believed inevitable. This has been challenged by Habr-Gama and her coworkers in Sao Paolo, Brazil. Her series lacks MRI staging and includes some early tumors, whereas CRT here is usually reserved for advanced cancers threatening the mesorectal margin on MRI, or with other adverse MRI features. The Brazil data, however, show that cancers which seem to have disappeared may indeed have done just that (complete clinical response CR or cCR), i.e., the patient may be cured. As many as 99/360 patients treated between 1991 and 2005 were clinical cCRs and a further 24 patients who had resections had no identifiable cancer in the specimen (ypT0N0). Only 2% of the 99 cCR patients observed without surgery have died of cancer in a follow-up extending for up to 10 years. Five percent regrowths detected during follow-up were all amenable to "delayed resection."

British surgeons have generally regarded the Habr-Gama series as interesting but without immediate relevance. Widespread CRT and mandatory involvement in MDTs does, in our opinion, make this viewpoint no longer tenable – at least for patients about to undergo APE with permanent colostomy. This operation is viewed with dread by many patients who might well prefer a surveillance option. Furthermore, the mandatory positive biopsy before APE is somewhat illogically scrapped if the tumor has "disappeared." Positive biopsy is unlikely in cCR cases because cancer often cannot be found in whole specimens when surgery is undertaken.

It is important that enthusiasm for the exciting possibilities that cCR opens up should be kept in proportion. Specialized primary surgery will continue to be the cornerstone of management, backed by specialized MRI selection for CRT plus histopathological audit to maintain standards. It is probable that 50–70% of patients are best treated by optimal surgery alone, and that most of the downstaged CRT cases will need surgery but will achieve clear margins when these appear threatened. In the short and medium term it is unlikely that more than around 10% of all rectal cancers will be in line for the nonsurgical option. Nevertheless, our fundamental understanding of modern cancer treatment for all solid tumors demands that this special group be properly investigated. Furthermore, if Habr-Gama's experience is confirmed, a significant minority each year may one day be spared the necessity for major surgery.

Summary

Rectal cancer is no longer a disease for the generalist. Rather it has become the paradigm and test bed for the future multidisciplinary specialist management of all solid tumors. The relative importance of surgical technique, modern RT, and the arrival of the new drugs represent one of the most fascinating and complex scenarios in modern medicine. Advances in surgery are individually small but together create one of the most spectacular improvements in actual cancer "cure" of the modern era. The challenge is to organize our cancer services so that all may benefit and so the other (so expensive) modalities may be tested against a standard (high quality) "product" standardized and audited oncological surgery.

Selected Readings

Adam IJ, Mohamdee MO, Martin IG, et al. (1994) Role of circumferential margin involvement in the local recurrence of rectal cancer. Lancet 344:707–711

Heald RJ, Moran BJ, Ryall RDH, et al. (1998) The Basingstoke experience of total mesorectal excision 1978–1997. Arch Surg 133:894–899

Hermanek P, Wiebelt H, Staimmer D, Riedl S (1995) The German Study Group Colorectal Carcinoma (SGCRC). Prognostic factors of rectal carcinoma - experience of the German Multicentre Study. Tumori 81:60–64

MacFarlane JK, Ryall RD, Heald RJ (1993) Mesorectal excision for rectal cancer. Lancet 341:457–460

Martling AL, Holm T, Rutqvist L, et al. (2000) Effect of a surgical training programme on outcome of rectal cancer in the County of Stockholm. Stockholm Colorectal Cancer Study Group, Basingstoke Bowel Cancer Research Project. Lancet 356:93–96

MERCURY Study Group (2006) Diagnostic accuracy of preoperative magnetic resonance imaging in predicting curative resection of rectal cancer: prospective observational study. BMJ 333:779

Quirke P, Scott N (1992) The pathologist's role in the assessment of local recurrence in rectal carcinoma. Surg Oncol Clin North Am 1:1–17

Stelzner F (1996) Das echte und das falsche Lokalrezidiv nach der Kontinenzresektion des rektumkarzinoms. Chirurg 67:611

Wibe A, Moller B, Norstein J, et al. (2002) A national strategic change in treatment policy for rectal cancer—implementation of total mesorectal excision as routine treatment in Norway. A national audit. Dis Colon Rectum 45:857–866

91 Adjuvant and Neoadjuvant Therapy for Colorectal Carcinoma

Anne Y. Lin · Deborah Schrag · W. Douglas Wong

Pearls and Pitfalls

Colon Cancer

- Adjuvant chemotherapy with 5-FU-based chemotherapy is used for the treatment of patients with Stage III colon cancer to minimize local recurrence and metastatic spread of disease.
- Combination regimens with oxaliplatin/5-FU/leucovorin (FOLFOX) have improved disease-free survival rates for patients with Stage III disease. The main side effect of oxaliplatin therapy is peripheral neuropathy.
- Novel targeted therapies with the monoclonal antibodies bevacizumab (anti-VEGFR) and cetuximab (anti-EGFR) are being investigated for use in the adjuvant setting.
- The risk of recurrence is approximately 20–25% for patients with Stage II colon cancer. There is an increasing trend towards treating Stage II colon cancer patients with adjuvant chemotherapy, particularly those with poor prognostic clinicopathologic features.

Rectal Cancer

- An adequate total mesorectal excision (TME) including circumferential margin is important for decreasing local recurrence rates.
- Adjuvant chemotherapy and radiation are recommended for Stages II and III disease.

Introduction

The risk of recurrence in colorectal cancer has decreased with optimal surgery and the addition of adjuvant and neoadjuvant therapy. However, even with an adequate resection for colorectal carcinoma, the risk of recurrence remains present. Adjuvant therapy is thus aimed at the subset of patients who may potentially harbor occult microscopic disease or who have deeper transmural extension of the neoplasm, in an attempt to minimize local recurrence and metastatic spread of disease. Adjuvant chemotherapy is the standard of care for Stage III colon cancer patients. Although controversial, there is an increasing trend toward treating Stage II colon cancer patients with adjuvant chemotherapy. For rectal cancer, adjuvant chemotherapy and radiation are recommended for Stages II and III disease.

Stage III Colon Cancer

5-Fluorouracil-based chemotherapy is currently the standard of treatment for patients with advanced-stage colon cancer. Historically, the added benefit of adjuvant chemotherapy for Stage III colon cancer was established in a series of trials by the National Cancer Institute Intergroup and the National Surgical Adjuvant Breast and Bowel Project in the 1980s. Since then, a 5-year follow-up has shown that levamisole-modulated 5-FU chemotherapy for Stage III colon cancers reduced recurrence and mortality (40% and 33%, respectively). An important finding from the Intergroup-0089 study showed that a 6-month regimen of leucovorin (LV)-modulated 5-FU is comparable to longer-duration therapy and to a levamisole-modulated 5-FU combination. 5-FU can be administered in a bolus or via an infusional fashion. Infusional therapy achieves a higher concentration of the drug with less toxicity. Intergroup 0153 showed that infusional 5-FU therapy was as effective as, but less toxic than, bolus 5-FU in patients with Stage III and high-risk Stage II disease. A preliminary report from a multi-center randomized trial showed a trend toward improved 5-year recurrence-free survival (RFS) and overall survival with less toxicity. Neutropenia and diarrhea were less frequent with infusional therapy; hand-foot syndrome, however, was seen more frequently.

An alternative means of administering 5-FU is via the orally active fluoropyrimidines, specifically capecitabine (Xeloda) and UFT. Capecitabine is activated by the enzyme thymidine phosphorylase within malignant cells. The X-ACT trial was a non-inferiority study that compared capecitabine to the 5-FU/LV Mayo Clinic bolus regimen. This study showed that oral capecitabine is equivalent to the intravenous regimen, with disease-free survival (DFS) as the primary endpoint. Although the incidence of hand-foot syndrome was greater in the capecitabine subgroup, and half of the group required a dose reduction, the overall incidence of adverse effects was less than with bolus 5-FU/LV administration. The NSABP C-06 study assigned 1,608 patients with resected Stage II or III colon cancer to oral UFT plus LV versus the Mayo Clinic 5-FU/LV bolus regimen and found comparable efficacy and toxicity.

As for combination adjuvant therapies, recent trials have examined the effect of adding oxaliplatin to 5FU/LV regimens, with 5FU/LV administered via an infusional (de Gramont) versus bolus (Roswell Park) method. The MOSAIC trial, for example, compares infusional 5-FU/LV versus infusional 5-FU/LV/oxaliplatin (FOLFOX4). Although there was no difference in overall survival, patients with Stage III disease in the infusional 5-FU/LV/oxaliplatin treatment arm had a significantly improved 4-year DFS (70% vs. 61%); this difference was not significant in patients with Stage II disease (85% vs. 81%). The NSABP C-07 study comparing bolus 5-FU/LV (Roswell Park) versus bolus 5-FU/LV/oxaliplatin (FLOX) showed an improvement in 3-year DFS in the bolus 5-FU/LV/oxaliplatin group (77% vs. 72%) for the overall group of patients with both Stage II and III disease. The National Comprehensive Cancer Network (NCCN) guidelines now include FOLFOX as an alternative to 5-FU/LV or capecitabine for Stage III colon cancer.

The primary side effect of oxaliplatin therapy is peripheral neuropathy. Ninety-two percent of patients who received FOLFOX in the MOSAIC trial experienced peripheral neuropathy; 12% had severe (grade 3) neuropathy. Although generally reversible, 4% had persistent grades 2 or 3 neuropathy at 18 months post-treatment. Other side effects of FOLFOX therapy include febrile neutropenia and severe diarrhea (2% and 11%, respectively). Bolus 5-FU/LV/oxaliplatin therapy is associated with more grade 3–4 diarrhea than infusional 5-FU/LV/oxaliplatin.

Another chemotherapeutic agent that has been the focus of many trials is irinotecan. The CALGB trial comparing bolus 5-FU/LV versus bolus 5-FU/LV/irinotecan (IFL) for adjuvant therapy in resected

Stage III disease showed greater toxicity and no clinical benefit for the irinotecan subgroup. The preliminary results for infusional 5FU/Folinic acid (FA) and irinotecan (FOLFIRI) versus 5FU/FA alone in the adjuvant setting for Stage III colon cancer showed no difference in DFS between the two groups. The NCCN guidelines advise against the use of bolus irinotecan in the adjuvant setting; final recommendations for infusional irinotecan are pending.

Novel targeted therapies such as bevacizumab, an antibody against the vascular endothelial growth factor receptor, and cetuximab, an antibody against the epidermal growth factor receptor, have been used successfully in metastatic colorectal cancer and are currently being investigated for use in the adjuvant setting. Current adjuvant trials underway include the following: NSABP C-08, which compares FOLFOX with and without the addition of bevacizumab in Stages II and III disease; Intergroup 0147 (ECOG/NCCTG), which compares FOLFOX versus FOLFOX, and cetuximab in patients with Stage III disease. As for side effects associated with these targeted therapeutic agents, bevacizumab has been associated with hemorrhage, thromboembolism, proteinuria, hypertension, and gastrointestinal perforation. Toxicities associated with cetuximab include an acneiform rash, malaise, and magnesium wasting.

Stage II Colon Cancer

While adjuvant therapy for Stage III colon cancer is clearly beneficial, the role of adjuvant therapy for Stage II colon cancer, with a 20–25% risk of recurrence, is less clear. A pooled analysis of Stage II colon cancer patients randomized to receive either adjuvant treatment with 5-FU/LV or observation showed no significant improvement in overall or event-free survival. The MOSAIC trial, which compared infusional 5-FU/LV versus infusional 5-FU/LV/oxaliplatin (FOLFOX4), showed no difference in overall survival or DFS in patients with Stage II disease. Based on a systematic meta-analysis of 12 randomized trials of 5-FU-based therapy, the American Society of Clinical Oncology (ASCO) reported no statistically significant improvement in overall or event-free survival. Because of the favorable prognosis of Stage II disease, i.e. 75–80% of patients never develop recurrent disease, larger trials are necessary in order to have adequate power to detect a less than 5% (2–4%) benefit. Preliminary results from the QUASAR trial, consisting of 3,239 subjects with colorectal cancer (91% with Stage II disease), showed a small but significant survival benefit in the adjuvant treatment group. This additional benefit, although small, may justify its use in selected high-risk Stage II patients. Individually customized treatment decisions that take into account risk factors and preferences are recommended in this circumstance. For example, consideration of adjuvant therapy may be warranted in patients with poor prognostic features, including inadequately sampled nodes (fewer than 12 nodes), poorly-differentiated histology, T4 lesions, obstructing or perforating neoplasms, venous invasion, and close, indeterminate, or positive margins. The importance of adequate lymph node sampling was demonstrated further in a recent study of patients with Stage II disease; the subset of patients with a greater number of nodes evaluated showed an improvement in overall 5-year survival. Identification of molecular characteristics, such as 18q loss of heterozygosity and microsatellite instability, may help stratify patients with Stage II disease into low-risk and high-risk subgroups. An ongoing trial ECOG E5202, incorporates not only patient stage (IIA versus IIB), but also tumor microsatellite instability and loss of heterozygosity at 18q into the stratification process for treatment with FOLFOX versus FOLFOX with bevacizumab. Assigning therapy based on molecular characteristics is a novel concept that will likely be the aim of additional future trials.

The MOSAIC trial, as previously mentioned, showed a slight improvement in 4-year DFS for patients with Stage II disease receiving infusional 5-FU/LV/oxaliplatin versus 5-FU/LV alone (85% vs. 81%). One may argue that this 4% benefit, in addition to the small benefit (2–4%) gained from adjuvant 5-FU/LV therapy compared with operation alone, provides an additional incremental benefit (up to 7%) with adjuvant treatment. The potential benefits, particularly in average-risk individuals lacking any adverse features, are limited, but for those with high-risk features (obstruction, perforation, and poorly differentiated histology), treatment may be worth considering. Our current recommendation is that the decision regarding adjuvant treatment of Stage II disease should be individualized after forthright patient-physician discussion of the potential benefits (up to 7%) versus risks of treatment-related mortality (<1%) and morbidity.

Rectal Cancer

Heald and colleagues introduced the concept of total mesorectal excision (TME) in rectal resection for improved local control and emphasized the importance of adequate circumferential, proximal, and distal margins. The introduction of adjuvant therapy for Stages II and III rectal cancer resulted in improvements in both locoregional control and overall survival. There are many trials historically evaluating postoperative and preoperative radiotherapy. At the time of introduction of TME, trials aimed at evaluating postoperative radiotherapy showed decreased local recurrence rates without survival benefit. The Swedish Rectal Cancer trial and the Dutch study were designed to examine the benefit of preoperative therapy, given the theoretical advantages of preoperative radiation, which include more tissue oxygenation, potential downsizing of the tumor, and decreased small bowel toxicity. The Swedish Rectal Cancer trial showed a significant decrease in local recurrence and improvement in overall survival with preoperative, short-course radiotherapy of 25 Gy in five fractions. Not all patients in this trial, however, had a standard TME resection. Thus, the Dutch study randomized patients to TME versus short-course radiotherapy followed by TME to assess the potential value of radiotherapy. Prior to initiation of the study, surgeons were trained to perform TME. Short-course radiotherapy, followed by TME, reduced 2-year local recurrence rates from 8% to 2%, but there was no difference in overall survival.

Similar attention was given to adjuvant chemoradiation during this time period. For example, trials by the GITSG and NCCTG showed improved overall survival for the subgroup treated with postoperative CMT. Thus, based on these trials, the NIH consensus statement in 1990 recommended treatment of patients with Stages II and III rectal cancer with 5-FU-based chemotherapy with radiation.

Multiple single-institution studies have demonstrated the potential benefits of neoadjuvant CMT, which provides complete or partial responders with improved resectability, as well as improved overall survival and recurrence rates. Recently, the German Rectal Cancer Trial, a randomized controlled trial, compared preoperative versus postoperative CMT. Patients in the preoperative group received 50.4 Gy in 28 fractions with continuous infusion 5-FU, followed by operative resection in 6 weeks' time. The postoperative group received an extra 5.4 Gy boost to the pelvis. Subsequent to surgery or radiotherapy, each group received an additional four cycles of bolus 5-FU. The preoperative CMT group showed several advantages compared with the postoperative subgroup, including a lesser rate of local recurrence (6% vs. 13%), less grades 3 and 4 toxicity including diarrhea (12% vs. 18%), a higher sphincter-preservation rate (39% vs. 19%), and a lower rate of anastomotic strictures (4% vs. 12%).

Although there are many benefits to preoperative therapy, there are potential limitations, which are related mostly to inaccurate preoperative clinical staging. A few examples are provided by data from the postoperative treatment subgroup: 18% were found to have pathologic Stage I disease; thus, they were overstaged and would have been overtreated with neoadjuvant therapy. Furthermore, another 10% were found to have metastatic disease at the time of the resection or thereafter, and therefore may not have benefited from neoadjuvant therapy. Despite these limitations, at the present time, neoadjuvant CMT has been embraced for the reasons listed above, which include increased sphincter-preservation rates, decreased bowel toxicity, and potential tumor down-sizing for improved operative control. One must be mindful, however, of the potential side effects of adjuvant therapy, including increased rates of bowel incontinence, as well as dissatisfaction with bowel function compared with the TME alone subgroup. Patients at potential risk of overtreatment include those with superficial T3N0 disease and adequate TME with at least 12 sampled nodes negative for metastasis, and those with disease in the proximal rectum. A subset of patients with favorable prognostic features, including pathologic as well as superficial radial extension on imaging by endorectal ultrasonography (<2 mm into perirectal fat), were found to have improved local control and RFS. A final recommendation for this subgroup will require randomized controlled trials, but subject recruitment may be difficult. More adequate staging techniques are needed before subjects will decide to have more limited treatment.

As for postoperative chemotherapy for rectal cancer, the optimal regimen still remains to be determined. Using data extrapolated from colon cancer trials such as the MOSAIC study, our standard is to give patients with clinical Stage III disease eight cycles of postoperative infusional 5-FU/LV/ oxaliplatin following neoadjuvant CMT and resection. For patients with clinical Stage II disease, our preference is for either 5-FU/LV versus 5-FU/LV/oxaliplatin or no treatment, based on absence or presence of favorable-risk characteristics. As in adjuvant treatment for Stage II colon cancer, the decision to treat remains controversial, and therapy needs to be tailored individually after patient-physician discussion of the benefits and risks of treatment.

Newer agents are being investigated for treatment of rectal and colon cancers. Preliminary results using capecitabine appear promising. Several current randomized trials are examining alternative agents, specifically irinotecan and oxaliplatin in conjunction with radiotherapy, for use in the neoadjuvant setting. Another trial compares capecitabine with infusional 5-FU in addition to preoperative radiotherapy. Several phase I and II trials have been performed using irinotecan-based therapy for locally advanced rectal cancer. The studies offer encouraging results and acceptable toxicity. Clinical studies using novel targeted therapies, specifically bevacizumab and cetuximab in combination with traditional cytotoxics, are underway, but none has yet been accepted as the standard of care.

Conclusion

Although this chapter has focused on adjuvant and neoadjuvant therapy for colon and rectal cancer, the importance of an adequate operative resection, for example TME, cannot be overemphasized. Our current regimen for adjuvant treatment of Stage III colon disease includes 5-FU/LV, capecitabine, or 5-FU/LV/oxaliplatin. For high-risk Stage II disease with poor prognostic features, our current practice is to consider these patients for adjuvant treatment with 5-FU/LV, capecitabine, or 5-FU/LV/ oxaliplatin. For patients with rectal cancer, our standard therapy is long-course preoperative chemo-radiation for patients with Stage II and III disease, followed by postoperative adjuvant chemotherapy.

Selected Readings

Colorectal Cancer Collaborative Group (2001) Adjuvant radiotherapy for rectal cancer: a systematic overview of 8,507 patients from 22 randomised trials. Lancet 358:1291–1304

Andre T, Boni C, Mounedji-Boudiaf L, et al. (2004) Oxaliplatin, fluorouracil, and leucovorin as adjuvant treatment for colon cancer. N Engl J Med 350:2343–2351

Benson AB, 3rd, Schrag D, Somerfield MR, et al. (2004) American Society of Clinical Oncology recommendations on adjuvant chemotherapy for Stage II colon cancer. J Clin Oncol 22:3408–3419

Cassidy J, Scheithauer W, McKendrick J, et al. (2004) Capecitabine (X) vs bolus 5-FU/leucovorin (LV) as adjuvant therapy for colon cancer (the X-ACT study): positive efficacy results of a phase III trial. J Clin Oncol (Meeting Abstracts) 22:3509

Chau I, Norman AR, Cunningham D, et al. (2005) A randomised comparison between 6 months of bolus fluorouracil/leucovorin and 12 weeks of protracted venous infusion fluorouracil as adjuvant treatment in colorectal cancer. Ann Oncol 16:549–557

De Gramont A, Boni C, Navarro M, et al. (2005) Oxaliplatin/5FU/LV in the adjuvant treatment of Stage II and stage III colon cancer: Efficacy results with a median follow-up of 4 years. In: ASCO Annual Meeting Proceedings, p 3501

Folkesson J, Birgisson H, Pahlman L, Cedermark B, Glimelius B, Gunnarsson U (2005) Swedish Rectal Cancer Trial: long lasting benefits from radiotherapy on survival and local recurrence rate. J Clin Oncol 23:5644–5650

Gray RG, Barnwell J, Hills R, et al. (2004) QUASAR: a randomized study of adjuvant chemotherapy (CT) vs. observation including 3238 colorectal cancer patients. In: ASCO Annual Meeting, p 3501

Haller DG, Catalano PJ, Macdonald JS, et al. (2005) Phase III study of fluorouracil, leucovorin, and levamisole in high-risk Stage II and III colon cancer: final report of Intergroup 0089. J Clin Oncol 23:8671–8678

Heald RJ, Husband EM, Ryall RD (1982) The mesorectum in rectal cancer surgery – the clue to pelvic recurrence? Br J Surg 69:613–616

Kapiteijn E, Marijnen CA, Nagtegaal ID, et al. (2001) Preoperative radiotherapy combined with total mesorectal excision for resectable rectal cancer. N Engl J Med 345:638–646

Lembersky BC, Wieand HS, Petrelli NJ, et al. (2006) Oral uracil and yegafur plus leucovorin compared with intravenous fluorouracil and leucovorin in Stage II and III carcinoma of the colon: results from National Surgical Adjuvant Breast and Bowel Project Protocol C-06. J Clin Oncol 24:2059–2064

Le Voyer TE, Sigurdson ER, Hanlon AL, et al. (2003) Colon cancer survival is associated with increasing number of lymph nodes analyzed: a secondary survey of intergroup trial INT-0089. J Clin Oncol 21:2912–2919

Mehta VK, Cho C, Ford JM, et al. (2003) Phase II trial of preoperative 3D conformal radiotherapy, protracted venous infusion 5-fluorouracil, and weekly CPT-11, followed by surgery for ultrasound-staged T3 rectal cancer. Int J Radiat Oncol Biol Phys 55:132–137

Minsky BD, Cohen AM, Kemeny N, et al. (1992) Enhancement of radiation-induced downstaging of rectal cancer by fluorouracil and high-dose leucovorin chemotherapy. J Clin Oncol 10:79–84

Minsky B, O'Reilly E, Wong WD, et al. (1999) Daily low-dose irinotecan (CPT-11) plus pelvic irradiation as preoperative treatment of locally advanced rectal cancer (meeting abstract). Proc Am Soc Clin Oncol

Moertel CG, Fleming TR, Macdonald JS, et al. (1995) Fluorouracil plus levamisole as effective adjuvant therapy after resection of Stage III colon carcinoma: a final report. Ann Intern Med 122:321–326

Moertel CG, Fleming TR, Macdonald JS, et al. (1990) Levamisole and fluorouracil for adjuvant therapy of resected colon carcinoma. N Engl J Med 322:352–358

NCCN (2006) Practice guidelines in oncology. Colon cancer 11:1010–1017

NIH consensus conference (1990) Adjuvant therapy for patients with colon and rectal cancer. JAMA 264:1444–1450

Poplin EA, Benedetti JK, Estes NC, et al. (2005) Phase III Southwest Oncology Group 9415/Intergroup 0153 randomized trial of fluorouracil, leucovorin, and levamisole versus fluorouracil continuous infusion and levamisole for adjuvant treatment of Stage III and high-risk Stage II colon cancer. J Clin Oncol 23:1819–1825

Quasar Collaborative Group (2007) Adjuvant chemotherapy versus observation in patients with colorectal cancer: a randomised study. Lancet 370:2020–2029

Sauer R, Becker H, Hohenberger W, et al. (2004) Preoperative versus postoperative chemoradiotherapy for rectal cancer. N Engl J Med 351:1731–1740

Saltz LB, N D, Hollis D, et al. (2004) Irinotecan plus fluorouracil/leucovorin (IFL) versus fluorouracil/leucovorin alone (FL) in Stage III colon cancer (intergroup trial CALGB C89803). In: ASCO Annual Meeting Proceedings

Scheithauer W, McKendrick J, Begbie S, et al. (2003) Oral capecitabine as an alternative to i.v. 5-fluorouracil-based adjuvant therapy for colon cancer: safety results of a randomized, phase III trial. Ann Oncol 14:1735–1743

Schrag D (2005) Improving rectal cancer outcomes with chemotherapy. Semin Colon Rectal Surg 16:162–169 van Cutsem E, Labianca R, Hossfeld D, et al. (2005) Randomized phase III trial comparing infused irinotecan/5-fluorouracil (5-FU)/folinic acid (IF) versus 5-FU/FA (F) in Stage III colon cancer patients (pts). (PETACC 3). J Clin Oncol (Meeting Abstracts) 23:LBA8

Wolmark N, Wieand HS, Kuebler JP, et al. (2005) A phase III trial comparing FULV to FULV + oxaliplatin in Stage II or III carcinoma of the colon: results of NSABP Protocol C-07. In: ASCO Annual Meeting Proceedings, p 3500

Willett CG, Badizadegan K, Ancukiewicz M, Shellito PC (1999) Prognostic factors in stage T3N0 rectal cancer: do all patients require postoperative pelvic irradiation and chemotherapy? Dis Colon Rectum 42:167–173

Part 8

Liver: Benign

92 Hepatitis

John J. Poterucha

Pearls and Pitfalls

- Increases in serum aminotransferases are indicative of hepatocellular injury, while increases in alkaline phosphatase suggest biliary injury, inflammation, or obstruction.
- Increases in serum bilirubin concentration can be secondary to intrahepatic cholestasis (hepatocellular pathology) or mechanical biliary obstruction.
- The best judge of hepatic function may be the prothrombin time (INR).
- Non-alcoholic fatty liver disease (NAFLD) is becoming a major cause of liver disease and cirrhosis.
- The most common causes of viral hepatitis are hepatitis A, B, and C.
- Hepatitis A infection is self-limited without chronic disease.
- Hepatitis B is transmitted by needle stick or sexual contact. Hepatitis B accounts for 40% of acute viral hepatitis and 15% of chronic viral hepatitis.
- Diagnosis of hepatitis B infection is made by hepatitis B surface antigen (HBs Ag).
- All healthcare workers should be immunized against HBV infection.
- Hepatitis C causes 20% of acute viral hepatitis, 60% of chronic hepatitis, and about 40% of all end-stage liver disease in the USA.
- Diagnosis of hepatitis C involves anti-hepatitis C viral antibodies (anti-HCV) or hepatitis C viral RNA (HCV-RNA).
- Sixty percent to 85% of persons with HCV infection remain chronically infected, of whom 20% will develop cirrhosis.

Introduction

There are many causes of liver injury and knowledge of the more common disorders is important to the surgeon. Hepatitis viruses are common causes of liver injury and their clinical importance should be recognized, not only because of their propensity for liver injury, but also because of the risk of transmission. The purpose of this chapter is to familiarize the surgeon with a practical approach to patients with liver disease with an emphasis on the agents that result in viral hepatitis. This chapter will be divided into four major sections:

A. Evaluation of the patient with abnormal liver tests
B. Viral hepatitis
C. Post-operative liver injury
D. Risk of surgery in patients with liver disease

Evaluation of the Patient with Abnormal Liver Tests

The evaluation of patients with abnormal liver blood tests hinges on many clinical factors including the patient's symptoms, age, risk factors for liver disease, personal or family history of liver disease, medications, and findings on physical examination. Because of these multiple factors, designing a standard algorithm for the evaluation of liver test abnormalities is difficult. It is important to understand the commonly used liver tests, the differential diagnosis of diseases characterized by increases in aminotransferases versus alkaline phosphatase, and evaluation of the jaundiced patient.

Commonly Used Liver Tests

Aminotransferases (ALT, AST): Aminotransferases (also referred to as transaminases) are enzymes located in the cytoplasm of hepatocytes and are therefore markers of hepatocellular disease. Injury to hepatocyte membrane allows these enzymes to "leak" out of liver cells, resulting in increases in serum within a few hours after liver injury. Aminotransferases consist of the alanine aminotransferase (ALT), also known in the past as serum glutamate pyruvate transaminase (SGPT) and aspartate aminotransferase (AST), or serum glutamate oxaloacetate transaminase (SGOT). ALT is more specific for liver injury than AST.

Alkaline phosphatase: In contrast, alkaline phosphatase is an enzyme in the hepatocyte membrane bordering bile canaliculi and is more representative of bile duct obstruction or inflammation rather than hepatocyte injury. Because alkaline phosphatase is also found in bone and placenta, an isolated increase in the enzyme should prompt further testing to see if the origin is from liver or other tissues; determination of alkaline phosphatase *isoenzymes* is one such way. Another marker of liver injury is serum gamma-glutamyltransferase (GGT), an enzyme of intrahepatic biliary canaliculi. Other than to confirm the hepatic origin of an increased alkaline phosphatase, GGT has little role in the determination of diseases of the liver, because its synthesis can be induced by many medications thus reducing its specificity for *clinically significant* liver disease. Alkaline phosphatase has to be upregulated and synthesized before it is released, and therefore, diseases characterized by acute biliary obstruction, such as might occur with a common bile duct stone, may not result initially in an increase in alkaline phosphatase.

Bilirubin: Serum bilirubin is measured in direct (conjugated) and indirect (unconjugated) fractions. Commonly occurring liver diseases generally lead to an increase in both direct and indirect fractions. Hepatocyte dysfunction or impairment of bile flow will cause hyperbilirubinemia that is usually $\geq$50% conjugated. Diseases characterized by overproduction of bilirubin, such as hemolysis or resorption of a hematoma, are characterized by hyperbilirubinemia that is $\leq$20% conjugated.

Prothrombin time and albumin: Prothrombin time (measured as international normalized ratio, INR) and serum albumin are markers of the synthetic function of the liver and are probably the best overall markers of severity of liver disease. Abnormalities in INR and albumin imply severe liver disease and should prompt immediate evaluation. Hepatocellular dysfunction is characterized by an inability to synthesize clotting factors despite adequate stores of vitamin K. A prolonged INR due to vitamin K deficiency may be produced by antibiotics associated with a prolonged period of fasting, malabsorptive disorders such as celiac disease, or severe cholestasis with an inability to absorb fat-soluble vitamins (e.g. vitamin K). Correction of the INR after administration of vitamin K documents vitamin K deficiency rather than impaired hepatocellular function.

Because serum albumin has a half-life of 21 days, decreases due to liver dysfunction are not apparent acutely; however, serum albumin can decrease relatively quickly in a patient with severe systemic illness such as bacteremia. These rapid decreases are likely secondary to cytokine release with accelerated metabolism of albumin. A decrease of albumin in a patient without overt liver disease should prompt consideration of albumin loss in the urine or gastrointestinal tract.

Hepatocellular Disorders

Diseases affecting primarily hepatocytes are said to cause "hepatitis" and are characterized by predominant increases in serum aminotransferases with normal or lesser increases in serum alkaline phosphatase. Hepatitis generally is subdivided based on disease duration into acute or chronic (duration arbitrarily defined as less than or greater than 3 months). Patients with acute hepatitis often have fatigue, nausea, mild upper abdominal pain, and jaundice; aminotransferases are usually >500 U/L (normal values are < 40–45 U/L). The abdominal pain of acute hepatitis is usually less severe than that of biliary duct obstruction. Increased liver tests or jaundice without a clear history of biliary pain is not an indication for cholecystectomy. The more common causes of acute hepatitis are listed in ❯ *Table 92-1.*

The degree and pattern of increases in aminotransferases may be helpful in the differential diagnosis of acute hepatitis. Acute hepatitis due to *viruses* or *drugs other than acetaminophen* generally produces increases in aminotransferase of 1,000–3,000 U/L. In general, ALT is greater than AST. ALT >5,000 U/L is usually due to acetaminophen hepatotoxicity, hepatic ischemia ("shock liver"), or an unusual virus such as herpes. The *hepatic ischemia* that occurs after an episode of hypotension, usually in patients with pre-existing cardiac disease, leads to very high serum aminotransferases that improve dramatically within a few days. Another cause of a short-lived increase in aminotransferases is transient bile duct obstruction, usually due to a stone. These increases can be as high as 1,000 U/L but improve within 24–48 h. Patients with transient bile duct obstruction usually have prominent abdominal pain. *Alcoholic hepatitis* is characterized by more modest increases in aminotransferase, always less than 400 IU and at times near normal. Patients with alcoholic hepatitis also usually have an AST:ALT ratio greater than 2 and frequently have an increases serum bilirubin out of proportion to the aminotransferase elevations.

◻ Table 92-1

Common causes of acute hepatitis

Disease	Clinical clues	Diagnostic tests
Hepatitis A	Exposure history	IgM anti-HAV
Hepatitis B	Risk factors	HBsAg, IgM anti-HBc
Drug-induced	Compatible medication/timing	Improvement after withdrawal from agent
Alcoholic hepatitis	History of alcohol excess, AST:ALT > 2	Liver biopsy, improvement with abstinence
Ischemic hepatitis	History of hypotension	Rapid improvement of aminotransferases
Acute duct obstruction	Abdominal pain, fever	Cholangiogram

See text for abbreviations.

◻ Table 92-2

Common causes of chronic hepatitis

Disease	Clinical clues	Diagnostic tests
Hepatitis C	Risk factors	Anti-HCV
Hepatitis B	Risk factors	HBsAg
Nonalcoholic steatohepatitis	Obesity, diabetes, hyperlipidemia	Ultrasonography, liver biopsy
Hemochromatosis	Arthritis, diabetes, family history	Iron studies, gene test, biopsy
Alcoholic liver disease	History, AST:ALT > 2	Liver biopsy
Autoimmune hepatitis	ALT 200–1,500, usually female, other autoimmune disease	Antinuclear or anti-smooth muscle antibody, biopsy

See text for abbreviations.

Diseases producing sustained (>3–6 months) increases in aminotransferases are said to be causing *chronic* hepatitis. In general, these increases in aminotransferase are more modest than those in acute hepatitis, usually 2–5 fold increased. Most patients with chronic hepatitis are asymptomatic, although some patients have fatigue and mild right upper quadrant pain. The differential diagnosis of chronic hepatitis is relatively lengthy, but the most important and common disorders are found in ❷ *Table 92-2.*

Risk factors for *hepatitis C* include a history of blood transfusions or intravenous drug use. Patients with *hepatitis B* may give a history of illegal drug use or frequent sexual contacts or be from a high endemic area such as Asia or Africa. *Nonalcoholic fatty liver disease (NAFLD)* is probably the most common cause of abnormal liver enzymes in the US. Patients with NAFLD usually have obesity, diabetes, and/or hyperlipidemia. Ultrasonography may show changes in echotexture of the liver consistent with fatty infiltration. A careful history will be necessary to help diagnose *drug-induced* or *alcohol-induced* liver disease. Most patients with *genetic hemochromatosis* have normal liver enzymes unless cirrhosis is present, although all will have excess hepatic iron deposition. Genetic hemochromatosis also causes diabetes, hypogonadism, and joint complaints. *Autoimmune hepatitis* may present as an acute or chronic hepatitis; patients usually have aminotransferases of 300–2,000 U/L, a bit greater than other chronic hepatidities. The presence of autoantibodies, hypergammaglobulinemia, and other autoimmune disorders are helpful clues to the diagnosis of autoimmune hepatitis. Low level positive antinuclear antibodies are very common in other forms of chronic liver disease and are therefore not pathognomonic of autoimmune hepatitis.

Cholestatic Disorders

Diseases that affect predominantly the biliary system are termed cholestatic diseases. These processes can affect the microscopic ducts (e.g. primary biliary cirrhosis), large bile ducts (e.g. pancreatic cancer causing common bile duct obstruction), or both (e.g. primary sclerosing cholangitis). In general, the predominant biochemical abnormality in these disorders is in alkaline phosphatase. Although diseases that produce elevations in bilirubin are often called "cholestatic," severe hepatocellular injury, such as occurs with an acute hepatitis, will also produce hyperbilirubinemia because of hepatocellular dysfunction. Common causes of cholestasis are illustrated in ❷ *Table 92-3.*

Large bile duct obstruction is often due to stones or benign or malignant strictures. Remember that acute large duct obstruction from a stone may produce early on, marked increases in aminotransferases,

◻ **Table 92-3**

Common causes of cholestasis

Disease	Clinical clues	Diagnostic tests
Primary biliary cirrhosis	Middle-aged female	Antimitochondrial antibody
Primary sclerosing cholangitis	Association with ulcerative colitis	Cholangiography (ERCP)
Large bile duct obstruction	Jaundice and pain	Ultrasonography, ERCP
Drug-induced	Compatible medication/timing	Improvement after withdrawal of agent
Intrahepatic mass lesions	History of malignancy	Ultrasonography, computed tomography
Infiltrative disorder	Features of sarcoid or amyloid	Biopsy

usually in the setting of biliary-type pain. Most patients with large duct obstruction will have dilated ducts on cross-sectional imaging such as ultrasonography, computed tomography, or magnetic resonance imaging. *Primary sclerosing cholangitis (PSC)* has a strong association with ulcerative colitis. Patients with PSC and PBC are often asymptomatic but may have jaundice, fatigue, or pruritus. *Primary biliary cirrhosis* (PBC) most commonly affects middle-aged women. *Intrahepatic mass lesions* should be considered in a patent with cholestatic liver test abnormalities and a history of malignancy. Any systemic inflammatory process such as infection or immune disorder may produce nonspecific abnormalities in liver tests, usually manifest by a mixed cholestatic (alkaline phosphatase) and hepatocellular (ALT or AST) pattern. NAFLD occasionally produces an increased alkaline phosphatase, while patients with alcoholic hepatitis commonly have an increased alkaline phosphatase.

Jaundice

Jaundice becomes evident visibly when serum bilirubin is >2.5 mg/dl. As noted above, it may be important to note whether the serum bilirubin is predominantly conjugated or unconjugated. A common benign disorder that produces an unconjugated hyperbilirubinemia (although not usually jaundice) is *Gilbert's syndrome*, which affects ~2% of the population. The total bilirubin is generally less than 3.0 mg/dl, while the direct will be 0.3 mg/dl or less. The bilirubin is generally greater in the fasting state or when the patient is ill. A presumptive diagnosis of Gilbert's disease can be made in an otherwise well patient with unconjugated hyperbilirubinemia, normal liver enzymes, and normal hemoglobin (to exclude hemolysis).

Patients with jaundice due to liver or biliary disorders have direct hyperbilirubinemia. The first goal is to differentiate intrahepatic diseases, such as alcoholic or viral hepatitis, from those with obstruction. Abdominal pain, fever, and/or a palpable gallbladder are suggestive of obstruction. Excess intake of alcohol, risk factors for viral hepatitis, a bilirubin greater than 15 mg/dl, and persistent markedly increased aminotransferases suggest that the jaundice is due to hepatocellular dysfunction. In patients with acute hepatocellular dysfunction and jaundice, improvement in bilirubin often lags behind improvement in serum aminotransferase. Computed tomography and ultrasonography are good initial tests to assess for obstructive causes of jaundice. Diseases characterized by large duct obstruction will generally exhibit intrahepatic bile duct dilatation. A common error is to attribute jaundice to extrahepatic bile duct obstruction or gallstones. Operations in patients with intrahepatic cholestasis are complicated commonly by worsening liver function, including life-threatening complications of portal hypertension. Sepsis can also produce jaundice by causing intrahepatic cholestasis.

Viral Hepatitis

Viral hepatitis is important both to surgeons and surgical patients, not only because hepatitis viruses result in clinically relevant liver disease, but also because of the risk of transmission. Viral infections are important causes of liver disease worldwide with five primary hepatitis viruses having been identified (hepatitis A, B, C, D, and E).

Disorders that cause hepatitis are characterized primarily by increases in aminotransferase (ALT and AST). Causes of hepatitis other than viruses include medications, nonalcoholic or alcoholic steatohepatitis, autoimmune hepatitis, or Wilson's disease. Non-hepatotropic viruses, such as cytomegalovirus or Epstein-Barr virus, can also result in hepatitis as part of a systemic infection.

It is useful to divide hepatitis syndromes into acute or chronic. Acute hepatitis can last from weeks up to 3–6 months and is often accompanied by jaundice. The symptoms of acute hepatitis are similar regardless of etiology and include anorexia, malaise, dark urine, fever, and occasionally abdominal pain. The abdominal pain accompanying hepatitis is located generally in the right upper quadrant of the abdomen, is usually mild and constant, and should not be confused with the more severe episodic pain associated with disorders of the biliary tract and pancreas. Chronic hepatitis is defined as the presence of hepatitis for more than 3–6 months. Patients with chronic hepatitis are often asymptomatic but may complain of fatigue. Occasionally, patients have manifestations of cirrhosis (ascites, variceal bleeding, or encephalopathy) as the initial symptoms of a chronic liver disorder. Each primary hepatitis virus causes acute hepatitis, but only hepatitis viruses B, C, and D result in chronic hepatitis (❷ *Table 92-4*).

Hepatitis A

Hepatitis A virus (HAV) causes about 30% of acute hepatitis in the US Acquisition of hepatitis A requires exposure to contaminated food or infected individuals. Groups at particularly high risk for acquiring hepatitis A include people living in or traveling to underdeveloped countries, children in day-care centers, homosexual men, and perhaps individuals ingesting raw shellfish. The incubation period for hepatitis A is 2–6 weeks.

The most important determinant of the severity of acute hepatitis A is the age at which infection occurs. Those infected when less than 6 years of age are often asymptomatic and if symptoms are present, rarely include jaundice. Up to 40% of individuals over 40 years of age have serologic evidence of a remote hepatitis A infection, yet neither the patient nor a parent will recall an episode of jaundice. Adults acquiring hepatitis A are much more likely than young children to have jaundice.

❏ Table 92-4

Comparison of the primary hepatitis viruses

	HAV	HBV	HDV	HCV	HEV
Incubation (days)	15–50	30–160	Unknown	14–160	14–45
Jaundice	Common	Common	Common	Uncommon	Common
Course	Acute	Acute or chronic	Acute or chronic	Acute or chronic	Acute
Transmission	Fecal-oral	Parenteral	Parenteral	Parenteral	Fecal-oral
Test for diagnosis	IgM Anti-HAV	HBsAg	Anti-HDV	Anti-HCV or HCV-RNA	Anti-HEV

See text for abbreviations.

Diagnosis of acute hepatitis A is made by the presence of IgM anti-HAV which appears at the onset of the acute phase of the illness and disappears in 3–6 months. IgG anti-HAV also becomes positive during the acute phase and persists for decades. A patient with IgG anti-HAV, but not IgM anti-HAV, has had an infection in the remote past or has received hepatitis A vaccine.

Hepatitis A is almost always a self-limited infection, although there may be a prolonged cholestatic phase characterized by persistence of jaundice for 1–3 months. Rarely, acute hepatitis A may cause fulminant hepatic failure and require liver transplantation. Hepatitis A does not result in chronic infection and should not be in the differential diagnosis of a chronic hepatitis.

Treatment of hepatitis A is supportive. Isolation of hospitalized patients is recommended, although viral titers are actually highest in the presymptomatic phase. Immune globulin should be administered to all household and intimate (including day-care) contacts within 2 weeks of exposure. Hepatitis A vaccine is recommended for individuals with contact to patients with hepatitis A, those planning prolonged stays in areas where hepatitis A is endemic, and persons with chronic liver disease.

Because HAV does not cause chronic infection, parenteral transmission (including that from needle-stick exposure) is rare. Hepatitis A, like any acute hepatitis, may result in jaundice, and the surgeon needs to differentiate the jaundice associated with acute hepatitis from that due to obstruction (see above).

Hepatitis B

Hepatitis B virus (HBV) is a DNA virus that causes about 40% of acute viral hepatitis and 15% of chronic viral hepatitis in the US. Most infected people living currently in the US are immigrants from countries in Asia and Africa with a high prevalence of hepatitis B who likely acquired hepatitis B perinatally or in early childhood. HBV may also be transmitted by needlestick exposure or sexual contact.

The incubation period after HBV infection ranges from 30 to 180 days. Clinical outcome varies. Acute hepatitis B in the adolescent or adult is icteric in 30%. Most patients recover after an episode of acute hepatitis B, although about 5% of infected adults will have persistence of HBsAg (see ❯ *Table 92-5* for a guide to hepatitis B serologic markers) for longer than 6 months and are termed chronically infected. The outcome of chronic infection is also variable. Some patients have normal liver enzymes, HBV DNA level < 20,000 U/ml, and a normal liver biopsy despite the persistence of HBsAg.

◻ Table 92-5

Hepatitis B: serological markers

Test	Significance
HBsAg	Marker for current infection
anti-HBs	Marker for immunity (resolved infection or immunization)
IgM anti-HBc	Suggests recent infection
IgG anti-HBc	Marker for remote infection
HBeAg and HBV-DNA level > 20,000 IU/ml	Marker for active viral replication (high infectivity)

HBsAg = hepatitis B surface antigen; Anti-HBs = antibody to hepatitis B surface; anti-HBc = antibody to hepatitis B core; HBeAg = hepatitis B e antigen; HBV-DNA = hepatitis B virus DNA.

Such patients are termed HBV inactive carriers and have an excellent prognosis. Individuals with abnormal liver tests and an HBV DNA level > 20,000 U/ml in the setting of chronic HBsAg positivity have chronic hepatitis B and are at much higher risk for developing cirrhosis and hepatocellular carcinoma. Spontaneous clearance of HBsAg occurs in 1–2% of chronically infected patients per year although is even less likely in those who have been infected since early childhood.

Seroconversion of hepatitis B antigen (HBeAg) positive to negative with development of antibody to hepatitis B e (anti-HBe) occurs in about 10% of chronic HBV patients per year and may be accompanied by a flare of disease. Patients with chronic hepatitis B who are HBeAg-negative but have HBV DNA > 20,000 U/ml (HBeAg-negative chronic hepatitis B), are often infected with pre-core or core promoter variants of HBV and may have a worse prognosis than those with wild-type virus.

In general, treatment is given to those patients with hepatitis B who are at risk for progression. Such patients include those with liver enzymes greater than twice the upper limit of normal and active viral replication as defined by HBV-DNA > 20,000 U/ml. Some treatment guidelines also recommend liver biopsy before treatment, especially in patients with only modest abnormalities of liver enzymes. Treatment for hepatitis B can be with pegylated interferon or one of the oral agents, lamivudine, adefovir, entecavir, and telbivudine. Predictors of greater likelihood of response include higher ALT, lower HBV DNA level, shorter duration of disease, and female gender. About 20–30% of patients treated with oral agents have seroconversion of HBeAg after 1–2 years of therapy; treatment should be continued for at least 6 months after seroconversion. Patients without seroconversion of HBeAg need treatment indefinitely. Seroconversion of HBsAg (i.e. cure) with the oral antiviral agents occurs only rarely and should not be considered a reasonable treatment goal.

HBV may be transmitted by needle-stick exposure. Patients with chronic hepatitis B (HBsAg-positive) who have HBV DNA levels > 20,000 IU/ml are at greatest risk for transmitting infection. Health care workers exposed to needles from HBeAg-positive individuals have a 30% risk of contracting hepatitis B if not already immune. All surgeons should receive the hepatitis B vaccine and verify immunity by measuring anti-HBs 6 months after vaccination and then every 5 years thereafter. Non-immune surgeons exposed to a needle-stick from a HBsAg-positive patient should receive hepatitis B immune globulin as soon as possible after exposure.

Surgeons should also be aware that hepatitis B can still be transmitted rarely by transfusion of blood products. It is estimated that one of every 63,000 units of blood transfused is tainted with hepatitis B. Surgeons may also transmit hepatitis B rarely to patients. Although routine hepatitis B testing of health care workers is not advised, individuals who perform invasive procedures and who do not develop anti-HBs after vaccination should know their HBsAg status, and if positive, the HBeAg and HBV DNA status. HBsAg-positive surgeons should seek counsel from their local medical society and be considered for therapy.

Hepatitis D

Hepatitis D (HDV or the "delta" agent) is a defective virus that requires the presence of HBsAg to cause disease. HDV infection can occur simultaneously with HBV (coinfection) or as a superinfection in persons with established hepatitis B. Hepatitis D is diagnosed by anti-HDV and should be suspected in a patient with acute hepatitis B or an acute exacerbation of chronic hepatitis B. In the US, intravenous drug users are the group of HBV patients at highest risk for acquiring HDV. Because hepatitis D requires the presence of HBsAg to cause disease, the general implications of hepatitis D to the surgeon are similar to those for hepatitis B.

Hepatitis C

Hepatitis C (HCV) is an RNA virus that infects about four million individuals in the US HCV causes 20% of acute hepatitis, 60% of chronic hepatitis, and about 40% of all end-stage liver disease in the US Clinically recognized acute hepatitis C is unusual, and the importance of hepatitis C lies in its propensity to cause chronic infection. Major risk factors for hepatitis C infection are intravenous drug use and blood transfusion prior to 1992.

The incubation period for HCV ranges from 2 to 22 weeks (mean 7 weeks). Most acute hepatitis C is asymptomatic and anicteric. Fully 60–85% of persons with HCV infection fail to clear the virus by 6 months and develop chronic infection. Up to 30% of patients chronically infected with HCV have persistently normal ALT values. Patients with chronic hepatitis C may have nonspecific symptoms such as fatigue and vague abdominal pain. Occasionally, patients present with extrahepatic manifestations such as vasculitis associated with cryoglobulinemia. Once HCV results in cirrhosis, symptoms are more common and include fatigue or complications of end-stage liver disease.

About 20% of patients with chronic hepatitis C develop cirrhosis over a 10–20 year period. A long duration of infection and alcohol abuse are risk factors for the development of cirrhosis. The rate of progression of hepatitis C is slow, with those patients developing cirrhosis generally doing so only after more than 15 years of disease. Patients with cirrhosis due to HCV are at risk for developing hepatocellular carcinoma and should undergo surveillance with ultrasonography every 6–12 months.

A guide to the interpretations of hepatitis C tests is found in ❯ *Table 92-6*. Antibody to HCV (anti-HCV) is not protective and indicates either current or resolved infection. Anti-HCV by enzyme-linked immunoassay (ELISA) is sensitive for HCV infection and is the screening test of choice in most laboratories. The specificity of the ELISA is improved with the addition of the recombinant immunoblot assay (RIBA). A positive RIBA indicates the presence of antibodies to HCV but still could represent a resolved infection. The presence of HCV-RNA by polymerase chain reaction is diagnostic of ongoing HCV infection. HCV-RNA level and genotype can also be obtained if therapy is being considered.

Therapy for hepatitis C with pegylated interferon and ribavirin for 6–12 months results in a sustained loss of virus response in about 50–60% of patients. Because of the multiple side effects of treatment and the relatively low response rates, treatment is generally recommended if a biopsy demonstrates substantial fibrosis or the patient has genotypes 2 or 3 (which are more likely to respond

◻ Table 92-6

Interpretation of anti-HCV results

Anti-HCV by EIA	Anti-HCV by RIBA	Interpretation
Positive	Negative	False positive EIA, patient does not have true antibody
Positive	Positive	Patient has antibody[a]
Positive	Indeterminate	Uncertain antibody status

See text for abbreviations.

[a]Remember that anti-HCV does not necessarily indicate current hepatitis C infection.

than genotype 1). Treatment is less likely to be effective or tolerated in patients with decompensated cirrhosis; such patients should be referred for liver transplantation.

Hepatitis C is spread parenterally and rarely can be spread by needle-stick exposure. Prospective studies demonstrate seroconversion rates of 0% to 11% after a needle-stick exposure from a hepatitis C-positive patient. Unfortunately, there is no hepatitis C vaccine available, and post-exposure prophylaxis has not proven beneficial. After exposure to a hepatitis C positive individual, HCV RNA should be determined in 2–4 weeks and anti-HCV in 3–6 months. In the unlikely event that hepatitis C transmission occurs, treatment with pegylated interferon and ribavirin may be offered.

There are case reports of transmission of HCV from surgeon to patients. Nevertheless, transmission is exceedingly rare, and there are currently no practice limitations for health care workers infected with HCV. Surgeons should also be aware that while blood product transfusion was a common cause of hepatitis C prior to 1990, the virus is now spread only rarely by blood transfusion. Estimates are that only one of every 103,000 units of blood transfused would be infected with HCV.

Hepatitis E

Hepatitis E causes large outbreaks of acute hepatitis in underdeveloped countries. Physicians in the United States are unlikely to see a patient with hepatitis E. A rare patient may become infected during foreign travel. Clinically, hepatitis E infection is similar to hepatitis A. Resolution of the hepatitis is the rule, and chronic infection does not occur.

Differentiation of viral hepatidities: Ordering tests for cases of presumed viral hepatitis can be confusing, but ❯ *Tables 92-7* and ❯ *92-8* give a practical guide for testing for patients presenting with acute or chronic hepatitis.

Post-Operative Liver Injury

Mild abnormalities in liver enzymes are common after general anesthesia. Most individuals undergoing abdominal operations will have decreased hepatic blood flow, which may contribute to these mild

◼ Table 92-7

Acute hepatitis: practical guide to ordering tests and interpretations

| Interpretation | Tests to order | | | |
	IgM anti-HAV	HBsAg	IgM anti-HBc	anti-HCV
Acute HAV	Positive	Negative	Negative	Negative
Acute HBV	Negative	Positive	Positive	Negative
Acute HBV[a]	Negative	Negative	Positive	Negative
Chronic HBV[b]	Negative	Positive	Negative	Negative
Acute or chronic HCV[c]	Negative	Negative	Negative	Positive
Exclude other causes[c]	Negative	Negative	Negative	Negative

See text for abbreviations.

[a]Occasionally patients with acute HBV will lack HBsAg.

[b]HBsAg without IgM anti-HBc is more suggestive of chronic HBV. Exclude HDV or other non-viral causes of acute hepatitis.

[c]Anti-HCV may not be positive in acute hepatitis C and, when present, may indicate chronic infection so other causes should be excluded.

abnormalities. A more severe acute hepatitis may occur after general anesthesia and is best described after the use of halothane but may also be seen with other inhaled anesthetic agents. Post-operative jaundice may be due to liver injury, although indirect hyperbilirubinemia occurs occasionally due to resorption of a large hematoma. Ischemic hepatitis only occurs after a sustained hypotensive episode and is characterized by marked increases in aminotransferases that improve relatively quickly but can be followed by jaundice.

Operations on Patients with Liver Disease

The alterations in hepatic blood flow that occur with general anesthesia can cause decompensation in patients with more severe forms of liver disease. Although good data about the risks of operation in patients with liver disease are lacking, the more severe the liver disease, the more likely that decompensation may occur. The type of operation may also be important, with the highest rates of decompensation occurring after abdominal or thoracic procedures; however, even relatively minor surgery such as umbilical herniorrhaphy in a patient with cirrhosis may result in worsening of liver disease. Patients with acute hepatitis, severe alcoholic hepatitis, and those with cirrhosis with evidence of hepatic compromise are at the highest risk of post-operative liver injury. In general, more severe forms of liver disease can be identified by the presence of laboratory parameters of abnormal liver function (hyperbilirubinemia, prolonged prothrombin time, or hypoalbuminemia), physical examination, or historical evidence of complications of portal hypertension (ascites, portal systemic encephalopathy, splenomegaly, or varices).

For patients with cirrhosis, outcomes after abdominal operations depend on the severity of liver disease as measured by the Child-Pugh score (see ❯ *Table 92-9*). Mortality rates of 10%, 30%, and 82%

❑ Table 92-8

Chronic hepatitis: practical guide to ordering tests and interpretation

Interpretation	Tests to order	
	HBsAg	anti-HCV
HBV	Positive	Negative
HCV	Negative	Positive
Exclude other causes	Negative	Negative

See text for abbreviations.

❑ Table 92-9

Child-Pugh classification of severity of liver disease

	1 point	2 points	3 points
Encephalopathy	None	Grade 1 or 2	Grade 3 or 4
Ascites	None	Mild	Moderate or severe
Bilirubin (mg/dl)	<2	2.1–3	>3
Albumin	>3.5	2.8–3.5	<2.8
Prothrombin time (INR)	<1.7	1.7–2.3	>2.3

Class A = 5–6 points, class B = 7–9 points, and class C = 10–15 points.

have been reported with patients with Child-Pugh class A, B, and C, respectively. Even patients with well-compensated cirrhosis are at risk for death after abdominal operations. Decompensation of the liver disease is even more common and consists usually of development or worsening of ascites, encephalopathy, jaundice, or bleeding. Ascites can be a particular problem after abdominal operations, because it can compromise wound healing. If advanced liver disease is noted at operation, stomas should be avoided if at all possible.

Complication rates after operations on patients with cirrhosis are high enough that nonoperative interventions are preferred if at all possible. In those situations where operative intervention is required, careful monitoring of mental status and fluid status in the postoperative period is especially important. Limiting the amount of sodium-containing intravenous fluids after operation will help prevent ascites.

Selected Readings

Centers for Disease Control and Prevention (1999) Prevention of hepatitis A through active or passive immunization: recommendations of the Advisory Committee on Immunization Practices (ACIP). Morbidity and Mortality Weekly Report 48(No. RR-12):1–54

Centers for Disease Control (1997) Immunization of healthcare workers: recommendations of the advisory committee on immunization practices and the hospital infection control practices advisory committee. Morbidity and Mortality Weekly Report 46(RR-18):1–42

Centers for Disease Control (1991) Recommendations for preventing transmission of human immunodeficiency virus and hepatitis B virus to patients during exposure-prone invasive procedures. Morbidity and Mortality Weekly Report 40(RR08):1–9

Friedman LS (1999) The risk of surgery in patients with liver disease. Hepatol 29:1617–1623

Ganem D, Prince AM (2004) Hepatitis B virus infection – natural history and clinical consequences. NEJM 350:1118–1129

Keeffe EB, Dieterich DT, Han SB, et al. (2004) A treatment algorithm for the management of hepatitis B infection in the United States. Clin Gastroenterol Hepatol 2:87–106

Lok AS, McMahon BJ (2007) AASLD practice guidelines: chronic hepatitis B. Hepatology 45:507–539

Poterucha JJ (2006) Approach the patient with abnormal liver tests and fulminant liver failure. In: Hauser SC (ed) Mayo Clinic Gastroenterology and Hepatology Board Review. Mayo Clinic Scientific Press, Rochester, pp 263–270

Poterucha JJ Chronic viral hepatitis (2006) In: Hauser SC (ed) Mayo Clinic Gastroenterology and Hepatology Board Review. Mayo Clinic Scientific Press, Rochester, pp 271–280

Schreiber GB, Busch MP, Kleinman SH, et al. (1996) The risk of transfusion-transmitted viral infections. NEJM 334:1685–1690

Strader DB, Wright T, Thomas DL, et al. (2004) AASLD guideline: diagnosis, management, and treatment of hepatitis C. Hepatology 39:1147–1171

93 Differential Diagnosis of the Liver Mass

Wei-Chen Lee · Miin-Fu Chen

Pearls and Pitfalls

- Currently, most liver masses are asymptomatic and are identified incidentally during survey for chronic liver diseases or other purposes.
- Many liver masses occur in cirrhotic livers secondary to chronic hepatitis B virus (HBV) and hepatitis C virus (HCV) infections.
- Abdominal ultrasonography is the most convenient imaging modality to screen patients at risk for liver masses and will differentiate cystic from solid tumors.
- Dynamic computed tomography (CT) is recommended to assess the liver tumor and remainder of the abdominal cavity simultaneously.
- CT, magnetic resonance imaging (MRI), and angiography can be valuable and complementary in the evaluation of liver masses.
- Tumor markers, such as α-fetoprotein (AFP), carcinoembryonic antigen (CEA), and carbohydrate antigen 19-9 (CA19-9), may help to narrow the differential diagnosis.
- Positron emission tomography (PET) has not proven useful or cost-effective for differentiating most liver masses.
- Liver biopsy is recommended only when operative intervention is not planned and a correct diagnosis would alter treatment planning.

Introduction

Currently, a majority of liver masses are asymptomatic and are diagnosed incidentally or during screening of patients with liver disease. Prior to the advent of ultrasonography, however, symptomatic or palpable large tumors were common. While identification of the presence of a liver mass is important, it is even more important to make a correct diagnosis.

Several benign and malignant liver tumors exist (❯ *Table 93-1*). The appropriate management of a liver mass necessitates an accurate differential diagnosis. Frequently, the diagnosis requires a thorough clinical history, physical examination, laboratory assessment, and imaging methods.

◘ Table 93-1

Classification of the common liver mass

Benign	Malignant
Hemangioma	Hepatocellular carcinoma
Focal nodular hyperplasia	Cholangiocarcinoma
Hepatocellular adenoma	Metastatic tumor
Simple cyst	Angiosarcoma
Polycystic liver disease	Cystadenocarcinoma
Cystadenoma	Epithelioid hemangioendothelioma
Abscess	
Angiomyolipoma	
Lipoma	
Inflammation pseudotumor	
Regenerative nodule	
Fat sparing	

Diagnostic Tools

Laboratory evaluation: Liver enzymes, alanine aminotransferase (ALT) and aspartate aminotransferase (AST), hepatitis B antigens, antibody to hepatitis C, AFP, and CEA all should be measured. HBVs and HCVs are both precipitating factors for hepatocellular carcinoma (HCC). In Southeast Asia, about 60% and 30% of patients with HCC are associated with chronic hepatitis B and hepatitis C infections, respectively. Thus, all the patients having liver tumors should have the profiles of virus infection to make a differential diagnosis. When present, AFP is a virtually diagnostic serum marker for HCC; however, only 65% of HCC patients have an increased serum level of AFP. CEA and CA19-9 are important markers of colorectal and other GI tract cancers, and increased values may indicate biliary or metastatic disease.

Liver ultrasonography: Because abdominal ultrasonography is both noninvasive and inexpensive, currently, it is the imaging method used most frequently to screen for liver tumors. Ultrasonography can effectively identify a liver mass of 5 mm and is valuable to differentiate cystic from solid lesions.

Dynamic computed tomography (CT): CT is the most effective tool to diagnose and evaluate liver masses. Neoplasms demonstrate a preference for arterial blood supply. This physiologic fact allows for differentiating characteristics on diagnostic imaging. Dynamic CT is performed at a time sequence when contrast medium is infused to obtain CT imaging in the arterial phase (25–30 s delay), portal phase (70–80 s delay), and delayed phase (10 min delay). Based on the vascular densities during these different phases, liver tumors can often be differentiated from one another.

Magnetic resonance imaging (MRI): MRI, a noninvasive examination, has a superior soft-tissue contrast and topographic accuracy. Contrast agents to be used with MRI have been developed to increase the accuracy of differential diagnosis. Superparamagnetic iron oxides (SPIO) are iron oxide particles that are taken up by the reticuloendothelial system. For liver imaging studies, intravenous infusion of SPIO reduces signal intensity of the liver parenchyma on T2-weighted images and help distinguish benign and malignant tumors.

Angiography: Angiography is an invasive examination that is used rarely, given the accuracy of noninvasive imaging. By analyzing blood supply and vascular pattern, differentiation of liver masses can be made. Furthermore, with the use of angiography combined with CT, smaller tumors can be identified more often.

Liver biopsy: When the entity of the liver masses cannot be determined by imaging studies, liver biopsy may be indicated; however, in patients with a worrisome lesion who are candidates for resection, biopsy is not necessary or recommended. Complications of biopsy such as intraperitoneal bleeding, intra-liver hematoma, bile leak, or malignancy seeding may occur. Therefore, liver biopsy is generally recommended only when operative resection is contraindicated and definite diagnosis is needed for other treatment planning, or when a lesion is not suspicious and a biopsy would prevent an operation.

Differential Diagnosis

Regenerative nodule: Liver cirrhosis results from hepatocellular necrosis, fibrosis, and regeneration. Because regenerative nodules are common in liver cirrhosis, the most important clinical problem is to distinguish a regenerative nodule from a small HCC. On liver ultrasonography, regenerative nodules are small, hypoechoic nodules. On dynamic CT, regenerative nodules do not enhance the arterial phase. On MRI, regenerative nodules are hypointense on both T1- and T2-weighted images. HCCs are typically hyperintense on T2-weighted images.

Fat sparing: Fat sparing is a focal area of normal liver parenchyma which is not occupied by fatty tissue in an otherwise fatty steatotic liver. On liver ultrasonography, the focal area is hypoechoic and, if one is not careful, can be mistaken for a small liver tumor.

Hemangioma: Hemangiomas, single or multiple, are the most common benign neoplasms of the liver. The sizes can range from several millimeters to more than 20 cm. Most hemangiomas are asymptomatic and are identified incidentally or during evaluation of patients with chronic HBV or HCV infection. Ultrasonography will show a hyperechoic mass, but is not always diagnostic. Non-contrast CT shows a hypodense lesion compared with the surrounding normal liver parenchyma; contrast-enhanced CT demonstrates peripheral, nodular enhancement on arterial and portal phases and is virtually diagnostic for hemangioma (❷ *Fig. 93-1*). For lesions less than 2 cm, CT may not show this typical pattern, and MRI can assist with the definitive diagnosis. On MRI, a hemangioma is typically hypointense on T1-weighted images and hyperintense on T2-weighted images.

Hepatocellular adenoma: Liver adenomas are rare tumors in the liver and occur predominantly in females who have taken contraceptive pills. Clinically, liver adenomas are identified incidentally or during evaluation of upper abdominal pain which can be due to intra-tumor bleeding. Liver ultrasonography demonstrates a well-defined, hyperechoic tumor. Hemorrhage within the neoplasm will result in a hypoechoic or heteroechoic pattern. Dynamic CT shows a hypervascular appearance with only slight peripheral enhancement on arterial phase and isodense or hyperdense on portal phase. On MRI, liver adenomas demonstrate hyperintense signals in both T1- and T2-weighted images; however, these imaging appearances are not specific. Liver biopsy may be needed to make a definite diagnosis and avoid the need for resection.

Focal nodular hyperplasia (FNH): FNH is a common benign tumor second in incidence to hemangioma. Liver ultrasonography may demonstrate either a hypoechoic or hyperechoic tumor, which is neither specific nor diagnostic. Dynamic CT will give a hypervascular lesion on arterial phase and isodense or hyperdense lesion on portal phase. Only 30–50% of FNH display the classic central scarring, which will have a linear, hypodense appearance on CT and help to make the diagnosis.

□ Figure 93-1
Dynamic CT of hemangioma. Dynamic CT demonstrates peripheral nodular enhancement on arterial phase

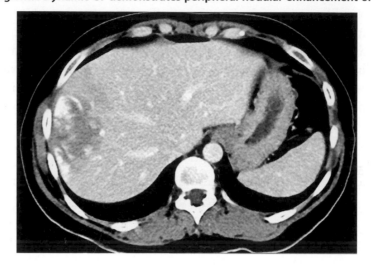

On MRI, liver FNH appear hypointense in T1-weighted images and hyperintense in T2-weighted images. If angiography is performed, it usually shows a large central arterial vessel.

Simple cyst and polycystic liver disease: Liver cysts are very common and range from asymptomatic lesions a few millimeters in size to large symptomatic lesions compressing adjacent structures. These cysts are the most common liver abnormality on imaging. Large cysts and polycystic disease may be palpable or cause abdominal pain. Liver ultrasonography or CT is diagnostic and demonstrates round, anechoic lesions with a smooth wall and posterior enhancement.

Abscess: Liver abscesses result from bacteria or parasites. Patients may present with fever and right upper quadrant pain. Ultrasonography demonstrates a round or oval liver lesion, mixed echogenicity on occasion with a fluid/debris level, and an irregular wall. Contrast-enhanced CT typically demonstrates a hypodense lesion with irregular, enhancing walls. Occasionally, gas bubbles or gas–fluid levels can be seen in the cystic lesion.

Angiomyolipoma: Angiomyolipomas are composed of variable amounts of fat, vessels, and muscle, and are seen commonly in the kidney, but only rarely in the liver. Because of the fat content within the mass, liver ultrasonography shows a hyperechoic tumor. On CT, angiomyolipomas are hypodense without contrast enhancement and heterogeneous with contrast enhancement. On MRI, they appear hyperintense on T1-weighted images but more heterointense on the T2-weighted images. Detection of the fatty component confirms the diagnosis.

Inflammatory pseudotumor: Inflammatory pseudotumors are unusual liver masses, typically identified incidentally. They consist of hepatocytes, fibroblasts, and inflammatory cells. Liver ultrasonography may show either hyperechoic or hypoechoic tumors. On dynamic CT, they appear hypervascular on arterial phase and isodense or hyperdense on portal phase. Inflammatory pseudotumors may mimic either benign or malignant neoplasms. Therefore, the differential diagnosis is arduous based on imaging studies alone, and liver biopsy may be necessary to make a definite diagnosis and avoid unnecessary hepatectomy.

Cystadenoma and cystadenocarcinoma: Cystadenomas and cystadenocarcinomas are rare cystic neoplsams in the liver originating from biliary epithelium. Liver ultrasonography demonstrates typically an anechoic cystic lesion with septations or papillary growths from the wall of the cystic area. CT may also demonstrate cystic lesion with septa or papillary growing. Cystadenomas and cystadenocarcinomas cannot be differentiated by imaging studies alone, and surgical resection is usually indicated.

Hepatocellular carcinoma (HCC): HCCs, single or multiple, are the most common primary malignancy in the liver. More than 60% of HCC occurs in cirrhotic livers highly associated with chronic hepatitis B and hepatitis C infections. The definitive diagnosis is assisted by laboratory assessment and imaging. A serum level of AFP >400 mg/ml in the setting of a suspicious lesion on imaging is virtually pathognomonic of HCC. When the serum level of AFP is <400 mg/ml, but two separate imaging modalities are highly worrisome, HCC is also assumed. Sonographic images of HCC are varied and depend on the size of the neoplasm(s). Small HCCs (<3 cm) are typically hypoechoic, whereas large HCCs are hyperechoic or heteroechoic. The lesions may also have a hypoechoic halo. On dynamic CT, HCCs are hypervascular on the arterial phase and hypodense on the portal phase (❯ *Fig. 93-2*). On unenhanced MRI or MRI enhanced with SPIO, HCCs are hypointense on the T1-weighted images but heterointense on the T2-weighted images. However, a mosaic pattern is common for HCC.

Choangiocarcinoma (CCC): CCC can be divided into central and peripheral types. Central types of CCCs are located most commonly at the liver hilum and cause obstructive jaundice and dilated intrahepatic bile ducts. In contrast, the peripheral types of CCC must be differentiated from other liver tumors. On ultrasonography, the lesion may be hypoechoic, isoechoic, or hyperechoic. On contrast-enhanced CT, peripheral CCCs are ill-defined and nonspecific. On MRI, they appear hypointense in T1-weighted images and hyperintense in T2-weighted images. All the findings of imaging studies, however, are nonspecific and nondiagnostic for peripheral CCCs. Liver biopsy may be needed to make a definite diagnosis.

Metastatic tumor: Metastatic tumors represent the most common malignant neoplasms in the liver. The colon, pancreas, stomach, and breast are the most common primary sites from which these hematogenous metastases arise. Metastatic tumors should be suspected when there are multiple liver tumors or when there is a history of a previous cancer.

Angiosarcoma: Angiosarcomas are rare primary hepatic malignancies and are the most common malignant mesenchymal neoplasm. Angiosarcomas are typically not encapsulated and involve the

◘ Figure 93-2
Dynamic CT of HCC. Dynamic CT demonstrates hypervascular tumors on arterial phase (a) and hypodense on portal phase (b)

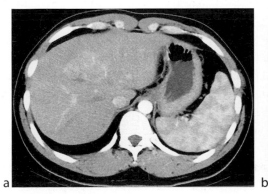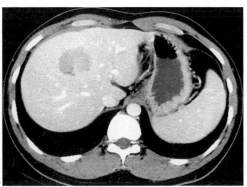

a   b

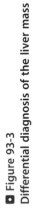 Figure 93-3

Differential diagnosis of the liver mass

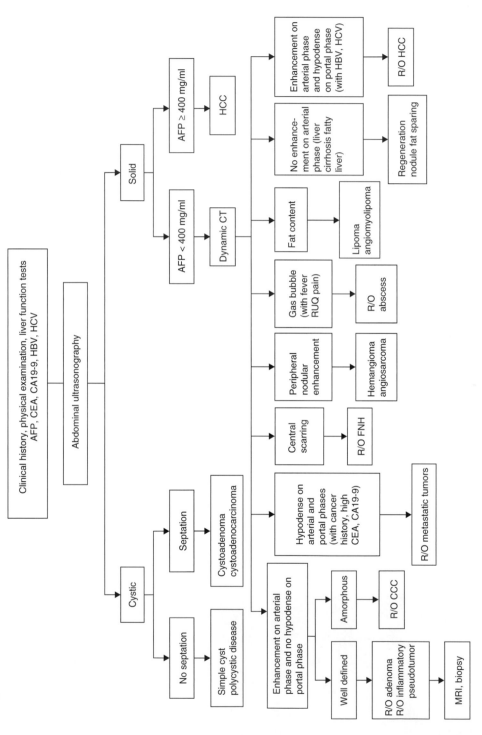

liver diffusely. Ultrasonography demonstrates multiple, ill-defined hyperechoic lesions. On contrast-enhanced CT, angiosarcomas have marked contrast enhancement and may mimic hemangioma closely; however, if intraperitoneal hemorrhage is present, angiosarcoma is highly suspected. On MRI, angiosarcomas are hypointense with focal hyperintensity on T1-weighted images and heterointense on T2-weighted images.

Conclusion

Liver masses are a common clinical problem and especially so with the increased use of modern imaging modalities. The appropriate clinical management relies on an accurate diagnosis. A thorough clinical history, laboratory data, and liver imaging can provide the definitive diagnosis in the majority of patients (❯ *Fig. 93-3*). Liver biopsy is reserved for select patients who are not candidates for resection, those in whom the diagnosis would preclude operative exploration, or when an exact diagnosis is necessary for treatment planning.

Selected Readings

Gibbs JF, Litwin AM, Kahlenberg MS (2004) Contemporary management of benign liver tumors. Surg Clin N Am 84:463–480

Hammerstingl RM, Schwarz W, Vogl TJ (2003) Contrast agents. In: Vogl TJ, Lencioni R, Hammerstingl RM, Bartolozzi C (eds) Magnetic resonance imaging in liver disease. Georg Thieme Verlag, Stuttgart/New York, pp 45–91

Lee WC, Jeng LB, Chen MF (2002) Estimation of prognosis after hepatectomy for hepatocellular carcinoma. Br J Surg 89:311–316

Lee WC, Jeng LB, Chen MF (2000) Hepatectomy for hepatitis B-, hepatitis C-, and dual hepatitis B- and C-related hepatocellular carcinoma in Taiwan. J Hepatobiliary Pancreat Surg 7:265–269

Yeh CN, Lee WC, Chen MF, Tsay PK (2003) Predictors of long-term disease-free survival after resection of hepatocellular carcinoma: two decades of experience at Chang-Gung Memorial Hospital. Ann Surg Oncol 10:916–921

94 Benign Hepatic Neoplasms

Juan Hepp

Pearls and Pitfalls

- Hepatic lesions are frequently identified incidentally on imaging performed for other purposes.
- With the exception of large lesions, benign hepatic neoplasms are typically asymptomatic.
- With current high quality imaging, it is possible to differentiate the majority of hepatic neoplasms as benign or malignant.
- Resection of indeterminant, worrisome lesions is generally preferred over biopsy.
- Hepatic hemangioma is the most common, solid lesion found in the liver.
- Focal nodular hyperplasia (FNH) does not require resection, but at the least, initial follow-up imaging is recommended.

Introduction

The more frequent use of imaging studies of the abdomen, especially ultrasonography (US), has lead to frequent consultation because of the finding of an (often) asymptomatic hepatic lesion. The lesion can be solid or cystic, benign or malignant, or a primary or secondary neoplasm. These patients should be evaluated with thorough clinical history and appropriate diagnostic studies. The most frequent benign solid and cystic lesions of the liver are listed in ❂ *Table 94-1*.

Hemangioma

The incidence of hemangiomas is approximately 5% in adults and 7% in autopsies, and they are the most frequently identified lesion in the liver. Hemangiomas are more frequent in women and adults. The most usual form are the capillary hemangiomas, typically small, followed by the cavernous hemangiomas, which can reach considerable size and are more likely to cause symptoms. Hemangiomas (❂ *Fig. 94-1A*) usually have characteristic features on imaging that allow a confident, non-invasive diagnosis (see Chapter 93). Grossly, these lesions are well delineated, and their macroscopic aspect is easy to recognize by the surgeon (❂ *Fig. 94-1B*). The hemangioma sometimes generates a fibrous plane in contact with the liver, facilitating its enucleation.

Symptoms arise typically from compression of adjacent organs or rapid enlargement due to intratumoral bleeding or thrombosis. Rupture with bleeding into the peritoneum is exceedingly rare, but when this occurs, the associated mortality is very high. Patient stabilization is vital in these

■ Table 94-1

Benign liver tumors

Origin	Denomination
Epithelial	
Hepatocellular	Focal nodular hyperplasia
	Hepatocellular adenoma
	Regenerative nodule
Cholangiocellular	Simple cyst
	Biliary cystadenoma
	Biliary adenoma
Mesenchymal	
Endothelial	Hemangioma
	Hemangioendothelioma

cases, and different methods can be used to obtain some stabilization, including arteriographic embolization, hepatic artery ligation, and perihepatic packing to control the hemorrhage and allow a resection under more appropriate conditions. The rarity of spontaneous rupture does not justify a preventive hepatic resection of even large but asymptomatic hemangiomas.

The literature mentions frequently the term "giant" hemangioma with no consensus regarding the size of the lesion. Hemangiomas with a diameter >4 cm are described as giant hemangiomas but do not imply any special therapeutic implications. The mass effect of large hemangiomas 20 cm or larger may produce discomfort, malaise, or obstructive symptoms and may be palpable on physical examination. Clear correlation of the symptoms with the lesion should guide the appropriateness of operative intervention. Laboratory work-up is typically normal, even for large hemangiomas. The Kasabach-Merritt syndrome, most commonly described in patients with thrombocytopenia and consumption coagulopathy secondary to skin and spleen hemangiomas, may occur rarely with liver hemangiomas. Very few cases have been described, and the treatment is enucleation or liver transplantation.

Imaging studies beginning with US usually make the diagnosis. Fortunately, good quality US and its adequate interpretation is usually sufficient for the diagnosis of hemangioma. Hyperechogenicity with well-defined borders is typical, and if Doppler exam is added, a greater vascular flow is appreciated easily. Typical CT findings suggesting hemangioma include a hypodense lesion in comparison with the surrounding liver parenchyma. After injecting intravenous contrast, the lesion fills irregularly from the periphery reaching the center after a few minutes. The enhanced lesion persists longer than the rest of the liver (❍ *Fig. 94-1*). This finding is typical of hemangioma. The specificity of MRI exceeds that of CT in the diagnosis of hemangioma. Disadvantages of MRI, however, include cost, availability, expertise, and contraindications in persons with pacemakers or metallic prostheses, and it may require sedation in claustrophobic patients. Both methods allow simultaneous evaluation of the remainder of the abdomen as well. MRI offers the advantage of use in patients with allergy to contrast media. Hemangiomas are characteristically hyperintense on the T2-weighted images; after administration of gadolinium, a peripheral filling lesion similar to CT findings is noted. Although hepatic scintigraphy with ^{99m}Tc-labeled red blood cells has diagnostic merit, this study has been supplanted by the previously described imaging methods. Selective arteriography of the liver shows a corkscrew aspect of the vessels and a cotton-like filling, both of which are very characteristic. This method is almost never required because of its cost and invasive nature.

◘ Figure 94-1
Central cavernous hemangioma. a. CT: note compression of hepatic veins. b. Left liver resection that includes the cavernous hemangioma and a smaller neighboring hemangioma

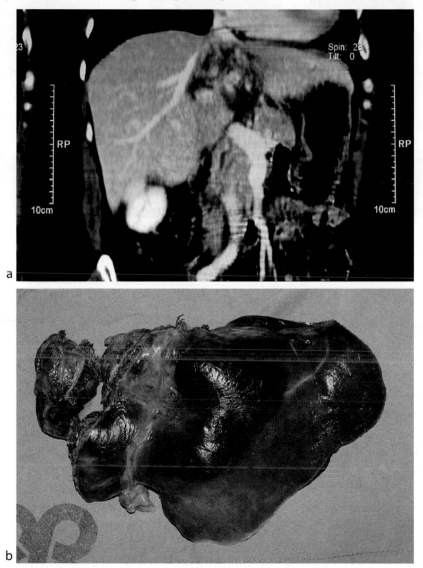

Biopsy of lesions suspicious for hemangioma is generally not advised due to the risk of complications and failure to exclude definitively a neoplasm. A biopsy of any focal liver lesion is useful only if it will change the therapeutic plan; otherwise, the lesion should be observed or resected.

For asymptomatic hemangiomas, once a confident diagnosis has been made, the therapeutic approach for the vast majority of these cases is periodic observation. Yearly follow-up of the lesion with US may demonstrate that the lesion does not grow and does not develop changes within the lesion. Complications developing from an asymptomatic lesion during follow-up are very unusual, not predictable, and do not justify resection.

Rarely, one may see a hemangioma that enlarges through the years, for instance, during pregnancy (❯ *Fig. 94-2*).

◘ Figure 94-2
Large right hepatic hemangioma that enlarged rapidly during pregnancy. a. CT; b. resected hemangioma

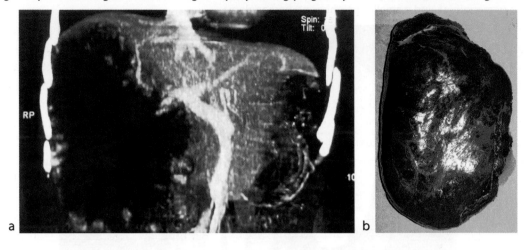

The indications for resection of hemangioma include symptomatic lesions or patients in whom the diagnosis is uncertain. Patient concerns, performance status, and other medical conditions also impact the decision for operative intervention. Some patients with a large hemangioma have been advised erroneously to undergo extirpation of the hemangioma because of symptoms not related to the neoplasm. In a very anxious patient in whom the lesion is easily resectable, the operative risk is relatively low, and if the patient understands the risks, resection may be appropriate. The majority of symptomatic, resected, or complicated hemangiomas are larger than 10 cm. The management of hemangiomas that measure ≥15 cm is controversial in otherwise asymptomatic patients. It seems reasonable to observe them periodically and carefully, and if there is any evidence of growth or symptomatology, to resect them.

Operative resection involves enucleation or formal anatomic resection, depending on the location and relationship to portal branches and hepatic veins. Operative approach, laparotomy, and laparoscopic approaches depend on the location, size, and characteristics of the lesion. Planning the resection will also depend on intra-operative findings. Sometimes a simple enucleation of a hemangioma that "hangs" from the liver will be possible; in other patients, the hemangioma may be a deep lesion that requires a surgeon expert in hepatic resections. Often a fibrous plane exists between the hemangioma and the hepatic tissue that facilitates a safe and easy enucleation. An especially useful tool is the ultrasonic dissector that facilitates enucleation of the hemangioma. Because hemangiomas are benign lesions, it is not necessary to resect margins of healthy liver. Full visualization and mobilization of the liver with early control of the vascular pedicles facilitates the resection. On occasion, a dominant hepatic artery or an arterial branch that feeds preferentially the lesion can be found.

Preemptive transvascular embolization of the hemangioma is not justified based on the low risk of spontaneous hemorrhage but has been very useful in the management of ruptured hemangiomas. It is not uncommon to find neighboring smaller hemangiomas when resecting a large one; however, they require no intervention, because they have an exceedingly small risk of becoming symptomatic. Postoperative complications are rare and are the same as those found in any hepatic resection.

Focal Nodular Hyperplasia (FNH)

FNH was first described in 1958. This lesion believed to be hormone-dependent is much more frequent in young women and has been related to the use of oral contraceptives. FNH can reach considerable size, yet most are asymptomatic and found only incidentally on an imaging procedure for another complaint. When symptoms do appear, they are secondary to its mass effect. Malignant degeneration or hemorrhage has not been described. FNH is a macroscopically well-defined lesion without a capsule arising within otherwise normal hepatic tissue. The lesion appears more pale than normal liver, has prominent vessels on its surface, and presents a somewhat lobulated aspect, with a firm, rubbery consistency (❯ *Fig. 94-3A*). Frequently, a central radial scar consisting of a vascularized fibrous septum is seen characteristically on imaging studies. Histologically, this lesion suggests a regenerative nodule with a predominance of Küpffer cells and biliary duct hyperplasia, thus differentiating FNH histologically from adenomas. Differentiating FNH from adenoma preoperatively on imaging studies, however, may prove challenging. Biliary scintigraphy with radiolabeled sulfur colloid shows a prominent uptake by the abundant Küpffer cells into the FNH, thereby allowing the differentiation from adenoma. Ultrasonography shows an echogenic lesion but only occasionally having the "characteristic" central, vascularized scar. CT and MRI show a homogeneous, vascularized lesion and, when present, outlining a radial central scar with a "cartwheel" aspect (❯ *Fig. 94-4*) that differentiates FNH from adenoma; however, smaller lesions usually lack the features. Arteriography is not recommended, but when done will show a well-vascularized lesion and, when present, the central, vascularized scar. Usually one of these techniques will permit a confident diagnosis. On occasion, however, a small lesion (<5 cm) can be seen in a central location. Biopsy is not recommended, because it will usually be inconclusive. In patients without substantive risk factors like cirrhosis or chronic viral infection, follow-up imaging in 3–6 months seems the best approach; if the lesion remains unchanged over time, a benign lesion seems most likely. Growth in size, however, warrants an aggressive approach. For the peripherally located, small lesions, a laparoscopic wedge excision may be the best approach unless FNH is highly suspected, in which case follow-up imaging surveillance seems best.

Treatment of known FNH is limited to observational surveillance and discontinuation of oral contraceptives in women. Because there is no worry of malignant degeneration or other complications within the lesion (bleeding, necrosis, abscess, etc.), there is no justification for resection unless there are symptoms related to its mass effect. Under these circumstances, the operative treatment consists of

◻ Figure 94-3
Focal nodular hyperplasia. a. External macroscopic view. Note uneven surface. b. Cut surface of resected tumor

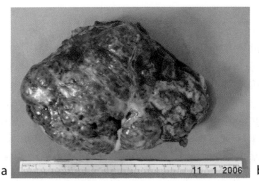 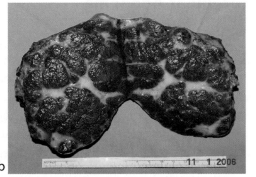

◩ Figure 94-4
a, b. CTs of focal nodular hyperplasia showing the typical central radial scar

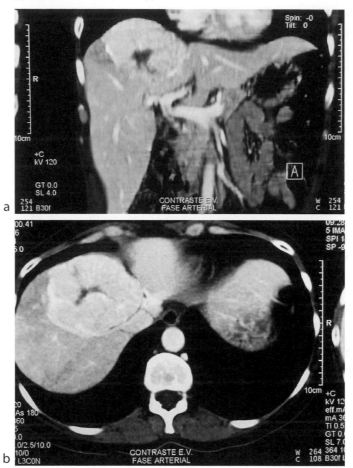

enucleation; there is no need to perform a wedge-type excision or formal anatomic resection of a known FNH. The vast majority of FNHs, however, are resected because of an uncertain diagnosis; in these cases, the resection is performed according to location and with oncologic intent.

Hepatocellular Adenoma

Hepatocellular adenomas (HA) are usually seen in young women and are associated with the use of hormones. These benign neoplasms are well-delineated, solitary, benign neoplasms of a few centimeters in size, yellow-pink in color, soft on palpation, and showing foci of hemorrhagic dots on the transected surface. Certain patient populations are predisposed to developing HA, including patients with galactosemia, type 1 glycogen deposits, Turner's and Klinefelter's syndromes, and most conspicuously, users of oral contraceptives, estrogens, androgens, danazol, clomiphene, and growth hormone. The relationship between HA and oral contraceptives, as well as with pregnancy, is well-described;

indeed, patients showing growth of an HA during pregnancy are well-documented, lending strong support to the association of HA and steroid sex hormones. A decrease in the size of the HA has also been described when oral contraceptives are discontinued.

The risk of developing HA in oral contraceptive users depends on the concentration of the estrogen, duration of use (more than 2 years), and the woman's age (>30 years of age). Overall, however, the risk is extremely low and must vary with individual genomic predisposition. Of concern, however, is that there is a greater risk of rupture and bleeding during pregnancy in patients with known HA. In addition, the co-existence of HA and the development of hepatocellular carcinoma has been postulated, although the evidence supporting a definite association is difficult to confirm. Histologically, HAs consist of a homogeneous population of hepatocytes that may contain abundant glycogen; a notable absence of the portal triads and biliary ducts and the presence of thin-walled blood vessels and peliosis are pathognomonic findings. Sometimes it can be very difficult to differentiate well-differentiated hepatocarcinomas from HAs.

Adenomas are usually asymptomatic but on rare occasions may present with rupture and massive bleeding. They are most often detected on imaging studies performed for other, non-specific abdominal symptoms that are difficult to relate to the lesion. Laboratory work-up for abnormalities in liver enzymes, tumor markers, or viral infection should be normal. Imaging studies are crucial for their categorization to differentiate HAs from FNH, hepatocellular carcinoma, or metastases; a scintigraphic study (with ^{99m}Tc colloid sulphur), as described previously in the differential diagnosis with FNH, may be useful. On US, HA appears as an echogenic lesion. On CT, it looks hyperdense prior to giving intravenous contrast and variable in intensity after contrast administration. On MRI, the HA is hyperintense on T1-weighted images, iso-intense or less prominent on T2-weighted images, and with the use of gadolinium, it becomes very prominent. Angiography is indicated rarely but will show a hypervascularized lesion with areas of hemorrhage and tortuous vessels. The diagnosis of HA is made usually by excluding other alternatives more pathognomonic on imaging. Differentiation from hepatocellular carcinoma is most problematic and may require resection to prove. Biopsy of the lesion, as mentioned in the description of FNH, is not indicated, because it is not helpful.

The appropriate treatment of HA is resection when there is risk of rupture, bleeding, or question of the diagnosis. The operative approach, laparotomy or laparoscopy, will depend on the location and characteristics of the lesion. Enucleation, wedge resection, or local ablation is usually sufficient. Although experience with alcohol injection or radiofrequency ablation is limited, these approaches seem reasonable in selected situations. Oral contraceptives must be stopped, and long-term follow-up with ultrasonography is recommended in patients in whom resection is not indicated.

Angiomyolipoma

This rare, benign neoplasm of mesenchymal origin is usually seen in the kidney but also rarely in the liver. Its relationship to tuberous sclerosis is not well-defined but appears to be real. The histologic characteristics consist of a mixture of lipomatous tissue, blood vessels, and smooth muscle in variable proportions. The tumor may be single or multiple and often reaches quite a large size. The pre-operative diagnosis can be difficult, but the MRI finding of a tumor full of fat is useful for diagnosis. Percutaneous biopsy has a poor yield and may suggest a sarcoma. The malignant potential

◻ Figure 94-5
Angiomyolipoma. a. CT demonstrating a vascular lesion with fatty infiltration. b. Cut surface of resected neoplasm

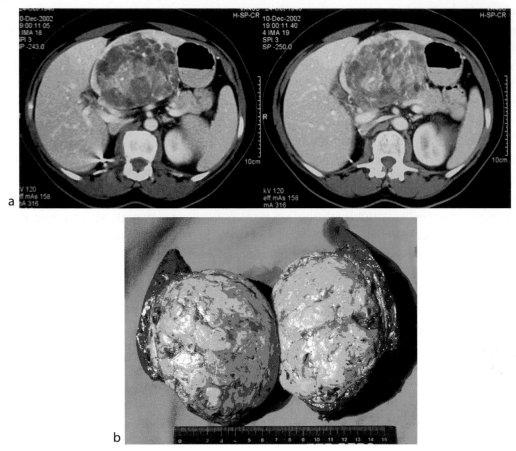

of this tumor is not clear. Given the rarity of this neoplasm and its diagnostic difficulty, it seems prudent to recommend resection (❯ *Fig. 94-5A, B*).

Inflammatory Pseudotumor of the Liver

This entity was described in the liver in 1953. This lesion presents as a well-defined mass with foci of hemorrhage and necrosis, a chronic inflammatory infiltrate, and proliferation of fibrous elements. Although often treated aggressively by resection, its natural evolution when diagnosed correctly is toward spontaneous regression. The pathogenesis has been attributed to an infectious origin with an intense inflammatory response; others have treated inflammatory pseudotumors with steroids. The diagnosis is based ultimately on the histology, and if suspected highly, a biopsy would preclude resection; however, as with all liver tumors, biopsy is fraught with the possibility of seeding if the tumor is malignant, and this possibility should be kept in mind when considering biopsy. Because of such concerns, resection is the usual approach to these unusual liver tumors.

Other Benign Tumors

There is a variety of other benign neoplasms in the liver, but each has an extremely low incidence, including biliary hamartoma, solitary fibrous tumor, benign mesothelioma, lipoma associated with myolipoma or angiolipoma, mesenchymal hamartoma, mixoma, and teratoma.

Incidentally Discovered Liver Lesions

With the widespread use of state-of-the-art imaging, the recognition of liver lesions has become relatively frequent. These abnormalities on imaging can cause great anxiety in the patient, and the clinician must present an organized, systematic approach to diagnosis and therapy. The first point is to differentiate cystic from solid lesions (see Chapter 93). Once a cystic lesion has been excluded, the next step is to determine whether this solid tumor is benign or malignant, because this may determine either resection versus observation or enucleation versus formal, anatomic resection. The patient's age, history, and clinical background becomes very important. The presence of other hepatic diseases, history of extrahepatic malignancies, neoplasias that could have given rise to a metastasis, alcoholism, trauma, viral infections, particularly hepatitis B or C, and the use of medications, mainly estrogens, contraceptives, or toxic drugs, may prove very important. Laboratory evaluation usually includes hepatic function tests and screening for the existence of markers of past or current hepatitis B or C infection. Tumor markers such as α fetoprotein and embryonic antigen are used selectively, based on the clinical history and characteristics of imaging. Imaging studies usually begin with US, but usually also require CT and/or MRI to make a more definitive diagnosis. Biliary scintigraphy may differentiate adenoma from focal nodular hyperplasia. Selective arteriography is used or indicated only infrequently but may be helpful to detect neovasculature characteristic of hepatocellular carcinoma.

In summary, the most common benign tumors of the liver are cavernous hemangioma, hepatocellular adenoma (HA), and focal nodular hyperplasia (FNH). Imaging studies usually allow a confident diagnosis of these three benign lesions. When there is question of the diagnosis, resection is usually indicated, because percutaneous liver biopsy risks seeding of the neoplasm if malignant. When the diagnosis is HA, we usually recommend resection, because HA is associated with the risk of bleeding, rupture, or potential malignant degeneration. Hemangiomas and FNH are managed by observation and have a operative indication only if they are symptomatic.

Small lesions (<2 cm) are difficult to characterize with imaging, and if there are no risk factors for neoplasia, we recommend a program of periodic surveillance, particularly if the lesion is difficult to access surgically. If the lesion increases in size, resection is usually necessary.

Selected Readings

Farges O, Daradkeh S, Bismuth H (1995) Cavernous hemangiomas of the liver: are there any indications for resection? World J Surg 19:19–24

Hoffman AL, Emre S, Verham RP, et al. (1997) Hepatic - angiomyolipoma: two case reports of caudate-based lesions and review of the literature. Liver Transpl Surg 3:46–53

Koea J, Broadhurst G, Rodgers M, McCall J (2003) Inflammatory pseudotumor of the liver: demographics, diagnosis and the case for nonoperative management. J Am Coll Surg 196:226–235

Kuo PC, Lewis WD, Jenkins RL (1994) Treatment of giant liver hemangiomas of the liver by enucleation. J Am Coll Surg 178:49–53

Nagorney DM (1995) Benign hepatic tumors: focal nodular hyperplasia and hepatocellular adenoma. World J Surg 19:13–18

Roocks JB, Ory HW, Ishak KG, et al. (1979) Epidemiology of hepatocellular adenoma. The role of oral contraceptive use. JAMA 242:644–648

Weimann A, Ringe B, Klempnauer J, et al. (1997) Benign liver tumors: differential diagnosis and indications for surgery. World J Surg 21:983–991

95 Hepatic Abscess: Current Concepts

William Sanchez M · Hernando Abaunza O

Pearls and Pitfalls

- Due to its dual circulation, the liver has a greater probability of developing abscesses of metastatic bacterial origin from other tissues.
- Over the past 30 years, the incidence of pyogenic liver abscess has increased, and the etiologies have changed.
- Risk factors for developing pyogenic liver abscesses include transplant patients, mainly liver transplants, immunosuppressive diseases, cancer, diabetes, biliary diseases, and other non-specific conditions such as old age, alcoholism, and the presence of infectious gastrointestinal diseases.
- Hospital mortality is increased in patients with pyogenic liver abscesses in the presence of cancer, hyperbilirubinemia, leukocytosis ($>20,000$ cells/mm^3), hypoalbuminemia, pleural effusion, intra-peritoneal perforation of an abdominal viscus, multiple small abscesses, and diabetes.
- Signs and symptoms are usually non-specific and are related to the local and systemic response to the infection.
- Treatment of pyogenic liver abscesses includes one or more of the following modalities: (1) antibiotic therapy, (2) percutaneous drainage, (3) operative drainage, and (4) hepatic resection.
- Current management of pyogenic liver abscesses involves drainage under image guidance.
- Amebic liver abscesses are more common in males than in females, are found rarely in children, and are usually present in young individuals with an incidence greater during the summer months in endemic areas. About 80% of amoebic abscesses present as a solitary lesion localized in the right lobe.
- Unlike pyogenic abscesses, amoebic abscesses present in a more subacute manner often with symptoms for weeks or even months.
- Serum antibodies, especially IgG, offer value (70–90%) for the diagnosis of amoebic liver abscesses.
- Treatment for amoebic liver abscess is based on therapy with metronidazole; success rates range from 40% to 90%.

Introduction

Hippocrates described liver abscesses and suggested that the nature of the drainage used could change the prognosis of this disease. In 1836, John Bright described the clinicopathologic manifestations, but it was Ochsner in 1938 who published his classic review of 47 patients, noting a mortality of 80%.

Because of its dual circulation, the liver has a greater probability of developing "metastatic" abscesses of hematogenous origin secondary to infections originating in other tissues. Traditionally, three types of liver abscesses have been described: pyogenic, amoebic, and hydatid. In the current world literature, there are reports of liver abscesses secondary to many of types of bacteria, fungi, and parasites. This chapter focuses on pyogenic and amoebic abscesses, because they account for more than 90% of all liver abscesses.

Pyogenic Abscess

Incidence: During the past 30 years, the incidence of pyogenic abscesses has increased in certain patient populations. The widespread use of hepatic ultrasonography and other modalities of non-invasive imaging has been an important contributing factor to the increase in the number of cases diagnosed and, therefore, in part to its greater incidence.

Other factors associated with this rise in incidence include the increasing use of chemotherapy for malignancies, immunosuppressive agents for organ transplantation, diseases such as AIDS which predispose to opportunistic infections, and a greater frequency of invasive procedures of the biliary tract. Other groups at increased risk include diabetics, alcoholics, those with other gastrointestinal bacterial diseases (appendicitis, diverticulitis, infectious colitis), and the ever-increasing elderly population. Hematogenous seeding of infectious agents overwhelm the phagocytic capability of Küpffer's cells and give rise to abscess formation.

Etiopathogenesis: The most common route for development of hepatic abscess is metastatic spread to the liver through the portal venous system (46%) from a source in the splanchnic system. Cholangitis, especially when associated with endoscopic instrumentation, biliary stones, neoplasms, or biliary stenosis, serves as the primary focus of infection leading to the formation of liver abscesses (38–50%). Finally, the source of infection remains unknown in a subset of patients with "cryptogenic" hepatic abscess in whom a hematogenous pathogenesis is suspected either via the hepatic arterial inflow or portal venous inflow.

Hepatic abscesses may be single or multiple (❯ *Figs. 95-1* and ❯ *95-2*) and thereby provide some clues to the etiopathogenesis. In nearly 70% of patients, involvement of the right lobe is attributed to the preferential flow of the mesenteric and portal venous flow. Involvement of the left lobe is associated more frequently with intra-hepatic stones (❯ *Fig. 95-3*).

Besides its association with diseases described traditionally, such as diabetes, cirrhosis, biliary stones, colonic diverticulitis, and appendicitis, pyogenic liver abscesses are also associated with other medical conditions of more recent development. Abscess formation secondary to radio-frequency ablation of malignant primary or metastatic neoplasms ranges between 1% and 6%.

A recent study of 603 patients with hepatocellular carcinoma treated with radio-frequency identified the risk factors associated with abscess formation to be pre-existing biliary abnormalities favoring ascending cholangitis, retention within the tumor of the ionized oil from the trans-arterial chemoembolization, and prior cryotherapy treatment. In itself, transarterial embolization of malignant liver neoplasias has a very low rate (<0.5%) of liver abscess formation, but when it occurs, the

■ Figure 95-1
Pyogenic liver abscesses. Pathologic specimen. Note multiple focus

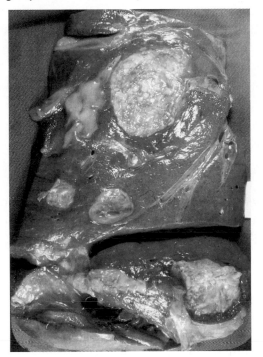

■ Figure 95-2
CT of pyogenic liver abscess. Note multiloculated abscess in segment II–III

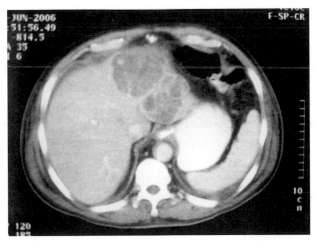

organisms are usually gram-positive bacterial infections; others have suggested that patients with bacteriobilia related to previous instrumentation or bilioenteric anastomosis are also at increased risk.

The immunosuppressed populations are most at risk of developing liver abscess. Hematologic malignancies predispose to the development of metastatic infectious processes such as splenic abscess, brain abscess, and hepatic abscess, and especially fungal abscesses, both before and during treatment.

◘ Figure 95-3
CT of multiple intrahepatic biliary lithiasis of left hepatic duct. Note presence of pyogenic liver microabscesses and atrophy

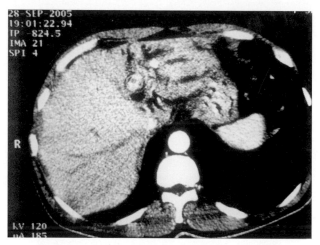

Similarly, approximately 1% of patients with HIV infection will develop some form of hepatic abscess; the susceptibility appears to vary with the degree of immune compromise. In liver transplant patients, cytomegalovirus (CMV) infection of the liver is characterized by the formation of diffuse parenchymal abscesses usually containing Küpffer cells infected with the virus. In addition, the presence of CMV infection associated with immunosuppression also favors the presence of invasive aspergillosis. When the CD4 count is >500, the organisms involved are generally gram-negative aerobes, mainly Klebsiella species, followed by *E. coli* and Pseudomonas; when the CD4 count is <200, abscesses have a mixed flora or are secondary to microbes such as Mycobacterium, Nocardia, Aspergillus, and other opportunistic species.

The post-transplantation population represents a somewhat unique group; not only are they immunosuppressed, but the liver graft has suffered an element of ischemic insult, and the biliary tree has been instrumented or become colonized with bacteria secondary to a bilio-enteric anastomosis. Transplant patients, particularly liver transplant patients, may develop liver abscesses (approximately 1–4%). Two factors have been associated with the predisposition to abscess formation: hepatic artery thrombosis (66%) and the use of biliary drainage catheters or biliary instrumentation resulting in bacteriobilia or especially cholangitis.

Finally, the etiology of cryptogenic abscesses that occur in 10–20% of patients with hepatic abscesses has not been established clearly. Some groups have suggested that these types of hepatic abscesses arise from small infarctions or areas of thromboembolism that become superinfected by microbes derived from bacteremias of the portal system, or possibly from defects in the reticuloendothelial system where there is a loss of the ability to clear opsonized particles from the circulation. Ultimately, abscess development depends on the interaction between the patient's immune system, the route of dissemination, and the virulence of the pathogen (❷ *Table 95-1*).

Mortality: Despite the fact that patients with pyogenic liver abscesses have highly debilitating diseases, advances in early diagnosis, less invasive treatments, and more sophisticated antimicrobial and supportive therapies have resulted in an overall decrease in mortality. Nevertheless, the following risk factors have been associated with increased hospital mortality: presence of malignancy, hyperbilirubinemia, increased

◘ Table 95-1

Pathogenesis of pyogenic liver abscesses

Dissemination route	Etiology	Causing microbe
Hepatic artery	Bacteremic infection	Gram (+) aerobes
		Gram (−) aerobes
Portal vein	Benign or malignant gastrointestinal disease	Gram (−) aerobes
		Gram (−) anaerobes
Biliary tract	Cholangitis (stones, stent, tumors, post-ERCP)	Gram (−) aerobes
		Gram (−) anaerobes
Round ligament	Umbilical piercing, umbilical catheter	Gram (+) aerobes
Liver parenchyma	Trauma, post radiofrequency	Gram (−) aerobes
Liver parenchyma	Transplant – arterial thrombosis	Gram (−) aerobes
		Cytomegalovirus
		Opportunistic germ
Mixed	AIDS, transplant, chemotherapy	Opportunistic germ
		Fungi
		Gram (−) aerobes
Continuity	Post-cholecystectomy, infection or perforation of neighboring organ	Gram (−) aerobes
		Gram (−) anaerobes
Cryptogenic	Unknown	Gram (+) aerobes
	Dental diseases?	Gram (−) aerobes

partial thromboplastin time, hypoalbuminemia <2.5 g/dl, leukocytosis (>20,000 cells/mm^3), and diabetes. One factor that increases mortality markedly is spontaneous abscess perforation which, though uncommon, occurs in approximately 5% of patients and is associated with abscess size >7.8 cm in diameter (P = 0.043), presence of intra-luminal gas (P < 0.001), and involvement of the left lobe (P = 0.018).

Clinical presentation: Overall, the male-to-female ratio for pyogenic liver abscesses has a slight predominance in males. Clinical signs and symptoms of pyogenic liver abscesses are usually non-specific and are related to the local and systemic response to the primary site of infection. Major symptoms include fever (80–100%) and abdominal pain, especially in the right upper quadrant (60–85%). Less common are nausea, vomiting, and weight loss. Physical findings vary widely and include right upper quadrant tenderness (50%), hepatomegaly (40%), and jaundice (30%). The presence of a pleural or pericardial effusion, ascites, or severe shock may be the initial manifestation of a severe complication of the liver abscess.

Liver abscesses caused by Klebsiella can be associated with endogenous endophthalmitis which, although uncommon, can progress rapidly to visual loss in spite of medical intervention. The main risk factor associated with this finding is a history of diabetes. Every patient with a liver abscess who complains of any ocular pain or visual disorders must be referred to the ophthalmologist immediately.

Standard laboratory tests reflect a generalized state of systemic infection. Leukocytosis is present in 60–70% of patients and is a poor prognostic factor when greater than 20,000 cells/mm^3. Other findings may include hypoalbuminemia, anemia, and abnormal liver function tests depending on the duration of the disease prior to diagnosis. Abscess cultures are positive in >70% of cases of which at least 50% are polymicrobial. Blood cultures are positive in 40% of cases.

Treatment: Treatment of pyogenic liver abscesses involves the following therapeutic modalities: (1) parenteral antibiotic therapy, (2) percutaneous drainage, (3) operative drainage, and/or (4) hepatic resection. Antibiotic therapy is the only constant treatment once the diagnosis is made, while selection of the other forms of treatment depends on the specific conditions of the patient.

One adverse prognostic factor associated with mortality is delay in starting antibiotic therapy. For that reason, once the diagnosis of a liver abscess is made, empiric treatment with parenteral, broad-spectrum antibiotics should be initiated until culture of the luminal content confirms the organism(s) involved, after which the antibiotic therapy can be focused on the organism(s) involved. Unlike amoebic liver abscesses that usually resolve with anti-amoebic treatment alone, pyogenic abscesses treated only with antibiotic therapy have an unacceptable mortality (20%). Some selected groups of patients may benefit from this single modality of therapy, usually involving patients with small single or multiple abscesses of biliary origin, children, CMV microabscesses, and those with a rapid clinical response to monotherapy without evidence of systemic infection. There is no exact duration of suggested antibiotic therapy in these select patients, and the decision to discontinue treatment is based on clinical improvement, absence of fever or leukocytosis, and resolution of the abscess on follow-up imaging studies.

The current gold standard for the management of pyogenic liver abscesses not amenable to treatment with antibiotic therapy alone is percutaneous aspiration with placement of a drainage catheter under image guidance. The best candidates are patients with single, well-defined abscesses <7 cm in diameter with no associated complications (bleeding, perforation) or signs of severe septicemia. In some patients, aspiration alone, in conjunction with effective antibiotic therapy, can prove successful; in one study of 115 patients with pyogenic liver abscess (averaging 7 cm in size) treated with antibiotic therapy and percutaneous needle aspiration alone, the treatment was successful in 98%, with an average of two aspirations per patient, and in half the one aspiration was enough to achieve abscess control.

If symptoms persist for 2 or 3 days after percutaneous treatment or if the overall status of the patient worsens without any changes in the imaging studies, operative drainage should be considered. Factors associated with failure of percutaneous drainage include multiple or multiloculated abscesses, size greater than 7 cm, viscous fluid or substantial necrotic material, intracystic bleeding, and perforation of the abscess. Liver abscesses associated with choledocholithiasis or biliary sepsis initially are managed currently with percutaneous catheter drainage, although on occasions there is a need for sphincterotomy, stenting, or nasobiliary tube placement. Although some groups have reported irrigation of the abscess cavity with antibiotics, this form of treatment is neither widely accepted nor usually needed.

Operative treatment is reserved currently for patients who do not respond to antibiotic therapy and percutaneous drainage or in patients with complications secondary to catheter placement (abscess rupture, intracystic bleeding, peritonitis). The selection of either a laparoscopic approach or an open technique depends on the experience of the surgical team and the specific situation. Hepatectomy or left lobectomy may be the first modality of treatment in patients of liver abscesses secondary to recurrent intrahepatic biliary lithiasis.

Amoebic Abscess

Pathogenesis: Colonic amoebiasis occurs worldwide, but developing countries have been identified as endemic areas, especially those located in tropical and subtropical regions. Amoebic infestation is associated usually with malnutrition and poor sanitary conditions. Nevertheless, with globalization of the population, symptomatic infections are found in practically all parts of the world. Approximately 10% of the world population is infected with some type of amoebas. In those countries where the incidence is high (Mexico, Brazil, Vietnam, Colombia), the rate of symptomatic infections ranges between 2% and 49%, of which only about 10% of colonized subjects develop some form of invasive amoebiasis. The primary extracolonic manifestation of amoebiasis is liver abscess; interestingly, a recent history of colonic dysentery is rare; indeed, the hepatic abscess may occur several years after the primary infection or even without any clinical history of colitis.

The cystic form of the parasite is in a vegetative state, and once swallowed, it remains in the colon and develops into its trophozoite form. This form can invade the colonic mucosa, giving rise to the typical flash-shaped ulcers. From there, the trophozoite form of the parasite can reach the liver via portal circulation, resist complement lysis along the way, and colonize and infect the liver parenchyma; abscesses form through the action of proteolytic enzymes that destroy the parenchyma, creating thrombosis and microabscesses that grow in size. Although grossly purulent, the luminal content usually remains sterile, except in about 20% of patients in whom bacterial superinfection may occur.

Mortality: Mortality in patients with amoebic abscesses depends on the virulence of the parasite, the host's immune status, and, especially, the presence of complications. In non-complicated cases, mortality is <5% but increases markedly to 11–40% when there are complications.

In a series of 503 patients from China with amoebic liver abscesses, 110 (22%) perforated, including 79 that perforated into the pleuropulmonary space, 15 into the subphrenic space, 11 into the peritoneal cavity, and 5 into other anatomic areas such as the pericardium, abdominal wall, and chest wall. Some 45% of patients with perforations into the abdominal cavity died compared with 14% of those who had perforations into a different anatomic site. Most abscesses in the pleuropulmonary and subphrenic spaces were managed satisfactorily with metronidazole and percutaneous drainage. Of 501 amoebic abscesses reported from Mexico with chest complications, 326 ruptured through the diaphragm. Treatment was with metronidazole plus emetine and drainage. Mortality in this group was 12%. In contrast, free perforation into the abdominal cavity is a strong predictor of mortality. Other predictors of poor prognosis include perforation into the pericardium, multiple abscesses, volume greater than 500 ml, encephalopathy, albumin < 2/dl, diabetes mellitus, and severe anemia.

Clinical Presentation: Amoebic liver abscesses are 10 times more common in males than in females and are found only rarely in children. Amoebic abscesses tend to occur in young individuals, and their incidence is greater during the summer months in endemic areas.

About 75% of amoebic abscesses present as a solitary lesion localized usually in the right lobe; however, in one series from India, the involvement was of the left lobe in a greater percentage of patients (❯ *Fig. 95-4*). Unlike pyogenic abscesses, amoebic abscesses are more subacute, and it may take weeks for symptoms to appear. At first, symptoms are non-specific and usually include fever (remitting or intermittent but generally not generally than 40°C unless there is bacterial superinfection) and localized epigastric abdominal and right upper quadrant pain. When the abscess lies adjacent to the diaphragm, there may be referred shoulder pain, cough, or even pleurisy; right pleural effusion is present in 25–50% of cases. Deep abscesses may present with only fever and no other associated signs or symptoms. Gastrointestinal symptoms may be present in about 25% of patients and include nausea, vomiting, abdominal distension, and diarrhea, but concomitant colitis is rare.

More than 50% of patients have anemia as a function of a chronic process and an increased sedimentation rate. Moderate leukocytosis and neutrophilia are present in about 70% of patients.

Figure 95-4
CT of amebic liver abscess. Note single abscess in segment II–III

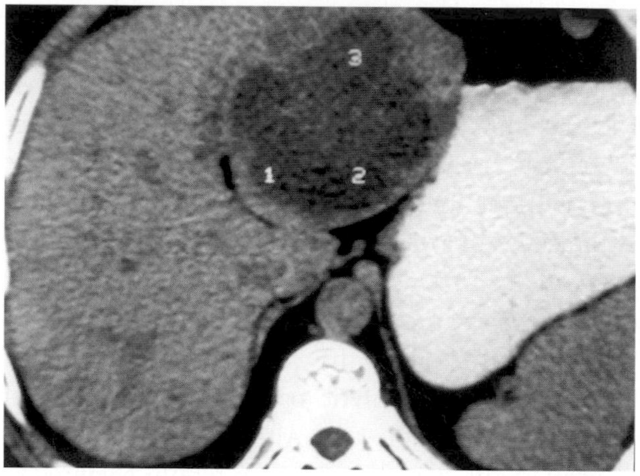

Liver function tests may be normal, but serum alkaline phosphatase and transaminase values may be increased slightly. Blood cultures, as well as cultures of the purulent, anchovy past-like intracystic material, are negative.

Indications, sensitivity, and specificity of the imaging studies are no different from those with pyogenic liver abscesses. Serum antibodies are of high, reliable diagnostic value for amoebic liver abscesses and are positive in 75% of patients in the acute phase and in >90% during the later phase. These tests remain positive for several months or even years afterward. Recent techniques of molecular biology directed at the serum, such as co-agglutination, ELISA, or polymerase chain reaction, may differentiate between recent and past infections, with reported sensitivities and specificities >90%. The co-agglutination test (Co-A) is a quick and easy way to determine the presence of circulating antigens in the serum of patients with amoebic liver abscess in 90% of cases, although there are problems with false positive results in patients with other parasitic or bacterial infections.

Treatment: The initial treatment of amoebic liver abscess involves a primary non-operative approach with antibiotics from the imidazole group, in particular metronidazole. The success rate with monotherapy ranges between 40% and 90%. Empiric response to the treatment with metronidazole also enables confirmation of the diagnosis of amebic liver abscess. There should be a rapid improvement of clinical symptoms, while radiologic changes become apparent only 7–10 days after the initiation of treatment. The radiologic signs of abscess and liver involvement disappear within 10–300 days, depending on the size and characteristics of the abscess. When there is no response to treatment with metronidazole, another possibility is to add chloroquine (600 mg/day for 2 days, followed by 300 mg/day for another 3 weeks) with or without paromomycin or diloxanide furoate. Dehydroemetine is considered the last line of treatment because of its high cardiac and gastrointestinal morbidity.

Percutaneous drainage with or without a catheter is performed only in patients who do not show any improvement with medical management and in other situations such as impending rupture, large left-lobe abscesses (>5–7 cm), suspicion of a bacterial superinfection, and ultrasonographic confirmation of a largely fluid collection. The success of the combined therapy is >90%; laparoscopic or open drainage is reserved for otherwise untreatable complications.

Considering that there is no animal reservoir or vector for Entamoeba histolytica, theoretically a vaccine could potentially eliminate intestinal infections and, consequently, amoebic liver abscesses. Immunologic assessments have shown that specific protection against amoebic infections is associated with the production of antibodies against the adhesion molecule lectin, an antigenic protein found in 95% of the infectious strains of Entamoeba histolytica. Experimental studies in animal models using immunologic therapies directed at galactose and N-acetyl-D-galactosamine, lectin, serine-rich proteins, cysteine proteases, lipophosphoglycanes, amoebapores, and protein 29-kDA have proven to be effective immunoprotection, thus constituting the future prophylactic treatments for Entamoeba histolytica infections, a disease that could be prevented by improving sanitation designed to avoid fecal contamination of water and food sources.

Selected Readings

Choi D, Lim HK, Kim MJ, et al. (2005) Liver abscess after percutaneous radiofrequency ablation for hepatocellular carcinoma: frequency and risk factors. AJR Am J Roentgenol 184:1860–1867

Chu KM, Fan ST, Lai EC, et al. (1996) Pyogenic liver abscess. An audit of experience over the past decade. Arch Surg 131:148–152

Haque R, Huston CD, Hughes M, et al. (2003) Current concepts: amebiasis. New Engl J Med 348:1565–1573

Huang CJ, Pitt HA, Lipsett PA, et al. (1996) Pyogenic hepatic abscess. Changing trends over 42 years. Ann Surg 223:600–607; discussion 607–609

Hughes MA, Petri WA Jr. (2000) Amebic liver abscess. Infect Dis Clin North Am 14:546–582

Kim W, Clark TW, Baum RA, Soulen MC (2001) Risk factors for liver abscess formation after hepatic chemoembolization. J Vasc Interv Radiol 12:965–968

Rahimian J, Wilson T, Oram V, Holzman RS (2004) Pyogenic liver abscess: recent trends in etiology and mortality. Clin Infect Dis 39:21654–1659

96 Portal Hypertension

Héctor Orozco · Miguel Angel Mercado

Pearls and Pitfalls

- Portal hypertension has various etiologies, each with a particular pathophysiology that may impact treatment options.
- Extrahepatic portal hypertension is secondary to portal thrombosis and is associated frequently with disorders of coagulation (protein C, protein S, or antithrombin III deficiencies).
- In hepatic cirrhosis, the obstructive process is intrahepatic, leading to increases in both vascular resistance and splanchnic vasodilatation.
- There is no specific prophylaxis that will prevent portal hypertension-induced variceal formation; however, for primary prophylaxis (to try to prevent variceal bleeding), the treatment of choice is β-blockade, although endoscopic treatment of varices may be considered.
- For secondary prophylaxis (recurrent bleeding), the first line treatments are β-blockade and endoscopic procedures with band ligation.
- Transjugular Intrahepatic Portosystemic Shunt (TIPS) is a second line procedure used in refractory patients after failed endoscopic therapy and as a bridge to hepatic transplantation.
- Surgical intervention may be recommended as a secondary prophylaxis in patients with early failure of medical management and good hepatic function (Child-Pugh A-B).
- Operative procedures that preserve prograde portal (hepatopedal) flow are the procedures of choice.
- Non-selective shunts are effective for control of hemorrhage, but the incidence of encephalopathy is high.
- In our experience, the distal splenorenal shunt is the preferred surgical option with reservation of extensive devascularization procedures for situations of inappropriate anatomy (splenic thrombosis).
- Liver transplantation is reserved for patients with refractory bleeding and poor liver function (Child-Pugh C).

Introduction

Increased pressure in the portal venous system is known as portal hypertension (PH). Normal total hepatic blood flow is about 2 l/min but comes from two sources; the hepatic artery contributes about 600–700 ml/min and the portal venous system about 1,300 ml/minute. The portal venous system supplies 75% of the oxygen delivery to the liver with the remainder from the hepatic artery.

PH is a combination of increased resistance at the hepatic sinusoidal level and an increase in total hepatic blood flow. The production of vasoactive substances at the hepatic sinusoids also contributes to these hemodynamic changes. In the setting of PH, there is also an increased pressure within the lymphatic system that can contribute to the development of ascites as well. The main consequences of PH are bleeding from gastro-esophageal varices and hypersplenism (leukopenia, anemia, and thrombocytopenia).

The most common conditions leading to PH in adults are alcohol abuse, viral infection-induced cirrhosis, and venous thrombosis, while in Africa, the Middle East, and South America, hepatic fibrosis due to schistosomiasis is equally common.

Etiopathogenesis

Intrahepatic PH: In most Western countries, the cirrhosis leading to intrahepatic PH is related either to alcohol abuse or viral hepatitis (usually hepatitis B or C) leading to cirrhosis. With increasing frequency, however, non-alcoholic steatohepatitis (NASH) is becoming a more common etiology of advanced cirrhosis (accounting for as much as 20% of all cirrhotics in the United States), probably related to the increased prevalence of obesity worldwide. Other more unusual etiologies include hemochromatosis, α-1 anti-trypsin deficiency, Wilson's disease, etc.

Extrahepatic PH: PH can occur from obstruction or thrombosis of venous inflow to or from the liver. The main causes of posthepatic, extrahepatic PH are obstruction of the hepatic veins, inferior vena cava, or both, as in the Budd-Chiari syndrome (hepatic outflow occlusive disease).

Prehepatic extrahepatic PH is due primarily to thrombosis of the portal vein. This disorder can occur in children with omphalitis; however, many of these children have idiopathic portal hypertension. Not infrequently, these patients will also have histologic and functional hepatic abnormalities even though the macroscopic features of the liver appear to be normal. It is possible that these children have idiopathic PH and that the portal thrombosis is only one of the stages of the disease.

Another cause of extrahepatic PH is thrombosis of the splenic vein, which leads to a segmental increase in extrahepatic venous pressure termed sinistral, or "left-sided" PH. This segmental PH occurs most frequently as a complication of pancreatitis, although other causes include pancreatic neoplasms or trauma. This segmental increase in venous outflow of the spleen leads to intrasplenic venous hypertension, which induces the development of venous collaterals of drainage through the stomach via the short gastric veins leading to gastric varices. Rare causes of prehepatic PH include iatrogenic or spontaneous arterio-portal fistulae that may occur after percutaneous hepatic biopsies, percutaneous biliary intubation, or secondary to visceral aneurysms. Finally, primary thrombosis may occur in the setting of thrombophilias such as deficiencies in Protein C, Protein S, and anti-thrombin III autoimmune pathologies (antiphospholid antibodies), and other hematologic abnormalities such as paroxysmal nocturnal hemoglobinuria. These abnormalities can cause both pre- and posthepatic PH.

For many years, the belief was that rupture of esophageal varices was the only cause of bleeding. Nowadays, we know that bleeding from gastric varices is also a frequent cause. In these patients, it is common to find a congestive gastropathy as well.

The portal pressure should be considered dynamic rather than static, because abrupt increases in pressure in the portal system are frequent. These increases are transmitted to the varicose plexus by everyday life activities such as sneezing, physical exertion, or defecation. Hemodynamic studies with a catheter in the portal vein demonstrate that the Valsalva maneuver can increase the portal pressure by 20–60 mm of pressure.

Clinical Manifestations

The main signs and symptoms suggestive of PH are abdominal collateral circulation, evidence of esophageal varices, abdominal ascites, and splenomegaly. In more recent times, endoscopic ultrasonography has been used to classify varices and identify collateral circulation. CT and Doppler ultrasonography may better define the areas of the hepatic or splenic helium; these two diagnostic methods have the advantage of being non-invasive.

The most severe consequence of PH is esophageal hemorrhage from the thin-walled esophageal varices. Nevertheless, not all patients with PH experience esophageal bleeding. Only 15–30% of all the patients with cirrhosis, PH, and esophagogastric varices will develop variceal hemorrhage.

Diagnosis

After a thorough clinical and physical examination, determination of underlying liver disease and defining the etiology for the PH (pre-, intra- or posthepatic) is imperative. Laboratory evaluation, radiologic imaging, and endoscopic means are the most fruitful. Angiographic studies, although invasive, are necessary occasionally for rare causes of PH (❷ *Fig. 96-1*). The goals are to define the presence/absence of hepatic parenchymal disease (e.g. cirrhosis; see Chapter 92), the site of portal venous obstruction (intrahepatic, hepatic venous outflow, extrahepatic portal system, etc.), and the presence or absence of esophageal, gastric, and/or small bowel varices.

Treatment

Surgical treatment of PH is usually indicated only in patients who have failed medical management, with the goal of avoiding recurrent bleeding. Operative intervention as prophylaxis in select, high-risk

◘ Figure 96-1
Extra hepatic portal hypertension with spontaneous spleno-renal shunt

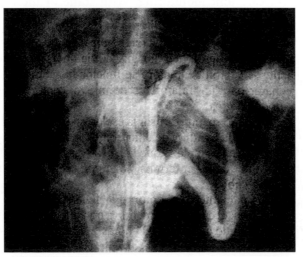

patients without prior complications has been advocated by some authors but remains highly controversial, and most studies of prophylactic operative decompression have not shown an advantage in overall survival. In contrast, prophylactic treatment for the patient with PH is based in the use of drugs such as β-blockers or those that modify the cardiac output, systemic blood pressure, and portal pressure. Several prospective studies have demonstrated the ability of β-blockers to reduce variceal bleeding complications compared with placebo. Currently, there are prospective studies suggesting the value of prophylactic endoscopic banding of the varicose plexus in patients without prior variceal hemorrhage; variceal banding is useful in patients with contraindications to or intolerance of pharmacologic prophylactic measures.

Treatment of PH is based on presence or absence of symptoms, etiology, extent of liver disease, and prior treatments. If varices are present, specific treatment should be considered, including pharmacologic therapy, sclerotherapy, or transjugular intrahepatic shunting (TIPS). Under conditions of active variceal hemorrhage, the options include emergency sclerotherapy, balloon tamponade, emergency TIPS, or surgical therapy (portosystemic shunts, devascularization procedures, or even hepatic transplantation).

Pharmacologic treatment: Several studies have demonstrated that vasopressin decreases the pressure of the portal system and produces constriction of the muscular esophageal walls with collapse of the gastroesophageal varices. Given the short half-life of vasopressin, continuous IV infusions are required.

The combination of nitroglycerin and vasopressin may help to control not only the portal hypertension but also will protect the patient with coronary artery disease from the cardiac side-effects of a vasoconstrictive agent. This treatment may have some adverse effects, such as lowering the blood pressure that may lead to other complications. Other drugs such as somatostatin or its homologues are relatively effective for the control of acute bleeding and appear equally effective as sclerotherapy and/or variceal banding in prospective controlled trials.

Balloon tamponade: A useful maneuver for controlling acute, severe bleeding from esophageal varices is to place a transoral balloon tamponade system such as the Blakemore-Sengstaken tube or the Minnesota tube. These tubes have an external balloon that applies pressure directly on the varices when the balloon is inflated in the gastric and/or esophageal lumen. Balloon tamponade is used only in the emergency situation when the bleeding cannot be controlled by other measures. Use of these tubes is limited and requires intensive care unit monitoring. With some of the newer techniques discussed below, balloon tamponade is used only rarely today.

Sclerotherapy and variceal banding: Endoscopic sclerotherapy and banding are effective in controlling acute variceal bleeding in up to 95% of patients. In addition, they also allow stabilization of patients who may require a more definitive procedure. Because recurrent variceal bleeding occurs in up to 40% of patients after sclerotherapy or variceal banding, the addition of pharmacologic treatment decrease recurrence of bleeding.

Transjugular intrahepatic shunt (TIPS): Placement of an intrahepatic shunt creating a fistula between a branch of the portal vein with a hepatic vein is accomplished through transjugular transhepatic venous approach and is known as a TIPS procedure. This procedure is carried out percutaneously under fluoroscopic control. The catheter is positioned retrograde into a hepatic vein; from this position and through this catheter, a needle is advanced through the hepatic parenchyma until an intrahepatic portal vein with adequate caliber is accessed. After that, this track is dilated, and an 8–10 cm circular metallic endoprosthesis is placed. This prosthesis/shunt allows decompression of the PH through the shunt into the low pressure vena cava.

Theoretically, TIPS is an ideal treatment option for decompressing the portal system in patients with poor liver function, abnormalities in coagulation, ascites, jaundice, and even encephalopathy, where operative risks would be substantial. Potential advantages of TIPS are that it avoids the need for an operative portosystemic shunt in the very high risk patients and does not alter surgical anatomy in candidates for a liver transplantation. Potential disadvantages of TIPS include the need for specialists in interventional radiology and the risks of encephalopathy or liver failure. Indeed, development of encephalopathy after TIPS may accelerate the need for liver transplantation. Other risks include the possibility of hepatic vein or portal vein thrombosis, which may lead to obstacles for future liver transplantation, or shunt occlusion which occurs in up to 30% of patients within the first year after placement. The use of "protected" or "coated" stents appears to decrease the incidence of stent occlusion.

Emergency surgical treatment: Operative intervention in patients who arrive in the emergency room with severe bleeding secondary to hepatic cirrhosis is associated with a very high mortality rate. Procedural options include portosystemic shunts (selective and non-selective) and devascularization procedures. Non-selective shunts offer excellent control of PH and ascites but have an increased risk of inducing or worsening encephalopathy. These procedures include end-to-end or side-to-side porto-caval shunts or the mesocaval shunt.

Devascularization procedures have been advocated by some for the emergent treatment of patients with bleeding. These procedures involve transmural or direct ligation of esophageal varices, transaction and reanastomosis of the esophagus to disrupt continuity of gastroesophageal varices, esophagogastric resections, and esophagogastric devascularization. While these procedures have some merit in the emergent management of patients with bleeding esophageal varices, the long-term outcome is much less favorable; surviving patients exhibit a high incidence of recurrent bleeding. In the emergent setting, operative intervention in patients with Childs C cirrhosis is contraindicated. These patients are best treated with nonsurgical methods described previously, including TIPS. On occasion, patients with prehepatic PH from schistosomiasis or portal venous thrombosis may benefit in the acute setting from an esophagogastric devascularization procedure such as the Sugiura-Futagawa operation.

In an elective setting in patients with preserved liver function and a patent, anatomically appropriate portal anatomy, the treatment of choice is total porto-systemic shunt via portacaval shunt (end-side or side-side), a side-to-side splenorenal shunt, or a mesocaval shunt. One operative procedure that may stop variceal bleeding is the small diameter mesocaval or portocaval "H" shunt with a small diameter graft. According to Sarfeh and colleagues, this type of "semi-selective" shunt is capable of partial decompression of the portal system without complete diversion of the hepatic portal flow. Probably the most attractive portal decompressive procedure is the distal splenorenal shunt, also called the Warren shunt. The "selective" distal splenorenal shunt is technically more demanding and time-consuming and is used rarely in the emergent setting.

Devascularization procedures, such as described by Sugiura and Futagawa, are successful in the management of acute variceal bleeding and have the advantages of a decrease in operative mortality, avoidance of encephalopathy induced by shunts, and do not require preoperative vascular imaging. In an elective setting, these procedures are best used in patients with schistosomiasis and not cirrhosis.

Selection of Patients for Elective Operative Management

The clinical evaluation of patients considered for operative intervention to correct complications of PH is critical. It is imperative to determine the underlying liver function, Childs class, MELD score, and other potential prohibitive comorbidities in all patients. Evaluation includes laboratory, endoscopic, and imaging tests.

Laboratory studies include the concentrations of serum glucose, urea, creatinine, and electrolytes, hematologic studies, complete liver function tests, coagulation parameters (prothrombin time), and platelet count. Endoscopic evaluation is also necessary to evaluate the presence of esophageal or gastric varices, congestive gastropathy, and any other gastric or duodenal abnormalities. Radiologic evaluation may include ultrasonography to assess liver parenchyma, hepatic vasculature, and direction of portal venous flow.

Once this preliminary evaluation has been completed, the next step is to decide which operative procedure is best suited to the patient. To facilitate this decision, angiographic studies are recommended that together are called hepatic panangiography. In the past, angiography included a celiac artery injection along with the venous phase to determine the patency and anatomy of the portal venous system; when appropriate, the vena cava and left renal vein was also imaged to determine its distance from the splenic vein. Currently, CT angiography and magnetic resonance angiography are often able to define satisfactorily the vascular anatomy without the invasiveness of angiography.

Hepatic venography can serve as an indirect evaluation of the hepato-portal flow; at the same time it is allows assessment of pressure gradients between the portal and systemic systems. The pressure measurements made are the wedge hepatic pressure, which estimates closely the portal vein pressure; the "corrected portal pressure" or transhepatic pressure gradient can then be calculated using the difference between the wedge pressure and the pressure in the inferior vena caval; normal "corrected" portal pressure is <5 mmHg.

In patients with chronic liver disease and PH with preservation of portal hepatic flow, a selective shunt is the preferred procedure. The "selective" shunts include the distal splenorenal or "Warren" shunt or alternatively an "H" type mesocaval shunt with a small diameter (8 mm) graft. In those patients with sinistral hypertension due to splenic vein thrombosis *without* liver disease, splenectomy is generally curative. When there is concomitant thrombosis of both splenic and superior mesenteric veins, the Sugiura procedure may be used, beginning with the abdominal approach, and 4–6 weeks later completed with the thoracic approach. A modification of the Sugiura-Futagawa procedure which we call "complete porto-azygous disconnection," involves an abdominal devascularization with subsequent endoscopic eradication of esophageal varices via banding.

Porto-systemic shunts: The non-selective porto-systemic shunts, such as the portocaval, central splenorenal, mesocaval with an "H" or "C" graft, and portorenal shunts decompress completely the portal system and control hemorrhage very effectively. But as a result of the extent of diversion of portal flow, these total shunts are associated with an increased risk of encephalopathy, because they divert essentially all portal venous flow away from the liver (❍ *Fig. 96-2*). To reduce this risk of encephalopathy, several authors have advocated the use of an intervening small diameter graft (<8 mm) to provide resistance to total diversion and to preserve at least some portal flow.

With the conventional, non-selective porto-systemic shunts, the risk of hepatic encephalopathy in the postoperative period can reach 40–50% in patients with compromised hepatic function (Childs B and C). In contrast, the selective porto-systemic shunts, such as the distal splenorenal shunt or Warren

◼ **Figure 96-2**
Porto-caval shunts. End to side (a) and side to side (b)

Porto-caval shunt end to side

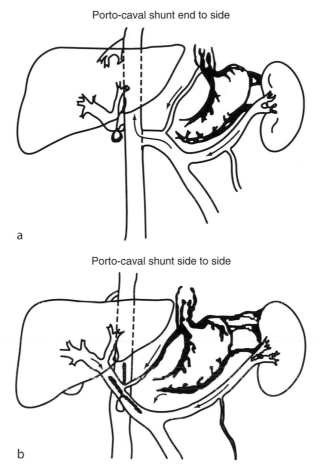

a

Porto-caval shunt side to side

b

shunt (❯ *Fig. 96-3*) decompresses the varices in the esophagogastric area without altering hepatic portal flow from the superior mesenteric vein (and gut blood flow), at least acutely. With longer follow-up, many patients will develop venous collateral connections with the pancreatic veins in an attempt to decompress the "preserved" portal pressure, thereby partially reversing the selective nature of the operation.

Budd-Chiari Syndrome: In patients with hepatic venous outflow obstruction leading to posthepatic PH in whom the inferior vena cava is not affected, a conventional non-selective porto-systemic shunt, such as a side-to-side portocaval or mesocaval "H" or "C" graft, will decompress the PH effectively. In contrast, when the hepatic hypertrophy of the caudate lobe causes compression of the inferior vena cava or when there is an inferior vena caval web or thrombosis, portocaval or mesocaval shunts are contraindicated, and alternatives such as a mesoatrial shunt with a graft must be considered. Some groups have shown that not every patient with Budd-Chiari syndrome requires operative intervention due to development of spontaneous portosystemic shunts in some patients. Surgical treatment was reserved for those patients with evidence of hepatic tissue necrosis on biopsy, which portends a poor prognosis without operative intervention. Conversely, others suggest that hepatic necrosis will develop

Figure 96-3
Distal spleno-renal shunt (Warren shunt)

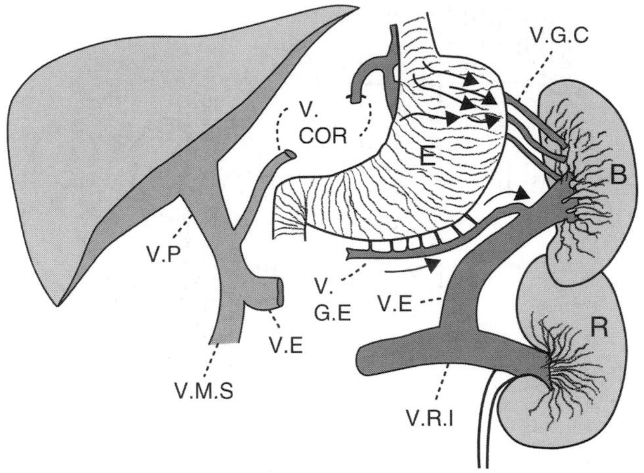

in most if not all patients with Budd-Chiari syndrome and recommend operative intervention to avoid eventual hepatic failure.

In the setting of acute, severe, hepatic necrosis, liver transplantation is necessary, however, due to the possibility of recurrent thrombosis, we recommend lifelong anticoagulation after transplantation for Budd-Chiari syndrome.

The most recent alternative to treat this problem is the placement of a TIPS. Endoluminal rechanneling of the hepatic vein with subsequent placement of a portoatrial expandable coated stent is another possibility.

Esophagogastric devascularization: When a porto-systemic shunt is contraindicated, esophagogastric devascularization (Sugiura-Futagawa) or complete porto-azygous disconnection may be considered. In the authors' experience of more than 1,000 patients with mean follow-up of 10 years, esophagogastric devascularization can be performed with low rates of postoperative morbidity and mortality. The mortality rate of 25% in the emergency setting is considerable compared with 2% in the elective setting. Postoperative encephalopathy occurs in less than 5% of patients and recurrent bleeding in 10%. Estimated 3-year survival is 85%.

The Sugiura-Futagawa procedure consists of an extensive esophageal and gastric devascularization from the area of the left inferior pulmonary vein of the thoracic esophagus to the lesser curvature of the stomach; this devascularization is completed with transaction of the lower third of the esophagus with reanastomosis, combined with splenectomy, pyloroplasty, and gastric devascularization. In general, this treatment approach is done in two stages. In young people with adequate hepatic function and PH without cirrhosis, this procedure can be done in one stage.

The authors have utilized a modification of the Sugiura-Futagawa technique. Instead of dissecting and devascularizing just the lesser curvature, the gastro hepatic ligament, left gastric (coronary) vein and artery, and all the structures to the abdominal esophagus and fundus and body of the stomach are divided (*Fig. 96-4*). In addition, the right gastric vein and artery are ligated in three different places along the lesser curvature with non-absorbable sutures. The major curvature of the stomach is completely devascularized except for the right gastroepiploic artery; this devascularization is done with preservation of the spleen. For the thoracic stage, the esophageal transaction was modified. Instead of transecting the esophageal mucosa in its entire circumference, as described by Sugiura, we

◻ **Figure 96-4**
Complete porto-azygous disconnection

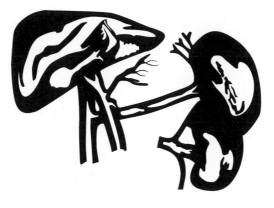

divide the anterior muscular layer, free the mucosa in its entire circumference, and perform a complete circular suture; in so doing, we ligate all the variceal plexus, diminishing the possibility of a postoperative esophageal fistula. The last modification is ligation of the right gastroepiploic vein distal to the pylorus. These modifications have been called a complete porto-azygous disconnection. Given the effectiveness of endoscopic obliteration of the esophageal variceal plexus, we now perform the abdominal phase of the complete porto-azygous disconnection and then perform endoscopic variceal banding instead of the traditional second stage, transthoracic operation.

Prevention and Treatment of Hepatic Failure After Operation

One of the major concerns in the operative management of patients with PH is hepatic failure after operation. Careful patient selection and preoperative preparation is essential. During the operation, it is important that hemodynamic stability be maintained. The procedure must be performed with meticulous dissection to avoid hemorrhage resulting in hypovolemia and hypoxia which may exacerbate any potential hepatic injury. Crystalloid administration must be controlled carefully during the operation to avoid fluid retention and promote or worsen ascites in the postoperative period. Frequently, colloid solutions or albumin are used postoperatively to avoid excessive administration of crystalloid. Narcotics, sedatives, or hypnotics are used with reservation, and high protein consumption is avoided in the early postoperative period. In some instances, oral or rectal lactulose and non-absorbable oral antibiotics (neomycin) are required to avoid hepatic pre coma or ammonium intoxication. In general, in well-selected patients with preserved hepatic function undergoing elective surgery for PH, it is rare that additional treatments for hepatic insufficiency are necessary.

Hepatic transplantation: Hepatic transplantation offers potential definitive treatment of hepatic cirrhosis, PH, and resulting bleeding varices. Hepatic transplantation is not indicated in patients with adequate hepatic function when their only problem is bleeding, given the limited organ availability and the favorable results of shunts and devascularization procedures in these patients. Other factors that influence the decision for hepatic transplantation are the etiology of the hepatic disease, organ availability, presence of a small hepatocellular carcinoma, and psychosocial factors of patients with alcoholic liver disease.

Selected Readings

Abraldes JG, Angermayr B, Bosch J (2005) The management of portal hypertension. Clin Liver Dis 9:685–713

García-Tsao G (2006) Portal hypertension. Curr Opin Gastroenterol 22:254–262

Henderson JM, Yang Y (2005) Is there still a role for surgery in bleeding portal hypertension? Nat Clin Pract Gastroenterol Hepatol 2(6):246–247

Klupp J, Kohler S, Pascher A, Neuhaus P (2005) Liver transplantation as ultimate tool to treat portal hypertension. Dig Dis 23:65–75

Mercado MA, Orozco H, Chan C, et al. (2004) Surgical treatment of non-cirrhotic presinusoidal portal hypertension. Hepatogastroenterology 51:1757–1760

Rosemurgy AX, Osborne D, Zervos EE (2005) Portal hypertension: the role of shunting procedures. Adv Surg 39:315–329

Vignali C, Bargellini I, Grosso M, et al. (2005) TIPS with expanded polytetracluoroethylene covered stent: results of an Italian multicenter study. Am J Roentgenol 185:472–480

97 Cystic Liver Diseases

Catherine Hubert · Laurence Annet · Bernard E. Van Beers · Yves Horsmans · Jean-François Gigot

Pearls and Pitfalls

- The most common cystic diseases of the liver are congenital liver cysts (CLCs), parasitic liver cysts, and cystic liver tumors.
- Appropriate diagnosis of the cyst is mandatory before treatment, since management options vary, ranging from observation to radical resection.
- Patient history, imaging studies, serological markers, and cyst-fluid analysis when a parasitic liver cyst has been excluded, are key factors for making an appropriate differential diagnosis of cystic liver disease.
- Uncertain diagnosis is often encountered between a complicated CLC and a neoplastic cyst.
- Liver cystadenoma is a rare but either overtly or potentially malignant lesion, requiring radical excision.
- A tailored surgical treatment is indicated for patients suffering from cystic liver lesions, ranging from fenestration to resection.
- Because the natural history of CLC is benign, treatment options should be discussed only when cysts are large in size or strategically located *and* when specific cyst-related symptoms or complications are present.
- The causal relationship between abdominal pain and the presence of a large CLC should always be questioned before surgical treatment.
- When doubt persists concerning supposed cyst-related abdominal pain from a large CLC, percutaneous cyst aspiration should be performed as a pretherapeutic test. If abdominal complaints resolve after percutaneous aspiration (and recur with cyst recurrence), symptoms can be reasonably attributed to the cystic disease. Otherwise, another cause should be searched for.
- Missing the diagnosis of liver cystadenoma and thus adopting a conservative treatment leads to recurrence, sometimes as a malignant lesion.
- Macroscopic and microscopic examinations of the cyst wall with routine frozen section are key factors during surgery to differentiate between benign complicated congenital and neoplastic liver cysts.
- The diagnosis of neoplastic liver cyst is a formal indication for surgical treatment, even if the patient is free of symptoms.
- Precise ultrasonographic classification of hydatid liver cyst allows the choice of a tailored treatment strategy.

Introduction

Cystic lesions of the liver are commonly encountered in clinical practice as a result of the patient's accessibility to modern noninvasive imaging techniques. Cystic liver lesions can be broadly divided into four categories: congenital, traumatic, parasitic, and neoplastic (❯ *Table 97-1*). Disease prevalence is broadly different for each type, with congenital liver cysts (CLCs) being the most frequent. The natural history and the risk of malignant transformation are completely different for the various types of cystic liver diseases. Appropriate diagnosis of hepatic cyst is thus essential to enable the physician to plan the correct treatment, which ranges from observation for asymptomatic CLCs to radical resection for cystic liver neoplasms. Differential diagnosis is based on the clinical history, imaging studies, and sometimes on sampling of intracystic fluid.

Classification of Cystic Liver Diseases

Congenital Liver Cysts

CLCs are cystic formations, containing crystal-clear fluid when uncomplicated, with no communication to the intrahepatic bile ducts. CLCs are considered to develop from dilatation of aberrant intrahepatic bile ducts during embryogenesis. Microscopically, CLCs are lined by a single layer of cuboid or columnar epithelium, resembling biliary epithelial cells. The small cysts are surrounded by normal hepatic tissue but large cysts can produce atrophy of the adjacent tissue. The disease is common with a prevalence of 1–5% in the general population, but is reported to be more frequent in women. The lesions may be solitary or multiple, vary from a few millimeters to several centimeters in diameter, and are usually unilocular. Few lesions are really huge in size or potentially responsible for producing

◼ Table 97-1

Classification of cystic liver diseases

• *Congenital liver cysts*
– Simple
– Polycystic disease
– Biliary hamartoma (microhamartoma, von Meyenburg complex)
– Ciliated hepatic foregut cyst
• *Parasitic liver cysts*
– Echinococcal cyst (hydatid disease)
• *Neoplastic liver cysts*
– Primary
• Cystadenoma
• Cystadenocarcinoma
• Cystic mesenchymal hamartoma
– Secondary
• Cystic metastases from sarcoma, melanoma, lung, breast, mucinous colorectal, neuroendocrine tumors
• Large necrosed primary tumors (hepatocellular carcinoma etc.)
• *Acquired liver cysts*
– Posttraumatic hematoma or biloma
– Liver abscess

symptoms. The natural history of CLC is benign regarding disease progression. Most CLCs, even large lesions, are discovered incidentally in asymptomatic patients and do not require any treatment.

Only 10–15% of large CLCs will become symptomatic or complicated. The most common symptoms are upper abdominal discomfort and pain. However, the causal relationship between abdominal pain or discomfort and a benign CLC should always be questioned and accepted only if the cyst is large enough and after other possible causes of the symptoms have been excluded. In cases of doubt, a percutaneous aspiration test should be used to ensure that symptoms resolve with cyst aspiration. In most cases, liver function is entirely normal. Complications of large CLCs are uncommon but include compression of adjacent organs (biliary tract, stomach, or duodenum), intracystic hemorrhage or infection, posttraumatic rupture and torsion of pedunculated cysts. Hemorrhage is the most common complication, revealed by sudden acute abdominal pain with tense and painful hepatomegaly. However, the frequent finding of brownish intracystic fluid suggests that subclinical hemorrhage is probably more frequent than previously thought. Spontaneous cyst infection is exceptional and is caused usually by repeated percutaneous drainage. The typical radiological appearances are modified in complicated CLCs, leading to difficulties in the differential diagnosis with cystic liver neoplasm. Indications for treating CLCs include highly and specifically symptomatic or complicated large cysts.

Polycystic Liver Disease

Adult polycystic liver disease (PLD) is a rare, inherited autosomal recessive disease, and is characterized by the presence of numerous cysts scattered throughout the liver parenchyma. However, liver failure is exceptional. It is generally accepted that hepatic cysts in patients with PLD result from cystic dilatation of biliary microhamartomas that originate from von Meyenburg's complexes. The disease prevalence in autopsy series is between 0.05% and 0.53%, with a female preponderance. The disease is usually associated with polycystic kidney disease (PKD) and coexistent cerebrovascular aneurysms are seen in up to 10–20% of the patients. The prognosis of PLD is usually related to end-stage renal insufficiency due to PKD and to the occurrence of cerebral hemorrhage. A routine search for intracranial aneurysms is thus advocated in PLD patients.

The clinical course of PLD is slowly progressive, with gradual increasing liver volume and compression of adjacent organs. Most PLD patients remain asymptomatic for a long period of time. When present, the commonest symptoms are related to gross polycystic hepatomegaly. These include chronic dull abdominal pain, abdominal discomfort, early satiety and supine dyspnea, leading to progressive physical disability in the individual's daily activities and professional life. Complications of PLD are uncommon, including acute intracystic hemorrhage and cyst infection, but are often severe with compressive complications such as biliary obstruction, portal hypertension, inferior vena caval compression, and hepatic venous outflow obstruction (Budd-Chiari syndrome).

Indications for surgery are restricted to selected patients with incapacitating or complicated polycystic hepatomegaly. The choice of surgical treatment is dictated by the cyst number, size, and distribution within the liver and by the complications of the disease. Our group reported a practical classification of PLD based on the number and size of the liver cysts and the amount of remaining normal liver parenchyma. Type I PLD includes patients with a limited number (< 10) of large cysts (> 10 cm), a situation that is quite similar to multiple CLCs with a huge dominant liver cyst. Type II

PLD is represented by patients with diffuse involvement of the liver parenchyma by multiple medium-sized cysts with remaining large areas of noncystic liver parenchyma on preoperative CT. Type III PLD is a severe form of PLD with massive, diffuse involvement of the liver parenchyma by small- and medium-sized liver cysts and only a few areas of preserved liver parenchyma between the cysts. To evaluate the results of surgical treatment, liver volumetry should be used from preoperative and serial postoperative abdominal CT.

Parasitic Hydatid Liver Cyst

The liver is commonly (60%) affected by hydatid disease. The disease is caused by *Echinococcus granulosus*, a tapeworm encountered in endemic countries such as the Mediterranean area (including North Africa, Spain, and Greece), the Middle East, Iran, the East of Europe, and in South American countries such as Argentina, Chile, and Uruguay. The disease has almost disappeared from other parts of the world such as Western Australia and New Zealand where sheep farming is common. The disease is seen all over the world because of increasing immigration and worldwide travel from high-risk regions. Humans are intermediate hosts after enteral ingestion of infective eggs from infested dogs. The parasite becomes encysted within the liver and develops a germinal membrane that is responsible for production of scolices, crystal clear hydatid fluid, and daughter cysts. With increasing-size, the host-compressed liver produces a reactive fibrous capsule encircling the hydatid liver cyst (HLC). The cyst is usually solitary and unilocular but may be multiple (25–30%) within the liver and the abdominal cavity or the lungs.

HLC is a slow-growing disease, remaining silent during a long clinical latency. Diagnosis is made on imaging and serologic studies, with a positive indirect hemagglutination test in more than 80% of the patients. A negative serological test does not rule out the diagnosis of echinococcosis, especially in patients with positive P1 or P2 erythrocytes serotypes. Eosinophilia is inconstant and liver tests are normal, except in cases of biliary complication. These lesions become symptomatic because of a space-occupying effect that produces abdominal pain or mass, allergic reactions, or more commonly, complications. HLC compresses progressively the surrounding intrahepatic parenchyma, blood vessels, and bile ducts. Biliary complications are common (10–30%), and may be caused by rupture of the cyst content into the biliary tree which, in turn, is responsible for bile-staining intracystic fluid, abnormal liver tests, obstructive jaundice, or cholangitis. Other complications include cyst infection, compression of the portal system or the liver outflow (Budd-Chiari syndrome), rupture into the pleural, pericardial cavity or the bronchial tree, perforation into adjacent viscus (stomach, duodenum, small intestine), spontaneous, or posttraumatic rupture in the peritoneal cavity. This last complication is the least frequent but the most severe complication of hydatid disease, causing secondary peritoneal implantations that are difficult to eradicate.

Surgical treatment is usually recommended in all operable patients because of the often complicated clinical presentation of the disease, despite its benign nature. The purpose of surgical treatment is to eradicate completely the parasites, to obliterate the remaining cyst cavity, and to treat associated complications. The sonographic classification reported initially by Gharbi and colleagues and later modified by the World Health Organization aims to predict the functional state of hydatid disease and facilitate patient selection for treatment (❯ *Table 97-2*).

◘ Table 97-2

Ultrasound (US) classification of hydatid liver cysts according to Gharbi et al. (1981) and WHO (2003)

Gharbi et al. (1981) classification	WHO (2003) classification	Ultrasound features	Parasitic activity status
–	CL	• Pure fluid collection, unilocular, no cyst wall, signs not pathognomonic for hydatid cyst	Active
Type I	Type CE 1	• Fluid collection with cyst wall, hydatid sand	Active
Type II	Type CE 2	• Multivesicular fluid collection, cyst wall, "rosette-like"	Active
Type III	Type CE 3	• Fluid collection with detached laminated membrane, "water-lily" sign, less round, decreased intracystic pressure	Transitional
Type IV	Type CE 4	• Heterogeneous hypoechoic or hyperechoic cyst contents, high internal echoes, no daughter cysts	Inactive
Type V	Type CE 5	• Thick calcified cyst wall, calcification partial to complete	Inactive

CL: cystic lesion; CE: *Echinococcus granulosus* cyst.

Neoplastic Liver Cysts

Liver cystadenoma is a rare cystic tumor (representing <5% of hepatic cysts), with a strong tendency to recur after incomplete excision and undergo malignant transformation into cystadenocarcinoma. The disease occurs more often in middle-aged women. Macroscopically, the lesion is a single, usually large, multiloculated cyst, containing mucinous PAS-positive fluid. Irregularities or septations within the cyst wall are present. Microscopic examination reveals a single layer of mucin-secreting cuboidal epithelium with vacuolated cells and often polypoid or papillary projections are observed. Some mucinous liver cystadenomas harbor an ovarian-like mesenchymal stroma. Liver cystadenomas are premalignant lesions, with malignancy occurring almost exclusively in preexisting cystadenomas and potentially affecting the entire cyst epithelium but more often involving only focal areas of malignant epithelial transformation. This feature explains why a needle biopsy can be falsely negative.

Liver cystadenoma is a slow-growing tumor. Symptoms are usually related to mass effects, including abdominal pain or discomfort. Extrahepatic or intrahepatic tumor compression may occur. Liver function tests are normal, but imaging studies and cyst fluid sampling are useful for diagnosis. Fine needle aspiration cytology (FNAC) examination and determination of CA-19-9 in the mucinous fluid can be suggestive of neoplastic liver cysts. Because of the malignant potential of liver cystadenoma, complete surgical excision is always indicated, even in asymptomatic patients. Indeed, partial excision exposes the patient to an almost constant risk of recurrence and further malignancy.

Other Uncommon Liver Cysts

Several liver diseases may appear cystic on imaging studies. Benign cystic conditions include posttraumatic liver hematoma or biloma, liver abscess, or cystic mesenchymal hamartoma. Previous history of right upper quadrant (RUQ) trauma directs the diagnosis to a traumatic origin. Additionally, the radiological aspect differs from that of true hepatic cysts, with the coexistence of nonliquefied liver hematoma forming a thick pseudocystic wall in cases of trauma. Liver abscess is suspected by the presence of high fever, chills, acute RUQ pain with elevated white cell count, and septicemia.

Radiologically, liver abscesses have a thicker, more irregular wall than simple cysts and often contain debris which produces internal echoes. On computed tomography (CT) and magnetic resonance imaging (MRI), prominent perfusion abnormalities are often observed in the adjacent liver parenchyma. The history and clinical examination should help to differentiate abscesses and primary liver cysts. Mesenchymal hamartoma is characterized by a complex cystic–solid imaging appearance, thick wall, and some enhancing internal stromal components. Acquired malignant cystic diseases include complete or partial necrosis of large primary tumors such as hepatocellular carcinoma or metastases from sarcoma, melanoma, lung, breast, and mucinous colorectal or neuroendocrine tumors. Central cystic degeneration or extensive tumor necrosis may result in a cyst-like appearance. However, with contrast-enhanced imaging, any central nonenhancing area is surrounded by peripheral nodular enhancement from viable tumor. Percutaneous biopsy of the thick cyst wall for histological examination will be helpful in obtaining a definitive diagnosis.

Characterization of Cystic Liver Lesions

An appropriate differential diagnosis among congenital, parasitic, and neoplastic cystic liver diseases is crucial, not only because of the differences in the natural disease history and malignant potential, but also for treatment planning. Characterization is based on patient's clinical history, blood samples, imaging studies, and often cyst-fluid analysis.

Clinical History

A history of travel from an endemic country favors a diagnosis of hydatid liver disease. A family history should be sought in patients suffering from PLD. A specific clinical background is encountered in case of traumatic liver pseudocyst and liver abscess. Otherwise, clinical history is of limited value in differentiating congenital from neoplastic liver cysts.

Blood Sampling

Serological tests, when positive, allow diagnosis of hydatid liver disease and an elevated serum Ca 19-9 is often encountered in overt or metastatic liver cystadenocarcinoma. Biological signs of infection and septicemia favor liver abscess. Elevated liver function tests are only predictive of biliary compression or intraductal migration of hydatid debris.

Imaging Studies

The typical radiological appearances are the cornerstone for characterizing cystic liver diseases. Percutaneous ultrasound (US) is the simplest and least expensive diagnostic imaging modality, but CT or MRI are increasingly used for differentiating hepatic cysts. Determining features for defining the cyst type include cyst number, density, septae and cyst wall thickness, and nodularity.

Congenital liver cysts appear as anechoic, hypodense avascular solitary lesions (❯ *Fig. 97-1*), with an imperceptible or thin wall, without focal wall thickening or nodularity, without septation or intracystic formation and containing homogeneous fluid with strong posterior acoustic enhancement on US. Homogeneous cystic lesions with low signal intensity on T1-weighted images and high signal intensity on T2-weighted images are typical MRI features. It is usually considered that CLCs do not demonstrate septations except false septations due to contiguous CLCs. The intracystic fluid becomes heterogeneous in cases of hemorrhage or infection. It may contain echoes on US, demonstrate fluid layering or increased density on CT scan (❯ *Fig. 97-2*) or appear hyperintense on T1-weighted images. The wall of a cyst complicated by hemorrhage or infection often becomes thick because of inflammation.

Hydatid liver cysts appear as a cystic lesion with a "double line" sign which reflects the pericyst and the laminate membrane of the cyst. Hydatid cysts contain homogeneous or heterogeneous fluid of variable density with internal daughter vesicles, "hydatid sand" and echogenic septa. Calcifications are observed in the hydatid cystic wall in 25% of the patients. CT and MRI demonstrate multiple septa and

◨ Figure 97-1
Uncomplicated congenital liver cyst: hypodense lesion, with a thin wall and a homogeneous cyst content

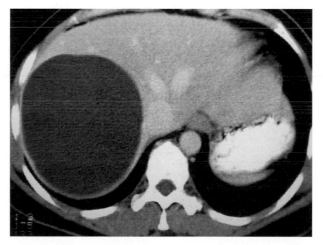

◨ Figure 97-2
Congenital liver cyst complicated by intracystic hemorrhage: hyperdense cyst content due to blood clots

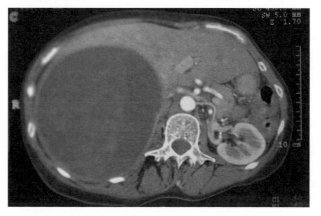

loculations, as well as daughter cysts (❂ *Fig. 97-3*). The wall of the HLC is often thick and markedly hypointense on T2-weighted images because of their fibrous content. The radiological aspect of HLC is quite typical. However, some young, unilocular echinococcal liver cysts, with echo-free intracystic fluid (named type I in the ultrasound GHARBI classification) may simulate a simple CLC. Classical distinctive characteristics of simple and hydatid cysts of the liver are presented in ❂ *Table 97-3*. Additionally, hydatid disease may have been contracted in an area where this parasitic infection is not endemic and calcifications, septations, and split-wall may be absent.

Liver cystadenoma or cystadenocarcinoma appears as multiloculated lesions containing heterogeneous mucinous fluid and numerous intracystic internal septations due to intracystic papillary projections from a thick and irregular cystic wall. Internal septations, cystic wall, and mural nodules are enhanced after intravenous administration of contrast medium (❂ *Fig. 97-4*). Sometimes, calcifications are seen in the septations and mural nodules. In cystadenocarcinoma, increased solid components within the cystic wall are observed. The distinctive characteristics of liver cystadenoma and CLC

❏ Figure 97-3
Hydatid liver cyst: heterogeneous cyst content with intracystic daughter cysts

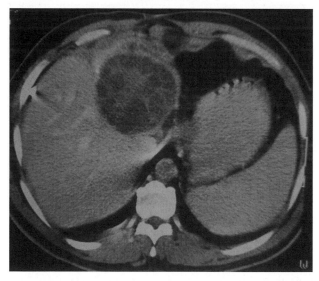

❏ Table 97-3
Distinctive characteristics between congenital liver cysts and hydatid liver cysts

	Congenital liver cyst	Hydatid liver cyst
History of stay in endemic countries	No	Yes
Blood samples		
Eosinophilia	Absent	Inconstant
Serological tests	Negative	Usually positive
Imaging features		
Septations	Absent	Common
Calcifications	Absent	Common
Split-wall	Absent	Common
Communication with biliary tree	Absent	Common

are listed in ❷ *Table 97-4.* In summary, any mural nodularity or irregular thickening, multiple septations, or a fluid level within a cystic mass are important criteria for an alternative diagnosis, such as hydatid or neoplastic cysts. However, despite the improvements in imaging techniques, the parasitic or neoplastic nature of an hepatic cyst still may be misdiagnosed, leading to inappropriate treatment exposing the patient to recurrence and reoperation.

Cyst-Fluid Evaluation

The features of cyst fluid are important in characterizing hepatic cysts: translucent fluid in congenital cysts, clear watery fluid in echinococcal cysts, and blood or mucoid contents in neoplastic cysts. However, in CLC complicated by bleeding or infection, the aspect of cyst fluid is brownish or bloody and may be confused with the one of neoplastic cysts. Percutaneous cystic aspiration with cytology and

◘ Figure 97-4

Liver cystadenocarcinoma: mural nodules within cyst wall with intracystic septations and heterogeneous cyst content

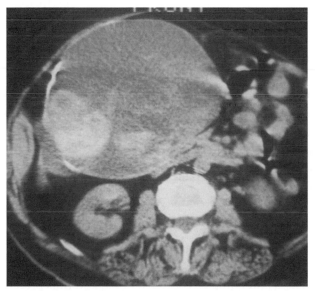

◘ Table 97-4

Distinctive characteristics between liver cystadenoma and congenital liver cysts (CLCs)

	Liver cystadenoma	Congenital liver cyst
Clinical history	Middle-aged women	All ages
Imaging studies		
Number of cysts	Unique	Unique or multiple
Presence of septations	Present	Absent
Presence of papillary projections	Common	Absent
Aspect of cystic fluid	Mucinous	Serous
Natural history		
Malignant transformation	Possible	Exceptional
Recurrence after partial excision	Common	Possible

◘ Figure 97-5

Macroscopic appearance of inner cyst wall at surgical exploration. a. Typical appearance of a congenital liver cyst: thin transparent cyst wall allowing visualization of liver parenchyma and vessels. b. Typical features of liver cystadenocarcinoma: thick cyst wall with papillary polypoid projections, vegetations and mucoid fluid within the cyst

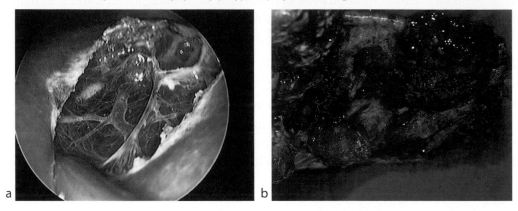

assays for carcinoembryogenic antigen (CEA) and CA-19-9 of the cystic fluid are useful in differentiating cystic hepatic neoplasms. However, when a resectable liver cystadenocarcinoma is suspected on imaging, fine needle aspiration biopsy should be avoided to prevent tumor seeding. Additionally, reactional changes to the cyst wall from bleeding or infection may also be confusing. Thus, great attention should still be paid to any unusual cystic fluid appearances and to careful inspection of the inner aspect of the cyst wall to exclude irregular and nodular areas (❷ *Fig. 97-5*). Such abnormalities should prompt the undertaking of multiple biopsies and frozen section examination to rule out a neoplastic liver cyst. Specimens should be of adequate size and several biopsies, particularly from areas of thickening or irregularity in the cyst wall, may be necessary. The importance of these issues is well illustrated by the series of Wellwood et al. in which the nature of two malignant cysts was not recognized during operation.

Treatment

Treatment options should be tailored to the type of liver cyst, and thus preoperative differentiation and correct preoperative diagnosis is crucial. The management of cystic liver diseases has recently benefited from progress in interventional radiology and laparoscopic surgery.

Congenital Liver Cysts

When indicated, treatment options for CLC include surgery or percutaneous ablative techniques. At present, no comparative study evaluating these approaches has been reported. A treatment algorithm for CLC is detailed in ❷ *Fig. 97-6*. The choice of treatment should be guided by cyst number and intrahepatic location, coexistent cyst complications, and patient risk factors. Surgical treatment includes fenestration techniques, which are usually performed through a laparoscopic approach that has become the gold standard minimally invasive surgical option. Large, superficial, accessible cysts on

■ Figure 97-6
Management algorithm in patients suffering from congenital liver cysts (CLCs)

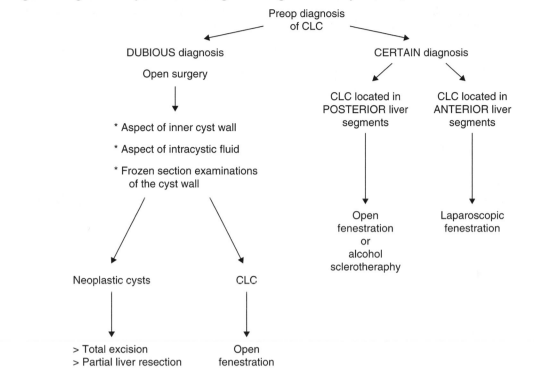

the liver surface (the cyst appearance should be carefully inspected on preoperative CT) and located in the anterior liver segments 2–6 are ideal indications for a laparoscopic approach. On the contrary, posterior or deep-sited cysts are difficult to approach laparoscopically. These last patients may be good candidates for percutaneous alcohol sclerotherapy or for an open surgical approach. Finally, CLC located in segment VIII are more prone to early cyst recurrence after a deroofing technique because the residual cyst cavity is immediately covered by the diaphragm unless an in situ omentoplasty is employed to obliterate the cystic cavity. Appropriate and meticulous surgical techniques should be used to achieve good results. These include a wide deroofing technique using harmonic shears, careful preservation of surrounding liver parenchyma to avoid bleeding, careful inspection of the fenestrated cyst wall for possible bile leakage during the procedure, and ablation of the cyst lining epithelium of the residual cystic cavity by the use of Argon Beam Coagulator. When using strict selection of patients and appropriate surgical techniques, definite success rate exceeding 90% can be obtained with no reported mortality and a complication rate <10–15%. An open procedure or conversion during laparoscopic approaches should be reserved to atypical CLC with a dubious preoperative diagnosis or when a neoplastic cyst cannot be ruled out during surgical exploration. Percutaneous cyst sclerotherapy with alcohol under US or CT guidance has been reported as another minimally invasive approach for treating CLC. While simple cyst aspiration is always associated with cyst recurrence, alcohol sclerotherapy is a very efficient technique. Repeat sessions of interventional procedures are usually needed with large cysts. However, a cystogram should be performed before alcohol sclerotherapy to exclude biliary communication, which is a contraindication for the technique. Successful results are achieved in 70–90% of patients, with no mortality and very low morbidity (<10%). Late cyst recurrence occurs in 0–15%.

Polycystic Liver Disease

The purpose of any treatment option is to reduce significantly (or to replace) the mass effect of the huge polycystic liver with minimal morbidity in order to achieve long-term relief of symptoms and to improve the patient's quality of life. Currently, the most appropriate therapeutic approach for PLD remains controversial and rests between laparoscopic or open fenestration approaches (2), open partial liver resection (8), and liver transplantation. A treatment algorithm for PLD patients is detailed in ❯ *Fig. 97-7*. Type I PLD should be considered for a laparoscopic approach, if dominant liver cysts are superficial and accessible. The fenestration technique is the same as that used for treating CLC. Percutaneous alcohol sclerotherapy should be reserved for high-risk patients, to contraindications of a laparoscopic approach of CLC, or for selective ablation of a deep-sited compressive dominant hepatic cyst.

The surgical management of type II PLD is more controversial, including open fenestration techniques with or without partial liver resection. Very few patients can be approached laparoscopically and only if dominant hepatic cysts are located in the anterior liver segments. The concept of fenestration is to unroof as many cysts as possible, starting from the superficial and then, stepwise, opening the deep-sited cysts, taking great care to avoid vascular and biliary tract injuries within the cystic septa. If two or more adjacent liver segments are spared by the disease, combined liver resection/fenestration can be chosen. In the limited reported clinical experience with open fenestration techniques in patients with PLD, the mortality was low (1–5%), but the complication rate was significant (40–50%), including ascites (50–70%) and biliary leaks. The purpose of liver resection is to achieve long-term relief from symptoms by inducing a significant reduction in the volume of massive cystic hepatomegaly. In the limited reported clinical experience, the mortality was 5–10% and the complication rate was not insignificant (50–60%).

Liver transplantation should be considered for diffuse forms of type III PLD without any segmental sparing as well as for patients with liver insufficiency, after recurrence following initial

◘ Figure 97-7
Strategy for treatment of highly symptomatic patients with polycystic liver disease

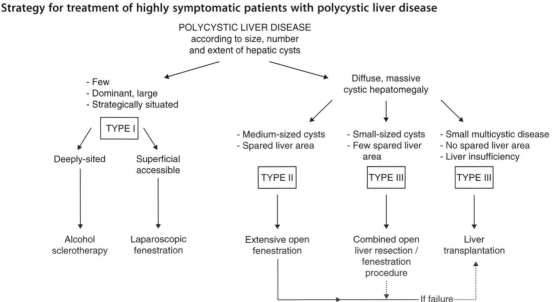

liver resection or in cases of end-stage PKD, combining in such cases, liver and kidney transplantation. Due to the complicated presentation of this benign disease and the significant complication rates of all types of surgical treatments of these difficult patients, each case must be discussed with a multidisciplinary team approach, including hepatologists, nephrologists, and liver and transplant surgeons.

Hydatid Liver Cysts

Until recently, only surgical treatment was effective for HLC. With the advent of percutaneous injection of scolicidal agents and laparoscopic surgery, the treatment strategy for echinococcal liver cysts has been challenged. The treatment algorithm for HDL is given in ❷ *Fig. 97-8*, according to the WHO disease classification which is a useful guide to the treatment decision-making process. Indications for surgery include large cysts with multiple daughter cysts, superficial liver cysts prone to rupture, infected cysts, cysts communicating with the biliary tree, cysts compressing adjacent organs, and extrahepatic cysts. Contraindications for surgery include elderly and high-risk patients, pregnancy, multiple deep-sited intraparenchymal cysts which are difficult to access, dead cysts, totally calcified cysts, and very small cysts.

The objectives of *operative management of HDL* include adequate exposure of the cyst, safe cyst decompression with prevention of intraperitoneal spillage, sterilization, and complete removal of parasitic cystic content, management of cysto-biliary communications, management of the residual cavity, and finally the detection and treatment of other abdominal lesions. Meticulous protection of the peritoneal cavity from spillage is crucial. When approached through a laparotomy, the operation begins by placing packs with hypertonic solution around the liver to absorb any inadvertent spillage of cyst content during the procedure. The cyst is decompressed partially with a trocar and the cyst content is aspirated as much as possible. then the scolicidal agent is instilled within the cyst to sterilize the parasite. Formalin is no longer used for sterilization of HDL content, due to the risk of biliary damage when a cyst-biliary communication exists. The most commonly used scolicidal agent is 20% hypertonic

❑ Figure 97-8
Strategy for treatment of hydatid liver cysts

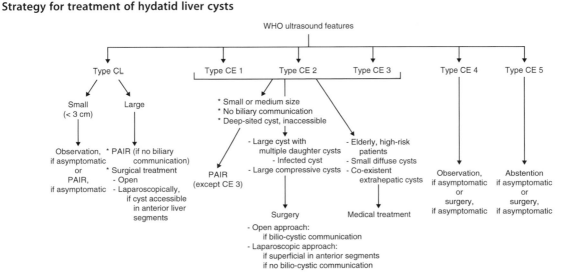

saline solution. Once the cyst is opened and deroofed, the germinal membrane and residual daughter cysts are removed and the inner host capsule is carefully inspected to exclude any biliary fistula. A methylene blue test is employed by cystic duct injection to detect occult fistula. Preoperative detection and treatment of cysto-biliary communications is essential to avoid occasional severe postoperative complications. If the bile duct is obstructed by hydatid material, surgical or endoscopic common bile duct clearance is performed with external or internal biliary drainage, associated with direct suture of the cysto-biliary fistula within the cystic cavity. In the few instances where the HDL communicates with a major hilar bile duct, a Roux-en-Y cysto-jejunostomy or an intracystic hepatico-jejunostomy may be necessary. Finally, the residual cystic cavity is obliterated by omentoplasty. Peritoneal drainage of the cystic cavity is always indicated.

More radical procedures can be used to manage the residual cyst cavity such as cysto-pericystectomy, by removing partially or completely the host-derived fibrous pericyst. This procedure is technically more demanding, but has the main advantage of avoiding entirely a residual cystic cavity and preventing disease recurrence. However, when HDL is closely adjacent or adherent to major intrahepatic vessels or biliary radicles, partial pericystectomy should be performed. If small parts of the pericyst are left in place, there is a risk of bile leak and sepsis. Formal liver resection is rarely indicated except in cases of severe parenchymal destruction. Surgical treatment of the echinococcal cyst carries a mortality rate of 1–4% and a complication rate of 20–30%. The most frequent postoperative complications are overlooked cysto-biliary communications or hydatid debris in the common bile duct, cyst cavity infection, pleuro-pulmonary complications and wound infection. Postoperative bile collection or chronic biliary fistula should be managed by endoscopic sphincterotomy and stenting. The long-term recurrence rate is approximately 5–10%. Cyst growth appears to be the best imaging marker for diagnosing locally recurrent disease during follow-up.

Laparoscopic management of HDL has been recently advocated as being able to fill all the objectives of surgical disease treatment. However, the limited area for surgical manipulation and the difficulty in controlling spillage during puncture and decompression are disadvantages of this approach. Treatment of biliary communication is also difficult by laparoscopic means and may lead to conversion to an open approach. Indications of laparoscopic surgery include type CE 1–3 HDL in an accessible location. Exclusion criteria for laparoscopic management include preoperatively anticipated biliary communication, deep intra-parenchymal cysts, a posterior inaccessible cyst, multiple (> 3) cysts, and cysts with thick and calcified walls. Conversion to open laparotomy is indicated in cases of unsafe exposure, unsatisfactory access, intraoperative bleeding, and spillage in the peritoneal cavity or intrabiliary cyst rupture. Postoperative morbidity in laparoscopic series is reported to be 8–25% (open series: 12–63%) with treatment-related mortality in almost 0%. The rate of short-term recurrence following laparoscopic treatment of HDL is reported to be 0–9%.

Percutaneous aspiration injection reaspiration (PAIR) technique, under US or CT guidance, is gaining acceptance as a minimally invasive treatment of this benign disease, because of its low morbidity and easy applicability, but selection of patients is of paramount importance. Percutaneous treatment is indicated for CE type 1 and 2 HDL, some groups of CE type 3 that do not contain solid material, suspect fluid collections (CL), and in patients with univesicular recurrent cysts and infected hydatid cysts. Contraindications include subgroups of CE types 3 and 4 and cysts that have ruptured into the biliary tree or the peritoneal cavity. There is a theoretical risk of dissemination, peritoneal spillage, and anaphylactic shock (0.1–0.2%). However, the mortality rate (0.9–2.5%) and the complication rate (15–40%) are low.

Medical treatment with Mebendazole or Albendazole is currently indicated for inoperable patients, multiple intra-abdominal, or combined intra- and extra-abdominal disease, multiple small liver cysts, and small central hydatid cysts requiring major hepatectomy as an alternative treatment procedure. Its use can be considered in the prevention and management of secondary hydatidosis, management of recurrent disease, in combination with surgery and interventional radiology, for pulmonary hydatid disease and for hydatid diseases in bones. A prospective controlled trial has demonstrated the efficacy of preoperative administration of Albendazole in preparation to surgery and may obviate the need for scolicidal agents with their inherent risks. Side effects of Mebendazole include nausea, abdominal discomfort, and occasional vomiting but are rarely serious. Hepatotoxicity, alopecia, and leucopenia have also been reported. Chemotherapy is contraindicated in large liver cysts, cysts with multiple septa-division, honeycomb-like cysts, superficial cysts prone to rupture, infected cysts, inactive cysts, calcified cysts, coexistent severe chronic liver diseases, bone marrow depression, and pregnancy.

Neoplastic Cysts

Complete excision of neoplastic liver cysts is required. Due to the potential for malignancy, partial excision exposes the patient to the risk of recurrence and further malignancy. Benign liver cystadenoma may be enucleated but the diagnosis of malignant transformation can only be made on final pathological examination. Radical liver resection should thus be preferred with adequate tumor-free margins. Long-term survival has only been reported after complete resection of neoplastic liver cysts.

Selected Readings

Devernis Ch, Delis S, Avgerinos C, et al. (2005) Changing concepts in the management of liver hydatic disease. J Gastrointest Surg 9:869–877

Gharbi H, Hassine W, Brauner MW, et al. (1981) Ultrasound examination of the hydatid liver. Radiology 139:459–463

Gigot JF, Jadoul P, Que F, et al. (1997) Adult polycystic liver disease: is fenestration the most adequate operation for long-term management? Ann Surg 225:286–294

Gigot JF, Métairie S, Etienne J, et al. (2001) The surgical management of congenital liver cysts: the need for a tailored approach with appropriate patient selection and proper surgical technique. Surg Endosc 15:357–363

Gil-Grande LA, Rodriguez-Caabeiro F, Prieto JG, et al. (1993) Randomized controlled trial of efficacy of albendazole in intraabdominal hydatid disease. Lancet 342:1269–1272

Horsmans Y, Laka A, Gigot JF, et al. (1996) Serum and cyst fluid CA 19.9 determinations as a diagnostic help in liver cysts of uncertain nature. Liver 16:255–257

Ishak KG, Willis GW, Cummins SD, et al. (1977) Biliary cystadenoma and cystadenocarcinoma. Report of 14 cases and review of the literature. Cancer 38:322–338

Que F, Nagorney DM, Gross JB, et al. (1995) Liver resection and cyst fenestration in the treatment of severe polycystic liver disease. Gastroenterology 108:487–494

Wellwood JM, Madara JL, Cady B, et al. (1978) Large intra-hepatic cysts and pseudocysts: pitfalls in diagnosis and treatment. Am J Surg 135:57–64

WHO Informal Working Group on Echinococcosis (2003) International classification of ultrasound images in cystic echonococcosis for application in clinical and field epidemiological settings. Acta Trop 85:253–261

98 Liver Transplantation for Budd-Chiari Syndrome

François Durand · Jacques Belghiti

Pearls and Pitfalls

- Budd-Chiari syndrome is almost always associated with underlying prothrombotic conditions such as myeloproliferative disorders.
- In cases where Budd-Chiari syndrome first presents with acute liver failure (rare presentation), emergency transplantation is the safest approach unless TIPS (trans-jugular insertion of a porto-systemic shunt) can be undertaken in specialist centers.
- In patients with a chronic presentation, of refractory ascites, that cannot be improved by medical management or TIPS, represents the main indication for transplantation. Chronic encephalopathy following TIPS or surgical portosystemic shunt may also be an indication for transplantation.
- Early mortality following surgical portosystemic shunt is not significantly lower than that of transplantation; however, transplantation offers better long term survival.
- Patients with an underlying prothrombotic state, which is not reversed by transplantation should receive long-term anticoagulation. Vitamin K antagonists are standard therapy.
- TIPS misplacement can produce major technical difficulties during transplantation. When there is a potential indication for transplantation, it is strongly recommended that extension of the shunt over the ostium of the hepatic veins or within the main portal vein is avoided.
- Concomitant portal and mesenteric vein thrombosis is usually considered a contraindication for transplantation.
- Mortality following transplantation for Budd-Chiari syndrome mainly occurs during the first 3 months after the procedure.

Introduction

Budd-Chiari syndrome is a rare condition defined as hepatic outflow obstruction at any level from the small hepatic veins to the junction of the inferior vena cava and the right atrium, regardless of the cause of obstruction. In most cases, outflow obstruction results from obliterative thrombosis involving main (right, median and left) through to small hepatic vein branches. In rare instances, hepatic outflow obstruction may result from a membranous web of the inferior vena cava, extrinsic compression or even from intraluminal invasion by a tumor.

Although in some patients, the first manifestation can be acute with rapidly progressive liver failure, Budd-Chiari syndrome is a chronic liver disease. Thrombosis does not abruptly involve all hepatic vein branches but rather progresses over time, involving an increasing number of vessels.

Chronic hepatic outflow obstruction results in sinusoidal dilatation, congestion and hepatocyte necrosis and predominates in the central areas of the hepatic lobules. Centrilobular fibrosis progresses over time and nodular regenerative changes result. A frequent finding is superimposed thrombosis of intrahepatic small to middle size portal veins.

More than 70% of patients with hepatic vein thrombosis are found to have an underlying prothrombotic state consisting of a myeloproliferative disorder and/or coagulation disorder. The list of the underlying prothrombotic states in patients with Budd-Chiari syndrome are shown in ❯ *Table 98-1*.

Natural History and Prognosis of Budd-Chiari Syndrome

The natural history of Budd-Chiari syndrome varies from patient to patient. Most patients, experience complications related to portal hypertension such as ascites or variceal bleeding before 40 years of age. In some patients, the disease first manifests as massive liver cell necrosis and liver failure, probably as a consequence of an abrupt extension of thrombosis to previously preserved hepatic vein branches or collaterals. In this latter group, the prognosis is considered to be especially poor and when encephalopathy is present.

After a first episode of decompensation, the progression of the disease is variable. It is generally easy to prevent recurrence of variceal bleeding with beta-blockers or endoscopic elastic band ligation. In some patients, ascites is controlled with standard therapy, however, others develop refractory ascites with subsequent malnutrition and muscular atrophy. Other complications such as liver insufficiency, jaundice and encephalopathy may occur in parallel with ascites.

Determining the prognosis for Budd-Chiari syndrome is difficult. Besides the variability in the natural history, the outcome is influenced markedly by the various therapeutic interventions and the experience and skilled use of these by the treating center. It has been shown that the prognosis is influenced significantly by the independent variables of encephalopathy, ascites, INR and serum bilirubin. A prognostic score has been derived to allow identification of three groups of increasing severity risk (❯ *Table 98-2*). The presence of portal vein thrombosis is associated significantly with a

◼ Table 98-1

Prothrombotic states in patients with Budd-Chiari syndrome and reversibility with transplantation

Predisposing factor	Reversibility with transplantation
Myeloproliferative disorders	
• Polycythemia vera	No
• Essential thrombocythemia	No
• Others rare disorders	No
Coagulation disorders	
• Factor V Leiden mutation	Yes
• Protein C deficiency	Yes
• Protein S deficiency	Yes
• Antithrombin deficiency	Yes
• Plasminogen deficiency	Yes
• Factor II mutation	Yes
• Antiphospholipid syndrome	No
Paroxysmal nocturnal hemoglobinuria	No
Behcet's disease	No
Pregnancy	–

◘ Table 98-2

Prognosis of Budd-Chiari syndrome according to risk score: (1.27 encephalopathy + 1.04 ascites + 0.72 INR + 0.004 bilirubin [μmol/l])[a] (Murad et al., 2004)

Group	Risk score	5-year survival	95% confidence interval
1	0 to 1.1	89%	79%–99%
2	1.1 to 1.5	74%	65%–83%
3	Over 1.5	42%	28%–56%

[a]Encephalopathy and ascites are scored 0 if absent and 1 if present; INR is scored 0 if lower than 2.3 and 1 if greater than 2.3.

poor outcome. Eventually, some patients may develop hepatocellular carcinoma (HCC) although its incidence is much lower than in patients with cirrhosis of other origin.

Overall, not all patients, even those with an "acute-like" presentation, have a poor prognosis in the short and medium term. Reliable prognostic indexes, which take into account the most recent therapeutic options (TIPS in particular) and the causative disease are lacking.

Treatments other than Transplantation

The treatment of patients with symptomatic Budd-Chiari syndrome has two objectives; namely, to prevent further thrombosis and to achieve liver decompression.

Lifelong anticoagulation is the key in preventing further extension of thrombosis, either to patent accessory hepatic veins (or collaterals) or to the portal vein where blood flow may be slowed or even reversed. Vitamin K-antagonists (warfarin and derivates) represent the gold standard for long-term anticoagulation. In the long term, patients with polycythemia vera or essential thrombophilia may benefit from hydroxyurea to reduce hematocrit or platelet count. It has yet to be determined whether antiplatelet treatment is as effective or even superior to vitamin K antagonists in those patients with essential thrombophilia.

For years, surgical portosystemic shunting has been the reference procedure for achieving liver decompression in patients who remain symptomatic despite medical management. It has been shown that surgical shunting improves survival for patients with Budd-Chiari syndrome of intermediate severity (class 2, ◗ *Table 98-2*). In contrast, there is no clear benefit for patients with mild (class 1) or high severity (class 3) compared to medical management alone. Surgery is limited by in-hospital mortality, which is as high as 20% and a 30% rate of shunt dysfunction, due to thrombosis or stenosis in particular. This morbidity and mortality has been an incentive for developing percutaneous techniques (stenting and TIPS) as an alternative to surgery. Even in cases of complete obstruction of the hepatic veins, it is generally possible to insert a TIPS by trans-hepatic puncture through a hepatic vein stump, towards the right branch of the portal vein. Recent studies suggest that the morbidity is lower than that of surgical shunt and that sustained improvement can be achieved. However, long term results have not been well assessed.

Indications and Timing for Liver Transplantation

Liver transplantation, being a demanding procedure, is only justified in patients with severe complications, which are refractory or not amenable to other therapeutic options except by a surgical shunt.

Surgical shunt carries early mortality and morbidity risks equal to or even greater than transplantation but with poorer long term results. Therefore, transplantation should be considered as a first line option in patients who otherwise could be potential candidates for surgical shunt.

Indications differ according to which patients have an acute or chronic presentation. In patients with an acute presentation, emergency transplantation may be justified by the occurrence of acute liver failure. Indeed, patients with high serum transaminases (over 10 times the upper limit of normal), an associated severe decrease in coagulation factors and who eventually develop encephalopathy have an especially poor prognosis with conventional therapy. "Rescue" TIPS possibly represents an alternative to transplantation in patients with acute liver failure and successful cases with longstanding improvement have been reported. However, TIPS placement is much more demanding in Budd-Chiari syndrome than in patients with cirrhosis. Only in a few centers are there sufficient technical skill in TIPS to allow the use of this technique in an emergency setting. Nonetheless, if TIPS placement is impossible due to technical reasons or if the patient continues to deteriorate despite a patent TIPS, emergency transplantation should be performed. In our experience, patients with an acute-like presentation and a failure in TIPS placement rapidly develop severe acidosis and multiorgan failure. Therefore, whatever the initial option that might be considered, acute liver failure in the context of Budd-Chiari syndrome should be managed preferably in a center where there is access to emergency transplantation.

In patients with a chronic presentation, refractory ascites and poor nutritional status resistant to non-surgical therapeutic options including TIPS, represent the main indications for transplantation. Similarly, patients with repeated episodes of hepatic encephalopathy or chronic encephalopathy following a surgical shunt or TIPS should be listed for transplantation. Patients with chronic encephalopathy should be transplanted within 3 to 6 months since neurological changes secondary to longstanding encephalopathy may not be fully reversible after transplantation. HCC is an extremely uncommon complication of Budd-Chiari syndrome but, on theoretical grounds, guidelines for transplantation should be identical to those patients with cirrhosis and HCC; a single nodule less than 5 cm or 2 or 3 nodules each less than 3 cm. However, many patients with chronic Budd-Chiari syndrome have large, hypervascular, regenerative nodules, with features indistinguishable from those of HCC. Therefore, the identification of one or several malignant nodules among a number of regenerative nodules may be impossible. Patients with large tumors at the time of diagnosis are unlikely to benefit from transplantation due to the high risk of tumor recurrence. Till date, it has been impossible to propose practical guidelines to screen for HCC and make a decision for transplantation in the setting of Budd-Chiari syndrome.

Irrespective of whether the initial presentation is acute or chronic, a stepwise therapeutic approach seems appropriate, beginning with less invasive options with progression to a more aggressive approach when there is insufficient response or lack of success. Liver transplantation represents the most aggressive therapeutic option, but it has demonstrated good long term results with an excellent quality of life in most cases.

Contraindications for Transplantation

Relative and absolute contraindications for transplantation may be related to the underlying causative disease of the Budd-Chiari syndrome or most frequently due to technical limitations.

Some patients with paroxysmal nocturnal hemoglobinuria may not be candidates for transplantation due to the poor prognosis of their underlying disease. Conversely, obvious or latent myeloproliferative disorders do not represent contraindications for transplantation since prognosis is good and does not preclude long term survival after surgery. Most inherited coagulation disorders result from the reduced synthesis of normal coagulation factors or from deficient coagulation factors by the native liver. These disorders are corrected by liver transplantation and do not represent a contraindication (❯ *Table 98-1*). Acquired disorders such as the antiphospholipid syndrome, in contrast, are not reversed by transplantation. However, long term anticoagulation following surgery is likely to prevent recurrence of thrombosis. Budd-Chiari syndrome due to underlying malignancy has to be recognized because it represents a definitive contraindication.

Portal vein thrombosis is observed in up to 20% of patients with Budd-Chiari syndrome. Transplantation can be considered in such cases since restoration of portal blood flow may be successful after thrombectomy. Conversely, an organized thrombus extending to splenic and mesenteric veins represents a contraindication since portal perfusion of the graft cannot be achieved. In such patients, caval transposition has been proposed as an alternative technique since the donor's portal vein can be perfused via a porto-caval anastomosis. Unfortunately, the results of this technique have been dismal due to the high operative risk and the persistence of portal hypertension.

Technical Aspects

The widely adopted "piggy back technique" (preservation of the native inferior vena cava with by end-to-side caval anastomosis) may be difficult to perform in patients with Budd-Chiari syndrome. Firstly, the caudate lobe is markedly enlarged and dense adhesions are frequent adjacent to the suprahepatic vena cava. Secondly, thrombotic changes commonly involve the inferior vena cava, precluding end-to-side anastomosis. Furthermore, most patients with Budd-Chiari have prominent collateral vessels due to marked portal hypertension, which is a significant source of blood loss. As a consequence of the compression of the enlarged caudate lobe, the pressure is usually higher in the inferior than in superior vena cava. The pressure gradient between the portal vein and the inferior vena cava is reduced, precluding the hemodynamic effect of a porto-caval shunt. In such cases, early institution of veno-venous bypass is recommended with the return canula sited in the territory of the superior vena cava since this is likely to be functionally superior to temporary porto-caval anastomosis. After total clamping, the native liver and retrohepatic vena cava can be removed *en bloc*, followed by the implantation of the graft using an end-to-end caval anastomosis. This "standard" technique is also applicable in patients with organized thrombus of the retrohepatic vena cava that is not amenable thrombectomy.

Previous end-to-side porta-caval or meso-caval shunts should be dissected carefully. Previous meso-atrial shunts are more difficult to deal with and should obviously be ligated before graft reperfusion to ensure adequate portal perfusion. As indicated previously, an increasing number of patients have had TIPS placement before transplantation. If there is proximal extension of the shunt over the junction between the ostium of the hepatic veins, it can be impossible to free the TIPS or stent from the wall of inferior vena cava and to perform partial clamping of the ostium. With distal extension to the confluence of the mesenteric and splenic vein, it may be similarly difficult to free the TIPS from the main portal vein. Either proximal or distal extension precludes the use of split or living donor grafts. Occasionally, some patients have undergone retrohepatic inferior vena cava stenting prior to transplantation. Stent extension within the right atrium can make it impossible to free or clamp the suprahepatic inferior vena cava.

Post Transplantation Management

Massive post operative ascites seems to be more frequent in patients with Budd-Chiari syndrome than in those with cirrhosis secondary to parenchymal diseases. The presence of refractory ascites before transplantation predicts persistent ascites after the procedure. However, there is no evidence that Budd-Chiari syndrome has a specific impact but careful management of fluid losses is often needed within the first weeks.

Immunosuppression regimens do not differ from those of other transplanted patients but it is generally recommended that patients with myeloproliferative disorders receive anticoagulation indefinitely, as the risk of hepatic artery thrombosis is higher than that of venous thrombosis. Anticoagulation is based on heparin or low molecular weight-heparin within the first few weeks followed by vitamin K antagonists with a target INR (International Normalized Ratio) of 1.5:3. Bleeding complications after transplantation seem relatively uncommon and are reported as less than 10%. As shown in ❯ *Table 98-1*, most inherited coagulation disorders are reversed by liver transplantation. However, there is lack of clear evidence that patients with Budd-Chiari syndrome due to coagulation disorders are no longer at increased risk of thrombosis after transplantation. Since Budd-Chiari syndrome is more likely to be due to the combination of several prothrombotic states, longstanding anticoagulation is recommended generally in this population.

In patients with underlying myeloproliferative disorders, a combination consisting of hydroxyurea and anti-platelet agents has been proposed as an alternative to long term anti-vitamin K therapy but their precise role is not yet determined.

Results of Liver Transplantation

Since Budd-Chiari syndrome is a rare condition, most publications on liver transplantation include a limited number of patients (❯ *Table 98-3*). The largest series at the present time, comes from a multi-center European study of 248 patients. This series shows that 5-year probability of survival approaches 70%. Early mortality (within the first 3 months) accounted for more than 70% of the post transplantation deaths, similar to that observed in patients transplanted for end-stage cirrhosis and poor nutritional status. Impaired renal function prior to transplantation and a past history of shunt have been found to be predictive of post transplantation mortality. One year survival may be as low as 60% in patients with a serum creatinine greater than 160 µmol/L before transplantation; suggesting that transplantation might be better performed before the occurrence of renal failure. The main causes of early mortality include sepsis, multiple organ failure and graft loss from hepatic artery thrombosis.

■ Table 98-3

Survival after transplantation for Budd-Chiari syndrome

Author/reference	Year	Patients	Survival 1-year	3-year	5-year
Halff et al. 1990	1990	23	69%	45%	45%
Jamieson et al. 1991	1991	26	69%	69%	50%
Shaked et al. 1992	1992	14	86%	76%	–
Srinivasan et al. 2002	2002	19	95%	95%	95%
Ulrich et al. 2002	2002	27	–	–	87%
Mentha et al. 2006	2006	248	76%	–	71%

Recurrence of Budd-Chiari occurs in less than 2% of cases. Portal vein thrombosis is also uncommon although the reported incidence of 7% appears higher than in patients transplanted for other chronic liver diseases. However, patients with persistent prothrombotic disorders are more likely to develop complex vascular diseases of liver graft in the long term (for e.g. nodular regenerative hyperplasia-like syndrome) and need to be investigated.

The prognosis of most myeloproliferative disorders associated with Budd-Chiari syndrome is good in the long term. The progression of these disorders does not seem to affect the results of transplantation, at least within the first 5–10 years. However, it can be suspected that the proper course of myeloproliferative disorders could have a deleterious impact in the very long term.

Organ Allocation and Prioritization

Previously asymptomatic patients presenting with acute liver failure secondary to Budd-Chiari syndrome have an especially poor prognosis, the course of the disease being comparable to that of acute liver failure due to other causes. It is accepted generally that if these patients meet the criteria for transplantation, they should be placed on an emergency list (UNOS status 1A).

In patients with a chronic presentation, an unresolved issue is whether MELD (Model End-Stage Liver Disease) score is appropriate for organ allocation. MELD which relies on serum bilirubin, INR and creatinine, is a robust marker of mortality within 3 months in cirrhotic patients. However, there are several limitations regarding the use of this score in Budd-Chiari syndrome. Firstly, the MELD score variables are different from the independent prognostic markers, encephalopathy, ascites, INR and bilirubin (❍ *Table 98-2*) identified in Budd-Chiari patients. Secondly, refractory ascites is a leading indication for transplantation in a Budd-Chiari syndrome. As shown previously, MELD underscores the disease severity in a number of patients with refractory ascites and a low serum sodium seems to be an important prognostic marker in this particular population. Thirdly, most patients with Budd-Chiari syndrome are placed on vitamin K antagonists thereby rendering the use of INR redundant. On the other hand, there is no clear evidence that for a given MELD score (and taking into account increased INR on vitamin K antagonists), patients with Budd-Chiari syndrome have an increased mortality risk when listed for transplantation. Therefore, up until the present, no specific score and no "extra" MELD points have been proposed for Budd-Chiari syndrome. A prospective validation is needed.

Selected Readings

Cazals-Hatem D, Vilgrain V, Genin P, et al. (2003) Arterial and portal circulation and parenchymal changes in Budd-Chiari syndrome: a study in 17 explanted livers. Hepatology 37:510–519

Durand F, Valla D (2005) Assessment of the prognosis of cirrhosis: Child-Pugh versus MELD. J Hepatol 42(Suppl):S100–107

Halff G, Todo S, Tzakis AG, et al. (1990) Liver transplantation for the Budd-Chiari syndrome. Ann Surg 211:43–49.

Jamieson NV, Williams R, Calne RY (1991) Liver transplantation for Budd-Chiari syndrome, 1976–1990. Ann Chir 45:362–365

Langnas AN, Marujo WC, Stratta RJ, et al. (1992) A selective approach to preexisting portal vein thrombosis in patients undergoing liver transplantation. Am J Surg 163:132–136

Mahmoud AE, Helmy AS, Billingham L, Elias E (1997) Poor prognosis and limited therapeutic options in patients with Budd-Chiari syndrome and portal venous system thrombosis. Eur J Gastroenterol Hepatol 9:485–489

Mentha G, Giostra E, Majno PE, et al. (2006) Liver transplantation for Budd-Chiari syndrome: a European study on 248 patients from 51 centres. J Hepatol 44:520–528

Molmenti EP, Segev DL, Arepally A, et al. (2005) The utility of TIPS in the management of Budd-Chiari syndrome. Ann Surg 241:978–981; discussion 982–983

Murad SD, Valla DC, de Groen PC, et al. (2004) Determinants of survival and the effect of portosystemic shunting in patients with Budd-Chiari syndrome. Hepatology 39:500–508

Murad SD, Valla DC, de Groen PC, et al. (2006) Pathogenesis and treatment of Budd-Chiari syndrome combined with portal vein thrombosis. Am J Gastroenterol 101:83–90

Salvalaggio PR, Koffron AJ, Fryer JP, Abecassis MM (2005) Liver transplantation with simultaneous removal of an intracardiac transjugular intrahepatic portosystemic shunt and a vena cava filter without the utilization of cardiopulmonary bypass. Liver Transpl 11:229–232

Shaked A, Goldstein RM, Klintmalm GB, et al. (1992) Portosystemic shunt versus orthotopic liver transplantation for the Budd-Chiari syndrome. Surg Gynecol Obstet 174:453–459

Srinivasan P, Rela M, Prachalias A, et al. (2002) Liver transplantation for Budd-Chiari syndrome. Transplantation 73:973–977

Ulrich F, Steinmuller T, Lang M, et al. (2002) Liver transplantation in patients with advanced Budd-Chiari syndrome. Transplant Proc 34:2278

Valla DC (2003) The diagnosis and management of the Budd-Chiari syndrome: consensus and controversies. Hepatology 38:793–803

99 Liver Hemangioma

Alexis Laurent · Alain Luciani · Daniel Cherqui

Pearls and Pitfalls

- Hemangioma is the most common benign liver tumor.
- Diagnosis is easy in most cases and relies on US for small lesions and MRI for large lesions.
- Most hemangiomas are asymptomatic and require no treatment.
- When present, symptoms include pain and discomfort and are related to the size of the lesion. Complications are very rare and include rupture, hemorrhage and consumptive coagulopathy.
- Indications for surgical resection are rare and include symptoms, complications or inability to exclude malignancy.
- Surgical techniques employed include enucleation and liver resection.
- When indicated, surgical intervention on these large lesions should be undertaken with caution and expertise since there is a risk of major intraoperative bleeding.

Introduction

Liver hemangioma (LH), also called cavernous hemangioma, is the most frequent benign liver lesion with a reported prevalence ranging between 1% and 10%. They are most commonly found in women, with a female/male ratio ranging from 3:1 to 5:1.

Pathology

LH are vascular tumors consisting of a cavity filled with blood. They have an unknown etiology although an association with estrogen therapy has been suggested. In 90% of the cases LH are solitary. They can be situated throughout the liver but classically are more often located in the right lobe.

The size of the lesions varies from a few millimeters to 30 cm or more. LH is referred to as "giant" when the size is greater than 10 cm. Lesions are well circumscribed and are often surrounded by a thin capsule. They can be seen at the surface of the liver but can rarely be pedunculated. In vivo, LH typically has a sponge consistency. When cut, the surface slice is red-brown and can include areas of hemorrhage or infarction.

Histologically, LH derives from the endothelial cells that line the blood vessels. They consist of multiple, large vascular channels lined by a single layer of endothelial cells and supported by collagenous walls. The vascular compartments are separated by thin fibrous septae and may contain thrombi. Large

LH may develop a collagenous scar or fibrous nodule as thrombosis occurs. Rarely, stromal sclerosis may be associated with the absence of vascular cavities (sclerosing LH) and there may be focal stromal calcification.

Diagnosis and Natural History

While most LH remain small and asymptomatic, occasionally they may enlarge and give rise to various symptoms. When observed, 80% of LH remain stable in size, 15% grow slowly over a long period of time and less than 5% enlarge rapidly over a few months.

Most frequent symptoms include pain, discomfort or the occurrence of a palpable mass. All others causes of abdominal pain should be excluded before symptoms can be considered to be related to LH. Pain can be due to capsular stretching, compression or displacement of surrounding structures or occurrence of a complication. Complications are very rare and include spontaneous rupture, intratumoral hemorrhage, thrombosis with infarction and consumptive coagulopathy (Kasabach-Merritt syndrome). Despite the high prevalence of LH, only about 30 cases of spontaneous rupture have been reported, which makes it an exceptional event.

Some studies have suggested that the lesion increases in size during pregnancy and estrogen therapy. It is for this reason that, as for adenoma, estrogen has been suggested to have a role in tumor growth.

Imaging

Typical LH usually present as asymptomatic incidentally discovered liver nodules on imaging studies, especially on ultrasonography (US). Typical US features are seen in small LH (<3 cm) and include the presence of a homogeneous well circumscribed hyperechoic lesion with subtle posterior acoustic enhancement (❯ *Fig. 99-1*).

◘ Figure 99-1
Typical small liver hemangioma on ultrasound: homogeneous well circumscribed hyperechoic with subtle posterior acoustic enhancement (arrow)

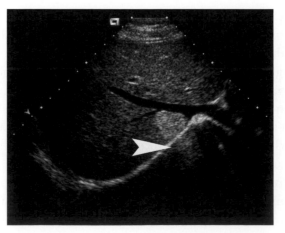

On CT scanning, hemangiomas usually disclose homogeneous hypodensity before injection. On dynamic contrast injections, lesions display early peripheral discontinuous, and progressive enhancement. On delayed phase imaging, the typical LH enhancement is complete (❯ *Fig. 99-2*).

MRI is the most sensitive and specific imaging technique for LH identification, with sensitivity and specificity figures above 90%. The main MRI features of LH include the combination of a well circumscribed lobulated lesion, showing major hyper-intensity on T2 weighted images (❯ *Fig. 99-3*). Following dynamic injection of gadolinium chelates, lesions behave similarly to CT with early peripheral,

▣ **Figure 99-2**
Typical liver hemangioma (arrowed) on CT: Hypodense lesion before contrast and centripedal filling after contrast with complete filling on delayed images

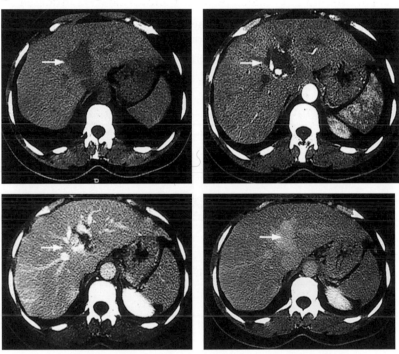

▣ **Figure 99-3**
Giant liver hemangioma (GLH) on MR: typical highly hyperintense image on T2 weighted image

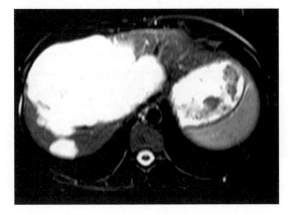

pseudo-nodular enhancement, leading to progressive and complete enhancement (❷ *Fig. 99-4*). Combining T2 and post-injection features, the respective sensitivity and specificity of MRI for the diagnosis of LH reach 98% and 99%.

However, atypical imaging presentations are possible. Giant hemangiomas present on US as large heterogeneous masses. On CT and MR, such lesions exhibit early, peripheral, globular enhancement and on delayed phases, fail to demonstrate complete enhancement (❷ *Fig. 99-5*). Rapidly filling LH, whether on CT or on MRI, display a complete, intense enhancement beginning on arterial phase imaging, and persisting on portal and delayed phases of acquisition. A differential diagnosis with secondary endocrine lesions should be considered, but the persistent enhancement on delayed phases

◘ Figure 99-4
Typical liver hemangioma (arrowed) on MR: Hypointense T1 lesion before contrast and centripedal filling after contrast with complete filling on delayed images (same case as in ❷ *Fig. 99-2*)

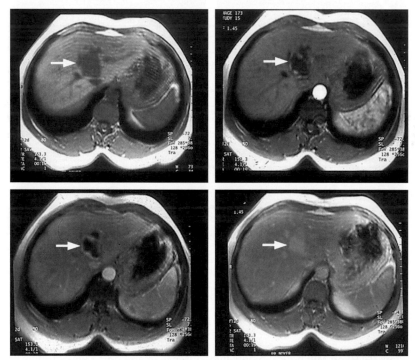

◘ Figure 99-5
Giant liver hemangioma (GLH) on MR: incomplete enhancement after IV contrast (same case as in ❷ *Fig. 99-3*)

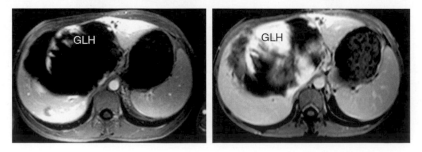

favors the diagnosis of LH. If calcification is present, this is usually situated peripherally. In this situation, definite diagnosis is rarely provided by imaging studies alone, as the normally observed high signal intensity of LH on MRI T2 weighted images can be hidden by the calcification. Sclerosing hemangiomas fail to show any of the characteristic features of LH and in particular lack their usual high signal intensity on T2 weighted images. Giant LH and rapidly filling LH and can by and large be diagnosed by specialized radiologists. The remaining atypical forms usually fail to be diagnosed confidently on imaging studies.

Imaging diagnosis is possible in more than 90% of LH. In specific cases, however, a definite pathological diagnosis may be desirable, principally in patients with a history of cancer. Fine needle aspiration has been used but it can be dangerous and has a low diagnostic yield. Surgical biopsy and frozen section during laparoscopy or laparotomy has been reported to have a better result and may avoid unnecessary resection.

Management

Once a diagnosis of LH has been established conservative management is the rule, because of their benign clinical course. Stability of the lesion should be established by repeated imaging at 3 months and at 1 year. Long term imaging surveillance is not justified when imaging is typical and the lesion is stable in size.

Cessation of estrogen therapy is controversial and only warranted in giant LH. Female patients should be informed of the possibility of growth in pregnancy. Radiotherapy and embolization have been proposed as a sole treatment or as a bridge to surgery but there are no data from reported series to substantiate this approach. Abscess formation has been reported following embolization. In exceptional cases of spontaneous rupture, emergency embolization prior to semi elective resection can be recommended.

There is no indication to consider resection of asymptomatic LH even when they are classified as giant. The only validated treatment is surgical resection but it is only indicated in three specific circumstances:

1. Giant LH with symptoms clearly related to the lesion
2. Complications of LH
3. Inability to exclude malignancy

Because only large and symptomatic LH should be resected, there is usually no place for a laparoscopic approach even although there has been an increasing trend in the use of this approach. Two types of resection technique can be considered. Some authors have described enucleation along the capsular plane since most LH are lined by a thin enclosing capsule. This is the procedure of choice when the capsular plane is easily found and it has been reported to be feasible in up to 60% of the cases. Temporary occlusion of the feeding arterial vessels may permit manual decompression of the lesion and facilitate enucleation. In other situations, such as when no plane is found or there is doubt regarding underlying malignancy, formal liver resection is indicated. Since surgery may be difficult for giant LH, and can carry a substantial risk of bleeding, such interventions should be performed by experienced hepatic surgeons. In these cases, vascular clamping of the liver inflow and total vascular exclusion should be used liberally. Exceptionally, giant non resectable and highly symptomatic LH have required liver transplantation but only 3 such cases have been reported in the literature.

◘ Figure 99-6
Liver hemangioma management algorithm

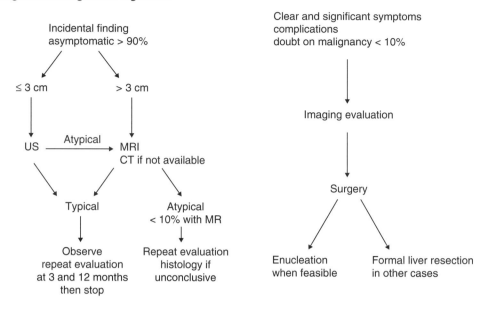

Conclusion

LH is the most frequent benign liver lesion but it is usually asymptomatic, follows a benign course, rarely enlarges and rarely gives rise to complication. Management of LH must follow strict rules (❷ *Fig. 99-6*). Diagnosis must be obtained by good quality imaging including ultrasonography for small typical lesions and MRI for larger or atypical lesions. Asymptomatic patients with typical LH do not require treatment and can be safely observed, even if the lesion is large. Surgical resection should only be proposed for the rare symptomatic or complicated LH and parenchymal preserving procedures such as enucleation should be preferred. However, major liver surgery may occasionally be required.

Selected Readings

Baer HU, Dennison AR, Mouton W, et al. (1992) Enucleation of giant hemangiomas of the liver. Technical and pathologic aspects of a neglected procedure. Ann Surg 216:673–667

Corigliano N, Mercantini P, Amodio PM, et al. (2003) Hemoperitoneum from a spontaneous rupture of a giant hemangioma of the liver: report of a case. Surg Today 33:459–463

Farges O, Daradkeh S, Bismuth H (1995) Cavernous hemangioma of the liver: are there any indications for resection? World J Surg 19:19–24

Gedaly R, Pomposelli JJ, Pomfret EA, et al. (1999) Cavernous hemangioma of the liver: anatomic resection vs. enucleation. Arch Surg 134:407–411

Gibney RG, Hendin AP, Cooperberg PL (1987) Sonographically detected hepatic hemangiomas: absence of change over time. Am J Roentgenol 149:953–957

Ishak KG, Rabin L (1975) Benign tumors of the liver. Med Clin North Am 59:995–1013

Motohara T, Semelka RC, Nagase L (2002) MR imaging of benign hepatic tumors. Magn Reson Imaging Clin N Am 10:1–14

Tepetes K, Selby R, Webb M, et al. (1995) Orthotopic liver transplantation for benign hepatic neoplasms. Arch Surg 130:153–156

Yamamoto T, Kawarada Y, Yano T, et al. (1991) Spontaneous rupture of hemangioma of the liver: treatment with transcatheter hepatic arterial embolization. Am J Gastroenterol 86:1645–1649

Yoon SS, Charny CK, Fong Y, et al. (2003) Diagnosis, management and outcome of 115 patients with hepatic hemangioma. J Am Coll Surg 197:392–402

Part 9

Liver: Malignant

100 Hepatocellular Carcinoma

Sheung Tat Fan

Pearls and Pitfalls

- Hepatocellular carcinoma (HCC) is the third leading cause of cancer-related death among males.
- Hepatitis B and C infections are the etiologic cause in the majority of patients.
- HCC is associated with a poor prognosis, because the tumor grows silently, spreads into luminal structures within the liver early, and being multicentric in origin, recurs frequently after the initial treatment.
- Planning of treatment depends on the extent of tumor spread, underlying liver function, remnant liver volume, and presence of concomitant medical disease.
- Liver transplantation and partial hepatectomy are effective treatment but are applicable in only 20% of patients. Combination therapy with radiofrequency ablation, transarterial chemoembolization, and/or intralesional alcohol injection together with close surveillance for recurrence are needed to attain long-term survival.
- Treatment of hepatitis B and C infection may reduce the incidence of HCC.
- Screening of high risk subjects, i.e. hepatitis B and C carriers, patients with cirrhosis, and family members of HCC, for detection of small tumors may improve the prognosis of HCC.

Etiology

Hepatocellular carcinoma (HCC) is a highly lethal disease. It is the third leading cause of cancer-related death among males. The incidence is increasing rapidly in Western countries. Hepatitis B virus is the major etiologic factor in most countries in Asia and Africa. In contrast, hepatitis C virus is the most important cause in Japan, America, and Europe. Most of the patients with hepatitis B in Asia develop the infection in the neonatal period, yet it takes about 30–40 years before the hepatitis B virus produces pathologic changes of cirrhosis, which predisposes to development of HCC. Thus, the peak age for incidence of HCC is in the sixth decade. In contrast, younger patients with hepatitis B virus who have normal liver or chronic hepatitis may also develop HCC. The mechanism of formation of HCC may be different between patients with normal liver, chronic hepatitis, and cirrhosis. Smokers and alcoholics have a higher incidence of HCC if they are chronic hepatitis B carriers. Food contamination by aflatoxin and water contamination by microcystin may increase the risk of hepatitis B carriers to develop HCC. For hepatitis C, it takes about 30 years for cirrhosis and HCC to develop after the infection. Cirrhosis of other etiologies also predisposes to the development of HCC.

Pathology

Grossly, there are three macroscopic types of HCC. The massive type occurs in patients at a younger age with a non-cirrhotic liver. The neoplasms are large with adjoining "satellite" nodules which represent spread from the main neoplasm (❯ *Fig. 100-1*). The cut surface is variegated due to necrosis and hemorrhage. The nodular type shows multiple grayish white, yellow, or brown nodules in a cirrhotic liver (❯ *Fig. 100-2*). The diffuse type is the least common (❯ *Fig. 100-3*), and grossly it may be indistinguishable from cirrhosis. Histologically, the liver is replaced by numerous small, disseminated tumor nodules. The disseminated type is missed frequently on imaging, but its presence should be suspected when major vessels are invaded.

HCC tends to invade luminal structures within the liver. Thus, branches of the portal vein, hepatic vein, bile duct, and lymphatics may be involved, with tumor spread from the terminal branches toward the major branch. The portal vein is involved most commonly by local invasion (❯ *Fig. 100-4*). The tumor grows in the portal vein against the blood stream. When segmental branches are reached, tumor fragments are dislodged, and emboli are disseminated to the adjacent liver segments. Such mode of spread accounts for the appearance of satellite nodules in the liver segments adjacent to the main neoplasm or contralateral liver when the bifurcation of the portal vein is invaded by HCC. Due to invasion into the hepatic vein, the lung is the most common site of extrahepatic spread. Peritoneal metastasis is unusual unless there is previous spontaneous rupture of HCC or puncture of a superficial HCC by biopsy needle.

The prognosis of HCC can be gauged by the histologic features. Neoplasms with evidence of invasion, e.g. lymphovascular permeation, liver invasion, invasion across tumor capsule, bile duct invasion, or microsatellite lesions, are associated with poor outcome. In contrast, solitary tumors without vascular invasion are associated with a relatively good prognosis.

◘ Figure 100-1
Massive type HCC. The adjoining nodule (arrow) represents spread from the primary neoplasm

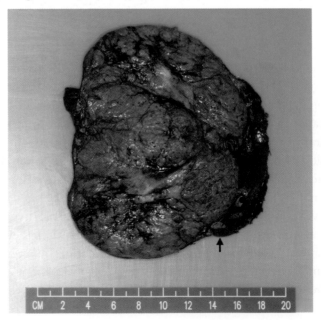

◘ Figure 100-2
Nodular type HCC in a liver explant

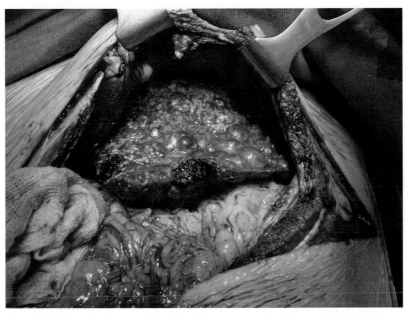

◘ Figure 100-3
Numerous tiny yellowish nodules. This is the diffuse type of HCC of a patient who was planned for liver transplantation. Because of the finding, liver transplantation was aborted

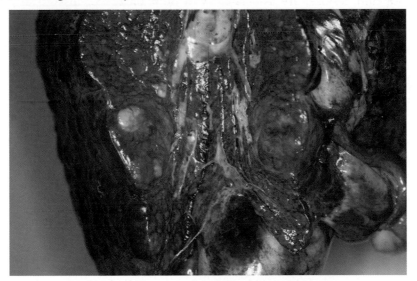

Presentation

HCC usually grows silently until it reaches a large size and causes symptoms of compression on adjacent viscera. Thus, the majority of patients with resectable HCC do not have symptoms. Most of the resectable tumors are detected on screening. Nevertheless, some patients do have an early symptom

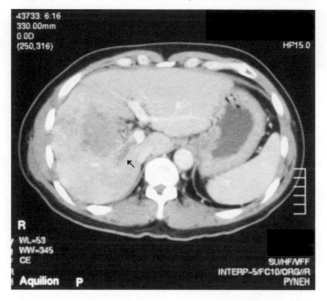

◘ Figure 100-4
CT of a patient with HCC. The right portal vein was invaded by direct extension of the tumor (arrow)

of distending discomfort which could be due to rapid tumor growth. Sudden epigastric pain may be due to intratumoral bleeding leading to distension of the liver capsule. Continuous intratumoral bleeding will lead to rupture of HCC (and hence shock and peritonitis), especially when it is superficial. Hemoperitoneum and spillage of cancer cells into the peritoneal cavity account for poor short- and long-term survival; however, a minor degree of hemoperitoneum may be found at laparotomy and is due to splitting of the liver overlying the rapidly expanding HCC rather than actual rupture of HCC. In such a situation, abdominal pain is less severe, hemodynamic disturbance is less obvious, liver function is less impaired, and the prognosis is not necessarily worsened.

In other cases, the presenting symptom is abdominal distension, possibly due to huge hepatomegaly or ascites. Sometimes, the patients present with hemoptysis, bone pain, or pathologic fracture. HCC may also produce a hormone-like substance and a para-neoplastic syndrome such as diarrhea, hypercalcemia, or polycythemia. Jaundice may be the first presentation (❯ *Fig. 100-5*) and may be due to compression or infiltration of the common hepatic duct by a large hilar HCC or tumor fragment dislodged from the intrahepatic duct into the common bile duct. In the latter situation, the patient may also present with acute cholangitis or pancreatitis.

Imaging/Diagnosis

The routine x-ray offers no role in diagnosis except in advanced stages when the right diaphragm is elevated. The majority of small HCC (<2 cm) are detected by ultrasonographic screening of patients with cirrhosis or hepatitis B carriers. On ultrasonography, small HCC appear as a hypoechoic, isoechoic, or hyperechoic lesion, whereas larger HCC are usually heterogeneous in appearance. Contrast-enhanced ultrasonography can improve detection of isoechoic tumors and can differentiate them from other hepatic tumors. The enhancement pattern is similar to that of computed tomography (CT) or magnetic resonance imaging (MRI).

☐ Figure 100-5

A large left liver HCC compressing on the common hepatic duct and portal vein (arrow). The patient presented with painless obstructive jaundice. At laparotomy, evidence of portal hypertension was also noted

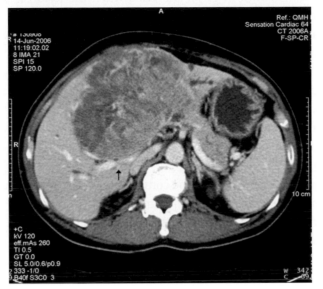

Contrast-enhanced CT and MRI are important diagnostic modalities in the recognition and staging of HCC. Contrast-enhancement in the arterial phase (about 30 s after contrast administration) and rapid washout in the portovenous phase (about 90 seconds after contrast administration) is the typical pattern of HCC. In addition, the topographic relationship of the tumor with major portal pedicles and hepatic veins is delineated clearly for planning of treatment. Hepatic angiography and porto-venography are performed rarely nowadays, because CT or MRI provides equally accurate assessment. Extrahepatic spread can also be delineated on CT or MRI. In case of doubt about the diagnosis and extent of spread, PET scans can be helpful, but both (18)F-FDG and ^{11}C-acetate should be used in the examination, because well-differentiated HCC are detected by ^{11}C-acetate radio-tracer, but not by (18)F-FDG; PET scan may replace bone scan in the evaluation of a patient with HCC for liver transplantation.

Serology Diagnosis

Serum alpha feto-protein (AFP) is a well established tumor marker used in the diagnosis of HCC. The serum level of AFP, said to be diagnostic for HCC, varies from center to center; however, a diagnostic level is meaningless, because the amount of AFP produced by the tumors varies widely and is not proportional to tumor size. About 20–40% of HCC, even when large, may not produce sufficient amounts of AFP to be detectable in blood. Perhaps a rising trend, even within the normal reference range, is an indication of a growing tumor. Falsely high AFP levels may be found in patients with hepatitis B virus reactivation or ongoing hepatitis C infection. Such a phenomenon must be borne in mind when interpreting the serum AFP level in a patient with HCC.

In Japan, AFP-L3 and des-gamma-carboxy prothrombin (a protein induced by vitamin K antagonist II, PIVKA-II) are also used widely for diagnosis of HCC. A number of other novel markers have also been developed to cover the deficiency of AFP. None has been established for routine use yet.

Tumor Biopsy

Cytologic or histologic confirmation of HCC is needed when the lesion is inoperable and when the imaging is inconclusive of HCC. Tumor biopsy is also needed when the serum AFP is not increased and when conservative or non-operative treatment is planned. Tumor biopsy, however, is not without risk. Hemoperitoneum, arteriovenous fistula, and hemobilia are serious potential complications of tumor biopsy and may cause hepatic decompensation and death. Tumor seeding into the peritoneal cavity or along the needle track may be seen if the patient survives long enough. In the presence of ascites, tumor biopsy is contraindicated. Therefore, the European Association of Study of the Liver suggested that tumor biopsy is not needed if two coincident imaging techniques have shown typical arterial hyper-vascularization or when arterial enhancement is seen in one imaging technique together with increased serum AFP > 400 ng/ml.

Apart from tumor biopsy, liver biopsy of the contralateral liver is also advocated for assessment of the extent of hepatic fibrosis, which may have prognostic value. Again, the procedure is invasive. A non-invasive ultrasonography (Fibroscan) has been developed for assessment of liver fibrosis and may provide useful information in the future.

Treatment

Both partial hepatectomy and liver transplantation are the effective treatments. Other treatments available currently include transarterial chemoembolization (TACE), radiofrequency ablation, and percutaneous alcohol or acetic acid injection.

Before a treatment plan is offered, multiple aspects of the following assessment must be made.

Tumor Status

The size and number of tumor nodules may be recognized by ultrasonography, CT, MRI, or PET scan. The proximity of the tumor to a major vascular pedicle and possible invasion is a concern for planning partial hepatectomy or radiofrequency ablation. Tumor invasion into the inferior vena cava or portal vein is a definite contraindication for operative exploration, but isolated portal vein thrombosis can be secondary to cirrhosis and portal hypertension. In the latter situation, liver transplantation is still possible. Ascites may be due to cirrhosis, but peritoneal spread may account for small amounts of fluid near the tumor. Blood clot adjacent to the tumor can be recognized by CT and is an indication of recent rupture and possible peritoneal spread. The sites of regional lymph node spread include the hepato-duodenal ligament, suprahepatic-subdiaphragmatic region, and behind the head of the pancreas. CT of the thorax or PET scan using dual radio-tracers is recommended for large HCC and those with hepatic vein invasion.

Liver Function Status

Assessment of liver function is mandatory to determine whether the patient can tolerate the proposed treatment. For partial hepatectomy, assessment of liver function is of paramount importance, because part of the uninvolved liver is removed with the tumor. For radiofrequency ablation, though a small part of the liver surrounding the tumor is ablated and little functional loss is anticipated, the systemic inflammatory response is sometimes excessive, and the patient may succumb to liver failure if the liver function is suboptimal. For TACE, the non-tumorous liver may also be affected by the treatment, and post-TACE liver failure may occur.

Liver function may be assessed by clinical examination. Presence of ascites, jaundice, and hepatic encephalopathy indicates that any treatment except liver transplantation is inappropriate. Laboratory assessment includes a platelet count, international normalized ratio (prothrombin time), and serum bilirubin and albumin levels. The Child-Pugh classification of liver function is a useful guide for partial hepatectomy, but it is important to note that two of the five parameters (ascites and encephalopathy) are not quantitative. In general, patients with Child-Pugh class A liver function are suitable candidates for partial hepatectomy. Child-Pugh B patients are borderline cases for local resection of a peripherally situated tumor. Child-Pugh C patients are definitely not candidates for partial hepatectomy. For other local treatments, Child-Pugh A and B patients may have low complication rates after the procedures, whereas Child-Pugh C patients represent a high risk; however, no detailed study has been carried out to date on the tolerance of cirrhotic patients to radiofrequency ablation and TACE.

Among Child-Pugh A patients, the actual liver function varies, and operative mortality may be as high as 13% after major hepatectomy. A better quantitative test of risk of postoperative liver failure is the indocyanine green (ICG) clearance test. The normal value is 10% retention at 15 min after intravenous administration of ICG. Major hepatectomy is still feasible if the ICG retention rate at 15 min is 14%. If blood loss is not excessive and blood transfusion not required, patients with 18% retention at 15 min may survive major hepatectomy.

Remnant Liver Volume Status

The survival of patients after partial hepatectomy or radiofrequency ablation depends upon the function and volume of the remnant liver. A remnant liver volume >30% is sufficient for postoperative survival; however, for patients with chronic liver disease, remnant liver volume >40% is needed. When the estimated remnant liver would be insufficient and the non-tumorous liver to be resected with the liver neoplasm is large in volume, portal vein embolization can be performed to induce liver atrophy of the resected side and hypertrophy of the remnant side. This procedure, however, is not applicable to patients with moderate or severe cirrhosis.

General Status

The purpose of assessment is to determine whether the patient has concomitant medical disease that makes the treatment dangerous. Patients with serious medical disease, e.g. recent myocardial infarction, stroke, uremia and severe chronic obstructive airway disease, are not candidates for partial hepatectomy or radiofrequency ablation via laparotomy. Presently, with better selection of patients, the operative mortality rate has been reduced markedly (<3%), but the complication rate remains high. Concomitant medical disease is the most important contributory factor to the high complication rate.

Partial Hepatectomy

Right or left hepatectomy is indicated when the tumor is confined to one side of the liver, when the remnant liver volume is sufficient, and when the liver function is optimal. For small tumors (<2 cm), the ideal treatment would be resection of the liver segment harboring the tumor together with the adjacent segments to eradicate possible spread from portal vein branches. It is also necessary to preserve non-tumorous liver. Currently, the principle of resection consists of removal of the tumor with a tumor-free margin of at least 5 mm, little blood loss, no blood transfusion, maximal preservation of non-tumorous liver, and preferably minimum manipulation of primary neoplasm (❯ *Fig. 100-6*). To reduce blood loss, intermittent inflow vascular occlusion can be employed, but the accumulated occlusion time should not exceed 120 min. Many hepatic surgeons believe that the best liver transection device is the ultrasonic dissector, despite its slowness. Other devices, e.g. harmonic scalpel, Tissue-Link, and others that deliver energy to coagulate the liver parenchyma, tend to induce liver necrosis and fail to identify clearly the intrahepatic portal pedicles and hepatic vein, which serve as important landmarks for safe and complete resection of hemiliver or liver segment.

The extent of hepatectomy is classified as major or minor, but there is no rigid rule of extent of hepatectomy. For example, a right hepatectomy can be carried out together with resection of a

◨ Figure 100-6

CT of a patient with right liver HCC. The arrow indicates the right hepatic vein invaded by HCC. Fluid collection outside the liver was also noted. The dotted line represents the line of liver transection. The operation was performed by the anterior approach, i.e. the liver transection was done without prior right liver mobilization to avoid dissemination of cancer cells into the systemic circulation

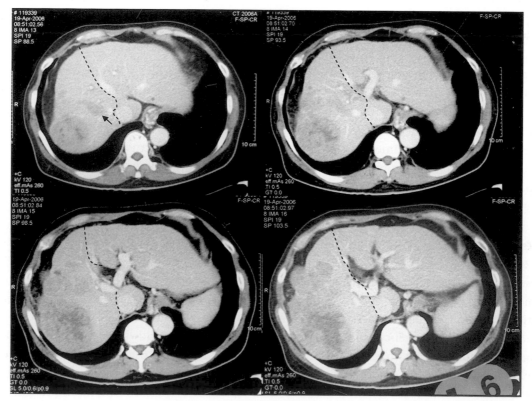

superficial tumor nodule in the left liver; the caudate lobe resection is included in a right hepatectomy. Segment V, VI, VII resection is performed to preserve segment VIII for a relatively small liver. Avoidance of blood loss and protection of the liver remnant from ischemic injury are the two important strategies to ensure postoperative survival. Meticulous attention to avoid bile leakage and bile duct injury is mandatory for success. In the latter situation, operative cholangiography is the prerequisite investigation.

Currently, partial hepatectomy for HCC can be performed with nearly 0% hospital mortality, about 30% complication rate, a 5-year survival of 49%, and a 10-year survival of 30%. Better survival rates are obtained for patients with TNM stages I and II (5-year survival of 80% and 60%, respectively).

Liver Transplantation

A remarkable advance has been the use of liver transplantation for selected patients with HCC arising in a cirrhotic liver. Liver transplantation is indicated for patients with Child-Pugh class B or C liver function and those without concomitant major medical diseases. Patients should be selected carefully based on formal radiologic criteria. Patients with solitary neoplasms < 5 cm or those with ≤ 3 tumors, each of which is ≤ 3 cm, are favorable candidates; this subset of patients has a 5-year survival of about 75–80%. Slight extension of the aforementioned criteria has been advocated recently to allow more patients to benefit from liver transplantation without jeopardizing the long-term survival rate. In contrast, use of liver transplantation for larger HCC or those with multiple satellite lesions is not indicated, because the survival is not better than after resective or ablative procedures. Nevertheless, whatever the selection criteria based on imaging, up to 25% of the patients have HCC recurrence after liver transplantation. The deficiency is that the size and number of tumor nodules do not reflect the actual pathologic features or biologic behavior. Well-differentiated HCC and those without vascular invasion have excellent prognosis after liver transplantation, but histologic information would not be available unless liver biopsy is performed or the explant is available. Recent research aims at identification of biologic markers of aggressiveness in patients' pre-transplant blood specimen that can predict post-transplant recurrence.

TACE

In this treatment of transarterial chemoembolization, a mixture of Lipiodol and a chemotherapeutic agent is administered into the artery feeding the HCC, followed by embolization and occlusion of the artery. Lipiodol has affinity for HCC and carries with it the chemotherapeutic agent in high local concentration directly to the HCC. Mixing of Lipiodol with the chemotherapeutic agent is by the syringe-pump method. Various combinations of chemotherapeutic agents have been advocated, but cisplatin appears to form a mixture with Lipiodol that is stable for 1–2 hours, which is more stable than the other chemotherapeutic agents. After injecting this mixture into the hepatic artery, the terminal branches of the feeding artery will be occluded, causing ischemia. Later, the chemotherapeutic agent will be released to act on the tumor. Subsequent embolization of the feeding artery is useful to prevent flushing away of the mixture by blood flow, but recent practice tends to omit the subsequent embolization, because the result appears to be equally satisfactory for small HCC without embolization and potentially harmful effects to the liver can be avoided.

TACE not only prolongs survival of patients with inoperable HCC, but it has also been used as a "bridge" or a means to "down-stage" the tumor to deceased donor liver transplantation. TACE is not effective against large HCC, however, and recurrence, especially at the periphery of the tumor, is frequent. The high recurrence rate may be due to stimulation of angiogenesis. Thus, an anti-angiogenesis treatment may be considered with TACE.

TACE is not without risk. Liver failure, liver abscess, and biloma are potentially lethal complications. Patients with Child-Pugh class C liver function tolerate TACE poorly. Thus, its role as a bridge to liver transplantation is applicable only in patients with Child-Pugh A and B cirrhosis. Overall, the 5-year survival rate of patients treated by TACE alone is about 20%.

Radiofrequency Ablation

This, non-resective treatment consists of insertion of an electrode into the tumor either percutaneously or transhepatically at the time of operation under CT or ultrasonography guidance; local heat is generated within the tumor during the subsequent delivery of energy via the electrode. The local temperature reaches 60°C, coagulating the tumor. RFA is most suitable for tumors $\leq$ 3–5 cm. Larger tumors can be treated by RFA, but preferably in several sessions to avoid excessive systemic inflammatory response. Percutaneous RFA, however, is not suitable for lesions near the bowel, diaphragm, and liver hilum. For these situation, an open approach is preferred, with the bowel or diaphragm packed away from the tumor before application of radiofrequency. For lesions close to the liver hilum, cold saline flushing of the common bile duct via cystic duct cannulation will decrease the injury to the hepatic duct. The reported mortality rate from RFA is low (<1%), but serious complications may occur, including liver abscess, hepatic duct damage leading to biloma, bowel perforation, gallbladder necrosis, hemoglobinuria, renal failure, and liver failure.

Overall, the 5-year survival of patients treated by RFA alone is about 33%. There has been an increasing tendency in recent years to treat potentially resectable HCC ($\leq$5 cm) by RFA. A randomized trial suggests that RFA for small HCC is as effective as formal operative resection.

Intralesional Alcohol Ablation

This treatment consists of injection of 95% alcohol into the tumor by percutaneous needle puncture under ultrasonography guidance. The mode of action is by drawing water from the cells leading to desiccation of the tumor. Although this approach is applicable to small tumors (<3 cm), the alcohol is less able to penetrate the tumor capsule, and therefore, may not finally treat the cancer cells that have invaded across the tumor capsule. Acetic acid is able to penetrate the tumor capsule and has been used to replace alcohol; however, the pattern of spread of alcohol and acetic acid across the lesion is unpredictable. Both treatments have been essentially replaced by RFA in recent years.

Other Treatments

Because the current treatments are not entirely effective and their applications are limited, new treatments are being developed. Recently investigated modalities include local radioisotope therapy (Yttrium 90, Iodine 131), TomoTherapy, and High Intensity Focused Ultrasound. The latter two modalities have the advantage of being totally non-invasive, but data are not yet sufficient to recommend them as routine procedures.

Choice of Treatment

Choosing the appropriate treatment for individual patients depends on the medical condition of the patient, size and location of the lesion(s), liver function, volume of the remnant liver, and availability of local expertise. Occasionally, the tumor can be downstaged by local or systemic chemotherapy and become resectable. Thus, young patients with good liver function free of concomitant medical disease should be offered aggressive treatment. Whatever the initial treatment, recurrence of HCC is common, and apart from liver transplantation, the incidence is as high as 60% in the first year. Combination of the aforementioned treatment modalities or their sequential use for recurrent HCC that developed during the course of the disease is the logical approach. For example, partial hepatectomy may be the first treatment. Subsequent recurrences can be treated by RFA, TACE, or even liver transplantation. The overall survival rate is improved if early recurrence is detected by careful surveillance and treated aggressively and promptly by the same or different modality.

Screening

Since the prognosis of HCC treatment depends on the tumor size and early HCC are asymptomatic, recent efforts to improve the overall outcome have targeted screening of the population at risk for development of HCC. The screened subjects are those with cirrhosis, hepatitis B or C carriers, and family members of HCC who are screened by ultrasonography and serum AFP measurement simultaneously at 6- to 12-month intervals. Both ultrasonography and AFP measurement are performed to compensate for deficiencies of each. The average size of HCC detected by such mode of surveillance is about 2 cm. Theoretically and ideally, about 90% of HCC can be detected by such screening. In practice, however, many early HCC are missed by this combination, especially in cirrhotic patients. More cost-effective surveillance methods are needed.

Prevention

Nationwide hepatitis B vaccination of children reduces the incidence of HCC among the population at risk. Treatment of hepatitis B by lamivudine and hepatitis C by interferon is beneficial in reducing the development of HCC among these patients. Recently, patients with HCC have been treated with lamivudine or interferon after the initial radical treatment, hoping to reduce the incidence of recurrence. The efficacy has not been confirmed yet, but this approach seems logical.

Selected Readings

Bruix J, Sherman M, Llovet JM, et al. (2001) Clinical management of hepatocellular carcinoma. Conclusions of the Barcelona-2000 EASL conference. European Association for the Study of the Liver. J Hepatol 35:421–430

Chen MS, Li JQ, Zheng Y, et al. (2006) A prospective randomized trial comparing percutaneous local ablative therapy and partial hepatectomy for small hepatocellular carcinoma. Ann Surg 243:321–328

Chien YC, Jan CF, Kuo HS, et al. (2006) Nationwide hepatitis B vaccination program in Taiwan: effectiveness in the 20 years after it was launched. Epidemiol Rev Jun [Epub ahead of print]

Lam CM, Fan ST, Lo CM, et al. (1999) Major hepatectomy for hepatocellular carcinoma in patients with an unsatisfactory indocyanine green clearance test. Br J Surg 86:1012–1017

Lau WY, Ho SK, Yu SC, et al. (2004) Salvage surgery following downstaging of unresectable hepatocellular carcinoma. Ann Surg 240:299–305

Poon RTP, Fan ST, Lo CM, et al. (2002) Long-term survival and pattern of recurrence after resection of small hepatocellular carcinoma in patients with preserved liver function: implications for a strategy of salvage transplantation. Ann Surg 235:373–382

Yang ZF, Poon RTP, To J, et al. (2004) The potential role of hypoxia inducible factor 1alpha in tumor progression after hypoxia and chemotherapy in hepatocellular carcinoma. Cancer Res 64:5496–5503

Zhu LX, Wang GS, Fan ST (1996) Spontaneous rupture of hepatocellular carcinoma. Br J Surg 83:602–607

101 Metastatic Cancer of the Liver

Matteo Donadon · Gareth Morris-Stiff · Jean-Nicolas Vauthey

Pearls and Pitfalls

- If untreated, patients with colorectal liver metastases have an overall 5-year survival < 5%, with a median survival of 12–15 months.
- Selected patients with colorectal liver metastases are candidates for curative hepatic resection with 5-year survival approaching 60%.
- Perioperative mortality and morbidity rates are <5% and 40%, respectively.
- Absolute contraindications for resection are peritoneal carcinomatosis, multiple extrahepatic sites of metastatic disease, and inability to achieve an R0 resection.
- Multiple but resectable hepatic metastases are not necessarily a contraindication to resection.
- Resectable lung metastases are also not necessarily a contraindication to resection.
- At present, the role of interstitial therapy should be confined to unresectable lesions
- Serum CEA levels are increased in 75% of patients with liver metastases and serve as markers of disease.
- Preoperative chemotherapy and portal vein embolization (PVE) are beneficial in potentially downsizing lesions in patients with initially unresectable disease to allow curative resection.
- Liver resection for hepatic metastases from neuroendocrine cancer and possibly breast cancer has a role, but no good data support resection of other metastatic neoplasms.
- Liver transplantation is generally not considered for unresectable hepatic metastases.
- Predictors of recurrence are R1 status, synchronous presentation of liver metastases with colon cancer, stage of colon cancer, size and number of metastases, preoperative CEA, and extrahepatic metastases.

Multidisciplinary Approach to Metastatic Cancer of the Liver

The liver is the most common site of metastases from a variety of primary cancers, particularly those originating from the gastrointestinal tract. In autopsy series of patients dying of neoplasia, hepatic metastases are found in up to 36% of patients, the most frequent primary sites being: colon and rectum, lung, pancreas, breast, and stomach. The prognosis of patients with untreated liver metastases is generally very poor, and if untreated, the majority of such patients succumb to their disease within 12 months of diagnosis.

The increase in diagnosis and recognition of the importance of close follow-up of gastrointestinal malignancies during the past decade has led to a corresponding increase in the identification of liver metastases. These lesions are now being detected at an earlier stage as a result of improvements in imaging techniques and an increased awareness of potential treatment options amongst the medical community. As a result, patients who until a few years ago were considered candidates only for palliative care are nowadays being offered a chance of cure, because of a multidisciplinary and multi-modality approach in which liver resection is the key.

Operative Resection of Colorectal Liver Metastases

Colorectal cancer is the second leading cause of cancer-related mortality worldwide, and every year more than 140,000 patients in the Unites States are diagnosed with this disease. Even though 85% of patients have neoplasms amenable to curative resection at the time of diagnosis, the disease recurs in more than half of the patients within 5 years. The most frequent sites of colorectal metastases are the liver, which accounts for 30–60% of colorectal metastases, and the lung, representing 20–30%. Up to 25% of patients have liver metastases detected at the time of diagnosis of the primary colorectal neoplasm (synchronous metastases), while the remaining 30% develop liver metastases after their initial diagnosis (metachronous metastases). Without treatment, the median survival of patients with colorectal liver metastases is 12–15 months, and the 5-year survival rate is less than 5%. Many treatment modalities have been investigated to prolong the survival of patients with colorectal liver metastases, but liver resection remains the only method associated with long-term survival.

Natural History of Untreated Colorectal Liver Metastases

The natural history of untreated colorectal liver metastases has been defined clearly by studies that examined the impact of operative treatment on survival in the era predating the use of systemic chemotherapy. Scheele et al. reviewed 1,209 patients with colorectal liver metastases and compared three subgroups of patients: 921 who underwent a debulking procedure, hepatic arterial infusion, or palliative care; 62 who were untreated; and 226 patients who underwent curative resection. Only the curative resection group had 5-year survivors with 5- and 10-year survival rates in this cohort of 40% and 27%, respectively. In another study, Scheele et al. showed that patients who underwent curative resection and were cancer-free at 5 years, had an 88% probability of being cancer-free at 10 years. This study provides the best presumptive evidence that operative resection for colorectal liver metastases can modify directly the natural history of disease and improve long-term survival.

Indications and Contraindications to Operative Resection

Traditionally, contraindications to resection of colorectal liver metastases have been unresectable liver disease and extrahepatic disease (❯ *Table 101-1*). In many studies, multiple hepatic metastases and the presence of bilobar disease were said to be associated with a worse prognosis, especially in patients with more than four hepatic metastases, because there was said to be a high risk of recurrence after operative resection. It is now recommended that patients with more than four hepatic metastases should undergo a thorough preoperative staging, and in this subset of patients, preoperative systemic chemotherapy should be considered, even if the disease is initially resectable. As such, the presence of multiple hepatic metastases is no longer considered an absolute contraindication to resection.

◘ Table 101-1

Contraindications to resection of colorectal liver metastases

Relative	Absolute
Extrahepatic metastases	Peritoneal carcinomatosis
Colonic recurrence	Multiple extrahepatic metastases
Solitary resectable peritoneal metastasis	Inability to perform hepatic R0 resection
Hilar lymph nodes metastases	

Another controversial area is the appropriateness of operative resection in patients with metastases in perihepatic lymph nodes, as their presence predicts a poor outcome after operation. Jaeck et al. showed recently that metastases in hilar and perihepatic lymph nodes have a worse impact on prognosis than multiple liver metastases, increase in serum carcinoembryonic antigen (CEA) level, or even solitary resectable peritoneal disease. Therefore there is currently no indication for routine resection of perihepatic lymph nodes in patients with colorectal liver metastases.

Several authors have reported long-term survival in patients with resectable extrahepatic metastases. Elias et al. showed a 5-year overall survival rate of 28% in patients with more than five hepatic metastases and multiple sites of extrahepatic disease. Other studies have shown that long-term survival can be expected after complete resection (R0 resection) of colorectal metastases to the lung, even when these metastases are present at the time of diagnosis of the primary colorectal tumor.

Diagnosis and Preoperative Work-Up

Patients with primary colorectal cancer should undergo follow-up examinations, which differ in intensity and in the imaging modalities used according to the preference of the treating physician. Most follow-up protocols consist of physical examination, colonoscopy, measurement of serum levels of CEA and CA 19-9, and abdominal computed tomography (CT). CEA may be of importance because the vast majority of patients with colorectal disease have an increase in serum CEA. After a curative colonic resection, levels fall to normal, and thus a secondary increase in serum CEA is indicative of recurrent or metastatic disease acting as a stimulus for radiologic localization. Increased serum levels of CEA are seen in greater than 75% of patients with colorectal liver metastases. Moreover, CEA represents one of the most important prognostic factors for long-term survival after resection of colorectal liver metastases. Recently, Adam et al. identified CA 19-9 as an important indicator of prognosis in patients undergoing hepatic resection; however, further confirmatory studies are necessary to support this finding prior to widespread implementation.

The preferred imaging modality for detection of colorectal liver metastases is CT, because it is available widely and allows simultaneous imaging of the thorax, liver, abdomen, and pelvis. We favor quadruple-phase (precontrast, arterial, portal, and delayed), multislice CT with rapid intravenous contrast injection (3–5 ml/s) and 2–5 mm cuts of the liver.

Fluorodeoxyglucose positron emission tomography (FDG-PET) has been used recently in the preoperative work-up of patients with colorectal liver metastases and has a role in selection of the best candidates for liver resection. A recent meta-analysis provided evidence that FDG-PET has greater sensitivity in the detection of colorectal liver metastases (95%) than helical CT (65%) or 1.5 T magnetic resonance imaging (MRI) (76%). The resolution of FDG-PET, however, remains inferior to that of CT or MRI, as does its specificity, especially in patients who have undergone preoperative chemotherapy; interpretation of results in this setting may be misleading.

Recently, the role of contrast-enhanced ultrasonography in the detection of colorectal metastases has been investigated. This new technique is promising, because it combines the well-established sensitivity of ultrasonography with the specificity of contrast examination, allowing further characterization of hepatic lesions. Furthermore, contrast-enhanced ultrasonography can be performed during intraoperative ultrasonography, now performed routinely during liver surgery, to give the surgeon an additional diagnostic tool in their diagnostic armamentarium.

Several groups have reported benefit from the use of intraoperative staging laparoscopy to minimize non-curative or "open and close" laparotomy rates which vary between 10% and 40%. This wide range probably reflects differences in the quality of the preoperative imaging work-up and also center-to-center variation in case-mix. Currently, we advocate laparoscopy in patients with advanced metastatic in whom hepatic injury from preoperative systemic chemotherapy is suspected.

Once patients have been diagnosed and a multidisciplinary decision is made that resection is appropriate, it is essential to ensure that they undergo repeat high quality imaging studies, with abdominal and pelvic CT (or MRI) within a month of the date of operation. A full cardiac and pulmonary work-up should be performed if past history and symptoms warrant. Baseline evaluation of hepatic function is mandatory before any hepatic resection to exclude dysfunction as a result of concomitant liver disease or side effects related to chemotherapy, because impaired hepatic function will have a negative impact in terms of a higher complication rate and may also limit the extent of the resection possible. In addition, candidates for extended resection, i.e., the removal of more than four adjacent segments, should undergo estimation of the future liver remnant (FLR) volume performed using CT volumetry of the liver.

Techniques for Resection

The current operative technique for liver resection is based on the segmental hepatic anatomy described by Couinaud in 1957. The surgical nomenclature used for anatomic resection is presented in ❯ *Fig. 101-1*. Non-anatomic resection, often referred to as atypical, wedge, or limited resection, consists of the removal of a part of the liver parenchyma without following the distribution of the portal vein branch that supplies the part of the liver being resected. Although some authors report a survival benefit for patients undergoing anatomic versus non-anatomic resection, no definitive evidence supports anatomic resection; long-term survival without local recurrence can be also achieved with nonanatomic resection even with minimal resection margins. Indeed, a recent multicenter analysis showed that the width of the negative surgical margin does not correlate with the probability of intrahepatic recurrence, only that the presence of a positive (versus negative) resection margin correlates with increased risk of intrahepatic recurrence.

Resection of hepatic colorectal metastases usually begins with a J-shaped incision in the right upper quadrant. After a full exploration of the peritoneal cavity, the liver is mobilized by dividing all the relevant supporting ligaments. The liver is inspected, palpated, and evaluated further by intraoperative ultrasonography. Transection of the liver parenchyma can be carried out with one or more of a number of different current instruments, including ultrasonic dissectors and radiofrequency coagulators (❯ *Fig. 101-2*), or with the more traditional crushing clamp technique. Generally, the resection is performed with control of the inflow (Pringle's maneuver) and sometimes of the outflow as well to reduce blood loss.

☐ Figure 101-1

Anatomic nomenclature of the liver based on the Brisbane 2000 hepatic resection nomenclature (Reprinted from Abdalla et al., 2004. With permission from Elsevier)

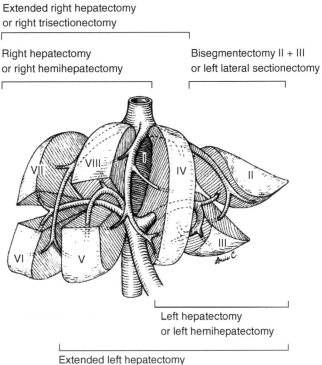

☐ Figure 101-2

Two-surgeon technique for hepatic parenchymal transection. The primary surgeon directs dissection with the ultrasonic dissector from the patient's left side and the secondary surgeon operates with the saline-linked cautery device from the patient's right side (Reprinted from Aloia et al., 2005. With permission from Lippincott, Williams & Wilkins)

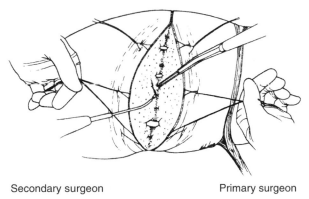

Perioperative Results

Liver resection is a well-established procedure that can be performed with mortality rates of less than 5%, with large centers now quoting rates of 1–2% and morbidity rates of less than 40%. The most powerful determinants of poor outcome after liver resection are preoperative cirrhosis or severe hepatic dysfunction, intraoperative bleeding, requirement for perioperative blood transfusions, insufficient remnant liver, and the development of postoperative infections. Indeed, these conditions can lead to hepatic failure, which although it occurs in fewer than 5% of patients, can have devastating consequences. Optimal patient selection, meticulous intraoperative technique, and careful postoperative management are essential to minimize surgical complications.

Long-Term Survival

❯ *Table 101-2* reports the main predictors of recurrence in major series of liver resection for colorectal metastases. Despite expanding indications for resection of colorectal metastases, overall 5-year survival is now reported to be as high as 58% in single and multi-institutional studies. The factors with the greatest influence on survival are margin status, stage of the primary colon neoplasm, preoperative plasma CEA level, size and number of hepatic lesions, and presence or absence of extrahepatic disease.

Surgical margin status is an important factor that influences long-term survival. Historically, a margin less than 1 cm was considered suboptimal, and some have even suggested that an anticipated margin less than 1 cm was a contraindication to resection. A recent study by Pawlik et al., however, showed that the width of resected margin (1–10 mm) did not affect local recurrence or survival, and indeed only the presence of a positive surgical margin (R1) was associated with an increased risk of recurrence (11%) and decreased survival (❯ *Fig. 101-3*). Thus, patients with an

◧ Table 101-2

Predictors of recurrence and long-term survival after resection for colorectal liver metastases

Author, year	R1 status	Synchronous presentation	Primary nodes +	Size of metastases	Number of metastases	Preoperative CEA	Extrahepatic disease	5-Year survival
Gayowski, 1994	+	+	+	−	+	−	+	32%
Scheele, 1995	+	+	+	+	−	−	−	40%
Nordlinger, 1996	+	+	+	+	+	+		28%
Jaeck, 1997	+	+	+	+	+	+	−	26%
Jamison, 1997	−			−	−			32%
Jenkins, 1997	+			−	−		+	25%
Elias, 1998	+	+	−	−	−	−	−	28%
Ambiru, 1999	+	−	+		+	+		23%
Fong, 1999	+	+	+		+	+	+	46%
Minagawa, 2000	−		−		+	−	−	38%
Figueras, 2001	+	−			+	+	+	53%
Choti, 2002	+	−	−	−	+	+		58%
Fernandez, 2004	−		−	−	+	−		58%
Abdalla, 2004	+	−		+	+			58%
Pawlik, 2005	+	−	−	+	+	+		58%

CEA, Carcino-Embryonic Antigen.

◘ Figure 101-3

Survival after curative resection for colorectal liver metastases stratified by margin status. No difference in survival was seen in patients with negative surgical margins, regardless of the width of the margin (Reprinted from Pawlik et al., 2005. With permission from Lippincott, Williams & Wilkins)

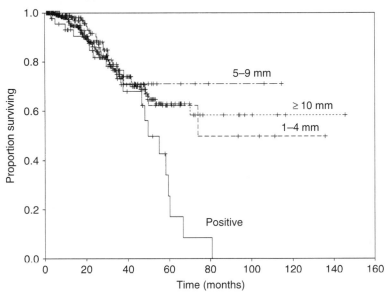

anticipated surgical margin <1 cm based on preoperative imaging or intraoperative findings could still undergo resection as long as negative margin is achievable.

Specific molecular markers have been linked with clinical outcome. In a recent study, our group demonstrated that human telomerase reverse transcriptase (hTERT) expression was associated independently with a worse prognosis after curative resection of colorectal liver metastases. In this study, hTERT-positive patients had a twofold increase in risk of death compared to hTERT-negative patients. This finding is important, because the use of molecular markers may prove useful to select high-risk patients who may benefit from preoperative systemic chemotherapy.

Follow-Up

After resection of colorectal liver metastases, patients should be followed carefully to allow for early detection of recurrence. Follow-up evaluations after resection of colorectal liver metastases probably should include CEA and CA 19-9 measurements, liver function tests, pelvic and abdominal CT, and chest radiography every 3–6 months. A colonoscopy is also mandatory every 1–3 year after resection of the primary colonic resection. This schedule should be continued at least for 5 years after liver surgery.

Selected patients can undergo re-resection for recurrent colorectal liver metastases, and such patients can experience long-term survival. Adam et al. showed 5-year overall survival rates of 32% after the third hepatectomy, with no increase in postoperative morbidity or mortality rates.

Methods to Improve the Resectability of Colorectal Liver Metastases

Several strategies are available to render initially unresectable colorectal liver metastases resectable.

Neoadjuvant Systemic Chemotherapy

The development of new, more effective chemotherapy agents, such as oxaliplatin and irinotecan, has led to more widespread use of chemotherapy for patients with colorectal liver metastases – both those with resectable and those with unresectable disease at presentation. Indeed, both drugs, which are commonly used in combination with 5-fluorouracil–folinic acid-based regimens, can downsize liver metastases and control extrahepatic disease sites effectively. The use of these agents in conjunction with advances in techniques of parenchymal transection have led to a change in the concept of unresectable liver metastases and has expanded the population of patients who are potential candidates for hepatic resection.

The indications for neoadjuvant chemotherapy are based on risk factors for disease recurrence. Factors considered are size and number of metastases, disease-free interval between diagnosis of the primary colorectal neoplasm and the metastases, and presence of extrahepatic disease.

The more widespread use of neoadjuvant chemotherapy has given rise to a clinical dilemma: to prescribe or not to prescribe preoperative chemotherapy in patients with resectable colorectal liver metastases? This dilemma is not merely academic, because recent reports indicate an increase in the risk of adverse events after hepatic resection in patients treated preoperatively with systemic chemotherapy. Hepatocellular damage, including hepatic steatosis and more importantly steatohepatitis, has been described in patients treated preoperatively with irinotecan (yellow liver syndrome) and a sinusoidal obstruction syndrome is being described with increasing frequency in patients treated preoperatively with oxaliplatin (blue liver syndrome). These chemotherapy-related hepatic injuries can reduce the regenerative capacity of hepatocytes in response to major hepatectomy through alterations of nuclear factors such as nuclear factor-kappa B, which may interfere with the priming phase of liver regeneration. Therefore, the use of neoadjuvant chemotherapy should be considered cautiously in patients with resectable disease at presentation, in whom chemotherapy-related intrahepatic complications could necessitate modification of the surgical strategy or even prevent resection as a treatment option.

Portal Vein Embolization and Two-Stage Hepatectomy

Portal vein embolization (PVE) is used before major and extended hepatic resection to induce atrophy of the liver parenchyma to be resected (the embolized lobe) and compensatory hypertrophy of the liver to be preserved (the remnant liver), thereby increasing the hepatic reserve of the FLR. First developed in Japan, PVE is now frequently used by many centers worldwide and contributes to improved resectability rates for patients with liver cancer.

PVE is usually performed via a percutaneous, transhepatic approach consisting of ultrasound-guided puncture of a portal branch followed by embolization of the entire hemi-liver to be resected. Embolization can be achieved with a variety of substances, such as 100% ethanol, ethiodized oil, and cyanoacrylate, none are superior to the others. PVE is a well-established and well-tolerated procedure. The indications for PVE are based on the calculated FLR volume and the presence or absence of underlying liver disease. The FLR is calculated as the ratio of the FLR volume to the total liver volume (TLV) as calculated by CT, using a formula extrapolated from the association between TLV and body surface area. This measurement allows for an estimation of the hepatic metabolic demand for each patient. The presence of underlying liver disease is another important factor to consider, because severely damaged livers may not have the capacity to regenerate. Both cirrhosis and severe steatosis have been found to impair liver regeneration after major hepatectomy. The use of PVE in these settings will allow hypertrophy of the remnant liver, albeit at a slower rate than for healthy liver, thus reducing the risk of subsequent hepatectomy.

Hypertrophy of the FLR after PVE is expected within the first month. The greatest increase in FLR occurs within the first 3 weeks, after which regeneration reaches a plateau. Hypertrophy of the nonembolized liver is regulated mainly by transforming growth factor-alpha, whose serum level has been reported as peaking at day 20 after PVE and thereafter reaching a plateau. Thus, 3–4 weeks should be considered the optimum time interval to assess the hypertrophy response to PVE. In addition to the absolute volume of hypertrophy, the rate of hypertrophy is important, and we desire a 5% increase within the first month after PVE.

There is little agreement on the minimal FLR volume needed to avoid the small-for-size syndrome. The surgical series published to date report different methods of measurement of liver volume and include patients with considerably different degrees of underlying liver disease. A functional residual liver volume of <20% is associated with an increase in postoperative morbidity. In general, for patients with a normal underlying liver, resection is acceptable when the functional residual liver volume is >20%. In patients with injured liver, >30% is required, while in patients with cirrhosis or steatohepatitis, more than 40% is desired.

The role of PVE in permitting an R0 resection in patients with multiple bilobar disease has been investigated recently by Jaeck et al. who proposed the novel approach of two-stage hepatectomy, via removal of metastases in the left liver during first-stage hepatectomy and removal of metastases in the right liver during the second-stage. The second stage can be performed with or without preoperative PVE, depending on the functional residual liver volume. This approach should be considered in patients not eligible for R0 resection performed within the context of a single procedure.

Interstitial Therapies

Interstitial therapies for colorectal liver metastases have been in use for many years. Ethanol injection, cryosurgery, and microwave ablation have been utilized for local control of disease, generally with only short-term success. Currently, the most commonly used interstitial therapy is radiofrequency thermal ablation (RFA), which requires placement of an electrode within the liver tumor under radiologic guidance (ultrasonography, CT, or MRI) and use of the electrode to generate thermal (radiofrequency) energy, which destroys the tumor. RFA can be performed percutaneously, laparoscopically, or during laparotomy.

While the use of RFA for liver metastases is reported to be effective and safe, there are currently no randomized data comparing resection and RFA. Abdalla et al. recently compared the results of operative resection versus RFA versus combined resection and RFA for colorectal liver metastases and found that recurrence was more common after RFA than after the combined procedure or resection alone (84%, 64%, and 52%, respectively). Moreover, true local recurrence (cut-edge of resected liver or RFA site) was more common after RFA than after resection (❷ *Fig. 101-4*). Consequently, the long-term survival rate was higher after resection than after local ablation (65% vs. 22%). Given these findings, operative resection should be considered the treatment of choice for colorectal liver metastases, and use of RFA should be restricted mainly to patients in whom resection is not feasible technically.

■ Figure 101-4

Overall survival of patients with colorectal liver metastases stratified by surgical treatment. Long-term survival was greatest in resected patients (Reprinted from Abdalla et al., 2004. With permission from Lippincott, Williams & Wilkins)

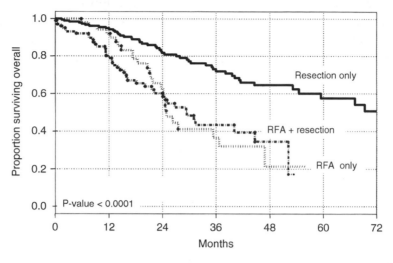

Adjuvant Systemic and Regional Therapy

Recurrence after hepatic resection for colorectal liver metastases will occur in up to 70% of patients at some point during the course of their disease. Systemic chemotherapy is advocated to minimize these recurrences and prolong survival; however, the optimal strategy for systemic chemotherapy is yet to be defined.

The use of hepatic arterial infusion (HAI) as adjuvant treatment after hepatic resection has been investigated in several studies. HAI is attractive theoretically, because it allows infusion of a high dose of cytotoxic agents directly into the liver for both resectable and unresectable disease. HAI requires implantation of a catheter in the distal gastroduodenal artery and a pump in a subcutaneous pocket. Catheter and pump are usually placed during a laparotomy or, more recently, laparoscopically. Several studies have reported benefits with HAI; however, a recent systematic review from the Cochrane Collaboration looked at seven randomized trials of HAI of 592 patients and failed to find improvement in long-term survival with HAI. The review concluded that HAI reduces the rate of intrahepatic recurrence but does not prevent systemic extrahepatic metastases. HAI has not been investigated definitively in patients with unresectable colorectal liver metastases, and the available results are controversial.

Major efforts in basic research are focusing on identification of molecular pathways of malignant growth that can be disrupted by new biologic agents. Inhibitors of epidermal growth factor receptor and vascular endothelial growth factor receptor are under evaluation currently in international clinical trials, and their use appears to produce a survival advantage. Indeed, a recent randomized trial showed that addition of vascular endothelial growth factor receptor inhibitor (bevacizumab) to the fluorouracil- and irinotecan-based therapy resulted in clinically meaningful improvement in survival in patients with stage IV colon cancer. Such randomized controlled trials will be required to define the optimal use of chemotherapy after hepatic resection for colorectal liver metastases.

Resection of Non-Colorectal Liver Metastases

It is now widely accepted that liver resection is the only potentially curative therapy for colorectal liver metastases. In contrast, liver resection for non-colorectal metastases is performed infrequently, even though such resectional therapy can be performed safely and with low morbidity and mortality. Published reports on this approach report a heterogeneous series of patients, and, thus, drawing any conclusions on the basis of these reports is difficult.

Metastases from Neuroendocrine Neoplasms

Resection of functioning neuroendocrine liver metastases (NLM) reduces endocrine symptoms and prolongs survival. NLM have two main distinguishing features that provide the rationale for treating these metastases with hepatic resection: NLM usually grow slowly, and the survival of patients with NLM is longer than that of patients with other kinds of liver metastases. Moreover, endocrine activity can interfere seriously with patients' quality of life and also reduce long-term survival. Survival rates after resection of NLM are respectably high. Sarmiento et al. reported a 5-year survival rate of 61%, and Jaeck et al. reported a 3-year survival rate of 91%. In addition, operative resection results in control of symptoms of NLM in up to 90% of patients, even in cases of nonradical resection.

Alternative therapies for NLM include transarterial embolization (because NLM are hypervascular neoplasms) and administration of somatostatin analogs. Results of transarterial embolization have been encouraging, and somatostatin analogs may also reduce the release of neuroendocrine factors.

Metastases from Breast Cancer

Metastatic breast cancer is a systemic disease, and liver metastases from breast cancer are generally considered a poor prognostic factor, associated with a median survival of between 5 and 12 months. Although the indications for hepatic resection for breast metastases need to be further clarified, operative resection of breast liver metastases should be considered, but only as part of a multidisciplinary approach based mainly on systemic chemotherapy. In highly selected patients with liver metastases from breast cancer, complete resection of liver metastases (R0) in association with systemic cytotoxic, hormonal, and biologic therapies can produce 5-year overall and disease-free survival up to 61% and 31%, respectively. The most important prognostic factor appears to be a long disease-free interval between diagnosis of the primary breast cancer and diagnosis of liver metastases. In these patients, multiple hepatic metastases should be considered a relative contraindication for liver resection, while the presence of extrahepatic localization remains controversial.

Metastases from Other Types of Primary Neoplasms

There are a few single-institution studies reporting limited survival benefits after resection of liver metastases from melanoma, sarcoma, gynecologic, gastric, and pancreatic cancers. Indications for resection for these types of metastases are extremely limited, and no sufficient data are available to make any recommendation. The presence of liver metastases from gastrointestinal neoplasms other than colorectal cancer is a manifestation of diffuse disease and is usually associated with a grim prognosis.

Hepatic Transplantation for Metastatic Cancer of the Liver

Some groups have advocated a role for liver transplantation in the treatment of unresectable metastatic cancer of the liver, especially for the less aggressive metastatic neuroendocrine neoplasms. A limited number of patients have undergone liver transplantation for non-neuroendocrine liver metastases. Results have been generally disappointing – few patients have survived beyond 3 years.

Currently, most authors agree that given the limited number of patients who can be treated and the high risk of recurrence because of the immunosuppressive therapy required after liver transplantation, liver transplantation has only a very limited role in the treatment of metastatic cancer of the liver. Moreover, the new, more aggressive, multimodality treatment strategies, such as neoadjuvant chemotherapy and two-stage hepatectomy with or without PVE, will allow us to offer hepatic resection with curative intent to more patients, meaning that fewer patients now have unresectable disease for which transplantation would even be considered.

Selected Readings

Abdalla EK, Vauthey JN, Ellis LM, et al. (2004) Recurrence and outcome following hepatic resection, radiofrequency ablation and combined resection/ablation for colorectal liver metastases. Ann Surg 239:818–827

Abdalla EK, Denys A, Chevalier P, Nemr RA, Vauthey JN (2004) Total and segmental liver volume variations: implications for liver surgery. Surgery 135(4):404–410

Adam R, Delvart V, Pascal G, et al. (2004) Rescue surgery for unresectable colorectal liver metastases downstaged by chemotherapy. A model to predict long-term survival. Ann Surg 240:644–658

Aloia TA, Zorzi D, Abdalla EK, Vauthey JN (2005) Two-surgeon technique for hepatic parenchymal transaction using saline-linked cautery and ultrasonic dissection. Ann Surg 242(2):172–177

Bipat S, van Leeuwen MS, Coman EFI, et al. (2005) Colorectal liver metastases: CT, MR imaging, and PET for diagnosis – meta-analysis. Radiology 237:123–131

Domont J, Pawlik TM, Boige V, et al. (2005) Catalytic subunit of human telomerase reverse transcriptase is an independent predictor of survival in patients undergoing curative resection of hepatic colorectal metastases: a multicenter analysis. J Clin Oncol 23:3086–3093

Hurwitz H, Fehrenbacher L, Novotny W, et al. (2004) Bevacizumab plus irinotecan, fluorouracil, and leucovorin for metastatic colorectal cancer. N Engl J Med 350:2335–2342

Madoff DC, Abdalla EK, Vauthey JN (2005) Portal vein embolization in preparation for major hepatic resection: evolution of a new standard of care. J Vasc Interv Radiol 16:779–790

Pawlik TM, Scoggins CR, Zorzi D, et al. (2005) Effect of surgical margin status on survival and site of recurrence after hepatic resection for colorectal metastases. Ann Surg 241:715–724

Scheele J, Stangl R, Altendorf-Hofmann A (1990) Hepatic metastases from colorectal carcinoma: impact of surgical resection on the natural history. Br J Surg 77:1241–1246

Scheele J, Stang R, Altendorf-Hofmann A, et al. (1995) Resection of colorectal liver metastases. World J Surg 19:59–71

Vauthey JN, Pawlik TM, Ribero D, et al. (2006) Chemotherapy regimen predicts steatohepatitis and an increase in ninety-day mortality after surgery for hepatic colorectal metastases. J Clin Oncol 24:2065–2072

Subject Index

Subject Index